D0998573

Rehabilitation of the Spine
SCIENCE AND PRACTICE

Rehabilitation of the Spine
SCIENCE AND PRACTICE

STEPHEN H. HOCHSCHULER, M.D.

Clinical Instructor
Division of Orthopaedic Surgery
University of Texas Southwestern Medical Center
Dallas, Texas
Co-founder, Texas Back Institute
Plano, Texas

HOWARD B. COTLER, M.D.

Associate Professor of Surgery
Department of Orthopaedics
University of Texas Medical School of Houston
Houston, Texas
Medical Director
Texas Back Institute
Houston, Texas

RICHARD D. GUYER, M.D.

Associate Clinical Professor
Division of Orthopaedic Surgery
University of Texas Southwestern Medical Center
Dallas, Texas
Medical Director of Research
Texas Back Institute
Plano, Texas

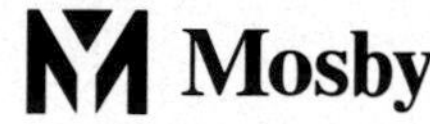

St. Louis Baltimore Boston Chicago London Philadelphia Sydney Toronto

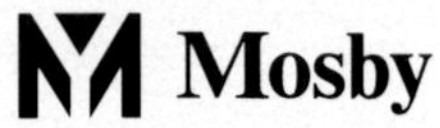

Dedicated to Publishing Excellence

Sponsoring Editor: James D. Ryan
Assistant Editor: Joyce-Rachel John
Associate Managing Editor, Manuscript Services: Deborah Thorp
Production Manager: Nancy C. Baker
Proofroom Manager: Barbara M. Kelly

Mosby-Year Book, Inc.
11830 Westline Industrial Drive
St. Louis, MO 63416

1 2 3 4 5 6 7 8 9 0 CL/MV 97 96 95 94 93

Library of Congress Cataloging-in-Publication Data

Rehabilitation of the spine : science and practice / [edited by]
Stephen H. Hochschuler, Howard B. Cotler, Richard D. Guyer.
p. cm.
Includes bibliographical references and index.
ISBN 0-8016-7195-7
1. Spine—Abnormalities. 2. Spinal cord—Abnormalities.
3. Spine—Diseases. 4. Spinal cord—Diseases. 5. Spine—Wounds and injuries. 6. Spinal cord—Wounds and injuries.
I. Hochschuler, Stephen H. II. Cotler, Howard B.
III. Guyer, Richard D.
[DNLM: 1. Spinal Diseases—rehabilitation WE 725 R345]
RD768.R42 1992
617.5′6—dc20 92-48185
DNLM/DLC CIP
for Library of Congress

DEDICATION

We dedicate this book to our families and teachers, who have encouraged and inspired us throughout our careers. Although our teachers are too numerous to name individually, we would like to make special mention of the following:

Charles Gregory, M.D., and Vert Mooney, M.D.—(S.H.H.)

Paul R. Meyer, Jr., M.D., Jerome M. Cotler, M.D., and James M. Hunter, M.D.—(H.B.C.)

Samuel Guyer, M.D., Richard H. Rothman, M.D., and Leon L. Wiltse, M.D.—(R.D.G.)

CONTRIBUTORS

Jean-Jacques Abitbol, M.D.
Assistant Professor of Orthopaedic Surgery
University of California at San Diego
University of California at San Diego Medical Center
San Diego, California

Charles K. Anderson, Ph.D.
Advanced Ergonomics
Dallas, Texas

Charles Aprill, M.D.
Spine Radiologist
Diagnostic Conservative Management, Inc.
New Orleans, Louisiana

Gunnar B.J. Andersson, M.D., Ph.D.
Professor and Associate Chairman
Rush University
Senior Attending Physician
Rush-Presbyterian-St. Luke's Medical Center
Chicago, Illinois

David F. Apple, Jr., M.D.
Associate Clinical Professor of Orthopaedic Surgery
Clinical Assistant Professor in Rehabilitation Medicine
Emory University School of Medicine
Medical Director, Spinal Center
Piedmont Hospital
Atlanta, Georgia

Andrew R. Block, Ph.D.
Director of Behavioral Medicine
Texas Back Institute
Plano, Texas

Richard S. Bockman, M.D.
Professor of Medicine
Cornell University Medical College
Head, Endocrine Service
Hospital for Special Surgery
New York, New York

Anna L. Bodenhamer, O.T.
Registered Occupational Therapist, Ergonomic Specialist
Director, Return to Work Program
Denton Regional Sports and Physical Therapy Center
Denton, Texas

G. Mitch Bogdanffy, M.S.
Research Associate
Texas Back Institute Research Foundation
Plano, Texas

Kathleen S. Botelho, P.T.
Senior Physical Therapist
Liberty Mutual Medical Service Center
Boston, Massachusetts

Aaron K. Calodney, M.D.
Assistant Professor
University of Texas Medical School at Houston
Director of Pain Management Center
Longview Regional Hospital
Houston, Texas

David M. Carpenter, M.S.
Director of Educational Programs
Center for Exercise Science
University of Florida
Gainesville, Florida

Catherine Carranza, O.T.R./L.
Injury Management Organization, Inc.
Carrollton, Texas

Tommy Clark, M.B.A.
Racine, Wisconsin

Michele Comer, P.T.
Quality Improvement Manager
Myofascial and Manual Therapy Institute
Richardson, Texas

Howard B. Cotler, M.D.
Associate Professor of Surgery
Department of Orthopaedics
University of Texas Medical School at Houston
Houston, Texas
Medical Director
Texas Back Institute
Houston, Texas

Rick B. Delamarter, M.D.
Assistant Clinical Professor of Orthopaedic Surgery
University of California at Los Angeles School of Medicine
Los Angeles, California

William H. Donovan, M.D.
Professor of Clinical Physical Medicine and Rehabilitation
Baylor College of Medicine
Medical Director
The Institute for Rehabilitation and Research
Houston, Texas

Charles C. Edwards, M.D.
Professor of Orthopaedic Surgery
University of Maryland
Director, Section of Spinal Surgery
University of Maryland Hospital
Baltimore, Maryland

W. Thomas Edwards, Ph.D.
Associate Professor and Director
Orthopaedic Research Laboratory
Department of Orthopaedic Surgery
State University of New York Health Science Center at Syracuse
Syracuse, New York

David F. Fardon, M.D.
Clinical Assistant Professor
University of Tennessee Hospital
Knoxville, Tennessee

Henry F. Farfan, M.D.
Orthopaedic Surgeon
Quebec, Canada

Sherlyn Fenton, O.T.R./L.
Assistant Director
Work Venture, Industrial Rehabilitation Program
Salem Hospital
Peabody, Massachusetts

Daniel N. Foster, M.S.
Laboratory Coordinator
Center for Exercise Science
University of Florida
Gainesville, Florida

Michael N. Fulton, M.D.
Adjunct Associate Professor
College of Medicine
College of Health and Human Performance
University of Florida
Gainesville, Florida
Orthopaedic Surgeon
Halifax Medical Center
Daytona Beach, Florida

Vance O. Gardner, M.D.
Associate Clinical Professor
Department of Orthopaedics
University of California—Irvine
Irvine Medical Center
Irvine, California

Steven R. Garfin, M.D.
Professor, Department of Orthopaedics
University of California at San Diego School of Medicine
Chief, Spine Service
University of California at San Diego Medical Center
San Diego, California

Paula J. Gilbert, P.T.
Physical Therapist
Texas Back Institute
Plano, Texas

J. Michael Graham, M.D., Ph.D.
Clinical Instructor
Division of Orthopaedic Surgery
Baylor College of Medicine
Northwest Spine Center
Houston, Texas

James E. Graves, Ph.D.
Assistant Scientist
Professor of Medicine and Exercise Science
University of Florida
Gainesville, Florida

Richard D. Guyer, M.D.
Associate Clinical Professor
Division of Orthopaedic Surgery
University of Texas Southwestern Medical Center
Dallas, Texas
Medical Director of Research
Texas Back Institute
Plano, Texas

Scott Haldeman, M.D., Ph.D., F.R.C.P.(C)
Associate Clinical Professor
Department of Neurology
University of California at Irvine
Irvine, California

Mark F. Hambly, M.D.
Northern California Spine Center
Sutter General Hospital
Sacramento, California

John Handal, M.D.
Assistant Clinical Professor
Department of Orthopaedics
University of Texas Southwestern Medical Center
Dallas Specialty Hospital
Dallas, Texas

David T. Hanks, Ph.D.
Clinical Psychologist
Texas Back Institute
Plano, Texas

Stephen H. Hochschuler, M.D.
Clinical Instructor
Division of Orthopaedic Surgery
University of Texas Southwestern Medical Center
Dallas, Texas
Co-founder, Texas Back Institute
Plano, Texas

Jerry Holubec, D.O.
Anesthesiology/Pain Management
Texas Back Institute
Plano, Texas

Mark W. Howard, M.D.
West Coast Spine Institute
Los Angeles, California

Valerie Shaw Jones, O.T.R./L.
Guest Lecturer at Boston University and Simmons College
Senior Occupational Therapist
Liberty Mutual Medical Service Center
Boston, Massachusetts

Thomas J. Kleeman, M.D.
Instructor in Surgery (Spine Fellow)
University of Maryland
Baltimore, Maryland

John P. Kostuik, M.D.
Professor of Orthopaedics—Neurosurgery
Department of Orthopaedic Surgery
The Johns Hopkins University
Baltimore, Maryland

Jeffrey A. Kozak, M.D.
Clinical Instructor
Division of Orthopaedic Surgery
Baylor College of Medicine
Fondren Orthopaedic Group
Houston, Texas

Martin H. Krag, M.D.
Associate Professor
Department of Orthopaedic Rehabilitation
University of Vermont
Burlington, Vermont

Edwin F. Kremer, Ph.D.
Assistant Adjunct Professor
Department of Psychiatry
Michigan State University School of Medicine
Lansing, Michigan
Program Director
Pain Rehabilitation Program
Mary Free Bed Hospital
Grand Rapids, Michigan

Stephen D. Kuslich, M.D.
Associate Clinical Professor
Department of Orthopaedics
University of Minnesota
Metropolitan Orthopaedic Associates
Minneapolis, Minnesota

Joseph M. Lane, M.D.
Professor of Orthopaedic Surgery
Cornell University Medical College
Chief, Metabolic Bone Disease/Orthopaedic Oncology Service
The Hospital for Special Surgery
New York, New York

Henry LaRocca, M.D. (Deceased)
Former Clinical Professor of Orthopaedic Surgery
Tulane University Medical School
New Orleans, Louisiana

Michelle Lazarski, P.T.
Supervisor, Physical Therapy Spinal Cord Injury Care Program
Thomas Jefferson University Hospital
Philadelphia, Pennsylvania

Casey K. Lee, M.D.
Professor, Orthopaedic Surgery
Department of Orthopaedic Surgery
New Jersey Medical School
Newark, New Jersey

Scott H. Leggett, M.S.
Director of Clinical and Research Programs
Department of Orthopaedics
University of California at San Diego
San Diego, California

Alan M. Levine, M.D.
Professor of Orthopaedic Surgery and Oncology
University of Maryland
Baltimore, Maryland

Thomas A. Lorren, P.T.
Pain Management Center
Longview, Texas

James W. Maxey, M.D.
Clinical Instructor of Surgery
University of Illinois College of Medicine at Peoria
St. Francis Medical Center
Peoria, Illinois

Mary Lynn Mayfield, R.N., B.S.N.
Education Coordinator
Return to Work Program
Texas Back Institute
Plano, Texas

Robert F. McLain, M.D.
Assistant Professor
Department of Orthopaedic Surgery
University of California at Davis
Davis, California

Michael S. Melnik, M.D., O.T.R.
Occupational Therapist
Exercise Physiologist
Minneapolis, Minnesota

Robert R. Menter, M.D.
Craig Hospital
Englewood, Colorado

Patricia McGauley Meyers, O.T.R./L.
Guest Lecturer
Boston University
Senior Occupational Therapist
Liberty Mutual Medical Service Center
Boston, Massachusetts

Nancy L. Meedzan, B.S.N.
Cardiac Rehabilitation Nurse
Liberty Mutual Medical Service Center
Boston, Massachusetts

Tammy Mondry, P.T.
Physical Therapist
Texas Back Institute
Plano, Texas

Pasquale X. Montesano, M.D.
Assistant Clinical Professor
University of California at Davis
Davis, California

Vert Mooney, M.D.
Professor of Orthopaedic Surgery
University of California at San Diego
Medical Director
University of California at San Diego Spine and Joint Conditioning Center
San Diego, California

Donna D. Ohnmeiss, M.S.
Research Associate
Texas Back Institute Research Foundation
Plano, Texas

Michael L. Pollock, Ph.D.
Director, Center for Exercise Science
Professor of Medicine and Exercise Science
University of Florida
Gainesville, Florida

P. Prithvi Raj, M.D.
Clinical Professor of Anesthesiology
The Medical College of Georgia
Medical Director
National Pain Institute of Georgia
Atlanta, Georgia

Ralph F. Rashbaum, M.D.
Clinical Instructor
Division of Orthopaedic Surgery
University of Texas Southwestern Medical Center
Dallas, Texas
Co-founder
Texas Back Institute
Plano, Texas

Wolfgang Rauschning, M.D., Ph.D.
Research Professor
Swedish Medical Research Council
Department of Orthopaedic Surgery
University Hospital
Uppsala, Sweden

Glenn R. Rechtine, M.D.
Clinical Associate Professor
University of South Florida
Tampa General Hospital
Tampa, Florida

Michael W. Reed, M.D.
Gulf Coast Hospital
Panama City, Florida

John J. Regan, M.D.
Clinical Instructor
Division of Orthopaedic Surgery
University of Texas Southwestern Medical Center
Dallas, Texas
Spine Surgeon
Texas Back Institute
Plano, Texas

Shelly Ritz, P.T.
Physical Therapist
Texas Back Institute
Plano, Texas

Jose E. Rodriguez, M.D.
Clinical Instructor
Department of Orthopaedic Surgery
Herman Hospital
Houston, Texas

Stephen L.G. Rothman, M.D.
Consultant Radiologist
Spinal Injury Service
Rancho Los Amigas Hospital
Rothman-Chafetz Medical Group
Torrance, California

Neil A. Schechter, M.D.
Private Practice
Georgia Spine Center
Staff, Cobb Hospital
Marietta, Georgia

Gary A. Schneiderman, M.D.
Assistant Clinical Professor
University of California at Davis
Northern California Spine Center
Sacramento, California

David K. Selby, M.D.
Clinical Professor of Orthopaedic Surgery
University of Texas Health Science Center
Dallas, Texas

J. Darrell Shea, M.D.
Medical Director, Lucerne Rehabilitation and Spinal Center
Orlando, Florida

Susan Simpson, P.T.
Physical Therapist
Texas Back Institute
Plano, Texas

Mary C. Sinnott, M.Ed., P.T.
Adjunct Instructor
Thomas Jefferson University
Temple University
Assistant Chief Physical Therapist
Thomas Jefferson University Hospital
Philadelphia, Pennsylvania

Pamela R. Snyder, B.S., P.T.
Physical Therapist
Director, Minnesota Lumbar Spine Clinic, Inc.
Minneapolis, Minnesota

William J. Stith, Ph.D.
Plano, Texas

Chester E. Sutterlin III, M.D.
North Florida Regional Medical Center
Gainesville, Florida

John S. Thalgott, M.D.
Clinical Instructor
Department of Orthopaedics
University of Nevada at Las Vegas
Las Vegas, Nevada

John J. Triano, D.C., M.A., Ph.D.(C)
Professor, National College of Chiropractic
Research Investigator
Hines Veterans Administration Hospital
Maywood, Illinois

Rocky S. Tuan, Ph.D.
Professor and Director of Research
Department of Orthopaedic Surgery
Thomas Jefferson University
Philadelphia, Pennsylvania

Heikki Vanharanta, M.D., Ph.D.
Professor of Physical Medicine and Rehabilitation
University of Oulu
Oulu, Finland

Eric J. Wall, M.D.
Resident, University of California at San Diego
San Diego, California

Stuart A. Weinerman, M.D.
Assistant Professor of Medicine
Cornell University Medical College
Assistant Attending
New York Hospital
New York, New York

Leon L. Wiltse, M.D.
Clinical Professor of Orthopaedic Surgery
University of California at Irvine
Staff, Long Beach Memorial Hospital
Irvine, California

Hansen A. Yuan, M.D.
Professor of Orthopaedic Surgery
State University of New York Health Science Center at Syracuse
Syracuse, New York

Jack E. Zigler, M.D.
Clinical Professor of Orthopaedics
University of Southern California School of Medicine
Chief, Spinal Injury Service
Rancho Los Amigos Medical Center
Los Angeles, California

FOREWORD

I very much appreciated being invited to write a foreword for this volume, since I deeply feel that frequent exchanges between the United States and France are necessary. Such a relationship is also in keeping with the history of our two countries. It is not well known that when a vote was taken to decide the official language in your young independent country, there was a majority of just one vote for English over French. But for that one vote this foreword would have been written in French!

I appreciate sharing the experience of so many authors in the United States through my familiarity with the American medical literature. The experience that has resulted in *Rehabilitation of the Spine: Science and Practice* coming from researchers at the Texas Back Institute is a good example of the much more advanced developments in this field in your country, the dissemination of which is very beneficial to other countries. One of the original aspects of the structure of this volume is its review of the physiopathology of various syndromes followed by a clinical study and a discussion of surgical treatment followed by information on rehabilitation, which is the book's main contribution. It is obvious that surgery is not always necessary to cure back pain, but it also appears that after successful surgical fixation of the spine, rehabilitation is as important as surgery in obtaining a good result. The follow-up rehabilitation and regular supervision, including permanent contact with the patient, is mandatory. This can be simple —for example, after a disc herniation—or this can be a long and difficult program—for example, tetraplegia due to spinal trauma, which will require an initial period of permanent control during the first several weeks, followed by regular contact with the patient (first monthly, then yearly, during which time both rehabilitation and social reintegration of the patient will be monitored.

This volume provides a full discussion of the whole panoply of spinal problems from the point of view of anatomy, evaluation, pathology, conservative care, and surgical treatment, as well as postoperative rehabilitation according to the principles of an array of rehabilitation programs.

Professeur R. Roy-Camille, M.D.
Hôpital Pitie-Salpetriere
Paris, France

PREFACE

When we originally discussed the creation of *Rehabilitation of the Spine: Science and Practice,* it was evident that while there are many treatises on the etiology and treatment of back pain, there have been very few dedicated to the rehabilitation of the spine. Patients suffering from various disorders of the spine are rarely cured of the ongoing disease process. Recognizing this poor cure rate, various caregivers have attempted to provide comfort, hope, and education in lieu of perfect restoration of function. Specifically, this work is dedicated to all those individuals suffering from spinal disorders, as well as the health care professionals who take care of these individuals.

With rapidly advancing technology, the interest in spinal disorders is increasing in geometric proportions. It is in the area of rehabilitation where the biggest progress has been seen. No longer is the patient treated with passive modalities such as heat and ultrasound, as was the case years ago, but is now being exercised back into health, whether treated conservatively or surgically. As life expectancy increases, so will the disorders of the spine. Most of the surgery we perform today will more than likely be superseded by less invasive and minimally invasive procedures of the 21st century and reliance more on rehabilitation.

The first portion of this text is divided into the basic sciences. The following sections deal with specific spinal disorders and their treatment, with or without surgery. We feel that the prominence of surgery in the treatment of spinal disorders will diminish as science and technology improves rehabilitation, and the prevention of spinal problems will take on a major role.

While the number of individuals are too numerous to list individually, we are most indebted to the authors who have provided their time and expertise and have made this volume come to fruition. Also we would like to especially thank Donna Ohnmeiss, without whom this work would not have been completed. Her endless hours of proofreading, editing, and coordinating timetables have been invaluable.

Stephen H. Hochschuler, M.D.

Howard B. Cotler, M.D.

Richard D. Guyer, M.D.

CONTENTS

INTRODUCTION

The American public and body politic justifiably are debating three central issues in health care: cost, quality, and accessibility. The reasons for this debate are apparent. In America, health care costs more than in any other nation: we spend approximately $2300 for every man, woman, and child; the next closest nation spends $1400 per capita. Moreover the costs are rising disproportionate to virtually all other inflationary indices. At the same time, the quality of service produced by these dollar expenditures is perceived to be less than optimal. Comparisons of standard health indicators demonstrate the United States does no better and, in some instances, less well than many other nations. Finally, this country, unlike most other industrialized nations, has limited access to health care; an estimated 37 million of our citizens have no health insurance.

What do these general concerns about American health care have to do with spinal disorders and particularly the rehabilitation of these disorders? A great deal insofar as spinal disorders are one of our society's more costly health conditions. Analyses done by my colleague Willy Cats-Baril and myself estimated that more than 60 billion dollars was expended on spinal conditions in fiscal 1990[2] (see Table). Our research and that of others indicate that at least 70% of these costs are attributed to those individuals who have extended disability.[1, 13] About one third of the costs are medical, the remainder are "indirect costs" and relate to lost work time and the costs of workers compensation, which for low back disorders alone is estimated to be in excess of 11 billion dollars in 1990.[14]

The potential future problem is even more ominous, when the growth in the spine-disabled population is calculated. Today, 2.5 million Americans are chronically disabled by back pain.[12] In previous decades the growth rate of disability has surpassed population growth by 14-fold.

Careful analysis of the spinal disabled reveals significant differences between them and the general population. Some of the differences are occupational: heavier job requirements, jobs that are repetitive and boring; some are psychosocial, such as poor relationships with fellow workers and employers and psychological dysfunction; and some are societal, for example, lower income and less education.[1, 4, 6]

A volume that brings together all of the expertise that lies behind these three statements and applies it to rehabilitation is both timely and useful. However, one should recognize the difference between known scientific fact and clinical belief. Not all perspectives promoted in this volume have been proved by rigorous outcome studies un-

TABLE.
Estimated Direct Costs of Spinal Disorders*

Services	1984 Cost	1990 Cost
Hospital inpatient	$ 4,462,770,000	$ 6,780,462,000
Outpatient and ER†	259,690,000	387,980,000
Outpatient diagnosis and therapeutic	1,010,590,000	2,000,000,000
Physician inpatient	1,075,750,000	1,707,080,000
Physician office, outpatient, and ER	1,048,120,000	2,411,690,000
Other practitioner	233,630,000	2,825,119,000
Drugs	121,340,000	191,697,000
Nursing home	2,933,520,000	4,952,394,000
Prepayment	501,530,000	615,080,000
Non–health sector goods and services	1,275,800,000	1,564,651,000
Total direct costs	$12,922,740,000	$23,536,153,000

*From Cats-Baril WL, Frymoyer JW: The economics of spinal disorders, in Frymoyer JW (ed): *The Adult Spine: Principles and Practice*. New York, Raven Press, 1991, pp 85–106. Used by permission.
†ER = emergency room.

equivocally demonstrating their efficacy.[3, 13] Despite the enthusiasm for functional testing, many of the costly devices advocated have yet to undergo the rigorous evaluation required. Although it seems attractive to remove a disc by the percutaneous route or to perform anterior and posterior fusions in patients with incapacitating symptoms, the data supporting these costly procedures remain unclear. Without such data, insurers, employers, and government will increasingly ask the questions: Is this diagnostic method or treatment one that has proven efficacy? Is the method cost-effective? Are there alternatives that will accomplish the same goal? Will we pay for it?

In my judgement, the topic of rehabilitation covered in this volume points us in the general right direction to be able to answer many of these questions affirmatively. When we have even more and definitive information, we will have made even greater strides in addressing how we can make one portion of American medical care both cost-effective and of the highest quality.

The Table shows only the direct medical costs of spinal disorders. The indirect costs (lost work time, compensation, etc.) are more difficult to quantify precisely. Our analysis[2] concluded that the probable indirect costs exceeded 30 billion dollars and the total costs quite likely exceeded 50 billion dollars.[1] The baseline 1984 data are from Grazier et al.[7] The 1990 figures and how they were compilated are derived from Cats-Baril and Frymoyer.[2]

An analysis of disability prevention and medical management of those with disability reveals a number of important features. First the success of a variety of prevention programs has been marginal.[4] The management of those with disability has enjoyed better success recently,[8, 9] but the results are often poor when ill-advised surgery is performed.[11] The prevalence of lumbar spine surgery is 10% in the permanently back-disabled population vs. 1% in the population as a whole.[6] We see wide variations in surgical rates, particularly spinal fusion, based solely on the community or region within which the patient lives. An amazing statistic generated by Deyo (personal communication, 1991) finds that the rate of lumbar spinal fusion in the Northeast is 3.5/100,000 population per annum vs. 35/100,000 in the West, yet the incidence and prevalence of spinal disorders is no greater.

The inescapable conclusion is that spinal disorders are very much a part of the broader context of the American health care dilemmas of cost and quality. What can we do about this dilemma as it relates to spinal disorders? An obvious area for fruitful endeavor is rehabilitation. This book brings together experts from diverse fields, all of whom have an interest in spinal rehabilitation applied not only to patients with chronic disability but also to those with more acute disorders. I am impressed by three major changes in knowledge that have affected how we treat and rehabilitate our patients during the past decade.

1. A body of epidemiologic information has evolved that most importantly emphasizes the essentially benign nature of most low back disorders, i.e., the natural history is favorable for recovery.[4] At the same time, disabling low back pain has been recognized as having a poor prognosis and requires aggressive intervention if function is to be restored.[8, 9]

2. We have moved from an attitude that emphasized rest and inactivity to one that promotes early function, activation, and exercise. A body of literature has accumulated that stands behind the clinical philosophy, including the beneficial effects of activity on virtually all connective tissues.[5] Some impressive results have been obtained in minimizing disability such as large-scale intervention studies conducted in Sweden.[10]

3. Our technological capabilities have vastly improved, particularly in the imaging of spinal disorders, spinal implants, and some measures of functional capacity. One of the dilemmas is the observation that our surgical success rates have not correspondently improved.

John W. Frymoyer, M.D.

REFERENCES

1. Bigos SJ, Battie MC: The impact of spinal disorders in industry, in Frymoyer JW (ed): *The Adult Spine: Principles and Practice*. New York, Raven Press, 1991, pp 147–154.
2. Cats-Baril WL, Frymoyer JW: The economics of spinal disorders, in Frymoyer JW (ed): *The Adult Spine: Principles and Practice*. New York, Raven Press, 1991, pp 85–106.
3. Deyo RA: Conservative therapy for low back pain: Distinguishing useful from useless therapy. *JAMA* 1983; 250:1057–1062.
4. Frymoyer JW: Back pain and sciatica. *N Engl J Med* 1988; 318:291.
5. Frymoyer JW, Gordon SL (eds): *New Perspectives in Low-Back Pain*. Chicago, American Academy of Orthopaedic Surgeons, 1989.
6. Frymoyer JW, Rosen JC, Clements J, et al: Psychologic factors in low-back pain disability. *Clin Orthop* 1985; 195:178.
7. Grazier KL, Holbrook T, Kelsey JL, et al (eds): *The Frequency of Occurrence, Impact, and Cost of Musculoskeletal Conditions in the United States*. Chicago, American Academy of Orthopaedic Surgeons, 1984.
8. Hazard RG, Fenwick JW, Kalisch SM, et al: Functional restoration with behavioral support: A one-year prospective study of patients with chronic low back pain. *Spine* 1989; 14:157.
9. Mayer TG, Gatchel RJ, Kishino N, et al: Objective assessment of spine function following industrial injury: A pro-

spective study with comparison group and one-year follow up. *Spine* 1985; 10:482.

10. Nachemson AL, Eek C, Lindstrom I, et al: Chronic low back pain disability can largely be prevented: A prospective randomized trial in industry. Presented at the 56th Annual Meeting of the American Academy of Orthopaedic Surgeons, Las Vegas, Feb 9–14, 1989.
11. Norton WL: Chemonucleolysis versus surgical discectomy: Comparison of costs and results in Workers Compensation claimants. *Spine* 1986; 11:440.
12. *Prevalence of Selected Impairment, United States—1977*. Hyattsville, Md, National Center for Health Statistics, DHHS Publication (PHS) Series 10, No 134, 1981.
13. Spitzer WO, LeBlanc FE, Dupuis M, et al: Scientific approach to the assessment and management of activity-related spinal disorders: A monograph for clinicians. Report of the Quebec Task Force on Spinal Disorders. *Spine* 1987; 12:1.
14. Webster BS, Snook SH: The cost of compensable low back pain. *J Occup Med* 1990; 32:13.

PART I

BASIC CONSIDERATIONS

1

Multidisciplinary Spinal Rehabilitation: Management by Objectives

Ralph F. Rashbaum, M.D.

Patients with work-related back pain are a population quite apart from those who have not sustained such an injury. They have been noted to be more resistant to prescribed treatment than noncompensable patients are and thus may require a more detailed treatment regimen to help ensure successful recovery to a productive life-style. Certainly all of the considerations applied to them will have equal applicability to the non–work-injured patient as well. In the past, it was the medical practitioner's perceived function to limit the suffering of his patient, as expounded in the Hippocratic oath. It was assumed that all pain sources were in fact similar, with acute and chronic pain both originating in tissue injury and the duration of time being the only variable distinguishing one from the other. It has now been recognized that acute pain represents actual tissue damage and that this should "heal" within a prescribed time. Chronic pain, on the other hand, has become more associated with a psychosocial response, no longer being totally determined by tissue injury, and so the application of treatment strategies normally accepted for acute pain syndromes are doomed to failure in a chronic pain population. It is with this in mind that treatment objectives must be rethought. Should only the complaints of pain be addressed and treatment directed toward alleviating it or should patients be encouraged to consciously "ignore" the pain since its purpose as once perceived as a signal of potential damage is no longer functional? Analgesics and marked reduction in physical activity of the injured segment appear appropriate, while on the other hand, for the chronic syndrome, these are not only inappropriate but are ultimately harmful to the patient as well, both physically and psychologically. Restoration of function rather than or in addition to alleviation of pain has become a treatment goal in many cases. It should be noted that these goals often coexist. We are now directing rehabilitation efforts toward reintegration of the impaired patient into the work force in a capacity in which he can perform, again not necessarily without the presence of pain.[5] Through education, reconditioning, retraining, workstation modification, and assistive work aids, attempts are made to return the injured worker to a productive life-style. Short of accomplishing this goal, equally important becomes the affirmation of disability and its quantification. Appropriate goal setting can then be placed around this lesser level of performance. This might also lead to decreased medical utilization, a benefit in its own right. Often an improved activity level, short of vocational participation but one that allows the patient to reintegrate into family activities, may also become a stated goal. The patient is taught to no longer allow the presence of pain to be a signal to use medication to extinguish that signal but that it is okay to hurt since he has learned that in spite of the presence of this signal he is quite capable of physical performance. The following bear consideration as they relate to injured patients and the application of rehabilitation efforts to return them to functional vocational participation.

In a commentary written by Bortz, he seems to advance the idea of the "disuse syndrome."[7] He equates the developing cultural sedentariness, a product of our automated society, as a source of "human ill-being." He describes the course of physical inactivity as leading predictably to deterioration of many body functions. Among them are cardiovascular vulnerability, obesity, musculoskeletal fragility, depression, and premature aging. He goes on to show that his proposed syndrome is experimentally reproducible and, more significant, that the clinical features are subject to both preventive and restitutive efforts that, as he states, are "happily cheap, safe, accessible, and effective." Cybernetic mechanics link optimal performance to regular use. For the musculoskeletal and cardiovascular systems, this implies physical work, as would cognition be implied in the central nervous system. In the musculoskeletal and cardiovascular systems, disuse leads to atrophy not only in the specific organ systems but, more universally, in an overall catabolism of body functions. Disuse of a muscle leads to structural loss of muscle fiber bulk,[50] in particular, slow twitch fibers, calcium resorption, and alteration in the number of membrane binding sites. Muscle catabolism that accompanies enforced bed rest causes a loss of 8 g protein per day.[45] At a functional level, there is disruption of the rhythmic process, loss of enzyme activity, or distortion of normal responses. These changes are assumed to be linked to the chemical pathways of energy generation. Again depression seems to be attendant to decreased activity. Peripheral and central nervous system catecholamine content is increased with physical activity.[11] The treatment program often prescribed for injured workers may actually be contributing to Bortz's disuse syndrome. Care providers have been guilty of applying treatment regimens for the sole purpose of pain control and, perhaps after achieving that goal, assume that the condition for which the patient was being treated is resolved. The patient has been characteristically released back to work. If the physician is not sure of the patient's performance capability, he is usually released to light, sedentary work. When told that there is no such job available, then the doctor, out of ignorance, frustration, or both, is apt to give a blanket work release. The resultant injury that usually follows such a situation is generally an aggravation of a previous injury and is most likely nothing more than the result of the worker being ill-prepared to meet both the physical and perhaps the emotional demands of returning to work. Invariably, work or any meaningful activity has not been engaged in for many months or even years in some cases. Worse still, body-altering surgery may have been performed, which usually has an impact on the ability to do a specific set of prior work tasks. Just how the surgery has had an impact on function must be identified and quantified so as to match the patient to a work situation in which he can reasonably be expected to participate without further ill effect. It is with this in mind that care providers must move away from subjective vocational decision making generally based on the degree of patient-reported pain to an objective determination incorporating both physical and psychological assessments. These assessments can guide the treatment program step by step and ultimately allow a matchup of the patient's maximum potential to the job market. It is now possible to determine specific job requirements by sending occupational therapists to the workplace. They can assess, with great accuracy, the physical demand characteristics of that job and make suggestions as to the possible workstation modifications. They can also show the patient how, through the use of assistive devices, proper lifting techniques, and perhaps the use of external supports, to engage in work activity safely and often without increased pain, thus reinforcing the fact that function can be restored and a productive life-style achieved.

As part of the multidisciplinary treatment team, the clinical psychologist can and should be involved early in the treatment program to determine whether psychosocial impediments exist that may prevent or delay reintegration back to the workplace. It has been shown that job dissatisfaction, boredom,[36, 53] and interpersonal difficulties with supervisors[6] are strong barriers to return to work and are often the most significant predictors of ultimate failure to accomplish this goal. These need to be addressed early so that patient resistance to or noncompliance with treatment and continuing complaints of pain are not thought to be organically based. This would prevent further need to define organic pathology with more invasive and more costly diagnostic testing. Unfortunately, too often in these situations one sees the treatment become more aggressive and usually result in an attempt at ill-advised surgery. Patients who do not "heal" in the time frame usually expected for their specific injury and thus who remain out of work have a good deal of time in which to advance pain behaviors. They play the invalid role to reinforce dependent posturing. They may become depressed, angry, withdrawn, and addicted and in general become emotional and economic drains on their families and society.[48] In essence, it needs to be determined what the patient seeks to gain from treatment. Is it merely to resolve the tissue injury and return to work, or is it perhaps to manipulate others and continue to play an invalid role? Without a knowledge of this psychopathology, treatment directed at observable tissue trauma is doomed to fail. In a study by Hazard et al.,[21] when asked to identify factors critical to their reemployment, those who participated with rehabilitation programs reported that for the most part psychosocial problems such as fear of reinjury, compensation issues, career employment dissatisfaction, and family discord were uppermost in their minds. It is then quite evident that the clinical psychologist should play a primary role in the management of the injured worker. The psychologist should be involved initially in patient management to help direct the team efforts over these identified and, it is hoped, not insurmountable obstacles. Certainly they would be able to direct treatment away from those efforts that could do little good and identify those with a potential for great harm. The psychologist with experience in behavior modification can help to teach the patient that work distraction can play an integral role in pain reduction. A consistent negative relationship between exercise and pain behavior has been observed.[20, 57] That is, the greater the activity level, the fewer pain behaviors observed. Here physical activity acted as a distractive mechanism, thus reducing or redirecting attention away from pain. Perhaps another explanation for both of these observations lies in the endorphin system. Stimulation of this neurohumoral system is brought about by increases in activity. These neurohumoral agents are reported to be very potent endogenous analgesics, often having 20 times the potency of exogenously administered morphine.[40] The often-held clinical assumption that increased activity for patients with chronic low back pain will increase pain was not borne out by Linton.[29] The frequently adhered to medical dictum that "if it hurts, don't do it," should not be applied in chronic pain states. The suggestion is made that decreased activity levels may not be directly related to nociception,[20] but rather to a variety of learned factors. Perhaps a stress-type reaction occurs where fear promotes anxiety and subsequent muscle tension so that the patient believes that participation in a given activity will promote more pain.[30] In these tension-induced states, Sarno postulates that the autonomic system becomes activated and this causes vasoconstriction of arterioles in skeletal muscle.[43] This would lead to relative ischemia and then to ischemic-induced pain. The skeletal muscles of endurance-trained athletes have increased capillary density, which leads to better muscle perfusion, decreased ischemia, and enhancement of recovery after muscle fatigue.[22] With patients who believe that activity will increase pain, it becomes apparent that unless this fear is allayed there will be a tendency to always use pain signals as a measure of when to quit activity. Attendant in the treatment of low back pain, whether acute or chronic, is the decision to impose bed rest or limitations of activity. This may be appropriate for brief periods in the case of low back strain or perhaps for a more protracted time in certain pain syndromes such as disc displacement. Deyo et al. have stated that in the former, 2 days' bed rest was equally as effective as 7 days,[15] but Waddell has chosen to restate this in another way.[51] He stated that 2 days of bed rest was less deleterious than 7 days. He goes on to state that even in the more serious condition of acute disc prolapse, there is little scientific or clinical evidence to support the value of prolonged bed rest. He was likely referring to a concept similar to the disuse syndrome. It is postinjury deconditioning that is frequently the major impediment of functional restoration, both from the physical or ultimately psychological basis.[41, 49] The physical rehabilitation process as it applies to a specific injury will progress through certain phases dependent upon the acute or chronic nature of the injury. With an acute injury, the initial phase of tissue repair necessitates decreased activity to allow healing of the damaged tissue. Bed rest, decreased movement of the injured part, and attention to pain relief become paramount. During recovery, the healing tissue will continue to consolidate when supported by the maintenance of strength and flexibility exercises.[44] The application of this philosophy becomes easily accepted when viewing the rehabilitation of the injured or operated knee where pain does not become the limiting factor of attempts to restore function. Why then should the situation as it relates to spinal injury be any different? Perhaps in the knee it is easier to identify the source of the pain, whereas in the spine, in over 80% of patients the painful pathology is not clearly identified. Thus more often than not it is the case that care providers do not know what type of spinal lesion is to be treated.

The next phase of treatment is restoration of function. This requires rebuilding muscular strength, with maintenance of improvement in flexibility, endurance, and coordination. Without this vital phase, a healed but physically weak area, when stressed again, will fail and result in pain. This may not represent a new injury but will often result in reinforcement of exaggerated pain behavior as well as reinforcement of the patient's fear that he will never be able to function productively again. Soon to follow is the disability process. This term indicates disability beyond that expected for a specific injury. The disability process implies that the injured worker has bought into some measure of suffering, a psychological condition, therefore an acquired psychopathology precipitated by a physical event, perhaps industry's equivalent of "combat fatigue syndrome." The patient who comes for evaluation is seeking two types of aid. Medical attention is sought to assess the potential for damage, but equally important and frequently overlooked is assurance as to the ultimate successful resolution of the problem such that it will not interfere with future endeavors. Those who have altered body function will draw upon past experiences or on what they have heard. They will tend to think the worst and remember a friend with a similar complaint who died with cancer or never recovered from the illness. Assurances need to be directed to both the patient and the patient's family since they will not want to provoke alarm or reinforce developing pain behaviors. Conversations with the patient and the family must not provoke anxiety through the use of terms such as "degenerative disc disease." This has a tendency to imply a disease process from which the patient may never recover, a condition that will continue to deteriorate with time and bring along with it worsening pain. By the same token, patients must not be dismissed by relating the injury to some mundane condition that in the patient's previous experience would be expected to resolve quickly. A previously thought muscle "sprain" that has healed quickly, when applied to a back injury, might impose a time frame for which this injury should heal. When healing does not occur as rapidly as expected, fear with all its attendant anxieties will replace patient confidence. When this is not addressed, pain behaviors ensue. The injured worker must be physically fit in order to compete economically. When this physical condition is jeopardized, then his future work is at risk. With this uncertainty, there is a move toward defensive posturing. Anything perceived as an additional threat, such as a late compensation check or harmless inquiry from the insurance company, can precipitate an unreasonable reaction, sometimes driving the patient to seek legal counsel. Litigation does not precede but tends to follow complications and dissatisfaction with medical care and insurance benefits.[28] A lack of sensitivity on the part of the employer can be perceived as a conspiracy to get the patient fired. This threat to economic well-being can precipitate more physical symptoms so as to reinforce the impression of disability, thus protecting economic survival.

The mere mention of surgery has been shown to result in higher claims costs.[28] There is also a fear, both real and imagined, that once returned to work, there may be a temporary decrease in the patient's productivity that results in termination, an economic disaster in two ways: first, an immediate cessation of weekly compensation checks since the insurance company is obligated only if the patient cannot work, and second, the significant likelihood that the patient would not be able to gain or retain other opportunity because of his work history. There does exist a sort of blackball system that excludes these people from other work unless they lie about previous injuries. It is easy to sympathize with employers who are in business for the "bottom line." That line has frequently been eroded due to some of the worker's compensation regulations. Not only does a previous back injury predict subsequent back injuries, but it is also strongly predictive of a higher subsequent claims cost. In an unpublished study, Kennedy found that when injured workers were told not to come back to work until they were 100% of their preinjury level and the doctor discharged the patients, this led to severe psychological and financial stress.[25] This ultimately led to 10 cases of total disability in the 200 cases reviewed. Kennedy went on to show that the presence of economic disincentives (receiving compensation or disability payments at or slightly below working wages) resulted in 6 cases of disability in the group of 200.

In normal subjects, there exists an imbalance between the strength of trunk flexor muscles and trunk extensor muscles, with the extensors being stronger in a ratio of 1.4 to 1.0.[47] It has also been shown that weak muscles are a contributing factor to low back injuries and subsequent low back pain.[2] Various authors have studied the relationship of trunk strength in normal subjects and patients with low back pain. Pederson et al. found no difference in back extensor strength between these two groups,[37] while Nachemson and Lindh found the difference to exist as it related to the duration of symptoms.[35] In those patients who had remained inactive for longer than 1 month, the values were lower in both flexors and extensors. Others have found that the extensors suffer the greatest loss in patients with chronic low back pain. The implication of this loss will become more apparent when considering the muscles needed to successfully perform work activity requiring either postural maintenance for extended periods of time or a significant lifting ability. One needs to consider the effects of postural stress in the causation of low back dysfunction and subsequent pain. The back extensor muscles play a key role in posture. DeVries studied back pain in patients and compared them with normal subjects by electromyelographic (EMG) analysis.[14] He noted differences in EMG fatigue patterns in subjects who were symptomatic vs. those without symptoms during prolonged postural stress. He suggested that this muscular deficiency was a causation of idiopathic low back pain and further suggested that this condition would be responsive to endurance exercise.[14] Magora, in studies of the association of low back pain and occupation, found postural stress to be a constant factor in the precipitation of low back pain, in particular where there was a prolonged maintenance of a particular posture.[31] If these two factors are considered together, that is, muscle insufficiency and postural stress, then it is relatively easy to see how certain work tasks could result in a greater incidence of low back pain and thus that frequent alterations of posture might be a simple means of decreasing this occurrence. Trunk strength is not the limiting factor as regards muscle function, but rather it is endurance that is the limiting factor. A muscle group may have a physical capacity to exert a force necessary to move an object one time, a function of that muscle strength, but it is a lack of endurance, affected by prolonged postural stress, that will ultimately precipitate an episode of low back pain. It is the inability of that muscle group to sustain repeated activity due to rapid fatigue that will lead to abnormal muscle substitution patterns with resulting low back dysfunction.[13] It is only a matter of time before the physical capacity of the fatigued muscle group is exceeded and unprotected stress applied to the spinal segment will result in low back pain. It becomes obvious that physical conditioning that encompasses both strength and endurance training becomes of particular importance in the prevention as well as the rehabilitation of low back injuries. Cady et al. assessed the effects of aerobic conditioning on a group of fire fighters over an 8-year period.[9, 10] They found that not only was the incidence of serious back injuries substantially reduced by conditioning, but that the time to convalesce from a back injury was decreased as well. The overall number of nondisabling back injuries did not change as a result of the program, but the number of disabling injuries was reduced by 50%. The frequency of this type of injury was ten times greater when comparing the most fit group with the least fit group. They concluded that the conditioning program must exert a protective effect against the occurrence of disabling back injuries and that when such an injury does occur, it serves to decrease the associated morbidity.

The positive effects of conditioning would also be borne out in a study by Browne et al.[8] in which a population of sedentary office workers, a much different population than in the study of Cady et al., were followed over a 5-year period after the initiation of an aerobic exercise program. Increased levels of fitness were associated with decreased disability costs and disability days. The American College of Sports Medicine issued a position statement in 1978 stating that workers whose jobs were considered physically demanding, i.e., material handlers, nurses, and truck drivers, should engage in an exercise program three to five times a week for 30 to 40 minutes to achieve an appropriate training effect and level of fitness.[3] Finally, in consideration of the positive effects of exercise is the observation that exercise brings with it a change to a healthier life-style. Those who exercise regularly seem to take a more active role in caring for themselves. They stop or decrease smoking and/or drinking, eat healthier foods, and tend to be thinner than those who do not exercise. The implications of these changes as they relate to both muscle and disc hygiene should be obvious. Spinal stability has been a well-appreciated factor in the precipitation of low back pain, in particular as it relates to abnormal alignment of a motion segment. Proper orientation of one segment with another is needed for normal motion to occur. Proper function of muscles is also required for motion. Shortening of these muscles due to disease or injury, whether iatrogenic (spinal surgery) or traumatic, will result in abnormal motion and subsequent deterioration of that motion segment or an adjacent segment. This results in dysfunction and ultimately precipitates pain. This leads one to postulate that stretching is needed in contracted areas as part of a rehabilitation effort, as well as reeducation of trunk muscles to impart a dynamic stabilizing force. Polatin et al. make a contrary observation that, however, is applied to a select group.[38] Patients who underwent spinal surgery, in particular, spinal fusions, showed a trend in that those with decreased mobility seemed to fare better as regards symptoms and return to work than did those whose mobility was greater or more nearly normal. Perhaps the resulting stiffness acts as a protective mechanism for the motion segment above the fusion, where physical stress would be shifted in an attempt to restore normal motion. One thing that does seem obvious is that pain relief derived from muscle stability is not a function of decreased load on the disc since the effect of these exercises would be to preload the spinal segment itself. There is strong evidence to support the need for adequate trunk mobility in normal subjects in an effort to prevent injuries. Flexibility of the lumbar spine supplies the mechanical advantage for function and efficiency.[17, 18] Pelvic motion is essential for bending and lifting activities.[17, 18] Movement of the spine, that is, loading and unloading, is necessary for the nutrition of the discs and synovial joints.[16] How should the rehabilitation effort as it applies to muscles of the back and/or those muscles needed for spinal stability during lifting be directed? Postural mechanisms have been alluded to as being causative of low back pain. These are postures in which the patient places the spine into a rather static posture such as increased lumbar lordosis. These natural postures cannot be altered by exercises devised to strengthen the abdominal muscles.[12] What then is the rationale for performing various exercises, and does their use make sense? It has been stated that strong abdominal muscles protect lumbar discs from excessive loads through the development of intra-abdominal pressure.[4] However, Jackson and Brown note that evidence fails to demonstrate a direct correlation of abdominal strength with increased intra-abdominal pressure.[23] Morris et al. stated that the activity required of the abdominal oblique muscles in developing an adequate intra-abdominal pressure during loading of the spine is only a sixth of that obtained by maximal voluntary contraction.[33, 34] Studies of patients with intractable back pain reveal that abdominal muscles maintain 80% of their normal strength.[5] One would assume that this would still be adequate to generate forces necessary to increase intra-abdominal pressure. It is the internal and external oblique muscles that generate intra-abdominal pressure, not the abdominal muscles as a unit. Intra-abdominal pressure is a reflex response, not a voluntary muscle contraction. In voluntary abdominal muscle contraction, the rectus abdominis and posterior spinal muscles are also active with resultant actual spinal compression. In the broadest sense, exercise was thought to bring about pain reduction in low back disorders by Williams, who advocated his flexion exercise regimen.[55, 56] This was thought to bring relief of pressure on the nerve root by opening up the neuroforamina. However McKenzie, a proponent of the opposite movement (extension), postulated that repeated extension exercises would cause a shift of nuclear material away from the posterolateral compartment and thereby decrease neural compression.[32] The question arises whether it is actually neural compression that is responsible for the patient's complaints. Certainly this could be argued for those pain syndromes that result in true radicular type pain. This, however, is a small segment of the population with dysfunctional low back pain. Acutely imposed nerve root compression does not cause pain but instead causes paresthesias. It is only after compression has resulted in edematous changes in the nerve root that pain is precipitated.[42] If one assumes that the ceasing compression of the nerve root must be of sufficient duration to allow for resolution of this edematous state, thus allowing inflammation to subside and the nerve root sensitivity to abate, could this really be expected to take place via repeated, temporary postural movements? It is very doubtful. Perhaps the proposed shift of nuclear material[46] upon extension could cause less distension of the annulus fibrosus with its outer third enervated by nociceptor fibers or result in a decrease in the stretch on these fibers as well as those in the posterolongitudinal ligament associated with repositioning of the disc brought about by extension maneuvers. The rationale for extension therapy, however, does rely on the following facts. The spine is able to withstand greater axial compression when normal physiologic curves are maintained.[24, 54] Extension unloads the discs and allows fluid influx. The disc needs low pressure to imbibe low-molecular-weight substances for nutrition.[27] The stronger the back muscles, the greater the ability to maximize lifting loads.[39] Those patients with chronic low back pain have significant loss of extensor power rather than flexor power when compared with normal subjects.[1] There is a profound decrease in extension muscle endurance as seen by EMG changes in patients with low back pain.[14] There exists a natural imbalance in normal subjects whereby the back extensor strength is greater than abdominal flexor strength.[47] Strong back extensor muscles protect the lumbar spinal ligaments in light and unloaded flexion activities.[26] One half of back extensor movement is produced by the erector spinae. The primary function of the spinal extensors is postural holding[33, 34] and eccentric control of trunk flexion. Extension of the spine is a complex movement in that many muscle groups are brought into play. Not only what would be considered most apparent, i.e., the back extensors, but also the hamstrings provide one third of the total extensor torque,[52] as well as the gluteus maximus, which is primarily involved in both hyperextension of the hips and trunk.[19] When loads are lifted from a flexed posture, it is these muscles that really supply the power for the lift.

In summary, in the rehabilitation of the spinal-injured worker, reasonable and attainable goals must be set. Activities should be directed toward those goals that establish a certain functional level. These goals, be they vocational or avocational, should be formulated with the patient's interest in mind. The anticipated level of participation should not be at a level greater than what has been achieved in the recent past. Function rather than pain relief is the primary goal. Pain is likely to diminish or resolve as function increases. Reassurances need be repeatedly given to the patient that "pain is okay." Care providers must be ever attentive in the initial rehabilitation visits to help patients through their bouts of fear and anxiety precipitated by this understandable increase in symptomatology and ultimately guide them into a productive and purposeful future. Thus, in order to meet the needs of the injured worker, a multidisciplinary team of specialists is essential for maximizing outcome.

REFERENCES

1. Addison R, Schultz A: Trunk strengths in patients seeking hospitalization for chronic low back disorders. *Spine* 1980; 5:539–544.
2. Alston W, Carlson KE, Feldman DJ, et al: A quantitative study of muscle factors in chronic low back syndrome. *J Am Geriatr Soc* 1966; 141:1041–1047.
3. American College of Sports Medicine: *Position Statement on the Recommended Quantity and Quality of Exercise for Healthy Adults*. Indianapolis, American College of Sports Medicine, 1978.
4. Bartelink DL: The role of abdominal pressure in reducing the pressure on the intervertebral disc. *J Bone Joint Surg [Br]* 1957; 59:718.
5. Berkson M, Schultz A, Nachemson A, et al: Voluntary strength of male adults with acute low back syndromes. *Clin Orthop* 1977; 129:84–98.
6. Bigos SJ, Spengler DM, Martin NA, et al: Back injuries in industry: A retrospective study. III. Employee related factors. *Spine* 1986; 11:252–256.
7. Bortz WM: The disuse syndrome. *West J Med* 1984; 141:691–694.
8. Browne DW, Russell ML, Morgan JL, et al: Reduced disability and health care costs in an industrial fitness program. *J Occup Med* 1984; 26:809–816.
9. Cady LD, Bishop DP, O'Connell ER, et al: Strength and fitness and subsequent back injuries in fire fighters. *J Occup Med* 1979; 21:269–272.
10. Cady LD, Thomas PC, Karwasky RJ: Program for increasing health and physical fitness of fire fighters. *J Occup Med* 1985; 27:110–114.
11. Corrosi H, Fuxe K, Hokfelt AG: The effect of immobilization stress on the activity of the central monoamine neurone. *Life Sci* 1968; 7:107–112.
12. Davies JE, Gibson T, Tester L: The value of exercise in the treatment of low back pain. *Rheumatol Rehabil* 1979; 18:243–247.
13. DeLateuer BJ, Lehmann JF, Fordyce WE: A test of the DeLorme axiom. *Arch Phys Med Rehab* 1968; 49:245–248.
14. DeVries HA: EMG fatigue curves in postural muscles. A possible etiology for idiopathic low back pain. *Am J Phys Med* 1968; 47:175–181.
15. Deyo RA, Diehl AK, Rosenthal M: How many days bed rest for acute low back pain? A randomized clinical trial. *N Engl J Med* 1986; 315:1064–1070.
16. Enneking WF, Horowitz M: The intra-articular effects of immobilization on the human knee. *J Bone Joint Surg [Am]* 1972; 54:973–985.
17. Farfan HF: Muscular mechanism of the lumbar spine and the position of power and efficiency. *Orthop Clin North Am* 1975; 6:135–144.
18. Farfan HF: The biomechanical advantage of lumbar lordosis and hip extension for upright activity. *Spine* 1978; 3:336–342.
19. Fischer FJ, Hortz JJ: Evaluation of the function of the gluteus maximus muscle. *Am J Phys Med* 1968; 47:182.
20. Fordyce W, McMahon R, Rainwater G, et al: Pain complaint–exercise performance in relationship in chronic pain. *Pain* 1981; 10:311–321.
21. Hazard RG, Fenwick JW, Kalisch SM, et al: Functional restoration with behavioral support: A one-year prospective study of patient with chronic low-back pain. *Spine* 1989; 14:157–161.
22. Hendriksson J, Reitman JS: Time course of changes in human muscle succinate dehydrogenase and cytochrome activities and maximum oxygen uptake with physical activity and inactivity. *Acta Physiol Scand* 1979; 99:91–97.
23. Jackson CP, Brown MD: Analysis of current approaches

and a practical guide to prescription of exercise. *Clin Orthop* 1983; 179:46–54.
24. Kapandji IA: *The Physiology of Joints,* vol 3. New York, Churchill Livingstone, 1979.
25. Kennedy WF: The industrial back injury. Submitted for publication.
26. Kottke F: Low back pain. *Arch Phys Med Rehabil* 1961; 42:426.
27. Kramer J: Pressure dependent fluid shifts in the intervertebral disc. *Orthop Clin North Am* 1977; 8:211–216.
28. Leavitt SS, Johnson MS, Beyer RD: The process of recovery: Patterns in industrial back injury. *Indust Med* 1971; 41:7–11.
29. Linton SJ: The relationship between activity and chronic back pain. *Pain* 1985; 21:289–294.
30. Linton SJ, Melin L, Gotestam KG: Behavioral analysis of chronic pain and its management, in Hersen M, Eisler R, Miller P (eds): *Progress in Behavior Modification,* vol 8, New York, Academic Press, 1984, pp 1–42.
31. Magora A: Investigation of the relationship between low back pain and occupation. III. Physical measurements: Siting, standing and weight lifting. *Indust Med Surg* 1972; 41:5–9.
32. McKenzie RA: *The Lumbar Spine. Mechanical Diagnosis and Therapy.* Waikanae, New Zealand, Spinal Publication, 1981.
33. Morris JM, Benner G, Lucas DB: An electromyographic study of the intrinsic muscles of the back in man. *J Anat* 1962; 96:509–520.
34. Morris JM, Lucas D, Bresler B: Role of the trunk in stability of the spine. *J Bone Joint Surg [Am]* 1961; 43:327–351.
35. Nachemson AL, Lindh M: Measurements of abdominal and back muscular strength with and without low back pain. *Scand J Rehabil Med* 1969; 1:60–65.
36. Niemcryck S, Jenkins C, Rose R, et al: The prospective impact of psychosocial variables on rates of illness and injury in prospective employees. *J Occup Med* 1987; 29:645.
37. Pederson OF, Peterson R, Staffeldt ES: Back pain and isometric back muscle strength of workers in a Danish factory. *Scand J Rehabil Med* 1975; 7:125–128.
38. Polatin PB, Gatchel RJ, Barnes D, et al: A psychosociomedical prediction model of response to treatment by chronically disabled workers with low-back pain. *Spine* 1989; 14:956–961.
39. Poulsen E: Back muscle strength and weight limits in lifting burdens. *Spine* 1981; 6:73–75.
40. Puig MM, Laorden ML, Miralles FS, et al: Endorphin levels in cerebrospinal fluid of patients with prospective and chronic pain. *Anesthesiology* 1982; 57:1.
41. Rose DL: The decompensated back. *Arch Phys Med Rehabil* 1975; 56:51.
42. Rydevik B, Brown MD, Lundborg G: Pathoanatomy and pathophysiology of nerve compression. *Spine* 1984; 9:7–15.
43. Sarno JE: Therapeutic exercise for back pain, in *Therapeutic Exercise.* Baltimore, Williams & Wilkins, 1984.
44. Selby DK: Conservative care of nonspecific low back pain. *Orthop Clin North Am* 1982; 13:427.
45. Seregon MS, Popov IO, Lebedeve AN, et al: Nutrition and metabolism during prolonged hypodynamic programs. *Kosm Biol* 1964; 13:79–93.
46. Shah JS: Structure, morphology and weakness of the lumbar spine, in Jayson M (ed): *The Lumbar Spine and Low Back Pain.* London, Pitman Medical, 1980, pp 359–405.
47. Smidt GL, Amundsen LR, Dostal WF: Muscle strength at the trunk. *J Orthop Sports Phys Ther* 1980; 1:165–170.
48. Sternbach RA, Wolf SR, Murphy RW, et al: Traits of pain patients: The low back loser. Presented at the 19th Annual Meeting of the Academy of Psychosomatic Medicine, San Diego, 1972.
49. Thomas LK, Hislop HJ, Waters RL: Physiologic work performance in low back disability. *Phys Ther* 1980; 60:407.
50. Tomasek RJ, Lund DD: Degeneration of different types of skeletal muscle fibers. *J Anat* 1973; 116:395.
51. Waddell G: A new clinical model for the treatment of low back pain. *Spine* 1987; 12:632–644.
52. Waters RL, Perry J, McDaniels JM, et al: The relative strength of the hamstrings during hip extension. *J Bone Joint Surg [Am]* 1974; 56:1592–1597.
53. Westrin CG, Hirsch C, Lindegard B: The personality of the back patient. *Clin Orthop* 1972; 87:209–216.
54. White AA, Panjabi M: *Clinical Biomechanics of the Spine.* Philadelphia, JB Lippincott, 1978.
55. Williams PC: Lesion of the lumbosacral spine. Part I. *J Bone Joint Surg* 1937; 19:343.
56. Williams PC: Lesion of the lumbosacral spine. Part II. *J Bone Joint Surg* 1937; 19:690–703.
57. Wynn-Parry CG: Pain in avulsion lesions of the brachial plexus. *Pain* 1980; 9:41–53.

2

*General Considerations: Stability, Flexibility, Strength, Cardiac Fitness, and Aerobic Capacity**

Stephen H. Hochschuler, M.D.

In the past, the rehabilitation of back disorders focused on pain reduction while attempting to attain the preinjury level of activities of daily living. The major emphasis was on the management of pain, not on function. In recent times, function and the sports medicine approach to rehabilitation have been more widely accepted. Consideration of overall fitness, not just abdominal strength and range of motion, has evolved.

In a recent policy statement, the American College of Sports Medicine (ACSM) recommended guidelines for exercise prescription.[1] These guidelines address the quantity and quality of training for the development and maintenance of cardiovascular fitness, body composition, strength, and endurance. It is my position that these same guidelines should be considered in the rehabilitation of spinal problems. Their recommendations include the following:

1. Frequency of training: 3 to 5 days per week.
2. Intensity of training: 60% to 90% of the maximum heart rate or 50% to 85% of the maximum oxygen uptake.
3. Duration: 20 to 60 minutes of continuous aerobic activity.
4. Mode of activity: those activities that use large muscle groups.
5. Resistance training: strength training to develop fat-free weight. The recommendation is for 8 to 12 repetitions of 8 to 10 exercises for the major muscle groups twice per week.

Rehabilitation in the 1990s includes cardiorespiratory fitness, muscular strength, endurance, and flexibility. The foregoing chapter will review programs for attaining these objectives. The purpose of this chapter is to emphasize the need to develop a level of overall conditioning and fitness. This not only increases one's level of general health and energy but also helps to develop specific physiologic adaptations necessary to reach a maximum level of performance and, perhaps more important, to reduce the risk of reinjury.

CARDIOVASCULAR FITNESS

Cardiovascular fitness is synonymous with cardiovascular endurance, aerobic capacity, and functional capacity. These terms relate to the ability of the heart, lungs, and blood vessels to acquire, transport, and deliver oxygen to the muscles. Oxygen is mandatory to release energy from fat, carbohydrate, and protein at the cellular level. This energy, in the form of adenosine triphosphate (ATP), is used to perform muscular work. ATP can be produced in muscles in either an anaerobic or aerobic process. The aerobic system uses oxygen to release the stored energy from the organic fuels with drastically improved efficiency.

Anaerobic metabolism can form ATP without the use of oxygen, primarily from the breakdown of carbohydrates. The catabolism of fat and protein requires sufficient oxygen to release their stored energy; thus they are not utilized as fuels in substantial quantities during anaerobic exercise.

Our bodies are constantly employing both energy systems to produce ATP. At rest, the delivery of oxygen is adequate to meet the body's energy demands, and the aerobic energy system is primarily engaged. As the body's need for energy increases to perform muscular work (the energy requirement for exercise intensity increases), the need for greater oxygen delivery to the exercising muscle occurs. There is a direct relationship between exercise intensity and oxygen demand. All individuals reach a point during exercise when the demand for oxygen exceeds the supply. This point, referred to as the anaerobic threshold, occurs when one is primarily limited to the breakdown of carbohydrates as the predominant fuel supply for ATP production. Concurrently, lactic acid, a by-product of anaerobic metabolism, accumulates in working muscle cells. This increased acidity results in a lower pH at the cellular level, which in turn inhibits ATP production and results in muscle fatigue and exhaustion.

*Published in part in Glisan B, Hochschuler SH: General fitness in the treatment and prevention of athletic low back injuries, in Hochschuler SH (ed): *Spinal Injuries in Sports*. Philadelphia, Hanley & Belfus, 1990, pp 31–42. Reprinted with permission.

Maximum oxygen uptake (Vo_2max) represents the maximal volume of oxygen transported to the exercising muscles.[1] Vo_2max is the objective measurement of aerobic capacity or cardiovascular fitness. The greater this value, the greater the level of cardiovascular fitness and potential exercise performance.

There are few studies investigating aerobic capacity and the incidence of back pain. Results from these studies do not clearly indicate the benefits of a cardiovascular fitness program to diminish back insults. One prospective study estimated Vo_2max by treadmill testing. No significant correlation between Vo_2max and the occurrence of back injuries was demonstrated.[3] This study, however, included a large number of subjects who smoked, which may have biased the results.

In a series of studies involving various cardiovascular measures, one investigator initially demonstrated a preventive value from increasing levels of physical fitness.[7] In a follow-up study, the same investigator demonstrated a 25% decrease in workers' compensation costs that appeared to be directly related to improvements in cardiovascular fitness and the initiation of a policy allowing for a more rapid return to work. This occurred while flexibility and muscular strength parameters did not significantly change.[8]

There is no conclusive evidence that cardiovascular fitness decreases the risk for back injury. Further research is warranted in this area. It is difficult to separate aerobic capacity from muscular endurance, strength, and other measures of general physical fitness due to their complex interrelationships. The end result may well be that increasing levels of all components of physical fitness (aerobic capacity, muscular strength and endurance, flexibility, and body composition) may be equally important in both decreasing the incidence of back injuries and assisting in the expeditious rehabilitation of an injury.

Five factors must be successfully structured to obtain optimal gains in cardiovascular fitness: type/mode of activity, intensity, duration, frequency, and rate of progression.

Type of Activity

To attain maximal gains in cardiovascular fitness, an activity must incorporate large muscle mass and be performed for a prolonged period of time in a continuous, rhythmic fashion. Exercise such as walking, swimming, jogging/running, cycling, and cross-country skiing usually meet the established criteria. Other activities such as hiking, figure skating, dancing, etc., can also significantly improve aerobic capacity if structured appropriately. Although less tedious than cycling or treadmill walking, these activities do not provide as great a control of exercise intensity and therefore should be employed cautiously in novices or rehabilitation participants until a base level of fitness is developed.

The back-injured patient must maintain cardiovascular fitness to avoid the deconditioning often associated with increased pain and depression. Specifically designed exercise protocols consistent with the patient's working diagnosis must be adhered to. In the case of a herniated disc, flexion exercises should be avoided. Bicycling in the upright position or swimming should be considered. In spondylolisthesis, extension exercises beyond neutral should be avoided and appropriate abdominal strengthening and dynamic stabilization instituted.

Rotation often exacerbates symptoms in the spine-injured patient. Rotational exercises should first be performed in an unloaded or slightly loaded position prior to more aggressive endeavors. Devices such as cycling equipment involving the upper part of the body or a standard treadmill provide cardiovascular exercise that has inherent rotational components and consequently should be employed cautiously.

Jogging and running warrant special attention. These activities transmit impact loading to the spine. These forces can be as much as three to four times the person's body weight. Jogging causes more vertical load than running and consequently may be more damaging to the spine. Hence, running might well be a better choice. Either may not be tolerated and hence should be prescribed cautiously. Lower-impact cardiovascular activities such as bicycling, swimming, walking, and stair climbing may indeed prove less hazardous and a better choice than jogging or running.

Exercise Intensity

To maximize gains in aerobic capacity, exercise intensity should correspond to 65% to 90% of an individual's maximal heart rate or 50% to 85% of his functional capacity (Vo_2max). This value varies depending on the patient's initial level of cardiovascular fitness. The greater the aerobic capacity, the greater his exercise intensity must be in order to achieve significant improvements in Vo_2max.

Provided that the total energy expenditure is the same, individuals may be able to exercise at lower intensities for a longer duration and obtain similar improvements in Vo_2max as they would exercising for a shorter time but at a greater intensity.[13, 30, 38] Exercise adherence is improved when subjects exercise at lower training intensities.[34] In addition, high-intensity training programs have been associated with a greater incidence of musculoskeletal injuries[24, 28] and cardiovascular symptoms.[12, 19, 31] Therefore, it appears advantageous to have patients exercise at lower intensities for longer durations. Exercise intensity may be monitored by a variety of techniques. The heart rate method will be discussed.

Generally, unless disturbed by environmental conditions, disease, or psychological stimuli, a direct relationship exists between heart rate and exercise intensity.[44]

Therefore, when exercising to increase aerobic capacity, the heart rate can be effectively utilized to prescribe and monitor exercise intensity.

The training heart rate can be accurately assessed during an exercise stress test on a bicycle or treadmill ergometer. When access or costs restrict performing these objective measures, a less sophisticated estimate may be calculated as below.

220 − (age/HR max) − resting HR* × % of HR max (range, 0.65 to 0.80) + (resting HR/target HR)

It is difficult to maintain the heart rate at exactly a specified value; hence a range of approximately ± 5 bpm is established, which is the target heart rate zone. The goal is to exercise at a work load that allows the patient's heart rate to plateau and remain within this range for the duration of the exercise session, excluding warm-up and cool-down.

Duration of Activity

To obtain maximal improvements in functional capacity, the duration of the exercise session, excluding warm-up and cool-down, can vary from 15 to 60 minutes. In general, the longer the duration of the exercise session, the greater the magnitude of improvement in V_{O_2} max.[1, 16, 19, 20, 26, 27, 41] Significant improvements in aerobic capacity have been demonstrated with high-intensity (greater than 90% maximum), short-duration (5 to 10 minutes) sessions. However, high-intensity sessions are associated with a greater risk of orthopedic injury and cardiovascular problems. Hence, for sedentary individuals, lower-intensity (40% to 70% of functional capacity), moderate-duration (20 to 30 minutes) exercise sessions are recommended. An individual should not experience undue fatigue an hour after an exercise session.[1] Lower-intensity exercises can be sustained for a longer duration with less fatigue. A low- to moderate-intensity and longer-duration exercise session is recommended for nonathletic adults when the goal is to improve aerobic capacity and not athletic performance.

A patient recovering from an orthopedic injury may not be able to tolerate even low-intensity and moderate-duration exercise. Repeated brief bouts of low-intensity exercise ranging from 15 to 20 seconds to 2 to 3 minutes may be appropriate initially until a base level of exercise tolerance is developed.

Frequency of Exercise

The general recommendation of the ACSM for training frequency is 3 to 5 days per week.[1] The greater the initial fitness level, the more frequently exercises can be performed. Frequency can vary from numerous daily exercise sessions of low intensity and short duration to three to seven single daily sessions per week. Training more frequently than 5 days per week is possible; however, 95% of the potential improvement in aerobic capacity is obtained in a jog/run program of 4 to 5 days per week.[29] The risk of orthopedic injuries increases exponentially with jog/run-type exercises following increased training frequency and duration. When exercise frequency exceeds 4 days a week, the participant is encouraged to employ "cross-training" techniques to minimize the potential for an overuse syndrome as well as to decrease the possibility of boredom.

Rate of Exercise Progression

Progression of aerobic exercise activities is highly dependent upon the health, age, functional capacity, and needs of the participant. Exercise progression is currently divided into three stages: initial, improvement, and maintenance.

Initial Conditioning Phase

A base level of conditioning is accomplished by initiating a low-level conditioning program that minimizes muscle soreness resulting from exercise. The length of time required to establish the base fitness level depends on an individual's adherence to the program. The initial conditioning phase consists of a 4- to 6-week period but may extend to as much as 10 weeks.

The initial exercise duration is typically no more than 10 to 15 minutes per session; however, for some patients, it is not uncommon to have total exercise sessions lasting 5 minutes or less. Exercise duration may be limited by local muscle fatigue, breathlessness, symptoms of cardiac disease (angina), or increased pain. Exercise prescriptions must be individualized.

Improvement Conditioning Phase

This phase differs from the initial phase in that individuals are progressed at a much quicker rate. The duration of exercise sessions is typically increased every 1 to 3 weeks. If the individual is not already exercising at an intensity that corresponds to 50% to 85% of his functional capacity, then this level should be accomplished within the improvement phase. The fitness level determines the progression of exercise intensity and frequency. The duration of exercise should be increased to 20 to 30 minutes before increasing the exercise intensity. Older patients may take longer to adapt to the stresses of exercise and thus may require a slower rate of progression.

Maintenance Conditioning Phase

Most individuals will obtain the greatest proportion of cardiovascular improvement within the first 6 months of a training program. The purpose of the maintenance phase is to maintain the improvements gained in the previous phases.

*The resting heart rate (HR) should be determined upon waking in the morning or while lying supine. The heart rate should be taken for 3 to 5 minutes and then averaged to determine the beats per minute (bpm). HR max = maximal predicted heart rate.

MUSCULAR STRENGTH

Muscular strength is defined as the maximal tension or force that can be generated by a muscle or group of muscles.[1] Maximal muscular strength is obtained from exercises of high resistance and low repetition. Muscular strength can be classified as static, dynamic, or explosive.

Static strength is the ability of a muscle to exert a maximal force for an extended period of time. A high level of static strength is required by a gymnast when performing movements such as the iron cross. Static strength requires isometric muscular contractions that generate muscle tension; however, there is little or no muscle shortening, lengthening, or joint movement. No external work is performed; however, internal muscular work is performed, which is reflected by the liberation of heat. Static strength may be assessed by a tensiometer or dynamometer.

Dynamic strength is the ability to repeatedly create forces to move or support a portion of the body weight for an extended period of time. This is exemplified by the repeated muscular contraction of the long-distance runner. Dynamic strength efforts use isotonic muscular contractions. The length of the muscles constantly varies from decreasing lengths (concentric contractions) to increasing lengths (eccentric contractions), both of which cause joint movement. Dynamic strength may be assessed by performing calisthenics or various forms of weight lifting, with cable tensiometers, or with dynamometers. An isokinetic dynamometer may also be used.

Explosive strength is the ability to exert a maximal, short burst of force. This type of strength is demonstrated by the shot-putter, who combines the explosive strength capabilities of various muscle groups to propel the shot into space. Explosive strength is essentially the same as muscle power. Power is defined as the amount of external work performed divided by time.[1, 36] Power is typically more important in pursuits when the velocity of force production, joint movement, and external work completed are key to successful performance.

MUSCULAR ENDURANCE

Muscular endurance is defined as the ability of a muscle or group of muscles to work at a less-than-maximal level for an extended period of time.[36] Improvements in muscular endurance are demonstrated from a conditioning program that applies low resistance and high repetitions against the muscle(s). The development of adequate levels of muscular endurance affords an individual the ability to perform repeated muscular contractions or work tasks for an extended period of time without undue fatigue. As muscular endurance increases, normally lesser improvements are seen in muscle strength and vice versa.

The development of strength and endurance is very specific to the muscle group trained and the type of contraction (i.e., isometric, isotonic, concentric, eccentric, etc.) and positions (joint angles) in which the muscle is trained. Even though some transfer of strength is demonstrated via isokinetic or isometric testing methods, if an individual trains in an isometric or isotonic manner, then he should be tested isometrically or isotonically, respectively.

THE KINETIC CHAIN

The human body is a conceptual kinetic chain consisting of many bones, joints, muscles, and connective tissues. A balance in the strength, endurance, and length of these tissues must be maintained to ensure proper motion, stability, and function. Often, if an imbalance of strength and/or length (tissue shortness, or hypomobility) exists on one side of a joint, there will be weakness and/or excessive muscle or connective tissue length (hypermobility) on the opposing side. When these conditions exist, the related joint is considered to be at risk of injury.

Under normal conditions, the trunk muscles, including the back extensors and flexors and lateral flexors and rotators, provide movement and stability to the trunk. When trauma has affected the musculotendinous unit or joint, changes in the muscle and/or connective tissue length, strength, or function associated with disuse and inhibition can occur. An accurate objective assessment of a patient's muscular strength vs. a normative data base is essential in rehabilitation. This information helps set goals.

Numerous investigators have attempted to identify the appropriate muscle agonist/antagonist strength ratios for the trunk.[5] There is great variation in the assessment of trunk muscle strength. This is associated with the variety of testing methods available (isometric, concentric, eccentric, and isokinetic). Most studies indicate that the peak torque ratios of the trunk muscles for healthy individuals (extensors to flexors) range from 1 to 2:1. The most commonly cited ratio is 1.3:1, which indicates that the trunk extensors are 30% stronger than the flexors. In the population with low back pain, ratios from 0.79 to 1.23 for extension/flexion have been reported.

Since the articulations of the back allow movement in multiple planes, it is important to look beyond just extension/flexion ratios and identify the ideal ratios for lateral flexion and rotation. The generally accepted ratio for lateral flexion and rotation is 1:1. Further studies are needed to analyze functional activities incorporating flexion/extension coupled with rotational and side-bending components.

Once muscle balance and strength have been assessed, the information must be integrated into a rehabilitation plan that includes specific strengthening and stretching exercises to correct imbalances. The information that follows highlights the pertinent relationships of the various muscle groups of the trunk and lower extremities to the pelvis.

Muscular Stability of the Vertebral Column

Stability of the trunk is provided by the anterior, lateral, and posterior musculature. Anteriorly these include the rectus abdominis and internal and external oblique muscles. The combined forces of these muscles act to oppose hyperextension of the vertebral column.[22] The anterior musculature assists in the maintenance of an ideal standing posture. Weakness or paralysis of these muscles may lead to excessive lordosis of the lumbar spine, thus increasing the potential risk for spinal injuries.

Posteriorly, the erector spinae, quadratus lumborum, intertransversarii, interspinalis, transversospinalis, and levator muscles function together to provide posterior stability for the vertebral column as well as opposition to the forces of gravity. They also function as antagonists to the anterior musculature. These major muscle groups are assisted by multiple other muscle groups including the neck, arms, buttocks, and legs to maintain an erect posture.[36] Therefore, appropriate strength of all these muscle groups is essential to maintain ideal posture.

Postural Alignment of the Lumbar Spine and Pelvis

The pelvis is the critical link joining the vertebral column to the lower extremities. During ambulation the mobile pelvis transmits the motion of gait to the vertebral column via strong ligamentous attachments to the lumbar spine.

The relationship of the pelvis to the spine is critical in the prevention and treatment of low back injuries. The pelvis may be tilted anteriorly or posteriorly in the sagittal plane. An extenuation of anterior pelvic tilt may result in hyperlordosis. This is caused by abdominal weakness and may be associated with contracture of the lumbodorsal fascia. A posterior tilt of the pelvis in the sagittal plane is often the result of lumbar or thoracic kyphosis and is associated with weakness of the paraspinal extensor muscles. Either of these sagittal-plane abnormalities changes the normal transfer of motion from the pelvis to the lumbar spine. This can accelerate the degenerative process involving the lumbar discs and facet joints. Critical to any rehabilitation program is an attempt to normalize the biomechanical relationship by balancing the strength and length of the appropriate trunk muscles.

Anterior Pelvic Tilt

Hip flexors, abdominals, hamstrings, low-back extensors, and gluteal muscles may be responsible for anterior pelvic tilt. Hip flexors insert along the anterior portion of the lumbar vertebrae and exert a forward and downward pull on the vertebrae. Excessive shortening of the hip flexors may be responsible for exaggerated anterior pelvic tilt. Although this situation may be counteracted by strong abdominal muscles, frequently the abdominal musculature is weak and elongated and thus contributes to hyperlordosis.[23] The elongated hamstring and gluteal muscles cannot counteract the hip flexors and create further pelvic tilt. Furthermore, adaptive contracture of the lumbodorsal fascia contributes to the problem. Treatment consists of a stretching program for the lumbodorsal fascia and hip flexors as well as strengthening of abdominal, gluteus maximus, and hamstring muscles to reduce excessive lumbar lordosis.

Posterior Pelvic Tilt

Posterior pelvic tilt causes a reduction in the lordosis of the lumbar spine commonly called "flat back." Contracture of the hamstrings and hip extensors with concomitant elongation of the hip flexors and back extensors predispose to this posture. A specific rehabilitation program consisting of hip flexor and back extensor strengthening along with hamstring, abdominal, and hip extensor stretching is recommended.

FLEXIBILITY

Empirical evidence suggests that generalized flexibility is essential for successful physical performance.[4, 10, 15, 17, 18, 32] Maintenance of flexibility is also apparently important in the prevention of injuries.[6, 17, 37]

Although flexibility is considered synonymous with range of motion, it is more correctly considered a combined result of the function of different anatomic structures. Muscles, tendons, ligaments, cartilage, joint surfaces, and synovial fluid all play a crucial role in joint mobility under both normal and pathologic conditions.[36]

Flexibility may be classified as static or dynamic. Passive motion to an anatomic end point is referred to as the static flexibility of a joint.[23] Dynamic flexibility, on the other hand, is the active range of motion that results from muscular contracture. Dynamic flexibility usually occurs through the midrange of motion and is not considered to be a reliable indicator of true joint motion. Dynamic flexibility is noted to increase physical performance while decreasing the risk of injury. For example, hamstring tightness places a runner at considerable disadvantage due to reduced knee extension, with a concomitant decrease in musculotendinous injury during activities.

When static or dynamic motion deficits are diagnosed, an effort to reestablish physiologic range of motion should be attempted. Hypermobility should be avoided. This is especially important in patients with spinal fusion, in whom an aggressive stretching program may cause hypermobility above or below the fused segment.

Neurophysiology

The muscle spindle and the Golgi tendon organ (found within the muscle tissue) are receptors that send vital sensory information regarding the position of joints and muscles as well as the degree of stretch experienced by these structures to the central nervous system (CNS). This information allows the complex interaction between agonist and antagonist groups to be formulated into purposeful motion. These receptors send vital sensory information via the neural afferent pathway to the CNS. The CNS processes the information and sends impulses via the neural efferent pathway[3] back to the agonist and antagonist muscles to provide them with information concerning the agonist muscle. The muscle spindles and the Golgi organs are both sensitive to changes in muscle length. The muscle spindle is responsible for what is called the "stretch reflex."[17, 32] The Golgi organ is also sensitive to changes in muscle tension. The interaction between these two receptors to control muscle length is quite complex. For example, when an agonist muscle (the hamstring) is stretched, the muscle spindles, because of their parallel arrangement to the muscle fibers, are also stretched, which causes them to send sensory information to the CNS that the muscle is being stretched. If the (hamstring) muscle and associated muscle spindles stretch too far or too fast, the agonist muscle (hamstring) will, through the stretch reflex (caused by the muscle spindles), stimulate the hamstring muscle to contract. The strength of this contraction will be proportionate to the degree and speed of the stretch. The greater the stretch and/or the faster the stretch, the greater the reflex contraction in the hamstring. This series of actions is executed as a safety mechanism designed to limit further stretching of the hamstring muscle.[39, 40] If the stretch is held for 6 to 10 seconds, the Golgi organs, being sensitive to the increase in muscle tension, will send their own impulses to the CNS, which will cause a reflex relaxation of the agonist (hamstring) muscle. This reflex reaction has been called the "inverse stretch reflex."[4] This protective mechanism allows the agonist muscle to be stretched in a relaxed fashion so that its extensibility limits are not exceeded, which reduces the potential trauma or damage to the muscle and related joint(s).

STRETCHING PROTOCOLS

There are different types of stretching exercise designed to increase flexibility. The oldest, termed "ballistic stretch," uses repetitive bouncing movements to elongate soft tissues.[15, 17] In contrast, "passive stretch" often requires another person utilizing external forces to elongate tissues.[4] "Static stretch" techniques are intended to elongate muscles and related tissue to a point of mild tension or mild discomfort. This position is then held for a specified time.[9, 11, 15, 17] Finally, "proprioceptive neuromuscular facilitation" (PNF) utilizes alternating submaximal muscular contractions with static stretching programs.[25, 32, 33]

Ballistic stretching has been abandoned due to the associated risk of joint and/or soft-tissue injury.[40] The rapid, forceful movements utilized in this technique elicit a vigorous stretch reflex from the muscle spindles[4] and a concomitant muscle contraction that may cause injury and should be discouraged. Correctly performed passive stretching, on the other hand, can be very effective in increasing range of motion. Care must be taken to minimize the risk of muscle or tendon injury due to an overly vigorous external force. Static stretching that is performed in a gentle fashion generates the least amount of muscle tension. When correctly performed, the spindle's stretch reflex is avoided, and the Golgi tendon organ is stimulated to cause muscle relaxation. This technique decreases the risk of soft-tissue injury and may be the safest.[4] PNF stretching techniques also use the Golgi organ's ability to override the muscle spindle's stretch reflex by eliciting the inverse stretch reflex mechanism and therefore are very successful in stretching contracted tissues.

Physiologic Response to Stretching

Although stretching programs are designed to increase the range of motion in specific muscles, often the connective tissue surrounding the joint is affected most significantly.[37] When a relaxed muscle is stretched, the most significant resistance to stretch is derived from the connective tissue in and around the muscle and not from stretching of the myofibrils.[2, 21, 35, 42] Often following trauma or surgery, pathologic changes occur in connective tissue in the form of scar formation, adhesions, and fibrotic contracture. Thus, stretching these contracted connective tissues may help to achieve the goal of improved range of motion.

The success of stretching protocols also depends on the mechanical behavior of connective tissues under a tensile stress. Connective tissue responds to stretch with both plastic and elastic properties.[36] In response to a tensile stress, the tissues initially respond in an elastic manner. Once the tensile stress is removed, the tissues return in springlike fashion to their prestretched length. The results of this form of stretching are temporary. If the tensile stretch is increased, however, plastic deformation may occur in the target tissue. When tensile load is removed, the tissue does not return to its prestretched length, and a more permanent clinical result is obtained. Those tissues that contain plastic elements are said to have a viscous property. In fact, connective tissues have both plastic and elastic components within their physiologic range. Therefore, connective tissues function as a viscoelastic material in which both elastic and plastic deformation occur, depending on the stretching technique and force used.[37, 43]

Successful tissue stretching therefore requires appropriate force and duration. In connective tissue models (tendon), the amount of time required to obtain tissue stretching varies inversely with the force used.[37, 42, 43] It has been observed that methods using long duration and low force result in greater long-term elongation of connective tissues than do those protocols in which high force and short duration are used. Because permanent elongation of muscle-tendon units is the goal of a stretching program, exercises that preferentially alter the plastic rather than the elastic elements should be promoted.

Clinical Guidelines for Stretching Exercises

A well-designed stretching program should include exercises for all major muscle groups. Specialized exercises should be undertaken for specific areas where contracture has been demonstrated. These exercises should be conducted slowly and gently and elongation of the specific structure carried to the point of mild tension or mild discomfort and held for 30 to 60 seconds. These may be repeated in sets three to four times in an effort to obtain the maximum increase in range of motion.

SUMMARY

In this chapter, we have attempted to review the preventive and therapeutic benefits of cardiovascular fitness, flexibility, muscle strength, and endurance. The emphasis in rehabilitation of spinal abnormalities has shifted from the management of pain to the development of function. Adherence to these fitness principles can speed the recovery of disabled individuals and potentially decrease the chance of recurrent injury.

REFERENCES

1. American College of Sports Medicine: Position statement on the recommended quantity and quality of exercise for developing and maintaining cardiorespiratory and muscular fitness in healthy adults. *Med Sci Sports* 1990; 22:265–274.
2. Banus MG, Zetlin AM: The relation of isometric tension to length in skeletal muscle. *J Cell Comp Physiol* 1938; 12:403–420.
3. Battie MC, Bigos SJ, Fisher LD, et al: A prospective study of the role of cardiovascular risk factors and fitness in industrial back pain complaints. *Spine* 1989; 14:141–147.
4. Beaulieu JE: Developing a stretching program. *Physician Sports Med* 1981; 9:59–69.
5. Beimborn DS, Morrissey MC: A review of the literature related to trunk muscle performance. *Spine* 1988; 13:655–660.
6. Bobath B: The treatment of motor disorders of pyramidal and extrapyramidal origin by reflex inhibition and by facilitation of movement. *Psychotherapy* 1955; 41:146.
7. Cady LD, Bischoff DP, O'Connell ER, et al: Strength and fitness and subsequent back injuries in firefighters. *J Occup Med* 1979; 21:269–272.
8. Cady LD, Thomas PC, Karwasky RJ: Program for increasing health and physical fitness of firefighters. *J Occup Med* 1985; 2:111–114.
9. Cornelius WL: Two effective flexibility methods. *Athletic Training* 1981; 16:23–25.
10. Cureton TK: Flexibility as an aspect of physical fitness. *Res Q Am Assoc Health Phys Educ (Suppl)* 1941; 12:382.
11. DeVries HA: Evaluation of static stretching procedures for improvement of flexibility. *Res Q* 1962; 33:222–228.
12. Firoelicher VF: Exercise testing and training: Clinical applications. *J Am Coll Cardiol* 1983; 1:114–125.
13. Gettman LR, Pollock ML, Durstine JL, et al: Physiological responses of men to 1, 3 and 5 day per week training programs. *Res Q* 1976; 47:638–646.
14. Glisan B, Stith WJ, Kiser S: Physiology of active exercise in rehabilitation of back injuries. *Spine State Art Rev* 1989; 3:139–152.
15. Harris ML: Flexibility: A review of the literature. *Phys Ther* 1969; 49:591–601.
16. Hartung GH, Smolensky MH, Harrist RB, et al: Effects of varied durations of training on improvements in cardiorespiratory endurance. *J Hum Ergol* (Tokyo) 1977; 6:61–68.
17. Holland GJ: The physiology of flexibility: A review of the literature. *Kinesiol Rev* 1968; 49–62.
18. Holt LE, Travis TM, Okita T: Comparative study of three stretching techniques. *Percept Mot Skills* 1970; 31:611–616.
19. Hossack KF, Hartwig R: Cardiac arrest associated with supervised cardiac rehabilitation. *J Card Rehabil* 1982; 2:402–408.
20. Jensen C, Fisher G: *Scientific Basis of Athletic Conditioning*. Philadelphia, Lea & Febiger, 1979.
21. Johns RJ, Wright V: Relative importance of various tissues in joint stiffness. *J Appl Physiol* 1962; 17:824–828.
22. Kareighbaum E, Barthelis KM: *Biomechanics: A Qualitative Approach for the Study of Human Motion,* ed 2. Burgess Publishing Co, 1985.
23. Kendall FP, McCreary EK: *Muscles: Testing and Function,* ed 3. Baltimore, Williams & Wilkins, 1983.
24. Kilbom A, Hartley L, Saltin B, et al: Physical training in sedentary middle-aged and older men. *Scand J Clin Lab Invest* 1969; 24:315–322.
25. Knott M, Voss DE: *Proprioceptive Neuromuscular Facilitation: Patterns and Techniques*. New York, Harper & Row, 1968.
26. Liang MT, Alexander JF, Taylor HL, et al: Aerobic training threshold. *Scand J Sports Sci* 1982; 4:5–8.
27. Milesis CA, Pollock ML, Bah MD, et al: Effects of different durations of training on cardiorespiratory function, body composition and serum lipids. *Res Q* 1976; 47:716–725.
28. Oja P, Teraslinna P, Partaner T, et al: Feasibility of an 18 month physical training program for middle-aged men and its effect on physical fitness. *Am J Public Health* 1975; 64:459–465.
29. Pollock ML: The quantification of endurance training programs, in Wilmore JM (ed): *Exercise and Sport Sciences Reviews,* vol 1. New York, Academic Press, 1973, pp 155–158.
30. Pollock ML, Dimmick J, Miller HS, et al: Effects of mode of training on cardiovascular function and body composition of middle-aged men. *Med Sci Sports* 1975; 7:139–145.
31. Pollock ML, Miller H, Janeway R, et al: Effects of walking on body composition and cardiovascular function of middle-aged men. *J Appl Physiol* 1971; 30:126–130.
32. Prentice WE: A comparison of static stretching and PNF

stretching for improving hip joint flexibility. *Athletic Training* 1983; 18:56–59.
33. Prentice WE: An electromyographic analysis of the effectiveness of heat or cold and stretching for inducing relaxation in injured muscle. *J Orthop Sports Phys Ther* 1982; 3:133–140.
34. Price C, Pollock ML, Gettman LR, et al: *Physical Fitness Programs for Law Enforcement Officers: A Manual for Police Administrators*. Washington, DC, 1978, US Government Printing Offices, Publication No 027-000-00671-0.
35. Ramsey R, Street S: The isometric length-tension diagram of isolated skeletal muscle fibers of the frog. *J Cell Comp Physiol* 1940; 15:11–34.
36. Deleted in proofs.
37. Sapega AA, Quedenfeld TC, Moyer RA, et al: Biophysical factors in range-of-motion exercise. *Physician Sports Med* 1981; 9:57–65.
38. Sharkey BJ: Intensity and duration of training and the development of cardiorespiratory endurance. *Med Sci Sports* 1970; 2:197–202.
39. Shellock FG: Physiological benefits of warm-up. *Physician Sports Med* 1983; 11:134–139.
40. Shellock FG, Prentice WE: Warming-up and stretching for improved physical performance and prevention of sports-related injuries. *Sports Med* 1985; 2:267–278.
41. Terjung RL, Baldwin KM, Codesey J, et al: Cardiovascular adaptation to 12 minutes of mild daily exercise in middle-aged sedentary men. *J Am Geriatric Soc* 1973; 21:164–168.
42. Warren CG, Lehmann JF, Koblanski JN: Elongation of rat tail tendon: Effect of load and temperature. *Arch Phys Med Rehabil* 1971; 52:465–474.
43. Warren CG, Lehmann JF, Koblanski JN: Heat and stretch procedures: An evaluation using rat tail tendon. *Arch Phys Med Rehabil* 1976; 57:122–126.

3

The Role of Education in the Treatment of Back Pain

Donna D. Ohnmeiss, M.S.

When the term "patient education" is used in relation to the treatment of patients with back pain, generally back schools come to mind. While back schools are commonly considered the educational component of treatment, a thorough education includes more. This is particularly true as we see changing roles in health care. In the past, the patient went to the health care provider to be cured, and the physician was primarily responsible for the patient's short- and long-term outcome. This model has been changing. For years now the general public has been taking on more responsibility for dental hygiene and thus a preventive role in dental problems. More recently changes have been observed in cardiovascular awareness and general fitness, with many individuals taking part in maintaining their health every day by exercising and monitoring their diets. In the area of back care, there is increasing emphasis on preventive actions, and once back pain has occurred, the care provider has taken on a role with patients that "I am not here to cure you, but to facilitate your efforts to improve your condition." Thus more responsibility has shifted to the patient. Fulfilling this role may greatly affect the patient's daily life-style, i.e., exercising; changing to a healthier diet; constantly being aware of posture, lifting techniques, and body mechanics; and depending on the patient's situation, possibly changing employment, household duties, and recreational activities. Patients need to have a better understanding of why it is important to make these significant life-style changes. Also, with more health-related information being easily available to the general public through television and magazines, there seems to be a general trend for many individuals to want to know more about their condition and treatment. For these reasons, the need for thorough patient education is increasing.

COMMUNICATION AND EXPECTATIONS

Good-quality patient education is an ongoing process that should incorporate all those involved with the patient's care, not just a back school session. The beginning of patient education is communication. Frequently this starts with the initial patient evaluation, including a discussion and explanation of the physical examination findings, plain films, and other evaluations that might be performed during the first office visit. Based on this information, a plan should be provided for the patient that includes the following:

- Medication (why prescribed, dosage, potential side effects)
- Radiologic evaluations prescribed (what type of evaluation, where to have it performed, time required, contraindications, modified diet required)
- Prescription of an exercise program (type of activities to perform and also those to avoid, duration, progression, warning signs as to when to cease an activity; it is particularly important to determine what activities the patient normally engages in at work and for recreation so that these areas can be adequately addressed)
- Physical therapy (why prescribed, general overview of what to expect, how to use prescribed modalities such as transcutaneous electrical nerve stimulation [TENS])
- General expectations (when to schedule the next appointment if not improved)
- Behavioral medicine evaluation (why prescribe, testing, counselling, family involvement)

Another area of patient education related to communication and motivation that may frequently be overlooked is providing the patient with feedback. It is expecting much on the part of patients to continue rehabilitation if they do not know how they are doing. Certainly patients know better than anyone if symptoms are resolving or not, but they need feedback concerning whether they are progressing as expected and if not, why, or if they are progressing better than expected, what the next step in their treatment is. When a patient is participating in a rehabilitation program, there needs to be objective measurement criteria established and the patient made aware of the results and plans for his program. This provides a basis for both the patient and the therapist to work from. The evaluations should be repeated at expressed time intervals and the results discussed with the patient so that he knows what progress has been made. This can serve to motivate the patient or help him accept changes in the program if satisfactory results are not being achieved.

BACK SCHOOLS

It is difficult to determine exactly when education became a part of treating patients with back pain. However, the term *back school* was first used by Fahrni in 1969 in Stockholm.[19] This concept expanded in Scandinavia. In 1977 Bergquist-Ullman and Larsson conducted a large-scale trial to evaluate the back school in an industrial setting and found favorable results.[1] Zachrisson Forssell provided a description of the back school in 1981.[20] Groups of six to eight patients received instruction from a physiotherapist in four sessions during a 2-week period. A visit to the patient's work site was also included if possible. From these roots many variations of back school have evolved. Most back schools do offer a base curriculum discussing general topics such as anatomy and body mechanics with individuals or small groups of patients with back pain. Other back schools have added relaxation therapy, diet and nutrition, and the performance of daily tasks. Back schools now may frequently encompass the performance of many physical activities.[15] This is also discussed by Fardon in Chapter 60. This broad use of the term *back school* may be better in that it tends to create a bridge between materials presented to the patient in a classroom setting and his active treatment program.

Another area of patient education deals with how to cope with pain. This education has taken on several forms. Frequently, relaxation skills are taught in a back school program. For patients who have difficulty relaxing due to muscle tension, biofeedback or sensory deprivation may be employed. All these techniques are directed at having the patient take measures to control his pain when it increases without relying upon the assistance of a health care provider or medication.

Often patients will have special, individual needs. Frequently these are related to work. In these cases, an occupational therapist can be of great help. He can discuss the job demands and postures required by the patient's occupation and provide input on how to modify the required activities or the job site to accommodate the patient. This sometimes requires the therapist to visit the patient's place of employment to determine whether the tasks can be performed in a manner that is not painful or harmful to the patient. Also, the therapist may be able to assist the patient with special needs encountered at home. This is particularly true when the patient is responsible for caring for others such as an infant. An experienced therapist can often provide specific suggestions for performing daily tasks related to child care. He will also be acquainted with assistive devices the patient may want to use while recovering from an injury. There are materials available to help provide specialized care to various patient populations with particular needs and interests. Some of these materials deal with pregnant patients,[13] ballet dancers,[3] athletes of many pursuits,[4, 8] equestrians,[14] and young patients.[5]

EFFECTIVENESS OF PATIENT EDUCATION

The effectiveness of back schools still remains controversial. While most agree with the concept, the reported outcome varies. This may be due to the fact that there is such great variation in the composition of back schools (number and length of sessions, program content, experience and skills of the instructor, emphasis on exercise, individualization of parts of the program, handout materials available, etc.), the groups being taught (patients with acute vs. chronic pain, education level, emotional status, pathology, etc.), and the evaluation parameters used (injury rate, length of follow-up, pain relief, perceived dysfunction, recurrence of symptoms, etc.).

The first attempt to evaluate the effectiveness of back schools was in 1977 when Bergquist-Ullman and Larsson conducted a large-scale trial at a car factory.[1] They found that a back school program reduced the incidence and cost associated with low back pain. Favorable results were also reported in a study comparing the results of patients who participated in the Swedish back school vs. a group of patients only performing the same exercises as the back school group, but not receiving instruction.[10] Sikorski also reported favorable results from patient education.[16] His program included not only general education but also specific advice based on the patient's symptoms, and a therapist visited the home or workplace to provide additional advice if the patient had significant problems at these locations. Patients felt that the education in back care was the most beneficial of the treatments provided (69%), exercise (64%) was second, while rest, immobilizers (corsets), and manipulation were less effective. Favorable results for back schools have been reported elsewhere.[7] A recent study evaluated the cost-effectiveness of a specialized back school for bus drivers.[18] Although the study was not particularly well designed, they found that the back school was not effective in reducing the incidence of injury; however, it was effective in reducing the number of work days lost due to injury. They also found the program to be cost-effective.

There have also been reports that back school was ineffective or not as effective as other treatments. Stankovic and Johnell reported that a "mini back school" was not as effective in treating patients as was the McKenzie protocol.[17] However, in their study, the back school consisted of only one 45-minute session discussing anatomy and spinal function, and patients were told not to exercise. This is quite different from what most describe as a back school. Other unfavorable results have also been reported.[2, 12]

With respect to the patient population enrolled in the

back school, a study by Julkunen et al. found that patients with chronic back pain who responded well to back school were emotionally well adjusted and had good cognitive capacity.[9] In contrast, those who responded less favorably were less well balanced emotionally and had less cognitive capacity.

The value of patients understanding their problems was identified in a study by Lacroix et al. that evaluated various factors in predicting outcome in patients with low back pain who received worker's compensation.[11] The possible factors they compared were orthopedic evaluation and prognosis, the number of nonorganic physical signs, Minnesota Multiphasic Personality Inventory (MMPI), age, education, English proficiency, and the patient's understanding of his medical condition as assessed by the Schema Assessment Instrument (SAI). They found that the only item correlating with return to work was the SAI. Among patients with a good understanding of their problem, 94% returned to work, while only 33% of those with a poor understanding returned to work. As these authors conjectured, it may be a matter of those patients who best understand their condition and treatment who tend to be more motivated to be compliant and thus have a successful treatment outcome. Interestingly, these authors also found a high correlation between English proficiency and high SAI score in predicting a good outcome. This may underscore the importance of making an extra effort to pursue better communication and education with patients having poor English skills.

The beneficial role of patient education was demonstrated in the reduction of medication used by patients with back pain in a special program.[6] Patients were educated on the type of drugs they were taking. This included the effects of the drugs, addictive properties, and side effects including behavioral changes. The main point emphasized during the program was education followed by putting the patient in charge of his medication usage. The strong emphasis on teaching the patient to be in control of his own condition, even to the extent of discouraging treatment aids such as TENS units, may account for the success rate maintained 12 months after discharge. This same concept may be applicable to patients with back pain in general. If patients learn that they can be in control of rather than controlled by their condition, the continual and sometimes increasing dependence on health care providers, pain-reducing devices, or medication can be ceased.

POTENTIAL PITFALLS IN PATIENT EDUCATION

Some of the same guidelines for providing effective education in a school classroom apply to patient education in a clinical setting. Even the best of intentions can go awry in the area of patient education if some simple guidelines are not followed. Great effort and expense can easily be wasted on colorful and informative educational materials if they are not created in a manner that is intelligible to the patient. The material should be in very simple vocabulary and include many illustrations. The education level to be targeted should be the lowest of the patient population frequently seen. Targeting to the average education level of a clinic will lead to the development of materials not useful to approximately half the patients being treated. Illustrations not only make the information easier to understand but can make it much more pleasing to look at than just reading large blocks of written text. Something frequently taken for granted is that the patient must be literate. Also, the patient's vision plays a role. The material should be in type large enough so that one does not have to strain to see it. This not only makes the information available to more people but also makes it more pleasant to read and thus more likely to be read by those exposed to it.

A barrier frequently encountered by many care providers is that some patients do not speak English. These patients come from a great many nationalities, the distribution of which varies from one location to another across the country. It is important for clinicians to recognize the language(s) frequently spoken by their patients and make efforts to have staff who can talk with these patients. Also, educational materials should be available in the languages spoken by groups often seen in the clinic. However, just translating text into a different language does not ensure that the patient can read and interpret it. Some of these patients may be illiterate in their native language or may have vision problems, or if the translator is not familiar with the medical terminology, the translations may be misleading. Thus it is very important to have someone not only very familiar with this particular population to verbally translate the materials but also who is familiar with various cultural beliefs, particularly in the area of medical treatment. In our clinic a large Hispanic population is seen. To accommodate the needs of this patient population, several staff members speak fluent Spanish, and written educational materials as well as videotapes for surgery and diagnostic procedures are available in both languages. Even patients who speak some English should be aware that bilingual materials are available and be given the choice of which they prefer to use. They may be able to understand the non-English version more easily than the English and thus gain more from it. It is very important for the patient to feel at ease with the person(s) providing education and not be embarrassed to ask questions or say that they are illiterate, need foreign language materials, have reading problems (poor vision, dyslexia, etc.), or do not understand some material presented to them.

One method of patient education that is becoming increasingly more popular involves the use of videotapes. This is very amenable to most patients since they are so familiar with watching television. However, the same rules hold true as for written material: keep it informative, but simple. At our institute, professional-quality videos have been produced that describe frequently performed diagnostic, injection, and surgical procedures. Each video lasts about 10 to 15 minutes. The patient and family members, if available, view the tape with a staff member. Although video educational materials are becoming more popular, this method opens the door for abuse on the part of educators. For example, most people could not conceive that students would learn much in a classroom if the teacher simply taped a series of lectures and, rather than teaching the class in person, would just play the tapes for students. Just as classroom students need contact with the educator, so do patients. The educator should be very familiar with the material on the tape and be available to explain or emphasize a point and answer questions viewers may have. When dealing with surgical patients, it is ideal to have the educator discuss the individual details of the patient's case including anything not covered on the tape. For example, a sample set of instrumentation or any device to be implanted should be available to the patient to look at and ask questions about. Videos may lose their effectiveness for patients with vision or hearing problems. Before sending an educational or exercise tape home with a patient, ask him whether a video player is available; like many things, if the educator takes this for granted, the patient may be embarrassed to indicate otherwise.

There are many booklets already prepared for educating patients with back pain. These provide a good starting overview but generally need to be augmented with information from the individual clinic the patient is visiting so that details associated with their care are delivered.

A potential source of great frustration for patients is that of inconsistent information being received from care providers. This problem is difficult to address if the patient is being seen by care providers who do not work together frequently. However, in many situations, physicians refer patients to the same team of therapists, and there should be good communication and understanding between them. Consistency in the information being provided to the patient can be greatly enhanced by the physician and the therapist having the same treatment philosophy, goals, and expectations in treating patients with back pain. Thus part of good patient education begins with care provider education.

METHODS OF DELIVERY

It certainly does not hurt to give the patient information in several forms such as in booklets, in videos, verbally, individually, in groups, and/or with family members present. It is important that the information be organized so that it does not become overwhelming or confusing. When receiving medical treatment and sitting in a doctor's office it is not unusual for one's mind to wander to other topics perhaps like who will take care of the family after surgery, what will happen to the work situation, the costs of treatment, and other personal concerns. Thus patients may miss part of the material being presented and will need to be exposed to it again.

Many educational programs are geared toward group education. This system has merit in that education can be delivered more cost-effectively to a group than to several patients individually, some patients may be more comfortable in a group setting, and they can often gain reassurance that there are others who are experiencing many of the same problems they have. However, there is also a need for individualized education. This lets patients know that their problems are the single focus of a health care professional for a period of time. Other advantages of individual education is that it can be tailored to suit the needs of that one patient. Perhaps he has special problems encountered in the workplace or at home not faced by other patients. Also, some patients may have individual problems or questions that they may feel embarrassed discussing in front of a group of strangers. Individualized patient education may include a designated visit to a staff educator but can often be handled simply by encouraging patients to ask questions to their physician, nurse, therapist or others who are already involved in their treatment.

In many cases, educating not only the patient but also those who live with the patient can also help contribute to good care. Family members can play a role in reinforcing the information delivered to the patient by the care provider and can also help see that the patient is following the prescribed course of home activity if the family members know what the patient should be doing.

SUMMARY

As patients are being expected to take greater responsibility for their health, they need to have a greater understanding of the importance of why making changes in their life-style (exercising, changing diet, not smoking, etc.) is important to their recovery and future prevention of back problems. They need someone to help them understand the relationship of discs, muscles, and other tissues related to their injury and recovery. Also, it is important to do away with the sometime deeply embedded notion that activity will lead to wearing away of tissues and thus inactivity is preventing future problems.

When patients are instructed, many of the same basic educational guidelines used in a classroom setting are applicable. The educational materials being presented need to be available on a level that is understandable to the patients and appealing to view, individualized attention should be available, patients should not only be allowed to ask questions but encouraged to do so, family involvement should be encouraged, and the educational sessions should not be overly lengthy as to extend beyond the patient's attention span. It is important to consider the patients being taught. This group can vary greatly from one center to another in terms of age, nationality, educational level, socioeconomic status, and job demands. Thus a detailed educational program that is effective at one center may not be appropriate at another. However, some of the same basic materials may be useful to provide a foundation for a program at another center if modifications are made to meet the specific needs of the new center's population. Designing a complete and effective patient education program can be time-consuming and costly; however, once good-quality materials are designed, they can generally be used for a long period of time with only occasional updates and modifications.

REFERENCES

1. Bergquist-Ullman M, Larsson U: Acute low back pain in industry. *Acta Orthop Scand* 1977; 170:1–117.
2. Berwick DM, Budman S, Feldstein M: No clinical effect of back school in an HMO: A randomized prospective trial. *Spine* 1989; 14:338–344.
3. Bryan N, Smith BM: The ballet dancer. *Spine State Art Rev* 1991; 5:391–399.
4. Cook T: The professional athlete. *Spine State Art Rev* 1991; 5:411–415.
5. Farrell JP, Drye CD: The young patient. *Spine State Art Rev* 1991; 5:379–390.
6. Gottlieb H, Alperson BL, Schwartz AH, et al: Self-management for medication reduction in chronic low back pain. *Arch Phys Med Rehabil* 1988; 69:442–448.
7. Hall H: The Canadian back education units. *Physiotherapy* 1980; 66:115–117.
8. Hochschuler SH (ed). *The Spine in Sports.* Philadelphia, Hanley & Belfus, 1990.
9. Julkunen J, Hurri H, Kankainen J: Psychological factors in the treatment of chronic low back pain. Follow-up study of a back school intervention. *Psychother Psychosom* 1988; 50:173–181.
10. Klaber Moffet JA, Chase SM, Portek I, et al: A controlled, prospective study to evaluate the effectiveness of a back school in the relief of chronic low back pain. *Spine* 1986; 11:120–122.
11. Lacroix JM, Powell J, Lloyd GJ, et al: Low-back pain: Factors of value in predicting outcome. *Spine* 1990; 15:495–499.
12. Lankhorst GJ, van de Stadt RJ, Vogelaar TW, et al: The effect of the Swedish back school in chronic idiopathic low back pain. *Scand J Rehabil Med* 1983; 15:141–145.
13. Prentice C, Canty AM, Janowitz IL: The pregnant patient and her partner. *Spine State Art Rev* 1991; 5:401–409.
14. Rashbaum RF: Soft tissue trauma in equestrian participation, in Hochschuler SH (ed): *The Spine in Sports.* Philadelphia, Hanley & Belfus, 1990, pp 180–191.
15. Robinson R: The new back school prescription: Stabilization training. *Spine State Art Rev* 1991; 5:341–355.
16. Sikorski JM: A rationalized approach to physiotherapy for low-back pain. *Spine* 1985; 10:571–579.
17. Stankovic R, Johnell O: Conservative treatment of acute low-back pain: A prospective randomized trial: McKenzie method of treatment versus patient education in "mini back school." *Spine* 1990; 15:121–123.
18. Verloot JM, Rozeman A, van Son AM, et al: The cost-effectiveness of a back school program in industry. *Spine* 1992; 17:22–27.
19. White LA: The evolution of back school. *Spine State Art Rev* 1991; 5:325–332.
20. Zachrisson Forssell M: The back school. *Spine* 1981; 6:104–106.

PART II
EVALUATION

4

Clinical Examination and Documentation

Jose E. Rodriguez, M.D.

The professional who chooses a career in medicine, besides being a person with technical skills, broad scientific knowledge, and wisdom, must have personal characteristics of warmth and humility, which serve to blend the art with the science of medicine.

Francis Peabody's classic essay entitled "The Care of the Patient" best describes what the practice of medicine is all about.

> The practice of medicine in its broadest sense includes the whole relationship of the physician with his patient. It is an art, based to an increasing extent on the medical sciences but comprising much that still remains outside the realm of any science. The art of medicine and the science of medicine are not antagonistic but supplementary to each other. There is no more contradiction between the science of medicine and the art of medicine than between the science of aeronautics and the art of flying. Good practice presupposes an understanding of the sciences which contribute to the structure of modern medicine, but it is obvious that some professional training should include a much broader equipment.
>
> The treatment of disease may be entirely impersonal; the care of the patient must be completely personal. The significance of the intimate personal relationship between physician and patient cannot be too strongly emphasized, for in an extraordinarily large number of cases both diagnosis and treatment are directly dependent on it, and failure of the young physician to establish this relationship accounts for much of his ineffectiveness in care of patients.
>
> What is spoken of as a "clinical picture" is not just a photograph of a man sick in bed, it is an impressionistic painting of the patient surrounded by his home, his work, his relations, his friends, his joys, sorrows, hopes and fears.
>
> Thus, the physician who attempts to take care of a patient while he neglects those factors which contribute to the emotional life of his patients is as unscientific as an investigator who neglects to control all the conditions which may affect his experiment. The good physician knows his patients through and through, and his knowledge is but dearly. Time, sympathy and understanding must be lavishly dispensed, but the reward is to be found in that personal bond which forms the greatest satisfaction of the practice of medicine. One of the essential qualities of the clinician is interest in humanity, for the secret of the care of the patient is in caring for the patient.

With the above essay, we do not have to go into further explanation of being well rounded as scientists, but it is most important to be a humanitarian. History taking is an art, and physical examination would be a technical skill. A precise and thorough history taking develops with experience and good knowledge of the medical science.

This chapter will concentrate on the physical examination of a patient with back pain, including musculoskeletal, neurologic, and mental appraisal. In general, physical examination of the cervical spine should include an examination of the head, neck, and upper extremities; examining the thoracic and lumbar spines should include a thorough evaluation of the chest, abdomen, and lower extremities (Table 4–1).

CERVICAL SPINE

The goals of the examination are to reproduce the patient's symptoms and identify the location of the problem. During the interpretation of symptoms, one must remember that the joints between C2 and C3 are the "headache joints" and the levels below C4 are the cause of shoulder and arm pain. Ideally, during the examination the patient should be sitting on an examining table or a high chair.

Inspection

Attention to the following must be noted:

A. Willingness to move the head and neck.
B. Position of the head.
C. Level and symmetry of the shoulders.
D. Contour of the neck from the side.
E. *Movements* of the neck. These must be *active*. Observe the range of motion (ROM) with the associated rhythm, degree of stiffness, and pain for each. Check whether the motion is smooth or halting.
   1. Flexion (chin to chest).—Normally, it is possible for the patient to make his chin touch his chest. This is usually the most uncomfortable movement for a patient with neck problems (Fig 4–1).

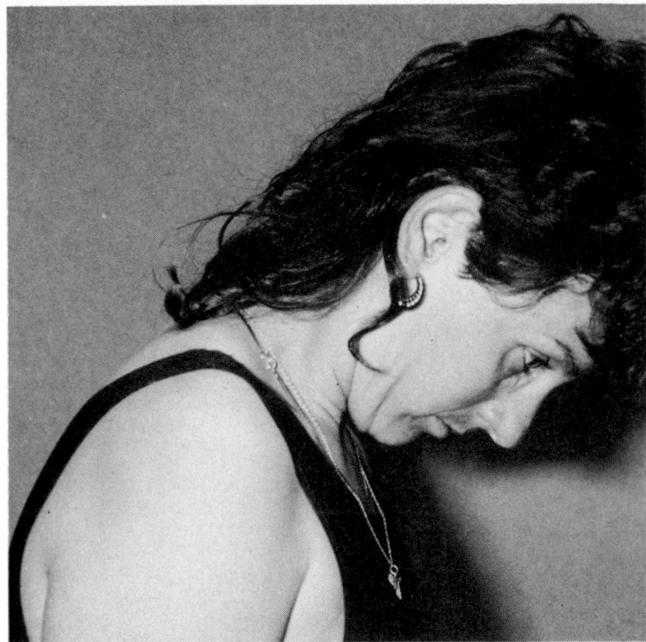

FIG 4-1.
Active flexion of the head and neck.

TABLE 4-1.
Subdivisions of Neurologic Examination

Mentation
Cranial nerves
Motor system
Sensory system
Reflexes
Cerebellar function

2. Extension.—This motion is restricted by disorders of the cervical spine. Normally, all vertebrae in the neck will move. Observe for dizziness. Fifty percent of the flexion/extension ROM occurs at the atlanto-occipital joint, and the other 50% is distributed along the remaining cervical segments (Fig 4-2).
3. Lateral flexion.—Patients are instructed to move the ear down toward the shoulder. Normal ROM is 45 to 50 degrees.
4. Rotation.—The patient is instructed to look over each shoulder. Normally, the chin aligns with the

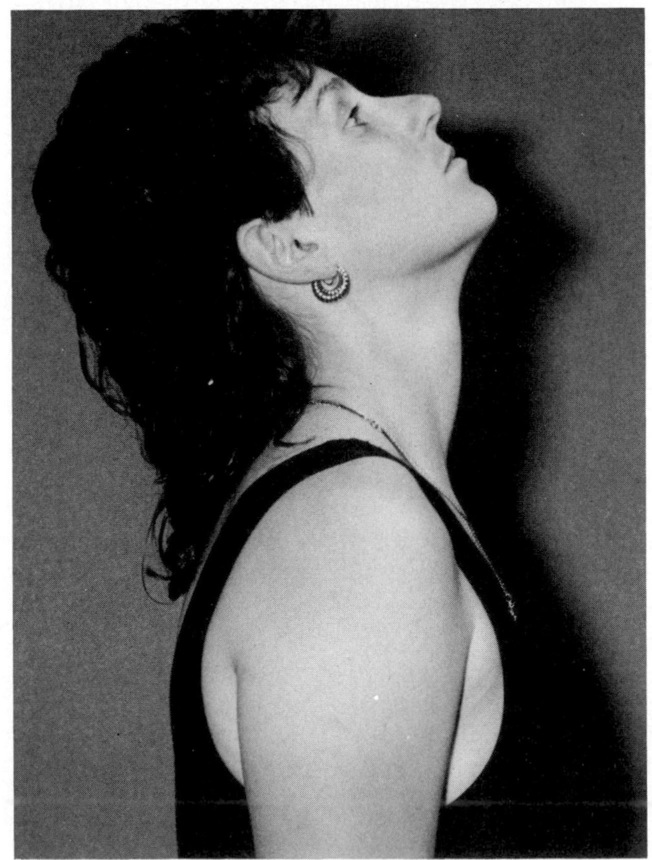

FIG 4-2.
Active extension.

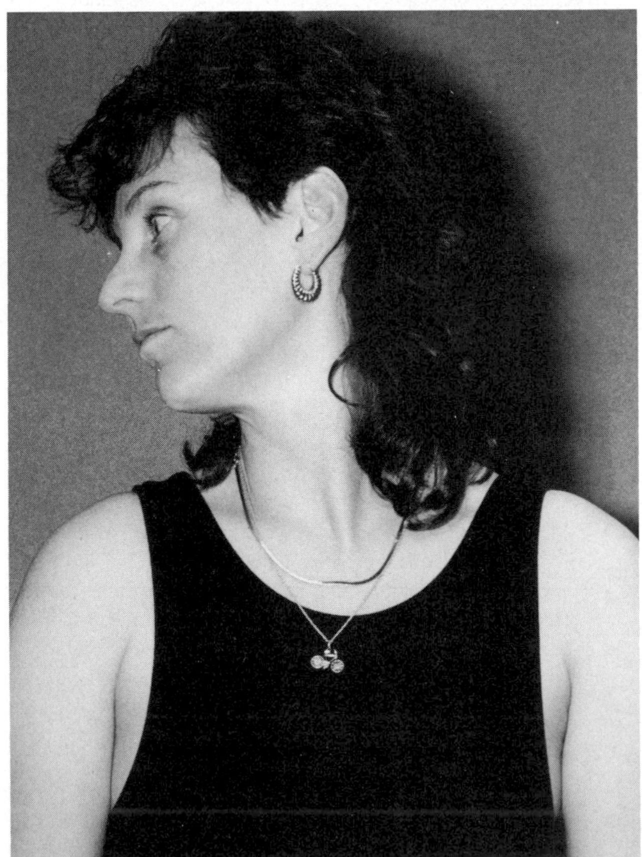

FIG 4-3.
Active rotation of the head and neck (anterior view).

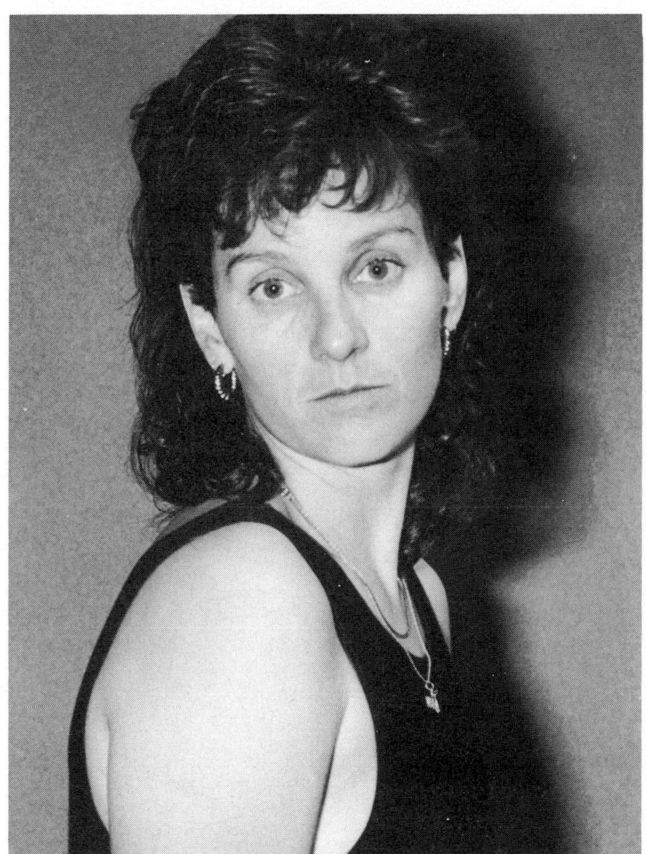

FIG 4–4.
Active rotation (lateral view).

shoulder (Figs 4–3 and 4–4). Fifty percent of this motion occurs at the atlantoaxial joint (C1–2), and the other 50% is evenly distributed among the remaining vertebrae.

Palpation

The objectives of this part of the examination are to determine the level of the lesion, the nature of the problem, and the mobility.

It is important to know the surface anatomy. Anteriorly, between the angle of the mandible and the mastoid process is the transverse process of C1, the hyoid bone at C3, thyroid cartilage at C4–5, and the first cricoid ring and carotid tubercle at C6. Posteriorly, the first large projection beneath the occiput is the spinous process of C2. The spinous processes of C3, C4, and C5 are difficult to palpate because of the cervical lordosis. The largest spinous process is C7, which is the most prominent. Methodically palpate from the occiput to the upper thoracic region by starting on the midline and then moving paramedially to detect pain, stiffness, or spasm.

Provocative Tests

On occasion, when palpation fails to reproduce the patient's pain, provocative tests are essential in achieving this objective.

1. Axial compression test.—The patient's head is slightly extended and laterally flexed followed by steady axial compression over the head (Fig 4–5). This first compresses mainly the facets and reproduces or increases facet symptoms or radicular symptoms if there is foraminal stenosis either by degenerative joint disease (DJD) or a herniated nucleus pulposus (HNP).
2. Quadrant test or Spurling maneuver.—This combines lateral flexion, rotation, and extension and causes further narrowing of the intervertebral foramina. It is a test for the mid and lower portions of the cervical spine (Fig 4–6).
3. Distraction test.—The head and neck are placed in neutral or slight flexion while the examiner pulls upward on the patient's head. This test usually alleviates local or radicular symptoms in patients with facet or foraminal involvement.
4. Lhermitte's sign.—This is more of a symptom than a sign. Patients develop a pain resembling a sudden electric shock throughout the body that is produced by flexing the neck *passively*. This may be positive after

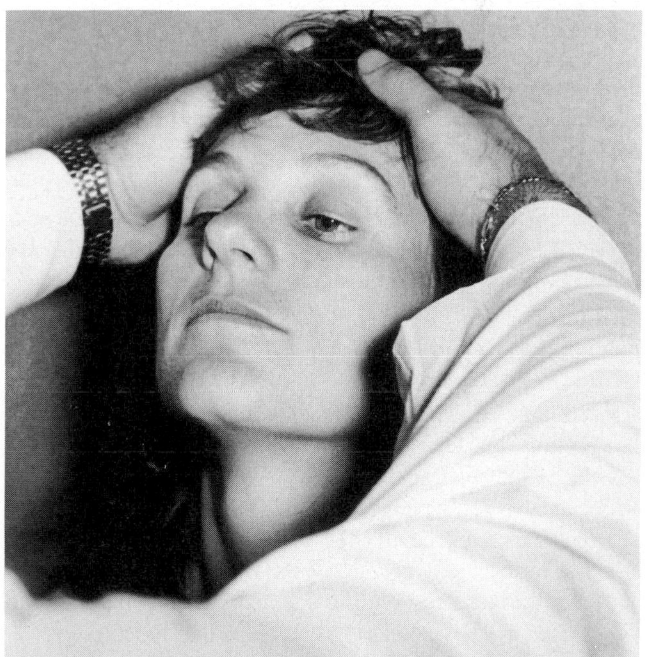

FIG 4–5.
Axial compression test, a provocative maneuver for facet and/or radicular symptoms.

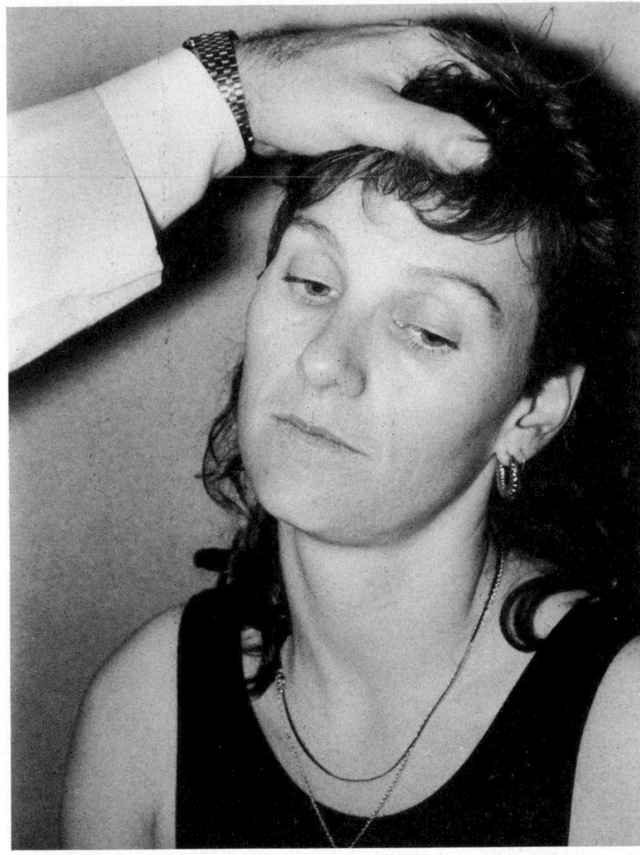

FIG 4–6.
Spurling maneuver, a provocative test for symptoms involving the middle and lower cervical spine.

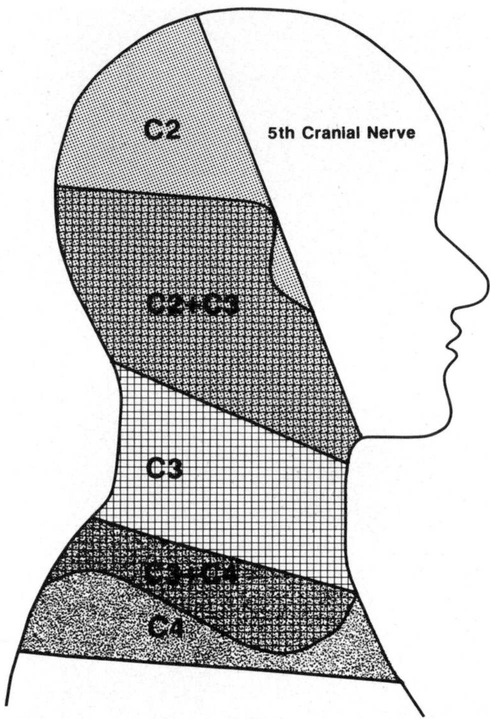

FIG 4–7.
Dermatomes of the skull and neck. Observe the overlapping of C2, C3, and C4 dermatomes.

trauma to the cervical cord, a tumor, multiple sclerosis, or cervical spondylosis.

5. Valsalva test.—This increases intrathecal pressure and is positive in patients with space-occupying lesions (tumor, HNP). The patient holds his breath and bears down as if moving his bowel.

Neurologic Examination

- C2 and C3 nerve root lesions may be suspected mainly by dermatomal distribution signs (Fig 4–7). Note the overlaps, especially of C2 and C3. These can also refer pain in the distribution of the trigeminal nerve, especially the ophthalmic branch.
- C4 root lesions produce pain and sensory changes along the corresponding dermatome and may be associated with weakness of the trapezius muscles.
- The C5 dermatome (axillary nerve) covers the lateral aspect of the arm.
- The C6 dermatome (musculocutaneous nerve) covers the lateral forearm.
- The C7 dermatome covers mainly the middle finger in its dorsal and palmar aspects.
- The C8 dermatome covers the ulnar aspect of the forearm and the ring and small fingers.
- The T1 dermatome (medial brachial cutaneous nerve) covers the medial part of the arm and the elbow.

See Figures 4–8 and 4–9 for dermatomes related to C5 to T1.

TABLE 4–2.
Motor Power Grading Table

Grade 0.—No muscle contraction.
Grade I.—Flicker or trace of contraction without movement, or contraction may be palpated in the absence of movement. There is minimal or no motion of the joints.
Grade II.—The muscle moves the part through a partial arc of movement with gravity eliminated.
Grade III.—The muscle completes the whole arc of movement against gravity.
Grade IV.—The muscle completes the whole arc of motion against gravity together with variable amounts of resistance.
Grade V.—The muscle completes the entire arc of motion against gravity and maximum amounts of resistance several times without signs of fatigue; this is normal muscular power.
S.—Spasm of muscle occurs.
C.—Contraction of muscle occurs.

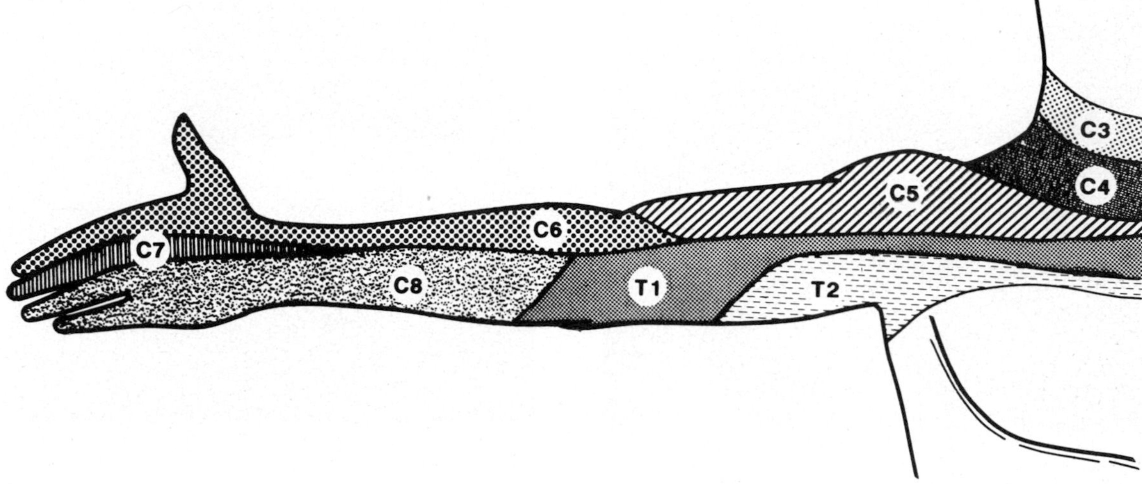

FIG 4–8.
C4 to T1 dermatomes (anterior view).

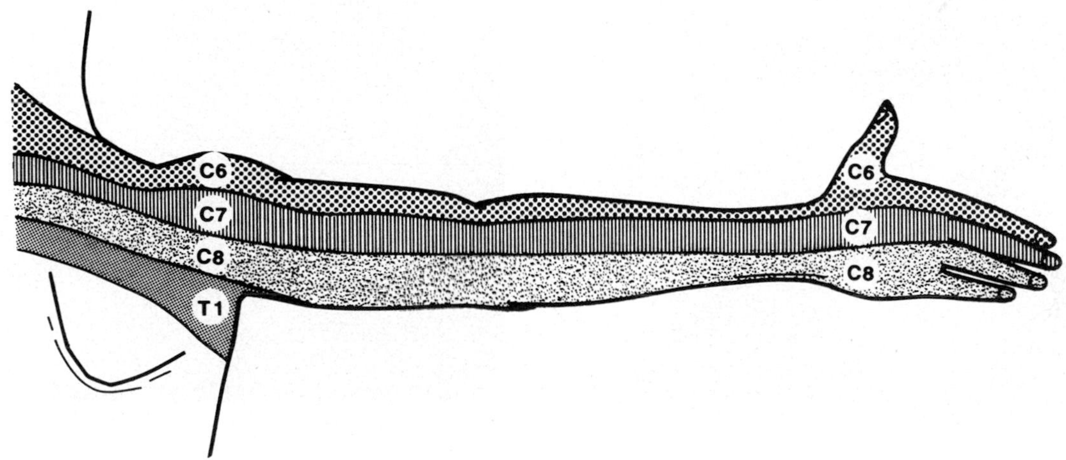

FIG 4–9.
C4 to T1 dermatomes (posterior view).

Motor Power

Table 4–2 presents a grading scheme for muscle power.

- C5: Axillary nerve with distribution to the deltoid muscle. The examination consists of resisting shoulder muscle function, especially abduction (Fig 4–10).
- C6: Musculocutaneous nerve with distribution to the biceps muscle. The examiner resists motion of the wrist extensors: extensor carpi radialis longus (ECRL) and brevis (ECRB), functions of flexion and supination (Fig 4–11).
- C7: Distribution to the triceps, wrist flexors, and finger extensors (Fig 4–12).
- C8: Distribution to the interossei, finger flexors (flexor digitorum perfundus [FDP]), and extensor pollicis longus (EPL).
- T1: Distribution to the interossei (Fig 4–13).

Reflexes

The stimulus is mediated through the deeper sense organs, which are considered proprioceptive in nature.

- Biceps C5: Relax the upper extremity and tap over the tendon in the antecubital fossa.
- Brachioradialis C6: Tap over the dorsoradial aspect of the distal third of the forearm (Fig 4–14).
- Triceps C7: Tap over the triceps tendon with the elbow flexed and relaxed (Fig 4–15).

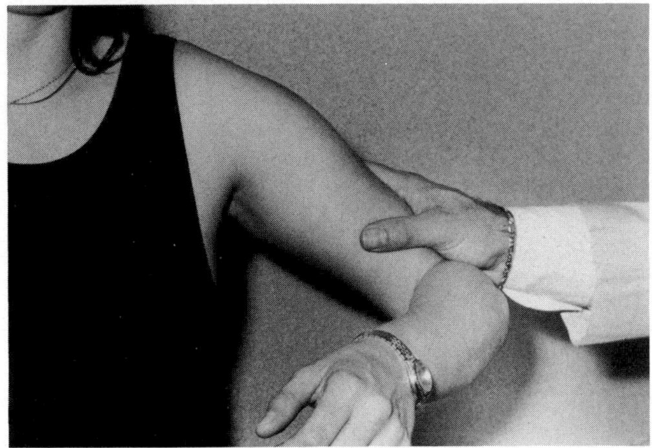

FIG 4–10.
Motor test for the deltoid muscle (C5).

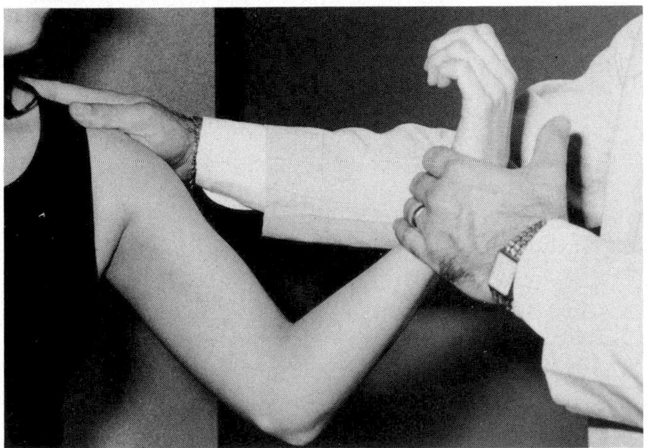

FIG 4–11.
Motor test for the biceps muscle (C6).

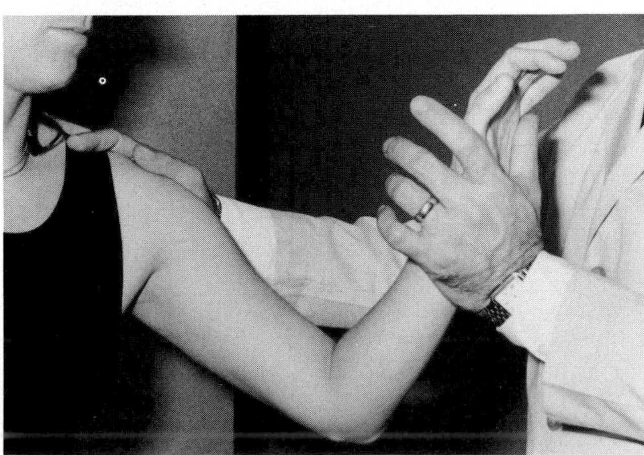

FIG 4–12.
Motor test for the triceps muscle (C7).

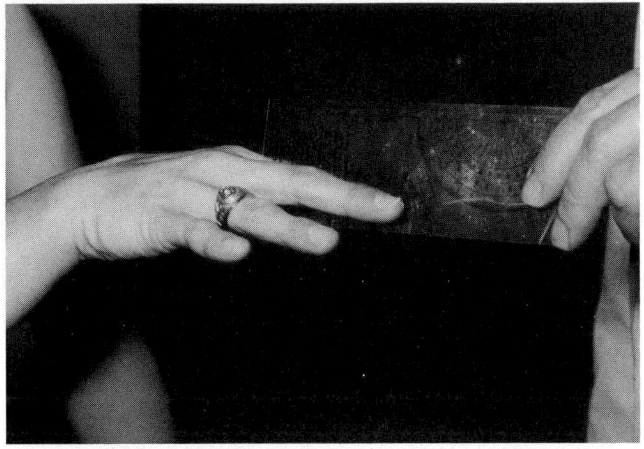

FIG 4–13.
Motor test for the interossei (T1).

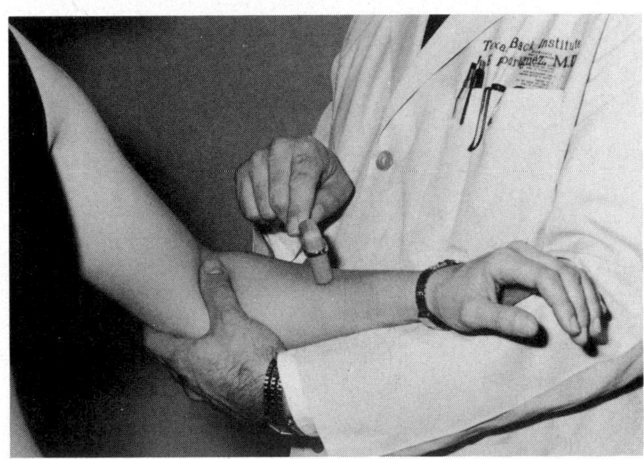

FIG 4–14.
Brachioradialis reflex (C6).

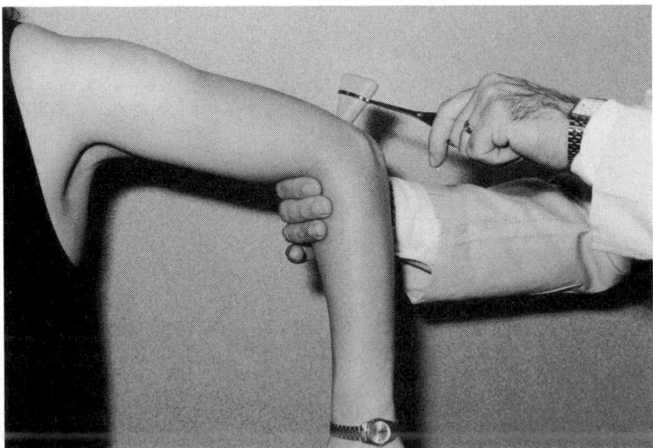

FIG 4–15.
Triceps reflex (C7).

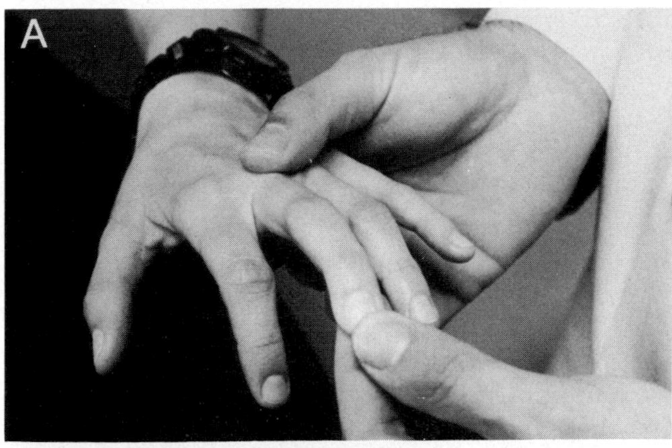

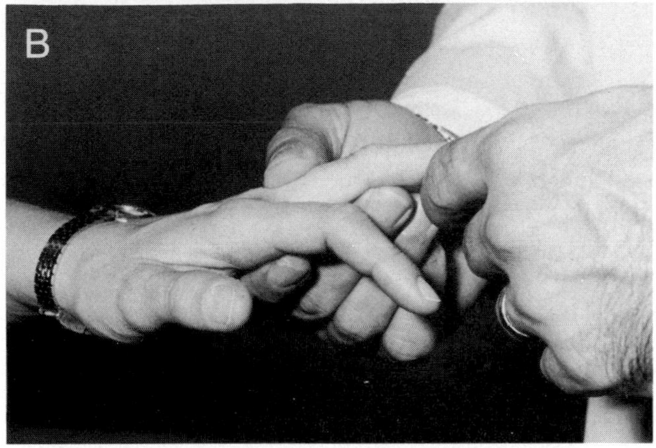

FIG 4–16.
A and **B,** Hoffman's sign maneuver. A positive sign indicates a pyramidal lesion above the C5 or C6 segments.

- Hoffman's reflex or sign: The examiner supports the patient's hand, dorsiflexed at the wrist to allow relaxation of the fingers. The middle finger is then partially extended at the metacarpophalangeal joint, and the middle or distal phalanx is grasped by the examiner's index and middle fingers. With a sharp flick of the examiner's thumb, the patient's nail is nipped or snapped to cause a forcible increased flexion of this finger followed by a sudden release. A positive sign would be present if the patient's thumb flexes and adducts and the index finger flexes simultaneously. The other fingers may flex as well. The sign is incomplete if only the thumb or the index finger respond. This sign indicates hyperactivity of the muscle stretch reflexes due to a lesion of the pyramidal system above the C5 or C6 segments (Fig 4–16).

THORACIC SPINE

It is important to understand that all the structures in the thoracic wall are potential sources of chest pain, particularly anterior chest pain, which commonly originates from the thoracic spine and is often overlooked by clinicians.

TABLE 4–3.
Chest Pain: Noncardiac

Thoracic Organs	Musculoskeletal	Abdominal Organs
Aorta	Cervical spine	Stomach
Pulmonary artery	Thoracic spine	Gallbladder
Pleura	Sternoclavicular joints	Pancreas
Mediastinum	Sternocostal	Duodenum
Esophagus	Costochondral	
Diaphragm	Scapulothoracic	
	Muscles	
	Skin	

Chest and chest wall pain can be musculoskeletal or visceral, local or referred. Medical training emphasizes assessing patients from the anterior position, but the posterior position is ignored (Tables 4–3 and 4–4). The spinal column must be examined from a posterior approach.

The most common cause of thoracic pain is dysfunction of one or more joint articulations, either the costovertebral joint, the facet joints, or both. Herniated discs in the thoracic spine are relatively uncommon and probably account for 1 in 200 protruded discs. The peak incidence occurs during the fourth decade of life and is usually more common below T8. Pain is the most common presentation, followed by sensory and motor disturbances.

Intercostal muscle strains may occur from prolonged stretching of these muscles, especially when lifting heavy objects down from an elevated position. For elderly people, coughing, sneezing, laughing, or lifting heavy objects should alert the physician to a musculoskeletal etiology.

Physical Examination

Inspection of the thoracic spine should include symmetry, scars, skin creases, and muscle spasm. This includes anterior, posterior, and side views of flexion, extension, and rotation.

Approximate ROM is flexion, 60 degrees; and extension, lateral bending, and rotation, 30 degrees each.

TABLE 4–4.
Musculoskeletal-Originated Chest Pain

Spinal Origin	Other
Cervicothoracic junction	Costochondritis
T4–12	Xiphodalgia
T12	Tumors
Twelfth-rib syndrome	Myofascial syndrome
Thoracolumbar junction	Rib fractures
Slipping-rib syndrome	Rib-tip syndrome
Disc herniation	Herpes zoster
	Muscle strain

Palpation

The examiner should try to identify muscle spasm not evident on inspection and also assess passive ROM, which may elicit pain at the extremes of the range. The spinous processes should be palpated proximally to distally, as well as the paravertebral region, where facet or costovertebral pain may originate.

Dermatomes

See Figures 4–17 and 4–18.

Reflexes

Superficial Abdominal Reflex

This is evaluated with the patient lying supine on the examining table. With the sharp end of the neurologic hammer, the physician strokes each abdominal quadrant and notes whether the umbilicus moves toward the stroked side. A lack of this reflex represents an upper motor neuron lesion. The upper abdominal muscles are innervated from T7 to T10, whereas the lower muscles are innervated from T10 to L1.

Superficial Cremasteric Reflex

This reflex is elicited by stroking the inner side of the upper part of the thigh with the sharp edge of a reflex hammer. If the reflex is intact, the ipsilateral half of the scrotum is pulled upward due to cremasteric muscle contraction (T12). Absence or a decreased reflex is indicative of an upper motor neural lesion if both muscles are involved and a lower motor neuron lesion between L1 and L2 if the problem is unilateral.

Beevor's Sign

This tests the integrity of the segmental innervation of the rectus abdominis and corresponding paraspinal muscles. This muscle group is segmentally innervated by the anterior primary division of T5–12 and sometimes L1. The patient is asked to perform a quarter sit-up with his arms crossed on the chest. While holding this position, observe the umbilicus, which should not move at all. If it does move, there is asymmetrical involvement of the anterior and paraspinal muscles. The umbilicus moves toward the strong or uninvolved side. This sign is positive in patients with poliomyelitis or myelomeningocele.

LUMBAR SPINE

This region of the spine not only provides support for the upper portion of the body but also transmits its weight to the pelvis and lower extremities. The upper portion of the lumbar spine is a transitional area between a relatively rigid thoracic cage and a significantly mobile lower lumbar segment. This transitional area is prone to injuries, especially those caused by axial loading (T11–L2).

The lumbar spine also transports the cauda equina to the lower extremities and provides mobility to the back.

See Table 4–5 for possible etiologies for low back pain.

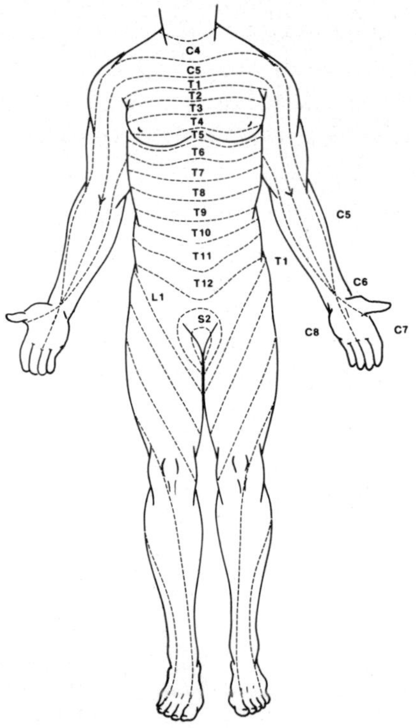

FIG 4–17.
Anterior thoracic dermatomes.

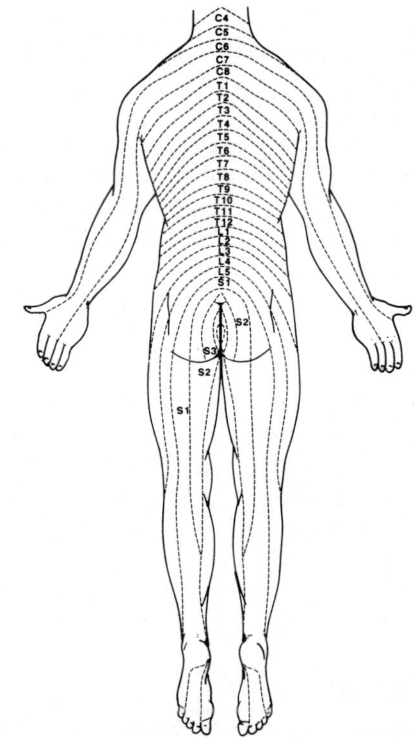

FIG 4–18.
Posterior thoracic and lumbar dermatomes.

TABLE 4–5.
Etiologies for Low Back Pain

Congenital disorders
Facet asymmetry
Transitional vertebrae
Sacralization of lumbar vertebrae
Lumbarization of sacral vertebrae
Tumors
Benign
Involving nerve roots or the meninges (neurinoma, hemangioma, meningioma)
Tumors involving vertebrae (osteoid osteomas, osteoblastomas, Paget disease)
Malignant
Primary bone tumors (multiple myeloma)
Primary neural tumors
Secondary tumors (metastases from the breast, prostate, kidney, lung, thyroid)
Trauma
Lumbar strain (acute or chronic)
Compression fracture (vertebral body, transverse process)
Subluxated facet joint (facet syndrome)
Spondylolysis and spondylolisthesis
Toxicity with heavy metal poisoning (radium)
Metabolic disorders (osteoporosis, hyperparathyroidism)
Inflammatory diseases
Rheumatoid arthritis
Ankylosing spondylitis
Degenerative disorders
Spondylosis
Osteoarthritis
Herniated nucleus pulposus
Spinal stenosis
Infections
Acute (pyogenic disc space infections)
Chronic (tuberculosis, aspergillosis, chronic osteomyelitis)
Circulatory disorders (abdominal aortic aneurysm)
Mechanical
Intrinsic (poor posture, poor muscle tone, unstable vertebrae)
Extrinsic (uterine fibroids, pancreatic carcinoma, pelvic tumors or infections, hip diseases, sacroiliac joint infections, lumbar scoliosis, pleurisy, gastric or duodenal ulcers, kidney diseases including nephrolithiasis, etc.)

Inspection

This includes skin evaluation for redness, ecchymosis, unusual skin marking like neurofibromas, hairy patches (faun's beard), and soft lipomas (fatty masses). Redness may be a sign of infection (cellulitis) or trauma. Ecchymosis is also associated with trauma. Neurofibromas, which are usually associated with "cafè au lait" spots, may impinge upon the spinal cord or nerve roots. Neurofibromas are also a cause of spinal structural deformities. Hair patches can be evidence of body defects like diastematomyelia or spina bifida.

Posture evaluation is an important part of the inspection. The shoulders and pelvis should appear level. The bony and soft-tissue structures on both sides of the midline have to be symmetrical. An unusual lumbar curve observed while the patient is standing may be due to a herniated disc, soft capsular or muscular injuries, scoliosis secondary to degenerative disease, and least common in the lumbar area, an idiopathic curve. The lower part of the spine should have a gentle lordotic curve, which can be absent due to muscle spasm. An increased or exaggerated lordosis is commonly associated with weak abdominal musculature. All the aforementioned characteristics should be checked while the patient is standing and walking.

Part of the inspection is passive and active ROM including flexion, extension, lateral bending, and rotation. The patient should be asked to try to touch her toes. The distance between the fingertips and the floor is measured or the angle between the lumbar spine and the lower extremities documented. *Flexion* is limited by the size and shape of the vertebral bodies. This motion involves *relaxation* and *stretching* of the supraspinous, interspinous, ligamentum flavum, and the posterior longitudinal ligament. Patients with muscle spasm may refuse to do this test (Fig 4–19).

Extension is measured by the approximate angle between the lumbar spine and the lower extremities. This motion involves *stretching* of the anterior longitudinal ligament and *relaxation* of the posterior ligaments. Patients

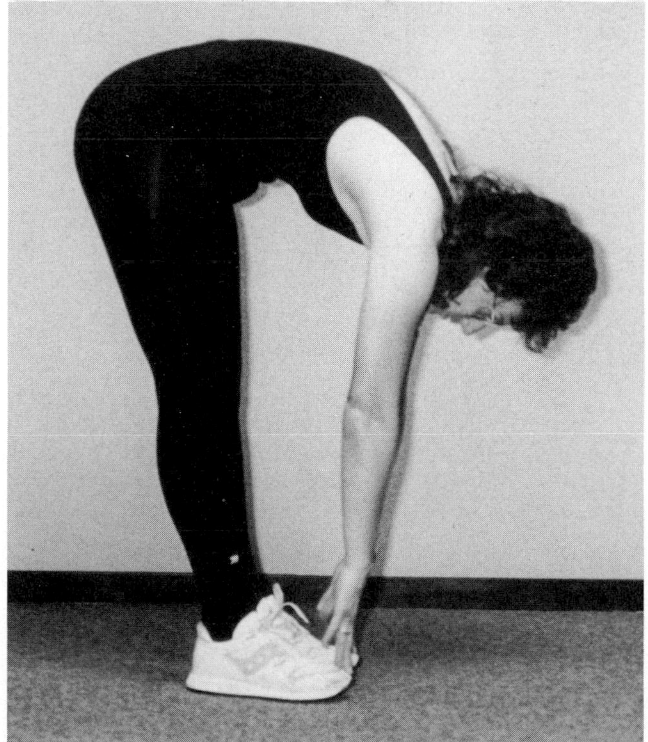

FIG 4–19.
Active flexion of the lumbar spine. Measure the distance between the fingertips and the floor.

with spondylolysis and/or spondylolisthesis may feel pain with extension and relief with flexion (Fig 4–20).

Lateral bending occurs by a combination of rotation and bending. This range is limited by the surrounding ligaments and facet capsules. This test is performed by the examiner stabilizing the pelvis and then asking the patient to bend as far as possible to each side. The arc of motion is noted and compared with the passive motion (Figs 4–21 and 4–22).

In a test of *rotation* the patient's pelvis has to be stabilized to prevent lateral bending. The patient is also asked to turn the trunk to each side. Active and passive ROM is documented and compared. Lateral listing of the patient may be a sign of a herniated disc or foraminal stenosis. In a posterolateral or foraminal herniation or in symptomatic unilateral foraminal stenosis, the patient will list the body to the contralateral side. A patient with a large lateral herniation will list to the ipsilateral side. In the former situation, the patient is attempting to increase the space available to the nerve by opening the foramina. In the latter,

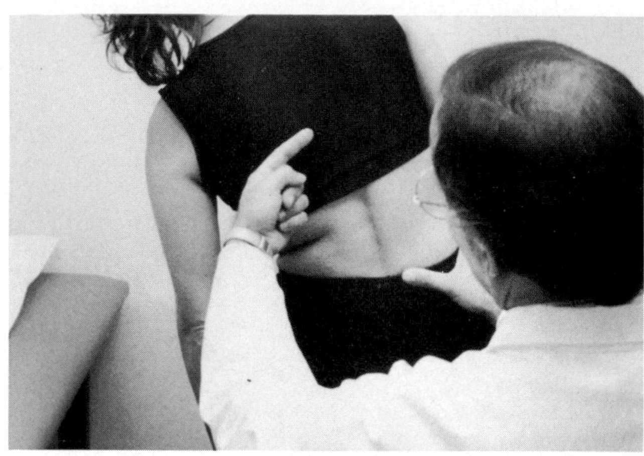

FIG 4–21.
Assessment of lateral bending of the thoracolumbar spine. Palpation of the iliac crest and the C4–5 interspace is done concomitantly for orientation purposes.

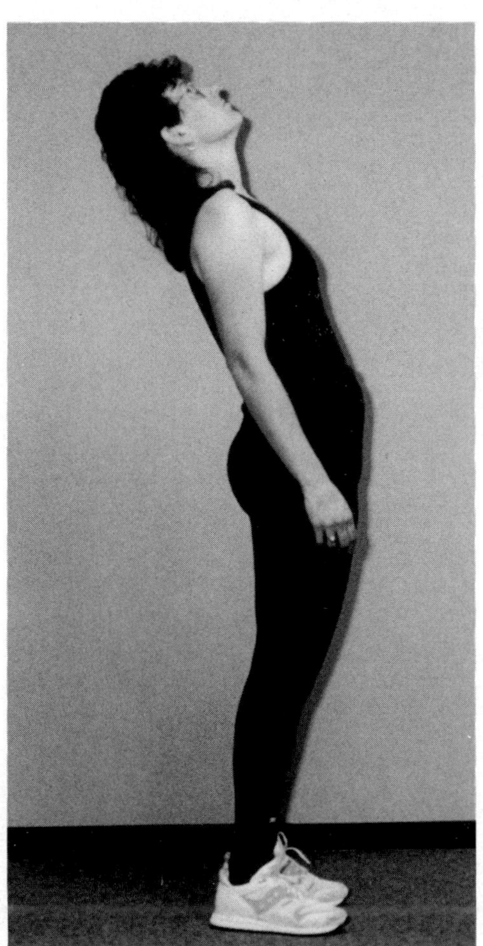

FIG 4–20.
Active extension of the lumbar spine.

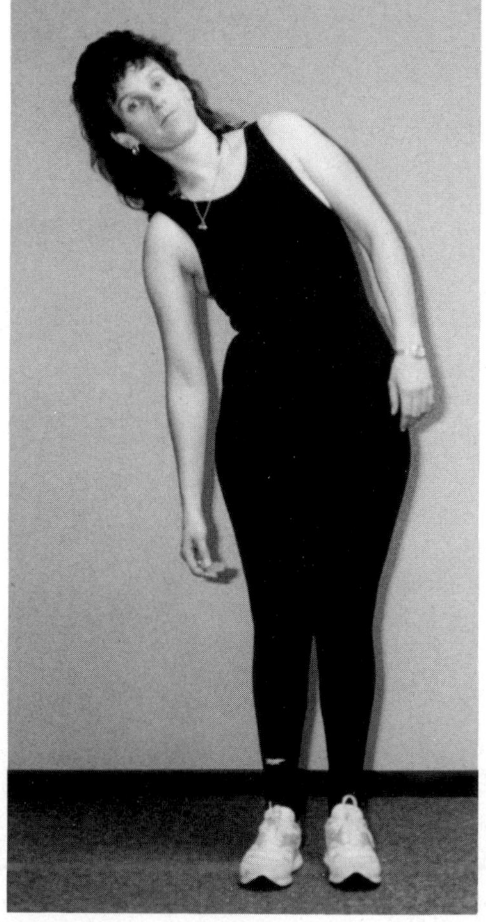

FIG 4–22.
Front view of active lateral bending.

the attempt is to relieve the nerve from external compression applied by a herniated disc.

Palpation

The examiner should methodically palpate the central and both paravertebral regions of the lumbar spine proximally to distally to try to identify tender points, crepitations, muscle spasm, fluctuation, or defects in the soft tissues or bones. For orientation, the physician should palpate the top of both iliac crests and, in the midline, the interspace at the same level of the crests. This usually is the L4–5 spinous interspace. This task may help in documentation of the approximate area where "pathology" was found during palpation (see Fig 4–21).

Gaps between spinous processes or the absence of any lumbar or sacral posterior elements is suggestive of spina bifida. A step-off from one spinous process to another is suggestive of spondylolisthesis.

Palpation of the sacrum and coccyx is as important as palpation of the lumbar spine. The coccyx can only be *fully* palpated through a rectal examination. Next palpate the *ilio lumbar* area where some ligaments are present. These are tender in post-traumatic and inflammatory conditions.

The ischial tuberosity and greater trochanter can be palpated better by flexing the hip to 90 degrees to try to locate tender points. The sciatic nerve can sometimes be palpated in thin people in the above-mentioned position. It lies between the ischium and the greater trochanter. If there is a radicular condition, palpation of the nerve may increase radicular pain (Fig 4–23).

Lipomas can be palpated near the spine (usually present paramedially) and iliac crests. The clunial nerves can be tender after blunt trauma to the gluteal region or crests, when surgical neuromas are formed by cutting the nerves during bone graft harvesting or biopsies of the crests.

The lumbar spine examination must include an evaluation of the abdomen and groin. Abdominal muscle tone can be palpated by asking the patient to do half a sit-up and noting any asymmetry in the muscle tone or deviation of the umbilicus to any of the abdominal quadrants (Beevor's sign described in the thoracic spine examination).

The umbilicus is usually at the L3–4 level; this is usually where the aorta divides into the common iliacs. Aortic aneurysms can usually be palpated above the umbilicus. In thin patients, the sacral promontory can be palpated below the umbilicus if the patient is relaxed and cooperative.

Neurologic Examination

If possible, observe the patient's gait. The patient's gait should be observed while she is walking on her toes and heels (this gives the examiner an idea of L5, S1 coordination and proprioception status). Ankle rises provide a good assessment of S1 function.

For the next part of the examination, have the patient sit upright with the legs dangling from the edge of the examining table. Each leg is gently raised individually to bring the knee into extension by pushing from the back of the heel. This test is the sitting root test (SRT), which is an indirect straight leg raise (SLR) test (Fig 4–24). In actual radiculopathy, both tests are positive within a 20- to 30-degree arc difference. A greater difference may indicate symptom magnification.

After the SRT, the deep tendon reflexes (DTR) of the patella and Achilles tendon are examined and any asymmetry in strength and briskness documented (Figs 4–25

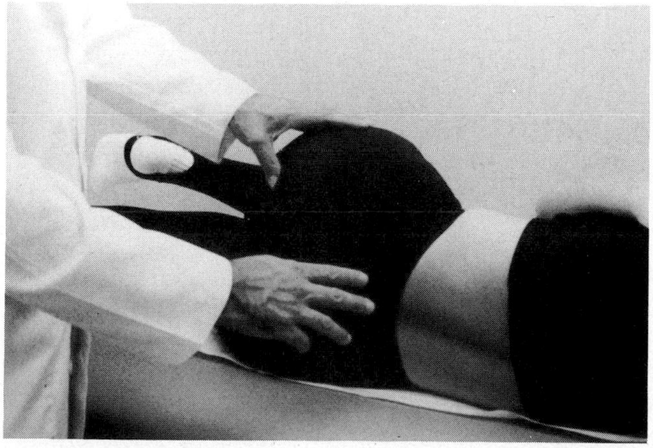

FIG 4–23.
Palpation of the "sciatic notch". The purpose of this test is to check for sciatic nerve radiculopathy.

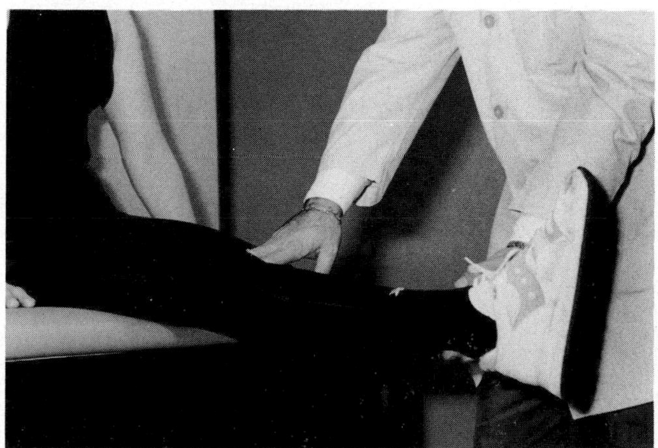

FIG 4–24.
Sitting root test, which is an indirect straight leg raising maneuver. In radiculopathies, this test is positive within a range of 20- to 30-degree arc difference.

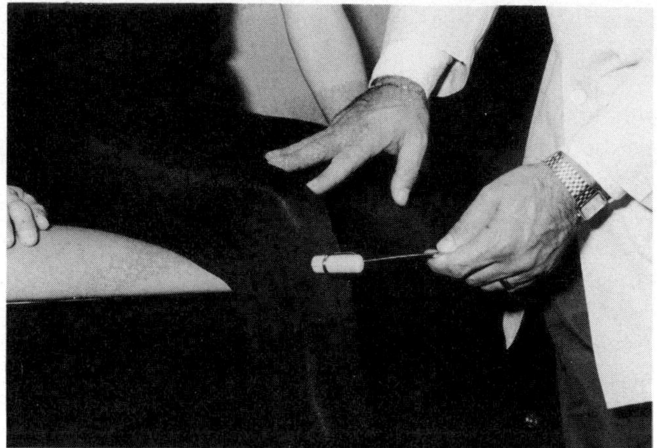

FIG 4–25.
Patella deep tendon reflex (L4).

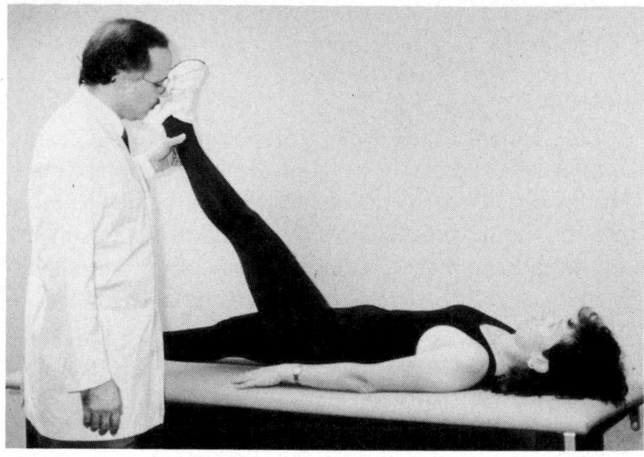

FIG 4–27.
Straight leg raising designed to provoke sciatic nerve radiculopathy.

and 4–26). The patellar reflex is L4, and the Achilles reflex is S1.

The patient is asked to lie supine on the examining table. Individual SLR or Lasègue's sign tests are performed by passively raising each leg and documenting the hip angle where *radicular* pain starts or increases (Fig 4–27). Back pain only during SLR does not make it a positive test, which is a common error made by physicians. The SLR and SRT are designed to reproduce or increase *radicular signs* involving the sciatic nerve. If pain or restriction is present, the location of the pain is ascertained, particularly contralateral radiation of pain, which is an indication of significant nerve root compression. With these tests, the L5 and S1 nerve roots move 2 to 6 mm at the level of the foramina. Whether this is a true sliding movement or passive deformation of the nerve in the foramina is still debatable. More important is the fact that when the SRT or SLR tests are performed in a situation where there is a three-dimensionally compromised canal or foramen, the involved nerve is subjected to a tensile or compressive force, or both, which it cannot accommodate without producing radicular symptoms. The L4 nerve root moves a lesser distance, and the more proximal roots show little motion. Thus, SRT and SLR tests are of more value in lesions of the fifth lumbar and first sacral nerve roots.

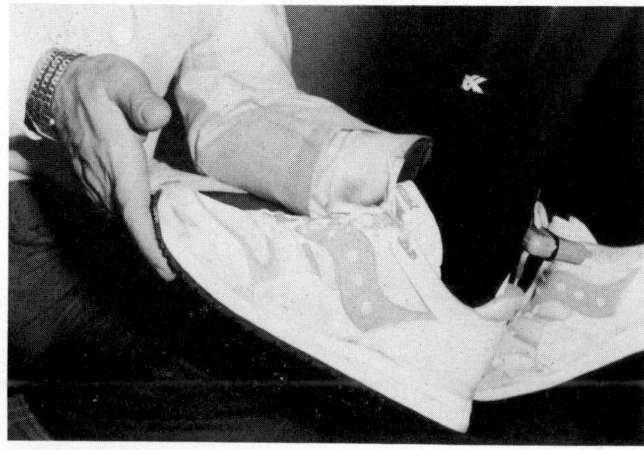

FIG 4–26.
Achilles reflex (S1).

Passive dorsiflexion of the foot at a point just a few degrees less than maximum SLR is also performed as a means of reproducing symptoms. If the patient does not experience pain during this test, then pain induced during the SLR is probably due to tight hamstring musculature. If the Lasègue test and the dorsiflexion maneuver are positive, the patient should be asked to locate, as closely as possible, the source of her pain, which may be anywhere in the lumbar spine or the course of the sciatic nerve.

Another method of identifying an irritated nerve in the lower lumbar area is to flex the hip so that a positive SLR is obtained by slightly extending the ipsilateral knee and applying finger pressure upon the tibial nerve in the popliteal fossa. This is known as the bowstring sign. While the patient is still in the supine position, a Patrick or Faber (eponym for flexion, abduction, and external rotation of the hip) test is performed, which is positive if there is hip or sacroiliac joint involvement. This test is performed by crossing one of the patient's legs over the other in a "figure 4" position (one foot over the opposite knee) and then pushing downward over the flexed knee (Fig 4–28). A negative test indicates a normal or asymptomatic hip or sacroiliac joint. Another test to determine pathology in the sacroiliac joint is the *pelvic rock test*. With the patient supine, the examiner places his thumbs over each anterior superior iliac spine (ASIS) and the palms over the iliac tubercles and forcibly compresses the pelvis toward the symphysis pubis. Pain in the sacroiliac joints makes the test positive.

To measure sacroiliac pathology, the *Gaenslen test* is

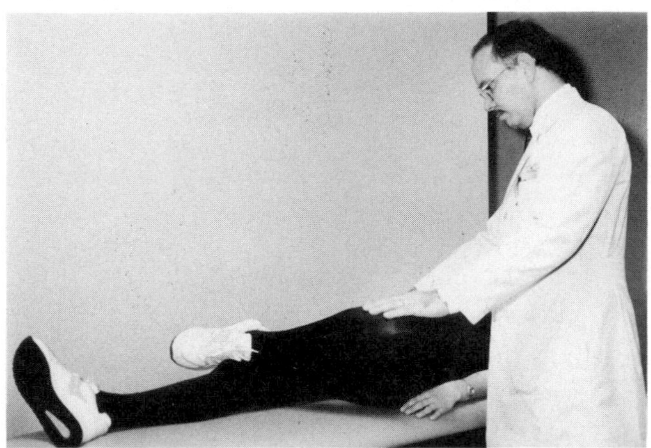

FIG 4–28.
Patrick's or Faber's maneuver, positive in hip and/or sacroiliac joint conditions.

performed. While the patient is still in a supine position, slide her to a position with one buttock over the edge of the table. The patient is asked to draw both knees toward the chest and then allow the unsupported leg to drop over the edge of the table while the other leg remains flexed. Complaints of further pain in the sacroiliac joint is another indication of pathology in this area (Fig 4–29).

The Kernig test is designed to stretch the spinal cord and reproduce pain. While the patient is lying supine on the examining table, have her place both hands behind the head and forcibly flex the neck. This test can elicit pain in the patient's cervical spine, lower part of the back, or the lower extremities, which is an indication of meningeal irritation or nerve root compression. This test is similar to Lhermitte's.

The Hoover test is designed to determine "symptom magnification." A patient who is trying to magnify symptoms may indicate that she is unable to raise the leg. As the patient tries to raise the leg in question, the examiner cups a hand under the heel of the opposite foot. Normally, when trying to raise a leg, downward pressure is applied on the contralateral leg. If no pressure is applied, this would imply that she is not really trying (Fig 4–30). Another method of determining exaggeration of symptoms is by performing the Burn's bench test. The patient is required to kneel on a bench with the knees and hips flexed and place her fingers on the floor. The kneeling position relieves stress on the lower part of the back and tension on the sciatic nerve, so patients with organic causes of low back pain are able to perform this test, whereas patients magnifying their symptoms will not perform the test adequately (Fig 4–31).

Another test done in the supine position is the Milgram test, which increases intrathecal pressure. The patient simultaneously elevates both legs with the knees straight, a few inches off the table, and tries to hold this position for at least 30 seconds. If the patient accomplishes the test without pain, intrathecal pathology is ruled out. If the patient cannot hold the position, is unable to lift her legs at all, or experiences pain during the maneuver, this suggests an intrathecal or extrathecal pathology.

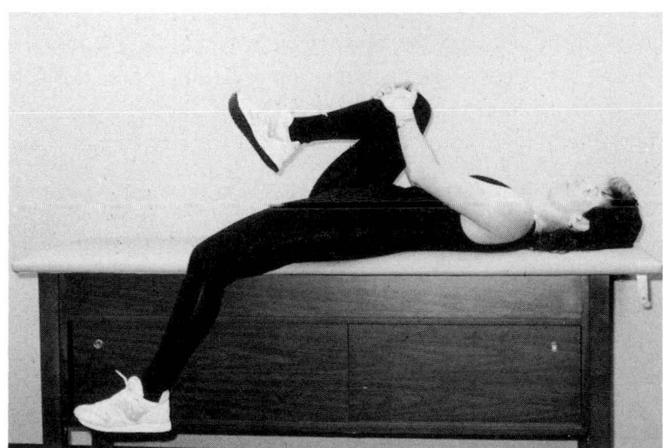

FIG 4–29.
Gaenslen's test to check for sacroiliac joint disease.

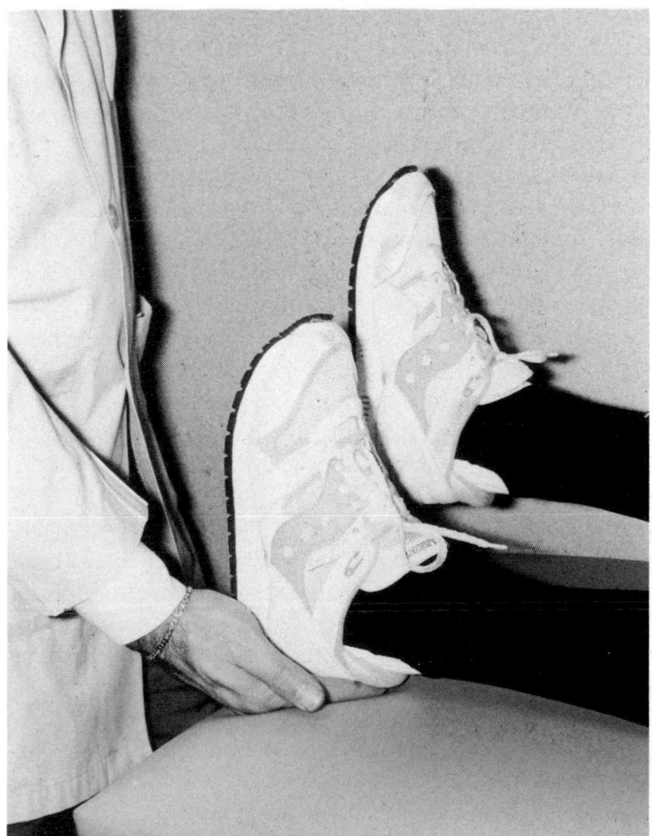

FIG 4–30.
Hoover test for diagnosis of patients with "symptom magnification."

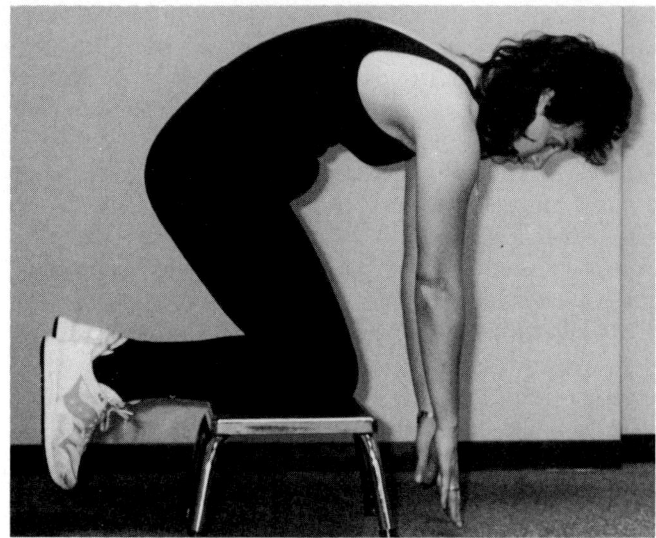

FIG 4–31.
Burn's bench test to rule out "symptom magnification" of lumbar etiology.

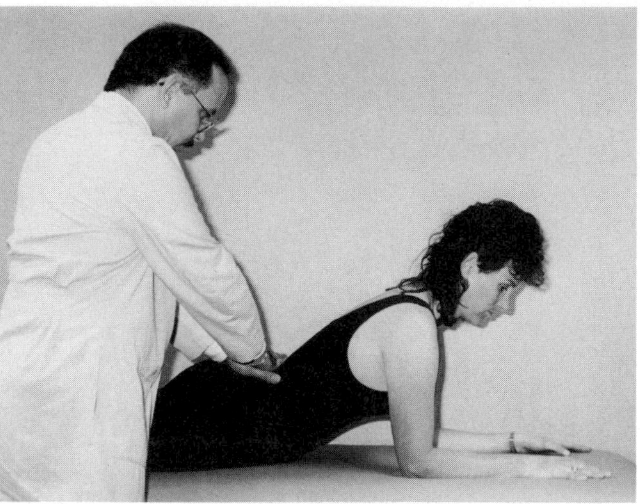

FIG 4–32.
Passive compression of the lumbar spine during active extension while in the prone position. Observe for possible aggravation of symptoms.

The Naffziger test is a compression test designed to increase intrathecal pressure by increasing the intraspinal fluid pressure, also in an attempt to elicit radicular symptoms. Both jugular veins are compressed until the patient's face begins to flush. The patient is then asked to cough; if this causes radicular pain, there is probably pathology pressing on the thecal sac. The Valsalva maneuver is a similar test, except that the patient bears down as if trying to move the bowels.

The patient is then asked to change to the prone position. Sometimes it is necessary to place a pillow under the hip for comfort. The examiner should observe the patient while she is turning over to evaluate the amount of guarding present in the low back region. The amount of guarding is an indication of the severity of the problem.

The amount of spasm in the paravertebral muscles should also be observed when the patient has reached the prone position, as well as whether a deformity or list present in the standing position has disappeared. Frequently, a lumbar list or spasm of the erector spinae muscles relaxes in the prone position. The existence of gluteal muscle atrophy should be noted and palpation of the spinous processes and iliac crests repeated. Areas of tenderness, deformities, or depression of the spinous processes should be noted. Superficial tenderness may be due to the presence of bursae over kissing spinous tips. If the pain appears to be deep upon palpation, there may be involvement of either the facet or disc. Look for radiation of the pain with any of the above maneuvers.

Areas found tender to passive compression are tested with the patient actively extending her back (Fig 4–32). This may cause aggravation of symptoms, and if so, this implies involvement of the articular facets or an extruded disc fragment. If the tenderness is relieved with extension, then instability of the disc unit is present. If the pain remains unchanged, then the test is indeterminate. A clinical suspicion of instability should be confirmed by dynamic roentgenography.

The femoral stretch test is conducted by passively extending the hip by flexing the ipsilateral knee to 90 degrees and holding and lifting the extremity from the ankle. A positive test response will cause radicular signs along the curve of the femoral nerve (L2–4).

Deep Tendon Reflexes

DTRs are usually tested with the patient in the sitting position. This includes the following:

1. Patellar reflex, which is mediated by the L2, L3, and L4 nerve roots. Clinically it is considered an L4 reflex. The reflex may be present even when the L4 root is totally cut because of its other innervation sources. With the patient relaxing the leg and dangling it off the examining table, the examiner taps over the patellar flexion (see Fig 4–25).
2. Tibialis posterior reflex, which is an L5 examination. Unfortunately it is difficult to elicit. The forefoot is held in eversion and dorsiflexion while the examiner taps over the tendon just proximal to its insertion into the navicular tuberosity.
3. Achilles or triceps surae reflex. The clinical neurologic level is S1 through the gastrocnemius muscle. The tendon is placed in slight stretch by dorsiflexing the foot passively and then tapping over the tendon (see Fig 4–26).

The reflexes are graded as absent, or 0, hypoactive, or 1+; normoactive, or 2+; and hyperactive, or 3+. This is usually determined by the examiner's experience or by comparison to the contralateral side.

Muscle Power

For gradings of muscle power, see Table 4–2.

A. Muscles examined in the sitting position:
   1. Iliopsoas (T12, L1, L2, L3): Main flexor of the hip. This is tested with the patient sitting on the edge of the examining table with her legs dangling. The contralateral pelvis is stabilized by placing one hand over the iliac crest. The patient is asked to actively raise her thigh from the table. The motion is repeated with the other hand over the patient's knee to provide resistance against the motion. This test is repeated on the opposite side, the findings compared, and strength documented.
   2. Quadriceps L2, L3, L4, innervated by the femoral nerve: These are better examined with the patient in the sitting position. The posterior aspect of the distal portion of the thigh is stabilized with one hand and the patient asked to actively extend her knee. The test is repeated with resistance provided by placing the other hand over the anterior aspect of the distal portion of the leg. The test is repeated on the opposite extremity and the results compared and documented.
   3. Tibialis anterior: Clinical test of L4 motor function, innervated by the deep peroneal nerve. To test, the patient is asked to dorsiflex and invert the foot while the examiner applies resistance with his hands over the dorsomedial aspect of the foot (Fig 4–33).
   4. Extensor hallucis longus: L5 motor function, innervated by the deep peroneal nerve. The patient is asked to dorsiflex the great toes while the examiner applies resistance with the thumbs over the dorsal aspect of the toes. The extensor digitorum longus and brevis, which are also innervated by the deep peroneal nerve, are examined as above.
   5. Peroneus longus and brevis: S1 function, innervated by the superficial peroneal nerve. The muscles are examined by securing the patient's ankle with the examiner's hands and having the patient plantar-flex and evert the foot while the examiner opposes the motion by pushing against the plantar and lateral aspect of the forefoot.

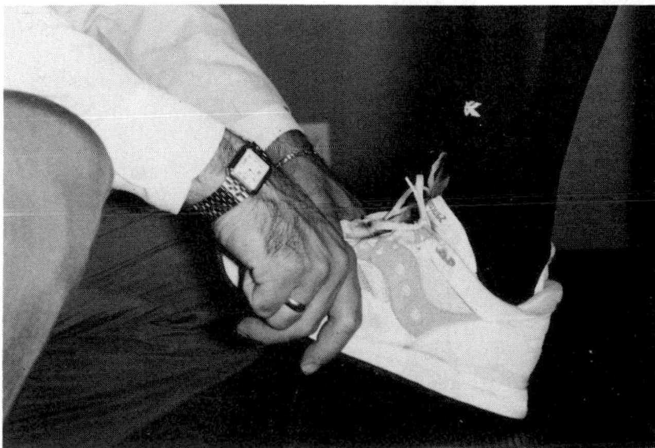

FIG 4–33.
Tibialis anterior muscle power test (L4).

B. Muscles examined in the supine position:
   1. Hip adductors group: Motor segments are L2, L3, and L4, innervated by the obturator nerve. This segment is tested as a massive group. The patient is asked to adduct the legs while the examiner places his hands between the patient's knees to apply resistance to the motion.
   2. Gastrocnemius-soleus muscles: Motor segments S1 and S2, innervated by the tibial nerve. This is a very strong group of muscles that has no legitimate manual examination. A way to assess the strength is by asking the patient to hold herself to the edge of the examining table with her hands, and then plantar-flex both feet and ankles against the examiner's hands, who applies resistance. Perhaps an even better way of evaluating this group of muscles is by asking the patient to perform 10 to 15 ankle raises while standing on one leg. This method can be included during the examination while the patient is standing.
C. Muscles examined in the lateral position:
   1. Gluteus medius: Motor segment L5, innervated by hip abduction. The patient is asked to abduct her leg while the examiner stabilizes the pelvis with one hand and applies resistance to the motion by placing the other hand over the lateral aspect of the leg and pushes downward (Fig 4–34). The patient is turned on the opposite side and the procedure repeated on the other extremity.
D. Muscles examined in the prone position:
   1. Gluteus maximus: Motor segment S1, innervated by the inferior gluteal nerve. The patient is asked to flex the knee and extend the hip. The examiner resists hip extension by pushing down on the posterior aspect of the thigh while simultaneously palpating the gluteus maximus for tone.
   2. Hamstrings muscles:
      a. Semimembranosus: Muscle segment L5, innervated by the tibial portion of the sciatic nerve.
      b. Semitendinosus: Also L5 and innervated by the other tibial portion of the sciatic nerve.

5

Lumbar Range of Motion

Paula J. Gilbert, P.T.

Optimal range of motion is a balance between mobility and stability. However, the majority of attention has been on the relationship between the flexibility of the lumbar spine in patients as compared with individuals with "healthy" spines. Spinal flexibility has become a consideration for pre-employment screening and disability ratings. Stretching the back has become incorporated into athletic and employment training programs. Although spinal range of motion receives much attention, there is still no general consensus as to the methods used to assess it or how values from various measurement techniques should be interpreted. Clinicians and researchers are continuously seeking tools with which to measure spinal range of motion in a manner that is easy to perform and cost-effective, yields valid results, and is meaningful in relation to the patient's condition. This chapter covers the physiologic movements of the spine, some of the techniques for measuring spinal range of motion, and their validity.

PHYSIOLOGIC MOVEMENTS OF THE LUMBAR SPINE

Knowledge of basic physiologic movements allows a more solid foundation from which to assess lumbar range of motion. Although there is a considerably large range of spinal mobility in the lumbar spine (approximately 55 degrees of lumbar flexion and 27 degrees of extension),[36] this net range is produced by small amounts of motion at each of the lumbar segments. The range and pattern of motion are dependent on the orientation of the facet joints and the elasticity, fluid content, and thickness of the intervertebral disc. The fundamental movements of the lumbar spine are flexion, extension, rotation, lateral bending, as well as components of axial compression and distraction.

Flexion

Straightening of the lumbar spine occurs during flexion.[9] This, if primarily seen in the upper and mid lumbar levels[5] (Table 5–1), may occur at the L4–5 level but not at the L5–S1 level.[46] Lack of motion at L5–S1 is related to zygapophyseal joint alignment. As the levels of the lumbar spine descend, the articular surfaces of the zygapophyseal joints, sagittal in orientation, become increasingly more frontal at the L5–S1 level.

TABLE 5–1.
Average Range of Motion (in Degrees) in Males 25 to 36 Years of Age*

	Lateral Flexion		Axial Rotation			
Level	Left	Right	Left	Right	Flexion	Extension
L1–2	5	6	1	1	8	13
L2–3	5	6	1	1	10	13
L3–4	5	6	1	2	12	13
L4–5	3	5	1	2	13	16
L5–S1	0	2	1	0	9	14

*Adapted from Pearcy M, Portek I, Shepherd J: *Spine* 1984; 9:294–297.

In the neutral standing position, the spine is lordotic. As forward flexion occurs, each of the lumbar vertebrae rotates from their lordotic position to a position in which the end plates of adjacent vertebrae become parallel.[9] Concomitant with anterior sagittal rotation, a small component of forward translation occurs as well.[46, 57] The L5–S1 surfaces account for more translation than flexion or rotation.[19, 32] During flexion, once the opposing zygapophyseal joints impact, the forward translation, or "shearing," is stopped. The tensile properties of the zygapophyseal joints, capsules, and the intervertebral joint ligaments resist anterior sagittal rotation, thus maintaining stability of the lumbar spine in flexion.[5]

Extension

Extension of the lumbar intervertebral joints involves posterior sagittal rotation and a small posterior translation.[5] The center of this rotation is slightly anterior to the disc nucleus. The movement of the joint is stopped when the inferior articular processes of the intervertebral joint fully contact the lamina of the vertebra below. If further extension with increasing load is applied, the upper vertebra then undergoes axial rotation.[60] The upper vertebra pivots on the impacted inferior articular process, and the opposite inferior articular process swings backward and strains its joint capsule.[5] L1–2 and L5–S1 have relatively greater range of extension (Table 5–1).[5] A greater amount of flexion/extension movement is possible at a joint if the disc is thick. This allows more movement to occur before the boney elements come in contact with each other and prevent further rotation. The degree of asymmetry between the anterior and posterior thickness of a disc will alter most patterns.[14]

Axial Compression

The movement occurring in the lumbar spinal segments while the person is in the upright position is axial compression. The intervertebral joints are designed as the principal weight-bearing components of the lumbar spine.[5] Interesting to note, during axial compression, the cartilaginous end plates are the first component of the spinal motion segment to show distortion by becoming convex under vertical compression.[8] The zygapophyseal joints are also reported to have some contribution in weight bearing.[12] Reported values for the amount of applied load the facet joints bear range from 40%,[31] to 28%, to "not very much."[39]

With axial compression of an intervertebral joint, the articular surfaces of the zygapophyseal joint slide past one another due to their parallel articular surfaces.[5] Obviously, with sustained axial compression, the disc may be narrowed, and the tips of the inferior articular processes of the facet joints (not the joint surfaces) may impact against the lamina of the vertebra below.[5] This has been reported to vary from 3% to 18% of the weight bearing in healthy joints[60] and 70% in pathologic discs,[1] with the highest estimates in the extended position.[29, 31, 35]

Axial loading of a lordotic spine also stretches or "energizes" the anterior longitudinal ligament, a ligament with reportedly little elasticity.[45] The tensile mechanism of this ligament under load imparts a "return to neutral" resilience once the load is removed.[1]

Axial Distraction

Although studies have reported relative separation of intervertebral joints with sustained axial distraction, the actual amount of movement appears to be negligible.[56]

Axial Rotation

Axial rotation produces torsion of the intervertebral discs and opposition of the zygapophyseal joints. Spinal rotation stretches the fibers of the annulus fibrosus that are angled toward the direction of rotation.[7, 15, 22] Likewise, the fibers angled opposite the direction of rotation are laxed.

The vertical axis of rotation of a lumbar vertebra passes through the posterior part of the vertebral body.[10] The posterior elements of a vertebra swing around this axis during rotation.[5] The center of rotation, however, changes not only with the direction of rotation but also with the degree of asymmetry and degeneration of the intervertebral joint.[14]

The contribution of weight bearing during axial rotation occurs principally from the facet joint and, to a lesser extent, from the intervertebral disc.[5] Since rotation about an axis results in more stress on the peripheral structures, lumbar rotation places a selective stress on the peripheral fibers of the annulus.[19]

Lateral Flexion

Lateral flexion, or side bending, involves a complex coupling of lateral bending and rotatory movements of the interbody disc and facet joints.[5] This combined motion pattern has been demonstrated by biplanar radiography of the lumbar spine.[46] In the erect position, lateral flexion causes vertebral bodies to rotate contralaterally.[19, 26] (Rotation in this sense refers to the direction of movement of the cephalic vertebral body on the more caudal vertebral body.)

FUNCTIONAL ASSESSMENT OF LUMBAR RANGE OF MOTION

Visual observation alone cannot be considered adequate in the evaluation of movement of the lumbar spine. However, a thorough clinical assessment that focuses on functional mobility is encouraged as a starting point for further assessment.

With all movements, the range, synergy, and quality of active movement is evaluated. The examiner should observe the body contours and bony prominences (including the spinous processes) for any localized restriction of movement, protective guarding, or painful arc of motion. As a general rule, facet joint restrictions are more noticeable in side bending; muscle tightness is proportionately more noticeable in forward bending.[21] The following assessments are all performed with the patient standing and were compiled from Grimsby, Svenson and Kelsey, and Paris.[19, 45, 52]

I. *Flexion.*—Viewed from the side and then behind the subject. Notice the characteristics of the motion.
   A. Smoothness vs. "hitches."
   B. Segmental contribution (including interplay of the cervical and thoracic spine and the pelvis).
   C. Lumbar lordosis reversal, nonreversal.
   D. "Listing" or swinging to one side.
   E. Disappearance of any scoliosis.
   Note: Quality of motion must be assessed in reference to quantity. For example, a subject with an extremely flexible hip girdle could overcompensate for a more rigid spine.

II. *Backward bending.*—Notice the characteristics of movements.
   A. Smoothness vs. hitches.
   B. Segmental contribution of other vertebral segments.
   C. L5–S1 extension can be affected more specifically with the subject being asked to actively push the buttocks posteriorly.

III. Side bending.—Note the characteristics of movements.
   A. Smoothness of the resultant "C" curve of the vertebral column (concavity toward the side one is bending). Any visual flattening or sharp angles to this "C" curve are noted.
   B. Some qualitative notations:
      1. With the feet placed approximately 6 in. apart the mid and upper lumbar movements are affected.
      2. With the feet more widely spread, the lower lumbar level is affected.
      3. Cranial-caudal direction of side bending is the usual test procedure in standing. To affect caudal-cranial movement, the subject can be positioned on a step stool with the lower extremity (of the side being tested) unsupported. The subject is then asked to "hip-hike" to effect caudal-cranial side bending.

IV. *Rotation*.—Notice the characteristics of the motion.
   A. Smoothness.
   B. Contribution of neighboring levels.
   C. A contralateral side bending (coupling) of the lumbar spine is the expected movement in the erect position. Note any flatness or sharp angles to this contralateral bending.

MEASURING METHODS

A measurement technique should meet three criteria:

1. The measurement procedure should be well defined (for example, clearly describe the position in which the patient is to be evaluated, i.e., standing, sitting, barefoot, lying supine; the verbal instructions used to direct the patient during testing; the length of time the patient is to maintain the desired position; the exact instruments used; the method of recording results; etc).

2. The measurement results should be reproducible. The evaluator should get the same results when testing the same subject repeatedly. Also, different evaluators should get the same results when testing the same subject by the defined evaluation protocol.

3. The measurements should be accurate—actually measure what the evaluator is trying to evaluate.[44] There is little information available that examines intratester and intertester reliability of range-of-motion measurements in patients with back pain[28] and in healthy subjects.[38] Also, further investigations addressing the reproducibility of some measurements are impossible since the testing procedure is not adequately discussed. The reported repeatabilities for specific assessment methods will be discussed later. Often accuracy is difficult to determine because there is no absolute method to exactly measure the property being evaluated. Generally, accuracy is determined by comparing a technique with a method that is well established or commonly used or by comparing it with an invasive procedure performed on a small group of subjects. In an attempt to assess accuracy, some measuring techniques have been compared with measurements of the lumbar spine obtained through radiographs; however, most have examined healthy subjects.[16, 30, 33, 41, 48, 54] It is important to note that repeatability should not be confused with accuracy. An evaluator may obtain the same result repeatedly; however, each time he may not be measuring the appropriate thing.

For measurements methods to be useful in a clinical setting, not only should they meet the criteria discussed above, but it is also desirable to have a normative data base with which to compare the measures obtained. This information provides a reference point to give the measurements more meaning. For example, just knowing a patient's range of motion in a given number of degrees is not as valuable as knowing whether this is nearly normal or greatly reduced as compared with a normal value. To compare patient data with asymptomatic population data (normative data), several factors must be considered. Not only should the normative value be known, but the associated standard deviation should also be known so that it can be determined whether a patient's range of motion is within a normal range.[49] Also, the patient's data should be compared with data collected from a comparable group based on age, sex, or other demographic characteristics that may affect the values obtained. For example, the biplanar x-ray study by Pearcy and Tibrewal provided normative range-of-motion data by using a group of 11 normal males 25 to 36 years of age.[47] It is doubtful whether this is an appropriate baseline with which to compare all patients.

Another issue that arises in the evaluation of patients is the relevance of the measure to clinical symptoms and an individual's overall condition. It is not possible to state with certainty whether any of the so-called normal values are applicable to a given patient, especially in the presence of pain. Even the American Medical Association (AMA) suggests that measurement of the lumbar spine is invalid for impairment inference if the subject is in acute pain.[13]

Sagittal Flexion/Extension

Observer error is particularly common in an examination of the spine, including measurement of trunk flexion.[42, 59] Numerous techniques have been developed to pursue objectivity; these include fingertip-to-floor distance, sit and reach, skin distraction test, standard goniometers, inclinometers, kyphometers, and computerized equipment. Subjective reports achieved through questionnaires make an effort to assess flexibility.[4] Lumbar motion testing has also taken a route of measurement through passive segmental palpation[18] and in vitro means.[54] The most recent method can evaluate coupling movements and involves two- and three-dimensional radiologic analysis.[51, 53] While the following does not include every testing device or method made available, the author has attempted to provide an overview of various methods.

Fingertip-to-Floor Distance

This evaluation is performed with the patient standing barefoot with his feet approximately shoulders' width apart. The patient bends as far forward as possible while keeping the knees straight. With the patient in the bent posture and the arms perpendicular to the floor, the distance from his middle finger to the floor is measured with a tape measure. The reported intratester and intertester variations for the fingertip-to-floor method are 76.4% and 83.0% respectively.[38]

Schober Flexion

With the patient standing in a neutral position, the top of the sacrum is marked. A mark is also made 10 cm above this one. With the patient in full flexion, the therapist measures the distance from the first mark on the sacrum to the upper mark. This provides a measure of flexion.

Schober's frequently referenced article included no data on consistency of results with repeated testing.[50] This technique was later changed to what is termed the "modified Schober" in which an addition mark was made 5 cm below a line connecting the dimples of Venus. The measurements were then made from this lower mark to the one made 10 cm above the line. The modified Schober's test for trunk flexion reported by Moll and Wright reported a standard deviation of 1.3 cm (differing from the original test of 3.3 cm).[41] Variation for the modified Schober test was reported to be 4.8%.[3] Macrae and Wright reported that the modified Schober method was closely correlated (.97) with flexion measurements made from bending radiographs.[33]

Kyphometer

This device is a protractor with a degree scale attached to two movable arms. The end of one arm is placed on the spinous process of L1 and the other arm at S1. The therapist takes an initial reading with the patient in the neutral position. The patient bends as far forward as possible, and the therapist takes another reading. The value of the first reading is subtracted from the initial value to obtain a measurement of the patient's flexion. This is a simple test to perform and is less cumbersome than evaluations using two inclinometers. It does require the therapist to be very familiar with the anatomy of the lumbar region for accurate placement of the device. Ohlen et al. reported the results of a study evaluating the Debrunner kyphometer (Protek AG, Bern, Switzerland).[43] They found the intraobserver coefficient of variation of lumbar flexion measurements to be 5.4% and that for extension to be 18%.

Inclinometer

Two inclinometers are frequently used for measuring lumbar spine range of motion. With the patient standing in the neutral position, one inclinometer is placed at the T12 spinous process and the other over the sacrum. The patient bends as far forward as possible, and readings are recorded from the two inclinometers. The sacral inclinometer value is subtracted from that of the one at T12. This removes the hip motion from the total motion, thus yielding the flexion of the lumbar spine. Lumbar extension is measured in a similar fashion. The inclinometers are placed at T12 and the sacrum with the patient in the neutral position. The patient is asked to extend as far as possible. The readings from both inclinometers are recorded, and the value from the sacral inclinometer is subtracted from the T12 inclinometer value to remove the motion attributed to hip movement. The remaining value is the patient's lumbar extension.

Mellin studied the Myrin inclinometer (OB Vinkelmatare Myrin, Lic Rehab, Solna, Sweden) commonly used in Scandinavia.[37] The average lumbar flexion measured on a group of 25 volunteers without back pain was 55 degrees, and lumbar extension was 19 degrees. He also reported that the intratester and intertester repeatability was .86 and .97, respectively, for lumbar flexion and .93 and .89, respectively, for lumbar extension.

An electronic inclinometer, the EDI 320 (Lumex Corp., Ronkonkoma, NY) has been developed to measure range of motion. This portable device automatically calculates the difference between readings taken in the neutral and the flexed or extended positions.

The inclinometer method, first described by Loebl[30] was later expanded and researched by Mayer and associates.[36] The inclinometer's reliability for testing lumbar flexion and extension remains in the forefront of clinically available measurement devices, a reflection of its related intratester and intertester reliability,[28] and has the AMA endorsement. Mayer reported that the overall results produced by the noninvasive inclinometer technique for lumbar flexion/extension were not significantly different from those obtained from the biplanar radiographic technique.[36]

The American Academy of Orthopaedic Surgeons (AAOS) has supported the use of a tape measure over the lumbar spine to measure forward flexion.[2] Recently, the AMA revised its guidelines and now recommends the use of the spinal inclinometer in measurements relating to functional impairment.[13] The AMA further states that a report utilizing the spinal inclinometer will take precedence over a report given by an alternate measuring technique. The AAOS and AMA fail to give validity and reliability references for their methods of spinal measurement[13]; however, these measurements have a great impact on the determination of impairment ratings.

Lateral Flexion

Inclinometer

With two inclinometers, lateral spinal flexion is measured in much the same manner as sagittal flexion. With the patient standing, one inclinometer is placed over the T12 spinous process and the other over the sacrum. The patient is asked to bend as far to the right as possible. Readings from the inclinometers are recorded while the patient is in this position. To obtain the patient's degree of lateral right flexion for the lumbar spine, the reading from the sacral inclinometer is subtracted from that of the T12 inclinometer. As with the sagittal measures, this is done to subtract flexion due to movement at the sacrum. The patient is asked to return to the neutral position and then to bend as far to the left as possible.

The data calculated from the Moll and associates' intertester reproducibility study by Merritt et al. was reported to have a coefficient of variance for right and left lateral flexion of 43% and 44%, respectively.[38] Mellin describes an alternative to the use of the Myrin inclinometer (commonly used in Scandinavia) for lateral bending. The shape of the base of the inclinometer, Mellin stated, was not appropriate for use on spinal sagittal curves.[37] After attaching the Myrin inclinometer to a plastic plate, Mellin reported intratester reproducibility of only .57 and .58 but intertester reproducibility of .86 and .91. This was consistent with reports from Kapandji[26] and radiographic studies by Pearcy and Tibrewal.[47]

Goniometer

The base of the goniometer is placed over the sacrum. The arm of the goniometer is positioned along the spine, perpendicular to the base, and a skin mark is placed at T12. The patient is asked to bend as far to the right side as possible. The upper part of the arm should be moved to remain over the T12 skin mark. The degree of movement of the upper part of the arm is recorded as the patient's right lateral flexion. Note that with this method there is no need to subtract movements since the base of the goniometer moves with the sacral motion. The base of the goniometer serves as a pivot point of the motion. To measure left lateral side bending, the process is repeated with the patient bending to the left.

Rotation

A rotometer was developed to measure left and right rotation of the spine with the subject in the seated position. This device is composed of a large protractor strapped to the patient's hips, and a belt is strapped to the patient at T1. The belt has a pointer attached that reaches to the protractor. At the beginning of the evaluation, the pointer is aligned with the "0" on the protractor. The patient is then asked to rotate to the right as far as possible. The therapist then records the number of degrees the pointer has displaced on the protractor as the patient's right rotation. The process is repeated with the patient rotating to the left. This is a somewhat cumbersome process, and the results may be influenced by rotation of the rib cage.[57]

Intertrial and interoperator reliability testing of the lumbar rotometer identified a maximum variation of 5 degrees in a range of 56 degrees, measurements that correlate well with cadaveric motion.[54]

Passive Mobility

Few studies have been published that deal with the reliability in evaluating passive mobility of the lumbar spine.[17, 20, 25, 34] However, clinicians trained in the techniques of specific mobility testing of the spine and who use them frequently are convinced of their reliability and validity.[18, 19, 25, 34, 45, 58]

There are several potential sources of inaccuracies of lumbar motion testing. The patient may be technically difficult to assess, subjects may fluctuate in their responses regardless of their cooperation and the skill of the examiner, or the motion (as in the spine) may be more difficult to measure even though both the instrument and examiner have been shown to be reliable.[6, 20]

Methods of Notation

Notation and recording spinal range of motion guide the ways in which the clinician reports logical and concise results to other disciplines.

When goniometers and inclinometers are used, the 0- to 180-degree system is recommended by the AAOS.[2] In the 0- to 180-degree system, the starting position for all movements is considered to be 0 degrees, and movements proceed toward 180 degrees. However, the starting position for some spinal patients is not exactly neutral (i.e., sometimes the patient is bent forward or listing).

Interestingly, the AMA writes in the *Guide to Evaluation of Permanent Impairment:* "Since a goniometer cannot be used to measure thoracolumbar rotation, reproducibility that satisfies validity criteria is impossible. Therefore, rotation is not measured."

Factors Affecting Movement

It is interesting to note that spinal range-of-motion findings are used as a partial basis for decisions regarding disability and compensation.[13] From a clinical point of view, for spinal flexibility to be meaningful there must be normative information. Consideration must be given to individual factors that affect spinal range of motion such as age, gender, obesity, and the ratio of standing height to sitting height.[41, 53]

Several studies have agreed that a general decrease in spinal range of motion occurs with aging.[3, 40, 53, 55] Conflicting reports exist regarding the importance of such factors in relation to flexibility. Troup et al. first intimated this difference when he found that lumbar range of motion changed significantly in males but not in females.[55]

SPINAL RANGE OF MOTION AND PAIN RELIEF

Little evidence exists to support the use of exercises to maintain or increase spinal range of motion as a protective measure, despite their popularity. Biering-Sorensen examined spinal flexibility in a large population and followed them for 1 year.[3] Males with greater flexibility experienced an episode of low back pain. Howell studied elite women rowers and found that the incidence of low back pain was greater in those who stretched their back regularly.[23] Kapp et al. performed a retrospective study on 67 patients with herniated nucleus pulposus.[27] Patients who regained lumbar extension reported relief of back pain. Some researchers are reporting that a general decrease in spinal mobility is associated with back problems,[3, 36] while others are reporting the opposite.[24] Still others report that a history of incapacitating back pain had no effect on spinal range of motion.[53]

Limited inferences can apparently be made from spinal measurement. However, limitation in the arc of motion does not identify the cause of dysfunction. Certain implications can be made about patient motion by comparing results from active and passive range-of-motion evaluations.[11] Active range of motion can reveal information concerning the capability of the neuromuscular complex to produce movement about a joint. Functional deficits in the neuromuscular pattern can include weakness or inappropriate activity of the antagonist. Active range of motion is the first step. Passive range of motion can yield information concerning joint and soft-tissue structures and their ability to allow motion.[11] Testing for "end feel" (the specific sensation transmitted to the examiner's hands at the end points of the movement) can also help determine what structures may be restricting motion.[19, 45]

Patient treatment is not based on any single piece of information but rather on information gained from all parts of the evaluation. Clinicians should avoid trying to base decisions on information simply because it is numerical without giving great thought as to the validity of the data. A differentiation between impression and measurement lays the groundwork for the development of scientific practice.[49]

OTHER CLINICAL CONSIDERATIONS

Frequently when patients are treated in an orthopedic setting, evaluations are based on comparing the performance of the injured limb with that of the other. This addresses performance variations attributable to age, sex, life-style, job demands, overall fitness level, and other individual factors. However, in the spine there is no opposite side with which results can be compared. This forces a much greater reliance on comparison to asymptomatic populations, which generally does not adequately address variation for individual factors.

Because there are difficulties with the use of traditional normal values and the use of the "contralateral spine" in spinal assessment, clinicians are challenged with setting alternative goals for the patient. These goals may be stated in functional terms. The clinician can identify functional activities deficient in the patient due to spinal dysfunction and predict basically the quantity of motion needed by the patient to gain function. In this way, goals are applicable and meaningful to the patient.

The use of functional activities to derive goals for joint motion allows the goals of treatment to be customized to the individual's performance and activity needs. Second, the use of functional standards permit more meaningful inference of range-of-motion measurements in the areas of evaluation and treatment. For example, 50 degrees of lumbar spinal motion might be determined to be required for a patient to lift a 30-lb child from the floor. But to perform this activity normally, the patient must also have adequate muscle power and the ability to avoid compensatory trunk movements. Such movements become habitual in patients with spinal joint restrictions. By focusing on functional goals, all three elements, motion, power, and posture, can be better considered by the clinician. The functional approach to treatment allows a better focus on strategies important to the patient and the existing problem rather than achievement of an arbitrary amount of movement.

The debate continues as to what spinal measurements should be performed and how they should be interpreted. It is evident, however, that without a scientific basis for the measurement and a well-described protocol for its performance, there can be no quality communication concerning the measurement.

REFERENCES

1. Adams MA, Hutton WC: The mechanical function of the lumbar apophyseal joints. *Spine* 1983; 8:327–330.
2. American Academy of Orthopaedic Surgeons: *Joint Motion Method of Measuring and Recording*. Chicago, American Academy of Orthopaedic Surgeons, 1965.
3. Biering-Sorensen F: Physical measurements as risk indicators for low-back trouble over a one-year period. *Spine* 1984; 9:106–119.
4. Bird HA, Eastmond CJ, Hudson A, et al: Is generalized joint laxity a factor in spondylolisthesis? *Scand J Rheumatol* 1980; 9:203–205.
5. Bogduk N, Twomey LT: *Clinical Anatomy of the Lumbar Spine*. New York, Churchill Livingstone, 1987, pp 58–71.
6. Boone DC, Azen SP, Lin CM, et al: Reliability of goniometric measurements. *Phys Ther* 1978; 58:1355–1360.
7. Broberg KB: On the mechanical behaviour of intervertebral discs. *Spine* 1983; 8:151–165.
8. Brown T, Hansen RJ, Yorra AJ: Some mechanical tests on the lumbosacral spine with particular reference to the intervertebral discs. *J Bone Joint Surg [Am]* 1957; 39:1135–1164.

9. Cailliet R: *Low Back Pain Syndrome,* ed 3. Philadelphia, FA Davis, 1980.
10. Cossette JW, Farfan HF, Robertson GH, et al: The instantaneous center of rotation of the third lumbar intervertebral joint. *J Biomech* 1971; 4:149–153.
11. Cyriax T: *Textbook of Orthopaedic Medicine. Soft Tissue Diagnosis.* New York, Casell, 1980.
12. Cyron BM, Hutton WC: Variations in the amount and distribution of cortical bone across the par interarticulares of L5. A predisposing factor in spondylolysis? *Spine* 1979; 4:163–167.
13. Engelberg A: *Guide to the Evaluation of Permanent Impairment.* Chicago, American Medical Association, 1988.
14. Farfan HF: *Mechanical Disorders of the Low Back.* Philadelphia, Lea & Febiger, 1983.
15. Farfan HF, Gracovetsky S: The nature of instability. *Spine* 1984; 9:714–719.
16. Fitzgerald GK, Wynveen KJ, Rheault W, et al: Objective assessment with establishment of normal values for lumbar spinal range of motion. *Phys Ther* 1983; 63:1776–1781.
17. Gonnella C, Paris SV, Kutner M: Reliability in evaluating passive intervertebral motion. *Phys Ther* 1982; 62:436–444.
18. Grieve GP: *Common Vertebral Joint Problems.* New York, Churchill Livingstone, 1987.
19. Grimsby O: Course notes. *Lumbar Spine.* 1990.
20. Hellebrandt FA, Duvall EN, Moore ML: The measurement of joint motion. Part II. Reliability of goniometry. *Phys Ther Rev* 1949; 29:302–307.
21. Hertling D, Kessler R: *Management of Common Musculoskeletal Disorders,* ed 2. Philadelphia, JB Lippincott, 1990.
22. Hickey DS, Hukins DWL: Relation between the structure of the annulus fibrosus and the function and failure of the intervertebral disc. *Spine* 1980; 5:106–116.
23. Howell DW: Musculoskeletal profile and incidence of musculoskeletal injuries in lightweight women rowers. *Am J Sports Med* 1984; 12:278–282.
24. Howes RG, Isdale IC: The loose back: An unrecognized syndrome. *Rheumatol Phys Med* 1972; 11:72–77.
25. Kaltenborn F, Lindahl O: Reproducibility of the results of manual mobility testing of specific intervertebral segments. *Swed Med J* 1969; 66:962–965.
26. Kapandji IA: *The Physiology of the Joints,* ed 2, vol 3. *Trunk and Vertebral Column.* London, Churchill Livingstone, 1974.
27. Kapp JR, Alexander AH, Turocy RH, et al: The use of lumbar extension in the education and treatment of patients with acute herniated nucleus pulposus. *Clin Orthop* 1986; 202:211–218.
28. Keeley J, Mayer TG, Cox R, et al: Quantification of lumbar function. Part 5: Reliability of range of motion measures in the sagittal plane and an in vitro torso rotation measurement technique. *Spine* 1986; 11:31–35.
29. Lin HS, Liu YK, Adams KH: Mechanical response of the lumbar intervertebral joint under physiological (complex) loading. *J Bone Joint Surg [Am]* 1978; 60:41–54.
30. Loebl WY: Measurement of spinal posture and range of spinal movement. *Ann Phys Med* 1967; 9:103–110.
31. Lorenz M, Patwardhan WC: Loadbearing characteristics of lumbar facets in normal and surgically altered spinal segments. *Spine* 1983; 8:122–130.
32. Lumsden RM, Morris JM: An in-vitro study of axial rotation and immobilization at the lumbosacral joint. *J Bone Joint Surg [Am]* 1986; 50:1591–1602.
33. Macrae IF, Wright V: Measurement of back movement. *Ann Rheum Dis* 1969; 28:584–589.
34. Maitland GD: *Vertebral Manipulation,* ed 4. London, Butterworth, 1977.
35. Markolf KL: Deformation of the thoracolumbar intervertebral joints in response to external loads. *J Bone Joint Surg [Am]* 1972; 54:511–533.
36. Mayer TG, Tencer AF, Kristoferson S, et al: Use of noninvasive techniques for quantification of spinal range of motion in normal subjects and chronic low back dysfunction patients. *Spine* 1984; 9:588–595.
37. Mellin G: Measurement of thoracolumbar posture and mobility with a Myrin inclinometer. *Spine* 1986; 11:759–762.
38. Merritt J, McLean T, Erickson R: Measurement of trunk flexibility in normal subjects: Reproducibility of three clinical methods. *Mayo Clin Proc* 1986; 61:192–197.
39. Miller JA, Haderspeck KA, Schultz AB: Posterior element loads in lumbar motion segments. *Spine* 1983; 8:331–337.
40. Moll JMH, Liyanage SP, Wright V: An objective clinical method to measure spinal extension. *Rheumatol Phys Med* 1972; 11:293–312.
41. Moll JMH, Wright V: Normal range of spinal mobility. *Ann Rheum Dis* 1971; 30:381–386.
42. Nelson MA, Allen P, Clamp SE, et al: Reliability and reproducibility of clinical findings in low back pain. *Spine* 1979; 4:97–101.
43. Ohlen C, Spangfort E, Tingvall C: Measurement of spinal sagittal configuration and mobility with Debrunner's kyphometer. *Spine* 1989; 14:580–583.
44. Oster C, Hanten W, Llorens L: *Introduction to Research.* Philadelphia, JB Lippincott, 1987, pp 32–55.
45. Paris S: Course notes. *The Spine, Etiology and Treatment of Dysfunction Including Joint Manipulation.* 1987.
46. Pearcy M, Portek I, Shepherd J: Three-dimensional x-ray analysis of normal movement in the lumbar spine. *Spine* 1984; 9:294–297.
47. Pearcy MJ, Tibrewal SB: Axial rotation and lateral bending in the normal lumbar spine measured by three-dimensional radiography. *Spine* 1984; 9:582–587.
48. Portek I, Pearcy MJ, Reader GP, et al: Correlation between radiographic and clinical measurement of lumbar spine movement. *Br J Rheumatol* 1983; 22:197–205.
49. Rothstein J (ed): *Measurement and Clinical Practice: Theory and Application. Measurements in Physical Therapy.* New York, Churchill Livingstone, 1985.
50. Schober P: Lendenwirbelsaule und Krezschmerzen. *Munch Med Wochenschr* 1937; 84:336–338.
51. Stokes IA, Wilder DG, Frymoyer JW, et al: Assessment of patients with low back pain and biplanar radiographic measurement of intervertebral motion. *Spine* 1981; 6:233–238.

52. Svenson B, Kelsey D: Course notes. *Medical Exercise Training*. Dallas, 1988.
53. Tanz SS: Motion of the lumbar spine: A roentgenologic study. *AJR* 1953; 69:399–412.
54. Taylor JR, Twomey LT: Sagittal and horizontal plane movement of the human lumbar vertebral column in cadavers and in the living. *Rheumatol Rehabil* 1980; 19:223–231.
55. Troup JDG, Hood CA, Chapman AE: Measurements of the sagittal mobility of the lumbar spine and hips. *Ann Phys Med* 1968; 9:308–321.
56. Twomey L: Sustained lumbar traction. An experimental study of long spine segments. *Spine* 1985; 10:146–149.
57. Twomey LT, Taylor JR: Sagittal movements of the human lumbar vertebral column: A quantitative study of the role of the posterior vertebral elements. *Arch Phys Med Rehabil* 1983; 64:322–325.
58. White AA, Panjabi MM: *Biomechanics of the Spine*. Philadelphia, JB Lippincott, 1984, p 84.
59. Wolf SL, Basmajian JV, Russe CTC, et al: Normative data on low back mobility and activity levels. *Am J Phys Med* 1979; 58:217–229.
60. Yang KH, King AI: Mechanism of facet load transmission as a hypothesis for low-back pain. *Spine* 1984; 9:557–565.

6

Evaluation by Functional Tests

Tom Lorren, P.T.

Function has been defined as "an action contributing to a larger action" and "the normal. . . contribution of a bodily part to the economy of the organism."[59] It has also been referred to as the "organism's ability to perform tasks involving homeostasis or manipulation of the environment."[38] In rehabilitation, the term "function" has been loosely used to delineate the movements and positions occurring as integral parts of daily life. This "function" is what we seek to restore to its normal state following injury by improving the resultant "dysfunction."

Despite the increasingly complex methods to evaluate patients with back problems, a detailed history and physical examination remain the basis for most diagnoses. The history and physical examination (with its reliance on the patient's self-report of pain) combined with information from imaging may elucidate some important components of the total patient assessment and treatment planning.

Relying on traditional methods of determining diagnosis and treatment identifies the need to objectively define nonspecific back pain in a clinically relevant way. Pain is the primary component of spinal dysfunction that prompts the patient to seek medical attention. However, in 88% of cases, specific anatomic pathology causing back pain cannot be identified.[60] This lack of a specific anatomic "pain generator" should not hinder the process of rehabilitation and the attendant evaluation of patient progress.

Due to the lack of visualization of the effects of treatment on structural components of the spine and the necessity to rely on the patient's report of pain to guide the treatment, focus tends to be on reducing symptoms. Pain often guides treatment selection and may be the determining factor in the patient's ability to return to a productive life-style. If clinicians rely on patient self-report, treatment will relate primarily to the pain sensitivity of the patient.[38] The majority of spinal pain occurrences are self-limiting,[46] and as Mayer and Gatchel have pointed out, "it is often not therapeutically productive to rely solely on self-reported pain as a means of determining the degree of severity of the problem or to gauge treatment progress."[38]

Pain may often be modulated through the use of passive modalities that provide relief on a temporary basis. This coupled with the body's own homeostasis will cause a general decrease in reported discomfort. Pain reduction as the only goal will often neglect the importance of activity and lead to the "deconditioning syndrome" or the loss of an individual's "physical functional capacity."[38] Deficits in physical functional capacity may play a substantial role in explaining a major part of the dysfunction and persistent pain in chronic back pain cases.[38] If function is not assessed and progress monitored, the patient may in fact be less able to tolerate activities essential to his life-style.

Activity-based programs are an essential part of rehabilitation. These programs combine pain-reducing modalities with increasing functional activity. Specific goals of improvement on quantitative physical function tests must be the objective guiding patient treatment. Objective measurements utilize quantitative data to show that function has been restored, even in the presence of pain.[40]

TYPES OF ASSESSMENTS

In the quest to overcome dysfunction and determine at what level an individual is capable of performing, there is a plethora of choices in the context of functional evaluation. Although there is a substantial behavioral component to function, the focus of this chapter is on physical functional tests. Some tests measure the performance of specific body parts (segments or muscles themselves or a specific group performance), while others measure the ability of a functional unit to work in concert with or to be substituted for other body functional units. All tests are somewhat related since the body functions as a whole. The advantage of isolated testing is that it allows a determination of an individual segment's ability to function. This isolation, for example, of lumbar range of motion from the rest of spinal range of motion, will focus the treatment on a specific dysfunctional area and allow its progress to be individually monitored in addition to its function in the spine as a whole.

Functional unit integration allows an evaluation of all units' performance in the completion of a task. An excellent example of this type of test is lifting. Failure to perform the task may stem from a breakdown in one or more individual segments. It may be that all individual components are functioning normally but not in concert. A combination of functional task integration tests with appropriate isolated segment testing can help determine dysfunction and guide treatment.

Physical functional tests primarily evaluate basic components related to daily activities. These components are range of motion of the spine and extremities, strength of specific muscle function units (such as hip extensors), endurance and fatigue of muscle function units, cardiovascular capacity, balance, and functional unit integration.

A key component in the assessment of function is the individual's effort. Functional assessment relies heavily on the subject's effort to produce a consistent maximal effort. This supposition greatly affects utilization of the data in a formalized treatment plan. The identification of inconsistent effort, through a process of testing and retesting, is considered an essential part of many functional assessments.

Inconsistent performance should not be considered a maximal effort, but neither should it be considered a concerted effort to lead the evaluation astray. These tests are not designed to identify malingerers. Deviations and apparent effort are rarely the result of conscious attempts by the patient to misrepresent true ability. The patient may at first produce submaximal effort due to factors such as unfamiliarity, inadequate instructions, fear of reinjury, pain, or anxiety. In tests requiring some skill to produce a desired result, "motor morons" may be unable to generate acceptable data if the necessary skill level is too great.

COMPONENTS TO ADDRESS

In evaluating functional performance, the search for relevant data must be preceded by identifying the reasons for the evaluation. This information will determine which function(s) are to be evaluated and the most appropriate test for doing so. Most commonly, the information sought is what the patient needs to do and what he can do. Functional assessments need to be broken into specific components to determine each component's ability to contribute to the whole. Within these assessment groups there are choices to be made regarding the complexity of the test, choice of movement, type of resistance, type of muscle contraction desired, plane of movement, method of restraint, segment to be tested, method of data acquisition, and most importantly, how to use the data to benefit the patient. When using mechanical or computerized testing equipment to guide a patient's treatment, the clinician relies on the accuracy of the machine and the ability to relate the information to functional ability. Any evaluation should meet the following criteria: safe, reliable, and reproducible; practical; predictive of ability; specific to the patient's needs; and ethical and legally defensible.[25]

Computers have become an integral part of daily life. It has reached the point that almost anything may be attached to a computer to generate "objective data." In the quest to perform evaluations at the state-of-the-art level, two obvious questions may be overlooked. Does the test need to be this complex and detailed? Are the data generated relevant?

There is no question that functional capacity testing provides objective information. However, frequently no one knows what it means or which information produced is the most relevant. For the most part, these tests do not always provide a complete overview of spinal function. For example, there is a 27% variability in dynamic strength unexplained when static strength measures are used.[13]

NORMATIVE/COMPARATIVE DATA BASES

In extremity testing, normative data comparisons invariably utilize the uninvolved extremity as the accepted "norm" for an individual. However, in the spine there is no comparable contralateral side. Therefore, for these tests to be useful, normative data bases need to be established.[41] To call these data bases "normal standards" is a misnomer. Individuals have wide ranges of "normal" due to anatomy, morphology, muscle fiber type, etc. The only true "normal" for the person being tested is himself. A better definition for these data bases would be comparative data. These data bases should not be used to determine normalcy but rather to set "standards of adequacy."[36] For a comparative data base to be useful, it must be standardized by age and sex. In addition, it must be activity specific. Without the differentiation at this minimal level, the data base may be too general to provide meaningful information. In this chapter, the author provides an overview of some of the evaluation devices available.

RANGE OF MOTION

Range of motion is one of the most easily obtained measures of function. In the American Medical Association (AMA) guidelines, it is the basis for determining a large portion of musculoskeletal impairment.[3] Originally, spinal range of motion was measured with a single-axis goniometer. Although useful for the extremities, this method assumed that the spine is a single unchanging fixed segment rotating about a single axis. Simple goniometric measurements look at areas, not segments. Hip and spinal motion could not be differentiated. Loebl described a method allowing the measurement of both the sacral (hip) and lumbar spine components separately during the same movement.[34] This was done by using an inclinometer (a measurement device utilizing a pendulum or other gravity-influenced indicator) to measure the degrees of motion in a plane perpendicular to the ground. This method required two inclinometers. The upper unit measured the gross motion, while the lower unit measured only the segment's movement on or below it. By subtracting the measurement of the lower unit from the upper one, the "true" lumbar range of motion was obtained. Due to some of the current technology's dependence on gravity for orientation, dual-angle inclinometry is generally sensitive to position. The tested individual must assume specific positions for the test to be performed correctly. In cases of severe impairment, this may pose some problems. Range of motion is the only standardized physiologic test available for the spine.[38]

Effort Validity

A proposed method of validating effort of lumbar flexion/extension range of motion is to do a supine straight leg raise (SLR). The theory is that the hamstrings are the primary limiter of anterior pelvic rotation.[40] It has been suggested that if true effort has been produced, the maximum SLR will be very close to the range of motion measured by the sacral component in the flexion/extension test. This proposition may have validity in individuals with range-of-motion limitations caused by nerve root tension. However, even compliant patients with back pain have difficulty in meeting this criteria. The primary problem appears to be that the two tests are performed in different positions. SLR is measured in a supine, "unloaded" position, while the sagittal mobility portion is rendered in a standing position. Patients with tissue intolerances to loading are loading their spine in the upright position. This loading combined with an anterior center of gravity shift causes increased symptoms with subsequent substantial limitation in the range of motion.

Equipment

Equipment to measure range of motion runs the gamut from the very simple to the very complex. The dual-inclinometer technique may be used with a simple bubble goniometer such as the MIE (Medical Research Limited, Leeds, UK). This technique requires the use of two inclinometers and subtracting the readings to derive the true motion. The Ortho Ranger (M.I. Technologies) is a small portable unit with a claimed error of 1%. It features finger-touch controls to "zero" the unit for baseline reference and "freeze," an end-range measurement to provide a greater degree of accuracy. While this unit allows the dual-inclinometer technique to be used by taking single measurements at the prescribed references, the operator must still subtract the numbers to arrive at a true segment motion.

The EDI 320 by Cybex (Lumex Corp., Ronkonkoma, NY) is also a small portable measurement device. This unit measures passive and active range of motion and also has "zero" and "freeze" functions. The key feature of this device is its ability to measure compound movements and automatically calculate the difference. This feature allows the user to do a two-inclinometer technique with a single device.

The Metrocom skeletal analysis system (Faro Medical Technologies, Lake Mary, Fla) is a three-dimensional digitizer capable of quickly measuring the entire human skeletal system. Originally developed as a scoliosis screening tool, the purpose was to be able to document changes in curvature without the need for constant exposure to x-ray radiation. With an electromechanical linkage connected to a pencil-like hand-held probe, the Metrocom digitizes palpable bony landmarks in a baseline starting position. The patient is instructed to move to the end range, where the landmarks are quickly redigitized. Since measurements are referenced to a position in space relative to the Metrocom, care must be taken not to shift body position. The Metrocom is capable of measuring according to the AMA guidelines for determination of impairment ratings. It also has the ability to determine limb length and x-ray angles. Options include measurement of the center of gravity and weight shifts from a quadrilateral force plate and an isometric strength testing device.

STRENGTH

Strength is defined as the ability of a muscle or muscle group to exert force.[5] Since force exertion is an essential basic component of functional ability, when patient complaints include a movement problem, muscle strength is generally a part of the problem.[4] Assessment of muscular strength can be divided into two fundamental types: localized (or isolated) segment testing and whole-body testing. An example of localized segment testing is measuring trunk extensor strength by a dynamometer with the patient in a seated position. Stabilization of adjacent segments in these situations is considered critical. With these measurement devices, the individual roles of the muscles need not be dissected. The localized spine measurements deal with a functional musculoskeletal unit and not the individual muscles.[36] Whole-body strength testing uses all muscle groups to complete a defined task such as lifting. Total-body task performance is considered to be a much more functional test.[38] Within these two fundamental assessment groups, strength is evaluated in two basic modes, static (isometric) or dynamic. Static testing is a method in which the muscle or muscle groups are evaluated by force production without movement. Dynamic testing allows movement of the muscle while being assessed. Both modes have advantages and disadvantages for evaluating function.

Isometric strength is a measure of the muscle's ability to produce a contraction at a fixed length. It is the oldest form of muscle strength testing and the best established. It is currently the only type of strength testing with published injury prediction rates.[44] From a clinical standpoint, isometric testing may be used more comfortably on patients who experience increased discomfort with movement. Dynamic testing may further be broken down into isotonic and isokinetic protocols. Isotonic testing provides a dynamic measure with a fixed resistance and variable velocity. This is represented by the daily occurrence of moving objects from one point to another. While picking up a box, the weight is fixed, but the velocity can be changed. Isokinetic testing is a dynamic measurement of the body's ability to apply force at a constant rate of speed. It is essentially the opposite of isotonics with respect to resistance and velocity. This application of force throughout a range of motion will give a proportional resistance to the muscle group throughout the different joint angles and result in optimal dynamic loading.[7] Isokinetics are only found in daily activity for a very limited time during movement. It is primarily a product of the clinician's need for a measurement tool to reduce variables. It has been suggested that isokinetic testing is not clinically useful since there are no naturally occurring isokinetic movements. Isokinetic testing is useful when creating an environment in which many parameters are kept constant with the patient being the variable. This allows an individual to be compared to himself or a representative group performing the identical test under identical circumstances. The performance in this situation is then used to make a generalization about the tested individual in comparison to known functional capabilities of the normative group. There is no machine-generated testing that can accurately predict function other than by inference. Ideally, testing should be done in a completely functional manner. However, this may not be feasible due to the complexity of motions and the contributions of the many variables playing a role in the final result. Isolated movements allow the examiner to more clearly identify the area of dysfunction but not to determine the ability of the individual to perform tasks. Functional testing allows a determination of the ability to perform tests with a specific load but does not identify specific deficits.

Within the context of dynamic movement, there are two more important muscle movement patterns. Both isotonic and isokinetic movements may have concentric and eccentric components. Concentric movement is a shortening contraction of a muscle, while eccentric movement is a "lengthening" contraction. Since daily activity requires both lifting and lowering movements, the importance of both contractions are easily realized.

It would be easy to assume that eccentrics is essentially the opposite of concentrics. In reality, there are several distinct differences. Greater muscle force is produced with eccentric contractions than with concentric ones.[15] As the velocity of the movement increases, concentric force decreases while eccentric force increases.[31] For the same work load, metabolic cost for eccentric work is less than for concentric.[6] Eccentric exercise has a greater mechanical efficiency than concentric exercise does as measured by electromyography (EMG) per unit tension.[30, 32] Eccentric exercise produces an increased load on the elastic components of the muscle being exercised.[54] Most muscle strains and tears occur during the eccentric phase of contraction.[21] Whole-body functional movements utilize a high degree of eccentrics against gravity, and it is important that this component be addressed prior to a return to activity. Mayer and Gatchel feel that two critical points appear to be established: that trunk muscle strength is an important factor in functional capacity of the lumbar spine and that because of the lack of visual feedback, mechanical devices to measure trunk strength directly are essential.[38] Trunk muscle strength testing requires relatively expensive machines to quantitate dynamic ability. Valid and reproducible measures must be complemented by an effort factor and must involve the use of a comparative data base.

Symptom-Limited (Submaximal) Testing

Isokinetic testing provides a procedure with minimal variables allowing the individual to be the main variable evaluated. This allows a measurement of consistency in patient performance that is based solely on the individual's previous contractions. A submaximum test is a method of obtaining data from an individual in an isokinetic mode that demonstrates maximum output before the onset of symptoms prevents the individual from going further. Generally, isokinetic testing is considered to be a maximum effort test. However, we have had success with establishing the maximum pain-free response in symptomatic patients. The patient is requested to slowly flex and extend within a comfortable range. If this does not produce symptoms, the patient is requested to progressively push harder and harder on both flexion and extension while verbally expressing the absence or onset of symptoms. At the onset of symptoms, the patient is requested to immediately stop. The greatest values generated are then used to establish a baseline to measure progress.

Normative Data

Localized segment testing by virtue of its reduction of variables has produced comparative data that serve as a baseline. Some of these "norms" have been devised on specific equipment and may have limited use. Generally, they do have overall applicability.

Range of motion in the localized-segment testing devices is the least accurate of all parameters. This is due to the extreme difficulty in maintaining an approximate body axis in line with a precise dynamometer axis. Although it is relatively precise, trunk range of motion from a testing unit is less accurate than trunk motion measured by a single-axis goniometer. A dynamic measurement of range of motion does, however, provide with some certainty the range of motion in which a patient is willing to function at a significant rate of speed. Normative values for total trunk flexion/extension range of motion are approximately 85 to 100 degrees.[17]

The peak torque-to-body weight ratio is a method of comparing an individual with a representative group. At 60 degrees per second, male body weight-to-flexion values in a standing position were reported to be about 95% and extension-to-body weight values to be up to 124%.[17] In females these values are 67% to 70% in flexion and about 95% of body weight in extension. A wide range of isokinetic peak torque-to-body weight ratios may be found among many populations.[17] As measured by torque production, men are stronger than women. However, when normalized to body weight, they may be equally strong.[27, 49]

Another common parameter used is the flexion-to-extension ratio. This ratio compares the force generation of the trunk flexors with extensors. It is a general rule that in normal individuals, extension is stronger than flexion at slow speeds. With isometric testing, healthy subjects' extension strength was greater than their flexion strength.[50, 55] This is felt to be indicative of normal muscle balance and the relationship of the agonist to antagonist complex. Beimborn and Morrissey reported that the peak torque extension-to-flexion ratio ranges between 1.0 and 2.0, with 1.3 being the most common.[8] In individuals with back problems, it is a decreased extensor strength that brings the flexion and extension measures much closer together.

Work

Work is defined as a force through a range of motion and is truly a quality measure. It has been described by some as area under the torque curve.[16] Although this definition serves to give a rough idea of effect in using the work values, the actual calculation of work is based on the torque-position overlay curve. This is a torque-to-position graph that has no time value. However, the concept of work as a volume for repetition does have merit in that it accurately conveys that a dip in the torque curve correlates to a decrease in work per repetition. Normative values for this complex parameter are difficult to establish and have been developed only on a limited basis. Some studies have shown that the best single indicator for prediction of performance by an individual is the ratio of work per repetition to body weight.[17] Many instruments require the individual to be in a standing position during testing. Others test in a seated position. In assessing the test information, it is important to know the body position since it will affect the results. Langrana and Lee in comparing sitting and standing measures found that motion was reduced in the seated position and flexion strength was twice as great as in standing.[33] They also found that sitting extension strength increased by 20%.

Endurance (Fatigue)

Muscular endurance has been defined as the ability of muscles to perform repeated contractions against a load.[7] With isokinetics this is usually determined by having the desired muscle group perform a series of actions against the dynamometer resistance until a predetermined force decay level has been reached. This predetermined level is usually established as 50% of the initial peak torque value. When this is compared with a previously established repetition norm, the method has been shown to be fairly reliable.[9] In the protocols commonly used for isokinetic trunk testing, it has been found that females may have better endurance than males.[33] Parnianpour et al. noted that the spinal task groups (flexors, extensors, lateral benders, axial rotators, and stabilizers) have a large amount of functional overlap and feel that altered kinematics due to muscle fatigue that could lead to nonoptimal loading of the elements may predispose these elements to injury.[45] The overlap indicates a need for coordination by the central nervous system. This coordination could be compromised by the onset of fatigue. The term *fatigue* was used to denote not only a decrease in power but a decrease or loss of protective function as well. Using a B200 (Isotechnologies, Hillsborough, NC) subjects were asked to repeat the test cycle as accurately and quickly as possible with maximum effort. If the typical endurance protocol of time to torque decay would have been used as the criteria, the results would not have indicated fatigue. Torque did not decrease, but velocity and range of motion decreased substantially in the primary plane of motion. The reduction of range of motion in the primary plane was coupled with increased motion in other planes. The authors felt that this was due to a loss of muscular coordination due to fatigue and may explain many injuries in the workplace.

Effort Validity

The unspoken promise of machine strength testing is that through the use of curve consistency the evaluator can determine whether or not an individual is giving a valid effort. The supposition is that inconsistency demonstrated by variations in the torque curves is indicative of unwillingness to produce useful data. Unfortunately, this is often carried to the illogical conclusion that inconsistency is the same as malingering. As was previously stated, this is an erroneous conclusion with the possibility of multiple factors producing the lack of a desired result. Despite this common misuse, curve analysis along with examination of work and other parameters as well as multiple-bout comparisons can provide good indications as to whether or not the data being collected are valid. The reliance on a battery of test protocols instead of a single bout ensures the best possible determination of data value.

Another commonly stated belief is that the use of torque curves in isokinetic testing is promising in the substantiation of diagnostic information.[50] However, there have been no torque curve interpretations found to be associated with specific pathology.[47]

Equipment

The Lido Back Unit (Loredan, Davis, Calif) is a sagittal unit capable of isokinetic testing (Fig 6–1). The unique feature of this system is the upper chest carriage that allows the unit to accommodate the spine's changing axis during dynamic movement. Dual actuators coupled with internal "soft stops" as well as external range-of-motion limiters provide patient control. The Lido also allows multipositional testing from full seated to full standing. Software provides an analysis of torque, range of motion, work, fatigue index, consistency, comparisons to body weight, antagonist muscle groups, and time events. Graphics display curve overlays, point modes, as well as three-dimensional curve analysis. Optional software allows the establishment of comparative data bases with research capability.

The B200 is a multiplanar testing unit that measures torques and position changes occurring about multiple centers. The B200 is able to test isometrically or isotonically and measures torques about all three axes simultaneously or in an isolated single axis. The patient stands on a platform with the pelvis stabilized and the shoulder harness arrangement holding the upper part of the trunk. The axes are located posterior to the lumbar segment. The electronically monitored hydraulic system prevents motion until a preselected minimal torque is produced, after which the acceleration of velocity is controlled only by the degree that the torque produced exceeds the preset minimum. The B200 is the only strength testing device that documents this change of patient's velocity to a movement. The unit does not do isokinetic testing. Proponents of this system state that its assessment is closer to real-world requirements of free movement. With isodynamic testing, the number of variables is felt by some to make clear-cut assumptions difficult. Effort validity and comparative data are provided in software available for the system that examines "physiologic" and "nonphysiologic" parameters. An example of a nonphysiologic parameter would be an individual who produces a velocity with a low resistance but a greater velocity when the resistance is increased. As a research tool and clinical test unit, the B200 provides a unique method of examining dynamic movement.

Cybex (Lumex Corp., Ronkonkoma, NY) produces two separate back systems, one for sagittal testing and one for axial rotation. Both of these units utilize isometric and isokinetic modes of testing and require the patient to be stabilized in order to produce valid measurements. The sagittal unit constrains the pelvis and lower extremities in order to isolate the lumbar spine muscle functional unit.

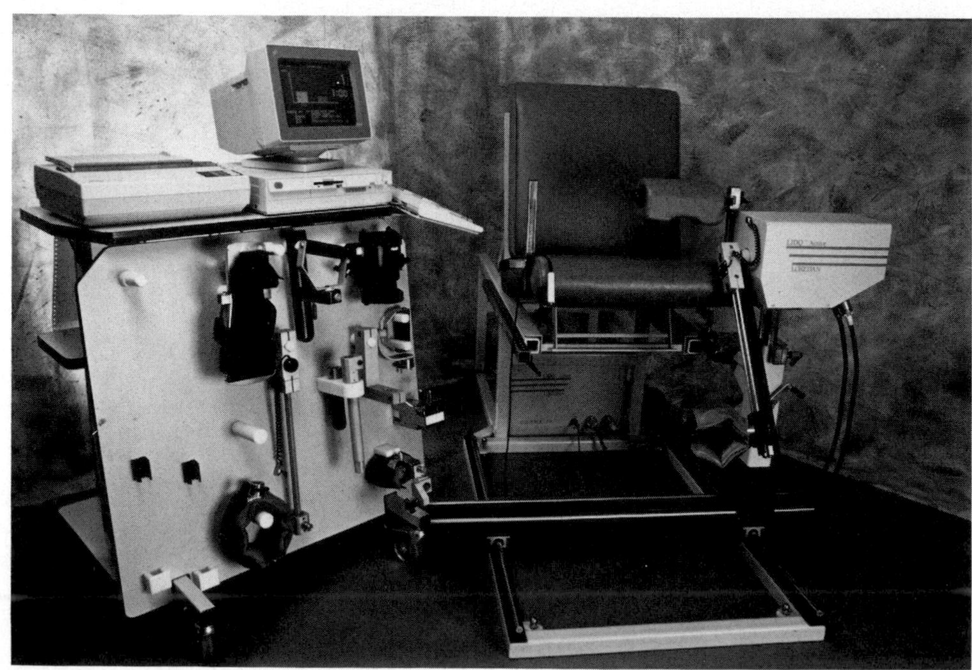

FIG 6–1.
The Lido back unit allows multipositional testing in the standing and seated positions.

Data are collected at any point in the range of motion at multiple speeds with gravity correction. The software calculates peak torque, acceleration time, work, power consumption, and curve variability. The torsional strength device measures the same parameters for the rotational movements. Test stabilization is provided by restraints as well as a seated position. Both units employ range-of-motion stops. Comparative data bases have been developed by the manufacturer.

Medx (Medx Corp., Gainesville, Fla) produces several systems for spinal testing and rehabilitation, including lumbar extension, torso rotation, cervical extension, and a lateral lumbar extension unit that allows the individual to test in both the vertical and horizontal positions. This lateral system is designed for use primarily in a research setting. The Medx systems allow static strength testing throughout the individual's available range of motion. They are characterized by complete stabilization to isolate the body segment being evaluated. Through use of a computerized program, the individual is tested at every 12 degrees throughout the range of motion.

Effort validity is determined by comparison to two static tests. Individuals providing a valid effort should be able to reproduce the curves and measures. Comparative data have been gathered on several groups.

Several manufacturers have introduced back attachments or attached units for the purpose of obtaining spinal test data from an existing multijoint testing unit. The testing is done in either the seated or standing positions for the back attachments and in the seated position only for the attached units. The attachment to these devices allows the introduction of eccentric modes into spine testing and allows the gravitational component to be eliminated through the use of a driven power system. Testing of extremely low levels of strength and motion is now possible. Since the development of these products is relatively new, comparative data have not yet been gathered.

Velocity

As the science of functional testing of the spine advances, it becomes apparent that a key component in the assessment of the trunk is the quantification of velocity. With spinal movement, there is force placed on the back as a result of trunk mass and acceleration. When the rate of movement of the spine is decreased, there is a reduction in trunk force. Changes in flexibility of the pathologic spine may be a resultant means to reduce the moment of force about the spine. In a study of normal persons and individuals with low back pain, the group with low back pain had a 50% reduction in flexion velocity when compared with normal individuals.[35] In hyperextension, the group with low back pain produced velocities that were less than 10% of the normal individuals.

The study of velocity and its effect on the spine is being advanced by several companies. The Lumbar Motion Monitor (LMM, Chattex, Hixson, Tenn) is a measurement system worn by the patient during task performance. Utilizing four potientiometers located in the lower unit, the computerized system looks at range of motion, acceleration/deceleration, and velocity. The LMM considers the lumbar region as a functional unit and does not differentiate individual segments. The compactness of the system and its freedom allows it to be utilized at the clinic or work site. Data analysis includes consistency of effort through curves and is backed by a comparative data base of 285 subjects. The system does measure true lumbar motion (as defined by dual inclinometry) and produces data that may be used in the evaluation of spinal impairment.

The CA-6000 Spine Motion Analyzer (Orthopedic Systems, Hayward, Calif) is a similar device with some distinct differences. The CA-6000 is smaller and lighter and has the capability of measuring the cervical spine. The three-dimensional system measures regionally through a cable attachment to a separate computerized system. Comparative data bases are being compiled, and the system is capable of rendering spinal ranges of motion that are useful for determining impairment ratings based on the AMA guidelines.

AEROBIC CAPACITY

The development of aerobic capacity is a must for the spine to function. Patients with chronic back pain have lower levels of aerobic capacity than do normal subjects.[48] Greater levels of cardiovascular fitness correlated well with decreased levels of self-reported pain and disability.

Aerobic capacity testing generally utilizes various devices such as treadmills and ergometers. The rested patient is exercised at a set initial work rate by utilizing a pulse monitor. Before beginning the test, a target heart rate is established at 80% to 85% of the estimated maximal heart rate. Individuals are screened to identify test contraindications such as a family history and elevated cholesterol levels. The test begins at a predetermined work rate and progresses through regular intervals until a predetermined heart rate is reached. At this point the result is expressed as the final work load, length of test, and the ratio of the final heart rate achieved to the target heart rate. Fatigue is defined as the patient's stopping due to fatigue before the target heart rate is reached. These tests are considered objective from the standpoint that heart rate is not considered to be under volitional control during exertion. In some cases, pain may cause an increased heart rate. Early extremity fatigue or an inadequate heart rate invalidates the test.

BALANCE

Sports rehabilitation specialists have long recognized the importance of retraining the body to regain the fine-tuned coordination with the central nervous system. In addition to motor control, this system is largely responsible for balance. The body maintains its balance through three essential components, all of which may be affected by a back injury. The first is sensory input, which is composed of visual, vestibulatory, and joint, muscle, and skin receptors. These help detect motions and the body's position in its environment. These deficits may be due to pathology or surgery. The second component, motor output, is the muscle response to the stimulus in maintaining the desired equilibrium. As has been mentioned previously, muscle strength is a key component to the restoration of function. The central nervous system is the final component of balance that selects and integrates the input to select the most appropriate musculoskeletal response.[43]

The vast majority of research in balance disorders has been done in the realm of vestibular and neurologic dysfunction. Some orthopedic studies have primarily investigated lower-extremity instability.[57]

Frequently, balance evaluation is assessed by the subject's ability to maintain an upright position. In spinal injuries, abnormal static postures as well as gait and movement deviations may create a new environment with which the body is not familiar. The alteration of movement may be retained long after the initial problem resolves. In addition, the lack of practice in activities of daily living may result in "clumsiness" in coordination and balance. The principle of balance analysis is the measurement of body weight distribution. This is generally tested in static and dynamic environments and is most often referenced by the location of the weight-bearing center of gravity.

When a person stands in place, the center of gravity periodically shifts from side to side and heel to toe; when walking, it shifts forward in smooth rhythmic movements. In normal adults, the anterior/posterior limits of stability are approximately 12 degrees of total arc (most forward to most backward), and the lateral limits are approximately 16 degrees.[43]

The assessment of balance in spinal orthopedics has been primarily done through visual assessment by the evaluator with augmentation from task completion tests. Equipment to assess this relatively new area is available, but the correlation to normal individual and to specific task performance is largely in the preliminary data collection stages.

Equipment

The MotionSpec (Baltimore Therapeutic Equipment Co., Hanover, Md) assesses such parameters as the speed of movement, the direction of movement, acceleration/deceleration, and a programmed sequence of starts and stops. The individual stands on a movable platform approximately 40 by 60 in. in size. As the platform moves, the patient's balance is challenged. Metal "shoes" provide the contact for precise measurement of the patient's foot movements and recovery times. The MotionSpec is capable of distances up to 20 cm, velocities up to 40 cm/sec, and accelerations up to 150 cm/sec. Specific comparative data with respect to the back have not yet been collected.

Balance Master System (NeuroCom International, Clackamas, Ore) offers a computerized system that evaluates input from a force plate. This allows evaluation of the center of gravity/mass, postural alignment, limits of stability, and rhythmic weight shifts. The software offers 26 standardized targets and the ability to customize specific patient targets. In addition, optional systems allow the clinician to examine not only static balance but dynamic balance as well. This is done through the use of a movable force plate. Target programs range from those that are responsive to patient movements to computer-driven surface movements that are unpredictable and force the patient to integrate and adjust in response. Surface conditions may be varied as well as pacing, limits of stability, center-of-gravity tracing, and audio cues. Specific back data have not been developed.

The Balance System (Chattex Corp., Hixson, Tenn) consists of four independent force transducers for the ball and heel of each foot. This small footprint (4 by 5 ft) system is computerized and has the ability to tilt the platform to assess dynamic conditions. In addition to establishing baselines, the Balance System tests for the absolute center of balance as it relates to heel/toe and left/right limits of postural stability as measured by postural sway within a specified percentage of body weight. A limited amount of comparative data has been established.

FUNCTIONAL UNIT INTEGRATION

The testing of functional unit integration allows the evaluation of all units' performance in the completion of a task. This integration is at the core of the concept of functional evaluation in human performance. The determination of functional unit integration is often the treatment focus of the injured worker. It is often difficult to determine how soon an injured employee should return to work.

Functional unit integration is increasingly being utilized prior to employment to determine at what physical level an individual can work. The assessment may use many techniques and systems, but the focus is always on functional unit integration capability. Of the many available assessment types, there are several distinct capability categories. With static evaluation, the individual is tested in various isometric positions with comparisons to some of the original hallmark research.[12] Dynamic testing is performed with movement but against a machine that measures output as well as provides a limitation of the variables such as speed and resistance. In functional capacity evaluations, the patient is given a battery of interrelated tasks to provide an overall assessment of capabilities.

Video analysis provides information by breaking down movements into components, and then the evaluator can determine forces as well as the quality of movement.

Lifting is integral to almost all functional task integration tests. It may be assessed by any of the methods as described above. Lifting is also of central focus in the assessment of spinal function as the most common issue in assessing ability.

Snook et al. divided the manual material handling into six basic tasks: lifting, lowering, pushing, pulling, carrying, and walking. They stated that almost every task in industry consists of a combination of two or more of these tasks.[53]

Drury et al. observed 2,000 different box handling tasks. The three most common tasks were lifting, lowering, and carrying.[18] A review of a 1982 survey compiled by the U.S. Department of Labor found that 75% of injuries were associated with an activity that featured lifting as opposed to placing, carrying, lowering, holding, pushing, and pulling.[58] Thirty-six percent of the injuries occurred because the object was too heavy, 34% occurred as a result of body movement or motion, and 24% were due to the lifted object being too bulky.

In assessing lifting capabilities, the maximal lift ability must not be used exclusively. In 1986, the Department of Labor published percentages in the *Dictionary of Occupational Titles*.[58] They defined lifting frequencies as the ability to produce the lift for a portion of the workday: occasional (lifting up to 33% of the day), frequent (34% to 67% of the day), and continuous (greater than 67% of the day).

Substantial research has focused on the development of mathematical models for predicting maximum loads that an individual could handle without injury.[44, 52] These models looked at task-related variables such as mass of the load, height of the lift, frequency of the lift, and the type and characteristics of the container. Worker-related variables included gender, age, aerobic and anaerobic capacity, endurance, strength, and anthropometric measures.[2]

The National Institute for Occupational Safety and Health (NIOSH) has published limits that provide assistance in determining whether the lift anticipated will generate unacceptable compressive forces.[44] These limits are based on load weight, the initial position of the load as related to the person, the vertical travel distance, and the frequency of the task. These factors are used to determine the maximum permissible limit (MPL), which is the limit at which most workers would not tolerate the compressive forces on the L5–S1 disc. Only 25% of males and fewer than 1% of females have the muscle strength capable of performing work above the limit.

NIOSH has also defined the action limit (AL) in terms of the disc compressive forces that may be tolerated by most healthy workers.[44] Greater that 99% of males and 75% of females can lift loads as defined by the AL. Tasks over the MPL are considered unacceptable, and tasks between the MPL and the AL are unacceptable without job screening or redesigning the tasks. Tasks that fall below the AL present a decreased amount of risk to workers. In testing of functional integration capability, the task defined should not ask individuals to perform duties that they may not be capable of, nor should it be so conservative as to put artificial limits on performance. An evaluation of the models listed in the *Work Practices Guide for Manual Lifting* found that they all predict lifting capacity with a reasonable degree of accuracy.[44]

STATIC TESTING

Static testing is the oldest and most established method of analyzing lifting capability. It is recognized by NIOSH as a method of identifying a worker who may be at risk for an overexertion injury.[44] The early research in lifting capacities focused on static strength as the measurement tool. The theory was that lifting capacity is a function of isometric back strength.[10, 12, 28]

The standard protocol for static lifting is based on work by Caldwell et al. and Chaffin.[10, 12] This protocol involves a five-second time frame with the maximum effort graduated over the first 2 seconds and held for the remaining 3. With this, Chaffin assessed isometric muscular strength in five different positions.[12] These positions and the isometric test itself are still considered standards and are commonly used. Static testing using these standards as a measurement of the strength capacity at a specific postural angle is therefore limited at retest or comparisons to that specific posture to ensure reproducible data.[12] The tested component was functional strength rather than isolating a given muscle. With this type of testing, the limiting factor may be something other than the spinal musculature, such as extremity pathology.

Comparative Data

The most commonly referenced comparative data for static lift testing are by Keyserling et al.[28] The static strength of 1052 male and 187 female healthy industrial workers was investigated. These data are useful in comparing how patients relate to a healthy industrial population. Any specific application beyond this group is not representative. However, other comparative data bases are available.[11, 14] Static lifting is safe, reliable, and practical. Although utilized as a predictor of lifting capabilities, dynamic testing may be a better predictor of this ability.

Equipment

The Isometric Strength Testing Unit (ISTU, Ergometrics, Inc., Ann Arbor, Mich) measures static lifting capacity using isometric principles as well push/pull and other upper-extremity functions. It has a platform and column with an attached strain gauge that may be disconnected for other uses. The computer and software utilize a biomechanical model based on postural assumptions, disc pressure measurements, and body segments that attempts to make a statement of an individual's risk of injury when a given isometric lifting force is exerted.

Effort is validated through the use of multiple trials and a coefficient of variation based on the force curve overlay. These validity measures are based on clinical observation and have not been published. Comparative data are referenced to the large data bases that exist as well as comparison of the individual to the *Work Practices Guide* as percent capable.

DYNAMIC LIFTING

Dynamic lifting offers many advantages over static testing for assessment of lifting capability. In addition to having an assessment that is closer to the actual task, dynamic lifting provides continuous information about an individual's ability to sustain motion through a range while under a load. It is less stressful and has been shown to better predict an individual's lifting ability.[1] The primary limitation for a static lift in determining capacity is its inability to take into account the dynamic portion of a task.[1, 26, 42]

Dynamic lifting is essentially an isotonic (isoinertial) function where a fixed external load is lifted through a defined distance. However, with the introduction of isokinetics, this additional method of testing has become a staple on most machines.

Isokinetic lifting is also a dynamic movement with the added ability to control the variable of velocity with its associated safety factor. The accommodating resistance also allows one to identify the maximum force capability of the individual. Isokinetic lifting is usually a component of a test and not the sole focus. Some data bases have been established by the manufacturers but are not as comprehensive as those for isometric testing.

As with other isokinetic systems, the manufacturers of isokinetic lift devices rely on reproducibility of data points as a verification of effort. This becomes somewhat more difficult in the trunk due to a lack of stabilization and posture control. The aspect of reproducibility becomes less of an effort factor and more of a skill parameter, and care should be taken to prevent too narrow an application.

Technology has now advanced to the point that manufacturers are able to reproduce the positive elements of lifting while minimizing the drawbacks. The use of active technology and three-dimensional tracking has the potential to greatly increase knowledge in this area.

Equipment

The Lido Lift (Loredan, Davis, Calif) is a unique lift analysis system that employs active technology allowing a measurement of lifting, lowering, lateral movement under load, work, power, and velocity for any movement within its workstation window (Fig 6–2). The software analyzes three-dimensional movement and provides multiple measurement of position and protocols to simulate most job tasks. Isokinetics as well as isometrics and isotonics provide comparative data bases. The Lido Lift has the ability to determine consistency based on the coefficient of variation and curve analysis. It includes boxes and lift attachments as well as two instrumented racks for repeatable task simulation. Safety is provided by overrides and a velocity brake that prevent injury if the user should drop the simulated weight.

The LiftStation (Isotechnologies, Hillsborough, NC) is a new system employing isometric technology and isotonics with the unique ability of enabling the user to directly attach the specific object that the individual will lift. This allows a direct re-creation of the lifting environment. There are protocols for standardized isometric as well as psychophysical tests. The data collected include weight, velocity, force, and consistency. The software provides a comparison to the NIOSH guidelines, makes lifting recommendations as per the *Work Practices Guides,* and relates recommendations to the *Dictionary of Occupational Titles*.

The Dynamic Lift (Baltimore Therapeutic Equipment Co., Hanover, Md) combines the concept of a weight stack with computerization (Fig 6–3). The software provides information on isometrics lifts, isotonic lifts, and push/pull movements. Safety features provide an automatic clutch to prevent a rapid weight drop. Comparative data are based on the NIOSH guidelines.[44]

Psychophysical Testing

The concept of maximal functional testing requires most patients to exceed their usual pain level. Assessing the maximal effort produced by patients with chronic pain does not take into account the functional qualities of muscle performance, which are limited by the individual's perception of pain. For patients with injuries or chronic pain, maximum efforts may increase their risk of further injury.[29] The assessment of a person's physical ability in relation to his perception of what is a tolerable limit should generally yield results more indicative of ability.[24] This output should be much more representative of the person's likely output in more general settings such as the job site or home. The term "psychophysical" denotes the fact that lifting capacity is influenced by the patient's self-report of maximum capability, discomfort, or perception of impending injury.[44] Psychophysical lifting is used to identify the maximum capabilities of the individual over a given period of time. As a protocol, it is adaptable to most of the lifting equipment described above.

The progressive isoinertial lifting evaluation (PILE) is designed to combine dynamic measurement with a built-in

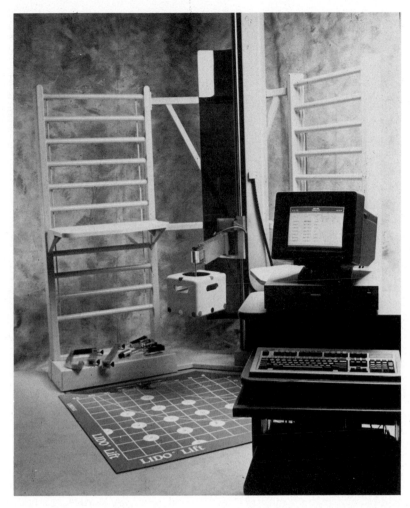

FIG 6–2.
A lift analysis system can be used to assess lifting, lowering, work, and velocity in a fashion simulating many job tasks.

effort factor in the quantification of lifting and lowering actions.[38] The PILE protocol involves lifting and lowering weights in a plastic box from the floor to the waist (0 to 30 in.). There is also a shoulder girdle and upper-extremity lift (cervical lift) from waist to shoulder height (30 to 54 in.). Lumbar and cervical tests are performed separately. Women begin with an 8-lb load, while men begin with a 13-lb load. Weight is increased every 20 seconds (5-lb units for women and 10-lb units for men). Lifting proceeds at a rate of four lifting and lowering movements in each 20-second interval. The subject progressively increases the weight lifted and total work performed until an objective end point is reached. This end point may be fatigue, aerobic capacity as defined by maximum heart rate, or a predetermined limit of 45% to 55% of body weight. However, there is some disagreement about the maximum acceptable lift weight.[20] A large difference in maximum acceptable lift was found among populations.[51] Lifting capability is maximum at floor level and decreases as the initial height of the load increases. The size of box has a significant effect on lifting. Increased box size is accompanied by a decreased lifting capability. If submaximal effort has been provided, the final heart rate will be low, with a discrepancy between the target heart rate and the final heart rate.

PILE tests are more expensive in terms of staff training and time for administration of the test. They are safe in that if the test is isoinertial, it presents dependable resistance to the force applied by the patient, thereby increasing the ability of the patient to proceed and avoid overexertion.[37] PILE tests do not have the ability to discriminate the weak link in the patient's biomechanical system.

FUNCTIONAL CAPACITY ASSESSMENTS

Functional capacity assessment (FCA) is a comprehensive physical task evaluation used to describe the various portions of an employee's job and his capabilities and limitations in performing those duties. It may contain components of all testing procedures previously described. For

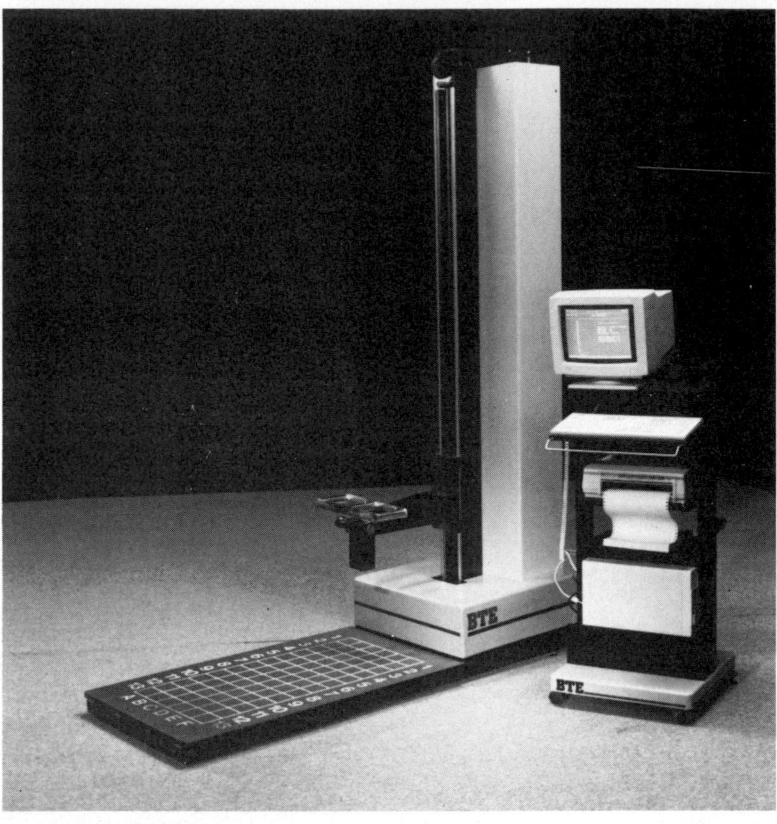

FIG 6–3.
A different type of lift analysis equipment combines the concept of a weight stack with computerization to assess lifting and compares performance with the NIOSH guidelines.

an FCA to be clinically relevant to the worker's employment, a work assessment and job site analysis must first be obtained. The work assessment is an interview process with the employee and the employer to determine the task requirement. The information is used to generate the baseline requirements for the task performance during the FCA. The job site analysis is an on-site visit of the employee's work environment. Additional information as to workstation design and materials placement is collected to help verify the work assessment information.

A musculoskeletal evaluation is done prior to the FCA to identify any interfering deficits and to ensure that the assessment is not contraindicated. Specific tasks performed include components of push/pull, lifting in various postures, carrying, kneeling, reaching, climbing, walking, sitting posture and tolerance, balance, and trunk stabilization. These tasks are timed to allow evidence of fatigue (if present) to be a limiting factor. The administering therapist will input additional information as to the patient's consistency, body mechanics, cooperation, and pace as well as any noted pain complaints and behavior. An Oswestry questionnaire may also be utilized as a report of the patient's determination of perceived disability.[19] A summary report of objective findings and observations as well as patient perceptions is provided to the medical care providers and necessary parties. Comparisons to known normative data may be made with recommendations pertaining to additional services and return to work.

The time required to administer an FCA may range from 2 hours to 2 days. The time spent is partially a function of the specific test protocol and whether a determination of performance and symptomatic levels the following day are of importance. The FCA clinically provides an assessment of job-related tasks by actually having the employee perform the tasks. In addition, there is an immediate determination of functional deficits for the treatment plan focus and a basis for impairment ratings and return-to-work decisions.

Equipment

Continued advances in technology have led to the full computerization of multiple task performance in one unit. This system, the Ergos Work Simulator (Work Recovery Centers Inc., Tucson) requires 400 to 600 ft^2 and an 8-ft-high ceiling. The system is fully computerized to ensure a controlled measurement. Five on-line computers are linked to a master computer, which allows assessment of three to five patients at the same time. The system is composed of five stations that measure individual components and repeatable factors for cross-reference of performance. The activities evaluated include lifting, pushing/pulling, trunk rotation, lift origin and destination, reaching, standing, stooping, bending, crouching, walking, climbing, balancing, carrying, grip strength, finger flexion, pinch strength, and wrist supination and pronation. Consistencies are maintained via a standardized assessment process that compares the patient's performance with previous and future employer requirements, the Department of Labor *Dictionary of Occupational Titles* classification system, NIOSH *Work Practices Guide for Manual Lifting,* and the *Methods Times Measurements* standards.

Optical Methods

Functional unit integration evaluation at its best would allow the patient to go about his specific task without impedance or restriction. Gracovetsky feels that some systems create difficulty by attempting to mechanically isolate the spine from the pelvis.[22] By using harnesses and belts and allowing movement only around a fixed axis of rotation, these machines interfere substantially with normal spine function. Currently, the least restrictive assessment mode is visual. In some video analysis systems, range of motion is assessed through simple photography of skin markers at specific locations on the patient. This is often supplemented with film or videotape. In more complex units, a computer-controlled video system focusing on light-emitting diodes rather than reflective markers has been used.[56] The limiting factors continue to be the relationship of the skin contour marking to that of the underlying spinal segment.[39] Although the motion of the skin does not precisely reconstruct the motion of the spinal segment, for certain types of exercises the markers do approximate the kinematics of the spine.[23]

The motion measurements that are the most precise are spinal flexion and extension. Lateral bending is reproduced without difficulty. Rotation as a component of lateral bending is noted but as a planar isolated movement limited by skin movement and the need to maintain the markers' visual connections with the camera. Extension is greatly compromised by skin motion.

Equipment

Spine Trak (Motion Analysis Corp., Santa Rosa, Calif) is a computerized video analysis system for the cervical, thoracic, and lumbar spines (Fig 6–4). Two cameras provide information from reflective skin markers during flexion, extension, and lateral bending. Velocity measurements as well as coefficients of variation are also obtained. The second camera is mounted overhead to provide information on components of rotation. Thc system has the capability for expansion through the addition of cameras, EMG equipment and force plates.

Lift Trak, also produced by Motion Analysis, is designed to analyze real-life lift performance in an uninhib-

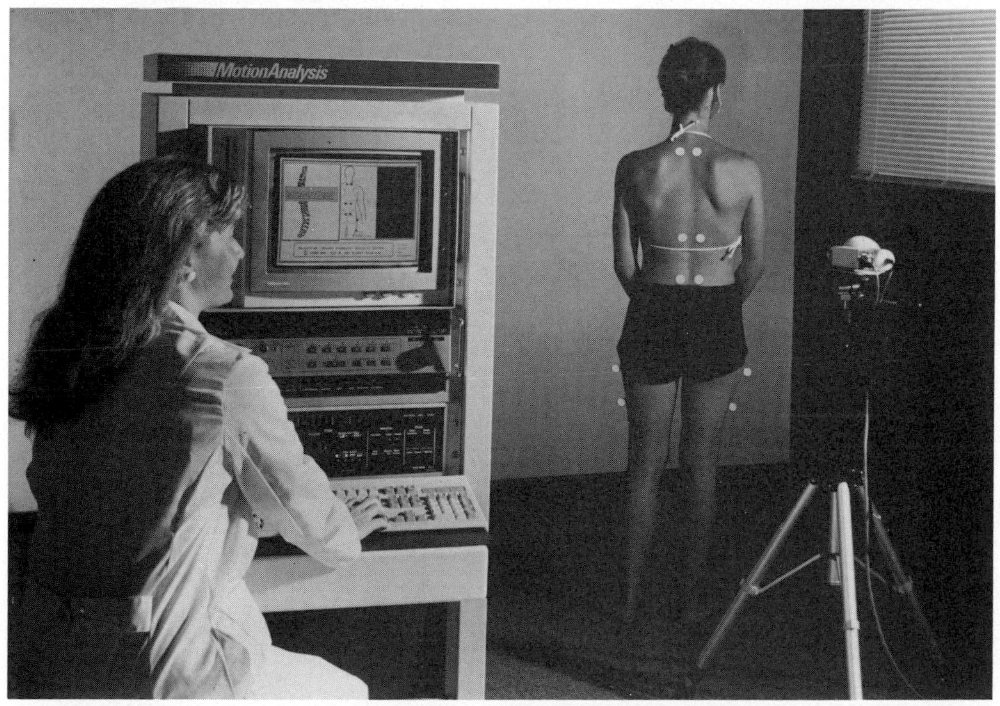

FIG 6–4.
Flexion, extension, and lateral bending can be assessed through the use of video analysis systems.

ited environment (Fig 6–5). By using biomechanical models, the inertial effect of the body as well as that of the load is calculated. Lumbar compressive forces and range-of-motion parameters are displayed to allow the examiner to modify postures and tasks to achieve the desired loads.

The Spinoscope (Spinex Medical Technologies, Montreal) obtains data from a dual-camera system while the activity of the multifidus muscles is recorded by using surface EMGs. The data are transmitted from the patient through the use of light-emitting diodes attached to the skin. When the patient bends forward, the motion of the marker in the sagittal plane produces information on intersegmental mobility and the reduction in lordosis. Through mathematical analysis, detailed information about the coordination of the spine, pelvis, and muscles is deduced. When compared with controls, a deviation may be interpreted as a loss of spinal function. The verification of effort is deduced through an analysis of coordination. Range of motion is under voluntary control and may be purposely limited. Coordination of the spinal segments is not easily controlled at the conscious level, which makes it a more attractive indication of performance. Data produced include analysis of motion as well as intersegmental mobility, torque, L5–S1 compression, velocity, power, and isometric and isokinetic forces. Comparative normal movements are based on experience with 800 subjects.

CONCLUSION

The goal of functional assessment has been to determine an individual's overall ability with particular reference to his demands. Despite the technological advances in equipment, the gold standard is still specific task performance. The current assessment tools yield pertinent data that, when combined, allow some reasonable assumptions to be made. However, methods for measuring talent, enthusiasm, motivation, and other personality parameters that greatly affect performance are either nonexistent or are not precise enough to allow definitive statements to be made. Strength testing has been a key component of functional testing and will likely continue to be so in the future. Comparative data are noticeably absent for all the main parameters and all the testing machines. This contributes to our lack of understanding of the relationship of one individual to another and the prediction of work performance in a specific task. The accurate assessment of effort for each parameter is essential to determine the value of the data collected. This determination has been only casually studied and has not been addressed by manufacturers. Continued research is needed to massively expand this important component.

Technology is currently much more advanced than the understanding of the data it generates. This "knowledge gap" must be closed in order to determine the significance of the information as well as its use in rehabilitation. An even greater discovery will be the determination of which data are useful. The field of rehabilitation medicine is notable for the dearth of research concerning measurements and outcome studies. It is our responsibility to pursue a valid determination of function.

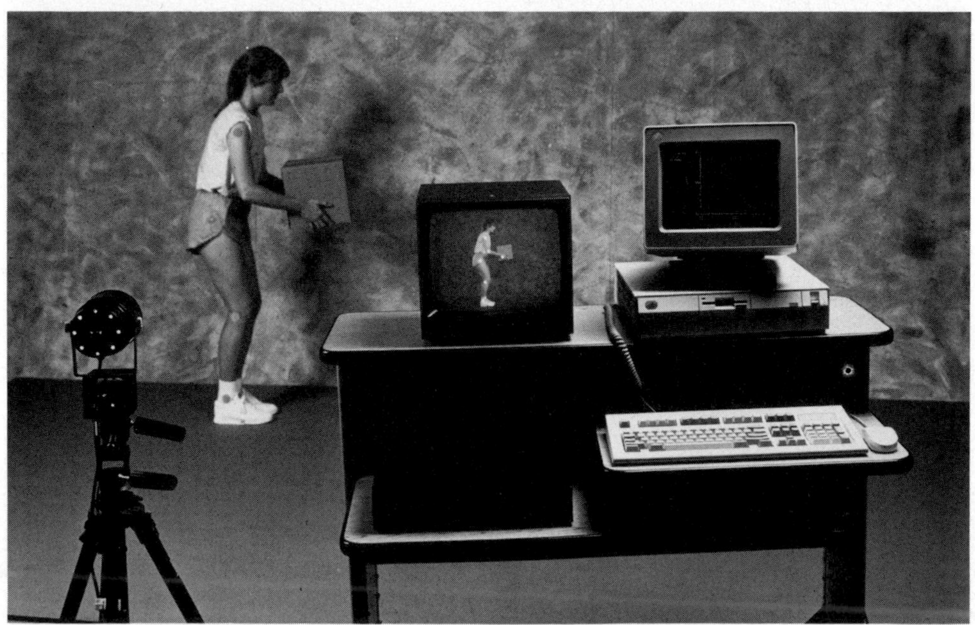

FIG 6–5.
Computerized biomechanical models are used to calculate load, range of motion, and forces on the spine during lifting tasks.

REFERENCES

1. Aghazadeh F, Ayoub M: A comparison of dynamic and static strength model for predication of lifting capacity. *Ergonomics* 1985; 28:1409–1417.
2. Aghazadeh F, Giang BC: Some considerations in the use of isometric, isoinertial and isokinetic strength models for predicting lifting capabilities. *Int J Indust Ergo* 1988; 2:101–110.
3. American Medical Association: *Guides to the Evaluation of Permanent Impairment,* ed 3. Chicago, American Medical Association, 1988.
4. Amundsen LR: *Measurement of Skeletal Muscle Strength: Instrumented and Noninstrumented Systems.* New York, Churchill Livingstone, 1990, pp 1–8.
5. Andersson GBJ: Evaluation of muscle function, in *The Adult Spine: Principles and Practice.* New York, Raven Press, 1991, pp 241–274.
6. Asmussen E: Positive and negative muscular work. *Acta Physiol Scand* 1953; 28:364–382.
7. Baltzopoulos V, Brodie D: Isokinetic dynometry, applications and limitations. *Sports Med* 1989; 8:101–106.
8. Beimborn DS, Morrissey MC: A review of the literature relating to trunk muscle performance. *Spine* 1988; 13:655–660.
9. Burdett R, Van Swearingen J: Reliability of isokinetic muscle endurance test. *J Orthop Sports Phys Ther* 1987; 8:484–488.
10. Caldwell L, Chaffin D, Dobos F, et al: A proposed standard procedure for static muscle strength testing. *Am Indust Hyg Assoc J* 1974; 35:201–206.
11. Chaffin D: Pre-employment strength testing: Updated position. *J Occup Med* 1978; 20:105–110.
12. Chaffin DB: Ergonomics guide for the assessment of human static strength. *Am Indust Hyg Assoc J* 1975; 36:505–511.
13. Chaffin D, Herrin G, Keyserling W: Pre-employment strength testing. *J Occup Med* 1978; 20:403–408.
14. Chaffin D, Herrin G, Keyserling W, et al: A method for evaluating the biomechanical stresses resulting from manual materials handling jobs. *Am Indust Hyg Assoc J* 1977; 38:662–675.
15. Chandler JM, Duncan PW: Eccentric vs concentric force velocity relationships of the quadriceps femoris muscle (abstract). *Phys Ther* 1988; 68:800.
16. Davies G: *A Comparison of Isokinetics and Clinical Usage and Rehabilitation Techniques,* ed 2. LaCrosse, Wisc, S & S Publishers, 1985.
17. Delitto A, Crandell CE, Rose SJ: Peak torque to body weight ratio in the trunk: A critical analysis. *Phys Ther* 1989; 69:138–143.
18. Drury C, Law C, Pawenski C: A survey of industrial box handling. *Hum Factors* 1982; 24:553–565.
19. Fairbanks JC, Davies JD, Coupel J, et al: The Oswestry low back pain disability questionnaire. *Physiotherapy* 1980; 66:271–273.
20. Garg A, Ayoub MM: What criteria exists for determining how much load can be lifted safely? *Hum Factors* 1980; 22:475–486.
21. Garret WE: Basic science of musculotendinous injuries, in Nicholas JA, Hershman EB (eds): *The Lower Extremity and Spine in Sports Medicine.* St Louis, Mosby–Year Book, 1986, pp 42–58.
22. Gracovetsky S: The spine as a motor in sports: Application to running and lifting, in Hochschuler SH (ed): *The Spine in Sports.* Philadelphia, Hanley & Belfus, 1990, p 11.
23. Gracovetsky S, Newman N, Asselin S: *The Problem of Non-invasive Assessment of Spinal Function,* section 1. Montreal, Diagnospine Research, 1989, p 7.
24. Hannson TH, Stanely JB, Wortley MK, et al: The load on the lumbar spine during isometric strength testing. *Spine* 1984; 9:877–884.
25. Herrin G: Occupational biomechanics: Simple/compound joint models including isometric lifting methods. Presented at a Sports Medicine for Working People conference, 1989.
26. Jiang B, Smith J, Ayoub M: Psychophysical modeling of manual materials handling capability using isoinertial strength variables. *Hum Factors* 1986; 28:691–702.
27. Kahanovitz N, Nordin M, Verderamer R, et al: Normal trunk muscle strength and endurance in women and the effect of exercises and electrical stimulation. Part II: Comprehensive analysis of electrical stimulation and exercises to increase trunk muscle strength and endurance. *Spine* 1987; 12:112–118.
28. Keyserling W, Herrin G, Chaffin D: An analysis of selected work muscle strength. Presented at the Human Factors Society 22nd Annual Meeting, Detroit.
29. Khalil TM, Goldberg ML, Asfour SS, et al: Acceptable maximum effort (AME), a psychophysical measure of strength in back pain patients. *Spine* 1987; 12:372–376.
30. Knuttgen HG, Bonde-Peterson F, Klausen K: Oxygen uptake and heart response to exercise performed with concentric and eccentric muscle contractions. *Med Sci Sports* 1971; 3:1–5.
31. Komi PV: Relationship between muscle tension, EMG, and velocity of contraction under concentric and eccentric work, in *New Developments in Electromyography and Clinical Neurophysiology.* Beauvechain, Belgium, Nauwelaerts Publishing Co, pp 596–606.
32. Komi PV, Kaneko M, Aura O: EMG activity of the leg extensor muscles with special reference to the mechanical efficiency in concentric and eccentric exercise. *Int J Sports Med Suppl* 1987; 8:22–29.
33. Langrana NA, Lee C: Isokinetic evaluation of trunk muscles. *Spine* 1984; 9:171–175.
34. Loebl W: Measurements of spinal posture and range of spinal movement. *Ann Phys Med* 1967; 9:103.
35. Marras WS, Wongsam PE: Flexibility and velocity of the normal and impaired lumbar spine. *Arch Phys Med Rehabil* 1986; 67:213–217.
36. Mayer TG: Assessment of lumbar function. *Clin Orthop* 1987; 221:99–109.
37. Mayer TG, Barnes D, Kishino N, et al: Progressive isoinertial lift evaluation I. A standardized protocol and normative database. *Spine* 1988; 9:993–997.

38. Mayer TG, Gatchel RJ: *Functional Restoration for Spinal Disorders: The Sports Medicine Approach*. Philadelphia, Lea & Febiger, 1988.
39. Mayer TG, Gatchel RJ, Kishino N, et al: Objective assessment of spine function following industrial injury: A prospective study with comparison group and one year follow-up. *Spine* 1985; 10:482–493.
40. Mayer TG, Kishino N, Keeley J, et al: Using physical measurements to assess low back pain. *J Musculoskel Med* 1985; 2:44–59.
41. Mayer TG, Smith S, Keeley J, et al: Quantification of lumbar function. Part 2: Sagittal plane trunk strength in chronic low-back pain patients. *Spine* 1985; 10:765–772.
42. Mirka G, Marras W: Lumbar motion response to a constant load velocity lift. *Hum Factors* 1990; 32:493–501.
43. Nashner LM: Sensory, neuromuscular, and biomechanical contributions to human balance. Presented at the American Physical Therapy Association Forum, Nashville, Tenn, June 1989.
44. National Institute for Occupational Safety and Health: *Work Practices Guide for Manual Lifting*. Cincinnati, US Department of Health and Human Services, 1981. Technical Report No. 81–122.
45. Parnianpour N, Nordin M, Kahanovitz N, et al: The triaxial coupling of torque generation of trunk muscles during isometric exertions and the effect of fatiguing isoinertial movements on the motor output and the movement patterns. *Spine* 1988; 9:982–992.
46. Roland M, Morris R: The natural history of low back pain. Development of guidelines for trials of treatment in primary care. *Spine* 1983; 2:141–144.
47. Rothstein J, Lamb R, Mayhew T: Clinical usages of isokinetic measurements. *Phys Ther* 1978; 67:1840–1844.
48. Schmidt A: Cognitive factors in the performance level of chronic low back pain patients. *J Psychosom Res* 1985; 29:183–198.
49. Smidt G, Herring T, Amunudsen L, et al: Assessment of abdominal and back extensor strength: A quantitative approach and results for chronic low back patients. *Spine* 1983; 8:211–219.
50. Smith S, Mayer T, Gatchel R, et al: Quantification of lumbar function. Part I. Isometric and multispeed isokinetic trunk strength measures in sagittal and axial planes in normal subjects. *Spine* 1985; 10:757–764.
51. Snook S: *The Design of Manual Lifting Tasks*. Bedforshire, England, The Ergonomics Society, 1978.
52. Snook S, Irvine C: Maximum acceptable weight of lift. *Am Indust Hyg Assoc J* 1967; 28:322–329.
53. Snook S, Irvine C, Bass S: Maximum weights and workloads acceptable to male industrial workers. *Am Indust Hyg Assoc J* 1970; 31:579–586.
54. Standish WD, Rubinovick RM, Aurwin S: Eccentric exercise in chronic tendinitis. *Clin Orthop* 1986; 208:65–68.
55. Thorstensson A, Nilsson J: Trunk muscle strength during constant velocity movements. *Scand J Rehabil Med* 1982; 14:61–68.
56. Thurston A, Harris G: Normal kinematics of the lumbar spine and pelvis. *Spine* 1983; 8:199–205.
57. Tropp H, Ekstrand J, Gilquist J: Stabilometry in functional instability of the ankle and its value in predicting injury. *Med Sci Sports Exerc* 1964; 16:64–66.
58. United States Department of Labor Employment and Training Administration: *Department of Labor Dictionary of Occupational Titles,* ed 4, supplement. Washington, DC, Government Printing Office, 1986.
59. *Webster's 7th Collegiate Dictionary*. Springfield Mass, G & C Merriam, 1970.
60. White AA, Gordon SL: Synopsis: Workshop on idiopathic low back pain. *Spine* 1982; 7:141–149.

7

Evaluation of Total-Body Impairment

Scott Haldeman, M.D., Ph.D., F.R.C.P.(C)

One of the primary legal and social characteristics of organized civilization is the development of a system to compensate individuals for injuries sustained as a consequence of negligence or actions by or on behalf of other individuals, corporations, businesses, governments, or other agencies.[1] Although references to compensation for injuries can be seen in ancient Roman law, the development of modern systems for compensation is generally considered to be rooted in 19th century Germany and England. In most of Europe the workmen's compensation system developed as part of an overall social security and welfare system that provided health care and disability compensation in one form or another for all citizens irrespective of the origin of an injury or illness. Although the assessment of costs may be divided between businesses, governments, and agencies depending on perceived responsibility, all citizens in fully socialized countries are considered eligible for compensation if they are unable to physically participate in some form of remunerative occupation. It therefore became necessary to assess the ability of injured or ill citizens to work and to determine residual functional impairment or disability.

Although the idea of disability compensation developed somewhat later and differently in the United States, there remains a basic premise that individuals with physical or mental incapacity for compensable employment should be supported by society. The 1908 Federal Employees Act and the subsequent passing of industrial injury and workmen's compensation acts in all states between 1914 and 1949 created the mechanism for compensation of workers injured while employed. The Social Security Disability Act in 1954 resulted in a system that would support individuals unable to obtain employment due to physical or mental disability that was not work related. In addition, a very complex legal tort system has been developed that allows individuals who have been injured as the result of negligence by others (auto accidents, product deficiencies, unsafe public places, etc.) to seek compensation based, in part, on the severity of the injury and the ability of the injured party to obtain remunerative employment. These laws have provided the basis for a social net that, imperfectly, is designed to prevent starvation and hardship by individuals who for one reason or another have an impairment in their ability to support themselves.

There are other social issues that require a determination of an individual's ability to perform certain functions. Vocational rehabilitation agencies require a detailed evaluation of an applicant's abilities and disabilities. Pre-employment screening always includes some assessment of work capacity. Disability insurance companies require an evaluation of policy applications. Similarly, many sports and recreational activities require an evaluation of a potential participant's ability to perform specific activities.

The assessment of ability, impairment, disability, or functional capacity in each of these situations inevitably begins with the physician who is required to make the initial evaluation. The report generated by a physician is then combined with assessments by vocational nurses or rehabilitation specialists, laboratory studies, and other information from coaches, coworkers, and employers. Legal or administrative decisions are then made on the basis of established rules, laws, or precedent. The increasing demand for these assessments has made it essential that physicians understand the various types of assessment and reporting requirements and be able to render an opinion on the ability or impairment of patients or applicants.

IMPAIRMENT VS. DISABILITY

Most texts, articles, and book chapters on this topic take considerable time to define and differentiate terms. Impairment is commonly described as a physical and mental limitation in function determined by a physician. Disability, on the other hand, is defined as the reduced capacity to meet certain work demands. The latter is commonly considered a legal term with factors such as age, sex, education, and prior work capacity taken into account. In reality it is very difficult to separate these terms, although each may be interpreted differently by different professions or agencies.

Other terms have also been introduced by legislative and administrative bodies, which further blurs the picture. Often specific agencies or laws have developed definitions for disability, impairment, handicap, loss of faculty, and disablement with attempts to differentiate among them. Unfortunately, definitions of the same terms by different agencies or laws may vary and even be in conflict. It therefore becomes important, although sometimes impossible, for physicians to understand what is actually meant by the terms they are required to address in a specific case.

This confusion has led most physicians to retreat into definitions that are often concrete but understandable. Hence, impairment has been defined in medical terms as "an anatomical or pathological abnormality leading to loss of normal bodily ability."[16, 41] Disability, in turn, is defined in social terms as the "diminished capacity for everyday activities and gainful employment" or the "limitation of a patient's performance compared to a fit person's of the same age and sex."[14, 41] Most administrative and legal decisions, however, do not make this clear definition. Such decisions take into consideration a physician's report, patient's statements, and the legal, regulatory, and social precedents as well as financial priorities. Each agency may assign different weighting to these factors. All the physician can do is provide an accurate and informative assessment of a patient or applicant. The physician's role is therefore to understand the type of information and conclusions that an agency requires and provide a report answering any questions that might be asked. Attempts to be more specific or advisorial or to advocate certain positions often lead to invalidation of a report.

THE COST OF DISABILITY

The past few decades have seen a rapid, almost exponential rise in the number of back pain disability claims. The number of people disabled by back pain, according to data from the U.S. National Center for Health Statistics, showed an increase of 168% between 1971 and 1981, which was 14 times faster than the population growth.[32, 33] Waddell and Main in the United Kingdom have noted a growth in the number of days of sick certification for back pain that is twice the growth of the number of days of sick certification for all forms of incapacity.[40] Berkowitz reports that expenditures for all forms of disability increased from $20 billion in 1970 to $169.4 billion in 1986.[5]

It is now estimated that medical costs make up only 33% of the total cost of workmen's compensation, with 67% being accounted for by disability payments.[25] In Britain, Fitton et al. noted that 65% of costs were for nontreatment sickness benefits.[17]

Each applicant for disability is inevitably assessed by a physician, and the growth in back pain disability has led to a similar growth in medical-legal costs. In California in 1986 there were 86,000 cases of workmen's compensation back injuries that were litigated at a cost of $395 million, $152 million of which was spent on medical-legal evaluations.[12] In 70% of cases, the extent of permanent disability was a major issue. According to the National Council on Compensation Insurance, back injuries are the most disputed of all claims by employers. Almost 6% of the total amount paid for permanent partial disability is consumed by medical-legal assessment and expert opinions.[8]

THE ACCURACY OF IMPAIRMENT RATINGS

One of the major problems and therefore cost factors in determining disability is the lack of consensus between medical-legal experts concerning the nature and extent of disability following an injury. Recent studies in California have focused on this issue.[11, 12] A single case was referred to 65 independent medical examiners (IMEs) with experience in disability rating. They were asked to estimate the level of disability. Table 7–1 illustrates the wide variation of opinion given the same data. After being supplied full consultation reports on specific patients, IMEs could differ by as much as 85 percentile points as to the degree of disability. To investigate this matter further, another set of IMEs were sent reports and asked to assess the level of work that could be performed by an injured worker. When asked whether an injured worker with a specific history, physical findings, and laboratory studies could perform activities that varied from heavy construction, warehouse work, building maintenance, nursing, bartending, or general office work, there was very little agreement between physicians given the same information (Table 7–2). A similar variation in the impairment rating of individual injured workers by different physicians was also noted in

TABLE 7–1.

Disability Rating of the Same Hypothetical Patient by 65 Independent Medical Examiners in a Specialty Dealing with Back Pain.*

"Assuming a 55-year-old person with uncomplicated laminotomy for the disc at L4–5 and a successful L4–S1 fusion, x-ray studies showing mild generalized osteoarthritis and narrowing at the L5–S1 disc space, and operative results considered 'good' 1 year postoperatively, what do you think the disability rating should be according to our California Disability Evaluation Schedule?"

No. of IMEs	Disability Rating Selected
2	0%
1	10%
4	15%
5	20%
20	25%
13	30%
16	50%
3	60%
1	70%
Total 65	

*From Clark WL, Haldeman S, Johnson P, et al: *Spine* 1988; 13:332–341. Used by permission.

TABLE 7–2.
Disability Rating (%) of 42 Case Reports Referred to Multiple Independent Medical Examiner: Difference Between High and Low Rating*

Difference (%)	No. of Cases
15	3
19–25	6
30–35	8
40–45	8
50–55	11
60–65	4
80–85	3

*From Clark WL, Haldeman S, Johnson P, et al: *Spine* 1988; 13:332–341. Used by permission.

West Virginia by Greenwood.[19] In the study by Clark et al., specific well-defined factors commonly associated with impairment or disability were developed.[12] When a rating system was developed with points given to specific factors that could be isolated from a report, the agreement between assessing physicians improved considerably (Table 7–3). In this study, it became evident that physicians could agree on basic facts from the history and physical examination but were not consistent in relating these factors to work capacity or disability. It was, however, possible to relate the average opinion of assessing physicians on disability to a point rating system in a linear fashion so that the end result was a similar degree of disability.

The American Medical Association (AMA) *Guides to the Evaluation of Permanent Impairment* have also relied on a factor point rating schedule based on clinical findings and diagnoses.[16] Although there is considerable controversy as the relative importance of the various factors used in the AMA guidelines and the failure to assign any value to patients' subjective complaints, these guidelines do have the advantage of reproducibility. If accurately and properly used, the AMA guidelines should produce relatively close agreement between physicians. This has been one of the bases of the popularity of these guidelines among so many of the state workmen's compensation agencies. The question remains, however, as to whether the AMA guidelines or, for that matter, any other system of rating impairment can accurately and fairly determine an injured worker's ability to perform specific forms of work.

TABLE 7–3.
Comparison of Current California and New Rating System with Updated Explanation*

Case No.	California Schedule	New System Second Trial
13	15	8
68	15	10
35	15	6
96	20	11
28	30	10
63	30	13
54	50	14
45	55	15
73	60	12
41	80	10

*From Clark WL, Haldeman S, Johnson P, et al: *Spine* 1988; 13:332–341. Used by permission.

FACTORS INFLUENCING THE ABILITY TO WORK

With the rapid increase in the cost of disability there has been a greater focusing of interest on factors that might influence an individual's ability to work. Recent studies in Britain[41–43] and California[11, 12] and ongoing studies in Vermont are attempting to define specific social, physical, and psychological findings that are associated with disability.

The California study surveyed 73 IMEs by submitting a list of 82 factors commonly found in reports and articles on disability.[12] The IMEs were then asked to rate these factors on a 5-point scale as to their relative importance in determining disability. Table 7–4 lists the results of the survey. Of particular interest was the high rating given to history and low rating given to x-ray findings and many commonly used tests.

It is not, however, necessary to rely completely on opinion when attempting to assess factors of disability. There is a growing body of research that gives some indication as to which factors are associated with a high incidence of impaired work capacity.

History of the Back Injury

One of the primary predictors of future back pain and disability is a past history of back pain and the chronicity of an episode of back pain. Leavitt, in reviewing Workers' Compensation Bureau (WCB) case files in California, found that a history of previous back injury was strongly predictive of a high cost in future injuries.[26] Dillane found that individuals with a history of back pain were four times more likely to have future episodes of back pain,[15] and Troup et al. found that such individuals were more likely to have persistent symptoms.[38] Andersson et al. noted that a person off work for 30 days had a 53% chance of returning to work within 10 days, but if the work loss was more than 90 days, the person had only a 16% chance of returning to work in the same period.[3]

Work Requirements

The relationship between the type of work and the incidence of back pain is beginning to evolve beyond the simple reporting of activities that cause injury. Chaffin and Park report the fairly obvious fact that lifting that approaches the maximum capacity for an individual is asso-

TABLE 7–4.
Weighting by Independent Medical Examiners (N = 73) of Initial List of Factors Considered in Disability Evaluation*

Weight†	Factor
History	
1.2	History of previous back surgery such as repeated surgery
1.5	History of previous back surgery such as failed fusion
1.5	History of previous back surgery such as disc space infections
1.6	History of previous back surgery such as laminectomy
1.6	History of previous back surgery such as fusion
1.7	Pain with sciatic radiation upon weight bearing
1.7	Heavy work involving lifting, bending, and twisting
1.7	History of previous back surgery such as response to previous surgery
1.8	History of previous back surgery such as chymopapain
2.1	History of previous back surgery such as kind and location of residual pain
2.4	Current back pain not relieved by treatment
Laboratory, roentgenogram, etc.	
1.2	Malignant tumor, primary or metastatic
1.6	Fracture-dislocation through the intervertebral disc
2.1	Positive bone scan
2.2	Positive brucellosis, typhoid, tuberculosis, or syphilis test
2.4	Spondylolisthesis
2.5	Osteoporosis—hormonal, corticoid
2.5	Cerebrospinal fluid protein content elevated
2.5	Elevated sedimentation rate or abnormal white blood count and differential
2.7	Disc narrowing increased over that usual for age
2.9	Old compressed fractures
3.0	Spondylolysis
3.6	Vertebral margin osteophytes
3.7	Asymmetrical sacralization/lumbarization
3.7	Abnormal facet tropism
4.2	Four lumbar vertebrae
4.3	Spina bifida occulta
Specialized tests	
1.8	Myelogram "positive"
1.9	Positive cystometrogram
2.1	CAT scan "positive"
2.4	EMG "positive"
2.5	Anatomically reasonable response to differential spinal anesthesia
2.5	Positive response to epidural steroid injection
2.7	Discogram "positive"
2.8	Positive response to facet block
3.0	Positive response to costovertebral joint block
3.1	Venogram "positive"
3.1	Positive "bicycle" test
3.2	Muscle spasm—by EMG?
4.7	Thermogram "positive"

*From Clark WL, Haldeman S, Johnson P, et al: *Spine* 1988; 13:332–341. Used by permission.
†A weighting of "1" indicates that the factor is considered very important; a weighting of "5" indicates that the factor is not considered important at all.

ciated with a high incidence of back pain.[10] Kelsey et al., on the other hand, associated frequent lifting of lesser weights, especially with twisting motions, with a markedly increased risk of back injury.[23] Increased risk of back pain has also been associated with continuous sitting or standing[27] and especially with the prolonged endurance of vibration.[18] It is now possible, epidemiologically, to rate different occupations as to their frequency and likelihood of injury.[13, 26] The issue of work requirements is not, however, clear-cut. Both Porter[35] and Bigos et al.[7] were unable to find any difference in the prevalence of back pain in employees doing light and heavy work in the same industry. There may be factors other than heavy work within a specific industry that are responsible for the increased risk of back pain disability.

Pain Symptoms

Although the primary complaint of patients with back impairment is pain, the determination or measurement of such pain and the factoring in of pain in impairment systems has proved almost impossible. The graded assessment by a physician of a patient's pain into mild, moderate, or severe by American Academy of Orthopaedic Surgeons (AAOS) guidelines[9] or as minimal, slight, moderate, or severe by the California system has proved to be of limited usefulness and bears little if any relationship to pathophysiologic changes. In reality, only the patient can assess the level of pain, but such self-assessment is always influenced by psychological, cultural, social, and at times, conscious bias. The AMA guidelines in the third edition address the issue of pain in the foreword.[16]

Although the importance of chronic pain was recognized, it was felt to be very difficult to include pain in a standardized impairment evaluation system. This text includes a special appendix on pain and concludes that little if any impairment exists in most instances of chronic pain syndrome. There is, however, a recognition that chronic pain may cause significant bio-psycho-social limitations in function resulting in both disability and handicap.

Attempts to measure pain by various rating scales and pain descriptions have not been of much value in the determination of impairment. Visual analogue scales[9] and such tools as the McGill Pain Questionnaire[30] give some idea of how patients perceive pain in reference to their past experience. These and similar tools may be of some value in monitoring a patient's progress during treatment but are of limited or no value in comparing the capacity of different individuals to perform a specific task. On the other hand, illness or pain behavior tests such as pain drawings,[36] assessment of nonorganic signs,[43] and assessment of somatic awareness[28] and depression[4] may provide information on how an individual is reacting to pain and how it is affecting his life.

Gross Spinal Function

The ability of the spine to perform its basic functions of movement and support has been a logical area for the assessment of ability and impairment. The primary assessment of function in the AMA guidelines has been range of motion. The most visible change in the third edition of the AMA guidelines has been an attempt to more accurately measure lumbar range of motion while still maintaining the importance of this parameter of function (Fig 7–1). The change from a goniometer to the double inclinometer in these measurements is a reflection of research by Mayer and his associates[22, 29] that demonstrated that the inclinometers more accurately differentiate spine motion from hip and shoulder motion. Very specific impairment values are given to reduced motion of the spine despite the fact that there is very little research that relates such restrictions to either impairment or disability.

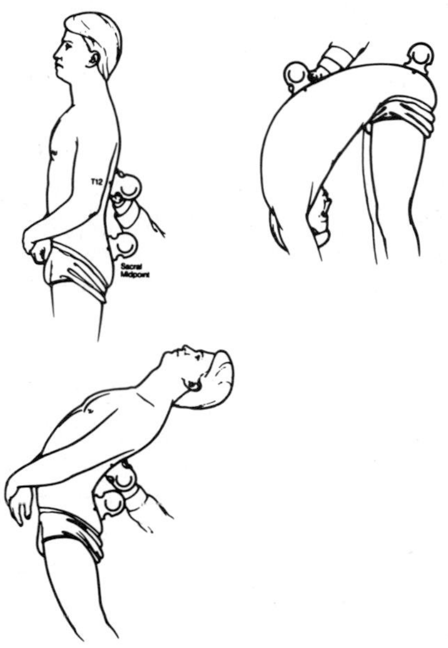

Sacral (Hip) Flexion Angle (Degrees)	True Lumbar Flexion Angle (Degrees)	Impairment of Whole Person (%)
45+	60+	0
45+	45–60	2
45+	30–45	4
45+	15–30	7
45+	0–15	10
30–45	40+	4
30–45	20–40	7
30–45	0–20	10
0–30	30	5
0–30	15–30	8
0–30	0–15	11

FIG 7–1.
An example of evaluating and rating lumbar range of motion according to the AMA guidelines. (From Engleberg AL (ed): *Guides to Evaluation of Permanent Impairment*, ed 3. Chicago, American Medical Association, 1988. Used by permission.)

In recent years there has been the development of a large number of commercially available strength and motion measurement instruments. The National Institute for Occupational Safety and Health (NIOSH) has developed a federal guide on manual lifting that attempts to establish maximum permissible lifting limits based on epidemiologic and biomechanic criteria, but these guidelines only apply to symmetrical lifting in the sagittal plane.[34] More recent studies on isometric, isokinetic, and isoinertial strength testing methods demonstrate that complex measurement of spine function in all three planes of movement is possible. There is, however, no standardization between the various testing methods. Furthermore, no relationship between these testing methods and fixed impairment has been established. The possibility that these tests may be of value in detecting whether an injured worker is exerting maximum effort during an assessment and thereby attempting to enhance or falsely claim impairment has been raised by Waikar et al.[44]

Neurologic Deficits

One of the most consistently measured and reported physical findings in a clinical examination of the spine is the presence or absence of neurologic deficits in the lower or upper extremities. The detection of neurologic deficits allows the physician to conclude that in all probability specific pathology or injury is present. This reduces the necessity of dealing with the all-illusive problem of rating the impairment caused by benign pain. The AMA guidelines put particular emphasis on sensory deficits, which are somehow perceived as legitimizing pain complaints in the extremities. It is, however, possible to have sensory and reflex deficits without pain or, for that matter, without detectable impairment of function.

Muscle weakness caused by neurologic injury, on the other hand, results in a well-defined and, to some extent, quantifiable impairment of function. The AMA guidelines have rated the loss of strength for each nerve root and given an assigned maximum value for such a loss (Fig 7–2). This has allowed for some discretion by examining physicians in determining the degree of maximum loss of function for a specific myotomal set of muscles. A similar impairment value has been assigned by the proposed California guidelines.[12]

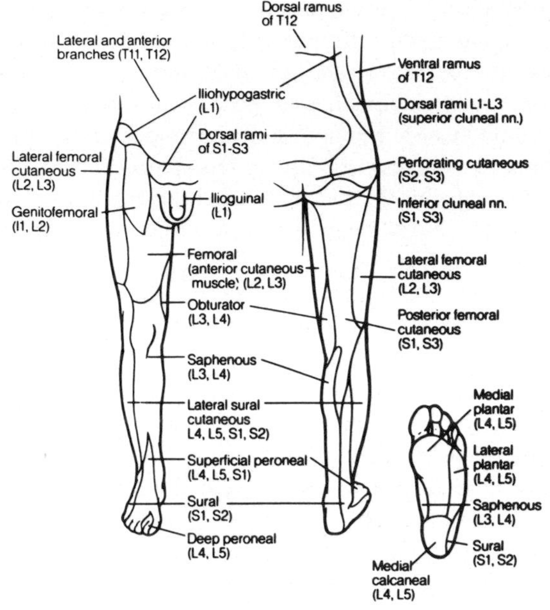

Nerve Root Impaired	Maximum Loss of Function Due Sensory Deficit, Pain, or Discomfort (%)	Maximum Loss of Function Due to Loss of Strength (%)	Impairment of Lower Extremity (%)
L3	5	20	0–24
L4	5	34	0–37
L5	5	37	0–40
L6	5	20	0–24

FIG 7–2.
The method of evaluating impairment due to neurologic loss according to the AMA guidelines. (From Engleberg AL (ed): *Guides to Evaluation of Permanent Impairment*, ed 3. Chicago, American Medical Association, 1988. Used by permission.)

Diagnosis

The fundamental goal of any clinical examination is to localize and define pathology, in other words, to reach a diagnosis. The diagnosis is often the one factor in a patient's assessment on which there is relative agreement. The Minnesota state workers' compensation system[31] and the AAOS 1966 manual for evaluating permanent impairment[2] both depend almost exclusively on the diagnosis for determining impairment. The AMA guidelines similarly give specific impairment ratings for spine fractures, disc herniations, spondylolisthesis, stenosis, and segmental instability.

Other systems such as the Social Security Administration disability program define impairment in terms of anatomic, physiologic, or psychological abnormalities determined by medically accepted clinical laboratory techniques. Under these rules, pain can only be considered for impairment purposes when objective findings can be documented that could reasonably be expected to produce the pain.[37, 39] The proposed California guidelines,[11, 12] on the other hand, give specific impairment values to the results of tests such as imaging and electrodiagnostic studies when such studies are accompanied by appropriate symptom patterns. One of the major problems in the diagnosis- and laboratory-based impairment systems is the breakdown in the relationship between pathology, symptomatology, and disability in patients with chronic pain[21] and even pain-free individuals.

Psychological Impairment

The final decision as to what an individual will or will not be able to accomplish in the presence of back pain is dependent upon the injured worker or sufferer of the pain. An extensive prospective study by Bigos and colleagues at the Boeing plant has shown that the strongest predictors of back pain reports and work loss or disability are psychosocial factors.[6, 7] They found a notable absence of correlation between physical variables such as strength, flexibility, and aerobic capacity and the incidence of back pain reports. They developed a so-called work Apgar model to assess an individual's satisfaction with his work environment and demonstrated a close relationship between this factor and future back pain reports. The importance of job stress and enjoyment in the incidence of back pain disability has been reiterated by other authors.[20, 45]

Other factors not directly related to functional or pathologic impairment may greatly influence an injured worker's likelihood of return to work. Litigation and the type of insurance coverage an individual has may have a great impact on the period off work. Greenwood noted that when treatment was reimbursed by the state insurance fund, workers were more likely to lose time from work than when treatment was reimbursed by the patient.[20]

WHOLE-BODY IMPAIRMENT

The inability to isolate and measure any single factor that will determine a person's ability or inability to perform certain tasks has led to the development of the concept of whole-body impairment. The AMA guidelines consider the body to be made up of a number of parts that contribute to the function of the body as a whole. It is assumed that the loss of function of one of the body parts does not mean that the whole person is impaired. The AMA guidelines then attempt to rate the value of a loss of a single part of the body in relation to the function of the whole person.

Unfortunately, the AMA guidelines bear little relationship to what the whole person is capable of doing when a single part is injured or deficient. There are numerous examples of severely impaired individuals climbing mountains, swimming long distances, and working in very strenuous jobs. At the same time, many injured workers have little or no ratable impairment under any of the diagnosis-related systems and yet feel and function as if they were totally disabled.

The California system attempts to approach the impairment rating process in a more global fashion. Rather than looking at pathology, it assesses an impairment or disability rating on the percentage of the work force from which an injured worker is excluded. Unfortunately, as mentioned earlier in this chapter, there is no means of determining this figure short of estimates by physicians, which have been demonstrated to be extremely inconsistent.

In practice, determining the impairment of a particular individual is an extremely complex and difficult process that often forces physicians to come to terms with their own biases and inadequacies. It requires an understanding of the law, societal and cultural differences, different work environments, psychology, pathology, and diagnostic methods, as well as methods of looking at functional capacity. Figure 7–3 gives a simple model that could be used by a physician assessing a patient for impairment.

The easiest of the three factors in this model for a physician to determine is the diagnosis of the presence or absence of structural pathology that may cause impairment. This has usually been accomplished during the initial evaluation and treatment of a patient, and all that is needed is a simple confirmation by the assessing physician of physical signs and test results. Functional impairment is more difficult, especially in a poorly motivated patient. Often, however, such functions as range of motion, straight leg raising, strength, neurologic deficits, and physical fitness can be determined. The use of expensive testing equipment to obtain absolute measures of function, however, must be viewed with skepticism due to the lack of a known correlation of these measures with impairment. Through the entire evaluation, pain and pain behavior as well as the psychosocial impairment of the injured worker must be assessed to determine whether these factors correlate with pathology and functional impairment. This is of special importance if the goal of assessment includes opinions concerning return to work or vocational rehabilitation.

The remainder of this chapter will deal with the manner in which these factors are incorporated into three of the most commonly used impairment rating systems in the United States.

AMA Guidelines

These guidelines are used more widely and have been the subject of the greatest amount of debate and revision of any of the systems in common use. Proper use of the guidelines rather than a cookbook approach can allow for a reasonably fair and accurate assessment of impairment. The actual numbers in the system, however, must be considered arbitrary and of value only to lawyers and administrators who are required to assign monetary or other benefits for specific injuries.

One can approach a patient undergoing assessment according to AMA guidelines by first looking for structural pathology and evidence of prior surgery. By reading the appropriate table, a percent impairment of the whole person is obtained.

The second step is a determination of functional impairment, which in the AMA guidelines, depends primarily on range of motion, straight leg raising, and motor and sensory neurologic deficits. There are very specific methods of measuring range of motion with the double incli-

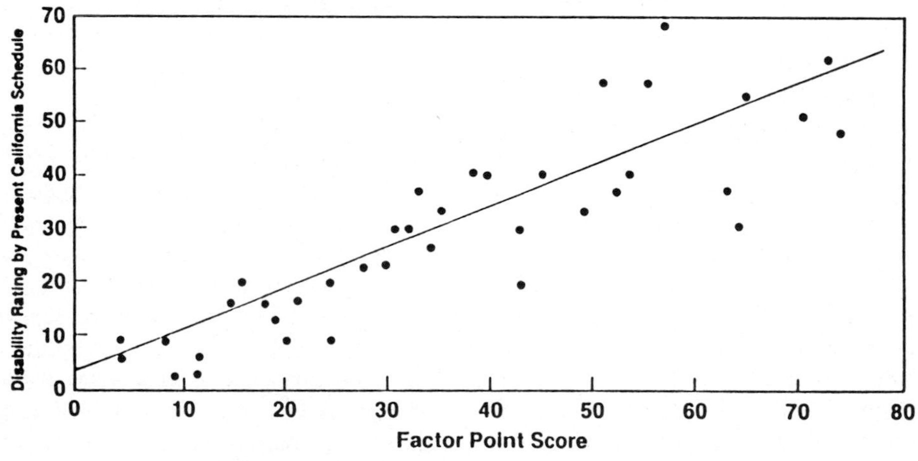

FIG 7–3.
A model for the assessment of impairment and disability.

nometer or goniometer methods, and specific numbers for percent impairment of the whole person can be generated. The assessment of motor and sensory deficits requires some degree of estimation of loss but gives a range of values that translate into percentages of impairment of the lower extremity, which in turn is convertible to percent impairment of the whole person.

Pain and psychosocial impairment get the least amount of emphasis in the AMA guidelines. It is, however, possible to take pain into account when assessing the residual symptoms associated with pathology and pain associated with sensory loss in radiculopathies. It is also possible to add a psychiatric impairment factor for such items as concentration, adaptation to stressful circumstances, etc., if these factors can be demonstrated.

California Guidelines

The current California guidelines require an assessment of the ability of an applicant to perform certain work-related activities. Although this process is notoriously unscientific and inconsistent, physicians can follow a rational method of reaching their conclusions in order to maintain credibility with the Workers' Compensation Appeals Board. The proposed new guidelines present a more structured approach that reaches the same average level of disability with a higher degree of consistency (Fig 7–4).

Under the current system, the assessing physician is required to list all objective findings, including physical examination findings, results of imaging, electrodiagnostic testing, and other laboratory results. These tests must be of sufficient consistency to reach a credible diagnosis. The proposed new system is very specific as to which examination findings and test results should be listed, how they should be interpreted, and what relative value of importance should be assigned to each positive finding. It is interesting to note that a review of multiple reports failed to reveal any information used by physicians to determine impairment that was not included in the listed factors.[11]

An assessing physician is then required to estimate the functional impairment of a patient by listing the type of work from which the injured worker is excluded. Although the current system does not list or recommend testing, cross-examination of physicians in deposition requires more than a simple estimation. Documentation of loss of motion, strength, aerobic fitness, or failure to tolerate a specific activity can assist in the justification for functional impairment. The proposed new guidelines again describe specific measures of function and recommend how such assessments should be made. In particular, lifting capacity and cardiovascular fitness are assessed.

The severity of pain and other symptoms are rated as minimal, slight, moderate, or severe depending on the degree to which they impair function. Psychological factors

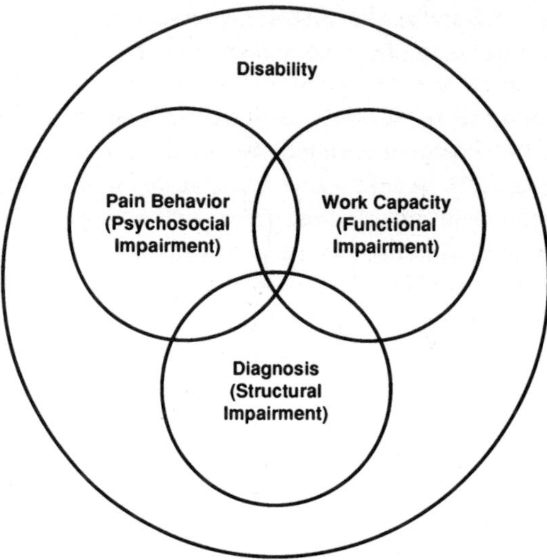

FIG 7–4.
Converting the impairment score to disability ratings (of 24 reports each rating by multiple IMEs and scored by the authors). (From Clark WL, Haldeman S, Johnson P, et al: *Spine* 1988; 13:332–341. Used by permission.)

of impairment are currently assessed by psychiatric consultation, which has its own specific rating system. The initial proposed guidelines[12] attempt to address the more simple psychosocial factors by including modifiers for nonorganic findings and assigning values for continuous or repetitive episodes of pain. Revision of these proposals[11] has again assigned these factors to psychiatric evaluation.

Social Security Administration

This is perhaps the most difficult of all the systems for this author to interpret. At the same time it leaves the greatest leeway for the physician to justify his opinion. Disability is defined as "the inability to engage in any substantial gainful activity, by reason of a medically determinable physical or mental impairment which can be expected to result in death, or has lasted, or can be expected to last, for a continuous period of not less than 12 months."

Since death is not an issue in most spine conditions and ongoing pain for 12 months, by definition, is chronic pain, applicants have to demonstrate a chronic, documentable inability to work. These regulations depend on the documentation of symptoms, signs, and laboratory findings. If the report by a physician is divided into its three components, it is possible to present information that can be evaluated with relative ease by the granting authority.

The diagnosis is dependent upon consistent clinical symptoms and physical examination findings with confirmatory imaging, electrodiagnostic, or other laboratory tests. Under the definition of symptoms the physician is required to list is the claimant's own perception of his physical or mental impairment. When combined with the examination of basic functions and supported by functional assessment tests, these claims can be confirmed or disputed. Psychological tests can be performed for psychopathology or nonorganic symptoms and malingering and the results and interpretation of these tests included in a report. When all this information is submitted, the ultimate psychosocial modifier, legislation and political policy decisions based on budgetary requirements, will determine a claimant's eligibility for Social Security disability.

CONCLUSION

The determination of impairment and ultimately disability as a result of spinal injuries has become a major issue affecting patients, physicians, and an increasing number of private and government agencies. It is becoming obvious that no single factor can be used as the determinant of spine impairment, and to date, no system has evolved that adequately allows for a fair, scientific, and rational approach to this problem. During the past decade, an almost exponential growth of disability related to back pain has made it imperative to develop new systems that are consistent among assessing physicians and relatively inexpensive. At the same time these systems should be able to differentiate between individuals who are totally disabled and require societal support, those who are partially disabled and require some form of compensation and retraining, and those who are able to return to their normal occupational and recreational activities. Ongoing research suggests that an approach that includes an assessment of pathology or structural impairment, an assessment of functional impairment, and an evaluation of psychosocial impairment is most likely to yield a valid system of determining impairment of the whole person and the ability to work.

REFERENCES

1. Allan DB, Waddell G: An historical perspective on low back pain and disability. *Acta Orthop Scand Suppl* 1989; 234:1–23.
2. American Academy of Orthopedic Surgeons: *Manual for Orthopedic Surgeons in Evaluating Permanent Impairment*. Chicago, American Academy of Orthopedic Surgeons, 1966.
3. Andersson GBJ, Svensson H, Anders O: The intensity of work recovery in low back pain. *Spine* 1983; 8:880–884.
4. Beck AT, Ward CH, Mendelson MM, et al: An inventory for measuring depression. *Arch Gen Psychiatry* 1961; 4:561–571.
5. Berkowitz M: *Measuring the Social Impact of Heart and Circulatory Disease Programs*. Santa Monica, Calif, Rand Corp, 1985.
6. Bigos SJ, Battie MC, Spengler DM, et al: A longitudinal prospective study of acute back problems. The influence of physical and non-physical factors (abstract). Presented at the International Society for the Study of the Lumbar Spine, Kyoto, Japan, May 1989.
7. Bigos SJ, Battie MC, Spengler DM, et al: A longitudinal study of work perceptions and psychosocial factors affecting the report of back injury. *Spine* 1991; 16:1–6.
8. Bureau of National Affairs: *Back Injuries: Costs, Causes, Cases and Prevention*. Washington, DC, Bureau of National Affairs, 1988.
9. Carlsson AM: Assessment of chronic pain. 1. Aspects of the reliability and validity of the visual analogue scale. *Pain* 1983; 16:87–101.
10. Chaffin DB, Park KS: A longitudinal study of low back pain as associated with occupational weight lifting factors. *Am Ind Hyg Assoc J* 1973; 34:513–525.
11. Clark W, Haldeman S: The development of guideline factors for the evaluation of disability in neck and back injuries. *Spine,* in press.
12. Clark WL, Haldeman S, Johnson P, et al: Back impairment and disability determination. Another attempt at objective, reliable rating. *Spine* 1988; 13:332–341.
13. David GC: UK national statistics on handling accidents and lumbar injuries at work. *Ergonomics* 1985; 28:9–16.
14. DHSS: *Handbook for Industrial Injury Medical Boards*. London, HMSO, 1986.
15. Dillane JB, Fry J, Kalton G: Acute back syndrome—a study from general practice. *Br Med J* 1966; 2:82–84.
16. Engelberg AL (ed): *Guides to the Evaluation of Permanent Impairment,* ed 3. Chicago, American Medical Association, 1988.
17. Fitton F, Temple B, Acheson HW: The cost of prescribing in general practice. *Social Science Med* 1985; 21:1097–1105.
18. Frymoyer JW, Pope MH, Clemens JH, et al: Risk factors in low back pain. *J Bone Joint Surg [Am]* 1983; 65:213–218.
19. Greenwood JG: Low back impairment rating practices of orthopaedic surgeons and neurosurgeons in West Virginia. *Spine* 1985; 10:773–776.
20. Greenwood JG: Work related back ache and neck injury cases in West Virginia. *Orthop Rev* 1985; 14:53–61.
21. Haldeman S, Shouka M, Robboy S: Computerized tomography, electrodiagnostic and clinical findings in chronic workers' compensation patients with back and leg pain. Presented at the International Society for the Study of the Lumbar Spine, Rome, May 1987.
22. Keeley J, et al: Quantification of lumbar function. Part 5: Reliability of range of motion measures in the sagittal plane and an in vivo torso rotation measurement technique. *Spine* 1986; 11:31–35.
23. Kelsey JL, Githens PB, O'Conner T, et al: Acute prolapsed lumbar intervertebral disc—an epidemiologic study with special reference to driving automobiles and cigarette smoking. *Spine* 1984; 9:608–613.
24. Klein BP, Jensen RC, Sanderson LM: Assessment of workers compensation claims for back strains/sprains. *J Occup Med* 1984; 26:443–448.
25. Leavitt SS, Johnston TL, Beyer RD: The process of recov-

ery: Patterns in industrial injury, Part I. Costs and other quantitative measures of effort. *Ind Med Surg* 1971; 40:7–14.

26. Leavitt SS, Johnston TL, Beyer RD: The process of recovery: Patterns in industrial back injury, Part 2. *Ind Med Surg* 1971; 40:7–15.
27. Magora A: Investigation of the relationship between low back pain and occupation. *Ind Med Surg* 1972; 41:5–9.
28. Main CJ: The modified somatic perception questionnaire. *J Psychosom Res* 1983; 27:503–514.
29. Mayer TG, Tencer AF, Kristoferson S, et al: Use of noninvasive techniques for quantification of spinal range of motion in normal subjects and chronic low back dysfunction patients. *Spine* 1984; 9:588–595.
30. Melzack R: The McGill pain questionnaire; major properties and scoring methods. *Pain* 1975; 1:277–299.
31. Minnesota Medical Association: *Worker's Compensation Permanent Partial Disability Schedule*. Minneapolis, Minnesota Medical Association, 1984.
32. National Center for Health Statistics: *Prevalence of Selected Impairments, United States, 1971*. Hyattsville, Md, DHHS Publication No (PHS) 75-1526, Series 10, No 99, 1975.
33. National Center for Health Statistics: *Prevalence of Selected Impairments, United States, 1981*. Hyattsville, Md, DHHS Publication No (PHS) 87-1587, Series 10, No 159, 1986.
34. National Institute for Occupational Safety and Health: *A Work Practice Guide for Manual Lifting*. Cincinnati, US Department of Health and Human Services, Report 81–122, 1981.
35. Porter RW: Does hard work prevent disc protrusion? *Clin Biomech* 1987; 2:196–198.
36. Ransford AO, Cairnes D, Mooney V: The pain drawing as an aide to the psychological evaluation of patients with low back pain. *Spine* 1976; 1:127–134.
37. Social Security Administration: *Disability Evaluation Under Social Security: A Handbook for Physicians*. Washington, DC, HEW Publication (SSA) 79–10089, 1979.
38. Troup JDG, Martin JW, Lloyd CEF: Back pain in industry—a prospective survey. *Spine* 1981; 6:61–69.
39. United States Department of Health and Human Services: *Report of the Commission on the Evaluation of Pain*. Washington, DC, US Government Printing Office, SSA Publication No 640–031, 1987.
40. Waddell G, Main CJ: Assessment of severity in low back disorders. *Spine* 1987; 12:632–644.
41. Waddell G, Main CJ, Morris EW, et al: Chronic low back pain, psychologic distress and illness behaviour. *Spine* 1984; 9:209–213.
42. Waddell G, Main CJ, Morris EW, et al: Normality and reliability in the clinical assessment of backache. *Br Med J* 1982; 284:1519–1523.
43. Waddell G, McCulloch JA, Kummell E, et al: Non-organic physical signs in low back pain. *Spine* 1980; 5:117–125.
44. Waikar AM, Schlegal RE, Lee KS: Strength tests for evaluation of low back injuries. *Trends Ergonom Hum Factors* 1986; 9:667–674.
45. Wood DJ: Design and evaluation of a back injury prevention program within a geriatric hospital. *Spine* 1987; 12:77–82.

8

Radiologic Imaging Techniques of the Spine

Charles Aprill, M.D.

> A little learning is a dang'rous thing;
> Drink deep, or taste not the Pierian spring:
> There shallow draughts intoxicate the brain,
> and drinking largely sobers us again.
>
> Alexander Pope, *An Essay on Criticism*[82]

A survey of the literature involving radiologic investigations of spine disorders will reveal reports of specific diagnoses defined by certain techniques. However, one can find other studies pointing out the poor predictive value of these same procedures.[36, 90] In this chapter, there will be no attempt to champion any specific technique. Rather, this work will survey a variety of methods for investigating the patient with complaints of pain presumably arising from a derangement of the spine. It will necessarily be incomplete. It is hoped that this survey will prompt the interested reader to a more in-depth study of those techniques found most applicable to his individual clinical practice.

Two categories of diagnostic investigation will be apparent. The *imaging* studies provide primarily morphologic information. Some of the invasive procedures may be referred to as *provocation/analgesic* tests.[62] These procedures provide information about morphology but by their nature provide insight into the association of deranged morphology and symptomatology.

The functioning spine is a segmented chain of bony elements with soft-tissue linkages and specific regional curves. The osseous components, vertebrae, are composed of cylindrical blocklike bodies anteriorly and rounded arches bearing several processes posteriorly. The soft-tissue linkages are the sites at which segmental motion occurs. The anterior component of the motion segment is the intervertebral disc, and the posterior component is the paired zygapophyseal joints. The anterior column and posterior elements form an osseoligamentous tunnel, the central canal, extending the full length of the spine. Paired lateral openings, root canals, are located at each segment below C1. These spaces serve as conduits for neural elements and major vascular plexuses. The chapter is divided into four major sections:

1. Segmentation and alignment
2. Anterior column
3. Posterior elements
4. Spaces and contents

SEGMENTATION AND ALIGNMENT

Segmentation

Basic to labeling of the spine is knowledge of the underlying pattern of regional segmentation. In the usual case, there are 7 cervical, 12 dorsal, and 5 lumbar segments that can be individually recognized on routine frontal and lateral radiographs. The five sacral segments form a bony conglomerate. Alterations of this standard pattern are quite common.

The presence of supernumerary ribs on the seventh cervical vertebra, "cervical ribs," is not rare. This represents "dorsalization" of the seventh cervical vertebra. This condition is recognized on routine frontal radiographs. Although usually of no clinical significance relative to the spine, it may be associated with syndromes involving compromise of the neurovascular bundle at the cervicothoracic junction. Apical tumors (Pancoast) may produce neck and arm symptoms simulating cervical pathology and can be recognized on frontal views.[61]

Failures of segmentation in the cervical spine are not uncommon. Congenital fusions (block vertebrae) are readily recognized on routine lateral radiographs. Failure of segmentation between the occiput and C1 (occipitalization of the C1 ring) is a significant anomaly.[51] It may be associated with abnormal enlargement of the dens and compromise of space available for the cervical cord. More common congenital fusions at the mid or lower cervical segments are significant in their frequent association with developmental narrowing of the central canal.[68]

The anomalies of segmentation in the lumbar area usually involve the junctional zones (thoracolumbar, lumbosacral). They result in an unusual number of lumbar-appearing vertebrae. An accessory rib on L1 or complete sacralization of L5 results in four lumbar-appearing vertebrae. Aplasia of the 12th rib or complete lumbarization of S1 results in six lumbar-appearing vertebrae. Although these conditions may be of little clinical significance, they can be a point of confusion if the segments are not labeled in a consistent manner. Consider the patient with complete sacralization of L5. The lumbosacral junction is anatomically the L4–5 segment. Herniation of the disc immediately above the lumbosacral junction represents pathology of the L3–4 disc. A myelographer, recognizing the anomaly, would report herniation at L3–4. The axial computed tomographic (CT) appearance of the lumbosacral junction provides no clue as to the segmentation anomaly. The interpreter of the CT scan, with no knowledge of the segmentation anomaly, might report the herniation to be at L4–5.

Asymmetrical fixation of the lumbosacral segment is a common normal variant and represents a partial transitional state. Such vertebrae bear a large transverse process on one side that articulates or is fused with the sacrum and a lumbar-type transverse process on the other side. L5 may be partially sacralized or S1 partially lumbarized. Knowledge of the spine segmentation pattern is essential to labeling of transitional segments (Fig 8–1). CT and magnetic resonance imaging (MRI) may not provide sufficient information for labeling.

The author follows simple rules when labeling diagnostic studies of the lumbar spine:

1. When there is an apparent anomaly of segmentation, review a frontal radiograph that includes all lumbar segments.
2. If the pattern is not clear, survey the entire spine. All humans have the same total number of vertebrae between the occiput and the first sacral segment, 24. The 24th vertebra is always labeled L5 (Fig 8–1), and the next caudad segment is S1. Accordingly, there can be no L6 vertebra (what would the L6 nerve innervate?). Similarly, the designation L4–S1 is improper (where is the L5 nerve?).

Partial transitional segments at the lumbosacral junction are considered to be of little clinical consequence. However, asymmetrical fixation alters the manner in which forces are distributed. This may result in structural adaptations and/or failure of specific components and cause a clinically significant condition. CT is particularly helpful in assessing the transitional lumbosacral segment (Fig 8–2).

Alignment

Alterations of alignment are far more common than segmentation variants but are also best demonstrated by the global view of the spine provided by routine radiographs. Scoliosis and the associated rotational deformities of the spine are quite complex, and the detailed analysis by routine film and planar imaging techniques (conventional tomography, CT, and MRI) are beyond the scope of this survey. Similarly, major fracture/dislocation will not be discussed.

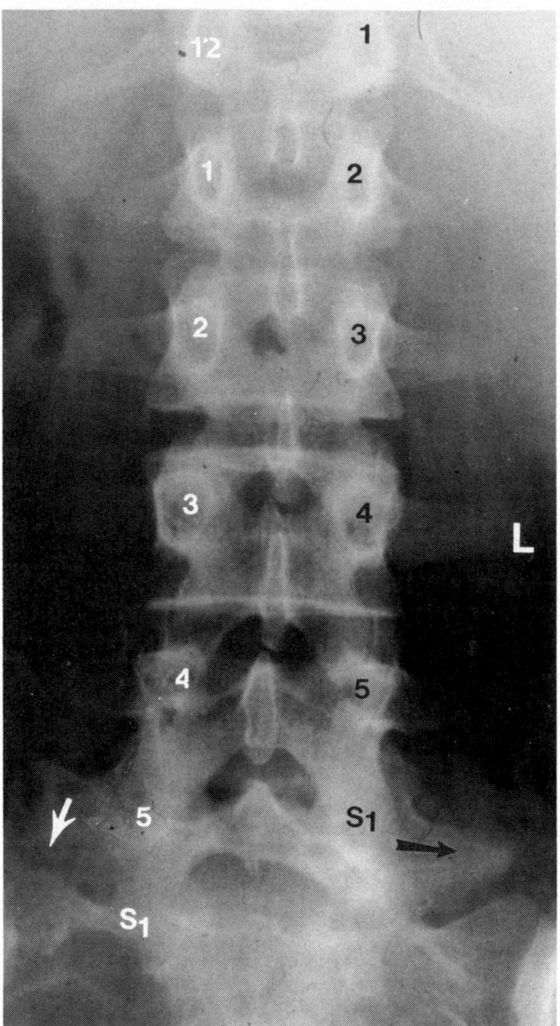

FIG 8–1.
Frontal radiograph of the lumbar spine with a segmentation anomaly: asymmetrical fixation of the lumbosacral segment. There is a lumbar-type transverse process on the left *(black arrow)* and a large process fused to the sacrum on the right *(white arrow)*. The labeling on the left *(black numbers)* is appropriate when the spine survey demonstrates a supernumerary rib on L1. The labeling on the right *(white numbers)* is appropriate when the spine survey demonstrates an usual cervical and dorsal segmentation pattern (7 cervical, 12 dorsal).

An important feature of alignment is the smooth lordotic curve characteristic of the normal cervical and lumbar spine. Proper exposure of lateral radiographs is necessary to ensure visualization of all segments. The junctional segments (C7–T1 in the cervical and L5–S1 in the lumbar region) are difficult to visualize in some patients. Evaluation is inadequate unless these segments are clearly demonstrated.

Alterations of the cervical lordotic curve are common and nonspecific. They may simply be the result of poor posture at the time of filming. It is imperative that radiographs be obtained with the patient in the neutral, true lat-

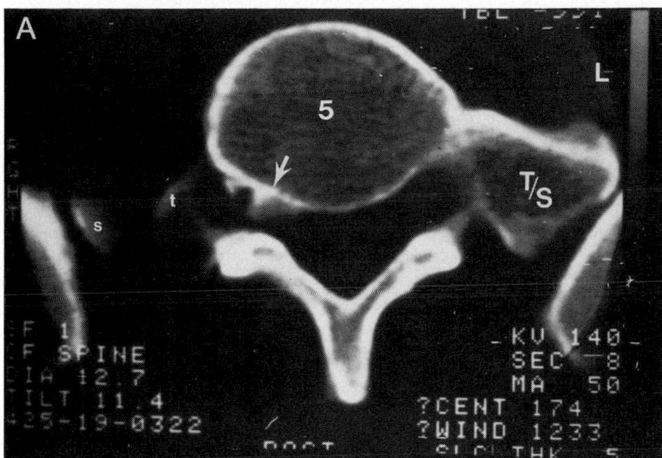

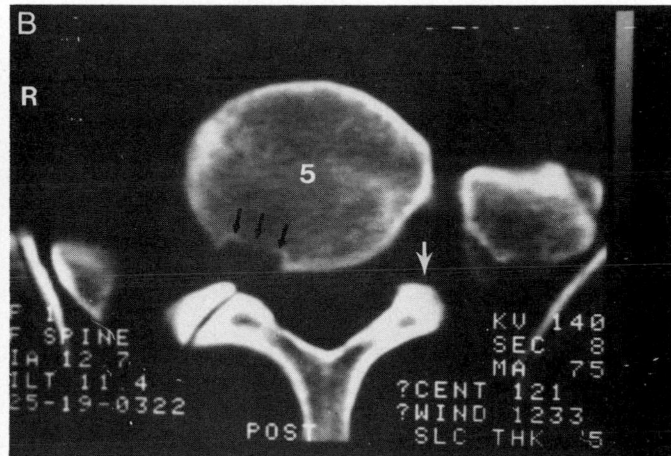

FIG 8–2.
Axial CT through the lower portion of the L5 vertebra. A frontal radiograph confirms the transitional L5 segment with a large transverse process fused to the sacrum on the left. **A,** large transverse process/sacral fusion *(T/S)* on the left. Note the smaller transverse process *(t)* separate from the sacral ala *(s)* on the right. A bony ridge has formed at the right posterolateral end plate and is projecting into the midzone of the L5–S1 root canal *(white arrow)*. **B,** section slightly below **A.** Note the small size of the articular processes on the left *(white arrow)*. This is common on the side of fixation. The articular processes on the right are normally developed. A notchlike defect in the inferior L5 end plate *(black arrows)* may represent the site of annular avulsion associated with chronic stresses. The marginal ridge seen in **A** conceivably represents the body's attempt to heal this lesion.

eral position. Reduction of the usual lordosis[96] or angular reversal of the cervical curve may be the result of soft-tissue damage (Fig 8–3). Persistent deformity following acceleration injuries (whiplash) is a poor prognostic sign, particularly in patients with pre-existing degenerative disease.[52] This combination favors early aggressive diagnostic evaluation.

Dynamic, flexion/extension radiographs of the cervical spine are commonly obtained in clinical practice. Their value is difficult to assess. The instantaneous axis of rotation of cervical segments has been carefully measured. It has been shown that by detailed analysis normal individuals can be differentiated from patients with neck pain on the basis of the position of the instantaneous axis of rotation.[1, 3] However, the technique is complex and not readily applicable to the routine clinical setting.

In the patient with upper cervical pain and cervicocephalgia, pathology at the C1–2 segment must be considered. Flexion/extension lateral radiographs are important in evaluating the C1–2 relationship. Separation of C1 from the anterior surface of the dens by only a few millimeters (in flexion) may reflect injury to the transverse ligament.[29] Open-mouth frontal views are also important in assessing the integrity of the dens and the relative position of C1.

CT scanning plays an important role in the assessment of C1–2 pathology. Because of the complex anatomy, some fractures may not be apparent on routine radiographs. Occult fractures may be obvious on axial CT (Fig 8–4). Rotation at C1–2 can be characterized by functional CT. Recent elegant studies have reported motion in normal subjects and patients with abnormalities.[21, 66] These highly specialized examinations should be reserved for those patients in whom there is strong clinical suspicion of dysfunctional movement at the C1–2 segment. Alterations of the lumbar lordosis may occur with a compression fracture or following surgery. In the absence of such specific pathology, reduced lordosis, as in the cervical region, is abnormal but nonspecific.

Flexion/extension radiographs are commonly obtained to assess "stability." Their predictive value is poor. There is an overlap in the range of motion of asymptomatic subjects and patients with documented instability.[37] Abnormal motion of the unstable spine may be restricted by pain and muscle spasm.[20, 33] Finally, the reliability of lateral radiographic measurement techniques has been questioned.[79]

Understanding patterns of segmentation and alignment is important in assessing individuals with complaints of spinal pain. The relative significance of any imaging finding can only be assessed in the light of accurate clinical correlation.

ANTERIOR COLUMN

Vertebral Bodies

The lateral radiograph demonstrates the unique configuration of the C1–2 complex and the C2 vertebral body. The C3 through C7 vertebrae have similar configurations on lateral radiographs. The appearance of the C3 through C6 vertebrae is similar on axial CT. The axial appearance of C7 is easily recognized by the absence of anterior tubercles on the transverse processes. The lumbar vertebral bodies are all similar in appearance on lateral radiographs.

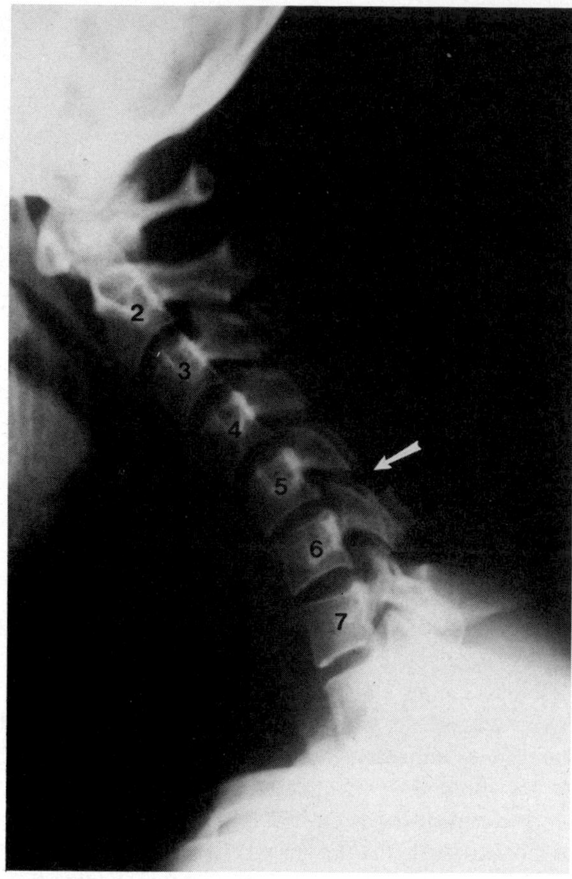

FIG 8–3.
Lateral radiograph of the cervical spine showing an angular kyphos deformity at C5/6 *(white arrow)* with no obvious fracture. The status of the posterior annulus, posterior longitudinal ligament, and capsular ligaments of the C5–6 facet joints cannot be determined, and further evaluation is warranted based on the clinical setting and symptomatology (see Fig 8–17,B).

Configuration of the L1 through L4 vertebrae is similar on axial CT. The transverse processes of L3 are usually the longest. In the axial plane, the configuration of L5 is characteristic with broad pedicles.

Routine radiographs are sensitive to distortions of vertebral configuration. Fractures, both acute and healed, are readily seen. The radiograph is less sensitive to pathology occurring within the vertebral bodies. Tumor (primary or metastatic) or benign bone destruction (infectious or metabolic) may alter bone density. However, such pathology may not be detected on routine film until the cortex of the body is involved. Radionuclide scanning is far more sensitive to intraosseous pathology but is nonspecific (Fig 8–5).

MRI is valuable in evaluating osseous pathology. It can detect alterations of the marrow space constituents associated with normal maturation. MRI may be the most sensitive method of detecting neoplastic and inflammatory disease.[7, 55]

End Plates

MacNab[48] described the appearance of bony flanges or ridges at lumbar intervertebral end plates. The "traction spur," seen as a small ridge near the end plate, has been suggested to be an indication of instability. Larger osteophytic ridges (claw spondylophytes) are suggested to be associated with chronic stresses at the annular/end plate insertion.[57] It is important to realize that these findings are related to the outermost fibers of the annulus and do not reflect the status of the nucleus (Fig 8–6). Massive proliferation of bone at the end plates is seen in patients with disseminated idiopathic skeletal hyperostosis.[71] The finding is unrelated to primary disc pathology. MRI is capable of detecting changes in the marrow space adjacent

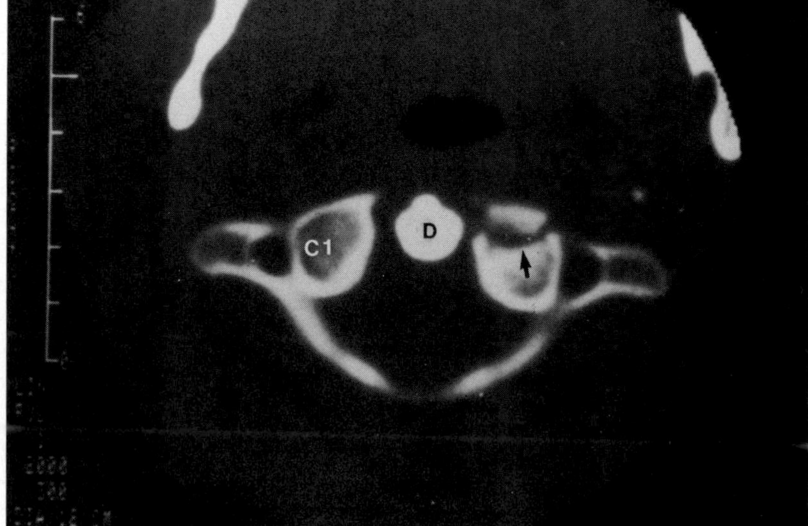

FIG 8–4.
Axial CT of the upper part of the cervical spine. A 1.5-mm section through the lateral masses of C1 shows a fracture *(black arrow)* on the left. The dens *(D)* is eccentric in its relationship to the lateral masses. Injury to the C1–2 ligamentous complex must be suspected.

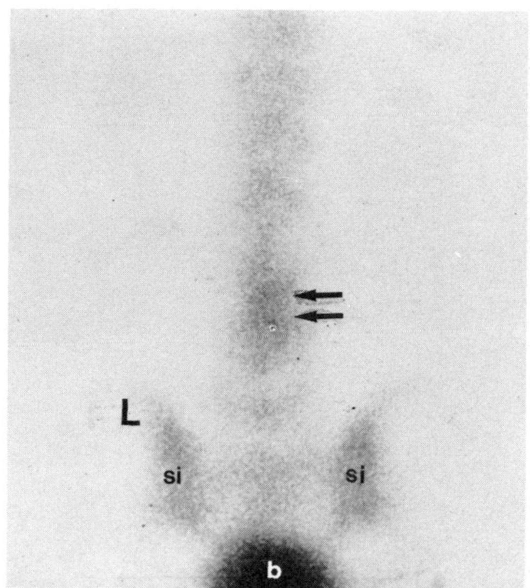

FIG 8–5.
Radionuclide bone scan, posterior view of the lumbar/lumbosacral region. There is normal accumulation of tracer in the bladder *(b)*. Activity in the sacroiliac joints *(si)* is symmetrical and normal. Activity in the midlumbar region *(black arrows)* is abnormal. The increased activity is in the region of the lower L3, upper L4 vertebral body. The scan image indicates a definite abnormality. A variety of clinical entities (osteomyelitis in the drug user, fracture in a trauma victim, incidental finding in a patient with large hypertrophic ridge formation at L3–4) may produce similar images.

to the end plates that reflect significant disc degeneration.[54]

Intervertebral Discs

Since the "dynasty of the disc" began (generally attributed to the paper of Mixter and Barr in 1934),[53] many practitioners base the worth of a diagnostic procedure on its ability to provide information regarding the status of the disc.

A primary indication for myelography over the past half century has been the assessment of patients with suspected disc herniation.[2] Diagnostic disc injection (discography) was developed specifically to address those patients in whom disc pathology was suspected clinically but not confirmed by myelography.[46] Among the first applications of CT and MRI to a study of the spine was evaluation of disc herniation.[23, 93]

Routine spine films provide no direct information about the intervertebral disc. Narrowing of the L4–5 motion segment has a slight positive correlation with an increased incidence of back pain.[34] Myelography provides only indirect information about the intervertebral disc. The myelogram can define extradural masses arising at the level of intervertebral discs. The addition of erect flexion and extension views provides some insight as to whether or not the epidural mass is fixed in size[94] (Fig 8–7). Integrity of the annulus and the specific position and configuration of the discal abnormality are left to speculation. Myelography is sensitive to masses that are in close proximity to the thecal sac. Accordingly, myelography will not effectively detect lateral herniations at any level in the spine and is relatively insensitive to central herniations at the L5–S1 segment because of the wide anterior epidural space. There have been numerous studies comparing CT and myelography.[15, 36, 69] For many practical reasons, CT is superior to myelography in assessing the intervertebral disc.

During the 1980s, the technology of CT matured. Current systems produce images of good spatial resolution. The major changes that have occurred in the last few years are related to speed of acquisition and processing. This technology has the advantage of familiarity and ready availability. The study is noninvasive but does involve radiation exposure. The number of segments evaluated in any survey is usually limited. Sections 4 to 5 mm in thickness are ideal to study the lumbar disc. The use of thin sections is not recommended in the lumbar spine because they are commonly associated with data starvation artifact and poor resolution. Thin sections (1.5 to 3.0 mm) are required to evaluate the cervical intervertebral discs. Thicker sections (4 mm or more) are unacceptable.

Images are acquired in the axial or transverse plane. CT provides direct visualization of the entire disc contour. The normal posterior annular contour of the upper four lumbar intervertebral discs is concave. The posterior margin of the L5–S1 disc is normally convex (Fig 8–8). The posterior contour of the normal cervical intervertebral disc is flat or slightly convex. The disc annulus may not be visible or may be seen as a very subtle convex zone of increased density at the disc space.

Abnormalities of disc contour may be classified as disc bulges or herniations. Disc bulge or protrusion of the annulus is a condition wherein the annular fibers are intact but have been weakened or stretched so that the disc margin projects beyond its usual confines. The most common example is the outward buckling of the annulus that occurs in spondylosis as a result of loss of disc height. The resulting circumferential protrusion is referred to as a diffuse annular bulge. Eccentric narrowing of the interspace results in bulging of only a portion of the disc annulus. Cadaveric studies suggest that large disc bulges are associated with concentric fissures in the outer margin of the annulus.[98]

Disc herniation implies a disruption of annular fibers and some displacement of discal tissue. Herniations may be divided into three types: prolapse, extrusion, and sequestration.

Prolapse refers to a contained herniation. The outermost fibers of the disc annulus remain intact and constrain abnormal annular or nuclear material. It is conceivable that

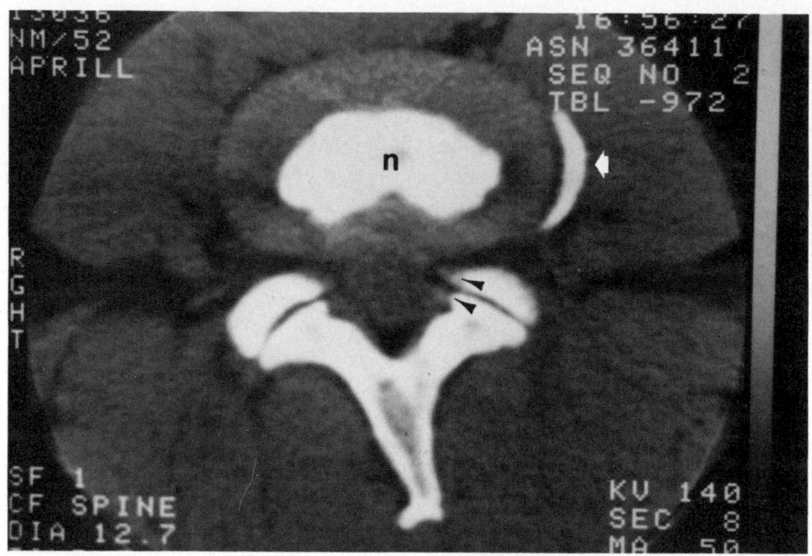

FIG 8–6.
Axial CT (postdiscography) at the L4–5 interspace. The pattern of contrast dispersal in the nuclear region *(n)* is normal, and contrast material does not extend into the annulus. The curvilinear zone of high density *(white arrow)* at the left lateral margin of the disc represents a moderate-sized spondylophyte. Small bony ridges are forming at the medial aspect of the left facet joint *(black arrowheads)*. These findings, in combination, suggest chronic left-sided stresses at this motion segment.

a condition exists wherein the annular fibers are stretched or weakened sufficient to allow a focal protrusion. The contour of the intervertebral disc would be abnormal, but the annular fibers would remain intact. Such a lesion would have an appearance identical to a small herniation (Fig 8–9). CT does not accurately assess the integrity of annular fibers.[92]

Disruption of the outermost annular fibers, including elements of the posterior longitudinal ligament, allows disc material to escape from the interspace. The result is disc *extrusion*. A mass of disc material projecting into the central canal a distance equal to half the sagittal diameter of the canal is likely to be an extruded fragment[32] (Fig 8–10).

Migration or displacement of extruded disc material is referred to as *sequestration*. Sequestered fragments are

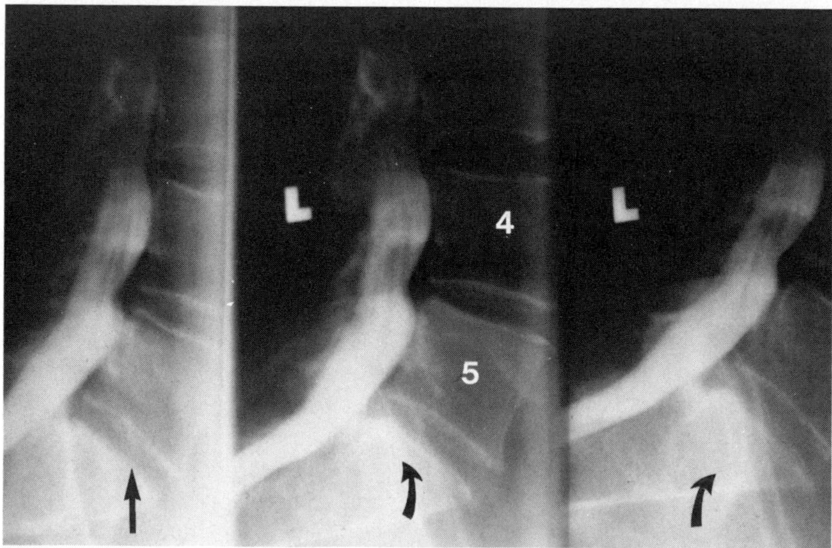

FIG 8–7.
Lumbar myelogram: erect lateral views in the neutral, extension, and flexion positions. The size and configuration of the extradural mass at L4–5 are relatively constant in these three positions.

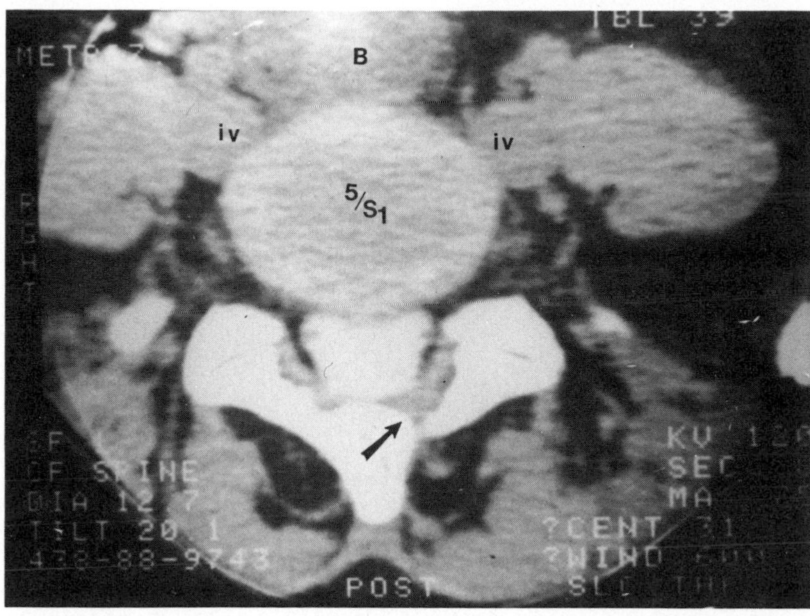

FIG 8–8.
Axial CT of the L5–S1 disc. This image was acquired several hours after lumbar myelography. Contrast material opacifies the thecal sac. The posterior disc margin is convex and projects into the central canal in the midline. This is the normal shape of the L5–S1 disc. Note the proximity of the iliac veins *(iv)* and loops of bowel *(B)* to the anterior margin of the disc. Asymmetry of the laminae and ligamentum flavum *(black arrow)* is a normal variant.

recognized by positions remote from the parent interspace (Fig 8–11). Cephalic or caudal migration may occur. When the abnormal mass lies behind the vertebral body near its midpoint, the differential diagnosis must include focal epidural hematoma. The CT appearance of a sequestered fragment and epidural hematoma may be identical.[45] When the sequestered fragment migrates laterally into the root canal, the differential diagnosis includes composite root sleeve anomaly,[67] primary neurogenic neoplasm, or metastatic tumor.[44]

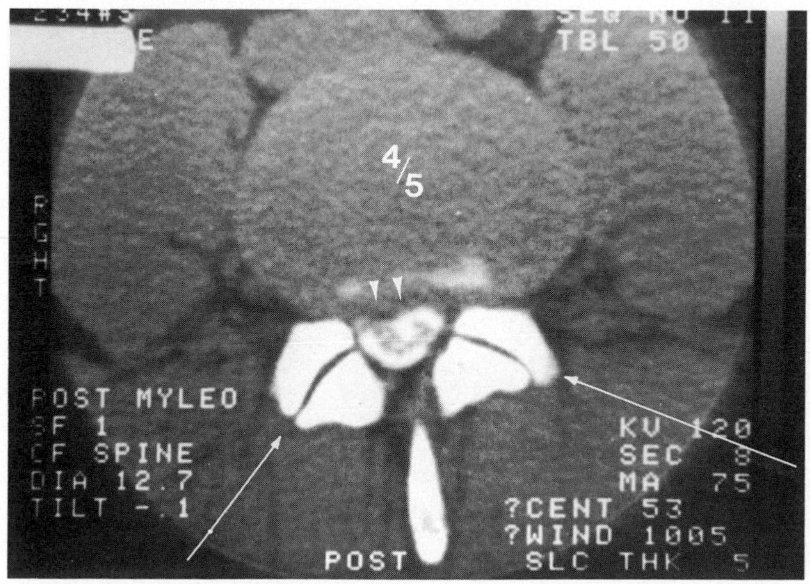

FIG 8–9.
CT of the L4–5 disc acquired after lumbar myelography. There is a definite impression on the right anterior aspect of the opacified thecal sac *(arrowheads)*. The disc contour is abnormal. CT does not differentiate between a focal disc bulge with intact annular fibers and a small contained herniation (prolapse). The scan also demonstrates asymmetry in the orientation of the facet joints (articular tropism) *(arrows)*.

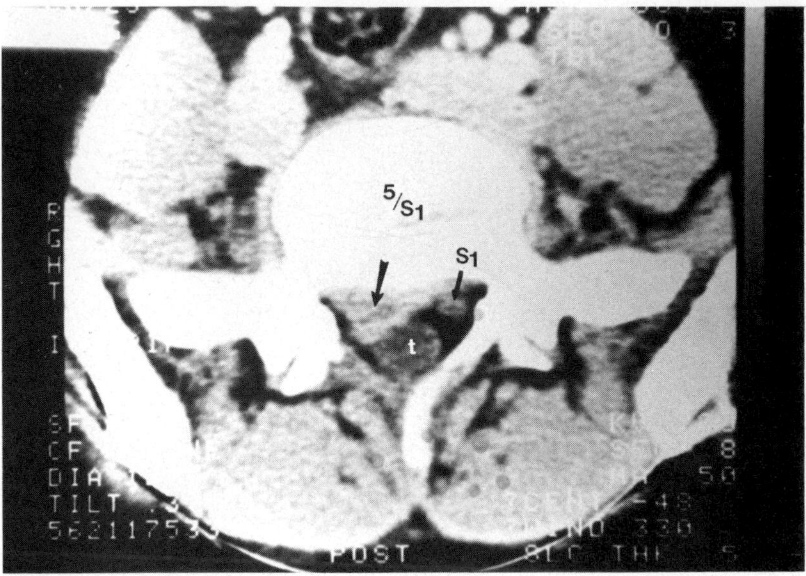

FIG 8–10.
Axial CT of the L5–S1 interspace: sections through the lower portion of the disc and the upper S1 end plate. A soft-tissue–density mass projects into the right anterior central canal *(large arrow)*. The mass does not affect the left S1 dural root sleeve and nerve *(small arrow)* but does slightly deform the right side of the thecal sac *(t)*. The right S1 dural root sleeve cannot be identified but is obviously displaced by the mass lesion. This image is typical of disc extrusion.

Modern systems can generate satisfactory reformatted images in multiple planes. Reformations of the axial data in both the sagittal and coronal planes can be useful in defining the size, shape, and position of disc fragments (Fig 8–12).

Large cervical disc herniations are easily recognized. Smaller lesions are difficult to visualize because of the relative paucity of epidural fat in the cervical region. The infusion of intravenous contrast material aids in definition of tissue planes. This may enhance visualization of small ex-

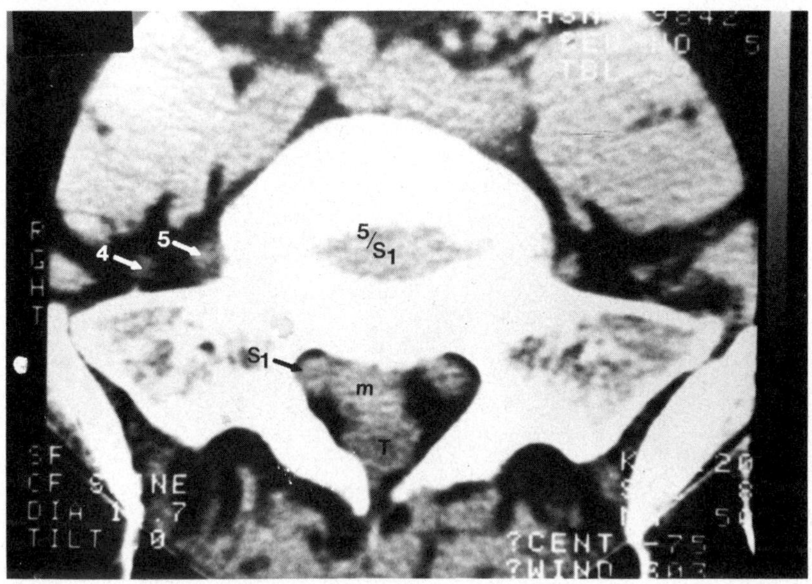

FIG 8–11.
Axial CT of a vertical gantry section through the L5–S1 interspace and upper sacral canal. The thecal sac *(T)* and the S1 dural root sleeves *(S1)* are identified. A soft-tissue–density mass *(m)* occupies the anterior epidural space immediately behind the S1 body. The mass was not connected to the disc space on review of adjacent images and represents a sequestered disc fragment that has migrated caudally. The L4 and L5 segmental nerves form the lumbosacral trunk and lie immediately anterior to the sacral alae.

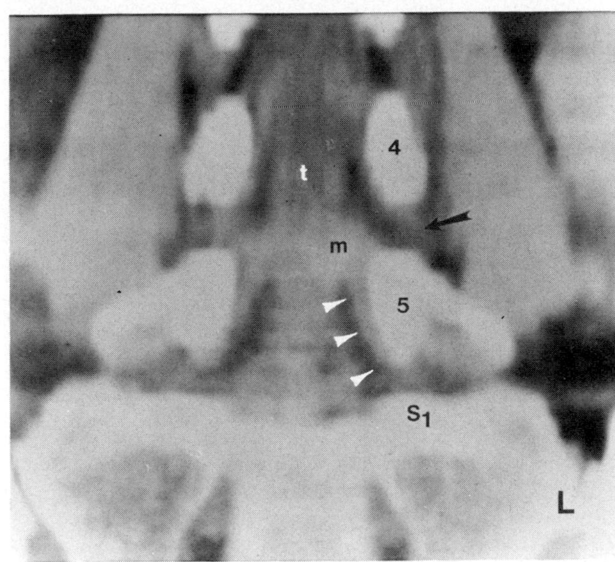

FIG 8-12.
Lumbar CT: coronal reformatted section through the anterior central canal. Left-sided herniation of the L4-5 disc is seen as an intermediate-density mass *(m)*. A lesion deforms the thecal sac *(t)* and compromises the left L5 segmental nerve *(arrowheads)* in the entrance zone of the L5-S1 root canal. The mass does not affect the L4 nerve *(black arrow)*.

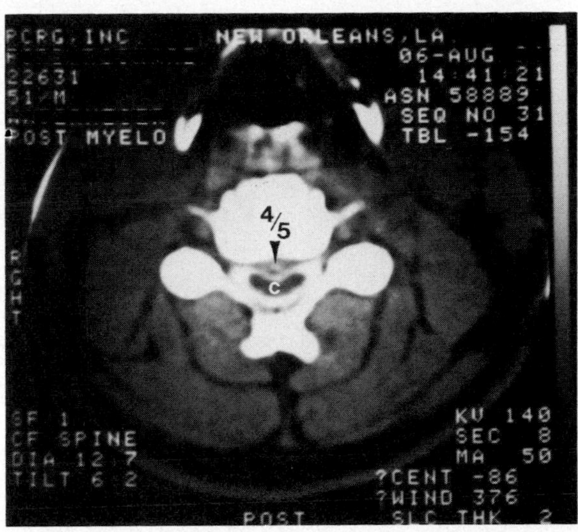

FIG 8-13.
Axial CT of the C4-5 motion segment acquired 4 hours postmyelography. A moderate-sized central disc herniation (prolapse) deforms the thecal sac in the midline *(black arrowhead)*. The cord *(c)* is deformed but not displaced. Symptoms include neck pain with no clinical manifestations of cervical myelopathy.

tradural lesions. However, pathologic impressions on the thecal sac are more conspicuous with intrathecal contrast enhancement (Fig 8-13). Posterolateral lesions result in asymmetrical filling of the dural root sleeves. Although this may be the result of posterolateral disc herniation, bony hypertrophy at uncovertebral articulations is a more common cause. The lowest cervical segment is difficult to adequately visualize by CT. The thickness of the shoulders in conjunction with the need to employ thin sections often results in "noisy" images. In stout patients, the lower two or three cervical segments may not be adequately visualized.

The development of surface coil technology in the mid-1980s[23] established MRI as a reasonable alternative to myelography and CT in the study of intervertebral disc disease. Despite rapid proliferation, the availability of MRI is still limited by comparison to the other techniques. MRI is noninvasive, does not involve ionizing radiation, and allows visualization of multiple segments. Images may be obtained directly in any desired plane of view. This technology is in rapid evolution. Clearly defined standards have not been established and have resulted in a variety of imaging protocols. This results in uneven technical quality and interpretation of the studies.

MRI can produce high-quality images of the intervertebral discs. Different chemical characteristics of tissues can be exploited by the use of a variety of pulse sequences. Spin-echo (SE) pulse sequences have been most commonly employed. SE T1-weighted images (repetition time [TR] 400-800/echo time [TE] 20-40) provide the best anatomic information. The spatial resolution of SE T1-weighted images is sufficient to evaluate disc contour (Fig 8-14).

The soft-tissue resolution of MRI provides direct visualization of internal disc structure. Good-quality SE proton-density and T2-weighted images (TR 1800-2000/TE 80-120) differentiate the nucleus from the outer ligamentous annulus of the normal disc. The intensity of signal is proportional to the water content of the proteoglycan matrix. The nuclear zone is seen as an area of high or bright signal in comparison to the low signal of the ligamentous annulus[39] (Fig 8-15). Reduction of SE T2 signal implies degradation of the nuclear matrix.[35]

SE T2 sequences require long acquisition times. The patients must remain still for periods in excess of 10 to 15 minutes. Patient movement can result in image degradation. A variety of techniques have been developed to address this problem.[64, 76] Gradient-echo (GRE) techniques are particularly effective. GRE images are acquired in much shorter time than standard SE T2 images. The shorter scan time reduces the likelihood of patient motion.

The contrast of GRE images is referred to as T2* (tee-two-star). The appearance is superficially similar to that of SE T2 images. Both sequences produce images demonstrating bright cerebrospinal fluid (CSF). The advantages of speedy acquisition and good quality have prompted some imagers to forego the longer, more troublesome SE T2 sequences.

However, the SE T2 and GRE images do not provide

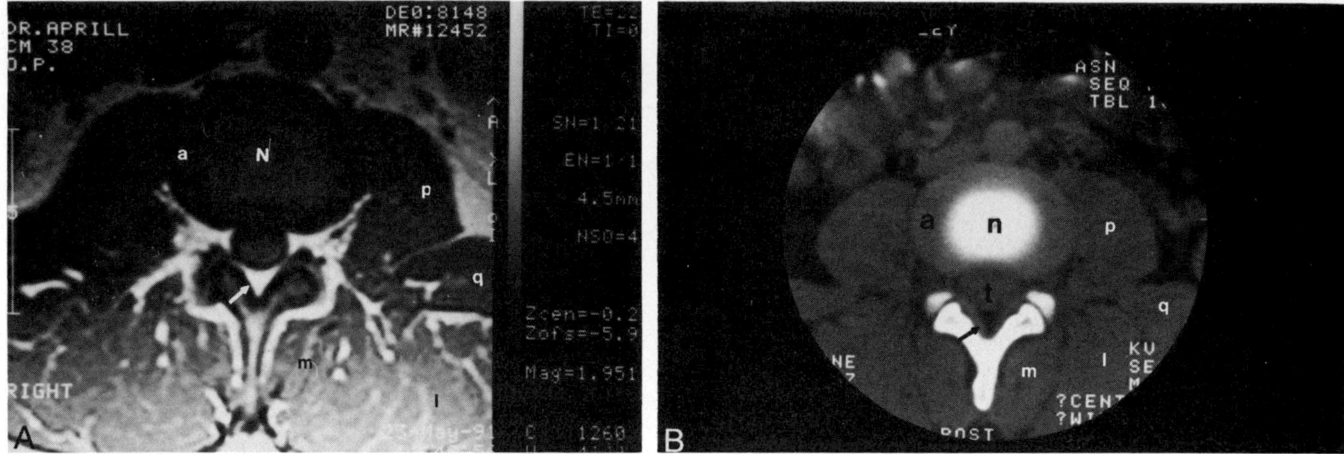

FIG 8–14.
A, lumbar MRI, 0.6 tesla, surface coil acquisition, SE T1 sequence (TR 780/TE 22), 4.5-mm thickness. A section through the L3–4 intervertebral disc shows normal disc contour. The outer annulus *(a)* is identified by its low signal. The disc margin is sharply defined. The nucleus and transitional zone *(N)* do produce some signal by virtue of the greater percentage of proteoglycans and higher water content. The resulting slightly gray appearance is barely discernible. The psoas *(p)*, quadratus lumborum *(q)*, multifidus *(m)*, and lumbar longissimus *(l)* can all be identified on this section. The posterior epidural fat pad *(arrow)* is identified on SE T1 images as a triangular zone of bright signal. **B,** axial CT at the L3–4 disc (postdiscography). The disc annulus *(a)* is relatively thick except at the posterior margin of the disc. The annulus has intermediate density on CT images. Contrast fills the nucleus *(n)*, which has a normal configuration. At this particular window/center setting, the contrast material can be differentiated from bone. However, the disc annulus and thecal sac *(t)* have very similar densities and are not easily differentiated. The posterior epidural fat pad *(arrow)* is recognized by the very low density of fat on CT images.

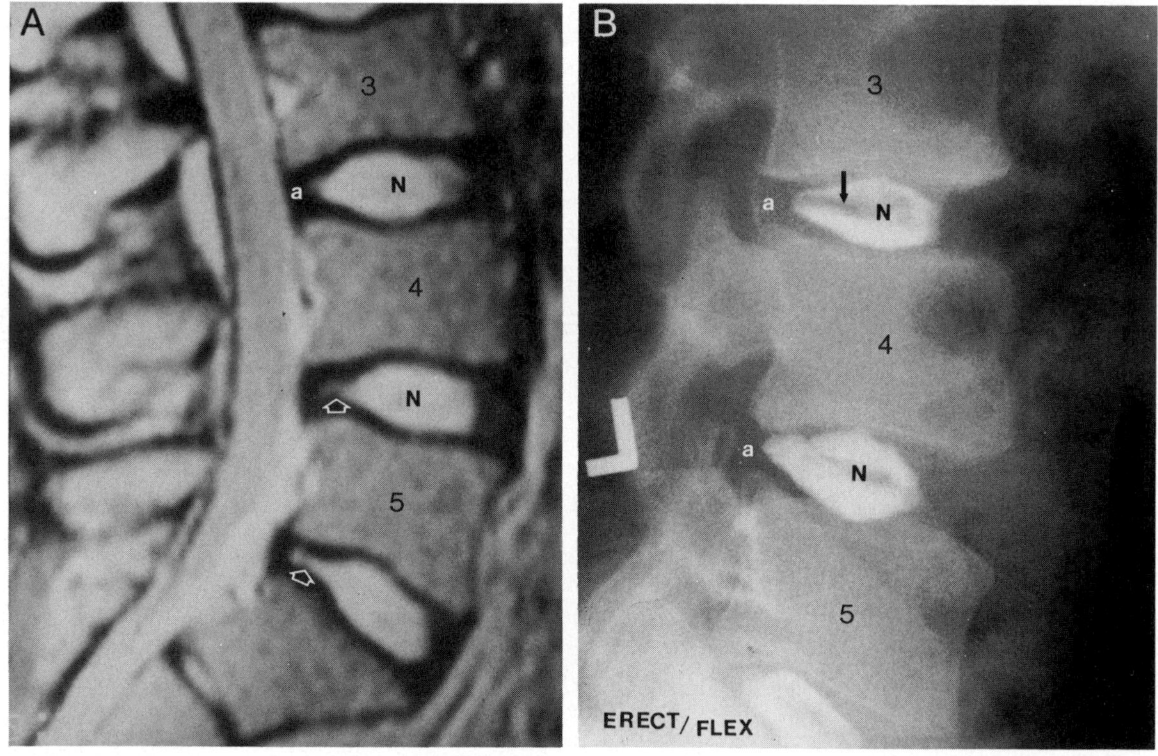

FIG 8–15.
A, sagittal MRI of the lower part of the lumbar spine, SE proton density (TR 1800/TE 40), 4.5-mm section thickness, 0.6 tesla. The nuclear signal is bright *(N)*. The outer annulus *(a)* is a continuous band of low signal, and the transitional zone *(arrows)* has an intermediate to bright signal at the margin of the nucleus. **B,** lateral view of the lumbar spine postdiscography. The nucleus *(N)* is opacified by contrast material. The outer annulus *(a)* is not directly visualized. The radiolucent line extending through the nucleus *(arrow)* represents a fibrous band within the structure of the nuclear matrix and is a normal finding. This film was obtained with the patient in the erect position and slightly flexed, which puts the maximum stress on the posterior nuclear-annular interface. This demonstrates the most posterior extent of the normal nucleus.

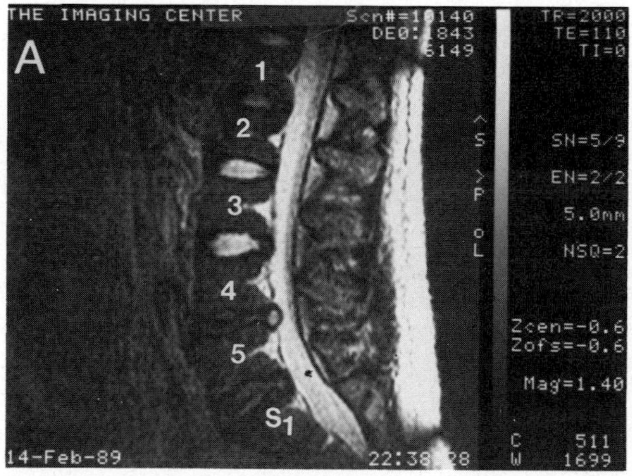

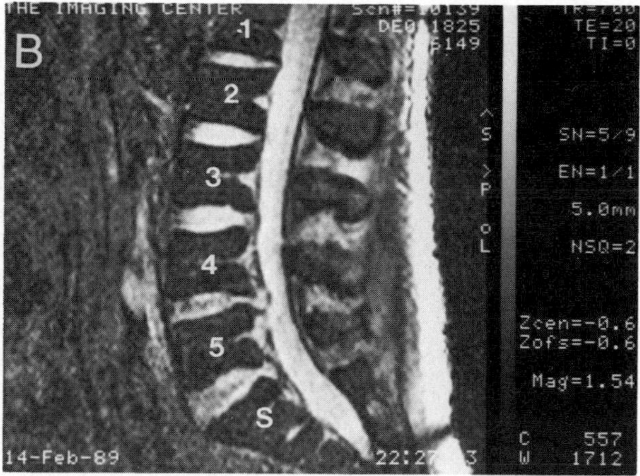

FIG 8–16.
Lumbar MRI, 0.6 tesla, midsagittal images, 5-mm thickness. **A,** SE T2 sequence (TR 2000/TE 110). A bright signal defines the nuclear zone of the normal L2–3 and L3–4 discs. The marked reduction of nuclear signal at L4–5 and L5–S1 reflects nuclear degradation. There is moderately large herniation at L4–5. The signal intensity within the herniated disc material is brighter than the "parent" nucleus. **B,** GRE image (TR 700/TE 20; flip angle, 30 degrees). Image contrast is similar to **A.** The signal intensity at the L4–5 and L5–S1 discs is much brighter than on the SE T2 sequence, and there is little difference in signal intensity between the prolapsed disc material and the "parent" nucleus. T2* contrast underestimates the severity of nuclear degradation. Compare the signal at L1–2. CSF is bright on both image sequences.

the same information about the intervertebral disc. The GRE images are not sensitive to subtle alterations of the nuclear matrix and will underestimate nuclear degradation (Fig 8–16). The signal intensity of herniated disc material may be brighter than that in the nucleus of the parent disc.[49] This phenomenon may reflect a local inflammatory process. It is not demonstrated on GRE images.

Visualization of the cervical cord and the ability to acquire direct sagittal images of good resolution are two advantages of MRI in the evaluation of cervical disc disease.

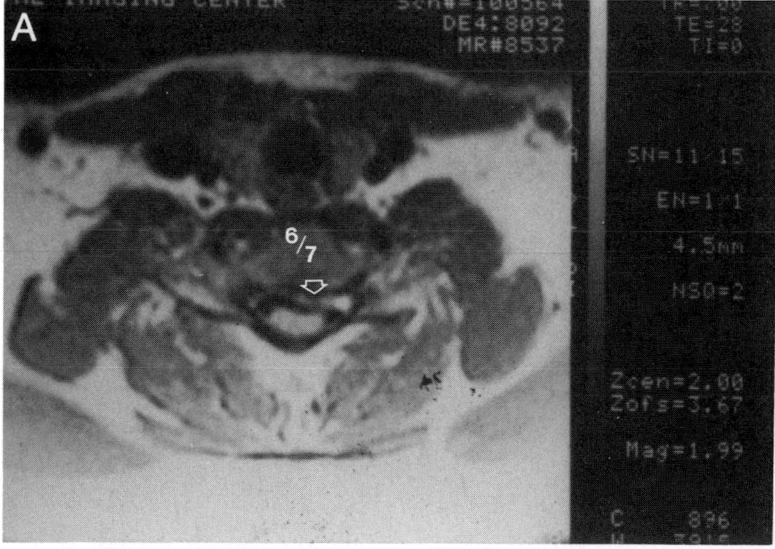

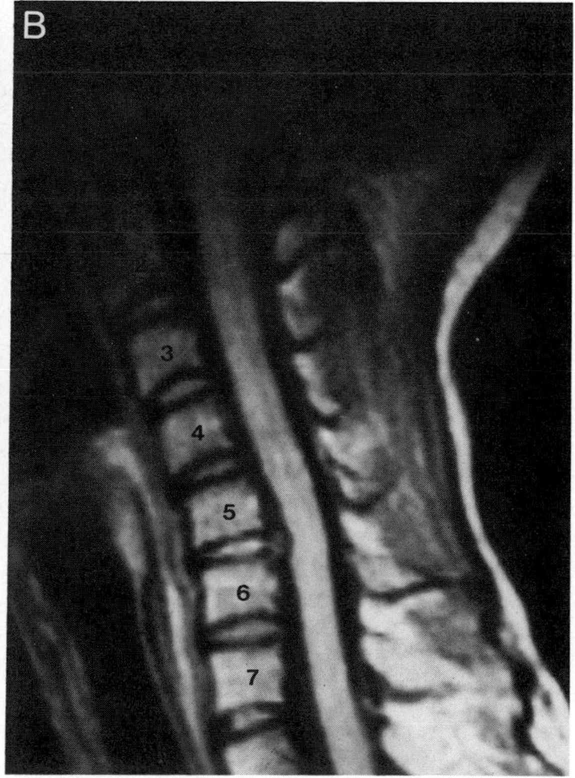

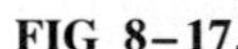
FIG 8–17.
A, cervical MRI, axial section through the C6–7 interspace, SE T1 (TR 700/TE 28), 4.5-mm thickness, 0.6 tesla. A moderately large left paracentral disc herniation *(open arrow)* deforms the left anterior thecal sac and displaces and slightly deforms the cervical cord. On SE T1 sequences, CSF has low signal, and the cord has intermediate signal. **B,** cervical MRI, midsagittal section, SE T1 sequence, 0.3 tesla. A moderately large disc herniation (prolapse) at C5–6 abuts and slightly deforms the anterior cervical cord. There is an angular kyphosis at C5–6 (same patient as in Fig 8–3).

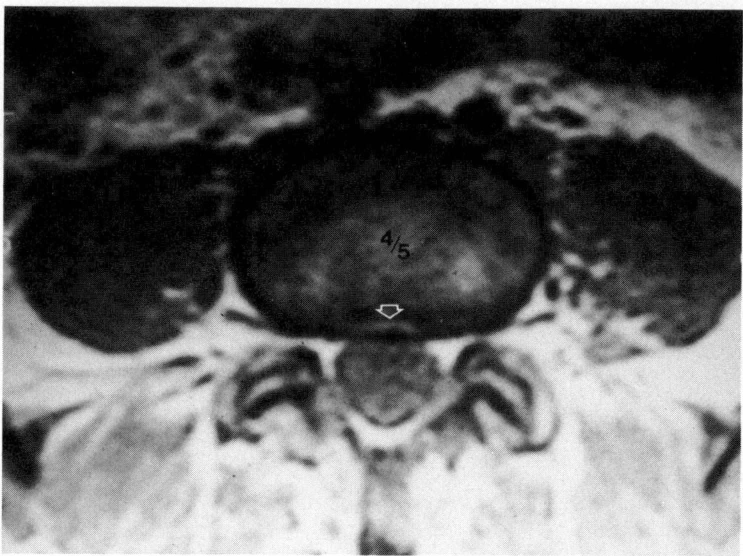

FIG 8–18.
Lumbar MRI, axial section through the L4–5 disc, SE T1 sequence. The linear zone of bright signal in the posterior of the annulus *(arrow)* represents a focal transverse fissure.

Herniations can be identified and their effect on the adjacent cord assessed noninvasively (Fig 8–17). GRE is effective in visualizing extradural pathology in the cervical spine.[26] The GRE technique is less effective in the evaluation of intradural disease.[84, 95]

Good-quality MRI of the cervical spine is difficult to obtain. Patient movement (physiologic or otherwise) often results in image degradation. The difficulty of differentiation of bony ridges from annular protrusion and the difficulty in assessing root canal stenosis by MRI are problems that may be resolved by continued improvement of the technology. However, these are areas in which CT scanning is effective and the studies are complementary.

Many patients present with neck and back pain complaints and no signs of nerve compression. Clinical studies suggest that the majority of back pain problems cannot be attributed to nerve compression.[31, 41] Such presentations suggest a somatic pain source. The disc annulus is innervated,[11] and pathology affecting the disc annulus must be considered a potential source of pain.

Pathoanatomic studies have shown that high-quality MRI can detect fissures in the annulus fibrosus in vitro.[98] Fissures of the disc annulus can be recognized in vivo[38] (Fig 8–18). The relative significance of these imaging findings with regard to back pain has not been definitely established. Enhancement of symptomatic annular tears or fissures following the infusion of gadolinium has been reported.[74] This invites speculation of inflammation, neovascularization, and/or invasion by granulation tissue in the damaged annulus as a cause of pain. This conjecture is

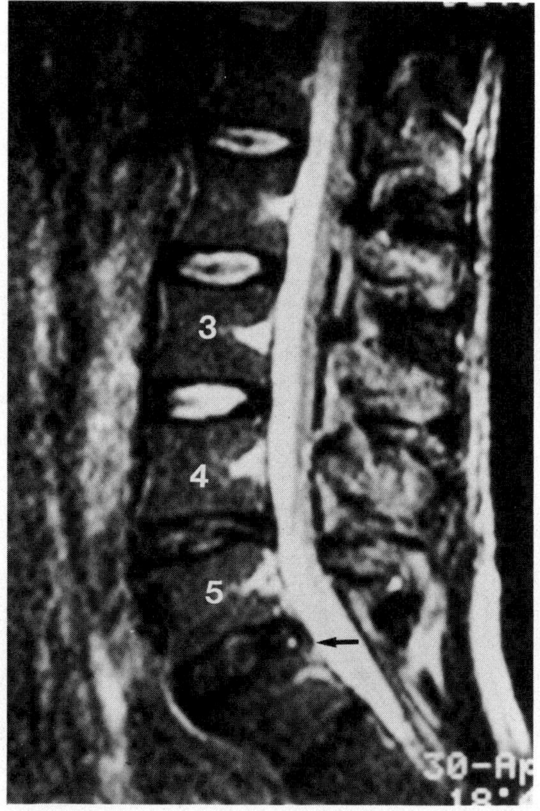

FIG 8–19.
Lumbar MRI, midsagittal section, SE T2 image (TR 2000/TE 120). There is normal signal intensity at the upper three lumbar discs and reduced signal intensity at the lower two lumbar discs. The area of bright signal (high-intensity zone) in the posteroinferior portion of the annulus of L5–S1 *(arrow)* represents a concentric annular fissure.

supported by the experimental demonstration of granulation tissue in traumatized discs.[58]

Some fissures are detected as zones of bright signal in the substance of the posterior part of the annulus on SE T2 images (Fig 8–19). This finding was recognized in 28% of 500 consecutive patients with complaints of back pain referred to the author's practice for lumbar MRI. Discography was performed on a small group of these patients. There was a strong correlation between the presence of a high-intensity zone in the disc annulus and reproduction of exact or similar pain on discography with a predictive value of 95%.[4] Diagnostic disc injection is the most accurate method of detecting and defining annular fissures. In a cadaveric study Yu et al. demonstrated that MRI performed under optimal conditions will detect only two thirds of the fissures that can be demonstrated by discography[97] (Fig 8–20). The accuracy of disc injection in defining the internal morphology of both normal and abnormal discs has been established.[27] Recent studies have reconfirmed the accuracy of postinjection imaging with both CT and MRI.[73]

Properly performed discography does not provoke pain in asymptomatic volunteers.[87] Studies of CT/discography indicate that deranged internal morphology can be quantified and that a correlation exists between the extent of annular disruption and the reproduction of pain by disc injection[85, 86] (Fig 8–21).

Diagnostic disc injection is a specialized technique. It involves radiation exposure. There is the risk of disc space infection and neural injury. The procedure is safe when performed by a knowledgeable, skilled practitioner. This examination should be reserved for those patients in whom symptoms are severe and the routine imaging procedures have not provided convincing evidence of abnormality (Fig 8–22). It is the only technique that can effectively differentiate between a symptomatic and asymptomatic degenerative disc.

CT/discography is the most sensitive method for diagnosing posterolateral herniation.[43] It is also helpful in the assessment of patients with disc herniation in whom chemonucleolysis and/or percutaneous diskectomy are being considered as treatment options.[24]

POSTERIOR ELEMENTS

Posterior Arch

A bony arch extends from each vertebral body. The base of the arch is formed by the vertebral pedicles. Paired laminae curve to merge in the midline. The laminae of adjacent segments are connected by the elastic ligamentum flavum. Together the laminae and ligaments form the posterior or ventral wall of the central spinal canal.

Each arch bears a number of processes. Paired transverse processes and a single posterior spinous process serve as attachment points for paraspinous muscles. Each

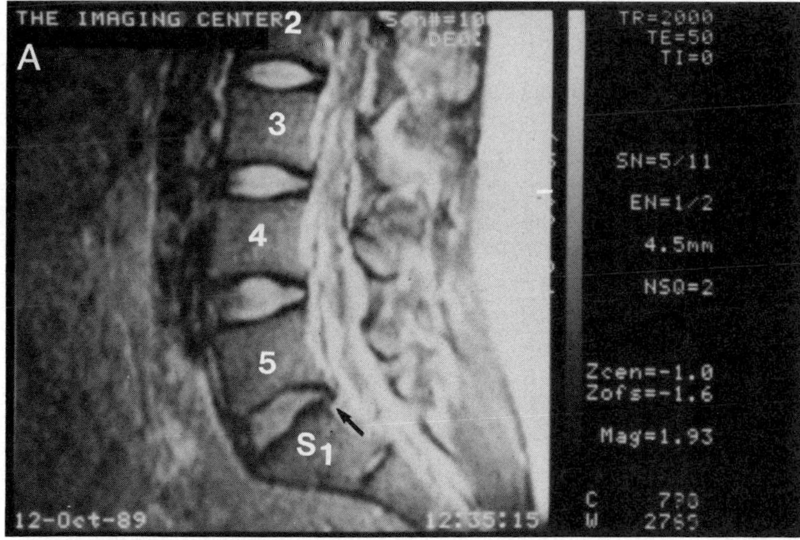

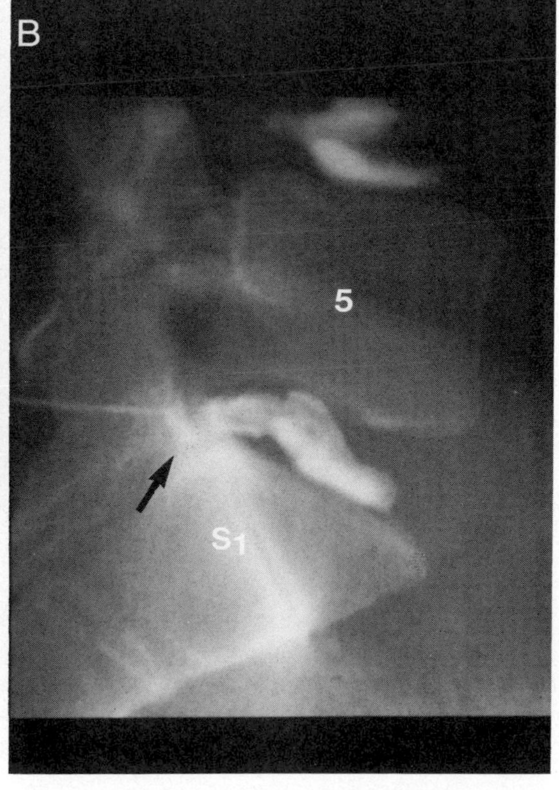

FIG 8–20.
A, lumbar MRI, midsagittal section, SE proton-density image. There is a very subtle decrease in signal intensity at the L5–S1 disc. The posteroinferior margin of the L5–S1 disc annulus is not continuous *(arrow)*. **B,** same patient as in **A.** In a lateral spot film obtained during L5–S1 disc injection contrast extends from the nucleus to the postero-inferior margin of the annulus *(arrow),* thus documenting the fissure suspected on MRI.

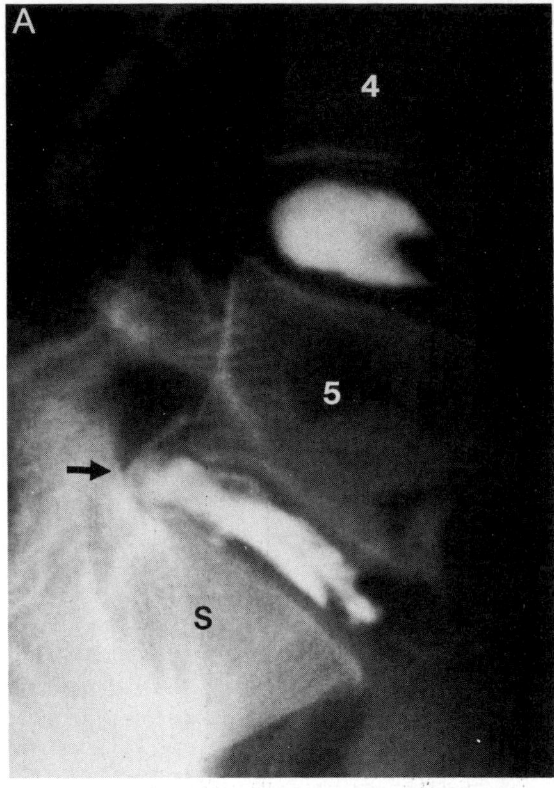

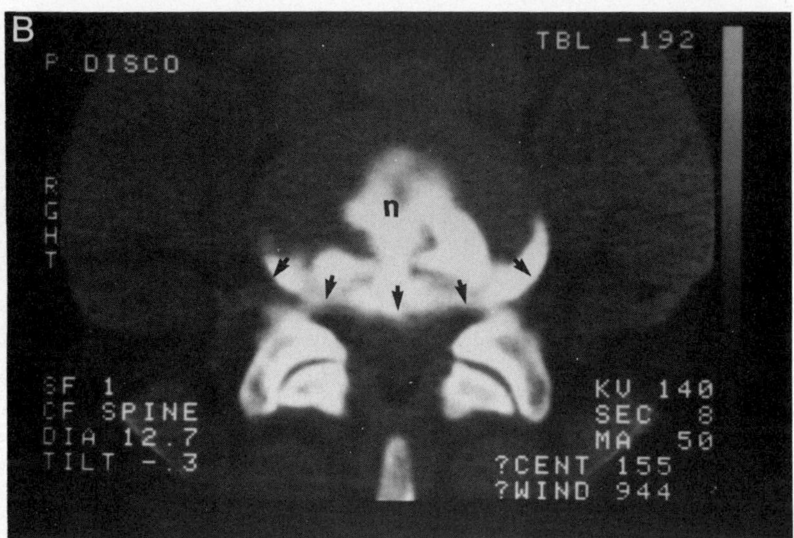

FIG 8–21.
A, lumbar discogram lateral spot film: normal nucleogram at L4–5. Distension did not provoke a pain response. The L4–5 nucleogram represents a type I pattern, as described by Adams, Dolan, and Hutton. The abnormal nucleogram at L5–S1 shows moderate nuclear disorganization and extensive posterior annular fissuring. Contrast material in the subligamentous space *(arrow)* defines the margin of the annulus. Disc injection provoked a concordant pain response. **B,** axial CT of the L4–5 disc postdiscography (different patient from **A**) shows a well organized central nuclear contrast collection and posterior midline and left paracentral radial fissuring extending to the outer margin of the annulus. The large circumferential subcapsular annular stain reflects widespread disruption of the annular fibers *(black arrows)*. There was a concordant pain response on disc injection.

arch possesses four articular processes. The superior articular processes of the lower vertebra are anterior to the inferior articular processes of the vertebra above.

The structure of the posterior arch is poorly demonstrated on routine radiographs. Conventional tomography does provide information regarding arch structure. CT provides the best visualization of these structures.

At each segment, the bony arch is continuous, and the processes are fairly symmetrical. Asymmetry of bony parts or disruption of the arch may be congenital or the result of acquired pathology. Specific features allow the characterization of lesions in some instances (Fig 8–23). Spondylolysis in the cervical spine is an uncommon lesion. It occurs most often at the C6 segment and is usually congenital. The common association of the primary arch defect with an occult spina bifida is characteristic of this lesion.

The clinical significance of any posterior arch abnormality will be determined by the alteration of form and/or function that results from the lesion. Spondylolysis at the L5 level is a common acquired lesion. It is usually asymptomatic. However, spondylolysis is always associated with a deformity of the configuration of the root canal. Instead of the usual vertical inverted teardrop configuration, the deformed canal is more oblique in orientation with vertical narrowing (Fig 8–24). The segmental neurovascular elements traversing the root canal are placed in a position of jeopardy. Superimposed disturbance of the segment by acute injury or chronic spondylotic pathology can result in the development of symptomatic lateral stenosis.

The articular processes vary in their orientation. The slope of the cervical processes favors rotation of the segment about a definable axis of rotation in flexion and extension.[1] The orientation of the lumbar processes serves to resist transverse rotation or torsion and forward displacements. It seems that the joints direct patterns of motion at each segment.

These joints are vulnerable to injury if subjected to forces that exceed tolerance. Chronic repetitive stresses may result in failure of the articular cartilage, eventual joint space narrowing, and hypertrophy and sclerosis of the articular processes, all features of degenerative osteoarthritis. As with the joints of the appendicular skeleton, this type of pathology is most often seen in older individuals. It does occur in younger individuals as a result of unusual stresses. The author has seen this phenomenon in young athletes (Fig 8–25) and as a result of subtle articular process fractures.

The joints may be injured by distraction with avulsion, disruption, or strain of the capsule. As a general

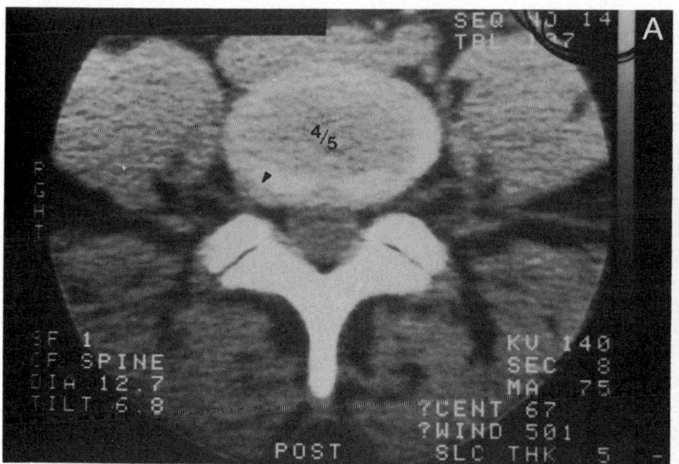

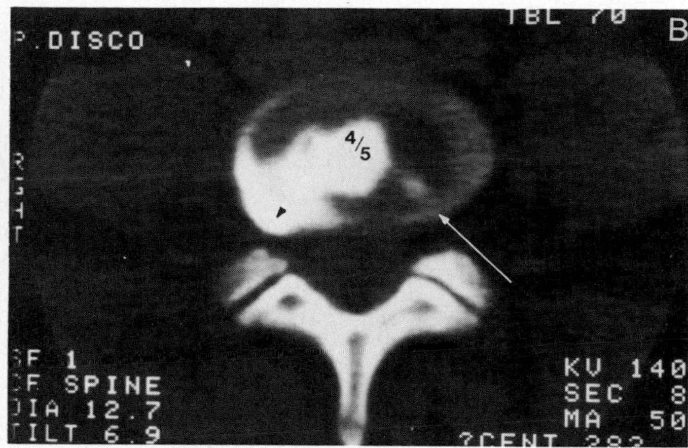

FIG 8–22.
A 42-year-old woman with a complaint of low back pain, right-sided with secondary pain in right hip/buttock and posterior aspect of the thigh. The pain is mechanical in character, and there is no clinical radiculopathy. **A,** axial CT through the L4–5 intervertebral disc shows slight asymmetry of the posterolateral disc margin and focal prominence of the disc annulus at the right posterolateral margin producing a slight mass effect in the midzone of the root canal *(arrowhead)*. **B,** axial CT, section through the L4–5 disc postdiscography. There is a fairly well organized central collection of contrast in the nuclear zone. A broad right posterolateral radial fissure extends to the outer annulus margin, and a concentric subcapsular fissure extends around the lateral margin of the disc. A focal prominence is evident in the midzone of the root canal *(arrowhead)*. Compare to **A.** The small collection of contrast in the left posterolateral part of the annulus is related to a 22-gauge needle tract *(arrow)*. An incidental finding is asymmetry of the posterior joint widths, wider on the right than the left. This finding suggests a probable torsion mechanism of segment failure.

rule, bone-detail CT images demonstrate fairly symmetrical joint width. Asymmetries of joint width can result from small degrees of rotation within the physiologic range. In such instances, several contiguous joints appear to be wider than their counterparts on the opposite side. Asymmetrical widening of an isolated joint (single segment) should raise the suspicion of a distraction injury (Fig 8–26).

Facet Joints

The joints formed by the opposing articular processes are officially known as "zygapophyseal joints."[59] The

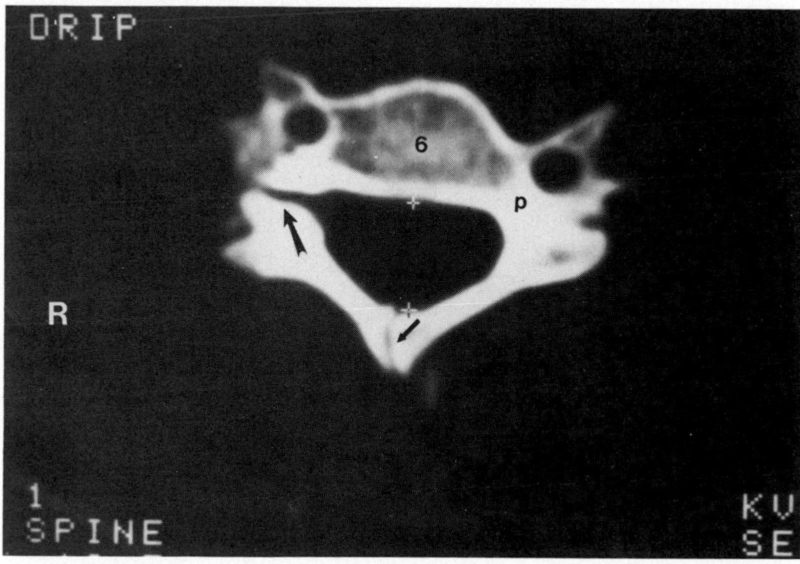

FIG 8–23.
Axial CT of the cervical spine, section through the midbody of C6. The linear zone of low density on the right side of the posterior arch *(large arrow)* represents a "spondylolytic" defect in the lower pedicle. The pedicle on the left *(p)* is normal. Occult spina bifida *(small arrow)* is a finding commonly associated with congenital spondylolysis.

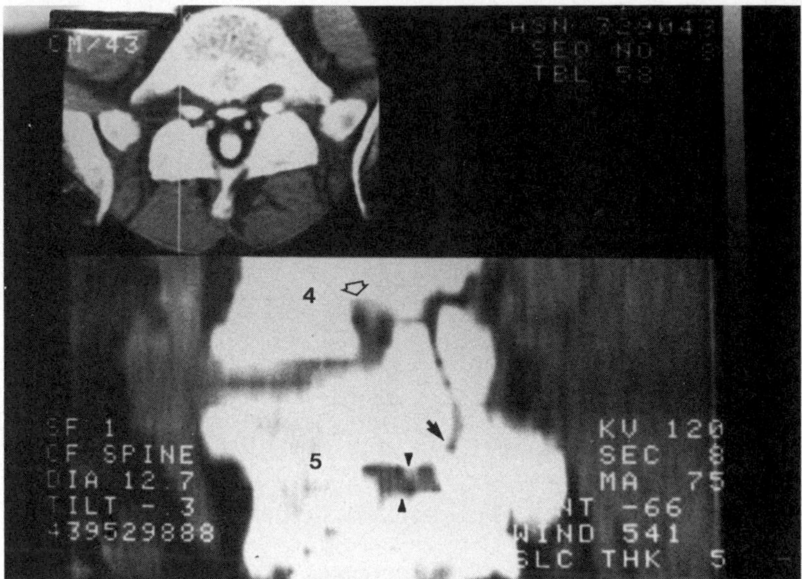

FIG 8–24.
CT of the lower part of the lumbar spine, right parasagittal reformation, section through the midzone of the root canals. The configuration of the L4–5 root canal *(open arrow)* is typical of the lower portion of the lumbar spine. The root canal at L5–S1 is vertically narrowed *(arrowheads)*. The vertical cleft in the pars interarticularis *(black arrow)* is the site of the defect in the pars interarticularis (acquired spondylolysis).

more familiar name, popularized in the American literature, is "facet" joints.

These articulations are true synovial joints. Each facet is covered by articular cartilage, and the joints are enclosed by a fibrous capsule. The anterior capsule is formed by laterally directed fibers of the ligamentum flavum.

The joints may be studied directly by arthrography, which is performed by directing a fine-gauge needle into the selected joint with fluoroscopic guidance. Small volumes (approximately ¼ cc) of contrast suffice to opacify the joint space. The appearances of the normal cervical and lumbar facet joints are similar. Capsular redundancies at the anterosuperior and posteroinferior aspects of the joints form articular recesses. A triangular "meniscoid" is

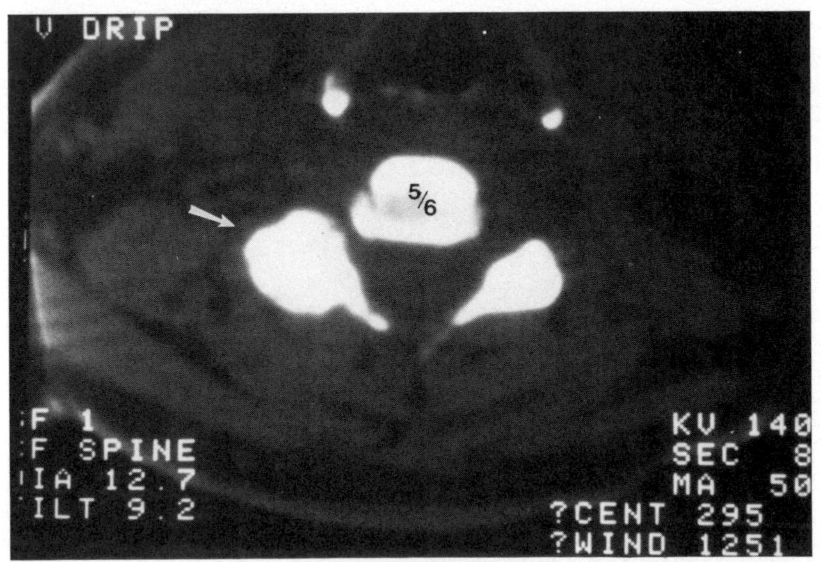

FIG 8–25.
Axial CT, section through the C5–6 interspace. This 35-year-old male physician, a weight-lifting enthusiast, has right neck pain on extension, right rotation, and right side bending. There is focal tenderness on the right at C5–6 but no radicular complaints. The scan demonstrates marked hypertrophy of the articular processes on the right *(arrow)* with moderate stenosis of the right root canal. The diagnosis is symptomatic osteoarthropathy and asymptomatic lateral stenosis.

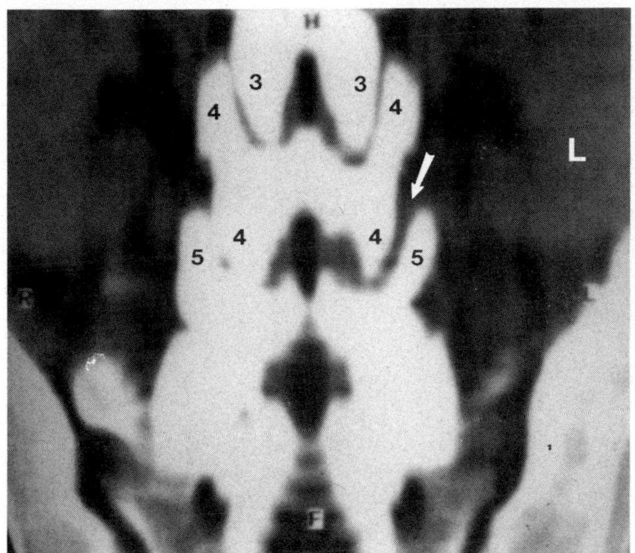

FIG 8–26.
Lumbar CT, coronal reformatted image, section through the midlumbar facet joints. The width of the joints at L3–4 is symmetrical. The L4–5 joint on the left *(arrow)* is wider than the right-sided joint. This isolated asymmetry may reflect pathologic distraction of the joint.

commonly seen in the superior recess of filled but undistended joints. As a general rule, the superior articular recesses are small by comparison to the inferior recesses. There are few published reports describing the performance and interpretation of cervical facet arthrography.[42] The author prefers the technique described by Okada.[60] A lateral approach to the cervical joints is both simple and safe.

The superior articular recess of the cervical joint projects into the superior aspect of the cervical root canal. It extends the full length of the articular process and lies immediately above but not in direct contact with the dorsal ganglion of the segmental nerve complex in the midzone of the root canal. Contrast material frequently extends medially from the inferior recess, between the laminae, and posterior to the ligamentum flavum. This pattern is common and was described by Okada.[60] It represents a normal variant. On occasion, contrast will extend across the midline and fill the opposite facet joint (Fig 8–27).

Although the lumbar facet joint has been the subject of many studies, there are relatively few papers devoted to the performance and interpretation of the arthrogram.[18, 47] A posterolateral approach is preferred. However, variations in the orientation and the overall configuration of the lumbar joints complicate the procedure. Axial CT scans help to determine the best approach. A direct posterior approach to the inferior recess may be required when the joint orientation is coronal. This orientation is common at the lumbosacral segment. Performance of arthrography in

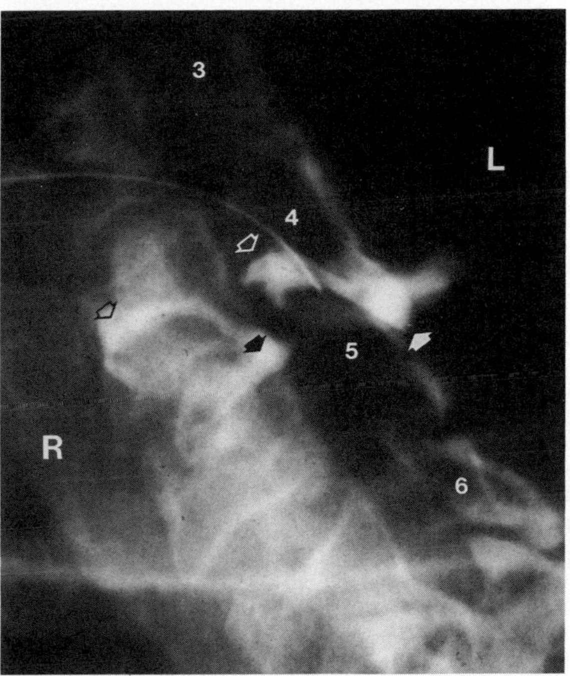

FIG 8–27.
Cervical facet joint arthrogram at C4–5, left posterior oblique view from the left side, with injection into the left-sided joint. The superior recess *(open white arrow)* and inferior recess *(solid white arrow)* are filled. The meniscoid in the anterosuperior recess is nicely demonstrated. The right-sided joint is also visualized *(black open* and *solid arrows)*. The arthrogram on both sides is normal. The right-sided joint filled from the left-sided injection. This cross-filling is a normal variant in the cervical region.

this circumstance requires technical precision and a detailed knowledge of the joint space.[78]

The superior articular recess of the lumbar facet joint lies immediately posterior and directly adjacent to the dorsal ganglion of the segmental nerve complex (Fig 8–28). The lumbar joints commonly "decompress" through the posteroinferior recess. Contrast will spread into the adjacent multifidus muscle. This does not represent rupture of the joint capsule but is simply leakage of fluid through a naturally weak area of the capsule. Arthrographic patterns have not been sufficiently well studied to draw any firm conclusions as to what is "normal" and what is "pathologic" (Fig 8–29).

Enlargement of the superior articular recess is an important observation. If the distended capsule projects into the root canal, it may act as a mass that mechanically stimulates the adjacent dorsal ganglion. Joint effusions may produce symptoms in this way.[19]

Although openings in the superior recess of lumbar facet joints have been reported, leakage by this route is rare. Disruption of the superior capsule would expose the contents of the root canal to joint exudates. Tears in the

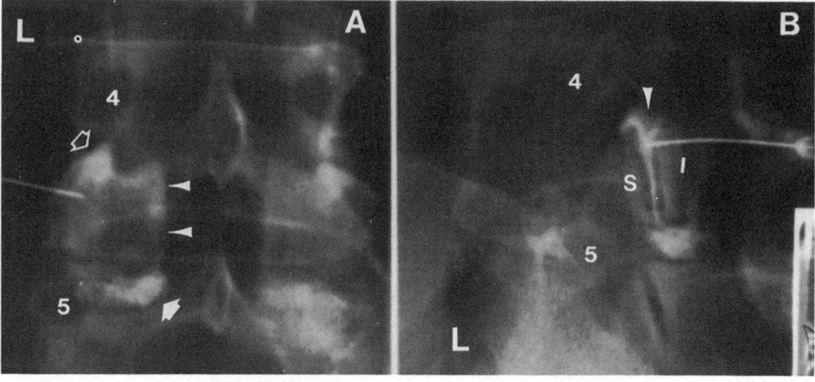

FIG 8–28.
Lumbar facet joint arthrogram at L4–5. **A,** prone view, left-sided joint injection. This normal arthrogram shows the superior recess *(open arrow),* inferior recess *(solid arrow),* and medial joint capsule *(arrowheads).* **B,** left posterior oblique view from the left, normal arthrogram. The midportion of the joint is interposed between the superior articular process of L5 *(s)* and the inferior articular process of L4 *(i).* The triangular "meniscoid" is evident in the superior articular recess *(arrowhead).*

medial capsular wall allow the escape of joint contents into the epidural space. Either condition may result in chemical stimulation of sensitive structures. These dispersal patterns are not observed on a routine basis, even with overdistension of the joints, and are considered to be pathologic by the author.

A facet syndrome remains undefinable clinically.[56] This should not be surprising in view of the variety of pathology that may befall the facet joints.

Osteoarthropathy involving the cervical and/or lumbar facet joints can be identified by imaging modalities. When symptomatic, these joints can be identified by careful manual examination. There is focal tenderness over the affected joint, and maneuvers to stress the suspected component are usually restricted and uncomfortable or painful. The arthrogram in such patients is usually abnormal. Injections commonly provoke familiar pain. Instillation of local anesthetic usually relieves the pain and local tenderness and results in improved movement initially. Many of these patients respond dramatically to intra-articular steroids. This particular facet joint syndrome, secondary to symptomatic facet joint osteoarthritis, is easily recognized.

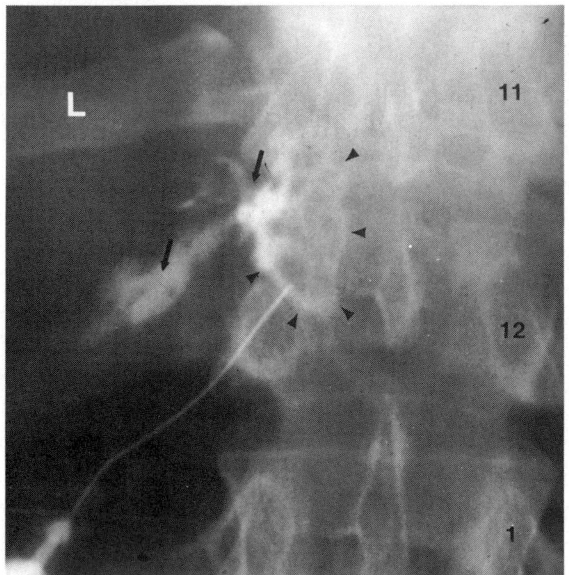

FIG 8–29.
Left thoracic facet joint arthrogram, T11–12, prone view. Contrast defines the normal joint space *(arrowheads).* Extension of contrast material laterally from the upper joint capsule *(arrows)* is remote from the needle insertion point and may represent disruption of the superior capsule.

Most patients do not present so clearly defined. Subjects suitable for investigation of the facet joints usually complain of mechanical pain (neck or back), with referred pain generally sclerotomal in character. Altered sensation in the extremities in the form of nondermatomal paresthesias is common. Facet joint pathology can result in true radicular pain with classic dermatomal distribution.

Careful manual examination will often reveal regions of reproducible tenderness, sometimes quite discrete. This is particularly common in the cervical region where the articular processes are more accessible to palpation. Maneuvers to mechanically stress the suspected component are often restricted and frequently uncomfortable or painful. The location of muscular tenderness is helpful in the evaluation of cervical facet joints. Symptomatic joints may produce tenderness in predictable zones.[6, 22]

The evaluation of lumbar joints is more difficult due to the inaccessibility of the articular structures and less predictable pain referral patterns with considerable overlap.[50]

Prior to injection, all imaging studies should be reviewed for anatomic alteration. All abnormal-appearing joints that might reasonably be associated with the expressed complaints should be studied. Initial evaluation should include the evaluation of multiple joints.

Arthrography is essential to verify intra-articular injection and study the joint space and capsular integrity. A volume of contrast material sufficient to opacify the joint space and demonstrate both the superior and inferior recesses is required. Often, .25 cc of contrast material is sufficient, particularly in the cervical region. On occasion, joints will accept and contain as much as 2.5 to 3 cc. Joint distension to evaluate pain response should be performed by the slow injection of a local anesthetic solution. Volumes of .50 to .75 cc are instilled slowly over a 10- to 20-second interval. The injection is interrupted when there is a pain response or an increase in resistance.

Patient response is observed and rated as with disc injections. A positive provocation response is only accepted if there is at least one negative response (internal control). If all studied components are provocation-positive, then this aspect of the study is indeterminate. A pain response occurring at the time of capsular penetration is commonly seen at joints that prove to be provocation-positive.

The analgesic effect is evaluated prior to discharge. A positive analgesic response includes improvement in the patient's self-rating of pain (visual analog scale), decreased tenderness at the primary site, and improved range of motion with decreased pain during the provocative maneuvers. Responses are rated as negative, partial, or complete.

A study in which one or more joints are clearly provocation-positive and analgesic-positive implicates those joints as participants in the chronic pain syndrome and invites a repeat evaluation. Repeat studies are necessary in order to identify placebo responders. The second study may be limited to those joints shown to be provocation-positive on the initial evaluation.

The efficacy of intra-articular steroids has not been resolved. It is difficult not to consider the instillation of a long-acting steroid suspension in joints that are provocation-positive on initial evaluation. Repeat steroid injections are rarely indicated and should be used judiciously.

Medial Branch Blocks

The zygapophyseal joints are innervated by the medial branches of the dorsal rami of the segmental nerve complex. Each joint receives sensory innervation from the nerve at that segment and a descending branch of the posterior ramus of the segment above. Target points for anesthetizing the medial branches have been described[9, 12] (Figs 8–30 and 8–31). Selected medial branch blocks are a rapid method of evaluating patients with potential facet joint problems. There is no provocation component. A positive study is based on the analgesic response. To be meaningful, very small volumes of local anesthetic are employed. One-half to ¾ cc of anesthetic (usually bupivacaine, 0.5%) is delivered slowly after the needle has been positioned at the target point. Slow injection (10 to 20 seconds) results in a relatively limited dispersal of the injected solutions (Fig 8–32).

It is now a matter of routine to perform medial branch blocks or formal facet arthrograms and intra-articular

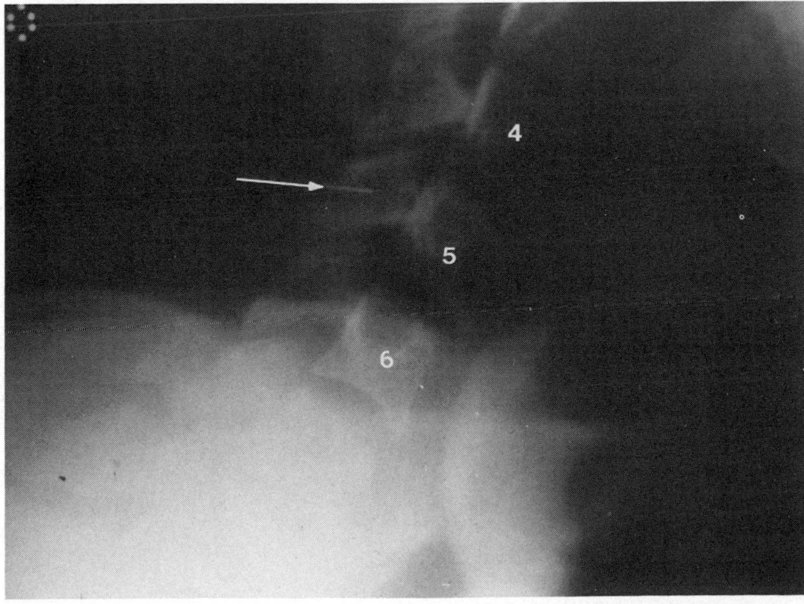

FIG 8–30.
Lateral cervical spine spot film. A needle *(arrow)* is in position for a C5 medial branch block, against the lateral aspect of the midpoint of the right C5 articular process.

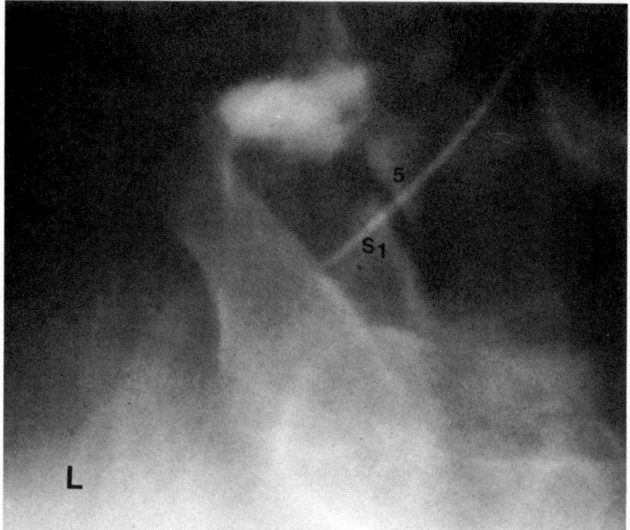

FIG 8–31.
Left posterior oblique view, lumbosacral junction, spot film. A needle is in position for an L5 medial branch block, and the tip of the needle lies against the lateral base of the S1 superior articular process *(S1)* at its junction with the sacral ala.

blocks on most patients referred for diagnostic disc injection. The combined studies provide insight into the prevalence of various isolated and combined lesions of the motion segment. A recent review of over 300 patients referred to the author's clinic for diagnostic evaluation of neck pain suggests that the incidence of symptomatic facet joints is quite high. In almost two thirds of the patients, the facet joints may be implicated as primary or secondary contributors to the chronic pain syndrome.[5]

Selective medial branch blocks are adequate if the treatment option to be exercised involves either radio frequency or cryoprobe medial branch rhizotomy. Formal facet joint injections are not necessary.

SPACES AND CONTENTS

The bony and soft-tissue linkages of the anterior column and posterior elements enclose a definable space. That space may be conveniently divided into the central canal and multiple laterally directed root canals.

Central Canal

The size and shape of the central canal are important features of the spine. Subjects with developmentally small canals have a reduced margin of safety in the event of any pathology that further compromises the available space. A reasonable assessment of the sagittal diameter can be obtained from lateral radiographs. The standard methods[40, 91] determine the distance from the midpoint of the posterior vertebral body to the nearest point of the corresponding spinolaminar line. Measurements in normal subjects and patients with symptomatic stenosis suggest that 14 mm is the lower limit of normal by this method.[14, 65] A second, or ratio, method compares the standard measured sagittal diameters with the anteroposterior width of the vertebral body measured through the midpoint.[83]

Absolute measurements may be misleading. Technical factors such as target distance and object film distance, which will vary with patient body build, result in variation of measurements. The Pavlov or Torg ratios are not influenced by technical factors and may indicate significant contraction of the central canal in patients with "normal" sagittal diameters determined by the standard method.

Accurate assessment of size and configuration of the central canal are best accomplished by axial CT. The bony limits as well as the soft-tissue components, which influ-

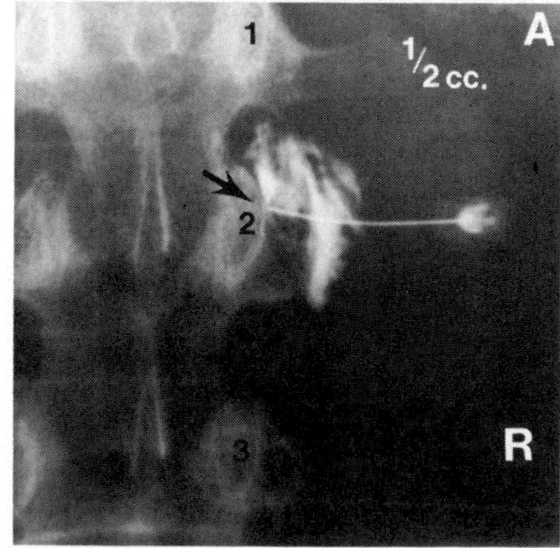

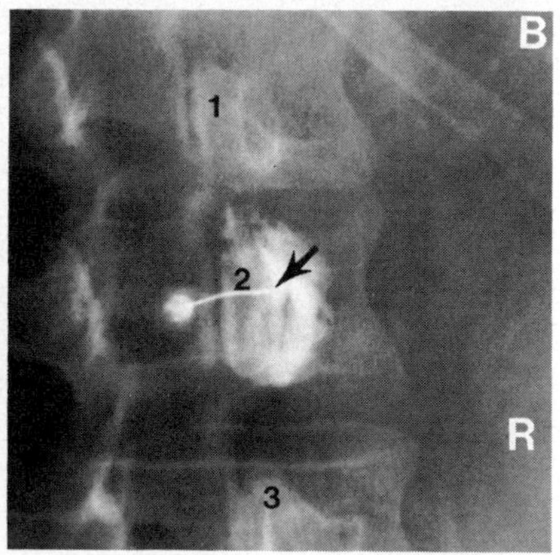

FIG 8–32.
Medial branch block to the right of L2. **A,** prone position. The needle tip is adjacent to the lateral base of the L2 superior articular process *(arrow)*. Contrast material, ½ cc, was instilled over a 10-second period. **B,** same patient, right posterior oblique view from the right with the needle tip at the target point *(arrow)*. The film demonstrates a limited dispersal pattern associated with slow injection. Contrast material lies immediately adjacent to the articular process in the region of the medial branch of the posterior primary ramus.

ence the size and configuration of the canal, are assessed. Both sagittal diameter and area can be accurately determined by CT.[28, 80] It is the cross-sectional area of the thecal sac that is critical in the evaluation of stenosis.[77] Myelography, CT scanning with intrathecal enhancement, and MRI all provide information regarding the size of the central canal and thecal sac.

MRI demonstrates the sagittal diameter of the central canal and defines extradural pathology quite well. Direct visualization of the cord is an added advantage in the cervical region (Fig 8–33). Cervical myelography is a static examination. The patient is maintained in the prone position with neck extended. A variety of extradural pathologies may be exaggerated in this position and result in focal narrowing of sufficient magnitude to block the flow of contrast material (Fig 8–34). It may not be possible to visualize segments above the level of block directly. The addition of postmyelography CT resolves this diagnostic problem because the contrast material usually traverses the zone of narrowing in sufficient quantity to be visualized on a postmyelogram CT scan.[30]

Formal myelography requires a volume of 10 to 15 cc of contrast material at a concentration of 240 to 300 mg/cc (iodine). Modern agents (iohexol and iopamidol) are safe but not without risk at these doses. Furthermore, cervical extension can be hazardous in the patient with a small canal, particularly when it is compromised by bony ridges and/or disc herniations or with superimposed instability and retrolisthesis.

Axial CT obtained immediately after the intrathecal injection of low volumes of contrast material (4 to 5 cc) into the lumbar cistern demonstrates excellent opacification of the subarachnoid space. The low-dose technique is adequate to visualize the thecal margins and dural root sleeve filling and to identify the cord and any intrathecal mass lesions. The use of this technique can eliminate the need for formal myelography in the study of cervical disease.

In the lumbar area, MRI defines extradural pathology quite well (Fig 8–35). However, axial images are not always reliable in assessing the size of the central canal and thecal sac. They are sensitive to motion degradation and do not define the bony margins of the central canal well. Axial CT is especially effective in defining the bony margins of the central and root canals and with intrathecal contrast enhancement accurately depicts the size (area) of the thecal sac (Fig 8–36). CT data are usually acquired with the patient recumbent in a comfortable position to reduce movement. It is a static examination. Lumbar myelography can be performed as a dynamic study. Patients can be brought to the erect position so as to apply an axial load on the spine. Flexion, extension, and side-bending films document the dynamic changes occurring as a result of extradural pathology (Fig 8–37).

The space that lies between the osseoligamentous boundaries of the central canal and the thecal sac is the epidural space. This is, in reality, a potential space because it contains large venous structures and varying

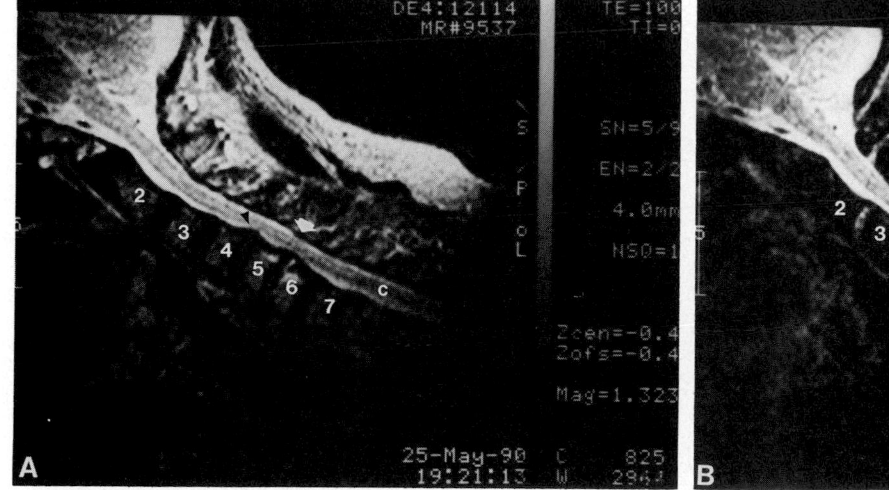

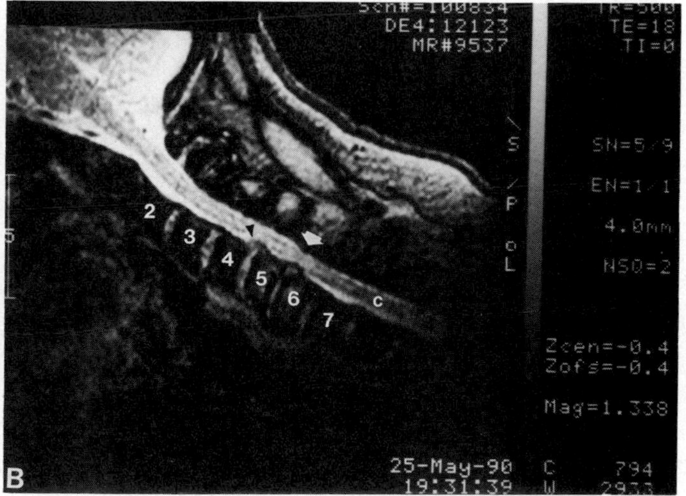

FIG 8–33.
MRI of the cervical spine, midsagittal section, in a 54-year-old male with severe neck pain and claustrophobia. Pain and fear result in patient motion artifact that degrades image quality. This is a common problem in a study of the cervical spine. **A,** SE T2-weighted images (TR 1700/TE 100), 4.0-mm thickness. **B,** GRE image (TR 500/TE 18; flip angle, 25 degrees), 4-mm thickness. Extradural disease at C4–5 and C5–6 is demonstrated on both pulse sequences. The stenosis is greatest at C5–6 *(arrow)* and is more conspicuous on the GRE sequence **(B).** There is no obvious cord compression. The images appear quite similar. However, all of the discs appear dark on the SE sequence; all appear bright on the GRE sequence. Note the difference in the appearance of the lesion at C4–5 on the two sequences *(arrowhead).*

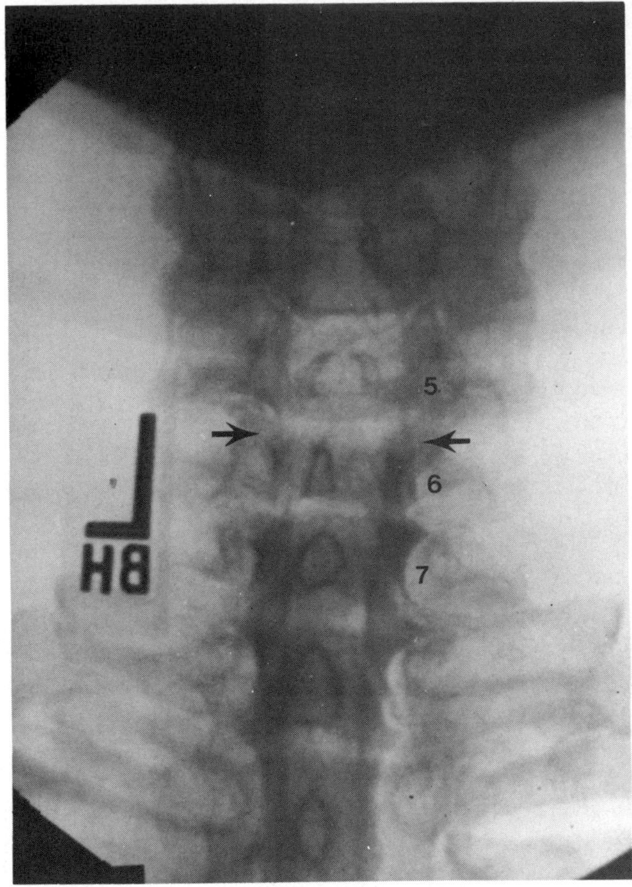

FIG 8–34.
Cervical myelogram, prone position, neck in extension, and the table tilted head down 15 degrees in the patient in Figure 8–33. The film demonstrates complete arrest of contrast flow at the C5–6 segment *(arrows)*. A myelographic block would not be expected purely on the basis of the MRI scan. Arrest of the contrast column prevents adequate study of the cervical cistern above the C5–6 segment.

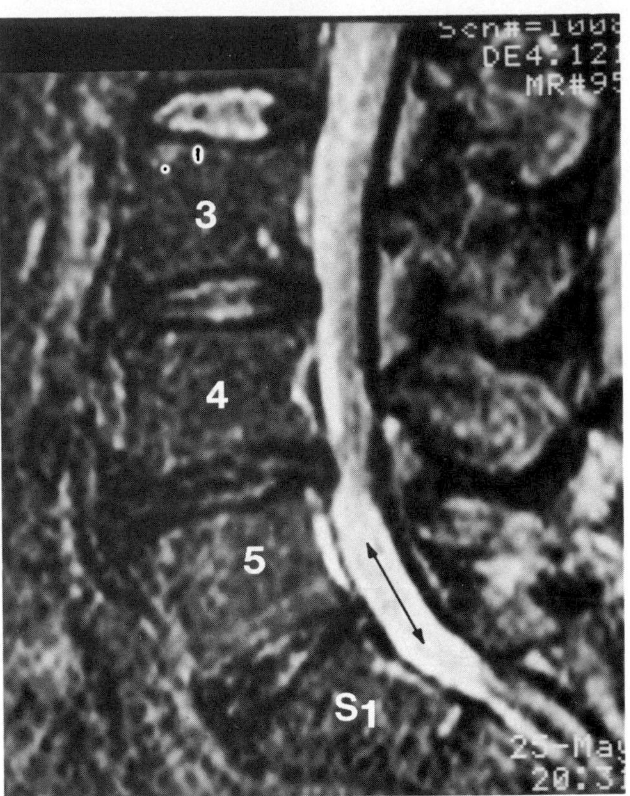

FIG 8–35.
Lumbar MRI, midsagittal section, SE T2-weighted image in a 51-year-old male with severe back and left leg pain. Multilevel disc degeneration can be seen. A diffuse annular bulge of the L4–5 disc deforms the thecal sac. Compression of the thecal sac prevents transmission of CSF pulsations. Bright "clear" CSF caudal to the disc protrusion *(double arrow)* implies significant stenosis.

amounts of fat running through loose areolar connective tissues.[63]

The veins of the epidural space are quite large.[16] The primary constituents of the internal venous plexus are the anterior internal vertebral veins that run longitudinally the length of the central canal in its anterolateral aspect. At the midbody level of each vertebra, there are a pair of basivertebral veins that serve as connections between the internal venous plexus and the blood pool of the marrow space. At each segment, radicular veins traverse the root canals connecting the internal to external vertebral plexus (Fig 8–38). These veins become conspicuous on CT scans during infusion of contrast (Fig 8–39) or on MRI scans following the injection of gadolinium.

In the cervical area, there is a relative paucity of epidural fat, and the venous syncytium is quite large (Fig 8–40). The veins are valveless and allow blood flow in any direction. The large complex of veins in the cervical region may serve to protect the thecal sac and cord from shocks during the wide range of motions occurring in the cervical region.

A fairly constant feature of the epidural space is a triangular fat pad at the posterior apex of the central canal. This triangular fat pad represents a relatively avascular space.

Epidural injections of local anesthetics and steroids have been employed in the treatment of a variety of painful spinal conditions. Although the indications may vary, there are numerous reports of favorable responses to such treatment.[25, 72, 75, 88] The anatomy of the epidural space suggests that these procedures are best performed by directing the needle into the midline, the least vascular region. Positioning is simplified by the use of fluoroscopy. The dispersal pattern seen with the injection of contrast material ensures proper needle position and documents the region affected by physiologic solutions (Fig 8–41). Injection into a venous structure and rapid clearance of the con-

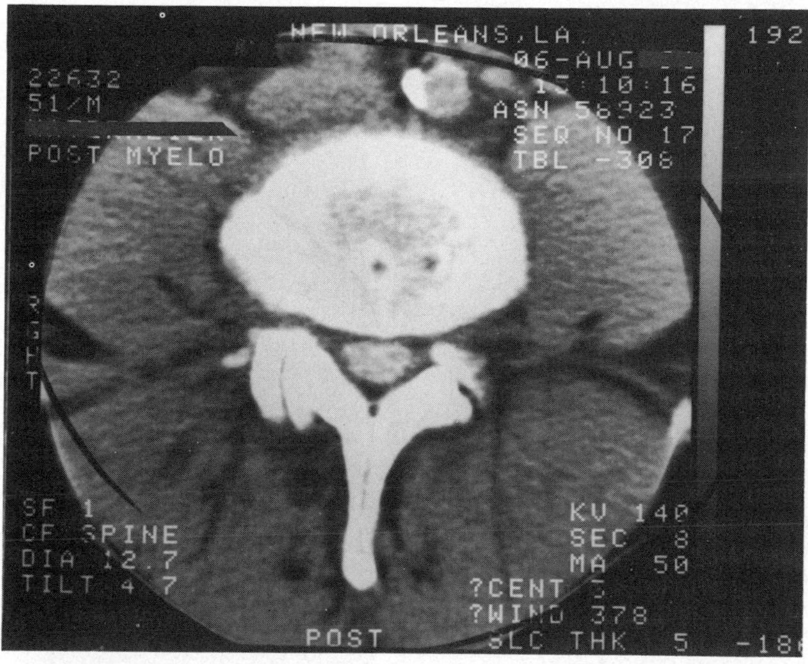

FIG 8–36.
Axial CT, section through the lower L4 end plate in the patient in Figure 8–35. The image was acquired 4 hours after lumbar myelography. Right-sided degenerative changes include end plate ridge formation and facet joint arthrosis. There is significant articular tropism. The central canal is small. The thecal sac is also small with no focal deformity.

trast material are recognized, and the procedure can be repeated at a different level. It has been suggested that the failure of epidural injections in many instances may be attributed to faulty needle position at the time of injection.[89] The standard "loss of resistance" or "hanging drop" techniques are not as reliable as direct visualization of the contrast dispersal pattern.

Root Canals

The root canals are short, tubular spaces that extend laterally at each segment. They are divided into an entrance zone and midzone. The entrance zone, which is a lateral extension of the central canal, contains the dural root sleeve and intrathecal rootlets of the segmental nerve complex. The midzone, which lies between the pedicles, contains the dorsal ganglion and ventral rootlets of the segmental nerve complex. Radicular veins and arteries accompany these neural elements.

Routine radiographs in the oblique projection demonstrate bony encroachment on the root canals. However, the planar imaging techniques, specifically CT and MRI, offer the best visualization of these spaces. CT is the modality of choice for studying osseous lateral stenosis because of its inherent sensitivity to bone pathology. Most stenoses can be identified in the axial plane (Fig 8–42). Complete evaluation requires reformation in the sagittal, parasagittal oblique, and/or coronal planes. MRI is not sensitive to lateral stenosis in the cervical spine but can be quite effective in demonstrating the lumbar root canal (Fig 8–43).

In the lumbar area, there is an ample quantity of perineural fat in the root canals. Subtle changes in the density of tissues in the root canal can be of great significance. Perineural induration, vascular congestion, or subtle annular protrusion may be recognized by a loss of detail and effacement of the anterior perineural fat (Fig 8–44). It is vascular congestion that may account for apparent enlargement of the dorsal ganglion in some instances.

When symptomatology involving an extremity suggests involvement of a specific neural element or when there are multiple anatomic abnormalities and the question arises as to which level of stenosis is functionally significant, a regional epidural injection (selective nerve block) may be employed.[17] The specificity of these procedures rests in the use of very limited volumes of local anesthetic. The primary diagnostic value is in the relief of radicular complaints following the precision injection of a small volume of physiologic solutions.

In the lumbar area, the extrathecal nerve traverses the upper portion of the root canal. The nerve and its investing membrane lie in close proximity to the medial inferior margin of the vertebral pedicle that forms the roof of the root canal. A safe needle position is lateral to the midpoint

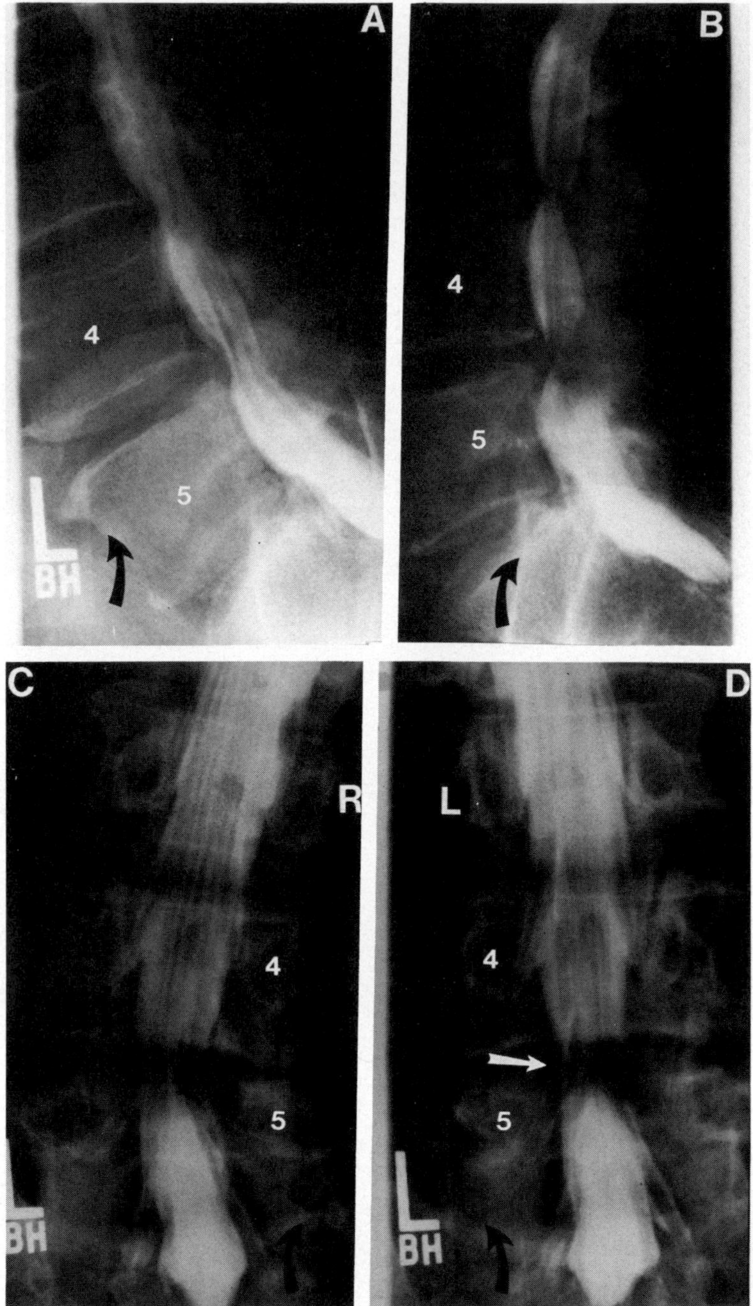

FIG 8–37.
Lumbar myelogram: dynamic study with an erect film of the patient in Figures 8–35 and 8–36. **A,** flexion. There are ventral impressions on the thecal sac at each of the four lumbar intervertebral disc spaces. The appearance of the central canal and thecal sac at L4–5 is not appreciably different from that noted on MRI (Fig 8–35). **B,** extension. There is severe narrowing of the thecal sac at the L4–5 level. In addition to the prominent ventral impression, there is now a significant dorsal mass effect associated with the posterior arch structures, with similar but less severe changes at L3–4. The degree of stenosis would not be demonstrated on prone myelography. **C,** right side bending. There is normal excursion and narrowing of the thecal sac at L4–5. Marked narrowing of the right-sided L4–5 interspace is present. The patient did not have any complaint with this maneuver. **D,** left side bending. There is limited excursion, narrowing of the thecal sac at L4–5, and a clearly defined angular deformity at the left L5 nerve *(white arrow)*. Severe back and left leg pain occurred with this maneuver.

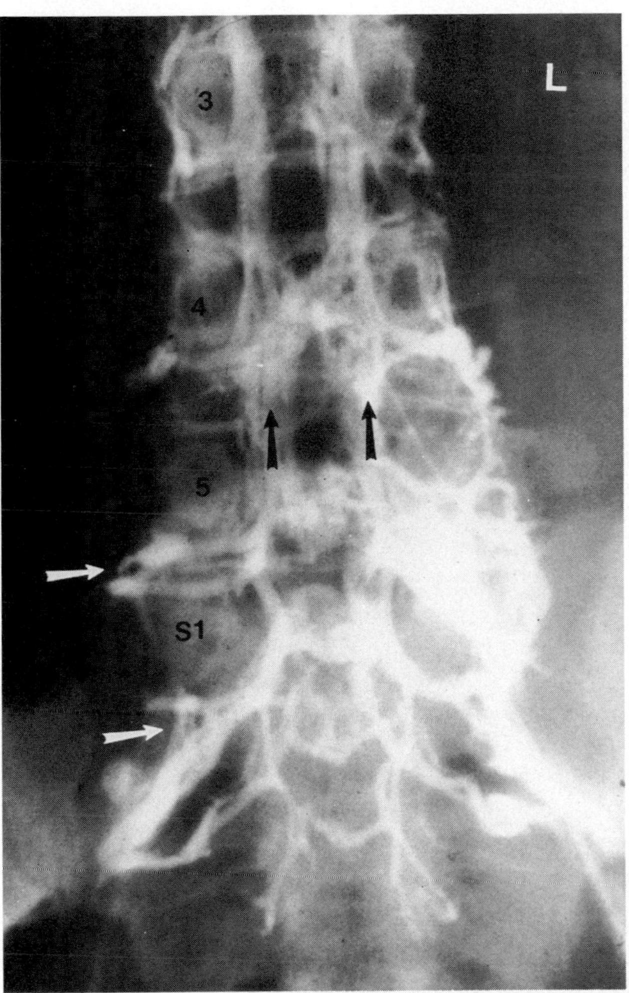

FIG 8–38.
Lumbar epidural venogram, frontal view. Anterior internal vertebral veins *(black arrows)* are the dominant longitudinal trunks. Transverse veins connect these with the basivertebral vein of each vertebra. Several radicular veins traverse each root canal *(white arrows)*.

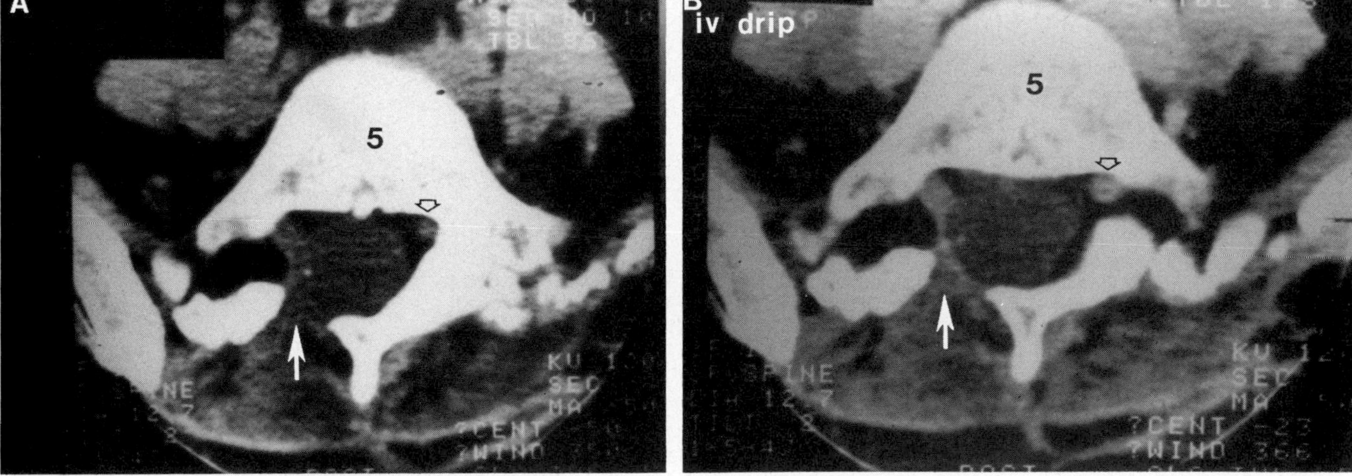

FIG 8–39.
Axial CT, section through the midbody of L5 after right subtotal laminectomy with posterolateral/intertransverse fusion. **A,** nonenhanced CT. The interface between the right side of the thecal sac and the epidural scar is indistinct *(white arrow)*. The left L5 dural root sleeve and contents occupy the entrance zone of the left L5–S1 root canal *(open arrow)*. **B,** same patient, axial CT during intravenous contrast infusion. The interface between the right side of the thecal sac and the epidural scar is clearly defined *(white arrow)*. Enhancement within the scar tissue redefines tissue planes distorted by surgery. Venous enhancement is apparent around the left L5 root sleeve *(open arrow)*. Compare with the unenhanced image. The apparent increase in size reflects the visualization of previously unseen radicular veins.

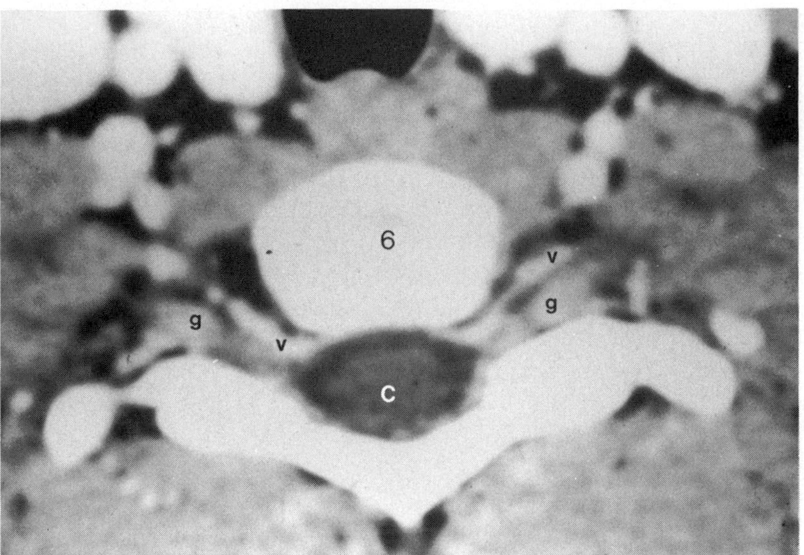

FIG 8–40.
Axial CT through C6. The image was acquired during a bolus injection of contrast material. Radicular veins *(v)* traverse the C6–7 root canals just anterior to the C7 nerves and ganglia *(g)*. There is slight enhancement of the cord, which allows it to be differentiated from the low-density CSF.

of the pedicle in the upper portion of the root canal. The lumbar segmental nerves follow an anteroinferior course. With care, a needle can be directed into a root canal without contacting the segmental nerve. It is essential to employ contrast material when performing regional epidural/selective nerve blocks.[81] Injection into a radicular vein would result in a false-negative block. Simple aspiration is not sufficient because the veins are small and there may be no return of blood on aspiration. The slow injection of solutions may be important in limiting the extent of fluid dispersal (Fig 8–45).

The cervical segmental nerves traverse the lower por-

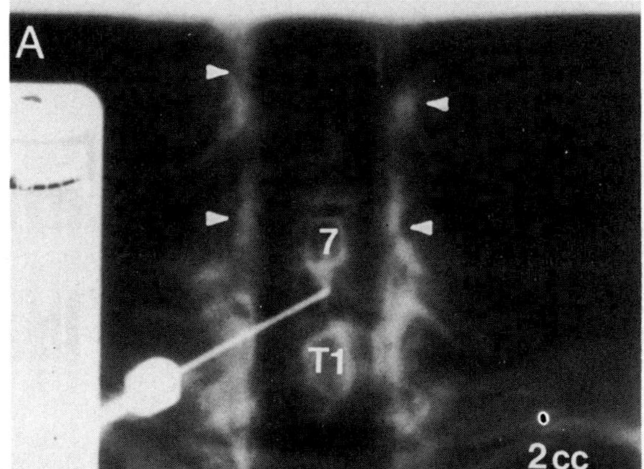

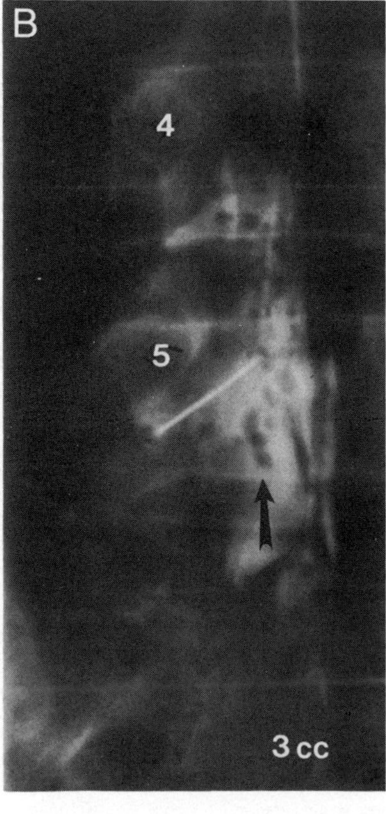

FIG 8–41.
Epiduragrams. **A,** cervical epidural injection, paramedian oblique approach to the epidural space at C7–T1, with the needle tip in the midline and 2 cc of contrast slowly instilled. There is dispersal in the epidural space *(arrowheads)* but no venous filling or subarachnoid opacification. **B,** lumbar epidural injection, paramedian oblique approach to the posterior epidural space at L4–5, with the final needle position in the midline. Injection of 3 cc of contrast material demonstrates epidural dispersal *(arrow)*. The 3-cc volume extends from the midbody of L4 to the upper part of the sacrum (two interspaces).

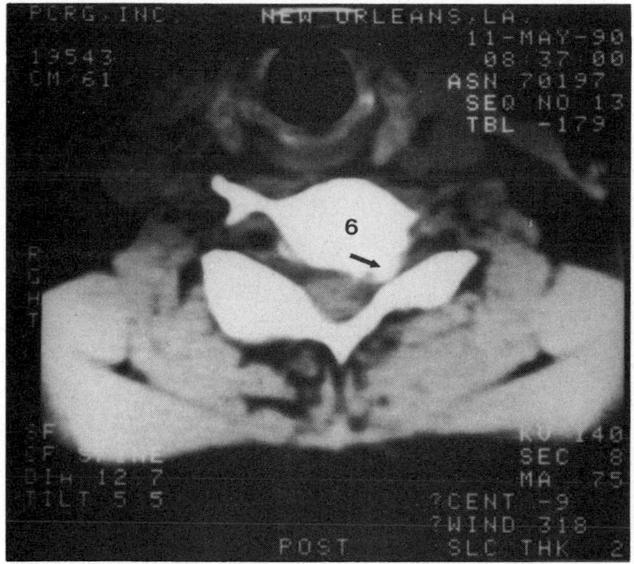

FIG 8–42.
Axial CT of the cervical spine, section through the C6 vertebra. Marked hypertrophy of the left uncinate process results in severe stenosis of the C6–7 root canal *(arrow)*. Despite marked hypertrophy of the right-sided articular processes, there is no lateral stenosis.

tion of the root canal. The dorsal ganglion lies in the small concavity in the anteroinferior surface of the superior articular process that forms the posterior wall of the cervical root canal. The root canal is directed anteriorly and inferiorly. The vertebral artery lies anterior to the segmental nerve. These anatomic features favor an anterolateral approach in the performance of selective cervical epidural/nerve blocks. The best needle position is posterior to the dorsal ganglion on the anterior surface of the superior articular process. As in the lumbar region, the use of contrast material is essential because of large periradicular veins. Proper positioning of the needle can be accomplished with minimal irritation of the segmental nerve. A satisfactory injection will outline the dorsal ganglion and epiradicular sheath with some flow medially into the epidural space (Fig 8–46).

General and selective epidural injections play a role in the diagnosis and treatment of spinal disorders. In patients

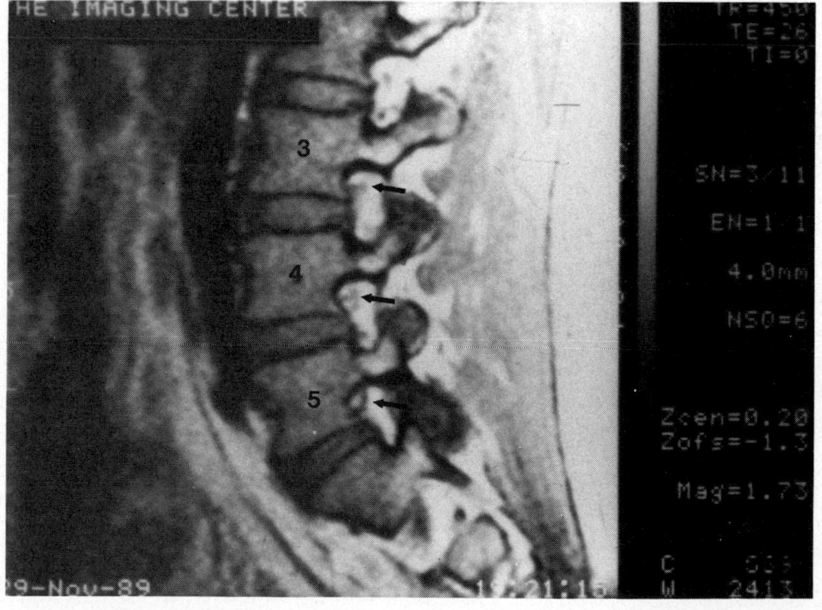

FIG 8–43.
Lumbar MRI, right parasagittal section through the midzone of the root canals, SE T1 image, 4-mm thickness. The image demonstrates normal configuration of the root canals in the sagittal plane. Neural and vascular structures are identified as areas of intermediate signal intensity *(arrows)* within the bright perineural fat.

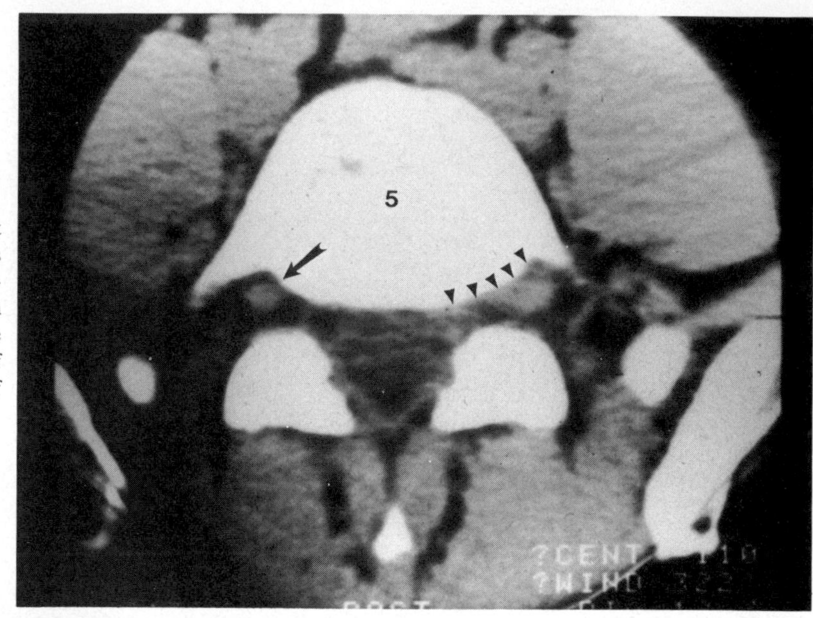

FIG 8–44.
Axial CT, section through the midzone of the L5–S1 root canals. The dorsal ganglion of L5 on the right *(arrow)* is surrounded by low-density perineural fat. The dorsal ganglion on the left is less distinct and appears larger. There is a loss of the low-density fat plane, with hazy intermediate density interposed between the ganglion and the margin of the vertebral end plate. This finding may be a reflection of perineural vascular congestion or induration *(arrowheads)*.

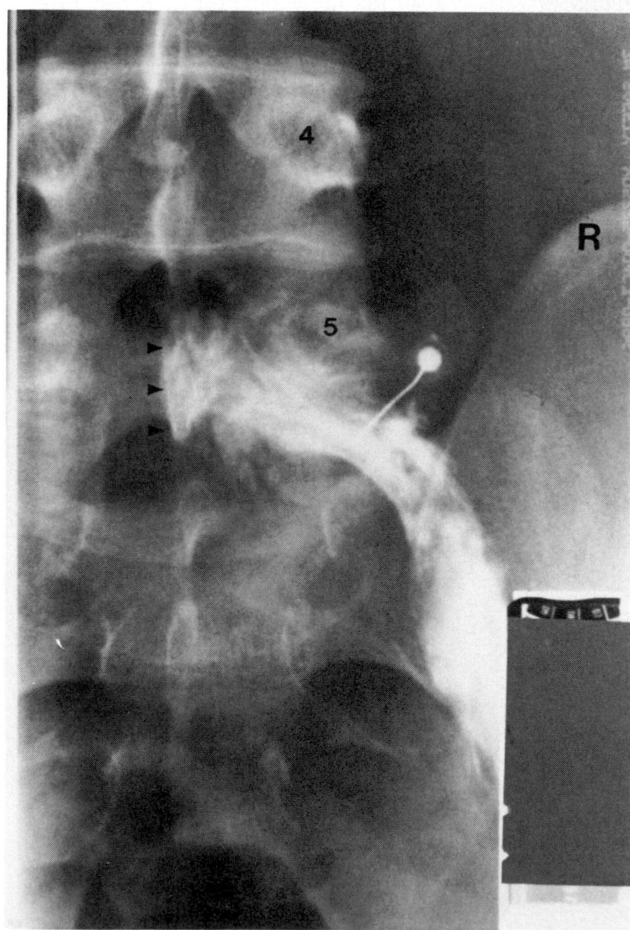

FIG 8–45.
Selective L5 nerve block/regional epidural injection with 2 cc of contrast material slowly instilled (20 seconds). Medial dispersal of contrast is arrested in the midline by the plica mediana dorsalis *(arrowheads)*. Distal flow opacifies the epiradicular sheath.

with nonspecific back pain, the response to epidural injections may be an aid in sorting out those patients whose problems are primarily psychological. Specialized epidural injection techniques[13] have been developed in this regard. In patients with unquestionable organic pathology, the epidural injection techniques can be effective in controlling pain sufficiently to allow patients to begin and continue rehabilitation programs (Fig 8–47).

CONCLUSION

The effective use of radiologic techniques in the diagnosis of spine disorders requires understanding the patient's specific complaints. The better that understanding, the more likely a physician is to choose an appropriate diagnostic study. The author has observed patients in whom an "exhaustive" and expensive workup did not address the patient's specific problem. Routine cervical spine radiographs, MRI, cervical myelography, and conventional CT from mid-C3 through mid-T1 provide no positive information in the patient with neck pain and headache resulting from C1–2 dysfunction. A careful history, examination, and recognition of altered C1–2 rotation should lead the diagnostic physician to specific studies such as functional CT and even arthrography in some instances (Fig 8–48).

Low back pain with radiation into hip/buttock region and lower extremity may arise from a number of sources. A commonly overlooked problem is symptomatic pathology involving the sacroiliac joints. Easily recognized in major trauma with disruption, the less severe derangements of these joints are underdiagnosed.[8] Complaints may be very specific but overlooked by a physician focusing on the back pain. The powerful imaging technologies of lumbar MRI and CT with or without myelography are attractive but will be negative or, worse, false-positive.

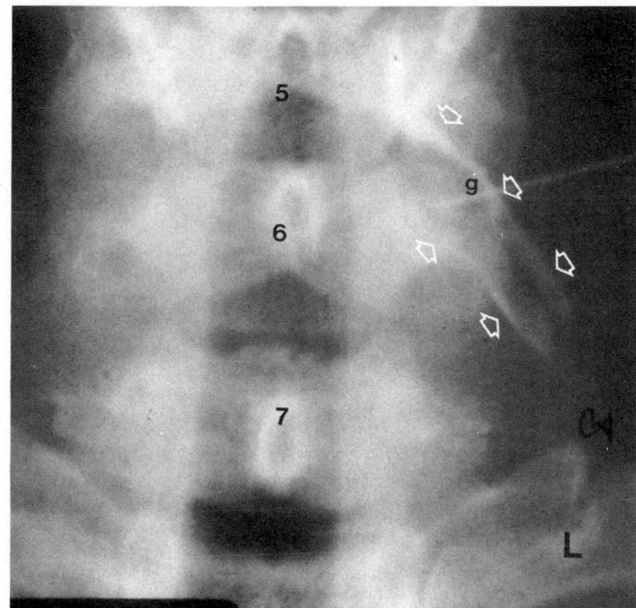

FIG 8–46.
Selective C6 nerve block/regional epidural injection: frontal spot film in a 38-year-old female with left C5–6 disc prolapse and C6 radiculopathy. The needle position is posterior to the dorsal ganglion and adjacent to the anterior surface of the C6 superior articular process. Contrast material opacifies the epiradicular sheath *(arrows)*. Localized swelling adjacent to the needle represents the dorsal ganglion *(g)*.

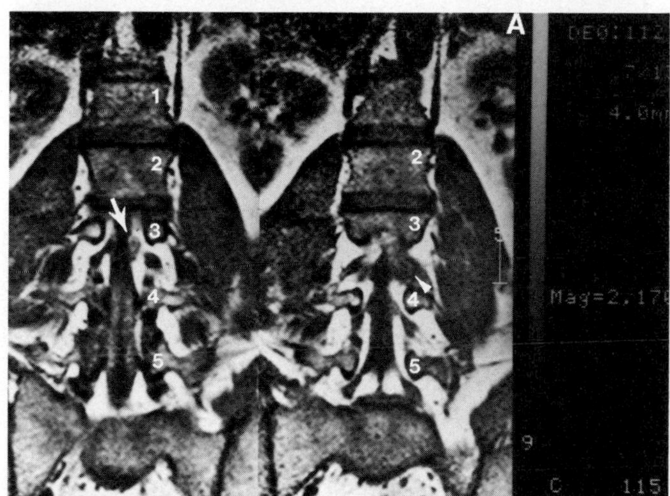

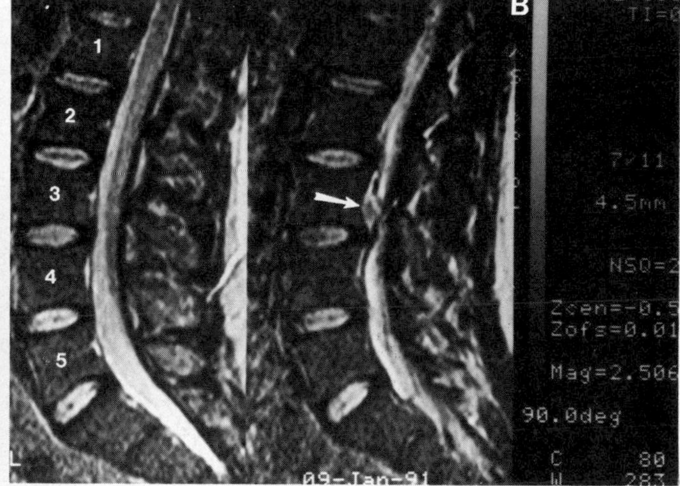

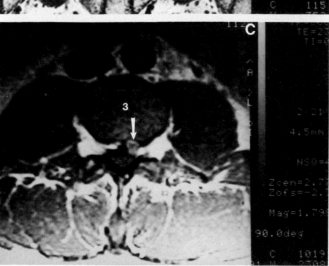

FIG 8–47.
Lumbar MRI in a 38-year-old male 48 hours after the acute onset of back pain and severe left sciatica. **A,** SE T1 coronal images through the mid-lumbar central canal. An oval mass of intermediate signal intensity *(arrow)* is interposed between the left side of the thecal sac and the L3 dorsal ganglion. A broad area of low-signal material virtually fills the left-sided L3–4 root canal *(arrowhead)*. **B,** SE T2 sagittal images. No abnormality is seen on the midline section, but there is reduced signal at the L3–4 disc. This left parasagittal section demonstrates an oval mass *(arrow)* of mixed signal intensity. An intermediate-signal nidus is surrounded by a zone of bright signal. **C,** SE T1 axial section through the lower part of the L3 vertebral body. A left-sided epidural mass *(arrow)* deforms the thecal sac. Even on a T1-weighted image, there appears to be a focal zone of intermediate signal (nidus) surrounded by an area of brighter signal. The diagnosis is a sequestered disc fragment and associated focal epidural hematoma. Complete recovery followed a regional epidural injection at L3 and dynamic lumbar stabilization training. The patient is asymptomatic and fully functional without further treatment at 10 months' follow-up.

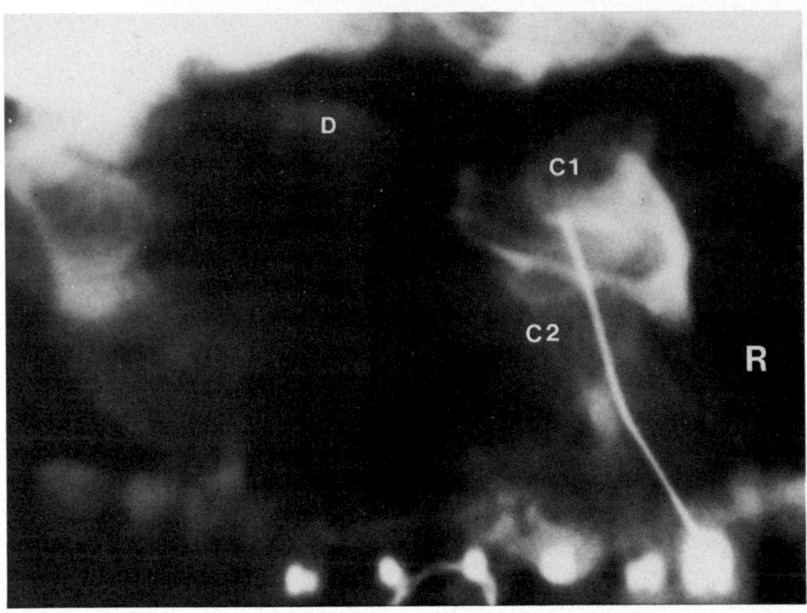

FIG 8–48.
Prone spot film of the upper portion of the cervical spine: C1–2 arthrogram in a 42-year-old male with complaints of severe persisting suboccipital/ occipital headache on the right and severe restriction of cervical rotation following a direct blow to right occipital region. The symptoms persisted for 2 years. "Conventional" workup was "negative." A focused examination demonstrated severe restriction of rotation at C1–2. Functional CT documented restricted motion on the right, but the arthrogram was normal. Distension provoked intense pain. An intra-articular block resulted in complete relief of pain but no improvement in motion. Osteopathic manipulation of C1–2 restored normal motion and relieved the pain. The patient completed a rehabilitation program and is functional at 1 year.

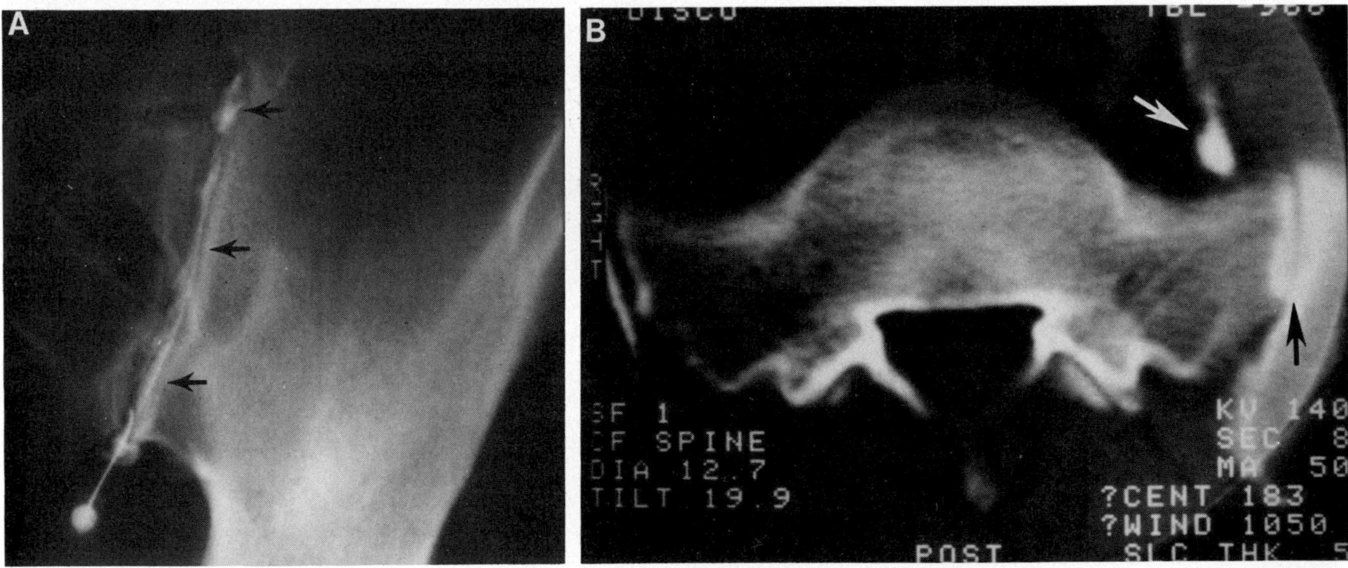

FIG 8–49.
A, right sacroiliac joint arthrogram, prone spot film. The needle enters the diarthrodial space at the bottom of the joint. At this point, joint orientation is parasagittal, and a direct posterior approach is successful. Contrast opacifies the entire sacroiliac joint *(arrows)*. A normal joint will accept approximately 1.5 cc of solution. **B,** axial CT following left sacroiliac joint arthrography. A diffuse haze in the left sacroiliac joint *(black arrow)* reflects residual contrast material. Ventral capsular disruption is evidenced by dispersal of contrast material into the immediate presacral space along the medial aspect of the iliopsoas muscle *(white arrow)*.

Careful attention to the complaints and appropriate examination will lead the physician to the sacroiliac joint. Arthrography is a developing technique for studying the sacroiliac joints. Ventral tears can be demonstrated (Fig 8–49). An analgesic block of the joint confirms the clinical significance of these anatomic findings. Appropriate *selection* of radiologic techniques requires an in-depth understanding of the specific complaints. The clinician must be aware of the capabilities and limitations of each technique. Proper *interpretation* requires knowledge of the gross[70] and clinical anatomy.[10] An accurate diagnosis is the result of careful clinical radiologic correlation.

REFERENCES

1. Amevo B, Worth D, Bogduk N: Instantaneous axes of rotation of the typical cervical motion segments: A study in normal volunteers. *Clin Biomech* 1991; 6:111–117.
2. Amundsen P: The evolution of contrast media, in Sackett J, Strother C (eds): *New Techniques in Myelography*. Hagerstown, Md, Harper & Row, 1979, pp 2–5.
3. Aprill C, Amevo B, Bogduk N: Abnormal instantaneous axes of rotation of the cervical spine in patients with neck pain. *Spine,* 1992; 17:748–756.
4. Aprill C, Bogduk N: High intensity zone: A diagnostic sign of painful lumbar disc on magnetic resonance imaging. *Br J Radiol* 1992; 65:361–369.
5. Aprill C, Bogduk N: The prevalence of cervical zygapophysial joint pain: A first approximation. *Spine,* 1992; 17:744–747.
6. Aprill C, Dwyer A, Bogduk N: Cervical zygapophysial joint pain patterns II: A clinical evaluation. *Spine* 1990; 15:458–461.
7. Avrahami E, et al: Early MR demonstration of spinal metastases in patients with normal radiographs and CT and radionuclide bone scans. *J Comput Assist Tomogr* 1989; 13:598–602.
8. Bernard T, Cassidy J: The sacroiliac joint syndrome, in Frymoyer J (ed): *The Adult Spine: Principles and Practice*. New York, Raven Press, 1991, pp 2107–2130.
9. Bogduk N: The clinical anatomy of the cervical dorsal rami. *Spine* 1982; 7:319–330.
10. Bogduk N, Twomey L: *Clinical Anatomy of the Lumbar Spine,* ed 2. Melbourne, Churchill Livingstone, 1991.
11. Bogduk N, Tynan W, Wilson A: The nerve supply of the human lumbar intervertebral disc. *J Anat* 1981; 132:39–56.
12. Bogduk N, Wilson A, Tynan W: The human lumbar dorsal rami. *J Anat* 1982; 134:383–397.
13. Cherry D, Gourlay G, McLachlan M, et al: Diagnostic epidural opioid blockade in chronic pain; preliminary report. *Pain* 1985; 21:143–152.
14. Countee R, Vijayanathan T: Congenital stenosis of the cervical spine: Diagnosis and management. *JAMA* 1979; 71:257–264.
15. Coin C, Chan Y, Keranen V, et al: Computer assisted myelography in disc disease. *J Comput Assist Tomogr* 1977; 1:398–404.
16. Crock H, Yoshizawa H: The blood supply of the lumbar vertebral column. *Clin Orthop* 1976; 115:6–21.
17. Cuatico W, Parker J, Pappert E, et al: An anatomical and clinical investigation of spinal meningeal nerves. *Acta Neurochir* 1988; 90:139–143.
18. Destouet J, Gilula L, Murphy W, et al: Lumbar facet joint injection: Indication, technique, clinical correlation, and preliminary results. *Radiology* 1982; 145:321–325.
19. Dory M: Arthrography of the lumbar facet joints. *Radiology* 1981; 140:23–27.
20. Dupuis P, Young-Hing K, Cassidy J, et al: Radiologic diagnosis of degenerative lumbar spinal instability. *Spine* 1985; 10:262–276.
21. Dvorak J, Penning L, Hayek J, et al: Functional diagnostics of the cervical spine using computer tomography. *Neuroradiology* 1988; 30:132–137.
22. Dwyer A, Aprill C, Bogduk N: Cervical zygapophyseal joint pain patterns I: A study in normal volunteers. *Spine* 1990; 15:453–457.
23. Edelman R, Shoukimas G, Stark D, et al: High resolution surface coil imaging of lumbar disc disease. *Am J Radiol* 1985; 144:1123–1129.
24. Edwards W, Orme T, Orr-Edwards G: CT/discography: Prognostic value in the selection of patients for chemonucleolysis. *Spine* 1987; 12:792–795.
25. El-Khoury G, Ehara S, Weinstein J, et al: Epidural steroid injection—A procedure ideally performed with fluoroscopic control. *Radiology* 1988; 168:554–557.
26. Enzmann D, Rubin J: Cervical spine: MR imaging with a partial flip angle, gradient-refocused pulse sequence: Part II. Spinal cord disease. *Radiology* 1988; 166:473–478.
27. Erlacher T: Nucleography. *J Bone Joint Surg [Br]* 1952; 34:204–210.
28. Eubanks B, Cann C, Brant-Zawadski M: CT measurements of the diameter of spinal and other bony canals: Effects of section angle and thickness. *Radiology* 1985; 157:243–246.
29. Fielding J, Cochran G, Lawsing J, et al: Tears of the transverse ligament of the atlas. *J Bone Joint Surg [Am]* 1974; 56:1683–1691.
30. Fink I, Garra B, Zabell A, et al: Computed tomography with metrizamide myelography to define the extent of canal block due to tumor. *J Comput Assist Tomogr* 1984; 8:1072–1075.
31. Friberg S: Lumbar disc herniation in the problem of lumbago sciatica. *Bull Hosp Jt Dis* 1954; 15:1–22.
32. Fries J, et al: Computed tomography of herniated and extruded nucleus pulposus. *J Comput Assist Tomogr* 1982; 6:874–887.
33. Frymoyer J, Hanley E, Howe J, et al: A comparison of radiographic findings in fusion and nonfusion patients, 10 or more years following lumbar disc surgery. *Spine* 1979; 4:435–440.
34. Frymoyer J, Newberg A, Pope M, et al: Spine radiographs in patients with low back pain. *J Bone Joint Surg [Am]* 1984; 66:1048–1055.
35. Gibson M, Buckley B, Mawhinney R, et al: Magnetic resonance imaging and discography in the diagnosis of disc degeneration. *J Bone Joint Surg [Br]* 1986; 58:369–373.

36. Haughton V, Eldevik O, Magnaes B, et al: A prospective comparison of computed tomography and myelography in the diagnosis of herniated lumbar discs. *Radiology* 1982; 142:103–110.
37. Hayes M, Howard T, Gruel C, et al: Roentgenographic evaluation of lumbar spine flexion-extension in asymptomatic individuals. *Spine* 1989; 14:327–331.
38. Herzog R: Magnetic resonance imaging of the spine, in Frymoyer J (ed): *The Adult Spine: Principles and Practice*. New York, Raven Press, 1991, pp 467–474.
39. Hickey D, Hukins D: Relation between the structure of the annulus fibrosus and the function and failure of the intervertebral disc. *Spine* 1980; 5:106–110.
40. Hinck V, Hopkins C, Savara B: Sagittal diameter of the cervical spinal canal in children. *Radiology* 1962; 79:97–108.
41. Horal J: The clinical appearance of low back disorders in the city of Gothenburg, Sweden. *Acta Orthop Scand Suppl* 1969; 118:1–108.
42. Hove B, Gyldensted C: Cervical analgesic facet joint arthrography. *Neuroradiology* 1990; 32:456–459.
43. Jackson R, Glah J: Foraminal and extraforaminal lumbar disc herniation: Diagnosis and treatment. *Spine* 1987; 12:577–585.
44. Kumar A, Kuhajada F, Martinez C, et al: Computed tomography of extracranial nerve sheath tumors with pathological correlation. *J Comput Assist Tomogr* 1983; 7:857–865.
45. Levitan L, Wiens C: Chronic lumbar extradural hematoma: CT findings. *Radiology* 1983; 148:707–708.
46. Lindblom K: Diagnostic puncture of the intervertebral discs in sciatica. *Acta Orthop Scand* 1948; 17:231–239.
47. Lynch M, Taylor J: Facet joint injection for low back pain. *J Bone Joint Surg [Br]* 1986; 68:138–141.
48. MacNab I: The traction spur: An indicator of segmental instability. *J Bone Joint Surg [Am]* 1971; 53:663–670.
49. Masaryk T, Ross J, Modic M, et al: High resolution MR imaging of sequestered lumbar intervertebral disc. *Am J Radiol* 1988; 150:1155–1162.
50. McCall I, Park W, O'Brien J: Induced pain referral from posterior lumbar elements in normal subjects. *Spine* 1979; 4:441–446.
51. McRae D, Barnum A: Occipitalization of the atlas. *Am J Radiol* 1953; 70:23–46.
52. Miles K, Maemares C, et al: The incidence and prognostic significance of radiological abnormalities in soft tissue injuries to the cervical spine. *Skeletal Radiol* 1988; 17:493–496.
53. Mixter W, Barr J: Rupture of the intervertebral disc with involvement of the spinal canal. *N Engl J Med* 1934; 211:210–215.
54. Modic M, et al: Degenerative disc disease: Assessment of changes in vertebral body marrow with MR imaging. *Radiology* 1988; 166:193–199.
55. Modic M, Feiglin D, Piraino D, et al: Vertebral osteomyelitis. Assessment using MR. *Radiology* 1985; 157:157–166.
56. Mooney V: Facet syndrome, in Weinstein J, Wiesel S (eds): *The Lumbar Spine*. Philadelphia, WB Saunders, 1990, pp 422–441.
57. Nathan H: Osteophytes of the vertebral column. An anatomical study of their development according to age, race, and sex with considerations as to their etiology and significance. *J Bone Joint Surg Am* 1962; 44:243–268.
58. Nguyen C, Ho K, Yu S, et al: An experimental model to study contrast enhancement in MR imaging of the intervertebral disc. *Am J Neuroradiol* 1989; 10:811–814.
59. *Nomina Anatomica,* ed 6. Edinburgh, Churchill Livingstone, 1989.
60. Okada K: Studies on the cervical facet joints using arthrography. *J Jpn Orthop Assoc* 1981; 55:563–580.
61. Page J, Olliff J: Value of anteroposterior radiography in cervical pain of nontraumatic origin. *Br Med J* 1982; 298:1293–1294.
62. Park W: Radiologic investigation of the intervertebral disc, in Jayson MIV (ed): *The Lumbar Spine and Back Pain,* ed 2. Bath, England, Pittman Medical, 1976, pp 185–230.
63. Parkin I, Harrison G: The topographical anatomy of the lumbar epidural space. *J Anat* 1985; 141:211–217.
64. Pattany P, et al: Motion artifact suppression technique (MAST) for MR imaging. *J Comput Assist Tomogr* 1987; 11:369–377.
65. Payne E, Spillane J: The cervical spine: An anatomicopathological study of 70 specimens (using special technique) with particular reference to problems of cervical spondylosis. *Brain* 1957; 80:571–596.
66. Penning L, Wilmink J: Rotation of the cervical spine. A CT study in normal subjects. *Spine* 1987; 12:732–738.
67. Peyster R, Teplick J, Haskin M: Computed tomography of lumbosacral conjoined nerve root anomalies. Potential cause of false-positive readings for herniated nucleus pulposus. *Spine* 1985; 10:331–337.
68. Prusick V, Samberg L: Klippel-Feil syndrome associated with spinal stenosis. A case report. *J Bone Joint Surg [Am]* 1985; 67:161–164.
69. Raskin S, Keating J: Recognition of lumbar disc disease: Comparison of myelography and computed tomography. *Am J Radiol* 1982; 139:349–355.
70. Rauschning W: *Clinical and Imaging Anatomy of the Lumbar Spine and Sacrum. Laseranatomy*. Video disc series. Metronics, Racho Palos Verdes, Calif, 1991.
71. Resnick D, Shapiro R, Wiesner K, et al: Diffuse idiopathic skeletal hyperostosis (DISH). *Semin Arthritis Rheum* 1978; 7:153–187.
72. Ridley M, Kingsley G, Gibson T, et al: Outpatient lumbar epidural corticosteroid injection in the management of sciatica. *Br J Rheumatol* 1988; 27:295–299.
73. Rosenbaum A, Yu S: MR/discography: A comparison of CT/discography and cryomicrotomes. Part II: Clinical applications. XIVth symposium neuroradiologicum. Proceedings. London. *Neuroradiology* 1991; 33(suppl):5–7.
74. Ross J, Modic M, Masaryk T: Tears of the annulus fibrosus: Assessment with Gd-DTPA enhanced MR imaging. *Am J Radiol* 1990; 154:159–162.

75. Rowlingson J, Kirschenbaum L: Epidural analgesic techniques in the management of cervical pain. *Anesth Analg* 1986; 65:938–942.
76. Rubin J, Wright A, Enzmann D: Lumbar spine: Motion compensation for cerebrospinal fluid on MR imaging. *Radiology* 1988; 167:225–231.
77. Schonstrom N, Bolender N, Spengler D: The pathomorphology of spinal stenosis as seen on CT scans of the lumbar spine. *Spine* 1985; 10:806–811.
78. Sellier N, Vallee C, Chevrot A, et al: Arthrographie articulaire vertebrale posterieure lombaire. *J Radiol* 1986; 67:487–506.
79. Shaffer W, Spratt K, Weinstein J, et al: The consistency and accuracy of roentgenograms for measuring sagittal translation in the lumbar vertebral motion segment. *Spine* 1990; 15:741–750.
80. Stanley J, Shabel S, Frey G, et al: Quantitative analysis of the cervical spinal canal by computed tomography. *Neuroradiology* 1986; 28:139–143.
81. Tajima T, Furukawa K, Kuramachi E: Selective lumbosacral radiculography and block. *Spine* 1980; 5:68–77.
82. *The Oxford Dictionary of Quotations,* ed 2. London, Oxford University Press, 1955, p 382.
83. Torg J, Pavlov H, Genuario S, et al: Neurapraxia of the cervical spinal cord with transient quadriplegia. *J Bone Joint Surg [Am]* 1986; 68:1354–1370.
84. Vandyk E, Ross J, Tkach J, et al: Gradient echo MR imaging of the cervical spine: Evaluation of extradural disease. *Am J Radiol* 1989; 153:393–398.
85. Vanharanta H, Guyer R, Ohnmeiss D, et al: Disc deterioration in low back syndrome. A prospective multicenter discography study. *Spine* 1988; 13:1349–1351.
86. Vanharanta H, Sachs B, Spivey M, et al: The relationship of pain provocation to lumbar disc deterioration as seen by CT/discography. *Spine* 1987; 12:295–298.
87. Walsh T, Weinstein J, Spratt K, et al: The question of lumbar discography revisited: A controlled prospective study of normal volunteers to determine the false-positive rate. *J Bone Joint Surg [Am]* 1990; 72:1081–1088.
88. Warfield C, Biber M, Crews D, et al: Epidural steroid injection as a treatment for cervical radiculitis. *Clin J Pain* 1988; 4:201–204.
89. White A, Derby R, Wynne G: Epidural injections for diagnosis and treatment of low back pain. *Spine* 1980; 5:78–86.
90. Wiesel SW, Tsourmas N, Feffer H, et al: A study of computer-assisted tomography I. The incidence of positive CAT scans in asymptomatic group of patients. *Spine* 1984; 9:549–551.
91. Wilkinson H, LeMay M, Ferris E: Roentgenographic correlation in cervical spondylolysis. *Am J Radiol* 1969; 105:370–374.
92. Williams A, Haughton V, Meyer G, et al: Computed tomographic appearance of the bulging annulus. *Radiology* 1982; 142:403–408.
93. Williams A, Haughton V, Syvertsen A: Computed tomography in the diagnosis of herniated nucleus pulposus. *Radiology* 1980; 135:95–99.
94. Wilmink J, Penning L: Influence of spinal posture on abnormalities demonstrated by lumbar myelography. *Am J Neuroradiol* 1985; 4:656–658.
95. Winkler M, Ortendahl D, Mills T, et al: Characteristics of partial flip angle and gradient reversal MR imaging. *Radiology* 1988; 166:17–26.
96. Winston K: Whiplash and its relationship to migraine. *Headache* 1987; 27:452–457.
97. Yu S, Haughton V, Sether L, et al: Comparison of MR and discography in detecting radial tears of the annulus: A postmortem study. *Am J Neuroradiol* 1989; 10:1077–1081.
98. Yu S, Sether L, Ho P, et al: Tears of the annulus fibrosus: Correlations between MR and pathologic findings in cadavers. *Am J Neuroradiol* 1988; 9:367–370.

9

Laboratory Testing

Richard D. Guyer, M.D.

Laboratory blood tests can be very helpful in directing the clinician to a correct diagnosis in the patient who presents with low back pain. While the vast majority of back pain complaints are related to mechanical etiologies such as lumbar strain syndrome, herniated nucleus pulposus, spinal stenosis, and other structural abnormalities, the remainder are related to underlying systemic illnesses that afflict 10% of patients presenting with low back pain.[14] Such testing can help to act as a screening modality as well as to make a specific diagnosis. As in all areas of medicine, the final diagnosis must be approached in a systematic fashion.

It has been suggested by Borenstein that one can distinguish five separate categories of nonmechanical back pain.[4] The first is related to those who present with fever and weight loss, including patients with vertebral osteomyelitis and malignant spinal tumors. Multiple myeloma is the most common primary malignant tumor affecting the spine, while metastases would be more common in older patients. The second group would be in those patients who present with night pain. Disorders in this group would include osseous and neural tumors of the spine[13] as well as paraspinal tumors. The third group would be those disorders characterized by morning stiffness. Stiffness that occurs from mechanical origin is generally of 1 hour or less, whereas that lasting for several hours is often a common symptom of a spondyloarthropathy.[4] Rheumatologic disorders can affect the axial skeletal spine as well as the sacroiliac joint. Included in this group are ankylosing spondylitis, Reiter's syndrome, psoriatic spondylitis, enteropathic spondylitis, and Behçet's syndrome. Patients who present with acute localized bone pain are in the fourth group. Grossly, these disorders cause a fracture or pain secondary to expansion of the bone. This group can be further categorized into those of abnormal mineral metabolism causing osteopenia such as osteoporosis, osteomalacia, hyperparathyroidism, or abnormal bone (Paget disease) and into marrow packing disorders in which bone cells are replaced with either inflammatory or neoplastic cells such as sarcoidosis and multiple myeloma. In addition, disorders that cause aseptic necrosis such as hemoglobinopathies may also cause localized bone pain. It is in this group especially that laboratory evaluation is extremely useful. Finally, visceral pain is the last category in which some intra-abdominal pathology refers pain into the lower part of the back. This can be either of a colic nature and relate to lesions of the ureter, uterus, colon, or gallbladder or of a throbbing nature and be associated with an abdominal aneurysm.[4]

SPECIFIC LABORATORY STUDIES

There are a plethora of tests that one may order, but only certain ones are indicated from results of the patient's clinical history and examination. The following represents the most common tests that can be utilized.

Complete Blood Count

The complete blood count (CBC) can detect anemias from systemic disease such as neoplasia, multiple myeloma, and hemoglobinopathies and can detect infections.

Erythrocyte Sedimentation Rate

This is a nonspecific test that indirectly reflects changes in concentration of serum fibrinogen and other acute-phase proteins. The erythrocyte sedimentation rate (ESR) is elevated with infection, neoplasia, and inflammatory disorders.[21] While it does not lead one to the proper diagnosis, this elevation is much like that of body temperature, which if elevated alerts the clinician to an abnormality, but not a specific one.

Chemistry Screen

Sequential multiple analysis by computer (SMAC) includes chemistry screening of electrolytes, renal function studies, liver function studies, bone chemistries, and glucose testing. Abnormalities in each of these studies refer to different problems that may be occurring in the patient:

- The fasting blood sugar level is helpful in alerting one to the diagnosis of diabetes as well as in directing one to the diagnose of a Charcot joint.
- Electrolyte abnormalities can occur secondary to endocrinologic disorders.

- Liver function studies can point to abnormalities primarily within the liver or bones.
- Renal studies, creatinine, and blood urea nitrogen (BUN) would indicate either primary or secondary renal disorders.
- Bone chemistries, including calcium, phosphorous, and alkaline phosphatase, would expose primary or secondary bone involvement from metabolic bone disease as well as neoplastic disorders.

This first line of blood testing is easily accessible to all laboratories. A second tier of testing, if those listed above are not helpful, will provide more specific information:

- Serum protein electrophoresis (SPEP) and urine protein electrophoresis (UPEP) are helpful in determining abnormalities in serum and urine globulin levels. These are found to be elevated in multiple myeloma.
- Human lymphocyte antigen B27 (HLA-B27) testing is useful for making a diagnosis of ankylosing spondylitis. HLA-B27 is present in greater than 90% of individuals with ankylosing spondylitis, but it is also present in 75% of patients with Reiter's syndrome, fewer than 50% of those with psoriatic arthropathy, and fewer than 50% of those with enteropathic arthropathy.[20]
- Immunoglobulin A levels are also found to be elevated in ankylosing spondylitis.[21]
- Acute-phase proteins such as a C-reactive protein are a nonspecific study, but the concentrations of these proteins are found to be increased in inflammatory disorders such as ankylosing spondylitis.[21]
- Immunoglobulin Aα_1 is an antitrypsin complex that has increased levels in myelomatosis and rheumatoid arthritis.[21]
- Latex fixation or rheumatoid factor is a test that is helpful in detecting underlying rheumatoid arthritis.
- Hemoglobin electrophoresis testing is helpful in exposing disorders such as sickle cell anemia or thalassemia.
- Homogentisic acid in the urine will elucidate the disorder of ochronosis.
- Urinary phosphate clearance and fluoride clearance are helpful in diagnosing fluoridosis.
- Endocrine disorders are easily detectable through a variety of hormonal assays. Thyroid function studies would determine hyperthyroidism associated with osteoporosis. Parahormone testing would evaluate hyperparathyroidism as well as hypoparathyroidism. Cortisol levels detect adrenal abnormalities.
- 25-Hydroxy-vitamin D levels will diagnose abnormalities with vitamin D metabolism and direct one toward underlying metabolic disorders.
- Spinal fluid analysis for cell count and protein and glucose concentrations is helpful in cases of infection and spinal tumors.

UTILITY OF LABORATORY STUDIES AND SPECIFIC DISORDERS

Fever and Weight Loss

Vertebral Osteomyelitis

Fortunately, this is a relatively rare condition occurring in 1% to 4% of all cases of pyogenic osteomyelitis.[25, 28] It is a disease that most commonly occurs in those patients over 50 years of age. Diabetics and intravenous drug abusers are at risk of developing this disorder. The lumbar spine is the most common site of spinal involvement, followed by the thoracic spine. The sedimentation rate is noted to be elevated in 73% of patients, and the white cell count is elevated in 35% of patients.[26] These studies are more confirmatory when used in conjunction with radiographic studies.

Spinal Epidural Abscess

This, again, is a rare condition in which diabetes mellitus is the most common underlying disorder.[26] This can be also associated with spinal surgery, lumbar punctures, and spinal anesthesia, with this group accounting for 14% to 22% of cases.[1, 6, 7, 16, 18] The white blood count is often normal, and blood cultures are positive only half of the time. However, the cerebrospinal fluid is found to be abnormal in 97% of cases.[6]

Pain With Recumbency

This would include both benign and malignant tumors of the spinal elements, including the osseous and neural structures, such as metastatic disease to the vertebral bodies and multiple myeloma. The spinal cord may be involved with benign tumors as well as malignant tumors. Ependymomas, meningiomas, neurofibromas, and schwannomas are the most common benign tumors that can present in this fashion.[13] In terms of osseous involvement, abnormalities can be seen in the mineral evaluation, including calcium, phosphorus, and alkaline phosphatase, as well as with serum protein electrophoresis as in multiple myeloma. Primary neural element tumors usually would not present with any significant abnormality other than abnormal spinal fluid analysis results, in which case the protein level is usually elevated to more than 100.

Morning Stiffness

The seronegative spondyloarthropathies comprise a group of conditions including ankylosing spondylitis, Reiter's syndrome, psoriatic spondylitis, enteropathic spondylitis, and Behçet's syndrome. Usually the patient presents with a history of prolonged morning stiffness lasting for more than 1 hour as well as pain in the sacroiliac region. Patients with Reiter's syndrome or psoriaticspondylitis may develop unilateral sacroiliac involvement and complain of unilateral back pain; they may also develop spondylitis without involvement of the sacroiliac joints. The pattern is different in those with ankylosing spondylitis and enteropathic spondylitis in that initially the sacroiliitis predominates and then the patient begins to develop more midline back pain as a result of the spondylitis. The clinician must be aware that each of these disorders also involves other organ systems and that ankylosing spondylitis will involve the eyes with uveitis and the heart with aortic insufficiency or conduction disturbances.[19] Reiter's syndrome also includes conjunctivitis, urethritis, and keratoderma blennorrhagicum. Psoriatic arthritis involves skin and nail changes, and finally, Crohn's disease and ulcerative colitis have intestinal manifestations that are more frequent when arthritis is noted.

Laboratory evaluation centers about the finding of the HLA-B27 antigen, which is present in approximately 90% of affected white patients vs. 8% of the general population. Seventy-five percent of those patients with Reiter's syndrome and fewer than 50% of those with psoriatic arthritis will have the antigen. Those with enteropathic arthropathy will be positive for HLA-B27 less than 50% of the time.[20] The ESR is usually elevated in the majority of patients with ankylosing spondylitis, and if there is active inflammation, the patient may have a mild normochromic, normocytic anemia and thrombocytosis. The only chemistry abnormality noted is in an occasional patient with an elevated serum alkaline phosphatase level.

Acute Localized Bone Pain

This group includes hematologic, metabolic, and endocrinologic disorders.

Hematologic Disorders

Hemoglobinopathies.—Because of the large amount of bone marrow found in the axial skeleton, hematologic disorders can result in low back pain. Hemoglobinopathies such as sickle cell anemia (hemoglobin SS) and sickle C hemoglobin disease as well as sickle thalassemia are the most common types and occur at a frequency of 1 in 625, 1 in 833, and 1 in 1667 black Americans, respectively. When back pain occurs with these disorders, it is during vaso-occlusive crises causing pain localized to the axial skeleton.[3] These patients are also susceptible to avascular necrosis, and since the hip is a very common site, the patient may present with pain localized to the hip, either anteriorly or posteriorly, which then radiates to the back. Laboratory studies would be accompanied by the finding of anemia with an abnormal hemoglobin electrophoresis result.

Myelofibrosis.—Myelofibrosis is a disorder resulting in metaplasia and fibrosis of the bone marrow. These patients can display extremity skeletal pain as well as axial pain. The latter is usually from compression fractures. Laboratory evaluation would include a CBC showing anemia and a blood smear showing the paucity of marrow elements on smear.[3]

Chronic Myelogenous Leukemia.—Patients with this disease develop back pain from infiltration of the bone marrow, which secondarily weakens the bone and causes compression fractures and neural impingement. Abnormalities may be seen in the white count, especially in the peripheral blood smear, which makes the diagnosis one of finding multiple myeloid lineage cells in varying degrees of maturation.

Acute Leukemia.—Low back pain is less common but can be due to leukemia infiltration of the bone marrow. Abnormalities would be seen in the white cell count and abnormal myeloid series in adults and lymphoblastoid series in children.[27, 29]

Lymphoma.—These include disorders such as Hodgkin's and non-Hodgkin's lymphoma. Approximately 15% of all lymphomas will affect predominantly the lumbar spine unless they are in the thoracic and cervical regions. These patients often complain of pain, especially with recumbency. Laboratory findings include anemia and an elevated sedimentation rate.[3]

Metabolic Disorders

Crystalline Deposition Disorders.—This group includes gout, pseudogout, and hydroxyapatite crystal deposition. Gout usually presents with a peripheral manifestation, and the uric acid concentration is elevated. The back is rarely involved in this disorder as well as in pseudogout and hydroxyapatite deposition.[15, 23, 31]

Hemochromatosis.—This is an inherited disorder with abnormal iron metabolism and excessive iron stores affecting multiple organ systems including the joints, liver, heart, and endocrine glands. This rarely affects the lumbar spine, and it is usually noted by disc calcification. The diagnosis is based on an elevated serum iron concentration with less than 60% saturation of the serum iron-binding protein transferrin. Elevated serum ferritin levels may also occur.[3]

Wilson's Disease.—This is an inherited disorder that results in enhanced copper accumulation and not uncommonly has lumbar spine involvement[22] resulting in pain and decreased range of motion. One may see abnormalities in ceruloplasmin levels.[17]

Alkaptonuria (Ochronosis).—This is a recessive-linked inherited disorder in which there is a deficiency of homogentisic acid oxidase that leads to the accumulation of homogentisic acid. This pigmentation is grossly black. The spine is typically affected, with pain in the morning not infrequent. The diagnosis is based on the finding of homogentisic acid in the urine.[3]

Fluorosis.—Patients with fluorosis may have vague complaints but with progression will complain of back pain and loss of motion.[5, 8] Laboratory findings reveal that urinary phosphate clearance is increased, as is urinary fluoride.

Osteopenic Disorders.—*Osteopenia* is a term used to describe the loss of bone mass. The most common causes for this are osteoporosis, osteomalacia, metastatic disease, and metabolic disorders. Osteoporosis is covered elsewhere in this text but is generally of the idiopathic or postmenopausal type. It is associated with spinal compression fractures (seen most commonly in the thoracolumbar spine area), hip fractures, and wrist fractures. The laboratory evaluation of these patients is most helpful, and the first line of screening would be a CBC, sedimentation rate, serum protein electrophoresis, thyroid function studies, and chemistry studies delineating liver functions, kidney function, calcium, phosphorus, alkaline phosphatase, and 25-hydroxy-vitamin D; a 24-hour urine calcium determination is carried out as well. This will help to eliminate thyroid disorders, gross gastrointestinal disorders, and renal disorders. If this initial screening does not detect any significant abnormalities, then one is dealing primarily with osteoporosis. If, however, there are significant abnormalities, then further evaluation would include specific endocrine studies, including cortisol levels and parathyroid hormone (PTH).[30]

Endocrine Abnormalities

Acromegaly.—The manifestations of this disorder are due to the overproduction of growth hormone. The spine is involved in approximately 50% of the patients, and manifestations include limited motion, kyphosis, and even spinal cord compression.[9] Laboratory testing would reveal elevation of growth hormone levels.

Hypoparathyroidism.—This is a disorder in which either PTH is underproduced or there is organ unresponsiveness. An ankylosing spondylitis–like syndrome has been reported in conjunction with this.[2, 12] Laboratory evaluation would show low levels of PTH, elevated blood levels of phosphate, hypocalcemia, and hyperphosphatemia.

Diabetes Mellitus.—Diffuse idiopathic skeletal hyperostosis can be associated with diabetes[30] and produce spinal stiffness, usually in the thoracolumbar area but also in the cervical region. The diagnosis of diabetes would be found in abnormal glucose determinations as well as glucosuria.

Visceral Pain

This would include disorders of the stomach, small intestine, kidney,[10] and female pelvic organs. Back pain may often be the only manifestation of the disorders, such as with a perforated ulcer of the stomach.[24] A careful history noting changes in gastrointestinal or genitourinary functions should lead to the correct diagnosis. Colicky or spasmodic pain is usually seen with disorders of the ureter such as from a stone, colon, or a gallbladder, while a throbbing pain can be seen in patients with an abdominal aneurysm.[11] Laboratory studies have little to add in the diagnosis of these various disorders since they are usually elucidated by physical and other specialized studies such as computed tomography (CT). Urinalysis will detect abnormalities of the urinary tract, and elevated BUN and creatinine levels may be found.

SUMMARY

In conclusion the vast majority of diagnoses can be made with a careful history, physical examination, and basic x-ray screening studies. If there are no obvious signs of systemic disorders or mechanical back pain, then the first screening studies should be a chemistry screen, CBC, and sedimentation rate along with hematologic screening studies, which might include an HLA-B27 determination and serum and urine protein electrophoresis if there is suspicion of a tumor. If one notes osteopenia on plain x-ray films, then further studies including endocrinologic studies, thyroid studies, and parathormone, cortisol, and 25-hydroxy-vitamin D testing would be indicated. While it is often tempting to order the entire battery of studies when the patient does not fit into a particular pattern, the clinician must be prudent and utilize these studies in a sequential fashion to maximize efficient care while minimizing excessive clinical waste and patient cost.

REFERENCES

1. Baker AS, Ojemann RG, Swartz MN, et al: Spinal epidural abscess. *N Engl J Med* 1975; 293:463–468.
2. Bland JH, Frymoyer JW, Newberg JH, et al: Rheumatic syndromes in endocrine disease. *Semin Arthritis Rheum* 1979; 9:23.
3. Bomalaski JS, Schumacher HR: Hematologic, metabolic, and endocrine diseases of the lumbar spine. *Semin Spine Surg* 1990; 2:106–120.
4. Borenstein D: Approach to the diagnosis and management of medical low back pain. *Semin Spine Surg* 1990; 2:80–85.
5. Bruns BR, Tytle T: Skeletal fluorosis reported two cases. *Orthopedics* 1988; 11:1083.
6. Coffman DM, Kaplin JG, Litman N: Infectious agents in spinal epidural abscesses. *Neurology* 1980; 30:844–850.
7. Danner RL, Hartman BJ: Updated spinal epidural abscess: 35 cases and review of the literature. *Rev Infect Dis* 1987; 9:265–274.
8. Fisher RL, Medcalf TW, Henderson MC: Endemic fluorosis of the spinal cord compression. *Arch Intern Med* 1989; 149:697.
9. Gellman MI: Cauda equina compression acromegaly. *Radiology* 1974; 112:357.

10. Gibson SM, Kimmel PL: Genetourinary disease affecting the spine. *Semin Spine Surg* 1990; 2:145–149.
11. Girodano JM: Vascular vs. spinal disease of back and lower extremity pain. *Semin Spine Surg* 1990; 2:136–140.
12. Gordan T, Eisenberg D: The endocrinologic association with autoimmune rheumatologic diseases. *Semin Arthritis Rheum* 1987; 17:58.
13. Guyer RD, Collier RR, Ohnmeiss DD, et al: Extraosseous spinal lesions mimicking disc disease. *Spine* 1988; 13:328–331.
14. Hadler NM: Regional back pain (editorial). *N Engl J Med* 1986; 315:1009–1012.
15. Hall MC, Selin G: Spinal involvement in gout. *J Bone Joint Surg [Am]* 1960; 42:341.
16. Hancock DO: A study of 49 patients with acute spinal extradural abscess. *Paraplegia* 1973; 10:285–288.
17. Henry TB: *Clinical Diagnosis and Management by Laboratory Methods,* ed 18. Philadelphia, WB Saunders, 1991, p 169.
18. Heusner AP: Non-tuberculous spinal epidural infection. *N Engl J Med* 1948; 239:845–854.
19. Hochberg MC: Ankylosing spondylitis. *Semin Spine Surg* 1990; 2:86–94.
20. Khan MA, Linden SM. Ankylosing spondylitis: Clinical aspects. *Spine State Art Rev* 1991; 3:529–551.
21. Malkiewitz A, Kushner I: Biochemical markers of inflammation in spondylitis. *Spine State Art Rev* 1991; 3:553–559.
22. Menerey KA, Eider W, Brewer GJ, et al: The arthropathy of Wilson's disease: Clinical and pathologic features. *J Rheumatol* 1988; 15:31.
23. Resnick D, Niwaygama G, Goergen TG, et al: Clinical, radiographic, and pathologic abnormalities in calcium pyrophosphate dihydrate deposition disease. *Radiology* 1977; 122:1.
24. Roberts IM: Gastrointestinal disorders presenting with back pain. *Semin Spine Surg* 1990; 2:141–144.
25. Ross PM, McGanity PJL: Vertebral osteomyelitis, pitfalls in diagnosis. *Infect Surg* 1984; 30:193–203.
26. Schwartz ST, Spiegel M, Ho G: Bacterial vertebral osteomyelitis in epidural abscess. *Semin Spine Surg* 1990; 2:95–105.
27. Spilberg I, Meyer GJ: The arthritis of leukemia. *Arthritis Rheum* 1972; 15:630–635.
28. Stauffer RN: Pyogenic vertebral osteomyelitis. *Orthop Clin North Am* 1975; 6:1015–1027.
29. Weinberger A, Schumacher HR, Schimmer BM, et al: Arthritis in acute leukemia: Clinical and histologic observations. *Arch Intern Med* 1981; 141:1183.
30. White TH: Osteopenic disorders of the spine. *Semin Spine Surg* 1990; 2:121–129.
31. Zwillich SH, Schumacher HR, Hoyt TS, et al: Universal spondylodiscitis in a patient with erosive peripheral arthritis and apatite crystal deposition. *J Rheumatol* 1988; 15:123–128.

10

Preoperative Diagnostic Studies

Jerry Holubec, D.O.

Physicians treating patients with back pain sometimes encounter frustrating cases. These are generally patients who have failed conservative treatment and for whom extensive, careful workup has failed to clearly identify painful pathology. The pain persists, and the patient continues to seek relief. The surgeon may still be hesitant to operate based on questionable pathology and needs more information in order to better make a decision concerning treatment. When dealing with patients with very chronic pain, the surgeon may also question the patient's psychological status, which would ultimately affect treatment outcome. Consequently, the surgeon may seek diagnostic input from an anesthesiologist or dolorologist in order to provide more insight into the pathogenesis of the patient's pain as well as help in determining the patient's potential response to surgery based on a differential sequential neural blockade. This diagnostic procedure monitors the patient's responses during a series of injections. Some of the injections should not have any effect on the patient's pain while others should block symptoms. Thus by carefully monitoring the patient's response to the type of injection being performed, one can determine whether the patient is providing the responses expected from each of the injections. It is important to remember that the results of this diagnostic procedure are just one piece of information and should not be the sole determinant of the patient's treatment plan. This information needs to be combined with results of physical examination findings, radiologic studies, and psychological evaluations when determining the appropriate treatment plan.

INDICATIONS

Patients with back pain for whom the etiology could not be clearly identified by routine diagnostic methods or those who present with recurrent pain after surgical removal of a lesion may be referred to an anesthesiologist/dolorologist for a differential sequential spinal block. This procedure can help to confirm suspected pathology, particularly in patients with radicular symptoms. It can also be valuable in patients who present with inconsistent physical findings and psychogenic pain or symptom magnification is suspected.

TECHNIQUE

Patient Preparation

The anesthesiologist/dolorologist must explain the procedure to the patient in such a manner that he responds freely and without coercion in order to eliminate bias. Unlike most diagnostic studies such as magnetic resonance imaging (MRI) or computed tomography (CT), the patient has an active role in the performance of the differential spinal block. Thus the procedure and the patient's role in it need to be clearly explained. The patient is told that an outpatient procedure called a differential sequential spinal block or pain study will be performed to help delineate the source of the pain. The patient's discomfort may originate from one of several pain generators: (1) the nerves coming out of the spinal cord, (2) mechanical instability of the lower part of the back, or (3) irritation caused by movement of the disc. The patient is instructed to have nothing to eat or drink after midnight prior to the procedure. Blood pressure, pulse, and oxygen saturation in the blood will be monitored. An intravenous catheter will be used for possible administration of medication. The patient will lie on his abdomen, and the back is cleansed with an antiseptic solution. Radiography will be used to guide needle placement, and only one injection will be felt; after that the only sensation will be pressure. The patient is then told that different medications will be injected and he will be asked whether the injection made the pain better, worse, or unchanged. The patient is informed that sometimes numbness is felt in the legs, and if this occurs he should let the physician know. It is emphasized that the numbness will resolve, but if back and leg pain continue along with the numbness, the physician needs to know this as well.

Many patients are concerned about giving a right or wrong answer to the pain-related questions as the medication is administered. It is explained to the patient that there are no right or wrong answers to the questions; what is of importance is how each injection affects his pain. Nothing is mentioned about the injection of local anesthetic.

Injection Technique

Upon the patient's arrival at the clinic, signatures on consent forms are obtained, and an intravenous catheter is started. The patient is placed in the prone position, and the lower part of the back is sterilized and draped. Under an image intensifier, the interspace of L2–3 or L3–4 is demarcated and infiltrated with 1.5% lidocaine solution. The method we use for performing differential sequential blockade is somewhat different from previously described procedures.[18, 25, 28] A 25-gauge needle is used in a bowed needle technique, and the subarachnoid space is penetrated.[14] The first solution injected into the subarachnoid space is the patient's own cerebrospinal fluid aspirated during the needle placement. After 2 or 3 minutes, the patient is asked, "Is your pain better, worse, or the same?" At this time, many patients will state, "My pain is fine," and again it is emphasized that the physician needs to know is whether the pain is better, worse, or the same. The next solution injected is 1 cc of normal saline without preservative; after another 2 to 3 minutes, the patient's pain is reassessed with the question: "Is the pain better, worse, or the same?" The third injection again consists of normal saline without preservative, and after another 3 minutes, the patient's pain is reassessed as before. The next solution injected is procaine and dextrose with cerebrospinal fluid. There is no hard and fast rule of how much procaine to inject; however, a tall individual would receive a dose of 50 mg procaine and 5 mg dextrose with a small amount of spinal fluid to make the solution hyperbaric. A small patient would receive 25 mg procaine with 5 mg dextrose and cerebrospinal fluid. Following this injection, the patient's pain is again assessed. The fifth injection, regardless of the patient's size, is 50 mg procaine and 10 mg dextrose in cerebrospinal fluid. After 3 minutes, the patient is asked to report whether the pain is better, worse, or unchanged. The last injection contains 100 mg procaine and 10 mg dextrose with spinal fluid. After this injection is complete, the needle is removed and the pain response assessed as before. The patient is then turned to the supine position and observed for approximately 15 minutes. During this time, the gurney can be tilted (Trendelenburg or reverse Trendelenburg) to yield a sensory block of approximately the T5 to T7 level with a total motor block of the lower extremities. The patient's pain is then assessed as before with delineation as to the level of the block.

INTERPRETATION OF RESULTS

There are three general responses to the differential sequential spinal blockade. The first group includes those patients who after injection of cerebrospinal fluid and the two normal saline injections report no pain relief whatsoever. After the injections of procaine, the patient typically states, "My pain is gone," or "I have no pain in my back (and/or legs)." It is to be noted that different types of nerve fibers may require similar and/or different concentrations of local anesthetic; therefore, sympathetic and sensory nerves may be blocked with injections of similar quantities and concentrations of local anesthetic.[8, 10, 20, 24, 25, 27] However, many other times, only the sympathetic nerves are blocked.

If the pain is not sympathetic in origin, it may continue. However, on the second and third injection of 50 mg procaine, 10 mg dextrose, and cerebrospinal fluid, the patient will say, "I don't have any pain whatsoever. My legs (and/or back) feel warm and tingly." This is gratifying for the anesthesiologist/dolorologist and for the spine surgeon as well because this response indicates that further diagnostic evaluation or intervention can be pursued. The pain is therefore interpreted on a sensory/motor basis.

The second group of patients will respond with comments indicating that some of the injections had a placebo effect (psychogenic mechanism). These patients classically, with injection of cerebrospinal fluid and again with normal saline, respond that the pain is gone. These patients do not report numbness because procaine was not injected. We do not know how patients will respond to the different solutions injected into the subarachnoid space; therefore, our preprocedure discussion with the patient includes the many responses he or she may have to the medications, i.e., pain with numbness of the leg, no pain with no numbness of the leg. Many patients provide responses that indicate that the injections had a placebo effect. These results are discussed with the spine surgeons. This does not necessarily rule out the existence of an organic pain generator; however, it may indicate a need for further psychological evaluation.

Patients in the third group remain very difficult diagnostic cases. Classically, these individuals will respond that every injection or solution either did not help them or helped them a little bit but they still have pain. We block these patients to T7 with a sensory block and a total motor block of the lower extremities. If the patient still has the pain, one can surmise that the patient has pain not originating in the lumbar spine. Several patients with encephalization[25] have had a motor block of the lower extremities with a sensory block to T7. When questioned whether they still had pain in their back or legs, they said "Yes." Many times this brings a sobering thought to patients when they realize that they are supposed to be numb and not feel any pain and yet they still have pain even with a block up to T7. For these patients, we strongly encourage counseling, psychological intervention, and possibly a lidocaine challenge test for this centralized pain state.*

DISCUSSION

After the differential sequential spinal block, we talk with the spine surgeons. If the differential spinal provided

*References 1, 2, 4–7, 11–13, 21, 22, 25, 26.

a placebo response from the patient, recovery expectations may not be fulfilled by having surgery even if a lesion is suspected.[9, 17, 18] This psychological element is important to the spine surgeon if he is to optimize the patient's total treatment. Patients who have a sensory block to approximately the T7 level—a total motor block of the lower extremities—and continue to experience pain in the lumbar spine are poor candidates for surgery. Their treatment program is directed toward psychological intervention and physical therapy rather than surgery. Like any other tool in the diagnostic armamentarium, the differential sequential spinal should not be employed as a definitive test with treatment decisions based solely on its findings. However, it can be combined with results from other evaluations to determine whether the patient is a candidate for further diagnostic tests and possibly surgical intervention or whether psychological intervention needs to be pursued rather than (or prior to) considering surgery.

BREVITAL PAIN STUDY

The use of Pentothal in a thiopental (Pentothal) pain study has been described by Krempen et al., who noted Walters as being the first to describe the procedure.[16] We have used this study in addition to the differential sequential spinal to help to better define the diagnosis in the surgical decision-making process. However with the barbiturate pain study, instead of using Pentothal, we use methohexital (Brevital). The main reason for this is that Brevital does not appear to concentrate in fat deposits to the extent that other barbiturate anesthetics do and has less protein binding. In addition, Brevital has less active metabolic by-products than Pentothal does during metabolization.[3, 15, 19, 23] All these factors lend to less time in the operating room and more time involving patient care. Also, patients tend to not have a hangover or drugged-out effect after undergoing a pain study with Brevital rather than Pentothal.

Describing the Pentothal pain study is sometimes like telling a patient that he is being given a "truth serum" to admit whether pain is really being experienced or not. However, if the physician tells the patient that he is going to have a Brevital or barbiturate pain study, the patient is less "offended" or guarded against having the test.

During the preoperative visit with the patient, the discussion of a barbiturate pain study or Brevital pain study is discussed to calm the patient's fears. The patient is informed that no needles are involved. Basically, an intravenous catheter is used, and medicine is delivered through this to relax the patient's muscles. Muscle testing is then performed. The test does not take very long to perform. The patient is told that he will be in a dreamlike sleep and then be taken to the recovery room. The question most frequently asked by patients is about the type of information this test will provide that other tests have not already provided. The most appropriate answer to this question is that no one study yields adequate information to totally determine the most appropriate course of treatment. The results of this study are combined with results from the differential spinal blockade, radiographic data, psychological evaluations, and physical examination findings. The patient undergoes a straight leg raising evaluation, and it is noted at what angle the evaluation causes grimacing or resistance to the test.

The patient is admitted to the hospital with the procedure being performed on an outpatient basis. The straight leg raising test is performed again immediately prior to the pain study. It is extremely important to understand that the patient will say that he has pain but there is no facial expression or resistance to the test. If there is only a verbal expression of pain, the patient is not appropriate for the pain study. The point at which the straight leg raise causes grimacing is recorded. The patient is preoxygenated by an anesthesiologist or a nurse-anesthetist and given approximately 80 to 100 mg of Brevital and, in many cases, 120 mg of Brevital intravenously or until the eyelid reflex is obliterated. Attention must be paid to the small window of decebration attained with Brevital. Constant testing for the eyelid reflex as well as facial grimacing or withdrawal from peripheral stimuli, such as a pinch in the trapezius or Achilles tendon must be performed. When a patient has no eyelid reflex but can respond to a painful stimulus, the straight leg raise test is performed again. It is noted at which angle the patient responds with a facial grimace or withdrawal from the test. The patient is then taken to the recovery room.

The Brevital pain study is very useful for patients who are thought to have a significant emotional component to their pain complaints. The basis for the Brevital study is that although the patient is decerbrated or unconscious under a light, general anesthesia, he is still able to react to a painful stimulus, such as a patient who has an eyelid reflex obliterated but still has a pain reaction to the painful stimuli as in a facial grimace. Generally, the results of the study are one of two outcomes.

The first group of patients is composed of those who experience pain at 30 degrees during the prestudy straight leg raise but, after administration of the Brevital, can perform the test through 80 or 90 degrees without facial grimacing. This outcome to the pain study is considered to be good objective evidence that an emotional functional overlay and coloring of the pain complaint exists. However, if after Brevital administration, the patient grimaces or withdraws from the straight leg test at an angle similar to that provoking this response prior to the Brevital study, this is considered to strongly indicate that the patient has an organic lesion. Therefore the patient's symptoms are caused by an organic lesion rather than emotional factors.

The Brevital or barbiturate pain study is best combined with the differential sequential spinal pain study. If the patient passes the differential spinal and passes the Brevital study, then the occurrence of a favorable surgical outcome, pending psychological tests, are very good. If the patient fails both these diagnostic tests, then the patient is considered a poor surgical candidate.

If the patient passes the differential spinal evaluation and fails the Brevital study, this indicates that the patient has a organic lesion, but emotional factors have a great impact on the patient's pain complaints. In this case, further psychological evaluation is needed. If the patient fails the differential spinal but passes the Brevital study, this is an indication that a central mechanism, most likely that of encephalization, is presenting itself.

As with any diagnostic test, the Brevital pain study is just one piece of information. It is best utilized in combination with the differential sequential spinal study and results of psychological testing.

REFERENCES

1. Awad EA: Interstitial myofibrositis: Hypothesis of the mechanism. *Arch Phys Med Rehabil* 1973; 54:440.
2. Boas RA, Covino RB, Shahnarian A: Analgesic response to IV lignocaine. *Br J Anaesth* 1982; 54:501–505.
3. Churchill-Davidson HC (ed): *Wylie & Churchill-Davidson's Practice of Anesthesia,* ed 5. Chicago, Mosby–Year Book, 1984, p 633.
4. Condouris GA: Local anesthetics as modulators of neuronal information, in Bonica JJ, Albe-Fessard DG (eds): *Advances in Pain Research and Therapy,* vol 1, New York, Raven Press, 1976, pp 663–667.
5. DeJong RH: *Local Anesthetics,* ed 2. Springfield, Ill, Charles C Thomas, 1977.
6. Dodd J, Craig EJ, Jessell TM: Neurotransmitters of neuronal monkeys at sensory synapses in the dorsal horn, in Kruger L, Liebeskind JC (eds): *Advances in Pain Research and Therapy,* vol 6. New York, Raven Press, 1984, pp 105–121.
7. Edwards WT, Habib F, Burney RG, et al: Intravenous lidocaine in the management of various chronic pain states. *Reg Anesth* 1985; 10:1–6.
8. Gasser HS, Erlanger J: The role of fiber size in the establishment of a nerve block by pressure or cocaine. *Am J Physiol* 1929; 88:581–591.
9. Ghia JN, Toomey TC, Mao W, et al: Toward an understanding of chronic pain mechanisms. *Anesthesiology* 1979; 50:20–25.
10. Gissen AM, Covino BG, Gregus J: Differential sensitivities of mammalian nerve fibers to local anesthetic agents. *Anesthesiology* 1980; 53:467–474.
11. Graubard DJ, Robertazzi RW, Peterson MC: One experience with intravenous procaine. *Anesth Analg* 1948; 27:222–226.
12. Hatangdi VS, Boas RA, Richards EG: Postherpetic neuralgia: Management with antiepileptic and tricycline drugs, in Bonica JJ, Albe-Fessard DG (eds): *Advances in Pain Research and Therapy,* vol 1. New York, Raven Press, 1976, pp 583–587.
13. Heavner JE, deJong H: Lidocaine blocking concentrations for B- and C-nerve fibers. *Anesthesiology* 1974; 40:228–233.
14. Holubec J: The bowed needle technique. Unpublished.
15. Hudson RJ, Stanski DR, Burch PG: Pharmokinetics of methohexetal and thiopental in surgical patients. *Anesthesiology* 1983; 59:215.
16. Krempen JF, Silver RA, Hadley J: An analysis of differential epidural spinal anesthesia and Pentothal pain study in the differential diagnosis of back pain. *Spine* 1979; 4:452–459.
17. Loeser JD, Bigos SJ, Fordyce WE, et al: Low back pain, in Bonica JJ (ed): *The management of pain,* vol 2. Philadelphia, Lea & Febiger, 1990, pp 1448–1483.
18. McCollum DE, Stephen CR: The use of graduated spinal anesthesia in the differential diagnosis of pain of the back and lower extremities. *South Med J* 1964; 57:410–416.
19. Deleted in proofs.
20. Nathan PW, Sears TA: Some factors concerned in differential nerve block by local anesthetics. *J Physiol* 1961; 157:565–580.
21. Peterson CG: Neuropharmacology of procaine. I. peripheral nervous actions. *Anesthesiology* 1955; 16:678–698.
22. Phero JC, DeJong RH, Denson DD, et al: Intravenous chloro-procaine for intractable pain. *Reg Anesth* 1983; 8:41.
23. *Physicians Desk Reference,* ed 46. Oradell, NJ, Medical Economics, 1992, pp 1248–1249.
24. Raj PP: Sympathetic pain mechanisms and management. Presented at the Second Annual Meeting of the American Society of Anesthesiologists, Hollywood, Fla, March 1977.
25. Ramamurphy S, Winnie AP: Diagnostic maneuvers in painful syndromes, in Stein JM, Warfield CA (eds): *Pain Management.* Boston, Little Brown, 1983, pp 47–59.
26. Schnapp M, Mays KS, North WC: Intravenous 2-chloro procaine in treatment of chronic pain. *Anesth Analg* 1981; 60:844–845.
27. Winnie AP: Anesthesiology and pain management. Presented at the 36th Annual Postgraduate Course in Anesthesiology, Snowbird, Utah, February 1991, pp 131–151.
28. Winnie AP, Collins VJ: The pain clinic. I: Differential neural blockade in pain syndromes of questionable etiology. *Med Clin North Am* 1968; 52:123.

PART III

PRACTICAL FUNCTIONAL ANATOMY AND EMBRYOLOGY

11

Embryology and Anatomy of the Spine

Robert F. McLain, M.D., Pasquale X. Montesano, M.D., and Wolfgang Rauschning, M.D.

GENERAL

The musculoskeletal and articular tissues of the human body take their earliest form during the second week of embryonic life and continue to mature and develop well into the second decade of postnatal life. The embryonic period is generally considered to begin during the second week following conception when the embryonic disc forms and continues until the eighth week of development. At the end of the eighth week all major internal and external structures are present in rudimentary form, and the developing human enters the fetal period. During fetal development the rudiments of organs and extremities grow, mature, and take on the form they will have at birth. The rate of body growth and weight gain is greatest during this period. Postnatal development of the musculoskeletal system involves the ossification of bones formed during the embryonic period, growth and elongation of musculoskeletal elements, and changes in shape and orientation to accommodate new forces and stresses produced by muscular growth and changes in physical activities.

The structures identified in the adult spinal column are derived from precursor elements that first appear during the embryonic period.[44, 45] These elements become apparent during the third week of development when the embryonic disc begins the process of gastrulation. The bone and soft-tissue elements of the spinal column are formed from the intraembryonic mesoderm, one of three component tissues found within the trilaminar embryonic disc. These three tissue precursors are identified as (1) the embryonic ectoderm, which gives rise to the outer epithelia and nervous system[24]; (2) the endoderm, which produces the visceral epithelia and internal organs; and (3) the intraembryonic mesoderm, from which are derived the axial and appendicular skeletons and their connective tissues, smooth and striated muscle, the hematopoietic tissues, and reproductive and excretory organs.[37]

The vertebral column forms around the notochord, which is formed from migrating mesenchymal (mesoblastic) cells. The notochord induces formation of the neural plate by the overlying ectoderm and then degenerates.[43] The paraxial mesoderm divides into paired segments along either side of the embryonic neural tube to form the segmented blocks of primitive connective tissue termed *somites*. Forty-two to 44 pairs of somites develop and eventually give rise to the bones of the skull and spine, their associated musculature, and the dermis of the overlying skin.

The developing vertebrae take form from three structural components: the centrum, neural processes, and costal elements. The central portion of the developing vertebral body is termed the *centrum*. The neural processes that will eventually form the neural arch arise on either side of the neural tube at the posterior margin of the centrum. Costal elements are present at all levels of the spinal column but form ribs only in the thoracic region. In the cervical region the costal element forms a small portion of the transverse process.

It is during this early developmental period that most vertebral defects are produced.[66] Once the embryonic period has been completed, the elements of the spinal column are in place, and the rest of the time until birth—the fetal period—is dedicated to the physical growth and remodeling of these structures. Events that occur during this embryonic period determine the complex anatomy of the adult spine and result in the numerous congenital defects that can affect it.

THE EMBRYONIC PERIOD

The beginning of the embryonic period is marked by the appearance of the amniotic cavity and development of a bilaminar embryonic disc.[37] The amniotic cavity appears at day 8 following conception (stage 5), coincident with the implantation of the developing blastocyst into the endometrium. As this cavity expands, the bilaminar embryonic disc is formed and consists of the embryonic epiblast on one surface and embryonic endoderm on the other. By day 14 (stage 6) the intraembryonic mesoderm has begun to form a third tissue layer in the embryonic disc[45] (Fig 11–1). The primitive streak initially forms as a midline thickening on the dorsal aspect of the disc at its caudal end. It elongates with the embryo in a craniocaudal direc-

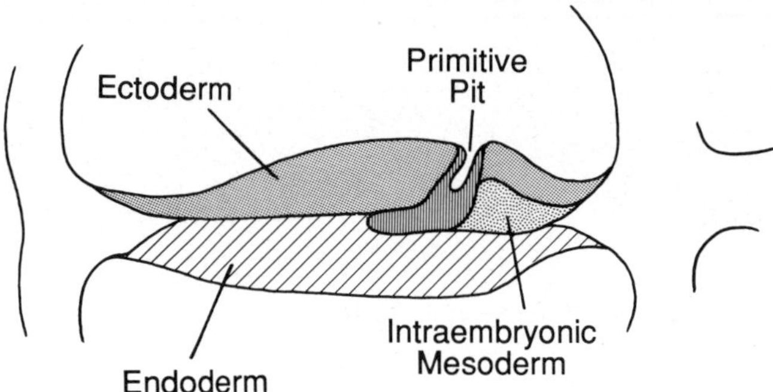

FIG 11–1.
Trilaminar embryonic disc during early notochord development. The drawing illustrates a midsagittal section at about 16 days. The notochordal process extends caudally from the primitive pit to lie in the midline between the embryonic endoderm and ectoderm.

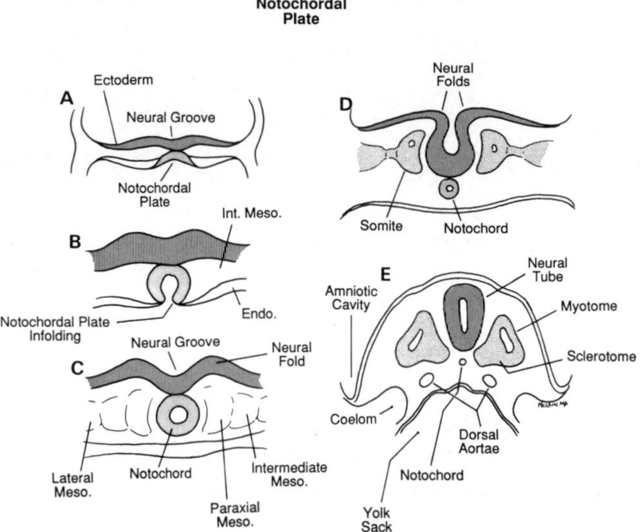

FIG 11–2.
Development of the notochord and neurenteric canal. **A,** a cross section through the embryonic disc at day 18 demonstrates the notochordal plate, a remnant of the notochordal process and primitive pit. **B,** as the embryo develops, the notochordal plate infolds to form a tube. **C,** the notochord induces the development of a thickened neural plate. At day 20, somites develop from the paraxial mesoderm. **D,** the invaginating neural groove forms two neural folds that fuse in the midline to form the neural tube. **E,** at 26 days, the neural tube has separated from the overlying ectoderm, and somites have differentiated into myotomic and sclerotomic portions. The intraembryonic coelom divides the lateral mesoderm into parietal and visceral layers. The notochord persists.

tion and forms a localized thickening at the cranial extreme called the primitive knot. The primitive streak gives rise to the intraembryonic mesoderm, the mesenchymal germ cells that will eventually produce the musculoskeletal system.[24] These mesenchymal cells migrate ventrally, laterally, and cranially between the two existing germ cell layers, the endoderm and ectoderm, to form a sheet of mesenchymal tissue on either side of the midline. The primitive knot gives rise to the notochordal process at about 16 days (stage 7), from which develops the notochord itself. The notochordal process runs longitudinally in the midline of the embryo between the two plates of mesenchyme. Once formed, this structure spontaneously degenerates to form the notochordal plate, which in turn infolds upon itself to form the notochord proper (Fig 11–2). Notochord development is usually complete by day 22 (stage 10).[44]

As the notochord develops, it induces the overlying ectoderm to form the neural plate. The ectodermal cells of the neural plate, the neuroectoderm, eventually give rise to the brain and spinal cord. The neural plate elongates cranially and caudally to extend along the notochord from its caudal tip to the primitive knot. At day 18 (stage 8) the plate begins to invaginate in the midline and forms two longitudinal neural folds on either side of the neural groove. By the end of the third week (stage 10) the neural folds have begun to converge and fuse dorsally to form the neural tube. This tube then separates itself from the surrounding ectoderm, the free edges of which overgrow the neural tube to form a continuous ectodermal layer over the dorsum of the embryo.

As the neural folds fuse and the neural tube separates from the overlying ectoderm, some neuroectodermal cells separate from the crest of each fold and begin to migrate laterally beneath the ectoderm. These neural crest cells are the precursors to the spinal ganglia and the ganglia of the autonomic nervous system, form the coverings of the spinal cord, and contribute to the formation of pigment cells and the adrenal medulla.[37]

Beginning about day 20 (stage 9) the paraxial mesoderm begins to form up into paired segments termed *somites* (Fig 11–2,D). These cuboidal tissue blocks form along either side of the neural tube and give rise to most of the axial skeleton, skeletal musculature, and the connective tissue of the skin. The somites form initially at the cranial end of the notochord, and subsequent pairs are added in a craniocaudal sequence until 42 to 44 pairs have been formed.[44] Because some of the most cranial somites degenerate before the most caudal ones form, they are never all visible at one time.

In all, 4 occipital, 8 cervical, 12 thoracic, 5 lumbar, 5 sacral, and 8 to 10 coccygeal pairs of somites form. The first occipital pair and 5 to 7 of the most caudal segments subsequently disappear. The remaining somites expand dorsally and medially to surround the notochord[20] (Fig 11–3). As the mesenchymal tissue condenses, alternating dense and loose zones appear, each set of dense and loose zones forming a single sclerotome (Fig 11–4). The densely cellular zone gives rise to two separate tissues. The cranial portion differentiates to form the early intervertebral disc, while the remaining caudal portion fuses with the loosely packed cells of the next most caudal zone

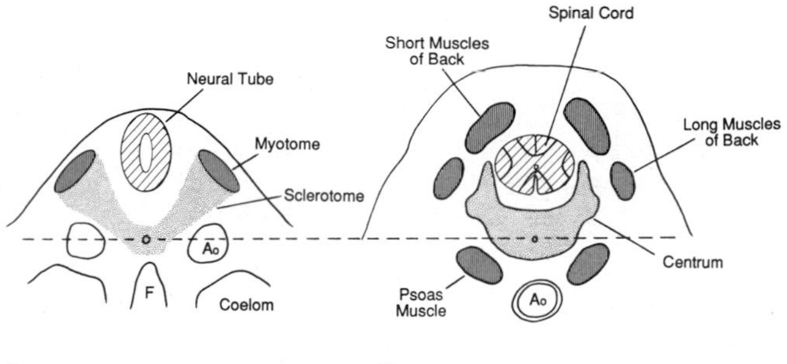

FIG 11–3.
Development of the dorsal musculature. **A,** day 26. Sclerotomic cells surround the notochord and trail behind the myotomic segments as they migrate dorsally and laterally. **B,** at 7 weeks, the myotomes have separated to form the major muscle groups of the trunk. *Ao* = aorta; *F* = foregut.

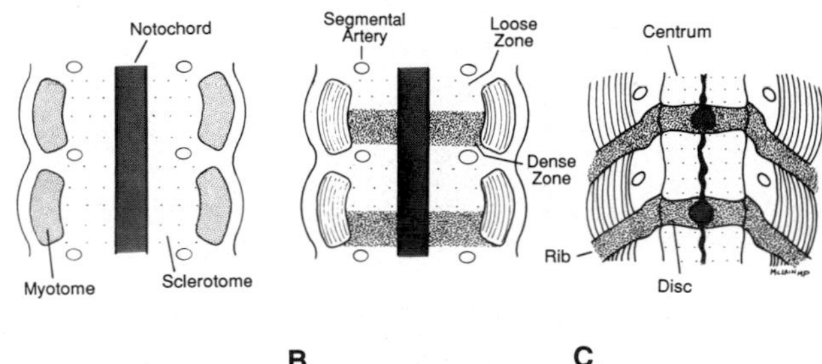

FIG 11–4.
Development of the vertebral centrum. **A,** a coronal section shows the early arrangement of the notochord surrounded by undifferentiated sclerotomic tissue. Two axial segments are illustrated. **B,** each sclerotome differentiates into loose and dense zones. **C,** as the notochord degenerates, the loose sclerotomic zones form the vertebral centra, while the dense zones contribute to the formation of ribs and neural arches, as well as form the intervertebral discs.

to form the centrum of the vertebral body. Abnormal segmentation may result in vertebral anomalies. Failure of normal segmentation may produce block vertebrae, unsegmented bars, or the Klippel-Feil syndrome.[22, 72]

In the past most authors subscribed to Remak's theory that these sclerotomies underwent resegmentation prior to forming the primitive vertebral elements of the centrum and intervertebral disc.[57] This theory has been refuted by more recent investigators,[44, 64, 65] who have demonstrated that the position of the segmental artery relative to the primitive segments varies both with time and with the distance from the midline of the section examined.

Although most of the notochord degenerates early in the embryonic period, notochordal rests persist within the tissues of the intervertebral discs. These remnants expand to form the nucleus pulposus.[54] While the remaining notochord usually degenerates completely, notochordal rests can be seen in some adults and occasionally give rise to a malignant tumor, the chordoma.[15, 36]

In the developing vertebra, the major portion of the vertebral body is derived from the mesenchymal centrum. This is consistent regardless of the vertebral level. The centrum gives off two dorsal prominences that form the neural processes (Fig 11–5). The neural processes extend dorsally on either side of the neural tube, eventually uniting and enclosing the tube later in the fetal period. The neural processes therefore give rise to the neural arch, spinous and transverse processes, and a portion of the vertebral body (Fig 11–6).

The costal elements first become apparent during the fourth week of development, with the thoracic elements differentiating into well-formed ribs by the beginning of the fetal period.[60] Costal elements are also found in the cervical, lumbar, and sacral vertebrae but contribute only to the transverse processes and sacral alae at these levels.[10] Occasionally, costal elements will continue to differentiate in the cervical or lumbar regions and give rise to fully formed cervical and lumbar ribs.[34, 61]

Chondrification

At about 6 weeks of development (stage 17) the process of chondrification begins (Fig 11–7), at which time the mesenchymal vertebral anlage is replaced by cartilage in anticipation of later endochondral ossification.[37, 44] The neural arches, including the pedicles, laminae, and transverse processes, are the first to be converted. The costal elements chondrify at 7 weeks (stage 19) and the centrum and the rest of the neural arches at 8 weeks (stage 23). Although some authors state that chondrification of the centrum starts from a single center,[23] others have observed that two centers of chondrification are seen in the mesenchymal centrum, one forming on either side of the notochord. These centers unite in the midline at the end of the embryonic period.[2, 42, 44, 62] Failure of one center to form or failure of the two centers to fuse has been suggested as possible causes of congenital deformities such as hemivertebrae or butterfly vertebrae.[7, 19]

THE FETAL PERIOD

At the beginning of the fetal period the embryonic forms of all essential internal and external structures can

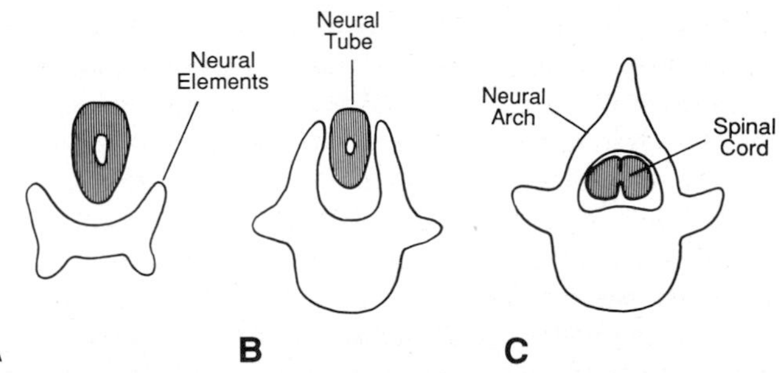

FIG 11–5.
As the vertebral centrum develops, the posterior elements take form from the neural processes. **A,** neural processes during early embryonic period. **B,** processes and neural tube at the beginning of fetal growth. **C,** neural arch prior to birth.

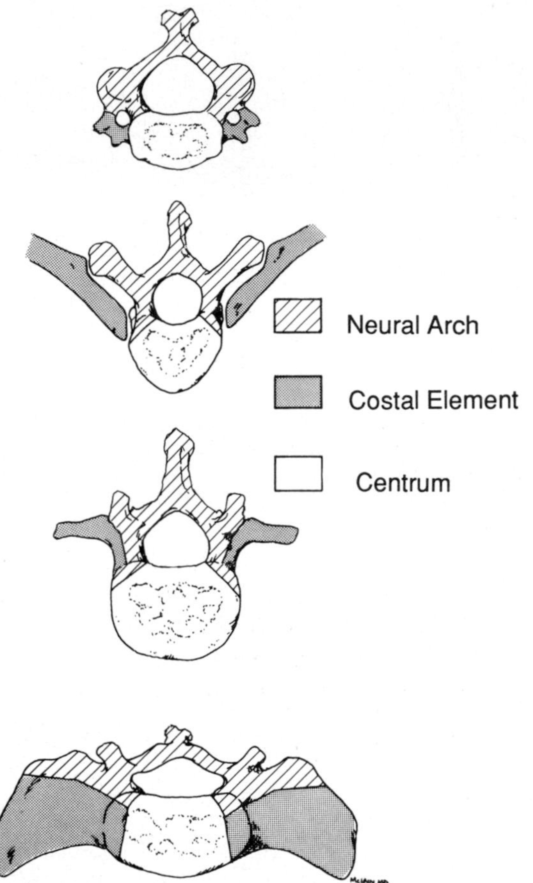

FIG 11–6.
Contributions of embryonic elements to parts of adult vertebrae. Cervical, thoracic, lumbar, and sacral vertebrae are illustrated.

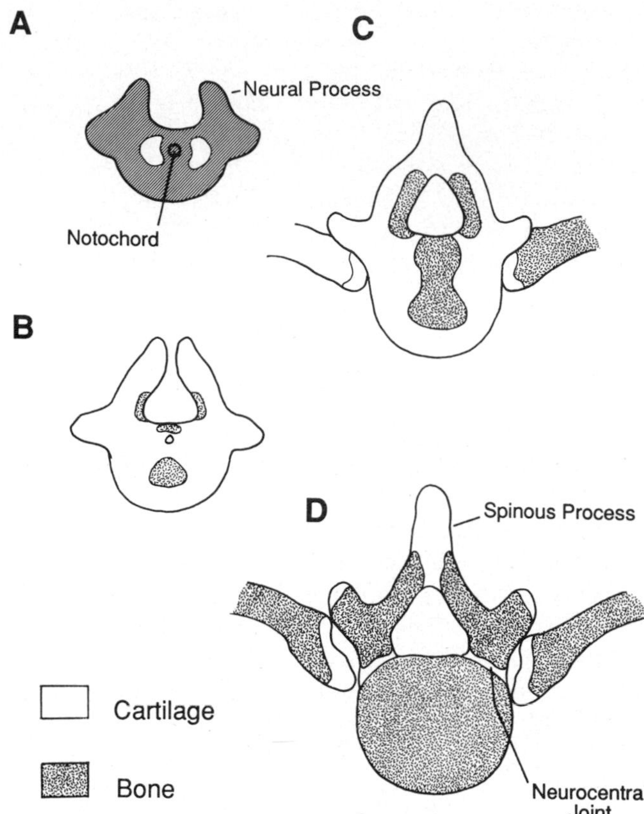

FIG 11–7.
Chondrification and ossification. **A,** the mesenchymal vertebrae begin to chondrify at about 6 weeks. **B** and **C,** early in the fetal period, the cartilaginous vertebra begins to ossify. Ossification centers first appear along the medial walls of the neural processes and as either a single or bipartite centers within the vertebral centrum. **D,** at birth, the vertebrae consist of three ossified portions—the centrum and each arch—connected by the cartilaginous neurocentral joints and the cartilaginous spinous process.

be identified. Development from this point on consists primarily of the maturation and growth of existing structures rather than the formation of new ones. The cartilaginous anlage formed during the embryonic period now begins the process of ossification.

Ossification

The neural arches and centra begin ossification at roughly the same time—9 weeks—but are not necessarily coordinated in the sequence they follow.[38, 41, 46] The neural processes begin to ossify along their medial walls prior to closure of the arches. The process continues until the pedicles, transverse processes, and laminae have all been ossified. By this time the neural processes have united and the spinous process has formed. This does not ossify until after birth. The general sequence of ossification in the neural arches is rostrocaudal.

Failure of the neural arches to unite normally results in a spina bifida deformity but does not result in myelodysplasia.[44] Meningocele and myelomeningocele are thought to result from events occurring early in the embryonic period, either from a failure of the neural tube to close or from injury to the neuroectoderm.[9, 14] Ossification of the centra begins in the thoracic region and progresses to the lumbar and then to the cervical regions. Two primary centers of ossification develop in the centrum initially—one dorsal and the other ventral.[64] These two centers fuse to form the single center seen at the end of embryonic development. If these centers do not fuse early, a coronal vertebral cleft may persist into fetal and even into postnatal life.[16, 56, 63]

The point at which the neural arch joins the vertebral body is termed the *neurocentral joint*. These cartilaginous synchondroses allow the vertebra to continue to grow and expand as a ring around the spinal cord. The neurocentral joints persist after birth but are usually obliterated by the age of 6 years.

Intervertebral Disc

The mesenchymal somites segment to form alternating dense and loose cellular zones that give rise to the precursor of the vertebral column. The cranial half of the densely cellular zone of each somite differentiates to form the intervertebral disc. Between weeks 6 and 8 of the embryologic period the disc matures from a broad band of uniformly cellular tissue into a nonuniform prototype of the adult disc. The peripheral tissues become more densely cellular and thickened, while the central tissues regress to a thin layer of cells across which the vertebral end plates can almost touch.[64] At the very center of this region a rest of notochordal cells may be seen. Over the next several weeks of embryologic and fetal development this notochordal tissue will proliferate and expand horizontally and longitudinally to form the early nucleus pulposus. The thickened peripheral tissues continue to mature into the annulus fibrosus.

During the fetal period, the delineation between the true notochord and the attendant perinotochordal tissues becomes blurred. Perinotochordal mesenchymal cells also contribute to the formation of the nucleus. The true notochordal cells undergo progressive mucoid degeneration and leave behind a less cellular tissue consisting of few notochordal cells, abundant mucoid substance, and a population of cartilage cells. By the age of 10 years the notochordal cells will all have disappeared, and the nuclear material will contain an increasing complement of fibrocartilage.[53, 54, 64, 66]

Spinal Cord

The tissue that will become the spinal cord is difficult to distinguish prior to the tenth week of development. The cells of the neural tube are not structured in a way that allows recognition of future cord elements prior to 6 weeks, and these elements slowly take form over the next 4 weeks. Nerve roots become visible during the seventh week. At 10 weeks the anterior and posterior horns of the spinal cord become easily distinguishable, as well as the spinal ganglia.

When the spinal cord initially develops, its caudal tip is level with the caudal end of the spinal canal.[4] Although the spine and cord grow synchronously during early development, the growth of the spinal column begins to outstrip that of the cord during the fetal period so that the tip of the cord may be found at progressively higher levels during development (Fig 11–8). At birth the tip of the cord is usually seen at the third lumbar level. This asynchronous growth continues so that at 2 to 3 months of age the cord ends at either the first or second lumbar levels. From this point the spine and cord grow at the same rate, and in adulthood the conus medullaris will still be found at this level in the majority of patients.[5]

Development of Primary Curves

The normal adult spine has four sagittal spinal curvatures (Fig 11–9). Of these, the kyphotic sacral and thoracic curves are considered primary because they develop before birth. These curves are thought to be the result of skeletal modeling due to the position of the fetus inutero.[46] The lordotic cervical and lumbar curves are generally thought to develop postnatally and are considered to be secondary. Depending on the in utero posture, however, some authors have identified the presence of cervical lordosis as early as 9½ weeks.[3, 45]

SPINAL ANATOMY

In order to construct a rational rehabilitation or surgical program for any patient, an understanding of spinal anatomy is needed. The following is a basic review of this anatomy; a more comprehensive discussion of specific topics is available in a number of texts.[12, 21, 26, 35, 50]

Bony Elements

The adult spine typically contains 7 cervical, 12 thoracic, and 5 lumbar vertebrae; the sacrum; and a variable number of coccygeal elements. Some individuals may have 1 more or 1 less thoracic or lumbar vertebra, but the missing element is often compensated by an additional vertebra in the adjacent segment.

Cervical Spine

The upper part of the cervical spine consists of three skeletal elements and their articulations: the occiput, at the base of the skull; the atlas, on which the occiput rests and articulates; and the axis, which contains the odontoid process about which the atlas rotates. The majority of craniocervical flexion, extension, and rotation is provided by these articulations.

Atlas

The first cervical vertebra, the atlas, is unique in several ways. The vertebra consists of a ring with broad superior and inferior articular facets and a rudimentary prominence for the spinous process. The vertebral body is absent, and the anterior ring articulates, instead, with the odontoid process from the axis below (Plate 1). The superior articular facets face cranially and somewhat medially to provide a broad contact area for articulation with the occipital condyles. The inferior facets are also concave and oriented caudally and medially to perch on the sloped "shoulders" of the axis below (Plate 2).

The posterior ring of C1 is narrow and rounded, with a small midline prominence that provides the origin for the suboccipital musculature. Extending laterally from the lateral mass, the transverse processes form the transverse foramen, through which the vertebral artery passes. At the junction of the posterior ring and the lateral masses a narrow groove is seen to cross the superior aspect of the ring. This groove transmits the vertebral artery from within the transverse foramen, over the dorsum of the C1 ring, and into the spinal canal. After passing through the transverse foramen of the axis, the vertebral arteries pass from these

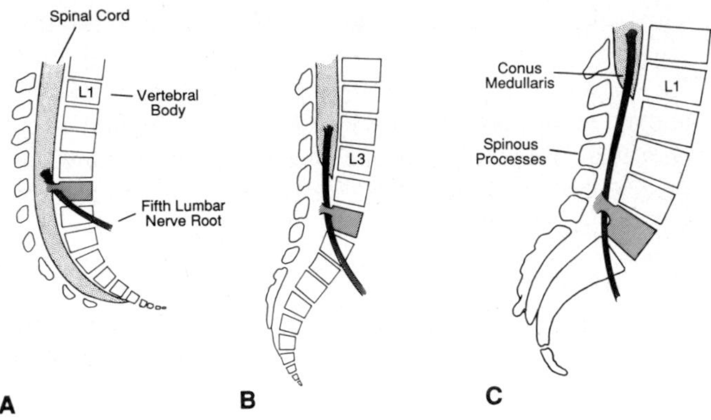

FIG 11–8.
Differential growth between the vertebral column and the spinal cord results in recession of the conus medullaris cranially during development. This results in formation of the cauda equina. **A,** spinal cord position during fetal period. **B,** position of conus medullaris at birth. **C,** position of conus at maturity.

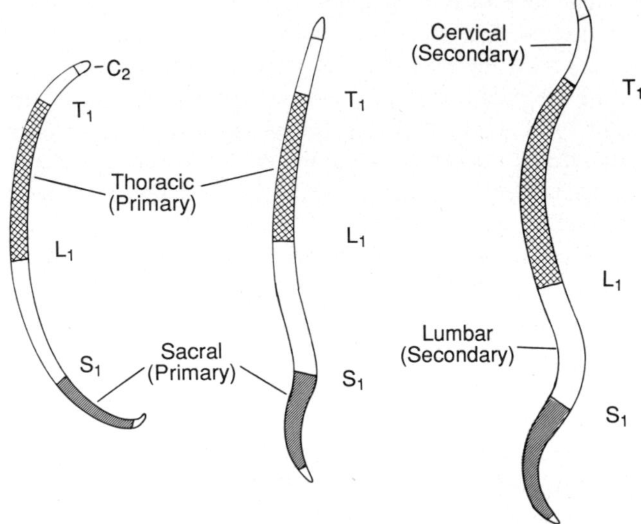

FIG 11–9.
Of the four significant curvatures present in the adult spine, two—the thoracic and sacral—are present in utero and are considered primary curves. As the individual grows and develops an upright posture, two secondary curves develop—the cervical and lumbar. Primary curves are kyphotic; secondary curves are lordotic.

grooves through the atlanto-occipital membrane. Because of their dorsal exposure, these arteries are at risk during dissection of the posterior ring, particularly if the dissection is carried laterally.

The anterior arch of C1 articulates with the odontoid process, and the semicircular depression formed by this articulation can be seen on the posterior aspect of the arch. Prominent tubercles on the medial aspects of the adjacent lateral masses represent the origins of the transverse ligaments, the dense ligaments that constrain the odontoid against the anterior ring (see Plate 1). The transverse ligaments along with the alar and apical ligaments are the primary stabilizers of the atlanto-axial articulation. Disruption of these restraints may lead to significant instability.[18, 69]

Axis

The C2 vertebra is uniquely constructed to control the rotational motion of the atlas above. The body of the axis provides broad convex facets superiorly on which the atlas may rotate and pivot, while the odontoid process provides a pivotal restraint that limits both anteroposterior and lateral translation and maintains axial alignment during rotational motions (Plate 3). The odontoid, representing the original centrum of the C1 vertebra, is bound to the anterior ring of C1 by the dense transverse ligaments and to the occiput by the superiorly oriented alar and apical ligaments.

The superior articular facets of the axis are located anterior to the vertebral canal and oriented upward and outward to provide a bearing surface for the inferior facets of the atlas. The inferior facets of the axis are located posterior to the vertebral canal and oriented in the plane more typical of cervical vertebrae. This shift of the weight-bearing axis from anterior to posterior may, in part, explain the tendency of the axis to fracture between the superior and inferior facets when exposed to excessive hyperextension.[69]

Subaxial Cervical Vertebrae

The third through sixth cervical vertebrae are fairly uniform in their construction and can be discussed in common terms. The seventh cervical vertebra is a transitional element, with a proportionally enlarged inferior end plate and an altered pattern of facet orientation to allow articulation with the subjacent thoracic vertebra.

The typical subaxial cervical vertebra consists of a relatively thin, small vertebral body with obliquely oriented pedicles giving rise to the lateral masses and their transverse processes. The posterior arch is characterized by narrow laminae flattened in the anteroposterior plane and by a prominent spinous process. The vertebral body is considerably wider than it is deep, with a somewhat kidney- or heart-shaped transverse cross section. As they progress caudally, the vertebral bodies gradually increase in size.

The spinous processes of the subaxial cervical vertebrae are usually bifid; the process of C7 is more prominent and easily palpable posteriorly, but it is not bifid. The transverse processes are each perforated to form the transverse foramen through which the vertebral arteries pass. These vessels generally bypass the transverse process of C7 and enter the foramen of C6 before passing cranially. Individual variation is considerable, and in some cases, vertebral arteries may not enter the transverse foramen until they reach the fourth cervical level.[51]

Thoracic Spine

All 12 thoracic vertebrae support ribs, although the last pair may be rudimentary. The ribs articulate with the vertebral bodies at paired demifacets located in the adjacent superior and inferior end plates and at concave, ventral facets located on the prominent transverse processes. The first rib articulates at a complete facet on the side of the first thoracic vertebra.

The vertebral bodies of the thoracic spine are heart shaped in cross section and intermediate in height relative to the cervical and lumbar segments. The pedicles join the body at the dorsolateral margin and are oriented in an anterior-to-posterior direction. The laminae are broad and gently sloping and give rise to superior and inferior articular facets that overlap each other like shingles on a roof. The spinous processes are long and triangular and oriented caudally at an acute angle from the vertebral arch.

The vertebral canal in the thoracic spine is considerably smaller and more rounded than in the cervical or lumbar regions. The narrow caliber of the vertebral canal puts the thoracic spinal cord at relatively increased risk of injury in the face of vertebral displacement or fracture.

Lumbar Spine

The lumbar spine consists of the five most caudal, presacral vertebrae. These massive, weight-bearing bones are characterized by their lack of costal facets, their stout transverse processes, and the broad, platelike spinous processes bound by thickened interspinous and supraspinous ligaments (Fig 11–10). In cross section, the lumbar vertebral bodies are slightly wider than they are deep and are slightly taller anteriorly than posteriorly. The pedicles take root from the posterolateral aspects of the vertebral body, are widely spaced, and are oriented progressively more obliquely as they approach the lumbosacral junction. This results in a gradually widening interpedicular distance when viewed in the anteroposterior plane. The vertebral canal diameter is increased distal to the thoracolumbar junction, but the canal is more triangular and partially occupied by the thickened ligamentum flavum (Plate 4). The pedicle is located in the superior third of the vertebral body, with the inferior vertebral notch somewhat larger than the superior one. Both contribute substantially to the intervertebral foramen.

The superior articular facets of the lumbar spine are concave and oriented in a superomedial direction so that they cup the inferior facets of the vertebra above. The inferior facets have a slightly convex articular surface that faces inferiorly and laterally. This orientation serves to limit vertebral rotation while maximizing flexion and extension in the anteroposterior plane.[35, 69]

Sacrum

The sacrum transmits the vertical loads of the spinal column to the pelvic ring through the sacroiliac joints.

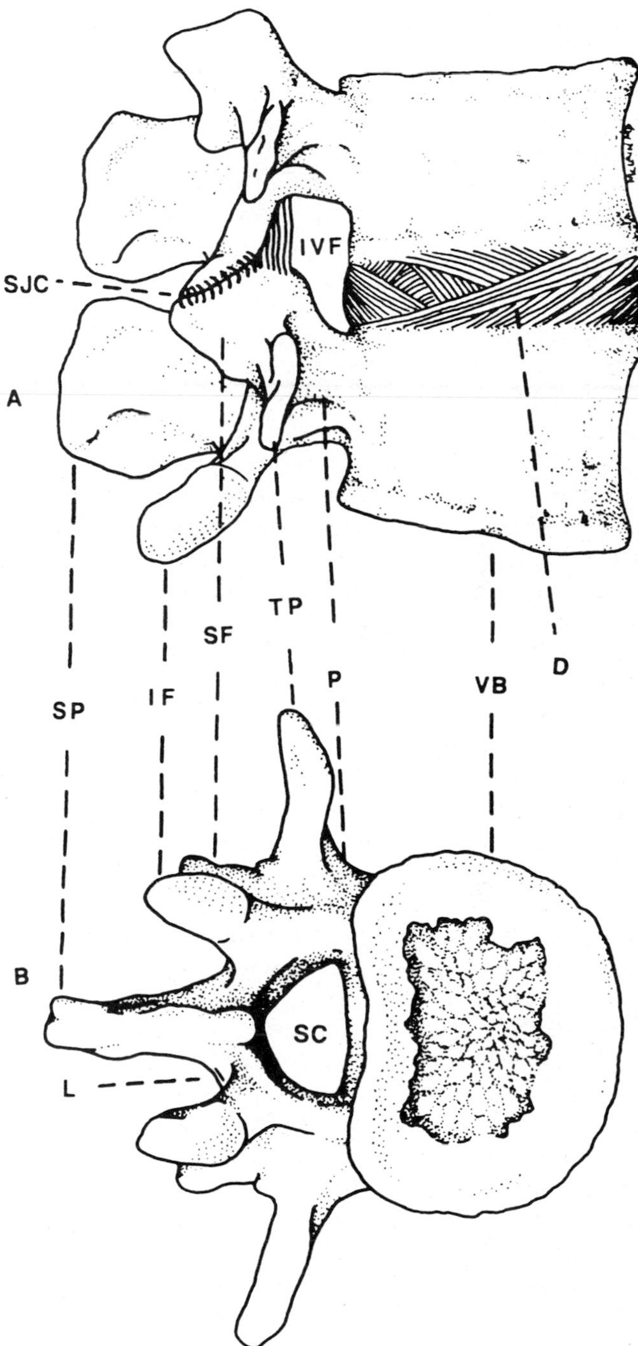

FIG 11–10.
Typical lumbar vertebra: **A,** lateral view; **B,** inferior view. *SP* = spinous process; *SJC* = synovial joint capsule; *L* = lamina; *SF* and *IF* = superior and inferior facets; *TP* = transverse process; *P* = pedicle; *SC* = spinal canal; *IVF* = intervertebral foramen; *VB* = vertebral body; *D* = intervertebral disc.

This broad, triangular element forms as a fusion of five embryonic sacral segments. The spinous processes fuse to form the midline sacral crest. The bone is flattened in the anteroposterior plane and concave anteriorly. The dorsal surface is perforated by the dorsal sacral foramina on either side of the median crest and by the sacral hiatus at its caudal extreme. The dorsal primary rami of the spinal nerves pass through the foramina. The sacral hiatus represents a failure of closure of the neural arch of the fifth and sometimes the fourth sacral vertebrae. This hiatus is contiguous with the epidural space. The terminal margin of the sacrum articulates with the coccygeal bones.

Intervertebral Foramen

Structures enter and exit the vertebral canal by way of the intervertebral foramen. This passageway is defined superiorly and inferiorly by the pedicles of the respective adjacent vertebrae (Fig 11–11). Its floor is provided by the articulation of the posteroinferior margin of the superior vertebral body, the posterosuperior aspect of the inferior vertebral body, and the posterior aspect of the interposed annulus fibrosus. The articular facets, pars articularis, and the ligamentum flavum combine to form the roof of the intervertebral foramen. Through this portal pass the spinal nerve and dorsal root ganglia, the recurrent sinuvertebral nerve, and the segmental arterial and venous branches[11, 52] (Plate 5).

The width and height of the intervertebral foramen may be compromised by spinal pathology. The foramen is oblong in shape, with a vertical diameter of between 12 and 19 mm and a transverse diameter of as little as 7 mm in the lumbar spine. Even with complete collapse of the disc there is ample height to avoid nerve root compression. However, since the diameter of the lumbar spinal nerve may be very near that of the normal foramen's transverse opening, there may be very little tolerance for stenosis in this plane.[30]

Articulations

The vertebrae of the spinal column articulate through an array of ligaments, facet joints, and the intervertebral discs. The interaction of these restraints dictates the capacity of each segment to rotate, flex, extend, or translate relative to its adjacent segments. Disruption of these elements, either through trauma or degeneration, may lead to pathologic motion and dysfunction.

The articular facets form true diarthrodial joints complete with articular cartilage, synovial membranes, and a thin joint capsule (Plate 6). These joints allow a certain amount of gliding motion permitting the articular facets to overlap each other somewhat during flexion, extension, or rotation. During some activities these joints may also be more or less load bearing, depending on their orientation.[29, 39]

A syndesmotic (ligamentous) articulation is formed between individual vertebral bodies by the anterior and posterior longitudinal ligaments and between the vertebral arches by the ligamentum flavum, intraspinous and supraspinous ligaments, and the intertransverse ligaments (Fig 11–12). These structures passively resist distraction of the vertebral elements as the column bends and twists in response to muscular or environmental forces.[69]

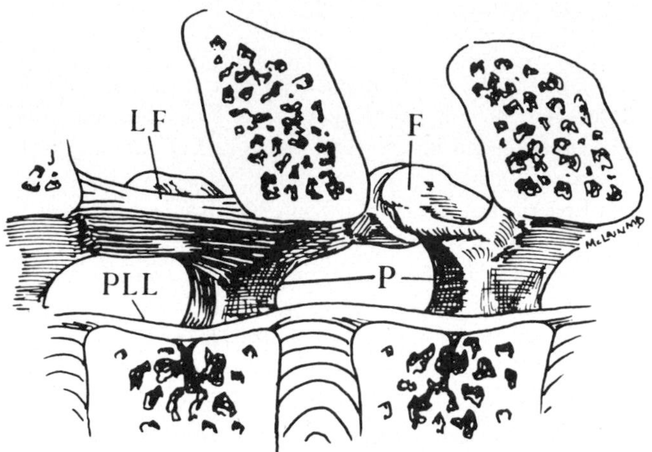

FIG 11–11.
Intervertebral foramen and structural boundaries as viewed from inside the spinal canal. *LF* = ligamentum flavum; *F* = facets; *P* = pedicles; *PLL* = posterior longitudinal ligament overlying the vertebral body.

The anterior and posterior longitudinal ligaments run the full length of the spinal column. The anterior longitudinal ligament is composed of three layers of longitudinally oriented fibers that provide tensile support to the volar surface of the spinal column.[48] These fibers are continuous with the anterior periosteum and are most densely attached along the anterior articular rim of the vertebral end plates. The deepest layer of fibers is short and crosses a single intervertebral disc between its origin and inser-

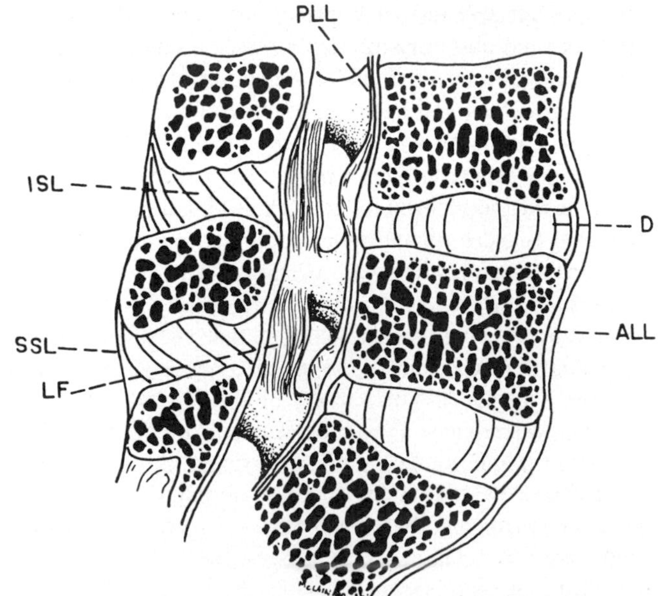

FIG 11–12.
Midsagittal section of the lumbar spine. *ISL* = interspinous ligament; *SSL* = supraspinous ligament; *LF* = ligamentum flavum; *ALL* and *PLL* = anterior and posterior longitudinal ligaments; *D* = intervertebral disc.

tion. The intermediate and superficial layers cross progressively greater distances. The result is a thick, densely adherent anterior ligament with considerable tensile strength.

The posterior longitudinal ligament is broad and uniform in the cervical and thoracic regions but becomes narrowed and segmentally irregular in the lumbar region, constricts to a narrow band between the pedicles, and fans out broadly over the intervertebral discs.[35, 50] The fibers of the posterior longitudinal ligament are interwoven with those of the posterior portion of the annulus. In contrast to the anterior ligament, the posterior ligament does not adhere to the vertebral cortex itself. Instead, it spans the concavity of the posterior vertebral cortex and allows the medullary vessels to enter and leave the vertebral body through the medullary sinus.[12, 50]

The posterior column articulation consists of a complex of ligaments spanning the interval between the laminae and the spinous and transverse processes of the adjoining vertebrae. The ligamentum flavum, which lies immediately dorsal to the spinal canal, takes its cranial origin from the volar surface of the lamina above and inserts on the upper margin of the lamina below (Fig 11–13). As a result, the ligamentum flavum is interposed between the contents of the spinal canal and the caudal rim of each lamina. If hypertrophied or redundant, it may contribute to cord compression or stenosis of the spinal canal (see Plate 4). It is thought that the elastic fibers contained within the ligamentum prevent it from becoming lax or redundant in hyperextension. Redundancy or protrusion of the ligamentum into the spinal canal is thought to contribute to neural compression in some cases of spinal stenosis.[39]

The interspinous and supraspinous ligaments bind the spinous processes together and provide significant tensile strength to the posterior column of the spine. These structures passively resist the natural flexion forces placed on the spine when erect. Following hyperflexion injuries, these elements may be disrupted and permit the spine to fall into a kyphotic deformity.[6, 13, 40, 69] The supraspinous ligament is thick and resilient and runs the length of the spine from the occiput to the sacrum. The interspinous ligaments are of little consequence in the cervical and thoracic regions but are more substantial in the lumbar spine where they bind the broad spinous processes of adjacent vertebrae together.

The intertransverse ligaments span the transverse processes of adjoining vertebrae. In the thoracic region they are difficult to distinguish from the paraspinous musculature, but in the lumbar spine they form a thin, membranous sheet that can be seen on dissection.

The strongest articulations of the spinal column are formed by the intervertebral discs (Plate 7). In aggregate, the discs make up approximately one fourth of the spinal column's length, one fifth of the length of the cervical and

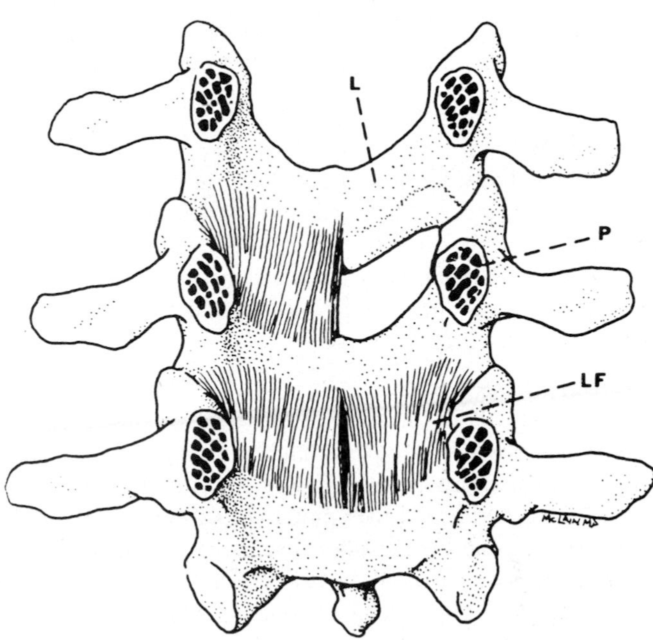

FIG 11–13.
Undersurface of the vertebral arch showing the attachment of the ligamentum flavum. *L* = lamina; *P* = pedicle; *LF* = ligamentum flavum.

thoracic segments, and nearly one third of the length of the lumbar spine.[1] Forming a fibrocartilaginous symphysis between vertebral end plates, the discs permit limited bending and rotation while restricting translation in all planes. They are composite structures made up of two tissues serving separate functions. The annulus fibrosus consists of concentric fibrous lamellae that encircle the gelatinous nucleus pulposus and firmly unite the vertebral end plates. These lamellae consist of collagen fibers embedded in ground substance and layed down in an alternating arrangement so that each layer of fibers runs at an oblique angle to the axis of the vertebral column. The orientation of fibers in adjacent lamellae is reversed so that fibers in one ring run at a 120-degree angle to those in the next.[52, 69] These fibers originate and insert in the cartilaginous end plate and take their firmest attachment from the outer bony ring of the vertebral apophysis.[8]

The annulus provides the mechanical strength of the intervertebral disc. The primary function of the annulus is to withstand tension by resisting internal tensile forces produced by expansion of the compressed nucleus pulposus and external forces produced by horizontal, torsional, and bending motions of the spinal column. Resistance to compressive forces is provided by the nucleus pulposus. The interface between the annular lamellae and the central nucleus is indistinct; the more central layers of the annulus have a higher glycosaminoglycan content and a lower collagen content, which gives a gel-like appearance similar to that of the nucleus.[47] These central tissues have significant hydrostatic properties capable of load and shock dispersal, while the outer tissues have little shock-absorbing capacity.[25, 49, 52]

Musculature

The stability of the spinal column in life is dependent on the musculature of the torso and proximal aspects of the limbs.[48] Contributions to spinal motion and posture are provided by the muscles of the abdomen, the thorax, the upper and lower limb girdles, as well as the musculature of the back itself (Fig 11–14).

Superficial Group

The superficial muscles of the back are primarily involved in suspension of the shoulder girdle from the thorax. The latissimus dorsi originates from the posterior thoracolumbar fascia and the spinous processes of the T7 to L5 vertebrae and the posterior iliac crest. It inserts into the bicipital groove of the humerus. The muscular portion of the latissimus covers the posterolateral aspect of the back below the scapula and is innervated by the thoracodorsal nerve. The trapezius originates from the spinous processes of the cervical and upper thoracic spines and forms a broad fan that narrows to insert distally over the scapular spine and distal end of the clavicle. The trapezius is innervated by the spinal accessory nerve and serves to elevate and stabilize the scapula during upper-extremity motion. Other muscles considered in the superficial group include the levator scapulae and the rhomboids major and minor, which function to elevate and adduct the scapulae.

Deep Group

The intermediate and deep muscles of the back originate from and insert on the axial skeleton itself. They serve to flex, extend, rotate, and stabilize the spinal column with respect to the pelvis and to position the head in space.

The deep muscles of the cervical spine include the splenius capitis and semispinalis capitis, large muscles originating from the spinous and transverse processes, respectively, of the cervical vertebrae and inserting into the occiput of the skull. The semispinalis lies just deep to the splenius, and both overlie the multifidus and semispinalis cervicis groups and the muscles of the posterior triangle of the neck. The muscles of the posterior triangle, the rectus capitis posterior major, rectus capitis posterior minor, obliquus capitis superior, and obliquus capitis inferior, serve to extend, rotate, or bend the head to the side. The rectus capitis posterior major and the obliquus capitis inferior both take origin from the spinous process of C2, while the rectus capitis posterior minor originates from the tubercle of the ring of C1 and the obliquus capitis superior takes origin from the superior aspect of the C1 transverse process. All except the obliquus capitis inferior insert on the occiput. The obliquus capitis inferior inserts, instead, on

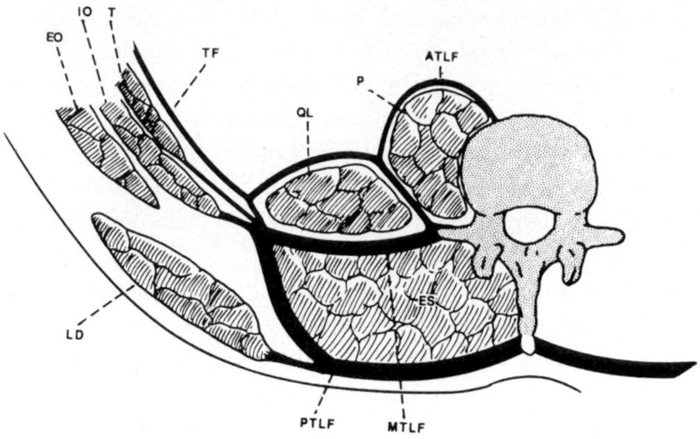

FIG 11–14.

Cross section of the dorsal musculature and associated fascia. *EO* and *IO* = external and internal oblique muscles; *T* and *TF* = transversus abdominis and fascia transversalis; *LD* = latissimus dorsi; *QL* = quadratus lumborum; *P* = psoas; *ATLF, MTLF,* and *PTLF* = anterior, middle, and posterior thoracolumbar fascia.

the transverse process of C1 just below the origin of the obliquus capitis superior.[58]

Below the cervical spine, the deep muscles tend to run contiguously between the thoracic and lumbar segments without interruption (Fig 11–15). Two groups of muscles can be defined within the deep layer. The erector spinae muscle group consists of the spinalis, longissimus, and iliocostalis muscles, which run from the sacrum and iliac crest to various insertions along the ribs and spinous processes. The transversospinalis group consists of the multifidus and the long and short rotators, muscles running between the transverse and spinous processes. The erector spinae group forms a broad muscle mass originating along the posterior surface of the sacral ala and iliac crest and from the spinous processes and supraspinous ligament along the thoracolumbar vertebral column. The spinalis muscle is the most medial of the erector spinae group. It runs cranially from the level of the second lumbar spinous process, with fibers originating at each level above and crossing several levels before inserting on a more cranial spinous process. The muscle consists of three different portions, thoracic, cervical, and capital, but these tend to run together and become indistinguishable. These muscles function to extend the spine and aid in lateral bending.[32]

The longissimus thoracis also serves to extend and laterally flex the spine. This is the longest muscle of the erector spinae group; it originates from the sacrum and lumbar transverse processes and inserts on the thoracic transverse processes and ribs. The iliocostalis lumborum is the most lateral of the erector spinae muscles and takes origin from the iliac crest and runs cranially to form two separate portions—a lumbar segment and a thoracic segment. The transversospinalis muscle group consists of the semispina-

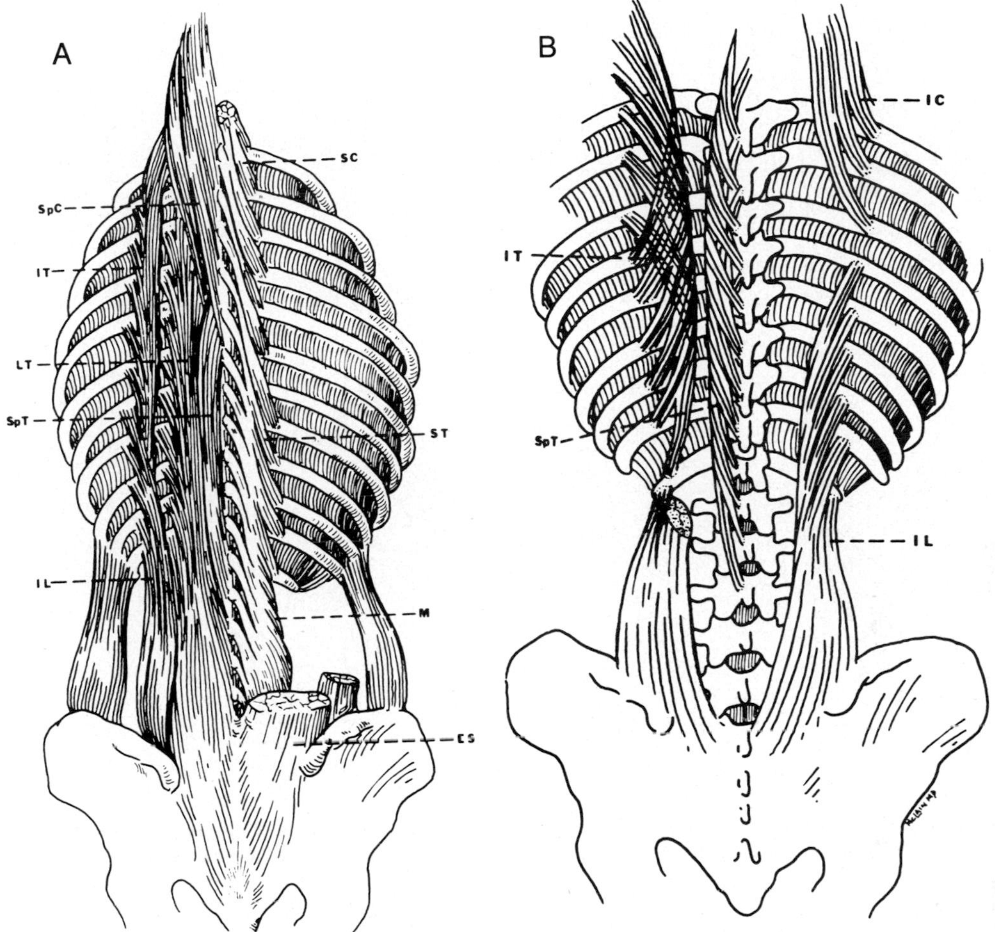

FIG 11–15.
Deep muscles of the back. **A,** intermediate layer of the deep musculature: *SpC* = splenius cervicis; *SC* = semispinalis capitis; *IT* = iliocostalis thoracis; *LT* = longissimus thoracis; *SpT* = spinalis thoracis; *ST* = semispinalis thoracis; *IL* = iliocostalis lumborum; *M* = multifidus; *ES* = erector spinae. **B,** erector spinae removed: *IT* = iliocostalis thoracis; *IC* = iliocostalis cervicis; *IL* = iliocostalis lumborum; *SpT* = spinalis thoracis.

lis, the multifidus, and the rotator muscles (Fig 11–16). The semispinalis muscles are restricted to the thoracic and cervical regions, while the multifidi and the rotators are found at all levels. These muscles originate from the transverse processes and travel variable distances to insert on spinous processes of the more cranial vertebrae. The semispinalis muscles take origin from the thoracic transverse processes and may cross five to seven superior segments before inserting into a cervical or thoracic spinous process. The multifidi act on somewhat shorter segments of the spine. These muscles are most prominent in the lumbar spine, take origin from the lumbar or thoracic mamillary processes, and insert into the spinous process two to four segments above.

The long and short rotators lay just deep to the multifidi, originate from the mamillary processes, and insert at the base of the spinous processes one or two segments above. These muscles provide postural support for the spine and assist in extension, lateral flexion, and rotation. Two other minor muscle groups also assist in postural support; the interspinalis muscles originate and insert on adjacent spinous processes, and the intertransversalis muscles bridge the gap between neighboring transverse processes.

The deep muscles of the spine are all innervated by the dorsal primary rami of their segmental spinal nerves. The exception is the intertransversalis group, which takes its innervation from branches of the ventral primary rami.[50]

Vascular Supply

The blood supply to the spinal column and the spinal cord is roughly segmental, although there is significant anatomic variability in the extent to which vessels overlap each other cranially and caudally. This variability is of primary concern when discussing the supply to the spinal cord. Ligation of dominant segmental arteries could curtail blood flow in watershed areas of spinal cord parenchyma and, at least theoretically, could result in cord ischemia.

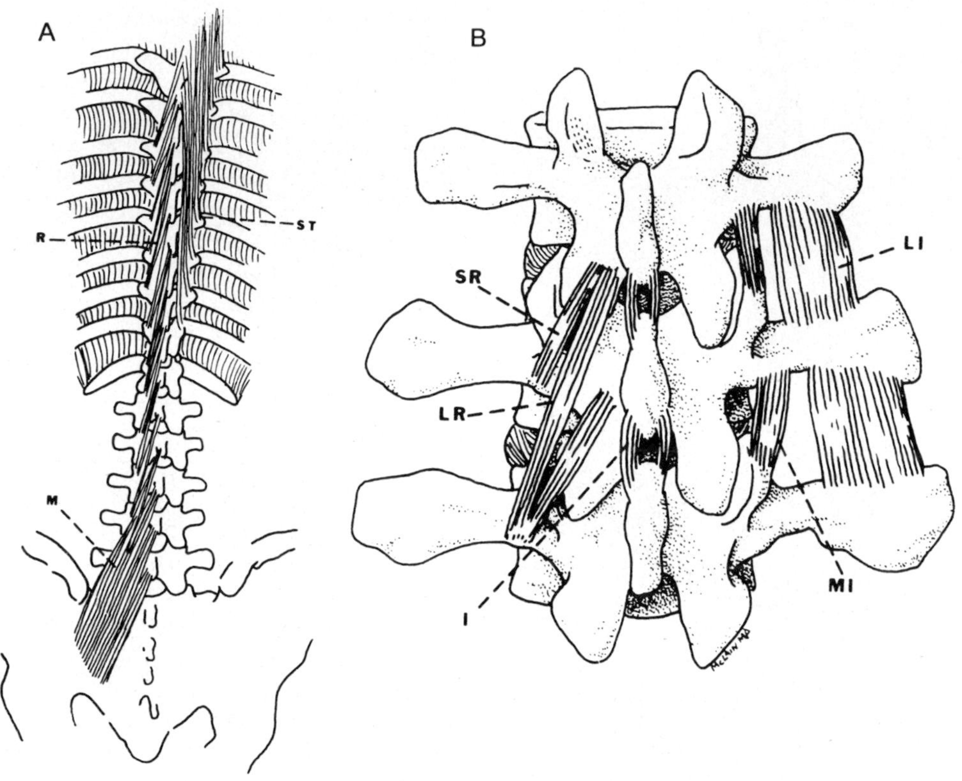

FIG 11–16.
Deep muscles of the back. **A,** deep layer. *R* = rotators; *ST* = semispinalis thoracis; *M* = multifidus. **B,** deep layer of the lumbar spinal musculature. *SR* = short rotators; *LR* = long rotators; *I* = interspinalis; *MI* = medial intertransversarius; *LI* = lateral intertransversarius.

Regional

The regional blood supply to the spinal column is provided by the vertebral arteries in the cervical spine and the segmental arteries in the thoracic and lumbar regions (Fig 11–17). The vertebral arteries arise from the left and right subclavian arteries, just distal to the takeoff of the carotid arteries. They pass superiorly between the anterior scalene and the longus colli muscles before entering the transverse foramen of the sixth cervical vertebra. Before exiting the cervical spine and passing out over the ring of C1, the vertebral arteries give off segmental branches at each cervical level. In the lumbar and thoracic spine the paired segmental arteries arise directly from the trunk of the aorta. These vessels anastomose to varying degrees with their neighbors, and their contributions to the blood supply may be asymmetrical. The largest of these segmental vessels, the radicularis magna, or the "artery of Adamkiewicz," usually takes origin from the left side between the T10 and L2 levels.[28, 31, 58] Its importance in the supply of the spinal cord is debated. The junctional zone of the thoracocervical spine, which commonly includes the lower two cervical and upper two thoracic vertebrae, is variably supplied by paired costocervical branches from the subclavian arteries.[50]

Local

Although the regional blood supply varies considerably from level to level, the local distribution is fairly uniform throughout the spine. Whether the regional supply comes from a segmental or vertebral artery, the local supply to the vertebra consists of four sets of nutrient vessels: anterior central, posterior central, prelaminar, and postlaminar.[12, 50] These vessels are derived from the dorsal branch of the lumbar or thoracic segmental arteries and directly from the vertebral arteries in the cervical spine.

In the thoracic and lumbar spine, the segmental vessels leave the trunk of the aorta and pass dorsolaterally to the level of the transverse process. As they pass laterally and dorsally, these vessels give off their first branches, the anterior central arteries, which penetrate the anterior cortex and supply the vertebral spongiosa.[17] At the level of the transverse process the segmental vessel divides into a dorsal and a lateral branch. The dorsal branch divides almost immediately. Before passing dorsally between the transverse processes the dorsal branch gives off the spinal artery, which passes through the intervertebral foramen into the spinal canal. Here the spinal artery trifurcates into the posterior central, intermediate, and prelaminar branches. The posterior central branch provides nutrient

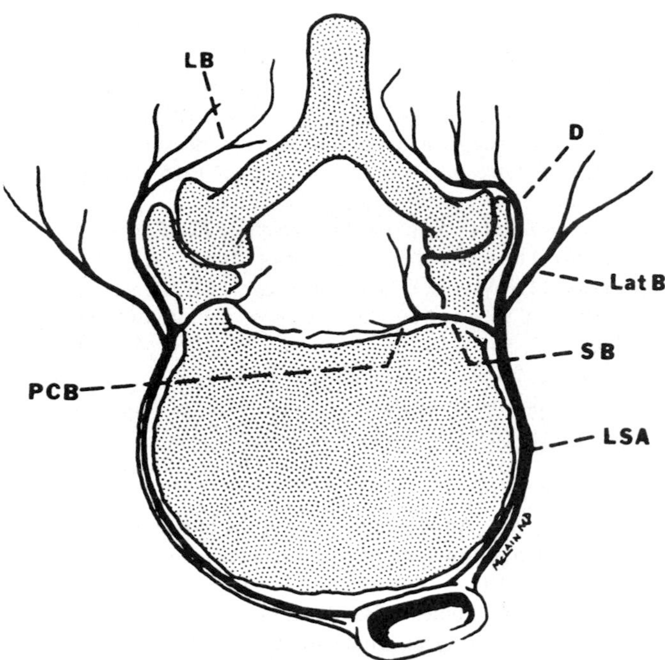

FIG 11–17.
Segmental vasculature of the spinal column and vertebral canal. *LSA* = lumbar segmental artery; *SB* = spinal branch; *Lat B* = lateral branch; *D* = dorsal branch; *LB* = laminar branch; *PCB* = posterior central branch.

vessels to the posterior portion of the vertebral body and to the posterior longitudinal ligament. The intermediate branch supplies the nerve roots and spinal cord. The prelaminar branch gives off nutrient vessels to the laminae and posterior elements as well as the epidural soft tissues.

After dividing from the spinal artery, the dorsal branch of the segmental artery passes posteriorly to supply the paraspinal musculature and the lamina and spinous processes. The dorsal branch divides into a medial and a lateral posterior branch, each of which give off numerous muscular branches. The medial (postlaminar) branch supplies the medial muscles of the back and the posterior vertebral arch, while the lateral branch supplies the main bulk of the back muscles.[50, 71]

The venous drainage generally follows the arterial pattern. The veins form both an internal and an external vertebral venous plexus, each with anterior and posterior ramifying networks. These vessels are broadly interconnected and lack valves, thus allowing retrograde flow during a Valsalva maneuver. This action is thought to play a role in the dissemination of infection and metastases from the pelvis and abdomen into the vertebral column.

Spinal Cord, Nerves, and Ganglia

The spinal cord in the adult enters the cervical spine through the foramen magnum superiorly and terminates at the thoracolumbar junction as the conus medullaris inferiorly. The cord has ample room in the cervical spinal canal, but as it enters the thoracic spine, the cord enlarges and the canal becomes smaller so that the cord is relatively tightly contained. At the thoracolumbar junction the conus ends, and the lumbar and sacral nerve roots continue caudally within the arachnoid space as the cauda equina (Plate 8). In the normal lumbar spine there is, again, ample room for the neural elements within the canal.

The conus medullaris contains the motor neurons and secondary sensory neurons associated with distal sacral function. This section of the cord is usually found at the first lumbar level but may descend below L2 in some cases or stop at T11 or T12 in others.[4, 5] This variability means that patients may sustain a conus medullaris injury with thoracolumbar fractures at levels other than the first lumbar vertebra.

The spinal nerves are formed from the combined dorsal and ventral nerve roots. The dorsal roots form as a coalescence of multiple rootlets emerging from the dorsolateral aspect of the spinal cord. Just prior to joining the ventral nerve root, the dorsal root develops a fusiform widening, the dorsal root ganglion. This ganglion contains the primary afferent neurons of the segmental spinal nerves and has been implicated as a source of back pain in some situations.[67, 68] The dorsal root then joins the ventral root, which emerges ventrolaterally at the same cord level and exits the intervertebral foramen as the spinal nerve.

Each of these spinal nerves gives off a recurrent branch, termed the *sinuvertebral nerve,* that is reflected back through the intervertebral foramen to supply afferent fibers to structures within the vertebral canal. As this nerve passes back through the foramen, just inferior to the vertebral pedicle it divides into superior and inferior branches. These branches then supply fibers to the posterior longitudinal ligament, the vertebral periosteum, the dura, and epidural vessels. These fibers run proximally and distally to anastomose with those of adjacent levels, thus providing a significant overlap of sensory elements.[55, 59, 70] Back pain produced by disc disruption or herniation is thought to be transmitted through the fibers of the sinuvertebral nerves.[50, 55]

Although a clear segmental distribution is usually claimed for the distributions of spinal nerves, anatomic studies have demonstrated a significant number of interconnections between adjacent nerves and between ventral and dorsal nerve roots.[27, 33]

REFERENCES

1. Aeby C: Die Alterverschiedenheiten der menschlichen Wirbelsaule. *Arch Anat Physiol* 1879; 10:77–113.
2. Angevin, JB: Clinically relevant embryology of the vertebral column and spinal cord. *Clin Neurosurg* 1973; 20:95–103.

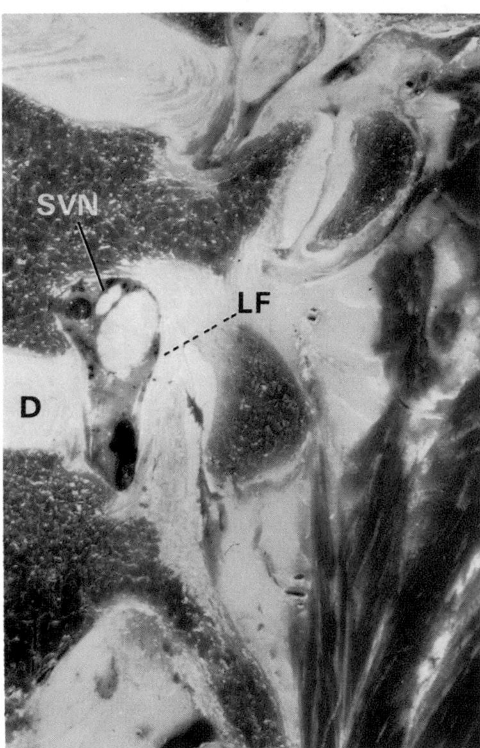

PLATE 5. Intervertebral foramen: parasagittal section through the lumbar pedicle. The spinal nerve can be seen as it exits the canal beneath the ligamentum flavum and inferior border of the pedicle. Segmental vessels and the sinuvertebral nerve pass through the volar foramen to the nerve. The relationship to the intervertebral disc is well demonstrated in this section. *SVN* = sinuvertebral nerve; *LF* = ligamentum flavum; *D* = intervertebral disc.

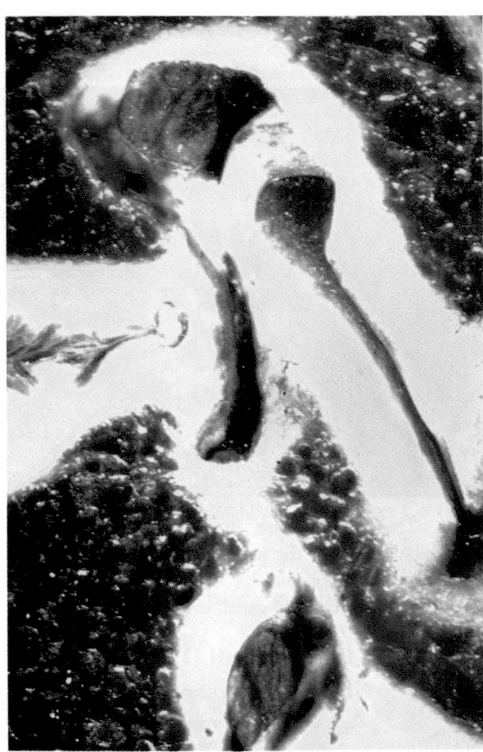

PLATE 6. Facet joint. The bulging facet capsule and intervertebral disc significantly restrict the area of the intervertebral foramen. The congruent articular surfaces of the inferior and superior facets of the adjacent vertebrae allow gliding motion of the joint during flexion and extension.

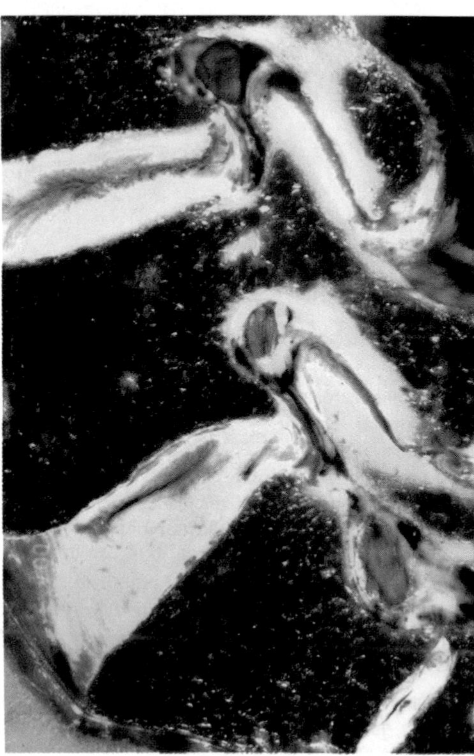

PLATE 7. A lumbar intervertebral disc cut in parasagittal section shows the laminar arrangement of the annulus fibrosus. The L5–S1 disc is significantly thicker anteriorly than posteriorly.

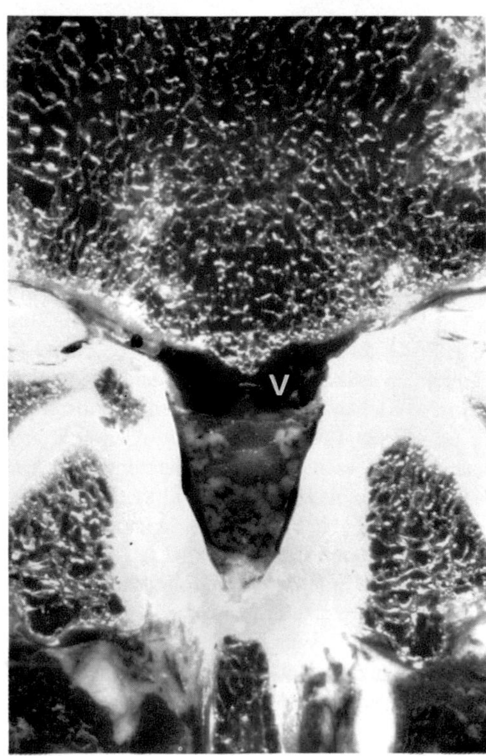

PLATE 8. Cauda equina. Paired nerve roots are seen within the dural sheath in the lumbar vertebral canal. A portion of the vertebral venous plexus is seen anterior to the cauda *(V)*.

44. O'Rahilly R, Benson DR: The development of the vertebral column, in Bradford DS, Hensinger RM (eds): *The Pediatric Spine*. New York, Georg Thieme, 1985.
45. O'Rahilly R, Meyer DB: The timing and sequence of events in the development of the human vertebral column during the embryonic period proper. *Anat Embryol* 1979; 157:167–176.
46. O'Rahilly R, Muller F, Meyer D: The human vertebral column at the end of the embryonic period proper. 1: The column as a whole. *J Anat* 1980; 131:565–575.
47. Panagiotacopulos ND, Pope MH, Block R, et al: Water content in human intervertebral discs. Part II: Viscoelastic behavior. *Spine* 1987; 12:918–924.
48. Panjabi MM, Goel VK, Takata K: Physiological strains in lumbar spinal ligaments: An in-vitro biomechanical study. *Spine* 1982; 7:192–203.
49. Panjabi MM, White AA: Physical properties and functional biomechanics of the spine, in White AA, Panjabi MM (eds): *Clinical Biomechanics of the Spine*. Philadelphia, JB Lippincott, 1990.
50. Parke WW: Applied anatomy of the spine, in Rothman RH, Simeone FA (eds): *The Spine,* ed 2. Philadelphia, WB Saunders 1982.
51. Parke WW: The vascular relations of the upper cervical vertebrae. *Orthop Clin North Am* 1978; 9:879–889.
52. Parke WW, Schiff DCM: The applied anatomy of the intervertebral disc. *Orthop Clin North Am* 1971; 2:309–324.
53. Peacock A: Observations on the postnatal structure of the intervertebral disc in man. *J Anat* 1952; 86:162–179.
54. Peacock A: Observations on the prenatal development of the intervertebral disc in man. *J Anat* 1951; 85:260–274.
55. Pedersen HE, Blunck CFJ, Gardner E: The anatomy of the lumbosacral posterior rami and meningeal branches of spinal nerves (sinuvertebral nerves). *J Bone Joint Surg [Am]* 1956; 38:377–391.
56. Reichmann S, Lewin T: Congenital cleft vertebrae in growing individuals. *Acta Orthop Scand* 1969; 40:3–22.
57. Remak R: *Untersuchungen uber die Entwickelung der Wirbelthiere*. Berlin, Reimer, 1885, pp 40–44.
58. Rickenbacher J, Landolt AM, Theiler K: *Applied Anatomy of the Back*. Berlin, Springer-Verlag, 1985.
59. Roofe PG: Innervation of annulus fibrosus and posterior longitudinal ligament. *Arch Neuropsychol* 1940; 44:100–103.
60. Sensenig EC: The early development of the human vertebral column. *Contrib Embryol Carnegie Inst* 1949; 33:21–41.
61. Sullivan D, Cornwall WS: Pelvic rib, report of a case. *Radiology* 1973; 110:355–357.
62. Tsou PM: The embryology of congenital kyphosis. *Clin Orthop* 1977; 128:18–26.
63. Tanaka T, Uhthoff HK: Coronal cleft of vertebrae, a varient of normal endochondral ossification. *Acta Orthop Scand* 1983; 54:389–395.
64. Uhthoff HK: In Uhthoff HK (ed): *The Embryology of the Human Locomotor System*. Berlin, Springer-Verlag, 1990.
65. Verbout AJ: A critical review of the "neugliederung" concept in relation to the development of the vertebral column. *Acta Biotheor* 1976; 25:219–258.
66. Walmsley R: The development and growth of the intervertebral disc. *Edinburgh Med J* 1953; 60:341–364.
67. Weinstein JN: Mechanisms of spinal pain. *Spine* 1986; 11:999–1001.
68. Weinstein JN, Pope M, Schmidt R, et al: Neuropharmacologic effects of vibration on the dorsal root ganglion. *Spine* 1988; 13:521–525.
69. White AA, Panjabi MM: *Clinical Biomechanics of the Spine*. Philadelphia, JB Lippincott, 1990.
70. Wiberg G: Back pain in relation to nerve supply of intervertebral disc. *Acta Orthop Scand* 1949; 19:211–221.
71. Willis TA: Nutrient arteries of the vertebral bodies. *J Bone Joint Surg [Am]* 1949; 31:538–541.
72. Winter RB: *Congenital Deformities of the Spine*. New York, Thieme-Stratton, 1983.

PART IV
BIOMECHANICS

12

Disc Biomechanics

William J. Stith, Ph.D.

The human spine contains 23 intervertebral discs, with the smallest discs in the cervical region and the largest in the lumbar region. A disc contains three integrated tissues: the annulus fibrosus, the nucleus pulposus, and the hyaline cartilage end plates. This chapter will review intervertebral disc anatomy with particular emphasis on structure and function. The facet joints will also be considered along with their role in disc function.

DISC ANATOMY/BIOCHEMISTRY

Annulus Fibrosus

The annulus is a complex of concentrically arranged lamellae of fibrocartilage with each lamella consisting of obliquely oriented collagen fiber bundles.[43] Each lamella runs a roughly parallel course with its directional arrangement of fibers alternating in subsequent layers.[4, 43] The collagen fibers within each lamella are arranged in parallel arrays at an angle of 60 degrees to the spinal axis and at about 120 degrees to fibers in adjacent lamellae so that alternate lamellae have their fibers roughly in register.[22, 41] The mean thickness of individual layers varies greatly throughout the annulus and is dependent on (1) the circumferential location (maximal at the lateral section), (2) the radial location (maximal at the inner part of the annulus), and (3) age (more than double in older spines, where values of 0.14 to 0.52 mm have been reported).[62]

The number of distinct layers in a disc usually varies between 15 and 25 and the number of fiber bundles from 20 to 62, with an average interbundle spacing of 0.22 mm.[62] The fiber bundles have been reported to vary in size from 10 to 50 mm.[43]

In any 20-degree sector of the annulus, at least 40% of the layers are incomplete. The parallel arrangement of the fiber bundles is often disturbed by irregularities of the laminae. The inclination of the fiber bundles can vary from 0 to 90 degrees near locations of irregularities. Considerable departure from the symmetry of the fiber bundles in successive layers is encountered in peripheral layers of the posterolateral section, where the maximum percentage of incomplete layers is found.[62] The anterior part of the annulus is almost twice as thick as the posterior portion.[3]

The inner third of fibers in the annulus attach to the end plates, and the outer two thirds attach to the intervertebral body, where the attachment is either into bone[35] or calcified cartilage.[25, 43] Nerve endings are reported to be present in the outer part of the annulus.[35]

The major component of the annulus is collagen, with three protein chains having high concentrations of the amino acids proline and hydroxyproline. These amino acids force the polypeptide chains into a left-handed helix, which greatly limits motion and thereby stabilizes the molecular structure.[26]

The collagen of the outer rim of the anterior part of the annulus is principally type I collagen and consists of the largest-diameter fibers (50 to 60 mm), which impart structure to the disc, with the strength of the disc dependent upon the concentration and stability of covalent bonds between collagen molecules in the fibrils.[22] The proportion of type II collagen within the smaller-diameter fibers (30 mm) increases from the outer layer of the annulus to the nucleus.[22, 43]

Studies have also shown the presence of elastic fibers in the annulus[13] that are restricted to the annular lamellae at the vertebral epiphysis and disc interface.[49] The elastic fibers branch and anastomose freely between the interlamellar collagen fibers, thus imparting a dynamic flexibility to the tissue.[49]

Nucleus Pulposus

The annulus blends into the nucleus gradually so that the two together may be thought of as a gradient of tissue rather than distinct entities. The nucleus accounts for 30% to 50% of the total disc area[21] and is a three-dimensional lattice gel system. The collagen fibrils of the nucleus are primarily type II collagen, which has the smaller-diameter fibrils.[22] The collagen fibrils are not arranged in any particular pattern and make up 15% to 20% of the nucleus.[21] The major constituents of the nucleus are proteoglycans, which through their fixed negative charge imbibe water and exert a high swelling pressure to keep the collagen network expanded. The concentration of proteoglycan also modulates the rate of fluid loss and the diffusion of larger solutes.[8]

In contrast to collagens, which are principally protein

in structure, proteoglycans are composed of a protein core to which polyanionic glycosaminoglycan chains of chondroitin sulfate and keratin sulfate are attached. The glycosaminoglycans are polysaccharides with one of the disaccharides always being an amino sugar (glycose amino) along with large carbohydrate polymers known as glycans. The proteoglycan monomers form large aggregates with hyaluronic acid, and the resulting complex is stabilized by a link protein.[8] The proteoglycans of the annulus, where they are present in much less concentration, are similar to those of the nucleus but have a higher proportion of proteoglycans capable of binding hyaluronate.[43] It appears that a large proportion of the proteoglycans of the nucleus are unable to form aggregates, possibly due to their lack of a hyaluronic acid binding region.[14]

While collagen acts to provide structure, proteoglycans act to impart function by allowing compression to squeeze fluid out and absorb some of the load. The interactive negative forces resist load by strongly repelling each other and resisting further deformation. After removal of the compressive force, the proteoglycans quickly expand to reabsorb the water lost.[93, 101] Studies in the rabbit intervertebral disc have shown that the swelling pressures are highest in the nucleus and lowest in the anterior part of the annulus.[34] The swelling pressure increases as charged density increases, with charged density dependent on the total concentration of proteoglycans and on the ratio of chondroitin sulfate (two charges per disaccharide) to keratin sulfate (one charge per disaccharide).[64]

Cartilage End Plate

This structure, which is composed of hyaline cartilage, is thicker and more calcified at the periphery than at the center.[22] One of its main functions is to act as a semipermeable membrane to facilitate fluid exchange between the disc and the vertebral body,[23] with the greatest exchange at the central portion of the end plate. Other functions of the end plate are to protect the vertebral centrum from pressure atrophy[50] and to confine the annulus and nucleus within their anatomic boundaries.[43]

DISC FUNCTION

The intervertebral disc acts to maintain a deformable space between the vertebral bodies so that flexibility of the spine can be achieved while also acting as a shock absorber to resist compressive forces.[4, 43]

This fibrous structure of the annulus is best suited to resist loads such as bending or tension that induce tension in the fibers; however, this tissue responds poorly to compressive forces. The nucleus, however, acts hydraulically to transform compression loads into radically directed tensile forces in the annulus.[29, 43]

Axial compression loading is the most common form of spine loading. The compressive forces are resisted by both the nucleus and the annulus, with intradiscal pressure increasing to approximately 1.5 times the applied load and hoop stress in the annulus to 3.5 times the applied pressure.[3, 57, 72] The hydration of the nucleus and annulus is proportional to the applied compression stress. At a given load, the osmotic swelling pressure developed by the proteoglycans balances the applied compression stresses.[5] A disc subjected to a load of 100 kPa (kilopascals) lost 8% of the fluid from the nucleus and 11% of the hydration in the annulus, with the dorsal aspect of the annulus losing more water than the other parts. Increasing the load to 200 kPa for 24 hours showed that water loss was not linearly proportional to load but was rate limited. Asymmetrical loading caused a 2% to 3% greater water loss in the annulus than with symmetrical loading. Symmetrical loading caused a 20 times greater increase in potassium over sodium in the disc with the greatest concentration seen in the nucleus.[56]

Studies on compression loading of pig discs have shown changes in water content of nucleus and in the inner layer of the annulus as the compression load was increased, but there were only slight changes in the outer layers of the annulus. The fixed charge density was found to increase up to five times for a 30-kg loaded disc. As the fixed charge density increases, further water loss is inhibited, and stability and the ability to provide support against a load are reinforced by suppression of water transport due to the high negative charge density.[76]

Most of the disc fluid loss occurs within the first few hours of compression loading. Fluid loss is reflected in decreased disc height, increased disc stiffness, and an increased radial bulge. The facet joints also act to absorb compression loading and thus protect the vertebral body and disc.[53] Before compression loading, there is little resistance in the joint, but after compressive loading in a simulated standing position, the joints resist an average of 16% of the applied compressive force with possible values as high as 70%.[1] Other values reported for facet loading have ranged from 2% to 13% depending on the decrease in the accompanying flexion rotation of the specimen.[53, 103] The facet pressure/load occurs as a result of muscle action to maintain the lumbar spine in an erect position while it is subjected to a flexion movement and axial compression. The facet pressure increases linearly with increasing flexion movement. Vertical facet load is transmitted by bony contact of the tip of the inferior facet with the lamina of the vertebra below. Involuntary, sudden extension of the lumbar spine can result in increased contact tip pressure and a concomitant decrease in disc pressure.[20]

The disc is the major load-bearing element in lateral and anterior shear, axial compression, and flexion. In lateral and anterior shear with high displacements, the facets may transmit part of the load. However, in posterior shear (extension and axial torque) the facets are the major load-bearing structure.[95]

Mechanically the disc may be regarded as a viscoelastic structure capable of maintaining very large loads without disintegrating. With static loading, the disc uses the creep mechanism to redistribute, equilibrate, and adapt the load through interaction of the nucleus and annulus to reach a steady state, which is particularly governed by the facet interaction. If a dynamic load is suddenly applied, the disc is first compressed and then begins to expand in the opposite direction, and the width increases; the disc then expands, the margins recede inward, and the vibrations die out. The disc thus acts as a shock absorber dampening oscillations. Failure can result when a dynamic load is applied to a disc that is already statically loaded to its elastic limit. The vibrations that occur can result in disc damage.[43] Disc prolapse will occur if weakness is already present at a specific site.[47]

Combinations of movements such as twisting, bending, and bending with rotation will result in increased stresses and strains on a disc, especially with a superimposed load, and are the most likely to result in disc injury.[24, 48, 70] It appears that the lowest two lumbar discs tolerate the greatest compressive loads, with the load at L5–S1 showing a possible 1.5 times greater load than that at L1–2.[46] Studies measuring disc pressure in vivo[67, 69] have shown, however, that the force acting on the L5–S1 disc in a subject lifting loads is 30% less than that obtained by using theoretical calculations. The difference may be due to absorption of part of the load by the walls of the abdominal cavity, which stiffen as the muscles contract in response to weight bearing. Increases in intradiscal pressure have also been recorded in coughing (40%), weight bearing (50%), trunk rotation (40%), stair climbing (40%), and slow walking (15%).[43]

Studies on porcine discs have shown significant differences in mechanical properties from tests performed on discs in living animals (in vivo) and those from deceased (in situ) animals.[52] After death there was a significant decrease in creep rate (greater than 25%), a significant increase in stiffness (greater than 30%), and a significant increase in viscosity (greater than 40%). During the breathing cycle, the relation between volume and pressure shows a considerable amount of hysteresis, which indicates variations in energy turnover. This energy may be transformed to spinal motion, modulating/augmenting the mechanical response of the disc through substantial flow, rearrangement of the collagen network, and/or volume changes within the disc. Pressure modulations within the disc may also play an important role in the functional and nutritive properties of the disc by enhancing the transport rates of solutes and metabolites.

DISC DEGENERATION

All discs show some degenerative changes with advancing age, and thus disc degeneration may be as unavoidable as aging.[44] One of the major changes in the disc is loss of water. The water constant of the nucleus drops from 85% to 90% at birth to 70% to 75% by the seventh to eighth decade.[19, 56, 73] The water content in the annulus drops from about 80% at birth to approximately 72% by the age of 30 years and then increases by about 5% to approximately 77% by the age of 80 years.[56]

Changes in morphology were assessed by both gross morphology and MRI.[96] This study and others indicated that disc degeneration became more frequent with age and that severe degenerative changes could be correlated with the loss of proteoglycans.[17, 21, 79, 98] The most common finding of early disc degeneration by MRI was infolding of the outer rim of the annulus. This process appeared to be caused by the radial infolding of the more central fibers of the outer part of the annulus toward the central nuclear complex, possibly due to the repeated axial loading on the progressively shrinking nucleus.[88] As the disc degenerates, there is a marked increase in fibrous tissue and degenerated cartilage cells in the nucleus and an obliteration of the lamellae of the annulus.[6] The cell number decreases in the central position of the nucleus, and a cell population is observed only in the region near the cartilaginous end plates.[74]

Proteoglycans are constantly being slowly turned over in the matrix, with the most active site of synthesis being the midannulus region. As viability of the cells decreases, the proteoglycan content decreases along with its mechanical function.[8] Concomitant with the decrease in water is the decrease in the ratio of chondroitin sulfate to keratin sulfate, with the greatest change observed in the nucleus.[2] Since keratin sulfate has a much lower fixed charge density, it would be expected to bind less water and therefore exert less swelling pressure. Thus not only is the concentration of proteoglycans decreasing but also their constituent species with a decreased water binding potential. As the nucleus solidifies, its ability to transfer compression loads into radially directed hoop stresses in the annulus also decreases. This is reflected by a decreased intradiscal pressure, which has been found to be inversely related to disc degeneration. Severely degenerative discs may have up to a 60% decrease in intradiscal pressure. Posture, muscle tone, spinal load, and intradiscal pressure are all related and are higher for in vivo studies than in vitro.[78] Consistent with the loss of intradiscal pressure has been the finding of inward bulging of the annulus in response to a mechanical load. It is postulated that the phenomenon of inward bulging over time could lead to lamellar disruption within the annulus.[89]

Degeneration of the inner and middle layers of the annulus was seen in specimens from the third decade of life, and swelling of fibers and separation of the fiber bundles were also observed in these specimens.[104] Irregularities in the annulus have been found to be greatest at the posterolateral region, where the greatest amount of layer interruption is also observed.[62] Proteoglycans and the intimate relationship between collagen fibers appear to give stability to the collagen fiber. In addition, the biaxial arrangements of the sheets place the strong axis of the sheets alternately and approximately at right angles to each other. With aging and the loss of proteoglycans, the spatial arrangement is altered with a loss of right-angle distribution. The result is instability, which may contribute to disc degeneration and clinical disc prolapse.[9]

Loading studies have shown that the maximum fiber strain is in the innermost annulus layer in the posterolateral region.[29, 91] Increases in type II collagen content in the annulus at the expense of type I[22] may lower the tensile strength of the annulus and make possible rupture of the thinner, more parallel posterior fibers of the annulus where loads may be six to seven times as great as the applied load, particularly if the disc is tilted backward.[71] A recent study showed that radiographically detectable lumbar degenerative changes were more prevalent and seemed to develop at a younger age in concrete reinforcement workers than in house painters. The pattern of degenerative changes was similar in the two groups, a finding that indicates that mechanical loading does not alter the degenerative changes but merely enhances their development.[82] Stresses in the disc resulting from heavy mechanical loading or degeneration from mechanical trauma may result in tearing of tissue, including cracks and crevices that progressively weaken the disc, thus making annular rupture possible.[12, 44, 87] Laboratory studies indicate that combined loading plus vibration can result in a motion segment suddenly buckling and lead to tracking tears from the nucleus through the posterolateral region of the annulus.[102] With aging there is a progressive increase in vertebral end plate concavity associated with decreased bone density. In the cancellous bone of vertebral bodies, a decrease in the number of support structures for end plates has also been observed.[99] As the end plate ages, there appears to be an increase in microscopic anomalies thought to be Schmorl's nodes. These anomalies have a random fiber orientation rather than the regular orientation seen in younger specimens, which should be more effective in withstanding nuclear pressure.[84] The end plate breaking point for those over 40 years of age is, on the average, approximately 50% of that for those under 40.[80] A significant effect of the aging process is the loss of blood vessels in the disc. By the age of 12 years the disc is largely avascular.[32] Nutrient transport in and out of the disc is primarily by passive diffusion, with sulfate and other negatively charged anions diffusing primarily from the periphery of the annulus, small unchanged solutes such as glucose and oxygen diffusing through the end plates and annulus, and small cations diffusing primarily through the end plates.[65, 100] Overall, about 40% of the bone-disc interface is permeable, with the central portion of the end plate being the most permeable.[65]

The disc and end plates are the principal medium through which axial compressive loads are transmitted through the lumbar spine. As the disc degenerates, more of the stress is transferred to the lateral aspect of the end plates.[58] Even with subfailure loading, microtrauma may be initiated with loss of end plate integrity and clinical function.[105] The end plate has been shown to fail under compressive loading before rupture of the annulus takes place.[60]

There appears to be, at least in laboratory studies, a close correlation between loading cycles to failure (fatigue strength) and the bone mineral concentration.[31] With increasing age and trauma there is calcification of the end plates, which can lead to obliteration of the disc space.[74]

Within the disc itself, the pH is already low, presumably due to lactic acid buildup from glycolysis taking place in the low oxygen tension of the disc.[18, 36, 65, 68] Calcification of the end plates can result in a decreased solute interchange, which can further compound the problem by lowering the pH. Lysosomal enzymes such as glycosidases, proteases, and sulfases are stimulated by an acid environment, with a pH of 5 being optimum.[26] Stimulation of the lysosomal enzymes may hasten the degradation or aging process inside the disc.[81] The outer rim of the annulus can be well nourished from peripheral blood vessels, but supply decreases rapidly within a few millimeters into the annulus. Thus steep gradients of oxygen and lactic acid develop across the disc, and cells within the inner part of the annulus, which are the most active in synthesizing proteoglycans, have the poorest nutrient supply in the adult.[8] Maximal cell density is determined by nutrient supply, with the exchange area and disc thickness being critical parameters.[92]

Nutrients reach the cells by fluid flow and diffusion, with both of these mechanisms affected by load and posture. Fluid flow is caused by pressure changes on the disc. High pressure causes fluid to be expelled from the disc, while low pressure allows the intake of fluid from surrounding tissue. Diffusion occurs in response to a chemical concentration gradient—nutrients in and waste products out.[44] Thus activity that results in spinal flexion can have an ameliorative effect on disc degeneration by increasing the flow of nutrients into the disc and waste products out. Increased activity results in increased aerobic metabolism in the outer part of the annulus and the central portion of the nucleus and brings about a reduction in lactate concentration.[40] A decrease in activity as a result of spinal fusion[39] has just the opposite effect. After 5 weeks' bed rest[59] the nucleus has been shown to decrease in size. In addition, physical and chemical factors such as vibration and smoking have been shown to decrease solute transport to the disc as well as lower the intradiscal oxygen tension[37, 38] which could result in an increased accumulation of lactate.

Oxidation of lipid can also occur in the disc and lead to an accumulation of brown deposit called lipofuscin, sometimes called the senile pigment/aging pigment.[7, 22, 94] The oxidation of lipid forms dialdehydes, which can react to cross-link collagen fibers and alter their mechanical properties as well as block their already slow turnover. Therefore, changes in diet and metabolism that deposit lipid in the disc may alter its mechanical properties and accelerate degeneration.[22] A recent study indicated that lipofuscin may be released from chondrocytes because of cell collapse as a result of an increase in metabolic cells in the nucleus, possibly as a response to aging.[45] However, no obvious correlation was found between the stage of disc degeneration and the incidence of pigment.

MRI is becoming more used to assess disc degeneration. It has been used to assess the effects of prolonged bed rest on the disc by showing a reduction in the nucleus.[59] It has also been successfully used to diagnose traumatic Schmorl's node formation in a patient following forced lumbar flexion that resulted in an injury.[55] MRI using gadolinium-diethylenetriamine penta-acetic acid (Gd-DPTA) has been used to assess diffusion into discs/peridiscal scar tissue. Gd-DPTA is a small molecule (molecular weight, 938) that does not cross intact cell membranes and can thus be used as a leak detector in damaged/degenerated vertebral end plates.[42, 85]

MRI and computed tomography (CT) studies on 330 lumbar discs have shown that disc degeneration was significantly more common at L4–5 and L5–S1 than at the other lumbar levels, with L3–4 being the next lumbar level most significantly affected.[16] The degeneration increased with age, with no significant difference noted by sex. Disc degeneration was found to occur in the absence of facet osteoarthritis. However, whenever facet osteoarthritis was present, disc degeneration was also present.

Disc degeneration with annular rupture can lead to leakage of nuclear contents. It is postulated that release of nuclear components may be important in the pathogenesis of back pain. An inflammatory response has been obtained from homogenized autogenous nucleus pulposus injected into the lumbar epidural space of dogs. This material was shown to irritate dura and nerve roots.[66] Enzymatic markers for inflammation (phospholipase A) have been found in human disc samples removed at surgery for radiculopathy due to lumbar disc disease.[86]

Laboratory studies have shown that nuclear extrusion is characterized by occasional loud popping sounds that occur in younger samples and appear to be characterized by extrusion of moist nuclear material into the defect.[63] Sealing of the defect was observed with both old and young nuclear gel, but without the pop in older samples. The sealing appeared fairly complete because normal pressure resistance was observed without leakage when saline was injected after completion of the loading cycles.

MRI studies performed on 246 patients with low back/radicular pain showed that even with significant dehydration and degeneration there is an almost two-thirds chance that there is no obvious displacement pathology with neural compression.[17] Disc protrusion is particularly rare in patients who are more than 60 years old, where an atrophied nucleus is usually present.[104]

DISC REPAIR

The disc appears to have a limited ability to resynthesize and repair its matrix. Chymopapain (0.125 nanokatal units) was injected into the intervertebral discs of rabbits.[54] One week after chymopapain treatment, the water and proteoglycan content was decreased in all disc tissues. In the anterior and posterior parts of the annulus, the proteoglycan content recovered after 12 weeks, but there was no recovery in the nucleus. The collagen content continued to increase up to the 12th week in the nucleus. In the anterior and posterior portions of the nucleus, noncollagenous protein recovered after 3 to 6 weeks, but there was no recovery in the nucleus. The intradiscal pressure was decreased at 1 to 6 weeks, but recovery was observed at 12 weeks. Other studies in dogs have reported that proteoglycan is regenerated in the nucleus 3 months after chymopapain injection.[10] In vivo studies on porcine discs[52] where scalpel cuts or a boring injury was made in the annulus resulted in a significant increase in viscoelastic properties (creep, etc.) similar to those associated with aging. Other studies in dogs have shown that by 24 months disc height, which had decreased 30% to 60%, was not significantly different from noninjected controls.[27] Laboratory studies on porcine discs have indicated that partial denucleation and acute chemonucleolysis produced biomechanical changes (decreased stiffness, increased creep) that were comparable to slightly degenerative, age-related changes seen in human discs.[51] Other studies have shown that the ability of the disc to resist loads is proportional to the amount of nucleus removed.[28]

Repair remodeling of components within the disc may follow Wolff's law, where structure may be dictated in response to stress, as has been shown in patients with scoliosis.[11] Collagen content as well as the ratio of type I to type II collagen in the annulus is increased on the concave side of the curve and decreased on the convex side, most noticeably in the outer part of the annulus. Collagen content is also increased in the nucleus, particularly in vertebrae located at apices of the curve.[11, 15] There were also significantly higher levels of aggregate and larger nonaggregating monomers similar to those seen in patients with cerebral palsy.[75] There may also be differences in proteoglycan components that represent a reparative/remodeling response by disc fibrocytes to the abnormal mechanical environment imposed by the scoliotic curve.[45]

When spines with a grossly degenerated disc were studied, the disc above the degenerated one but not the degenerated one itself was rich in new collagen, primarily type I, in both the nucleus and annulus. This is interpreted that the normal disc may be able to compensate in some ways for the defective disc below.[33]

The annulus appears to only have a limited potential for healing. In a patient with a tear in the posterior part of the annulus, there appeared to be a loss of collagen and an increase in proteoglycan and water around the tear that were not apparent in the remainder of the disc.[83] These results were similar to results in rabbits with surgically induced ventral disc herniation. After injury there was metaplasia into fibrocartilage, originally from cells along the margins of the annular wound, with proliferation of cells changing the entire disc space into fibrocartilage. The water content initially fell and then rose rapidly again before showing a gradual loss over an extended period. Proteoglycan levels paralleled changes in water content. The hyaluronic acid content decreased rapidly after herniation, but there was no change in the size of the proteoglycan monomers.[61]

Recent studies that used a stab wound into the disc of dogs have found that only the superficial portion of the annulus healed with a thin layer of fibrous tissue and that the deeper layers did not heal.[30] MRI studies have also shown some healing of dog annulus by fibrous tissue.[90]

Another study was made in sheep where a cut was made in the outer part of the annulus and the inner third of the annulus and nucleus left intact. At subsequent sacrifice of the sheep, progressive failure of the inner portion of the annulus was seen in all sheep at 4 to 12 months after the surgery. Although the outermost rim of the annulus showed the ability to heal, the defect induced by the cut led initially to deformation and bulging of the collagen bundles and eventually to inner extension of the tear and complete failure.[77] A recent study on mature canine disc components in tissue culture has indicated that cell proliferation may be induced by different growth factors, with the nucleus and transition zone responding more than the annulus.[97]

Care must be exercised in extrapolation from animal data to man when considering disc behavior in vivo, not only because of the possible differences in disc structural components but also the orientation of the disc in bipedal man vs. primarily quadrupedal animals. Consequently, the orientation and magnitude of forces affecting the disc will differ.[43]

CONCLUSION

The components of the intervertebral disc, annulus fibrosus, nucleus pulposus, and vertebral end plates, all act in concert to stabilize the spine and absorb and distribute load while allowing the spine to flex, extend, or rotate. Rotary motion is restricted by the two facet joints connected to each disc (three-joint complex). The nucleus plays a crucial role in shock absorption by transferring axial compression forces into radially directed hoop stresses in the annulus. This function is provided by proteoglycans, which bind water and collagen to provide structure. Even though the disc components turn over slowly, they must be replaced by cells located primarily in the inner part of the annulus. These cells must receive adequate nutrition, which comes primarily by diffusion through the end plates. Flow of nutrients into the disc and waste products out is aided by movement that flexes the spine. Excessive mechanical loading or repetitive dynamic loading can lead to end plate fracture with subsequent calcification and decreased transport of nutrients. Increasing age may intensify these effects. Impairment in the ability of the nucleus to uniformly transfer forces can result in the annulus absorbing larger loads with possible rupture in the posterolateral sections where fibers are thinner and fewer in number. End plate fracture usually occurs before annular rupture. A failure of disc components may result in the degeneration of adjacent structures such as facet joints, which may have to absorb increasing proportions of the spinal load.

REFERENCES

1. Adams MA, Dolan P, Hutton WC, et al: Diurnal changes in spinal mechanics and their clinical significance. *J Bone Joint Surg [Br]* 1990; 72:266–270.
2. Adams P, Muir H: Quantitative changes with age of proteoglycans of human lumbar discs. *Ann Rheum Dis* 1976; 35:289–296.
3. Akeson WH, Woo SLY, Taylor TKF, et al: Biomechanics and biochemistry of the intervertebral discs: The need for correlation studies. *Clin Orthop* 1977; 129:133–140.
4. Ashman RB: Disc anatomy and biomechanics. *Spine State Art Rev* 1989; 3:13–26.
5. Ashton-Miller JA, Schultz AB: Biomechanics of the human spine and trunk. *Exerc Sport Sci Rev* 1988; 16:169–204.
6. Bahk YW, Lee JM: Measure set computed tomographic analysis of internal architectures of lumbar disc. *Invest Radiol* 1988; 23:17–23.

7. Banga I: Investigations of fluorescent peptides and liposomes of human intervertebral discs relating to atherosclerosis. *Atherosclerosis* 1975; 22:533–541.
8. Bayliss MT, Johnstone B, O'Brien JP: Proteoglycan synthesis in the human intervertebral disc. *Spine* 1988; 13:972–981.
9. Bernick S, Walker JM, Paule WJ: Age changes to the annulus fibrosus in human intervertebral discs. *Spine* 1991; 16:520–524.
10. Bradford DS, Cooper KM, Oegema TR: Chymopapain, chemonucleolysis, and nucleus pulposus regeneration. *J Bone Joint Surg [Am]* 1983; 65:1220–1231.
11. Brickley-Parsons D, Glimcher MJ: Is the chemistry of collagen in intervertebral discs an expression of Wolff's law? *Spine* 1984; 9:148–163.
12. Brown T, Hansen RJ, Yorra AJ: Some mechanical tests on the lumbosacral spine with particular reference to the intervertebral disc: A preliminary report. *J Bone Joint Surg Am* 1957; 39:1135–1164.
13. Buckwalter J, Cooper R, Maynard J: Elastic fibers in human intervertebral disc. *J Bone Joint Surg Am* 1976; 58:73–76.
14. Bushell GR, Ghosh P, Taylor TKF, et al: Proteoglycan chemistry of the intervertebral discs. *Clin Orthop* 1977; 129:115–123.
15. Bushell GR, Ghosh P, Taylor TKF, et al: The collagen of the intervertebral disc in adolescent idiopathic scoliosis. *J Bone Joint Surg [Br]* 1979; 61:501–508.
16. Butler D, Trafimow JH, Andersson GBJ, et al: Discs degenerate before facets. *Spine* 1990; 15:111–113.
17. DeCandido P, Reinig JW, Dwyer AJ, et al: Magnetic resonance assessment of the distribution of lumbar spine disc degenerative changes. *J Spinal Disorders* 1988; 1:9–15.
18. Diamant B, Karlsson J, Nachemson A: Correlation between lactate levels and pH in discs of patients with lumbar rhizopathies. *Experientia* 1968; 24:1195–1196.
19. Durning RP, Murphy ML: Lumbar disc disease: Clinical presentation, diagnosis, and treatment. *Postgrad Med* 1986; 79:54–74.
20. El-Bohy AA, Yang KH, King AI: Experimental verification of facet load transmission by direct measurement of facet lamina contact pressure. *J Biomech* 1989; 22:931–941.
21. Eyre D, et al: Intervertebral disc, in Frymoyer JW, Gorden SL (eds): *New Perspectives on Low Back Pain.* Park Ridge, Ill., American Academy of Orthopaedic Surgeons, 1988, pp 131–214.
22. Eyre DR: Biochemistry of the intervertebral disc, in Hall DA, Jackson DS (eds): *International Review of Connective Tissue Research.* New York, Academic Press, 1979, pp 227–290.
23. Eyring EJ: The biochemistry and physiology of the intervertebral disc. *Clin Orthop* 1969; 67:16–28.
24. Farfan HF: *Mechanical Disorders of the Low Back.* Philadelphia, Lea & Febiger, 1973.
25. Francois RJ: Letter. *Spine* 1982; 7:522–523.
26. Gamble JG: *The Musculoskeletal System.* New York, Raven Press, 1988, pp 57–80.
27. Garvin PJ, Jennings RB: Long term effects of chymopapain on intervertebral disc of dogs. *Clin Orthop* 1973; 92:281–295.
28. Goel VK, Nishiyama K, Weinstein JN, et al: Mechanical properties of lumbar spine motion segments as affected by partial disc removal. *Spine* 1986; 11:1008–1012.
29. Goel VK, Weinstein JN, Patwarchan AG: Biomechanics of intact ligamentous spine, in Goel VK, Weinstein JN (eds): *Biomechanics of the Spine: Clinical and Surgical Perspective.* Boca Raton, Fla, CRC Press, 1990, pp 97–156.
30. Hampton D, Laros G, McCarron R, et al: Healing potential of the annulus fibrosus. *Spine* 1989; 14:398–401.
31. Hansson TH, Keller TS, Spengler DM: Mechanical behavior of the human lumbar spine II: Fatigue strength during dynamic compressive loading. *J Orthop Res* 1987; 5:479–486.
32. Hassler O: The human intervertebral disc: A micro-angiographical study on its vascular supply at various stages. *Acta Orthop Scand* 1970; 40:765–772.
33. Herbert CM, Lindberg KA, Jayson MIV, et al: Changes in the collagen of human intervertebral discs during aging and degenerative disc disease. *J Mol Med* 1975; 1:79–91.
34. Hirano N, Tsuji H, Ohshima H, et al: Analysis of rabbit intervertebral disc physiology based on water metabolism: I. Factors influencing metabolism of the normal intervertebral discs. *Spine* 1988; 13:1291–1302.
35. Hirsh C, Inglemark B, Miller M: The anatomical basis for low back pain. *Acta Orthop Scand* 1963; 33:1–17.
36. Holm S, Maroudas A, Urban JPG, et al: Nutrition of the intervertebral disc: Solute transport and metabolism. *Connect Tissue Res* 1981; 8:101–119.
37. Holm S, Nachemson A: Nutrition of the intervertebral disc: Acute effects of cigarette smoking: An experimental animal study. *Ups J Med Sci* 1988; 93:91–99.
38. Holm S, Nachemson A: Nutrition of the intervertebral disc: Effects induced by vibration. *Orthop Trans* 1985; 9:451.
39. Holm S, Nachemson A: Nutritional changes in the canine intervertebral disc after spinal fusion. *Clin Orthop* 1982; 169:243–258.
40. Holm S, Nachemson A: Variations in the nutrition of the canine intervertebral disc induced by motion. *Spine* 1983; 8:866–874.
41. Horton WG: Further observations on the elastic mechanism of the intervertebral disc. *J Bone Joint Surg [Br]* 1958; 40:552–557.
42. Hueftle MG, Modic MT, Ross JS, et al: Lumbar spine: Postoperative MR imaging with Gd-DPTA. *Radiology* 1988; 167:817–824.
43. Humzah MD, Soames RW: Human intervertebral disc: Structure and function. *Anat Rec* 1988; 220:337–356.
44. Hutton WC, Adams MA: The biomechanics of disc degeneration. *Acta Orthop Belg* 1987; 53:143–147.
45. Ishii T, Tsuji H, Sano A, et al: Histochemical and ultrastructural observation on brown degeneration of human intervertebral disc. *J Orthop Res* 1991; 9:78–90.
46. Jaeger M, Luttman A: Biomechanical analysis and assess-

ment of lumbar stress during load lifting using a dynamic 19-segment human model. *Ergonomics* 1989; 32:93–112.
47. Jayson M, Barks JS: Structural changes in intervertebral discs. *Ann Rheum Dis* 1973; 32:10–15.
48. Jensen GM: Biomechanics of the lumbar intervertebral disc: A review. *Phys Ther* 1980; 60:765–773.
49. Johnson EF, Chetty K, Moore IM, et al: Distribution and arrangement of elastic fibers in intervertebral discs of adult humans. *J Anat* 1982; 135:301–309.
50. Kazarian L: Biomechanics and injury classification. *Exerc Sport Sci Rev* 1981; 9:297–352.
51. Keller TS, Hansson TH, Holm SH, et al: In vivo creep behavior of normal and degenerative porcine intervertebral disc: A preliminary report. *J Spinal Disorders* 1989; 1:267–278.
52. Keller TS, Holm SH, Hansson TH, et al: The dependence of intervertebral disc mechanical properties on physiologic conditions. *Spine* 1990; 15:751–761.
53. Kim YE, Goel VK: Effect of testing mode on the biomechanical response of a spinal motion segment. *J Biomech* 1990; 23:289–291.
54. Kitano S, Tsuji H, Hirano N, et al: Water, fixed charge density, protein contents, and lysine incorporation into protein in chymopapain digested intervertebral disc of rabbit. *Spine* 1989; 14:1226–1233.
55. Kornberg M: MRI diagnosis of traumatic Schmorl's node. *Spine* 1988; 13:934–935.
56. Kraemer J, Kolditz D, Gowin R: Water and electrolyte content of human intervertebral discs under variable load. *Spine* 1985; 10:69–71.
57. Kulak RF, Belytschoko TB, Schultz AB, et al: Nonlinear behavior of the human intervertebral disc under axial load. *J Biomech* 1976; 9:377–386.
58. Kurowski P, Kubo A: The relationship of the intervertebral disc to mechanical loading conditions on lumbar vertebrae. *Spine* 1986; 11:726–731.
59. Le Blanc AO, Schonfeld E, Schneider VS, et al. The spine: Changes in T2 relaxation times from disuse. *Radiology* 1988; 169:105–107.
60. Lin HS, Liu YK, Adams KH: Mechanical response of lumbar intervertebral joint under physiological (complex) loading. *J Bone Joint Surg [Am]* 1978; 60:41–55.
61. Lipson SJ, Muir H: Proteoglycans in experimental intervertebral disc degeneration. *Spine* 1981; 6:194–210.
62. Marchand F, Ahmed AM: Investigation of the laminate structure of lumbar disc annulus fibrosus. *Spine* 1990; 15:402–410.
63. Markolf K, Morris J: The structural components of the intervertebral discs. *J Bone Joint Surg [Am]* 1974; 56:675–687.
64. Maroudas A: Nutrition and metabolism of the intervertebral disc, in Ghosh P (ed): *The Biology of the Intervertebral Disc*. Boca Raton, Fla, CRC Press, 1988.
65. Maroudas A: Nutrition and metabolism of the intervertebral disc, in White AA, Gordon SL (eds): *Symposium on Idiopathic Low Back Pain*. St Louis, Mosby–Year Book, 1982, pp 370–390.
66. McCarron RF, Wimpee WM, Hudkins PG, et al: The inflammatory effect of nucleus pulposus: A possible element in the pathogenesis of low-back pain. *Spine* 1987; 12:760–764.
67. Morris JM, Lucas DB, Bresler B: Role of the trunk in stability of the spine. *J Bone Joint Surg [Am]* 1961; 43:327–351.
68. Nachemson A: Intradiscal measurements of pH in patients with lumbar rhizopathies. *Acta Orthop Scand* 1969; 40:23–42.
69. Nachemson A: Lumbar intradiscal pressure: Experimental studies on postmortem material. *Acta Orthop Scand Suppl* 1960; 43:1–104.
70. Nachemson A: Some mechanical properties of the lumbar intervertebral discs. *Bull Hosp Jt Dis* 1962; 23:130–143.
71. Nachemson A: The influence of spinal movements on the lumbar intradiscal pressure and on the tensile stresses in the annulus fibrosus. *Acta Orthop Scand* 1963; 33:183–207.
72. Nachemson A: The load on lumbar discs in different positions of the body. *Clin Orthop* 1966; 45:107–122.
73. Naylor A, Happey F, MacRae T: Changes in the human intervertebral disc with age: A biophysical study. *J Am Geriatr Soc* 1955; 3:964–973.
74. Oda J, Tanaka H, Tsuzuki N: Intervertebral disc changes with aging of human cervical vertebra: From the neonate to the eighties. *Spine* 1988; 13:1205–1211.
75. Oegema TR, Bradford DS, Cooper KM, et al: Comparison of the biochemistry of proteoglycans isolated from normal, idiopathic scoliotic and cerebral palsy spines. *Spine* 1983; 8:378–384.
76. Ohshima H, Tsuji H, Hirano N, et al: Water diffusion pathway swelling pressure and biomechanical properties of the intervertebral disc during compression loading. *Spine* 1989; 14:1234–1244.
77. Osti DL, Vernon-Roberts B, Fraser RD: Annulus tears and intervertebral disc degeneration. *Spine* 1990; 15:762–767.
78. Panjabi M, Brown M, Lindahl S, et al: Intrinsic disc pressure as a measure of integrity of the lumbar spine. *Spine* 1988; 13:913–917.
79. Pearce RH, Grimmer BJ, Adams ME: Degeneration and the chemical composition of the lumbar intervertebral disc. *J Orthop Res* 1987; 5:198–205.
80. Perey O: Fracture of the vertebral end plate in the lumbar spine: An experimental biomechanical investigation. *Acta Orthop Scand Suppl*, 1957, p 22.
81. Pope M, Wilder D, Booth J: The biomechanics of low back pain, in White AA, Gordon SL (eds): *Symposium on Idiopathic Low Back Pain*. St Louis, Mosby–Year Book, 1982, pp 252–295.
82. Riihimaki H, Mattsson T, Zitting A, et al: Radiographically detectable degenerative changes of the lumbar spine among concrete reinforcement workers and house painters. *Spine* 1990; 15:114–119.
83. Roberts S, Beard HK, O'Brien JP: Biochemical changes of intervertebral discs in patients with spondylolisthesis or with tears of the posterior annulus fibrosus. *Ann Rheum Dis* 1982; 41:78–85.
84. Roberts S, Menage J, Urban JPG: Biochemical and struc-

tural properties of the cartilage end plate and its relation to the intervertebral disc. *Spine* 1989; 14:166–174.

85. Ross JS, Delemarter R, Heuftle MG, et al: Gadolinium-DPTA enhanced MR imaging of the postoperative lumbar spine: Time course and mechanism of enhancement. *Am J Radiol* 1989; 152:825–834.
86. Saal JS, Franson RC, Dobrow R, et al: High levels of inflammatory phospholipase A_2 activity in lumbar disc herniations. *Spine* 1990; 15:674–678.
87. Sandover J: Dynamic loading as a possible source of low back disorders. *Spine* 1983; 8:652–658.
88. Schiebler MC, Camerino UJ, Fallon MD, et al: In vivo and ex vivo magnetic resonance imaging evaluation of early disc degeneration with histopathologic correlation. *Spine* 1991; 16:635–640.
89. Seroussi RE, Krag MH, Muller DL, et al: Internal deformations of intact and denucleated human lumbar discs subjected to compression, flexion, and extension loads. *J Orthop Res* 1989; 7:122–131.
90. Sether LA, Nguyen C, Yu S, et al: Canine intervertebral discs: Correlation of anatomy and MR imaging. *Radiology* 1990; 175:207–211.
91. Shirazi-adl A: Strain in fibers of a lumbar disc. *Spine* 1989; 14:96–103.
92. Stairmand JW, Holm S, Urban JPG: Factors influencing oxygen concentration gradients in the intervertebral disc. *Spine* 1991; 16:444–449.
93. Stevens RL, Ryvan R, Roberston WR, et al: Biological changes in the annulus fibrosus in patients with low back pain. *Spine* 1982; 7:223–233.
94. Taylor TKF, Akeson WH: Intervertebral disc prolapse: A review of morphologic and biochemical knowledge concerning the nature of prolapse. *Clin Orthop* 1971; 76:54–79.
95. Tencer AF, Ahmed AM, Burke DL: Some static mechanical properties of the lumbar intervertebral joint, intact and injured. *J Biomech Eng* 1982; 104:193.
96. Tertti M, Paajanen H, Laato M, et al: Disc degeneration in magnetic resonance imaging. *Spine* 1991; 16:629–634.
97. Thompson JP, Oegema TR, Bradford DS: Stimulation of mature canine intervertebral disc by growth factors. *Spine* 1991; 16:253–264.
98. Thompson JP, Pearce RH, Schechter ME, et al: Preliminary evaluation of a scheme for grading the gross morphology of the human intervertebral disc. *Spine* 1990; 15:411–415.
99. Twomey LT, Taylor JR: Age changes in lumbar vertebrae and intervertebral discs. *Clin Orthop* 1987; 224:97–104.
100. Urban JPG, Holm S, Maroudas A, et al: Nutrition of the intervertebral disc: Effect of fluid flow on solute transport. *Clin Orthop* 1982; 170:296–302.
101. Urban JPG, McMullin JF: Swelling pressure of the lumbar intervertebral disc: Influence of age, spinal level, composition, and degeneration. *Spine* 1988; 13:179–187.
102. Wilder DG, Pope MH, Frymoyer JW: The biomechanics of lumbar disc herniation and the effect of overload and instability. *J Spinal Disorders* 1988; 1:16–32.
103. Yang KH, King AI: Mechanism of facet load transmission as a hypothesis for low back pain. *Spine* 1984; 9:557–565.
104. Yasuma T, Koh S, Okamura T, et al: Histologic changes in aging lumbar discs. *J Bone Joint Surg [Am]* 1990; 72:220–229.
105. Yoganandan N, Maiman DJ, Pintar F, et al: Microtrauma in the lumbar spine: A cause of low back pain. *Neurosurgery* 1988; 23:162–168.

13

Spinal Instability

John Handal, M.D., and David Selby, M.D.

The spinal segment is a three-joint mechanical structure. The spine provides a stable support for the extremities, the head, and loads applied to the torso. The in vitro stability is made more rigid by the spinal musculature. That is, an in vitro spine will buckle with an axial load of only 4 kg.[60] The limits of stability should provide rigid enough support yet allow the flexibility of normal activities. Beyond these limits lies instability. This chapter will consider the definition, criteria, components, and classification of clinical spinal instability.

SPINAL STABILITY VS. INSTABILITY

There are several definitions of spinal stability and instability.[31, 74] Spinal stability in mechanical terms refers to an unchanged stiffness to an applied load. Instability is a change in stiffness to an applied load. This stiffness may increase with less motion, as seen in late spinal stenosis, or may decrease with increased motion as in spondylolisthesis. The American Academy of Orthopaedic Surgeons' glossary on spinal terminology states, "Segmental instability is an abnormal response to applied loads, characterized by motion in motion segments beyond normal constraints."[5]

A second term to be defined is clinical instability. "Clinical instability is the loss of the ability of the spine under physiologic loads to maintain its pattern of displacement so that there is no initial or additional neurologic deficit, no major deformity, and no incapacitating pain."[96] The difference between segmental instability and clinical instability is in the applied loads. The term *clinical instability* refers to failure under physiologic loads. The definition also encompasses the clinical entities of neurologic deficit, deformity, and pain.

Segmental instability is a mechanical definition. The definition of segmental instability can also be applied clinically. However, in the clinical scope, segmental instability has only a very narrow view. For example, a nonprogressing spondylolisthesis in an asymptomatic patient represents a segmental instability. Segmental instability gives clinical instability its mechanical criteria. In the case of spondylolisthesis, criteria for segmental instability are met, but not the criteria for clinical instability. This patient is not clinically unstable because of the absence of pain, neurologic deficit, or major deformity. Therefore, this clinically stable patient does not require surgical treatment. However, through fibrosis, ligament hypertrophy, and abnormal musculature, this patient's spondylolisthesis has reached clinical stability.

COMPONENTS OF CLINICAL INSTABILITY

The previous example of spondylolisthesis has illustrated that treatment is indicated when a patient meets the criteria of clinical instability. The components of clinical instability are mechanical instability, pain, deformity, and neurologic deficit. These components bear delineation. The spine can be divided into regions: the upper cervical (C0, C1, C2), the lower cervical (C2–T1), the thoracic (T1–L1), the lumbosacral (L1–S1), and the sacroiliac regions. The mechanical criteria of instability for each spinal subdivision are based on normal kinematics of the forces, coupled with spinal motion. Kinematics is the study of motion characteristics of rigid bodies, with no consideration of the force involved.[96] Clinical instability brings the physician beyond the diagnostic images back to the patient. An understanding of clinical instability comes through its four components: pain, neurologic deficit, deformity, and mechanical instability.

Pain

Pain is an unpleasant sensory and emotional experience associated with actual or potential tissue damage.[5] Spinal pain can originate from many causes. It can be visceral (i.e., retrocecal appendicitis or from pelvic inflammatory disease) or vascular (i.e., aortic aneurysm).[14] The scope of this chapter is limited to intrinsic spinal structures as a cause of spinal pain. Spinal pain is of two types: somatic and radicular.[54, 55] Somatic pain arises from an innervated, anatomic structure (i.e., disc, facet joint, ligaments). The cause of somatic pain is any pathologic process occurring in that structure that results in stimulation of nocioceptive or pain-sensitive structures.[55] This process, be it mechanical, chemical, or both, can have many etiologies. An example is posterior element instability secondary to capsular laxity of the facet joint.[56] Facet pain in the instability phase of the degenerative cascade of

Kirkaldy-Willis[56] is one example of somatic pain. Apophyseal joint pain has been experimentally reproduced in the cervical and lumbar vertebrae[6, 26, 65] (Figs 13–1 and 13–2). Through noxious stimulation of the facet joint in normal individuals, the pain patterns of somatic pain can be seen. Although not as precise a pattern as a dermatome, these patterns give the clinician a clearer understanding of what the patient is describing. Discogenic pain is another example of somatic pain. Primary disc pain[28] is pain mediated through nerve endings in the annulus fibrosus. The process causing this pathologic state is mechanical and/or chemical. The chemical process can be direct irritation of the nocioreceptor in the annulus. Substances such as prostaglandin E, histamine, and postassium are known direct-contact irritants.[83] Neuropeptides such as substance P (SP) and vasoactive intestinal peptide (VIP) have been implicated in mediating the pain response associated with discography. SP, VIP, and others have been identified by radioimmunoassay in the outer portion of the annulus.[48] Experimental study of the disc through discography found elevated concentrations of VIP and SP in the dorsal root ganglion. When discography was performed on herniated discs, SP levels alone were elevated; those of VIP were not.[83] This differential effect of discography on an injured disc and SP is suggestive of a chemical mechanism of low back pain. A mechanical process can contribute to discogenic pain through radial tears.[28] These tears, which originate essentially from the nucleus, allow physical communication between the chemically pathologic state of the nucleus and the innervated outer rim of the annulus. A radial tear alone may not change the load characteristics of the disc; however, this mechanical defect has allowed potentially irritative substances to reach the nocioreceptors of the outer part of the annulus. The disc, although not mechanically affected, can be a source of somatic pain via a chemical process. A nonprolapsed or internally disrupted disc is symptomatic through these processes. Discogenic pain is somatic pain, and a patient's description of somatic pain is not a precise one. The patterns of somatic pain are not dermatomal but do overlap; however, understanding somatic pain allows a clinician to understand the patient. Somatic pain is real, has an anatomic basis, and is a clinical entity. To find its origins, it must be tested for correctly. Finally, the pathologic mechanisms causing somatic pain seem somewhat less obvious, or is it that clinicians try to diagnose somatic pain by studies for radicular pain? Instead, the diagnosis of somatic pain should be based on studies that examine the structures that cause it. Myelography, computed tomography (CT), and other canal studies are insensitive to the diagnosis of somatic pain. An evaluation of somatic pain in the absence of neurologic signs is accomplished through provocative testing (i.e., discography)[83, 89] and diagnostic blocks (i.e., selective nerve root injection and facet blocks).[48, 63] These diagnostic studies are based on the principle that an abnormal structure is a cause of pain that when stressed should reproduce the pain. Anesthetizing it with local anesthesia should relieve the pain. Infiltration of the apophyseal joint or dorsal root ganglion with local anesthesia and subsequent relief of pain implicate that structure as the source of the pain. Similarly, discography and disc infiltration with a

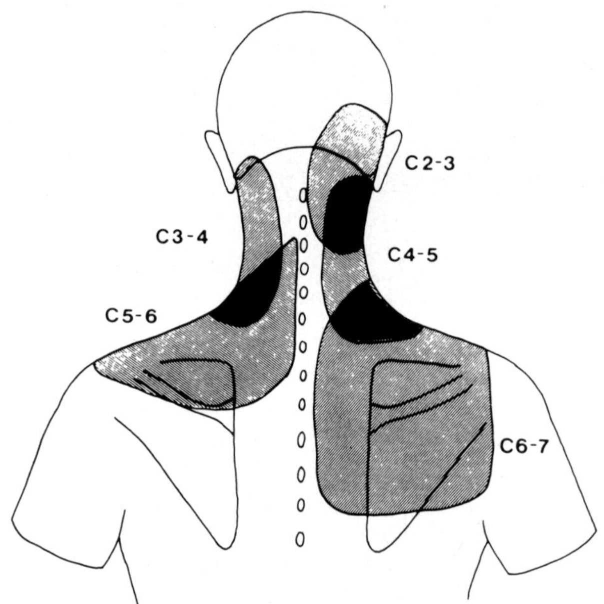

FIG 13–1.
Composite map of the characteristic distribution of pain from zygapophyseal joints at the segments C2–3 to C6–7. (From Dwyer A, Aprill C, Bogduk N: *Spine* 1990; 15:453–457. Used by permission.)

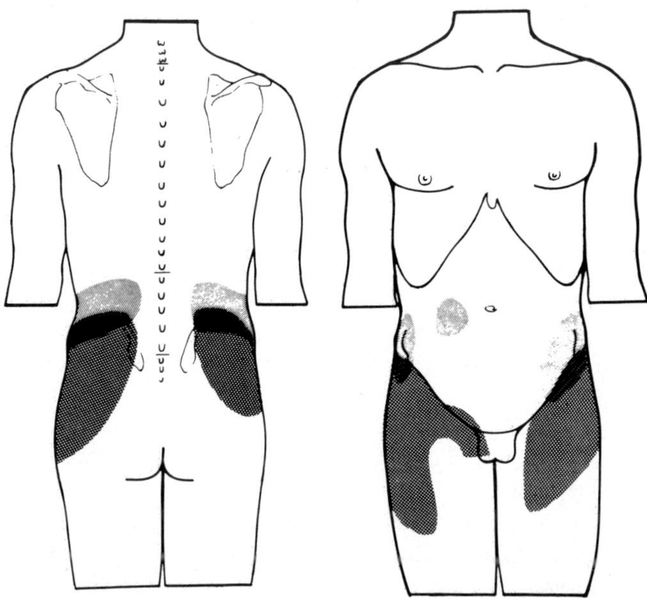

FIG 13–2.
A composite map of the characteristic distribution of pain from lumbar zygapophyseal joint injection. (From McCall I, Park W, O'Brien J: *Spine* 1979; 4:441–446. Used by permission.)

local anesthetic can identify the disc as a source of somatic pain through provocation and block. The origins of somatic pain can only be correctly diagnosed through the use of the appropriate diagnostic studies.

Radicular pain is referred pain from a particular nerve root that radiates from the spine into the dermatome of that root.[90] Anatomically, radicular pain is referred from the postganglionic ventral rami to the extremity. This well-recognized entity is a common explanation for referred pain into the distal end of the extremity. Myelography gave this entity its radiographic image.[69] Experimental studies on nerve compression[62] and nerve traction have reproduced paresthesias, pain, and numbness[84]; however, radicular pain should not be exclusively thought of as a mechanical event. Venous obstruction[62] and chemically mediated inflammatory processes[87, 91] have been implicated as causes of radicular pain. The diagnosis of radicular pain is made through an examination of the ventral rami. The ventral rami have both motor and sensory fibers. Radicular pain with motor weakness (motor nerve involvement) is well evaluated by electromyography (EMG). Correlation of spinal imaging studies such as CT, magnetic resonance imaging (MRI), and myelography with the EMG study and the patient's symptomatology is diagnostic of this problem. Radicular pain in the absence of motor weakness (i.e., sensory nerve involvement only) is diagnosed by spinal imaging studies such as myelography, CT, and MRI correlated with the patient's symptoms and selective nerve root injection. With only sensory involvement of the ventral rami, the EMG may have normal results. EMG is a diagnostic study of the motor neuron component of the ventral rami and is positive in the face of motor neuron denervation. Nerve root infiltration with local anethesia is more sensitive in the diagnosis of sensory radiculopathies.[20]

Pain is a common sign of instability.[71] The instability can be diagnosed if the clinician understands the somatic and radicular pain being described. Finally, pain is multifactorial in origin. Spinal pain has a physical measure (i.e., instability) and a psychological dimension. In the evaluation and treatment of spinal pain both organic (instability) and nonorganic (psychosocial, economic) factors must be taken into consideration. Both have a significant impact on the outcome, so they must be considered together when a treatment plan is formulated.

Mechanical Instability

The second component of clinical instability is mechanical. Mechanical elements of instability are kinematics of the functional spinal unit and the forces applied to the unit.

Kinematics

The spine can be divided into different sections based on its kinematic behavior. In this section the focus will be on kinematic criteria for the upper cervical region (C0, C1, C2), the lower cervical region (C2–T1), and the lumbosacral region (L1–S1). Kinematic criteria are expressed in single planes of motion; however, spinal motion is coupled.[28, 95]

Coupling means that a primary movement of the spinal segment is accompanied by a secondary simultaneous and involuntary movement.[97] As seen in Figure 13–3, segmental motion is not a single-plane rotation about one of the three axes of the spine[97]; translation also occurs. Translation is defined as "movement such that all particles in the body at a given time have the same direction of motion relative to a fixed point."[97] The coupled motion of translation and rotation do not occur about a single axis. Figure 13–3 depicts all motions occurring. As a result of

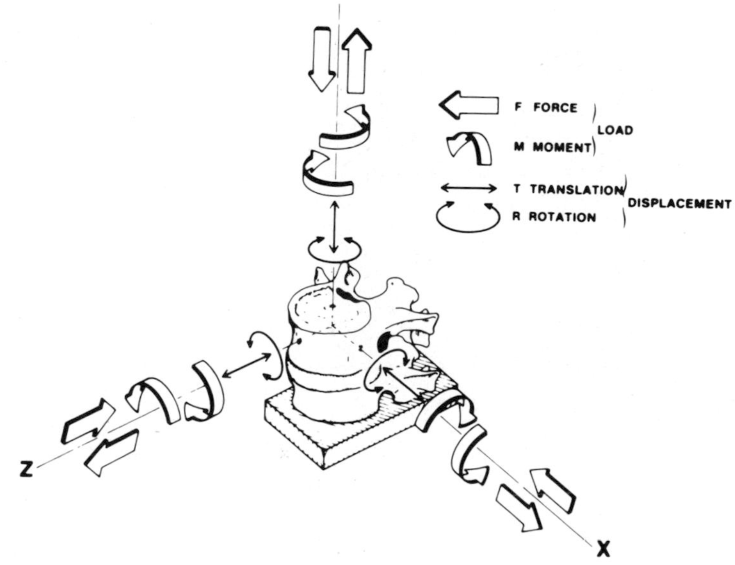

FIG 13–3.
A composite diagram of the spinal motions. (Adapted from White A, Panjabi MM: *Spine* 1978; 3:12.)

summation of these forces, the axis of rotation changes its center at every point in the line of motion. This leads to the concept of instant axes of rotation (IRA), which is defined as follows: for every instant of a rigid body in plane motion, there is a line in the body.[28] The IRA has been defined in the lumbar spine for both normal and degenerative lumbar spines.[18, 96] In the normal spine the IRA is relatively symmetrical and located in the middle column portion of the disc (Fig 13–4). With minor degeneration of the disc, the IRA becomes more erratic rather than increasing motion (Fig 13–5,A and B). As degeneration continues, the length of the IRA gets longer (more motion). Finally, in the end stages of degeneration, motion segment stiffness increases, and the length of the loci decreases (Fig 13–5,C and D). The centrode pattern of degeneration gives rise to two concepts: (1) changes in the IRA are clinically apparent by plain radiography, and (2), when apparent, it is diagnostic of a dominant lesion.

Knutsson first documented instability associated with disc degeneration. It was concluded that anterior displacement of greater than 3 mm is plain x-ray evidence of disc degeneration.[57] Hagelstem later identified patients with dynamic retrolisthesis to have significant degenerative changes in the disc.[47] MacNab included "the traction spur" in the radiographic criteria of instability[64] (Fig 13–6). The horizontal traction spur arises from outer annular fibers in the anterior or lateral position of the vertebra. The spur denotes segmental instability; however, the spur may be an asymptomatic finding and is not diagnostic of disc degeneration. In an attempt to measure flexion-extension motion, Dupuis et al.[22] assigned points of reference to the vertebral body. Horizontal and angular displacement was measured (Fig 13–7),[22] and this displacement identified the segment with abnormal motion and the specific area of the spinal segment responsible for the motion. This area was termed the "dominant lesion."[22] Freiberg used dynamic studies including traction/compression radiographs to document instability.[34] Although these methods describe segmental instability, they oftentimes do not correlate well with clinical symptoms. The presence of these motion abnormalities on plain x-ray studies has been shown in asymptomatic populations as well as symptomatic individuals.[36, 52, 86]

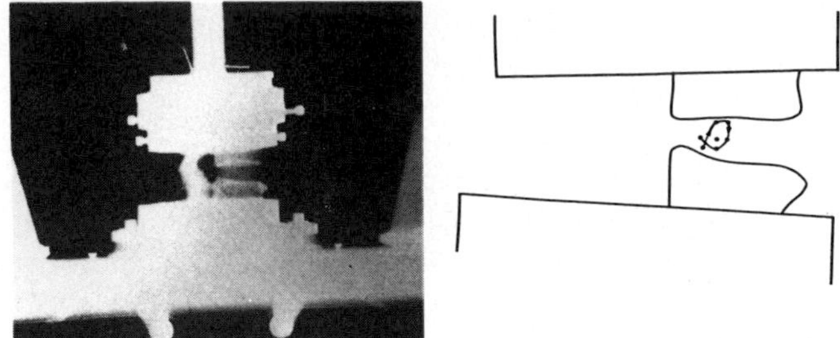

FIG 13–4.
Normal disc specimen by discography and instant axis of rotation, radiograph and centrode. (From Gertzbein S, Seligman J, Holtby R, et al: *Spine* 1985; 10:257–261. Used by permission.)

In an effort to correlate pathophysiologic changes with

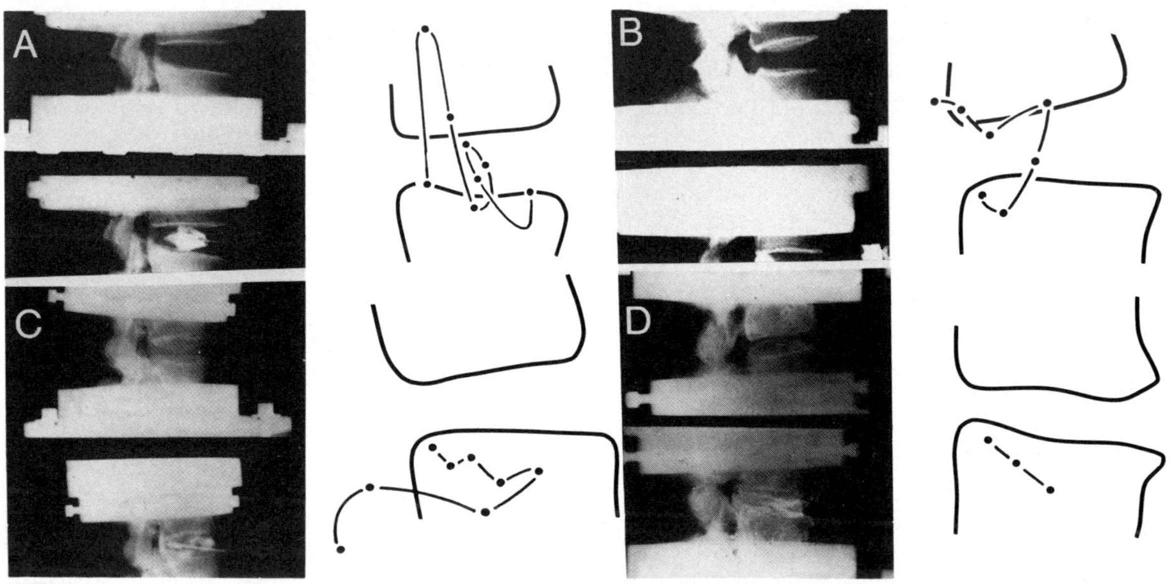

FIG 13–5.
A, minor degenerative disc disease. *Left,* radiograph and discogram. *Right,* instant axis of rotation. **B,** mild degenerative disc disease. *Left,* radiograph and discogram. *Right,* instant axis of rotation. **C,** moderate degenerative disc disease. *Left,* radiograph and discogram. *Right,* instant axis of rotation. **D,** severe degenerative disc disease. *Left,* radiograph and discogram. *Right,* instant axis of rotation. (From Gertzbein S, Seligman J, Holtby R, et al: *Spine* 1985; 10:257–261. Used by permission.)

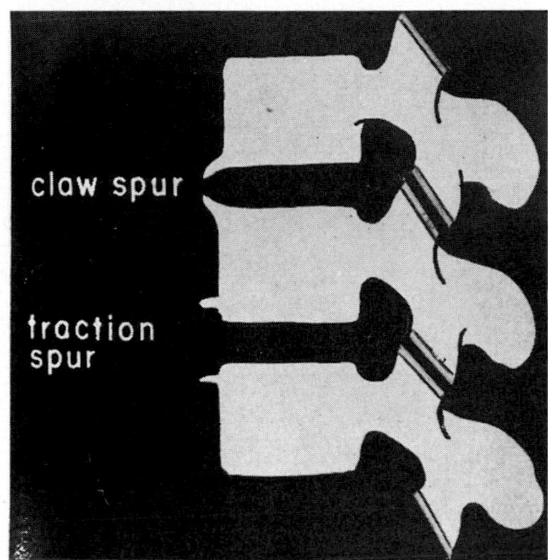

FIG 13–6.
The traction spur of MacNab. (From MacNab I: *J Bone Joint Surg [Am]* 1971; 53:663–670. Used by permission.)

TABLE 13–1.
Checklist for the Diagnosis of Clinical Instability in the Lumbar (L1–5) Spine*

Element	Point Value†
Cauda equina damage	3
Relative flexion sagittal-plane translation > 8% or extension sagittal-plane translation >9%	2
Relative flexion sagittal-plane rotation <−9%	2
Anterior elements destroyed	2
Posterior elements destroyed	2
Dangerous loading anticipated	1

*From Posner I, White AA III, Edwards WT, et al: *Spine* 1982; 7:374–388. Used by permission.
†A total of 5 or more equals clinical instability.

instability, Posner et al.[75] studied displacement vs. load. Stabilizing components were sequentially transected in posterior-to-anterior and anterior-to-posterior directions. For both flexion and extension an almost linear relationship exists between the amount of translation (z-, x-axis motion) and the number of ligamentous restraints sequentially cut.[21] Based on the pattern of ligamentous injury of the displacement, Posner et al. developed a checklist for lumbar instability from L1–5 and L5–S1. Tables 13–1 and 13–2 are the lumbar spine checklist and point values assigned to each parameter. A total score of 5 or more indicated segmental instability. Two elements of this checklist bear further explanation, cauda equina damage and dangerous loading anticipated. The loads applied in instability testing and assumed in the definition of clinical instability are physiologic. At times, the physiologic loading may rise dangerously high. An example would be competitive weight lifters. Cauda equina damage will be discussed in the section on neurologic deficit.

Regarding the cervical spine, similar checklists have been compiled. As in the lumbar spine, these checklists are a compilation of kinematic (motion) criteria, load, and neurologic injury. Because of anatomic and functional differences, the cervical spine is divided into upper (C0–2) and lower (C2–T1) divisions.

The occipitoatlantoaxial (C0, C1, C2) complex is a complicated series of articulations with three basic functions: first, it is a transitional zone between the multiple lower cervical segments and the fixed skull; second, it supports the skull throughout the range of motion; and third, it protects the spinal cord.[91] The motions of this segment are flexion-extension[25] and axial rotation.[23] These motions of translation and rotation occur about the z- and x-axes of the spine. Based on these and other studies,[24, 95] criteria for C0, C1, C2 instability is shown in Table 13–3.[51]

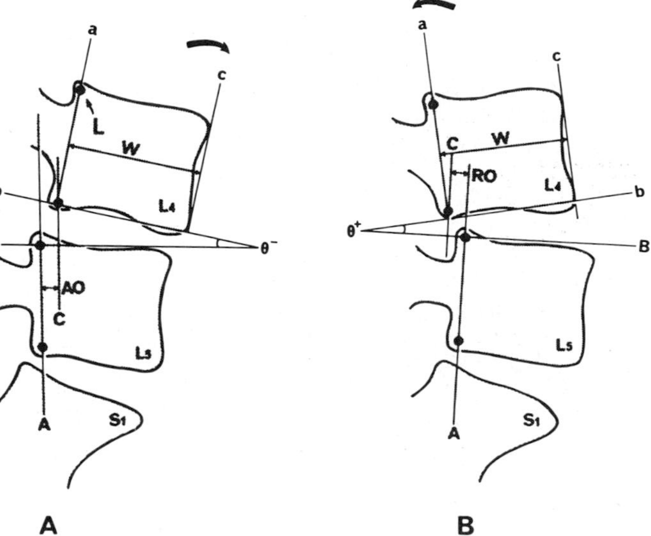

FIG 13–7.
Calculation of the percentage of horizontal displacement and angular displacement on flexion extension views. (From Dupis P, Yong-Hing K, Cassidy J, et al: *Spine* 1985; 10:262–276. Used by permission.)

TABLE 13–2.

Checklist for the Diagnosis of Clinical Instability in the Lumbosacral (L5–S1) Spine*

Element	Point Value†
Cauda equina damage	3
Relative flexion sagittal-plane translation > 6% or extension sagittal-plane translation >9%	2
Relative flexion sagittal-plane rotation <1 degree	2
Anterior elements destroyed	2
Posterior elements destroyed	2
Dangerous loading anticipated	1

*From Posner I, White AA III, Edwards WT, et al: *Spine* 1982; 7:374–388. Used by permission.
†A total of 5 or more equals clinical instability.

TABLE 13–3.

Criteria for C0–2 Instability*

>8 degrees	Axial rotation of C–C1
>1 mm	C0–1 translation
>7 mm	Overhang of C1–2 (total right and left)
>45 degrees	Axial rotation of C1–2 to one side
>4 mm	C1–2 translation
<13 mm	Posterior body of C2–posterior ring of C1
Avulsed transverse ligament	

*From Hohl M, Baker H: *J Bone Joint Surg [Am]* 1964; 46:1739. Used by permission.

Peculiar to the C0–2 complex is the importance of vertical translation, or y-axis motion. This can occur normally with C1–2 rotation.[25] Vertical translation of a significant degree can result in basilar invagination, which commonly occurs in disease states such as rheumatoid arthritis, trauma, and tumor. There are several methods described to measure basilar invagination (Fig 13–8). McGregor's line[66] is "the line drawn from the upper surface of the posterior edge of the hard palate to the caudal point of the occipital curve in the true lateral x-ray." A measurement of the tip of the odontoid process of 4.5 mm above this line is considered abnormal.[12] Chamberlain's line extends from the "dorsal lip of the foramen magnum to the dosal margin of the hard palate." This determination is made on a lateral radiograph of the skull. Normal position of the dens in relation to this line is between 1 mm below and 0.6 mm above Chamberlain's line, with standard deviations of 3.3 and 3.5 mm, respectively.[67] McRae's line is drawn from the anterior lip of the foramen magnum to the posterior lip of the foramen magnum. This determination is also made on lateral radiographs. Presumably, if the tip of the odontoid translates vertically above McRae's line, there would be symptomatic basilar invagination.[19] The digastric line (Fig 13–9) is drawn "between the two digastric roots, which lie in the lateral part of the base of the skull." This line is the cephalad limit of the odontoid process. There are many variables that render measurement of these lines less than reliable. The use of these lines for the diagnosis of basilar invagination must be complemented by documention of neurologic deficit and clinical correlation.[50, 61]

Segmental motion in the lower part of the cervical spine can be measured in a similar fashion as elsewhere in the spine. Each spinal unit of the lower part of the cervical spine (C2–T1) is anatomically distinct. As such, the patterns of motion of these spinal segments are unique. Flexion-extension motion in the lower part of the cervical spine is a coupling of translation and rotation, that is, in flexion the superior vertebra rotates anteriorly and translates forward. An arch of motion is created throughout the entire range. This arch was termed "the top angle" by Lysell.[61] The acuity of the top angle is flattest at C2–3 and deepest at C6–7. The top angle has been found to decrease in association with disc degeneration.[61] Direct measurement of z-axis motion indicates that the upper limit of normal is 2.7 mm of translation. Because of differences in x-ray

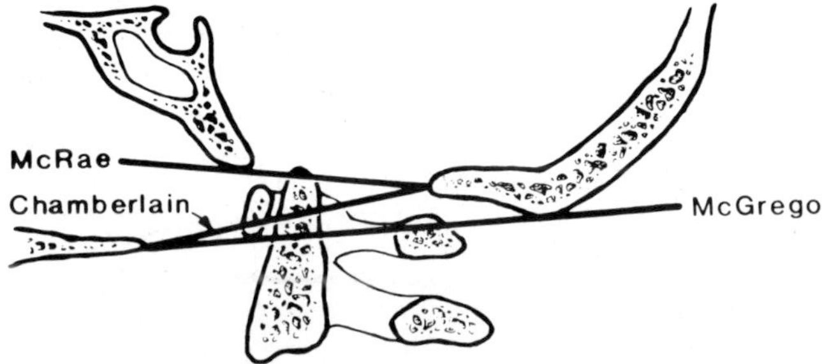

FIG 13–8.
Measurements of basilar invagination.

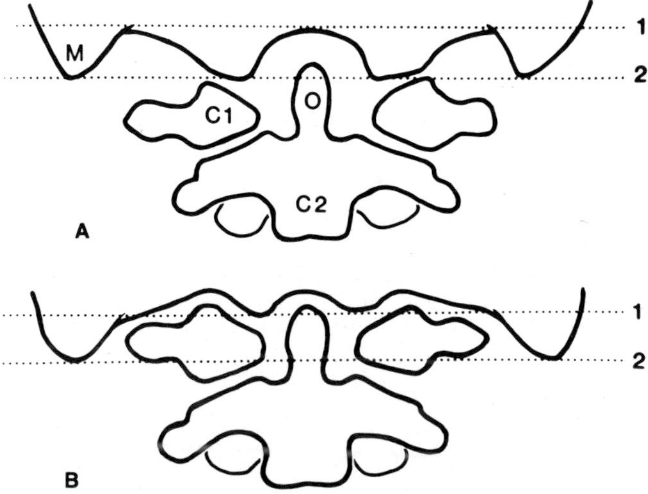

FIG 13–9.
The digastric line. **A,** normal. **B,** basilar invagination.

magnification error, 3.5 mm is suggested as the upper limit of normal.[95]

Further, range-of-motion studies found the greatest motion in the C5–6 segment. As elsewhere, correlating motion with degeneration in the spinal segment has proved inconclusive.[9, 33, 46] Peculiar to the lower part of the cervical spine is that motion decreases with age.[79] With this decrease in motion is found an increase in cervical symptomatology, i.e., neck, arm, upper trunk pain.[94]

In an effort to study displacement patterns in motion segments subjected to different loads, sequential sectioning of the ligaments of the segment was done.[81] This study of z- and x-axis motion resulted in a checklist (Table 13–4). Based on these criteria, a score of greater than or equal to 5 points is equivalent to segmental instability.[81] To define y-axis motion, White and Panjabi developed the stretch test[95] to measure vertical translation. This test is accomplished through cervical halter traction application. Incremental loads up to 33% of body weight or 65 lb are applied. Lateral radiographs are checked prior to addition of the axial load, and neurologic status is monitored throughout the entire study. From a study of eight normal subjects, an abnormal stretch test result is indicated by interspace separation of greater than 1.7 mm.[30] In the acute clinical situation, a carefully monitored stretch test employing displacement in the axial direction is reported to be safer than the potentially hazardous horizontal displacement.[2]

Forces

The second component of mechanical instability is force. Force, usually measured in newtons, is any action that tends to change the state of rest or motion of a body to which it is applied. The different types of singular forces experienced by the spine under physiologic conditions are compression, tension, torsion, and shear. Because of the coupled motions of the spinal segment, these forces are not experienced as a single vector of force. Under physiologic loading, the final force is usually a result of different single forces.

Torsion.—Torsion is a type of force applied by a coupling of forces parallel and directed opposite each other about the long axis.[95] Torsional stresses applied to a spinal segment are resisted mainly by the disc and the facet joints. The other elements of the functional spinal unit (i.e., end plates, vertebral bodies, ligaments) play a role in resistance to torsion, but that role is small: approximately 10% of the overall torque strength of the spinal segment is provided by these structures.[2, 30] Between the facet joints and the disc lies 90% of the torsional strength.[30] The facet joints can be divided by their function under applied torsion (y-axis rotation). The compression-side facet is termed the *working facet.*[30] The tension facet is termed the *working facet ligament*[30] (Fig 13–10). The working facet plays a significant role in resisting torsion under load because this facet is under compression (i.e., the compression facet). Approximately 60% more torsional strength in the functional spinal unit is resisted by the compression facet.[2] An in vitro study of L4–5 after partial, unilateral, and bilateral facetectomy demonstrated increasing instability with torsional load. With progressive removal of the compression facet an increasing degree of torsional rotation was found.[41]

The remaining torsional strength lies in the disc, which has been experimentally shown to resist about 40%

TABLE 13–4.

Checklist for Determining Stability/Instability of the Lower Part of the Cervical Spine*

Element	Point Value†
Anterior elements destroyed or unable to function	2
Posterior elements destroyed or unable to function	2
Relative sagittal-plane translation >3.5 mm	2
Relative sagittal-plane rotation >11 degrees	2
Positive stretch test	2
Medullary (cord) damage	2
Root damage	1
Abnormal disc narrowing	1
Dangerous loading anticipated	1

*From White AA, Southwick, WO, Panjabi MM: *Spine* 1976; 1:6–15. Used by permission.
†A total of 5 or more equals instability.

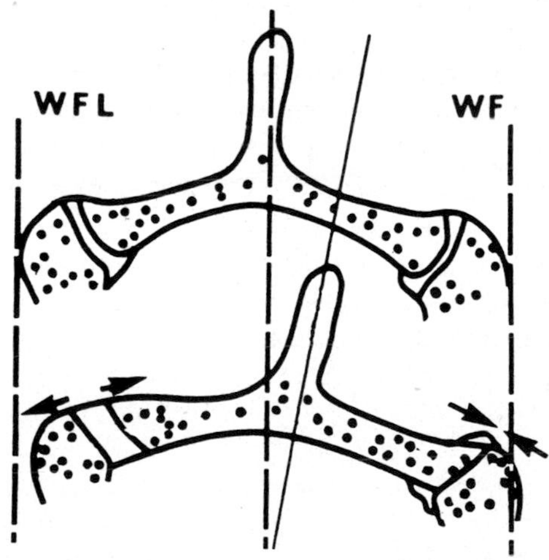

FIG 13–10.
The facet articular processes are forced into rotation. The compression facet or working facet *(WF)* and the tension facet or working facet ligament *(WFL)* are depicted. When the articular processes are forced together by rotation, there is deviation from the normal resting alignment. Sufficient compression and deviation of articular processes from their normal position during rotation can gap the working facet ligament (tension facet). As much as 5 to 10 mm of gapping on the tension facet has been observed prior to failure. (From Farfan H, Cossette J, Robertson G, et al: *J Bone Joint Surg [Am]* 1970; 52:468–497. Used by permission.)

to 50% of the torque of the whole normal functional spinal unit.[19] At the L5 level, torsion is additionally resisted by the iliotransverse ligament. This short ligament connects the transverse process of L5 to the pelvis and provides additional antitorsional strength to the L5–S1 level. Because of this, the most suspectible joint to torsion is the L4–5 one followed by the L5–S1.[29] In fact, L4 has the greatest mobility in the lumbar spine.[4] Physiologic torsion and abnormal torsional motion have been implicated in motion segment degeneration.[29, 30, 41] In vitro, the annular tears of a degenerated disc have been reproduced by torsional loading. Interestingly, these tears occurred in the outer part of the annulus, and disc herniation was not produced with pure torsion alone.[30]

Torsion appears to have its greatest endurance effect on the disc. The facets are also affected by torsion. Increased stresses in the facet are seen secondary to disc degeneration and applied torsion.[2] The angle of facet rotation in the normal lumbar spine is 1.2 degrees, which suggests that only small additional torque is needed to produce injury in a completely rotated lumbar spine.[2, 41] Facet articular cartilage injury of the compression facet would occur with minimal increases beyond full torque. Cartilage injury of the compression facet would occur with minimal increases beyond full torque. With cartilage injury and degeneration come increases in mobility. Indeed, degenerated spinal segments increase in rotational mobility.[2, 30, 41] Increases in rotational mobility would account for the shift from the facets to the disc for torque resistance. This was observed by Farfan et al.[30] in degenerated segments.

Compression.—Compression, measured in newtons, is "the normal forces that tend to push together material fibers."[27] Compressive loads affect the facets, discs, and vertebral end plates. Compression occurs along the y-axis.

The disc is the major compression-bearing component of the spinal segment. With in vitro compression loading, a sequence of events occurs: a radial bulge in the annulus increases in intradiscal pressure, with resultant vertebral end plate deformation. Increasing compression to failure results in end-plate fracture rather than disc failure (herniation).[73]

Compression does play a role in disc failure/herniation, but not as a pure force. Disc herniation has been produced by a combination of forces. In vitro, disc herniation has been produced by compression with rotation[43, 59] and compression with hyperflexion.[1]

End-plate failure depends on the load and the status of the disc. End-plate failure under compression can be of three patterns: central, peripheral, or entire end-plate failure. In central fractures, Schmorl's nodes occur usually when the nucleus is normal. The pressure within the nucleus places the annulus under tension and the central end plate under compression. At failure, a fracture will occur in the central end plate.[73, 77] In a degenerated nucleus, the forces are transmitted directly to the annulus. At failure, fracture occurs along the periphery. In general, with higher than physiologic loads, fracture of the entire end plate occurs.[73, 77]

The role of the facet in compression is position dependent. In the neutral position, the lumbar facets carry about 8% of the compressive loads. With extension, compressive load sharing increases to 30%, and with flexion the load decreases.[77, 82]

Shear.—Shear is a force parallel to the surface on which it acts. Shear is not a pure physiologic load but is usually the combined result of other loads. The facet and the discs play important roles in shear. The facets are estimated to resist approximately one third and the disc two thirds of the shear forces. The load distribution is rate dependent. With rapid loading the distribution is one third for the facet and two thirds for the disc. With slower loading and time, load shearing increases on the facets.[15]

Tension.—Tension is a normal force that tends to elongate the fibers of a material. Tension loads are a ligament function. The posterior column ligament complex allows normal motion, restricts the limits of that motion, and protects the spinal cord at high loads and fast speed (i.e., fractures). These ligaments are implicated in iatrogenic instability and deformity by their absence or failure.

Deformity

The third component of clinical instability is deformity. Spondylolisthesis, scoliosis, and kyphosis, common structural deformities of the spine, can be present with clinical instability. Spondylolisthesis is discussed elsewhere in this volume. This section is devoted to sagittal-plane deformity.

Kyphosis is an increased convexity in the curvature of the spine in the sagittal plane.[85] Through use of the Cobb method, sagittal-plane deformity can be measured[13]; however, this method may not always provide an accurate assessment of the curve for certain pathologic conditions, that is, Cobb's method may not represent an actual arch. It does reflect changes in the end vertebral bodies rather than changes within the curve itself (Fig 13–11).[88] Therefore, for a focal kyphosis (i.e., fractures) Cobb's method is quite valid. For longer curves (Scheuermann's disease), the length and width of the curve must be part of the determination for an accurate assessment. The cervical and lumbar portions of the spine are normally lordotic. A 5-degree or more fixed posterior angulation in these regions is considered a kyphotic deformity.

The spinal segment can be divided into three columns: anterior, middle and posterior.[16, 17] The anterior column consists of the anterolongitudinal ligament, anterior two

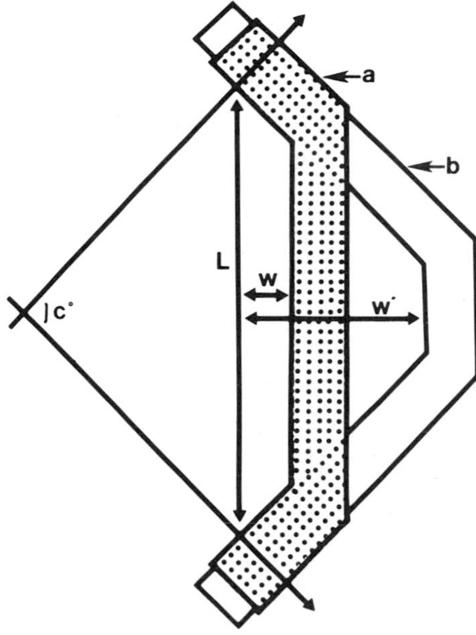

FIG 13–11.
The two spinal curves *(a* and *b)* represented by this schematic drawing are obviously quite different in magnitude. However, if Cobb's method is used to measure the deformities, the degree of curvature (*c* degree) are identical. The difference in the curves are more accurately reflected when the length of the curve *(L)*, and their respective widths (*w* and *w'*) are taken into consideration. (From Voutsinas S, MacEwen G: *Clin Orthop* 1986; 210:235–242. Used by permission.)

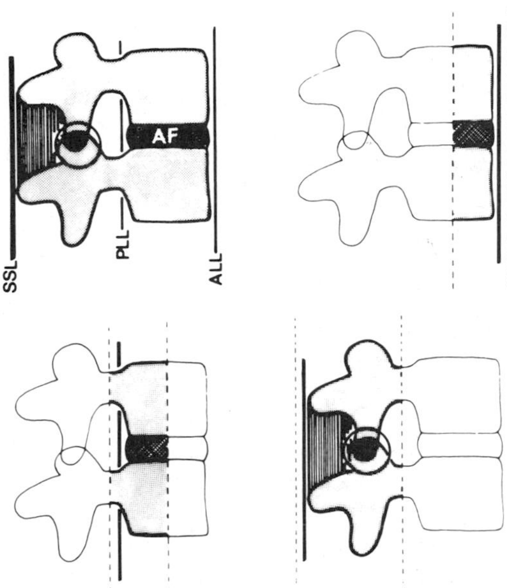

FIG 13–12.
The anterior, middle, and posterior columns are illustrated. (From Denis F: *Spine* 1983; 8:817–831.

thirds of the vertebral body, and anterior two thirds of the intervertebral disc. The middle column consists of the posterior third of the vertebral body, posterior third of the intervertebral disc, and posterolongitudinal ligament. The posterior column is the remaining posterior element of the spine and lies posterior to the posterolongitudinal ligament (Fig 13–12). Kyphosis is initiated or progresses with failure of the anterior and middle columns under compressive loads (i.e., fractures) or failure of the posterior column under tension (Fig 13–13).[98]

Mechanically, the changes in stresses within the column are directly proportional to the bending moment applied. With column failure (fracture), the biomechanical consequence is a change in position of the center of gravity (applied moment or force) with respect to the failed segment. This results in an increase in the flexion bending moment and a greater propensity for kyphotic deformity. White and Panjabi have constructed a mathematical model of this problem for the thoracic spine (Fig 13–14).[95] With this model they found increases in bending moments due to vertebral body wedging. Further, increases were greater for less kyphotic thoracic spines. This model infers a greater risk of developing a kyphotic deformity in a preinjury, relatively straight thoracic spine. However, the authors did not provide clinical documentation of this.

Neurologic Injury

The fourth component of clinical instability concerns neurologic injury. Clinical instability includes initial and/or additional neurologic deficit. This statement demands questioning. First, can medullary or root damage occur without instability? Second, is neurologic deficit evidence of instability?

Neurologic injury can occur without instability. Goseh et al. have shown in animal studies that medullary damage can occur with intact supporting structures.[44] This entity of neurologic deficit and an intact supporting structure occurs in humans. An example is cervical spondylitic myelopathy, which is a case of mechanical stability and progressive neurologic deficit. Here, neurologic injury is a function of canal size: a canal size of 10 mm in the presence of osteophytes is likely to be associated with cord compression.[99]

The developmental sagittal diameter is seen in Figure 13–15. A developmental anteroposterior diameter (DAD) of 10 to 13 mm may be considered premyelographic; 13 to 17 mm, a tendency for symptomatic spondylosis; and greater than 17 mm, less prone to develop spondylitic disease. The spondylitic anteroposterior diameter (SAD) measures the sagittal distance from the posterior osteophyte to the posterior portion of the lamina (Fig 13–15).[95]

As has just been discussed, evidence of neurologic injury is not necessarily associated with instability. However, in general it is felt that for traumatic lesions and tumors, neurologic deficits are associated with mechanical instability. Injuries to the cervical spine are an illustration

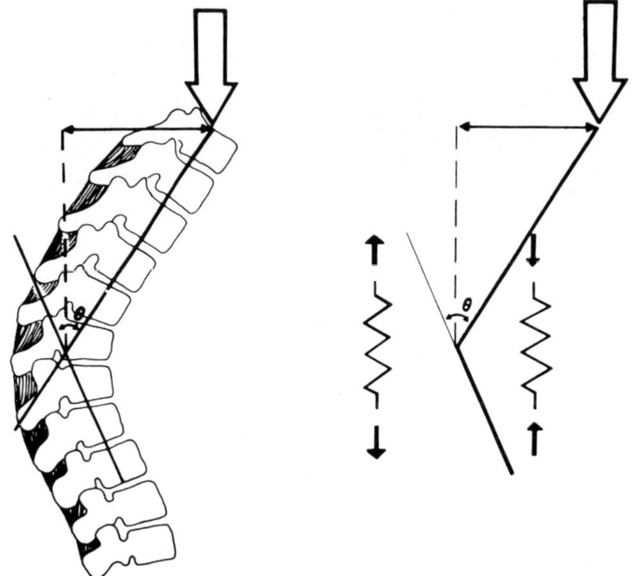

FIG 13–13.
On the *left* there is a kyphotic deformity showing a Cobb angle of 58 degrees. Vertically directed physiologic forces shown by a large *arrow* work at a moment arm at a certain length. On the *right,* the deformity is depicted schematically, showing that the posterior elements resist tensile loading. The anterior elements resist compressive loading. Factors tending to contribute to kyphosis include (1) an increase in physiologic load *(white arrow),* (2) an increase in moment arm, (3) weakening of the posterior elements, and (4) weakening of the anterior elements. (From White A, Panjabi MM: *Clin Orthop* 1977; 128:8–17. Used by permission.)

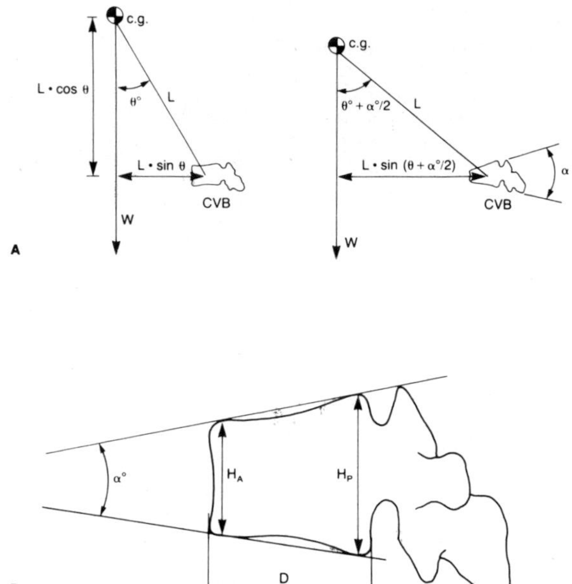

FIG 13–14.
A model to analyze the effect of vertebral wedging on the bending moment in the thoracic spine. **A,** on the *left* is the model before injury, which defines the relationship between the center of gravity *(c.g.)* of the trunk and the center of the vertebral body (CVB). *L* is the distance between the two centers, and θ is the angle formed by the small c.g.-CVB line with the vertical line of gravity. The model after wedging of α° is seen on the right. Note that there is an increased lever arm of the trunk c.g. with respect to the vertebra. **B,** the vertebral wedging may be defined by the wedge angle α° or by the anterior body height ratio. The relationship between the two parameters is depicted. (From White A, Panjabi MM: *Clinical Biomechanics of the Spine*. Philadelphia, JB Lippincott, 1990, p 157. Used by permission.)

of the issue of neurologic deficit and instability. There is no direct correlation between the amount of displacement and neurologic injury[7, 8]; however, a more significant correlation between neurologic deficit and high-energy injuries was found. Overall, fractures of cervical vertebral bodies are associated with a 3% incidence of neurologic deficit. In this group is a subgrouping of patients with vertebral body fractures plus posterior element damage; there is a 61% incidence of associated neurologic deficit.[37]

The authors believe that for an injury to result in neurologic deficit, the stability of the spine must have been compromised. Clinical instability is assumed to exist; thus an instability must be documented or ruled out.

LUMBAR INSTABILITY

A classification scheme of lumbar instability has been proposed by Frymoyer and Selby.[38] This classification is based on six different types of pathologic conditions, which are listed in Table 13–5.

Degenerative instabilities have been subclassified into primary and secondary instabilities[76] (Table 13–6). Axial rotational instability most commonly affects the L4–5 level. It is difficult to say whether axial rotational instability is a separate entity from translational instability, that is, in and of itself axial rotational instability may not represent a pure subset of instabilities; however, it does occur commonly with degenerative spondylolisthesis. With this instability, radiographic evidence of rotation includes malalignment of the spinous processes on anteroposterior radiographs and rotational deformity of the pedicles. Identifying the rotational component of the instability has implications in stabilization because if a rotational component can be identified, derotation alone may decompress the nerve root. Farfan has proposed rotation facet fusion. In older patients, it is recommended that it be supplemented with transverse process fusion.[28]

Translational instability caused by degenerative spondylolisthesis is common. Anterior translation of a vertebral body of greater than 3 mm is felt to be diagnostic of this problem. Other radiographic signs include narrowing of the disc space and traction spurs. At particular risk are females and diabetics.[78] Stabilization through transverse process fusion has been recommended for neurologically intact patients.[32, 42] In patients who are neurologically involved, decompression and fusion as opposed to decompression alone have yielded improved results.[32]

Retrolisthesis instability most frequently occurs at the

TABLE 13–5.
The Lumbar Spine Segmental Instabilities*

I. Fractures and fracture-dislocations
II. Infections involving anterior columns with:
  A. Progressive loss of vertebral body height and deformity despite antibiotic treatment
  B. Progressing neurologic symptoms despite appropriate antibiotic treatment if accompanied by criterion IIA
III. Primary and metastic neoplasms with:
  A. Progressive loss of vertebral body height and deformity
  B. Progressing neurologic symptoms if symptoms are not the result of direct tumor involvement of the spinal cord, cauda equina, or nerve roots but result from the conditions of IIIA
  C. Postsurgical—following resection of neoplasms
IV. Spondylolisthesis
  A. Isthmic spondylolisthesis
    1. L5–S1 progressive deformity in a child, particularly when accompanied by the radiographic risk signs of Wiltse. Rarely an unstable lesion in the adult
    2. L4–5 probably an unstable lesion in the adult
V. Degenerative
VI. Scoliosis—any progressive deformity in a child further subclassified per the Scoliosis Research Society

*From Frymoyer J, Pope M, Wilder D (eds): *The Adult Spine*. New York, Raven Press, 1990. Used by permission.

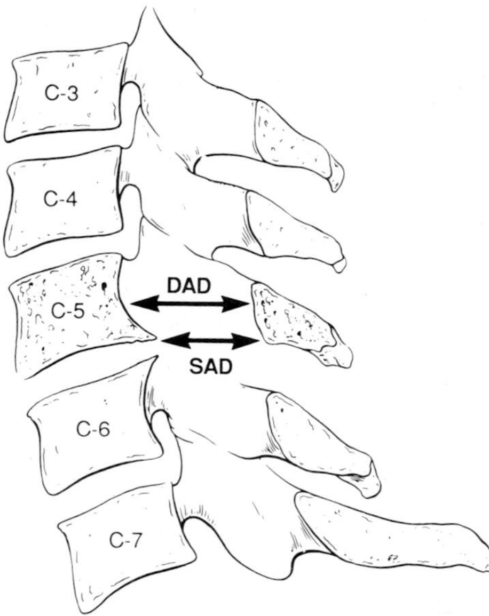

FIG 13–15.
The developmental anteroposterior diameter *(DAD)* and the spondylitic anteroposterior diameter *(SAD)*. (From White A, Panjabi MM: *Clinical Biomechanics of the Spine*. Philadelphia, JB Lippincott, 1990, p 288. Used by permission.)

L5–S1 level and is frequently associated with symptoms of the root below the involved level. Fusion in flexion by using distraction fixation has been advocated.[80] Decompression has been recommended when the retrolisthesis is associated with nerve entrapment and stenosis.

The fourth type, degenerative scoliotic deformities, may involve single or multiple levels. Nerve root entrapment may occur on the concave side of the curve. Nerve root involvement in the late stages of this deformity may involve multiple levels. Selective nerve root infiltration with lidocaine is helpful in deciding which levels to decompress. Decompression and fusion of the appropriate levels are the recommended treatment.

TABLE 13–6.
The Lumbar Spine—Degenerative Segmental Instabilities*

Primary instabilities
  Axial rotational instability
  Translational instability
  Retrolisthetic instability
  Progressing degenerative scoliosis
  Disc disruption syndrome
Secondary instabilities
  Post–disc excision—subclassified according to the pattern of instability as described under primary instabilities
  Post–decompressive laminectomy
    Accentuation of pre-existent deformity
    New deformity, i.e., no deformity existed at the time of the original decompression. Further subclassified as for primary instabilities
  Post–spinal fusion
    Above or below a spinal fusion, subclassified as for primary instabilities
    Pseudarthrosis

*From Frymoyer J, Pope M, Wilder D (eds): *The Adult Spine*. New York, Raven Press, 1990. Used by permission.

Type 5 internal disc disruption is a contained, nonprolapsing disc disease diagnosed by discography. Anterior interbody fusion is the current recommended surgical treatment. It has been questioned whether a disrupted disc causing this syndrome is an instability.[38]

Secondary instability follows disc excision, decompression laminectomy, and/or spinal fusion. These are iatrogenic instabilities. Instability following disc excision is estimated to occur in approximately 20% of patients.[38] It may take the form of a primary instability such as axial rotation, translation, or even retrolisthesis. The diagnosis is made by flexion/extension films in the late postoperative period. Most commonly this will occur at the L4–5 level. Instability following decompressive laminectomy is commonly associated with degenerative spondylolisthesis. The most common problem is increasing deformity after decompression. This increasing deformity is commonly related to the preoperative extent of the deformity, the patient's age, whether or not the disc has been excised, and the amount of facetectomy.

Since its introduction, spinal arthrodesis has been one of the most important and commonly employed operations of the spine[3, 49] and has been recommended in the treatment of spinal instability. In addition to the therapeutic benefits of spinal fusion, long-term liabilities have been documented. These late sequelae include excessive motion,[72] spinal stenosis,[10, 27] and degenerative changes.[11, 53] These changes have been observed in adjacent levels above and below spinal fusions and are related to stress concentrations at the interface of fused and unfused mobile segments of the spine. Frymoyer et al.[38, 39] estimated the incidence of instability following spinal fusion to be 20%.[38] Based on a follow-up of 10 years or more, Lehmann et al. found that 45% of patients had a positive Knutsson sign and 4% required fusion for progressive pain and deformity at the L3–4 level.[58] Surgical treatment of instability following spinal fusion can be accomplished by either anterior interbody or posterior intertransverse process fusion. Prior to extending a spinal fusion to an adjacent segment, clear documentation of post–spinal fusion instability must be made. Finally, because there are biomechanical and clinical data to support increases in shear stresses of adjacent mobile segments, the authors suggest fusing them to normal segments. These increased stresses on an adjacent degenerated segment would only serve to accelerate the cascade of degeneration within that segment.

Common operations of the spine including discectomy, laminectomy, and spinal fusion have been efficacious in the treatment of spinal disorders. They are commonly employed and in general are considered commonplace in the armamentarium of spinal surgeons. It is the commonplace nature of these operations that detracts from their long-term disabilities. Secondary iatrogenic instabilities such as instability following disc fusion, decompression laminectomy, and spinal fusion, including pseudarthrosis, are late sequelae of these commonplace operations. Clear documentation and understanding of the instability in the spinal motion segment allow the spinal surgeon to institute these surgical measures with the least amount of long-term morbidity.

SUMMARY

Instability is a spectrum. Clinical instability is the loss of the ability of the spine under physiologic loads to maintain its pattern of displacement so that there is no initial or additional neurologic deficit, major deformity, or incapacitating pain. Clinical instability takes into account the anatomic and biomechanical factors and draws them into a clinical setting. It is the entity of clinical instability that when documented requires treatment. It has been the purpose of this chapter to provide guidelines for the diagnosis of this problem.

REFERENCES

1. Adams M, Hutton W: Intervertebral disc—A hyperflexion injury. *Spine* 1982; 7:184–191.
2. Adams M, Hutton W: The relevance of torsion to the mechanical derangement of the lumbar spine. *Spine* 1981; 6:241–248.
3. Albee F: Transplantation of a portion of the tibia into the spine for Pott's disease: A preliminary report. *JAMA* 1911; 57:885.
4. Allbrook D: Movements of the lumbar spine column. *J Bone Joint Surg [Br]* 1957; 39:339.
5. American Academy of Orthopaedic Surgeons: *A glossary of Spinal Terminology*. Chicago, American Academy of Orthopaedic Surgeons, 1985.
6. Aprill C, Dwyer A, Bogduk N: Cervical zygapophyseal joint pain patterns II. A clinical evaluation. *Spine* 1990; 4:441–446.
7. Barnes R: Paraplegia in cervical spine injuries. *J Bone Joint Surg [Br]* 1948; 30:234.
8. Betson T: Fractures and dislocations of the cervical spine. *J Bone Joint Surg [Br]* 1963; 45:21.
9. Blanchard R, Kottke F: The study on degenerative changes of the cervical spine in relation to age. *Bull Univ Minn Hosp* 1953; 24:470.
10. Brodsky A: Post-laminectomy post-fusion stenosis of the lumbar spine. *Clin Orthop* 1976; 115:130–139.
11. Capen D, Garland D, Waters R: Surgical stabilization of the cervical spine. A comparative analysis of anterior and posterior spine fusions. *Clin Orthop* 1985; 196:229.
12. Chamberlain W: Basilar impression (platybasia): A bizarre development anomaly of the occipital bone and upper cervical spine with striking and misleading neurologic manifestations. *Yale J Biol Med* 1939; 11:487–496.
13. Cobb R: Outline for the study of scoliosis. *Instr Course Lect* 1948; 5:261.
14. Cope Z: *The Early Diagnosis of the Acute Abdomen,* ed 14. Oxford, England, Oxford Medical Publications, 1972, pp 48–78.
15. Cyron BM, Hutton WC: Articular tropism and the stability of the lumbar spine. *Spine* 1980; 5:168–172.
16. Denis F: Spinal instability as defined by the three column spine concept in acute spinal trauma. *Clin Orthop* 1984; 189:65–76.
17. Denis F: The three column spine and its significance in the classification of acute thoracolumbar spinal injuries. *Spine* 1986; 8:817–831.
18. Dimnet J, Fischer L, Carret J: Radiographic studies of later flexion in the lumbar spine. *J Biomech* 1978; 11:143–150.
19. Dolan K: Cervical basilar relationship. *Radiol Clin North Am* 1977; 15:155–166.
20. Dooley J, McBroom R, Taguchi T, et al: Nerve root infiltration in the diagnosis of radicular pain. *Spine* 1988; 13:79–83.
21. Dunsker S, Colley D, Mayfield F: Kinematics of the cervical spine. *Clin Neurosurg* 1977; 25:174.
22. Dupuis P, Yong-Hing K, Cassidy J, et al: Radiologic diagnosis and degenerative lumbar spinal instability. *Spine* 1985; 10:262–276.
23. Dvorak J, Hayek J, Zehnder R: CT—Functional diagnosis of the rotatory instability of upper cervical spine. *Spine* 1987; 12:726–731.
24. Dvorak J, Panjabi M: Functional anatomy of the alar ligaments. *Spine* 1987; 12:183–189.
25. Dvorak J, Panjabi M, Gerber M, et al: CT—Functional

diagnosis of the rotatory instability of upper cervical spine I. Experimental studies on cadavers. *Spine* 1987; 12:197–205.

26. Dwyer A, Aprill C, Bogduk N: Cervical zygapophyseal joint pain patterns I. A study in normal volunteers. *Spine* 1979; 15:453–457.
27. Eismont F, Simeone F: Bony overgrowth as a cause of late paraparesis after scoliosis fusion. *J Bone Joint Surg [Am]* 1981; 63:1016.
28. Farfan H: A re-orientation in the surgical approach to degenerative lumbar intervertebral joint disease. *Orthop Clin North Am* 1977; 8:9–21.
29. Farfan H: *Mechanical Disorders of the Low Back*. Philadelphia, Lea & Febiger, 1973, pp 61–93.
30. Farfan H, Cossette J, Robertson G, et al: The effects of torsion in the lumbar intervertebral joints: The role of torsion in production of disc degeneration. *J Bone Joint Surg [Am]* 1970; 52:468–497.
31. Farfan H, Gracovetsky S: The nature of instability. *Spine* 1984; 9:714.
32. Fidler M, Plasmans C: The effect of four types of support on segmental mobility of the lumbosacral spine. *J Bone Joint Surg [Am]* 1983; 65:943–947.
33. Fielding J: Normal and selected abnormal motion of the cervical spine from the second cervical vertebrae based on cineroentgenography. *J Bone Joint Surg [Am]* 1964; 46:1779.
34. Freiberg O: Lumbar instability: A dynamic approach by traction, compression and radiography. *Spine* 1987; 12:119–129.
35. Frymoyer J: The role of spine fusion. *Spine* 1981; 6:289.
36. Frymoyer J, Newberg A, Pope N, et al: Spine radiographs in patients with low back pain: An epidemiologic study in men. *J Bone Joint Surg [Am]* 1984; 66:1045–1055.
37. Frymoyer J, Pope M, Wilder D: Segmental instability, in *Lumbar Spine*. Philadelphia, WB Saunders, 1990, pp 612–636.
38. Frymoyer J, Selby D: Segmental instability: Rationale for treatment. *Spine* 1985; 10:280–286.
39. Frymoyer JW, Hanley EN, Howe J, et al: A comparison of radiographic findings in fusion and non-fusion patients ten or more years following lumbar disc surgery. *Spine* 1979; 4:435–440.
40. Gertzbein S, Seligman J, Holtby R, et al: Centrode patterns and segmental instability in degenerative disc disease. *Spine* 1985; 10:257–261.
41. Goel V, Goyal S, Clark C, et al: Kinematics of the whole lumbar spine—the effect of discectomy. *Spine* 1985; 10:543–554.
42. Goldner J: The role of spine fusion: Question 6. *Spine* 1981; 6:293.
43. Gordon S, Yang K, Mayer P, et al: Mechanism of disc rupture: A preliminary report. *Spine* 1991; 16:450–456.
44. Goseh H, Gooding E, Schneider R: An experimental study in cervical spine and cord injuries. *J Trauma* 1972; 12:570–575.
45. Gregerson G, Lucas D: An in vitro study of the axial rotation of the human thoracolumbar spine. *J Bone Joint Surg [Am]* 1967; 49:247–262.
46. Hadley H: Anatomic radiographic studies: Development in the cervical region, in *The Spine*. Springfield, Ill, Charles C Thomas, 1956.
47. Hagelstem L: Retroposition of lumbar vertebrae. *Acta Chir Scand Suppl* 1949; 143:31–49.
48. Helbig T, Lee C: The lumbar facet syndrome. *Spine* 1988; 13:61–64.
49. Hibbs R: An operation for progressive spinal deformity. A preliminary report of three cases from the service of the Orthopedic Hospital. *N Y State Med J* 1911; 93:1013.
50. Hinck V, Hopkins C, Savara B: Diagnostic criteria of basilar investigation. *Radiology* 1961; 76:572–585.
51. Hohl M, Baker H: The atlanto-axial joint. *J Bone Joint Surg [Am]* 1964; 46:1739.
52. Howorth B: Low back ache and sciatica: Results of surgical treatment. *J Bone Joint Surg [Am]* 1964; 46:1485–1499.
53. Hunter L, Braunstein E, Bailey R: Radiographic changes following anterior cervical spine fusion. *Spine* 1980; 5:399.
54. Kelgren J: Distribution of pain arising from deep somatic structures with charts of segmental pain areas. *Clin Sci* 1939; 4:35–46.
55. Kelgren J: Observations on referred pain arising from muscle. *Clin Sci* 1938; 3:175–190.
56. Kirkaldy-Willis W: *Managing Low Back Pain,* ed 2. New York, Churchill Livingstone, 1988, pp 24–36.
57. Knutsson F: The instability associated with disc degeneration in the lumbar spine. *Acta Radiol* 1944; 25:593–609.
58. Lehmann TR, Spratt KF, Tozzi JE, et al: Long term follow-up of lower lumbar fusion patients. *Spine* 1987; 12:97–104.
59. Liu Y, Goel V, Dejong, et al: Torsional fatigue of the lumbar intervertebral joints. *Spine* 1985; 10:894–900.
60. Lucas D, Bresler B: *Stability of the Ligamentous Spine*. San Francisco, Biomechanics Laboratory, University of California, 1961, Report 40.
61. Lysell E: Motion in the cervical spine. *Acta Orthop Scand Suppl* 1969; 123:1.
62. MacNab I: *Backache*. Baltimore, Williams & Wilkins, 1977.
63. MacNab I: Negative disc exploration. *J Bone Joint Surg [Am]* 1971; 53:891–903.
64. MacNab I: The traction spur, an indicator of segmental instability. *J Bone Joint Surg [Am]* 1971; 53:663–670.
65. McCall I, Park W, O'Brien J: Induced pain referral from posterior lumbar elements in normal subjects. *Spine* 1979; 4:441–446.
66. McGregor M: The significance of certain measurements of the skull and the diagnosis of basilar impression. *Br J Radiol* 1948; 21:171–181.
67. MacRae D, Barnum A: Occipitalization of the atlas. *Am J Radiol* 1953; 70:23–46.
68. Merskey H: Pain terms: A list with definitions and notes on usage. Recommended by IASP subcommittee on taxonomy. *Pain* 1979; 6:2549–252.
69. Mixter WJ, Barr JS: Rupture of the intervertebral disc with involvement of the spinal canal. *N Engl J Med* 1934; 211:210–215.

70. Murphy R: Nerve roots and spinal nerves in degenerative disc disease. *Clin Orthop* 1977; 129:46–60.
71. Paris S: Physical signs of instability. *Spine* 1985; 10:277–279.
72. Pearcy N, Burroughs S: Assessment of bony union after interbody fusion in the lumbar spine using a biplanar radiograph technique. *J Bone Joint Surg [Br]* 1982; 64:228.
73. Perey O: Fracture of the vertebral endplate in the lumbar spine—an experimental investigation. *Acta Orthop Scand Suppl* 1957; 25.
74. Pope M, Panjabi M: Biomechanical definition of spinal instability. *Spine* 1985; 10:255–256.
75. Posner I, White AA III, Edwards WT, et al: A biomechanical analysis of the clinical stability of the lumbar and lumbosacral spine. *Spine* 1982; 7:374–389.
76. Riggins R, Kraus J: The risk of neurologic damage with fractures of the vertebrae. *J Trauma* 1977; 17:126.
77. Rollander S, Blair W: Deformation and fracture of the lumbar vertebral end-plate. *Orthop Clin North Am* 1975; 6:75.
78. Rosenberg N: Degenerative spondylolisthesis: Predisposing factors. *J Bone Joint Surg [Am]* 1975; 57:467.
79. Schoening H, Hannan V: Factors related to cervical spine mobility, Part I. *Arch Phys Med Rehabil* 1964; 45:602.
80. Selby D: Internal fixation with Knodt's rods. *Clin Orthop* 1986; 203:179–184.
81. Sher A: Anterior cervical subluxation: An unstable position. *AJR* 1979; 131:275.
82. Shirazi-Adl S, Shrivastava S, Ahmed A: Stress analysis of the lumbar disc body unit in compression: A three dimensional non-linear finite element study. *Spine* 1984; 9:120.
83. Simmons E, Segil C: An evaluation of discography in the localization of symptomatic levels of discogenic disease of the spine. *Clin Orthop* 1975; 108:57–69.
84. Smyth M, Wright T: Sciatica and the intervertebral disc. *J Bone Joint Surg [Am]* 1959; 40:1401–1418.
85. *Stedman's Medical Dictionary,* ed 22. Baltimore, Williams & Wilkins, 1972, p 674.
86. Stokes I, Wilder D, Frymoyer J, et al: Assessment of patients with low back pain by biplanar radiograph measures of intervertebral motion. *Spine* 1981; 6:233–240.
87. Triano J, Luttges M: Nerve irritation: A possible model for sciatic neuritis. *Spine* 1982; 7:129–136.
88. Voutsinas S, MacEuen G: Sagittal profiles of the spine. *Clin Orthop* 1986; 210:235–242.
89. Walsh T, Weinstein J, Spratt K, et al: Lumbar discography in normal subjects. *J Bone Joint Surg [Am]* 1990; 72:1081–1088.
90. Watkins R, Collis J: *Lumbar Discectomy and Laminectomy.* Rockville, Md, Aspen Systems, 1987, pp 15–26.
91. Weinstein J: *Future Directions in Low Back Pain Research.* NIH/AAOS Workshop, AAOS Publishers, 1989.
92. Weinstein J, Claverie W, Gibson S: The pain of discography. *Spine* 1988; 13:1344–1348.
93. Werne S: Studies in spontaneous atlas dislocation. *Acta Orthop Scand Suppl* 1957; 23:1.
94. White A, John R, Panjabi M, et al: Biomechanical analysis of clinical stability in the cervical spine. *Clin Orthop* 1975; 109:85.
95. White A, Panjabi M: *Clinical Biomechanics of the Spine,* ed 2. Philadelphia, JB Lippincott, 1990, pp 85–126.
96. White A, Panjabi M: *Clinical Biomechanics of the Spine,* ed 2. Philadelphia, JB Lippincott, 1990, pp 227–373.
97. White A, Panjabi M: The bone kinematics of the human spine. *Spine* 1978; 3:12.
98. White A, Panjabi M, Thomas C: The clinical biomechanics of kyphotic deformities. *Clin Orthop* 1977; 128:8–17.
99. Wolf V, Khilani N, Malis L: The sagittal diameter of the bony cervical spinal canal and its significance in cervical spondylosis. *Mt Sinai Hosp* 1956; 23:283.
100. Yang K, King A: Mechanism of facet load transmission as a hypothesis of low back pain. *Spine* 1984; 9:557–565.

14

Cervical Spine Implants

Chet Sutterlin, M.D., and James Maxey, M.D.

The spine surgeon is currently exposed to an expanding array of devices designed for fixation and stabilization of the cervical spine. These implants vary in their ability to counteract the deforming forces to which the spine is exposed. In order to determine the potential clinical usefulness of each implant several logical steps are necessary. First, the goals for use of the device must be outlined as clearly as possible. Generally, these are to obtain reduction, restore alignment, provide stability, and promote arthrodesis, depending on the particular pathologic process that has compromised spinal function. Of course, a primary concern is to preserve neurologic function, and it is assumed that if a cervical device is chosen for use, its particular risk to neural, vascular, and other nearby structures is appreciated. Second, a scheme for characterization and classification of spinal instability assists in the organization of thought processes so that the proper implant may be chosen to realize the goals outlined above. Third, the choice of a particular device for obtaining cervical spinal stability should result from knowledge of the characteristics of an array of implants that can accomplish the aforementioned goals. A number of devices may be appropriate for use in fixation of a particular instability pattern. Biomechanical testing can elucidate which device or devices are best for that application.[2, 31, 39, 41] Studies have been performed in vitro on mammalian, human cadaveric, and plastic spine models.[17] In addition, some studies have been designed for in vivo evaluation of the effects of various methods of spinal fixation on the biomechanics of the resultant spinal fusion.[45] Fourth, the surgeon should be familiar with reports on use of the device in human subjects. Clinical trials provide information on the utility of an implant's use in humans to realize the goals outlined previously.[7, 9, 44] These clinical trials are also necessary to reveal the nature and frequency of complications that may result from use of the device.

Our purpose in writing this chapter is to review the biomechanical data that are currently available for various methods of fixation of the cervical spine. An attempt is made to discuss cervical stabilization as it relates to the etiology of instability by pathologic processes. However, the majority of biomechanical data have been collected by simulating acute traumatic instabilities of the cervical spine. It may be appropriate at times to apply the results of such tests to other clinical situations, such as instability produced by neoplasm, infection, or degenerative, rheumatologic, or postsurgical iatrogenic disorders. Where specific biomechanical testing of instability created by such situations is modeled, it will be presented. In addition, an attempt is made to present data on testing of specific regions of the cervical spine that possess unique anatomy, kinematics, and mechanical characteristics. Those regions are the occipitocervical junction, the atlantoaxial complex, the middle and lower portions of the cervical spine (C2–7), and the cervicothoracic junction. Our review indicates the majority of testing has been done on the middle and lower parts of the cervical spine.

TRAUMA

Classifications of Injury

Investigations into the determinants of spinal stability and instability have led to a more precise understanding of this concept. A grasp of the material is necessary to provide insight into the mechanical nature of the cervical spine as well as of cervical spine implants. White et al. performed in vitro flexion and extension tests in eight human cadaveric lower cervical spines (C2–7) with sequential sectioning of ligaments and facet joints to better define instability.[40] They concluded that instability existed if (1) all anterior and posterior ligaments were disrupted, (2) 3.5-mm displacement existed on lateral radiograph, or (3) 11 degrees of angular difference existed between motion segments. From these findings they later proposed a systematic approach for evaluating and treating lower cervical spine injuries.[41, 42] In addition, criteria were also established for instabilities of the occipitoatlantoaxial complex (Occ–C2).[41] Because it is recommended that the spinal surgeon consider these points when evaluating patients with cervical injury, the criteria for occipitocervical instability (Table 14–1) and the checklist for the diagnosis of middle and lower cervical instability (Table 14–2) developed by White and Panjabi are presented. For a more de-

TABLE 14–1.
Criteria for C0–2 Instability*

>8-degree axial rotation of C0–1 to one side
>1-mm C–C1 translation
>7-mm overhang of C1–2 (total right and left)
>45-degree axial rotation of C1–2 to one side
>4-mm C1–2 translation
<13 mm from the posterior body of C2 to the posterior ring of C1
Avulsed transverse ligament

*From White AA, Panjabi MM: *Clinical Biomechanics of the Spine*, ed 2. Philadelphia, JB Lippincott, 1990, p 285. Used by permission.

tailed description the reader is referred to the most recent edition of White and Panjabi's text.[41]

One of the largest clinical series for evaluating cervical instability is that of Bohlman.[6] He reviewed clinical and pathologic data on 300 patients and identified four distinct groups: (1) atlanto-occipital (Occ–C1), (2) atlantoaxial (C1–2), (3) lower cervical injuries (C3–7), and (4) injury in patients with ankylosing spondylitis. Three types of displacement were outlined: (1) minimal posterior subluxation (2 to 3 mm), (2) moderate anterior subluxation (3 to 5 mm), and (3) anterior dislocation (one-half vertebral body). In general, posterior cervical fusion was recommended for dislocations and corpectomy with anterior fusion for compressive fractures.

TABLE 14–2.
Checklist for the Diagnosis of Clinical Instability in the Middle and Lower Portions of the Cervical Spine*

Element	Point Value†
Anterior elements destroyed or unable to function	2
Posterior elements destroyed or unable to function	2
Positive stretch test	2
Radiographic criteria	4
Flexion/extension radiographs	
Sagittal-plane translation >3.5 mm or 20% (2 points)	
Sagittal-plane rotation >20 degrees (2 points)	
or	
Resting radiographs	
Sagittal-plane displacement >3.5 mm or 20% (2 points)	
Relative sagittal-plane angulation >11 degrees (2 points)	
Abnormal disc narrowing	1
Developmentally narrow spinal canal	1
Sagittal diameter <13 mm	
or	
Pavlov's ratio <0.8	
Spinal cord damage	2
Nerve root damage	1
Dangerous loading anticipated	1

*From White AA, Panjabi MM: *Clinical Biomechanics of the Spine*, ed 2. Philadelphia, JB Lippincott, 1990, p 314. Used by permission.
†A total of 5 or more equals instability.

Allen et al.[1] reviewed 165 patients with closed indirect injuries to the lower part of the cervical spine and developed their mechanistic classification wherein each group contained a spectrum of anatomic damage from least to most severe. Each group was thus a phylogeny, and those identified were distractive flexion, compressive extension, compressive flexion, vertical compression, distractive extension, and lateral flexion mechanisms with rotation providing a supplemental or lateralizing force. Neurologic injury was shown to be a function of the type and severity of spinal column injury. The authors find this mechanistic system most useful when choosing a cervical spine implant for reconstitution of stability, maintenance of alignment, and thus, promotion of fusion and protection of neurologic function.

Biomechanics

With regard to injuries to the cervical spine, the optimal situation would be to have a system for classification of cervical traumatic pathology by readily obtainable radiologic studies that would lead to an understanding of the existing anatomic as well as biomechanical deficiency. A rational treatment plan would follow. Those injuries that would heal reliably by nonoperative means would be treated so. Those that needed surgical stabilization would require not only an understanding of the mechanics of the injury but also an understanding of the mechanical characteristics of the various fixation methods available. Therefore, for each stage of severity for each specific mechanism of injury, a rational choice of one or more methods of stabilization would be evident with results that should be highly predictable with regard to maintenance of reduction and attainment of fusion. Such a situation does not exist at the time of this writing.

However, significant contributions have been made. Allen et al. reported on a mechanistic classification of closed, indirect fractures and dislocations of the lower portion of the cervical spine in 1982.[1] This work serves as an adequate starting point to achieve the aforementioned idealistic situation, and some biomechanical studies have been designed by modeling the specific injuries described in the classification of Allen et al.[12, 36, 38]

Lower (and Middle) Cervical Spine Injuries

Ulrich et al.[38] utilized ten human cervical spines for testing. They isolated the C5–6 functional unit devoid of muscular tissue and applied a flexion-distraction–type load to the specimen. The tilt angle and displacement were measured via transducer, a dorsal ligamentous injury was created, and then the C5–6 unit was repaired by various methods and the measurements repeated after each step. Comparative data were thus available for angular and translational motion. Five methods of stabilization were employed: (1) anterior H-plate, (2) posterior Arbeitsgemeinschaft für Osteosynthesefragen (AO) hook plate, (3) posterior interspinous wiring, (4) combined H-plate and AO hook plate, and (5) combined H-plate and interspinous wiring. The stabilization methods were again tested after complete discoligamentous disruption (simulating a distractive flexion stage 4 lesion according to the classification of Allen and associates). Their results indicated that

> complete discoligamentous severance of the specimen with exclusive anterior H-plate fusion produced the lowest degree of stability (Fig 14–1). The instability produced by posterior ligamentous severance (alone) can obviously be compensated to some extent by anterior fixation, but the posterior methods of fixation produce a higher degree of primary stability (Fig 14–2).

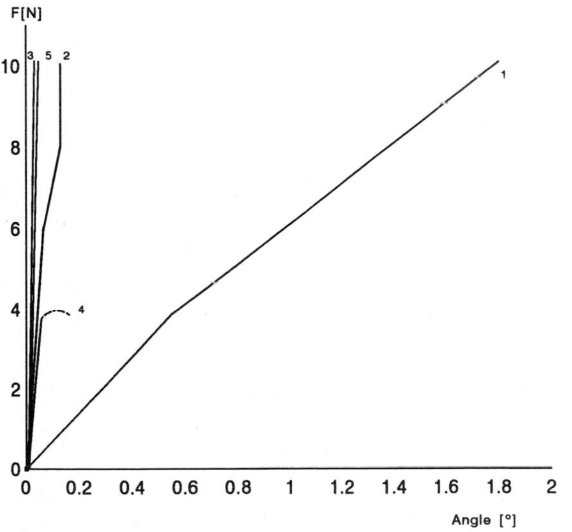

FIG 14–1.
Load displacement curve for *complete discoligamentous instability*. *1,* anterior H-plate; *2,* posterior hook plate; *3,* combined anterior H-plate/posterior hook plate; *4,* posterior sublaminar wiring; *5,* combined anterior H-plate/posterior sublaminar wiring. (From Ulrich C, Worsdorfer O, Claes L et al: *Arch Orthop Trauma Surg* 1978, 106:226–231. Used by permission.)

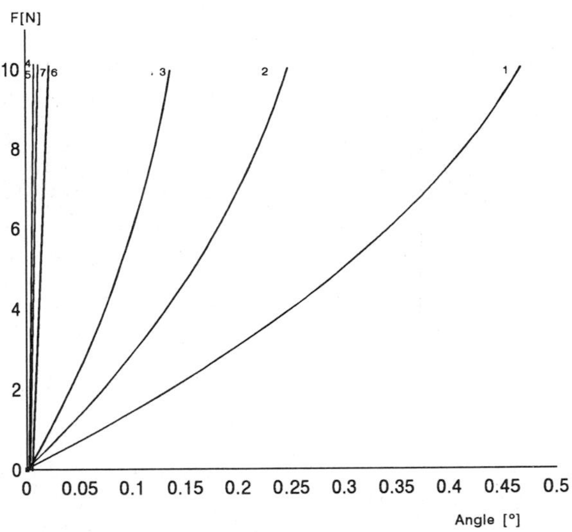

FIG 14–2.
Load-displacement curve for exclusive *posterior ligamentous severance*. *1,* posterior instability; *2,* intact motion segment; *3,* anterior H-plate; *4,* posterior hook plate; *5,* combined posterior hook plate/anterior H-plate; *6,* combined posterior sublaminar wiring/anterior H-plate; *7,* posterior sublaminar wiring. (From Ulrich C, Worsdorfer O, Claes L et al: *Arch Orthop Trauma Surg* 1978, 106:226–231. Used by permission.)

Sutterlin et al.[36] wished to investigate a *specific* lesion. We chose the most common phylogeny in the series of Allen et al., the distractive flexion lesion, and reproduced a stage 3 (DSF3) injury, or bilateral facet dislocation. We stabilized the bovine model of C4–5 discoligamentous injury by five individual methods *without* combined procedures. The fixation techniques chosen dorsally were (1) Rogers' wiring (Fig 14–3), (2) sublaminar wiring (Fig 14–3), (3) Bohlman's triple-wire technique (Fig 14–4), (4) an AO hook plate (Fig 14–5), and (5) a Caspar plate anteriorly (Fig 14–6). An M.T.S. 858 hydraulic materials testing device was used to apply a compressive, torsional, and flexural load to the intact and surgically stabilized specimen while data were collected to evaluate stiffness as well as simultaneous anterior and posterior strain in both a single and a multiple functional spinal unit (FSU) model. Static and cyclical tests were performed. Our findings agreed with but expanded on those of Ulrich et al.[38] All posterior wiring techniques restored stability in the DFS3 injury to that of the intact spine or better by reducing both ventral and dorsal strain with flexural loading (Fig 14–7). Of the four posterior techniques, the AO hook plate was the most effective at reducing anterior and posterior strain. The anterior Caspar plate was quite effective at reducing anterior strain but was *grossly inadequate* at preventing posterior strain in this type of injury when faced with a flexural load.

The same protocol was repeated in a human cadaveric model and the same pathologic lesion (DFS3) created.[12] In addition, the posterior Roy-Camille plate and combined procedures were investigated. The results verified conclusions from the previous experiment and confirmed the validity of utilizing the bovine spine for modeling the human situation (at least for this specific injury and these stabilization methods). In addition, Dr. Coe concluded that the combined anterior and posterior plating techniques "should be limited to injuries with significant anterior instability."

Other studies are either more clinically oriented* or, when biomechanical in nature, have a less well defined in-

*References 5, 8, 10, 13, 18, 29, 30, 35, 37.

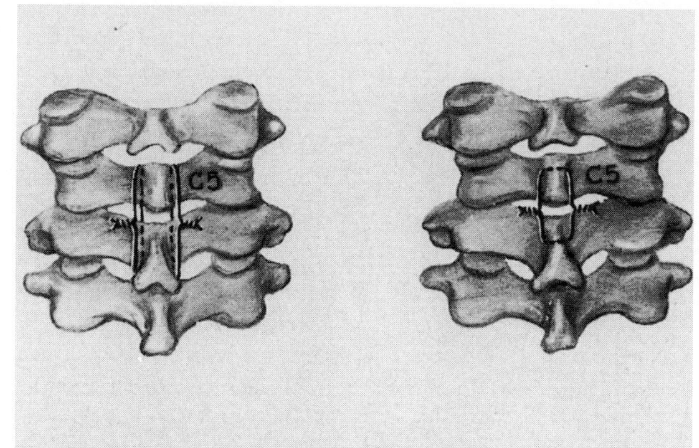

FIG 14–3.
On the *left,* a C5–6 sublaminar wiring technique is illustrated. The Rogers' wiring method is demonstrated on the *right*—two wire twists were used in order to achieve symmetrical tension across the involved vertebral levels. (From Sutterlin CE, McAfee PC, Warden KE, et al: *Spine* 1988; 13:795–802. Used by permission.)

jury model. However, their observations provide useful additional information and should be reviewed for a more complete appreciation of the subject. Investigations of anterior[46] and posterior[15, 19–21, 28, 43] techniques are referenced. Other than the experiments described previously, studies that compare stabilization methods for specific traumatic injuries of the cervical spine (i.e., based on the classification of Allen et al.) are nonexistent.

In summary, biomechanical evidence suggests that dorsal ligamentous injuries, when severe enough to require surgical stabilization, are most *effectively* fixed by a posterior procedure. Plates and screws are more effective than wires. The nature of the risks, potential complications, and technical difficulties in the two basic techniques is a matter of which the surgeon should be keenly aware. Injuries to the vertebral body that impair its ability to resist compressive loading are best fixed by restitution of this load-bearing capacity by corticocancellous bone grafting with or without anterior plating. This situation becomes more urgent when anterior decompression of the spinal cord is required. An anterior corticocancellous graft alone may suffice if the dorsal ligamentous structures are intact, especially if supplemented by halo vest fixation. If ventral decompression of the cord is required and the dorsal ligaments are incompetent, then grafting alone is inadequate and should at least include halo vest protection. Grafting and plating improve stability but are still inadequate to resist flexion forces when the dorsal ligaments are incompetent (except the possibility of adequate stability provided by a rigid anterior plate/screw junction such as that designed by Professor Morscher) and should probably be protected by some sort of brace. And finally, combined anterior and posterior stabilizing procedures are best indicated in this situation if one wishes to avoid use of the halo vest.

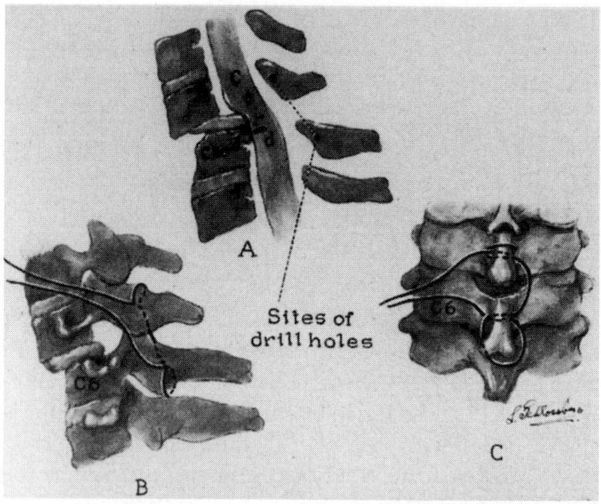

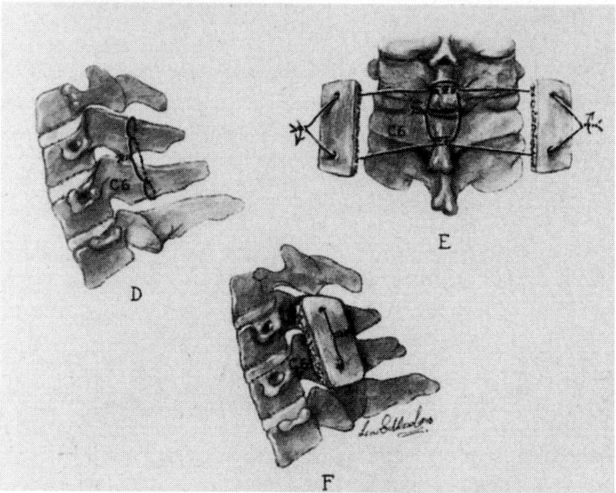

FIG 14–4.
Triple-wire technique. **A–C,** a posterior midline tethering wire (20 gauge) is passed through and around the base of the subluxed spinous processes in initial stabilization of a distraction-flexion stage 3 injury. **D–F,** two lateral wires are used to compress two large corticocancellous iliac strut grafts against the individual lamina. Note that the illustrations demonstrate the fixation methods for a C5–6 injury, but the bovine functional spinal unit used for the experimental protocol was C4–5. (From Sutterlin CE, McAfee PC, Warden KE, et al: *Spine* 1988; 13:795–802. Used by permission.)

The Occipitoatlantoaxial Complex

Fewer published works exist with regard to biomechanical studies on traumatic injuries to the occipitoatlantoaxial complex as compared with the middle and lower parts of the cervical spine. Most of the recent investigations are described only as abstracts at the time of this writing.

Hanson et al.[23] performed Gallie fixation and Magerl transarticular screw fixation on the C1–2 unit of four human cadaveric spines and measured their stiffness in flexion and rotation. They did not describe destabilization of

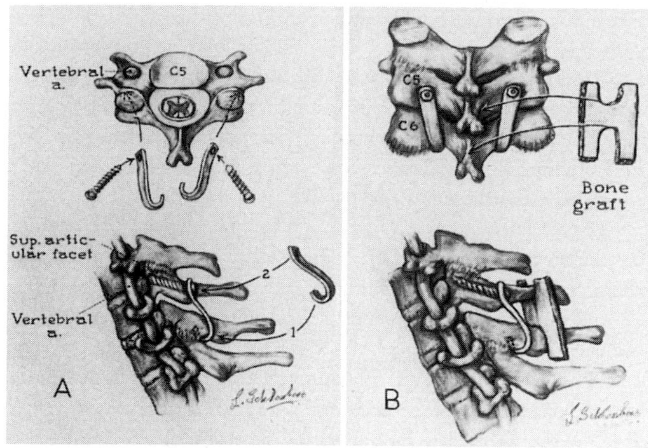

FIG 14–5.
The posterior AO hook plates with two cortical screws and posterior interspinous bone block are illustrated. The recommended angle of insertion and bicortical contact of the laterally directed screws are demonstrated. The exit point of the screws is adjacent to the foramen transversarium in close proximity to the vertebral arteries. (From Sutterlin CE, McAfee PC, Warden KE, et al: *Spine* 1988; 13:795–802. Used by permission.)

the spine in their methods but found that the Magerl technique was stiffer than that of Gallie. They concluded that the Magerl technique is more demanding and not meant to replace the Gallie fusion; in situations where the Gallie technique cannot be used (congenital absence of the dorsal arch of C1 or C2, too narrow a canal for passage of sub-

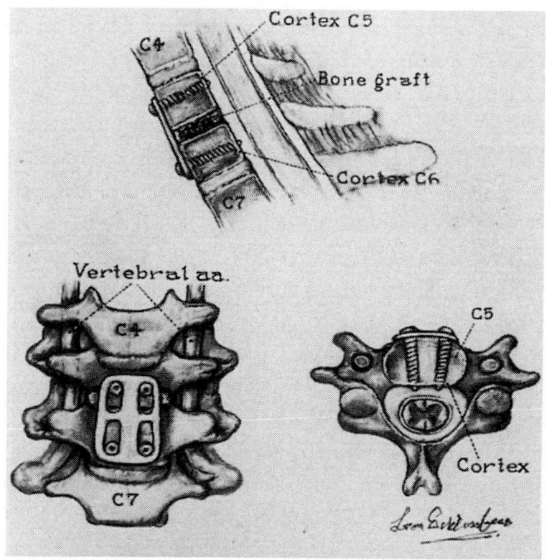

FIG 14–6.
The Caspar trapezoidal anterior plate stabilization technique is demonstrated. A Robinson tricortical iliac bone graft was used to replace the disrupted intervertebral disc at the level of subluxation. Care was taken to ensure that the four cortical screws obtained maximum stability by obtaining purchase of the posterior vertebral body cortices through actual entrance of the spinal canal, as is recommended. (From Sutterlin CE, McAfee PC, Warden KE, et al: *Spine* 1988; 13:795–802. Used by permission.)

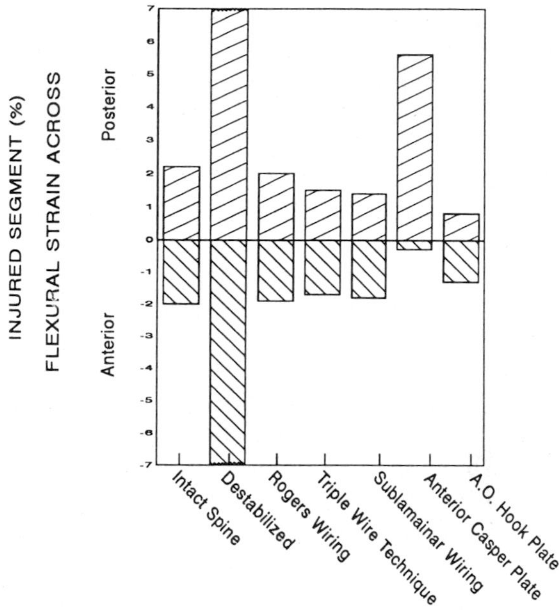

FIG 14–7.
The flexural strains across the C4–5 vertebrae are demonstrated—the anterior column strains are compressive, and the posterior column strains are tensile. Overall, the most successful construct in reducing anterior and posterior strains with flexion loads was the AO hook plate followed by all three posterior C4–5 wiring techniques ($P < .05$). Caspar anterior plating was actually the most effective in reduction of anterior strain because the plate and anterior bone graft act as a block to prevent compression. However, Caspar anterior plate instrumentation permitted unacceptably high tensile strain to be transferred to the posterior elements (the C4–5 posterior facets could distract apart). (From Sutterlin CE, McAfee PC, Warden KE, et al: *Spine* 1988; 13:795–802. Used by permission.)

laminar wires) or where Gallie fusion has failed (pseudarthrosis), the Magerl method of C1–2 fixation provides a useful adjunct.

Grob et al.[22] created a more specific C1–2 ligamentous injury and tested the ability of Magerl, Gallie, and Brooks fixation techniques to resist flexion, extension, bilateral rotation, and bilateral lateral bending displacements in six human cadaveric spines. They found that in general the techniques were equivalent in their ability to resist flexion and extension, but for rotation and lateral bending the Magerl method was better than the Brooks and Gallie techniques.

Smith et al.[34] utilized ten bovine spines and modeled a type II odontoid injury by resection of the base of the dens. They tested flexion, extension, torsion, and anteroposterior shear forces in calf spines fixed by six posterior techniques: (1) midline sublaminar wiring, (2) Gallie, (3) Brooks, (4) Magerl, (5) Clark, and (6) Clark supplemented by polymethylmethacrylate (PMMA). Again, the Magerl technique (along with the Clark technique supplemented by PMMA) provided superior immediate stability.

Crisco et al.[14] described a novel approach for assessing the immediate ability of fixation methods to stabilize the acutely injured spine by measuring micromotion between the dorsal arch of C1 and the dorsal bone graft block attached to C2. They postulated that decreased strain at this location should correlate with more favorable healing and subsequent fusion. Pure moments in flexion, extension, bilateral rotation, and bilateral lateral bending were applied to ten human cadaveric spines with specific ligamentous injuries to the C1–2 complex that was subsequently stabilized by four methods: (1) Gallie, (2) Brooks, (3) Magerl, and (4) Halifax techniques. Their data showed that Magerl screw fixation and Halifax clamps decreased micromotion between the dorsal arch of C1 and the bone graft block better than the Brooks technique did, with the Gallie method being the least effective. Other reports of C1–2 or occipitocervical fixation methods by posterior[11, 25–27, 32, 33] as well as anterior[3, 4, 16, 24] techniques are referenced but are more often clinically oriented and contain few if any biomechanical data.

In summary, it appears that for obtaining maximal stiffness of the atlantoaxial construct, Magerl's transarticular screw technique is recommended. However, standard wiring techniques (Brooks) can provide fixation with stiffness approaching that of the Magerl method. When dorsal elements are lacking, when stenosis prohibits the passage of sublaminar wires, or when a previous fusion with wiring has failed, then the Magerl technique presents a very useful option. There are no biomechanical data available for a comparison of other dorsal fixation methods, for a comparison of methods of dorsal fixation to the occiput, or for a comparison of anterior fixation techniques of the occipitoatlantoaxial complex.

REFERENCES

1. Allen BL, Ferguson RL, Lehmann TR, et al: A mechanistic classification of closed indirect fractures and dislocations of the lower cervical spine. *Spine* 1982; 7:1–27.
2. Ashman RB, Bechtold JE, Edwards WT, et al: In vitro spinal arthrodesis implant mechanical testing protocols. *J Spinal Disorders* 1989; 2:274–281.
3. Barbour JR: Screw fixation in fracture of the odontoid process. *South Aust Clin* 1971; 5:20.
4. Bohler J: Anterior stabilization of acute fractures and non-unions of the dens. *J Bone Joint Surg [Am]* 1982; 64:18.
5. Bohler J, Gandernak T: Anterior plate stabilization for fracture-dislocations of the lower cervical spine. *J Trauma* 1980; 20:203–205.
6. Bohlman HH: Acute fractures and dislocations of the cervical spine. *J Bone Joint Surg [Am]* 1979; 61:1119–1142.
7. Buckman PM: Spine instrumentation and the FDA: What spine surgeons should know. *J Spinal Disorders* 1989; 2:292–295.
8. Callahan RA, Johnson RM, Margolis RN, et al: Cervical facet fusion for control of instability following laminectomy. *J Bone Joint Surg [Am]* 1977; 59:991–1002.
9. Callahan TJ: The process of FDA approval of a spinal implant: Governmental perspective. *J Spinal Disorders* 1989; 2:288–291.
10. Capen DA, Garland DE, Waters RL: Surgical stabilization of the cervical spine: A comparative analysis of anterior and posterior spine fusions. *Clin Orthop* 1985; 196:229–237.
11. Clark CR, White AA: Fractures of the dens. A multicenter study. *J Bone Joint Surg [Am]* 1985; 67:1340.
12. Coe JD, Warden KE, Sutterlin CE, et al: Biomechanical evaluation of cervical spinal stabilization methods in a human cadaveric model. *Spine* 1989; 14:1122–1131.
13. Cooper PR, Cohen A, Rosiello A, et al: Posterior stabilization of cervical spinal fractures with subluxation using plates with screws. *Neurosurgery* 1988; 23:300–306.
14. Crisco JJ, Panjabi MM, Grob D, et al: Biomechanical evaluation of four upper cervical spine fixation techniques by bone graft micromotion (abstract). Presented at the 18th Annual Meeting of the Cervical Spine Research Society, San Antonio, Tex, 1990, Paper 23, pp 58–59.
15. Cusick JF, Yoganandan N, Pintar F, et al: Biomechanics of cervical spine facetectomy and fixation techniques. *Spine* 1988; 13:808–812.
16. Esses SI, Bednar DA: Screw fixation of odontoid fractures and non-unions (abstract). Presented at the 18th Annual Meeting of the Cervical Spine Research Society, San Antonio, Tex, 1990, Paper 9, pp 35–36.
17. Fidler MW: Posterior instrumentation of the spine. An experimental comparison. *Spine* 1986; 11:367–372.
18. Gassman J, Seligson D: Anterior cervical plate. *Spine* 1983; 8:700–707.
19. Gill K, Scott P, Corin J, et al: Posterior plating of the cervical spine: A biomechanical comparison of different posterior fusion techniques. *Spine* 1988; 13:813–816.
20. Goel VK, Clark CR, Harris KG, et al: Evaluation of effectiveness of a facet wiring technique: An in vitro biomechanical investigation. *Ann Biomed Eng* 1989; 17:115–126.
21. Goel VK, Clark CR, Harris KG, et al: Kinematics of the cervical spine: Effects of multiple total laminectomy and facet wiring. *J Orthop* 1988; 6:611–619.
22. Grob D, Crisco J, Panjabi M, et al: Comparative in vitro evaluation of the multidirectional stability of three dorsal atlanto-axial fusions (abstract). Presented at the 17th Annual Meeting of the Cervical Spine Research Society, New Orleans, 1989, Paper 31, pp 71–72.
23. Hanson P, Sharkey N, Montesano PX: Anatomic and biomechanical study of C1, C2 posterior arthrodesis techniques (abstract). Presented at the 16th Annual Meeting of the Cervical Spine Research Society, Key Biscayne, Fla, 1988, Paper 47, pp 100–101.
24. Harms J: Anterior plate for occipitocervical fixation and fusion (lecture), in *A.O. North American Spine Course*. Vail, Colo, 1989.

25. Holness RO, Huestis WS, Howes WJ, et al: Posterior stabilization with an interlaminar clamp in cervical injuries: Technical note and review of the long term experience with the method. *Neurosurgery* 1984; 14:318–322.
26. Itoh T, Tsuji H, Katoh Y, et al: Occipito-cervical fusion reinforced by Luque's segmental spinal instrumentation for rheumatoid diseases. *Spine* 1988; 13:1234.
27. Mitsui H: A new operation for atlanto-axial arthrodesis. *J Bone Joint Surg [Br]* 1984; 66:422–425.
28. Montesano PX, Juach E: Anatomic and biomechanical study of posterior cervical spine plate arthrodesis (abstract). Presented at the 16th Annual Meeting of the Cervical Spine Research Society, Key Biscayne, Fla, 1988, Paper 12, pp 39–40.
29. Murphy MJ, Daniaux H, Southwick WO: Posterior cervical fusion with rigid internal fixation. *Orthop Clin North Am* 1986; 17:55–65.
30. Oliveira JC: Anterior plate fixation of traumatic lesions of the lower cervical spine. *Spine* 1987; 12:324–329.
31. Panjabi MM: Biomechanical evaluation of spinal fixation devices: I. A conceptual framework. *Spine* 1988; 13:1129–1134.
32. Rogers WA: Treatment of fracture-dislocation of the cervical spine. *J Bone Joint Surg* 1942; 24:245–258.
33. Roosen K, et al: Posterior atlantoaxial fusion: A new compression clamp for Lam. Osteosynth. *Arch Orthop Trauma Surg* 1982; 100:27–31.
34. Smith MD, Kotzar G, Yoo J, et al: A biomechanical analysis of atlantoaxial stabilization methods using a bovine model (abstract). Presented at the 17th Annual Meeting of the Cervical Spine Research Society, New Orleans, 1989, Paper 36, p 81.
35. Stauffer ES, Kelly EG: Fracture-dislocations of the cervical spine: Instability and recurrent deformity following treatment by anterior interbody fusion. *J Bone Joint Surg [Am]* 1977; 59:45–48.
36. Sutterlin CE, McAfee PC, Warden KE, et al: A biomechanical evaluation of cervical spine stabilization methods in a bovine model. *Spine* 1988; 13:795–802.
37. Tippets RH, Apfelbaum RI: Anterior cervical fusion with the Caspar instrumentation system. *Neurosurgery* 1988; 22:1008–1013.
38. Ulrich C, Worsdorfer O, Claes L, et al: Comparative study of the stability of anterior and posterior cervical spine fixation procedures. *Arch Orthop Trauma Surg* 1987; 106:226–231.
39. White AA: Clinical biomechanics of cervical spine implants. *Spine* 1989; 14:1040–1045.
40. White AA, Johnson RM, Panjabi MM, et al: Biomechanical analysis of clinical stability in the cervical spine. *Clin Orthop* 1975; 109:85–96.
41. White AA, Panjabi MM: *Clinical Biomechanics of the Spine,* ed 2. Philadelphia, JB Lippincott, 1990.
42. Whitehill AA, Southwick WO, Panjabi MM: Clinical instability in the lower cervical spine: A review of past and current concepts. *Spine* 1976; 1:15–27.
43. White R, Reger S, Weatherup N, et al: A biomechanical analysis of posterior cervical fusions using polymethylmethacrylate as an instantaneous fusion mass. *Spine* 1983; 8:368–372.
44. Whitecloud TS: Clinical trials for spinal implants. *J Spinal Disorders* 1989; 2:285–287.
45. Whitehill R: Laboratory evaluations of cervical internal fixation devices: In vitro testing. *J Spinal Disorders* 1989; 2:282–284.
46. Whitehill R, Reger SI, Kett RL, et al: Reconstruction of the cervical spine following anterior vertebral body resection: A mechanical analysis of a canine experimental model. *Spine* 1984; 9:240–245.

15

Thoracic and Lumbar Spine Implants

Martin Krag, M.D.

Rapid development is one of the major characteristics of the spinal implant field, especially in the past 5 to 10 years. This has resulted largely from our improved understanding of spinal biomechanics as well as technical advances in radiographic imaging, implant design, and surgical and anesthetic techniques. Reviewed here are the major biomechanical issues of spinal implants organized primarily by the site of attachment to the spine and with an emphasis on those attaching by screws through the pedicle since this is the area in which the most development has occurred recently. These have been reviewed in further detail elsewhere.[51, 85, 157]

SPINOUS PROCESS

The earliest spinal implants, wires and sutures, were attached to the spinous processes as reported by Hadra in 1891[58, 59] and Lange in 1910.[97, 98] Since these implants can only sustain tensile loads, their applications are limited. For example, they are sufficient for fixation of reduced bilateral facet dislocations or incomplete chance fractures. However, if resistance to other loads is needed (e.g., compression resistance for burst fractures or anterior shear resistance for large articular process fractures), then spinous process wires are not sufficient (analogous to olecranon or patellar wiring without the longitudinal pins).

Plates bolted to the spinous processes have also been used.[125, 148, 159, 160] Although these can withstand longitudinal compressive and anterior shear forces to some extent, failures frequently occurred, especially through the development of kyphosis. This was probably due to insufficient strength of the spinous processes and the relatively poor resistance to flexion caused by the posterior placement of the spinous process bolts.

FACET JOINTS

Placement of screws across the facet joint is quite different from placement across the pedicle (see the later section on attachment through the pedicle). The former actually spans the joint, and any screw placement into the pedicle is really incidental. The functional purpose of this screw is to immobilize the joint. In contrast, a transpedicular screw is intended to provide a rigid "grip" or attachment to a single vertebra. To these screws are then attached the components (e.g., rods or plates) that span the joint(s) to provide immobilization.

The use of facet screws was first reported in the 1940s by Toumey[151] and King[77] and later by others.[13, 150] Boucher[20] and later Magerl[111, 113] each reported screw orientations different from the original (see Fig 15–1). Although these screws can resist shear loads along the plane of the facet joint, they resist flexion only poorly because their effective length *d* (in Fig 15–1) is short. Thus, anterior load-bearing capacity must be present to prevent kyphosis. Mechanical testing[65] on intact specimens (anterior load bearing by discs is present) has shown the effectiveness of this fixation method.

LAMINAE AND ARTICULAR PROCESSES

Until recently, the vast majority of spinal implants were attached to the laminae and articular processes, most commonly in the form of Harrington compression or distraction rods. The compression rods are almost equivalent mechanically to spinous process wires, not only because they require bony structures to resist all loads other than tensile but also because they tend to produce increased compressive forces. In some cases this can produce undesired results such as an increase in the amount of canal encroachment from burst-fracture bone fragments.

The structure of distraction rods[62, 63] is simple, but their biomechanics is not. Figure 15–2 illustrates rod placement in the lordotic lumbar area, although the principles are the same in the thoracic area as well. Initially, before distraction is accomplished (Fig 15–2,A), there is no contact between the rod and the spanned laminae. Ratcheting out of the upper hook produces not only distraction (thus the name "distraction rod") but also flexion (since the flexion/extension axis of rotation is anterior to the rod). This continues until enough flexion has occurred that the central portion of the rod contacts the laminae of the spanned vertebrae (Fig 15–2,B). Further flexion is resisted by the bending stiffness of the rod. The flexion produced can result in a troublesome "flat back."[24, 49, 96, 119, 161]

To prevent a "flat back" the rods can be prebent into

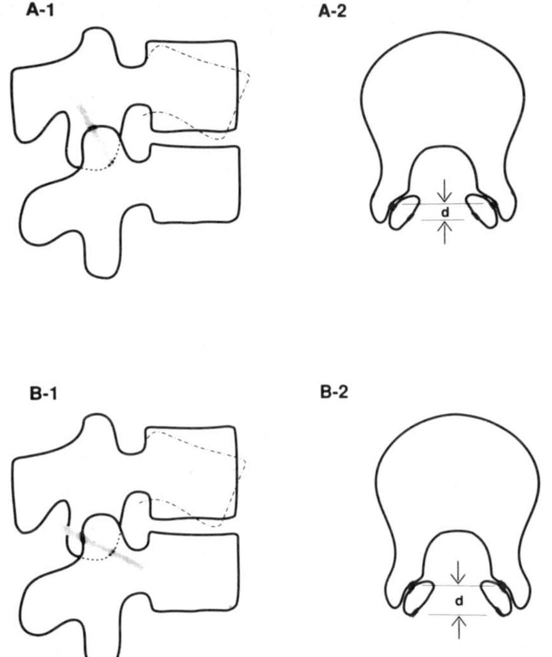

FIG 15–1.
Facet joint screws. **A,** method of Toumey[151] and King.[77] Resistance to flexion is fairly small (shown in **A-1**) because the effective length of screw resisting this is very small (*d* in **A-2**). **B,** method of Boucher.[20] Length *d* is greater here than in **A-2,** but it is still quite small. (Courtesy of C. Herndon, 1990.)

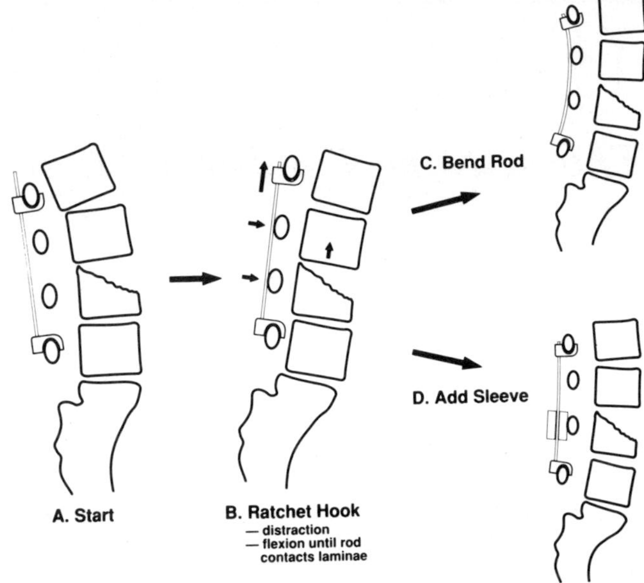

FIG 15–2.
Distraction rod. See the text for a description. (Courtesy of C. Herndon, 1990.)

lordosis (see Fig 15–5,C), but this can cause the rods to "flip" (rotate 180 degrees about an axis passing through the upper and lower hooks). This can be prevented by using square-ended rods and square-socketed hooks[30] or by wiring the rods and square-socketed hooks to the spinous processes or laminae.[36] An alternative is to place a spacer between the unbent rod and the lamina of the central vertebra.[40, 41]

One of the major loads resisted by these rods and hooks is a flexion moment *M* (Fig 15–3). This is accomplished (Fig 15–3,A) by a posteriorly directed force *F* at each hook and an anteriorly directed force *2F* at the middle of the rod. If the rod length is increased (from *2d* to *2D* in Fig 15–3,B), the hook force is correspondingly decreased (from *F* to *f*) since the moment is constant. Thus, the tendency for a hook to break off an articular process is reduced. By similar reasoning, with a long rod there will also be less stress on the ratchet-rod junction (assuming that the distance from the hook to the ratchet-rod junction is kept constant). These biomechanical advantages of this "long-rod" technique[6, 72] are somewhat offset by the biological disadvantage of a larger number of motion segments being spanned.

The placement of wires or flexible tape around longitudinal rods, with or without terminal hooks, has been described by various authors.[53, 106, 107, 126] As shown in Figure 15–4, because such wires or tapes can slide along or rotate about the rods,[85] this technique is useful primarily for "long-segment" implantations (i.e., those involving

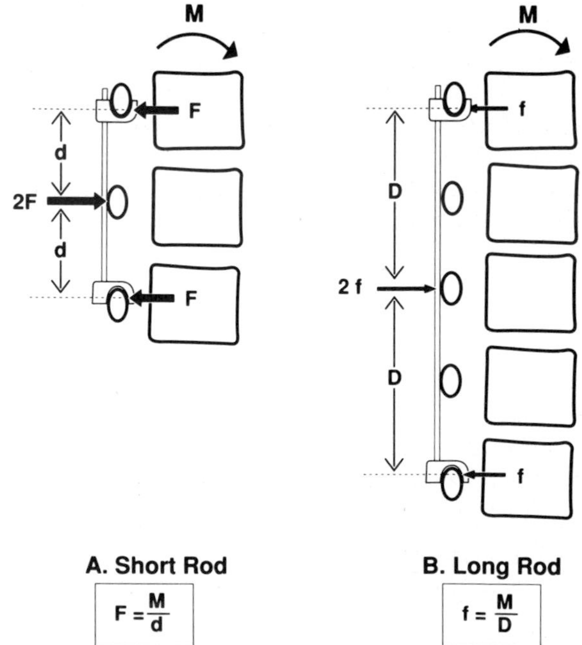

FIG 15–3.
Short vs. long rod. **A,** for a short rod, flexion-resisting forces *F* on the hooks are large because length *2d* is small. **B,** for a longer rod, greater length *2D* causes the hook forces to be reduced to *f* because the bending moment *M* is unchanged. (Courtesy of C. Herndon, 1990.)

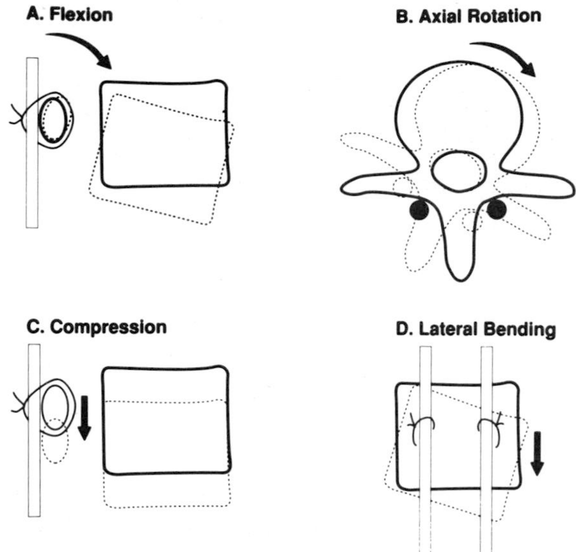

FIG 15–4.
A circumlaminar wire fails to control a variety of motion types. (Courtesy of C. Herndon, 1990.)

multiple motion segments)[92] in which only flexion-extension or lateral bending control is needed.

ANTERIOR IMPLANTS

Anterior implants that are simply interposed between adjacent vertebrae depend upon compressive forces to keep them properly positioned and require intact bony or ligamentous structures to resist all loads other than axial compressive loads. If the implant is keyed into place,[54] some shear resistance is provided, and if it has a porous structure that allows bony ingrowth,[54, 76, 153] even further resistance is eventually provided.

To provide improved initial strength, various anterior implants have been attached to the vertebral bodies by means of transversely oriented screws (Fig 15–5). The use of only a single upper and single lower screw to attach a single rod[46, 61, 73, 137, 138] does not provide much resistance to anterior shear or to flexion (Fig 15–5,A). The addition of a second rod (Fig 15–5,B)[75, 82–84] partially controls flexion, but if the screws are all parallel, there is little resistance to anterior shear (screw-bone friction only). However, if the screws are placed obliquely, substantial anterior shear resistance develops (similar to the resistance to lateral shear by obliquely positioned transpedicle screws, as shown in Fig 15–7 below). Adding a transverse connector between the rods,[28, 37] shown in Figure 15–5,C, provides even further resistance. Such a transverse connector is probably more important for these vertebral body screws than for transpedicular screws (see the section "Transverse Connectors," below) because the former are less effective in resisting flexion moments, which probably are the largest loads to which the screws are subjected.

Instead of rods as the longitudinal elements, plates have also been used. One approach has been to attach a single plate to two or more vertebrae above and below the lesion by means of a single screw per vertebra.[60] Further strengthening has been achieved by using two such plates rather than just one.[57] Yet another approach has been to use specially designed plates that allow two or more screws per vertebral body.[15, 18, 25, 70, 163] Various other devices also have been tried.[70, 124, 127, 156]

THROUGH THE PEDICLE INTO THE VERTEBRAL BODY (TRANSPEDICLE)

This method provides, for the first time, a strong grip on the vertebra that resists loads of any type, not just a few special types. Harrington and Tullos[64] first reported on this for spondylolisthesis reduction, and Roy-Camille and Demeulenaere developed the first really practical method,

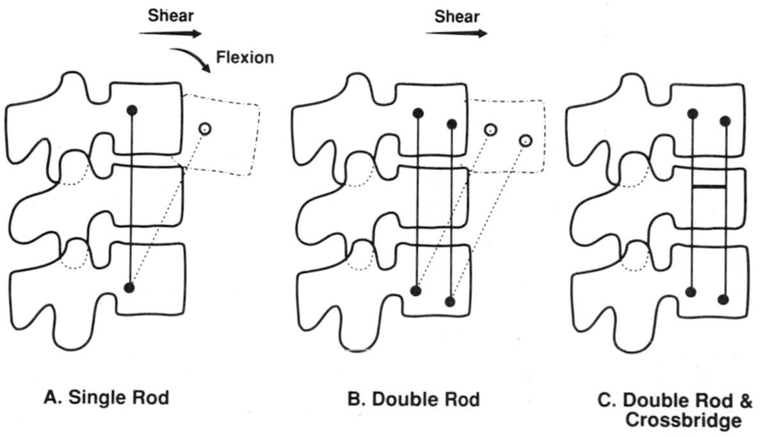

FIG 15–5.
Anterior screws and rods (or plates). **A,** a single rod allows anterior shear and flexion. **B,** a double rod controls flexion but still allows anterior shear. **C,** a transverse connector prevents both. (Courtesy of C. Herndon, 1990.)

TABLE 15–1.
Pedicle Diameter and Distribution by Size

Level	Mean (mm)	SD (mm)	n	Distribution (%)					
				3–3.9 mm	4–4.9 mm	5–5.9 mm	6–6.9 mm	7–7.9 mm	8–19.4 mm
T9	6.88	2.23	14	14	7	14	21	7	35
T10	7.47	2.24	18	11		11	39		39
T11	7.83	1.56	22			14	18	14	55
T12	7.63	1.79	24			21	21	12	46
L1	7.01	1.84	22	9		18	18	14	41
L2	8.67	0.64	14					7	92
L3	9.30	1.51	24				8	12	79
L4	11.03	1.36	24						100
L5	15.15	1.97	20						100

which consisted of longitudinal plates through which the screws passed.[131] A number of biomechanical issues are relevant to this attachment method.

Screw Design

Most studies of this topic have been done in nonvertebral bone specimens.* Only one of these studies (Decoster et al.[29]) systematically varied pitch, minor diameter, and major diameter in a way that allowed isolation of these variables. Martin et al.[115] emphasized the extent to which screws through plates were subjected to flexural loads (caused by cantilever bending); they also stated that resistance to this was an important design feature to prevent screw breakage. Insufficient attention to this loading mode is probably an important cause of the high rate of transpedicle screw breakage seen in some clinical studies.[68, 131, 136, 147, 158]

Studies relevant to transpedicle screw design have been both morphometric and biomechanical. Concerning the former, the initial report that provided the size distribution on pedicle diameter (Table 15–1)[92] emphasized the importance of preoperative computed tomographic (CT) scanning to detect excessively small pedicles. Subsequent reports,[14, 17, 139, 142, 165] have confirmed and extended these results, as well as those of Saillant.[139] Concerning the biomechanical studies,[47, 92, 100, 104, 143, 145] only one of these[92] has studied the major variables (pitch, minor diameter, and tooth profile) in a way that allows their isolation. In that study, pullout strength was measured for eight different screw types, each of which had a 6-mm major diameter. The important results were (1) 2-mm pitch threads were either no stronger (two of three subgroups) or only moderately stronger (21% in one subgroup) than 3-mm pitch; (2) the "V" and buttress tooth profile were the same in strength; and (3) although the deeper-threaded screws were somewhat stronger for pullout strength (the 3.8-mm minor diameter was 19% to 26% stronger than the 5.0-mm minor diameter), they were less than half as strong in bending. This is because the bending strength varies as the third power of the minor diameter ($[3.8/5.0]^3 = 44\%$), while pullout strength varies with the major diameter, which was constant in this study.

The role of osteopenia in determining screw strength has not been thoroughly studied, but a number of studies have already been completed.[22, 26, 71, 166, 167]

Fatigue strength is an important characteristic of screw performance, particularly for transpedicle screw–based implants, since this seems to be the most common metallurgical failure mode. The importance of minor diameter has been clearly shown by Liu et al.,[104] who reported a 104% increase in fatigue life as a result of a 27% increase (from 3.0 mm to 3.8 mm) in minor diameter ($1.27^3 = 2.04$). A lack of significant differences in minor diameters (the values of which were not reported) may explain why no differences in fatigue life were seen between the seven screw types studies by Geiger et al,[47] even though they did differ in major diameter. These authors as well as Ashman et al.[12] did note the importance of stress risers, which was also noted in whole-implant fatigue testing of the Vermont Spinal Fixator (VSF),[91] which was incapable of producing failure of the articulating clamp but could only produce failure at the first thread (a known stress riser). The reduction in screw fatigue life caused by bending of the screw was emphasized by Hsu et al.[68] and measured by Moran et al.[120]: a 50% decrease was produced by a 30-degree bend of the screw.

The importance of flexural loading (cantilever beam bending) for transpedicle screw breakage is worth emphasizing: insufficient attention to this has probably been an important cause of the high rate of screw breakage seen in some clinical studies.[68, 131, 136, 147, 158] Under optimal circumstances, the screws used to attach a longitudinal plate to a tubular bone are exposed predominantly to tensile loads and are shielded (by the friction between plate and bone) from loads transverse to the screw (i.e., flexural

*References 5, 16, 29, 34, 66, 81, 109, 115, 140.

loads). Although this is not necessarily true for screws through plates applied to tubular bone,[115] it is probably much less true for those applied over the irregular surface presented by multiple facet joints, even if they are trimmed as flat as possible.[66] This is partially due to the fact that each vertebra is only held against the plate by a single screw, in contrast to tubular bone applications with multiple screws per bone fragment. Probably the most effective method to deal with this problem is to develop a screw that is sufficiently resistant to flexural loads. One major difficulty with this is that at the present time we do not know the magnitude of the loads to which the screws are exposed in vivo. Even very extensive fatigue testing will only characterize the screw mechanically; it will not presently allow us to predict in vivo behavior. Only after there has been built up enough clinical experience with devices that have known mechanical characteristics will we be able to make such predictions.

Screw Placement

Entry Site and Orientation

Roy-Camille and colleagues have popularized the "straight-ahead" orientation[131, 136] (Fig 15–6, left), which has been adopted by a number of others.[102, 105, 121, 146, 147] Using this orientation to place such a screw through the center of the pedicle, the entry point must be sufficiently medial that it is directly below the center of the inferior articular process of the vertebra above. This virtually guarantees that this articular process will strike the uppermost screw of the implant when trunk extension occurs. How clinically important this is has not been established, but certainly it does not seem to be an optimal arrangement.

To overcome this problem, Magerl[110–113] and others* have used an "inward" or anteromedial screw orientation (Fig 15–6,B). The entry point can thereby be more lateral, along a longitudinal line tangent to the lateral cortex of the superior articular process and thus away from the inferior articular process.

The modification introduced by Magerl was extended by Krag et al.[95] who described an "in-and-up" orientation. The entry site is as far lateral as in the Magerl method, but is somewhat lower along a transverse line between the upper two thirds and lower third of the transverse process. The orientation is still medially angulated (along the pedicle axis) but also inclined as cephalad as possible without penetrating the superior end plate.

This doubly angulated placement provides three advantages. First, it allows the dorsally protruding screw to be out and down, further away from the facet joint above it. This may be more important than implant stiffness as a way of preventing degeneration of this facet joint (see also the section "Implant Stiffness" later in this chapter). Second, this placement provides a longer and thus stronger screw-bone interface[90] (see the section "Depth of Insertion," later in this chapter). Skinner et al.[145] have shown that angulation alone does not affect the strength; it is the increased length allowed by the angulation that produces the increased strength. Third, the convergence of each bi-

*References 2, 3, 31–33, 52, 92, 94, 155.

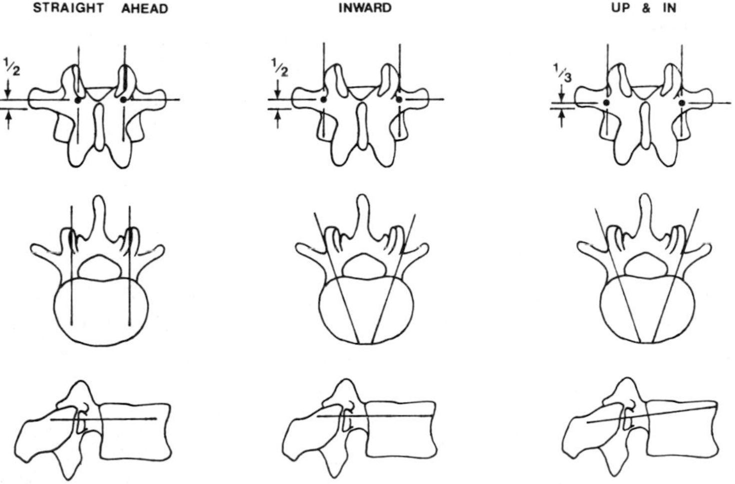

FIG 15–6.
Entry point and orientation alternatives for transpedicle screws. **A,** "straight ahead." The entry point is the intersection of a transverse line that bisects the transverse process and a longitudinal line that bisects the facet joint. Screw orientation is parallel to the sagittal plane and to the end plates. **B**, "inward." The entry point is more lateral, and the longitudinal orientation is anteromedial along the pedicle. The longitudinal line is along the lateral aspect of the facet joint (superior articular process). **C,** "up and in." The entry point is both more lateral and lower (more caudad). The transverse line divides the upper two thirds and lower one third of the transverse process. The orientation is still anteromedial but also anterocephalad (up and in), although not enough to intersect the superior end plate.

lateral pair of screws allows each vertebral body to provide an "intrinsic transverse connector" effect[89] (Fig 15–7) that resists lateral displacement of the upper vertebra relative to the lower, even without the addition of an implanted transverse connector.

In the sacrum, transpedicle screws can be placed not only anteromedially, as for the thoracic and lumbar vertebrae, but also anterolaterally into the ala. Relevant anatomic data have been reported by Dohring et al.[35] as well as others.[9, 43, 118] Biomechanical data have been reported by Zindrick et al.,[166, 167] who concluded that anterolateral were stronger than anteromedial screws for pullout testing, but no right-left comparison was performed, and interspecimen variation was large. Jacobs et al.[71] compared pullout strength from each of three screw orientations: anterolateral, anterior, and anteromedial. The strongest was the anteromedial. From the author's laboratory, Dohring et al.[35] reported testing that used flexion loading (believed to be more clinically relevant) and direct right-left comparison, which showed that the two screw orientations are equal at lower loads (0.1-degree screw rotation) but that the anteromedial orientation is stronger at higher loads (1.0-degree screw rotation).

To define the entry point for transpedicle screw placement, one can use posterior bony landmarks alone as an entry point guide, perform a laminotomy to assist in seeing or feeling the medial pedicle cortex, or use intraoperative radiography. The first method is constrained by anatomic variability, and the second method involves dissection, which might otherwise be unnecessary. Thus, in the author's opinion, the third method is preferred.

If screws are to be placed "straight ahead," an anteroposterior (AP) view along the intended screw path makes good sense. But if the screws are to be placed obliquely ("inward" or "up and in"), the AP view can be misleading (Fig 15–8,A). Evidence for this is the high "miss" rate (screw out of the pedicle) reported by the following authors when using this view: Robbins et al. reported 28.8%[128]; Roy-Camille, 13.5%[130]; Saillant, 10%[139]; and Weinstein et al., 21%.[155]

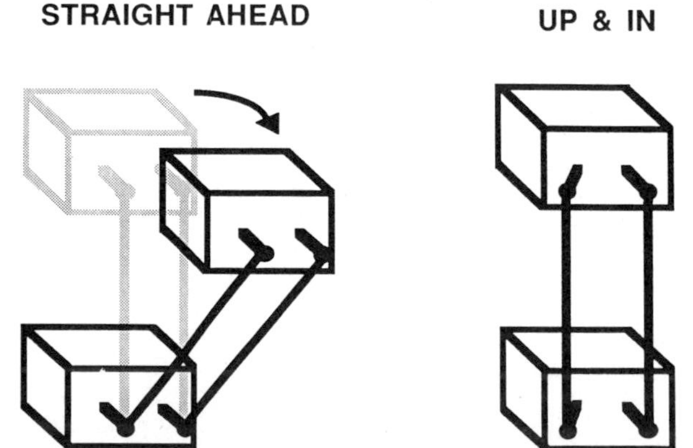

FIG 15–7.
A straight-ahead orientation of the screws causes them to be parallel, and thus lateral shifting meets with little resistance (friction between the screw and bone). An up-and-in orientation allows the vertebral body itself to function as a transverse connector.

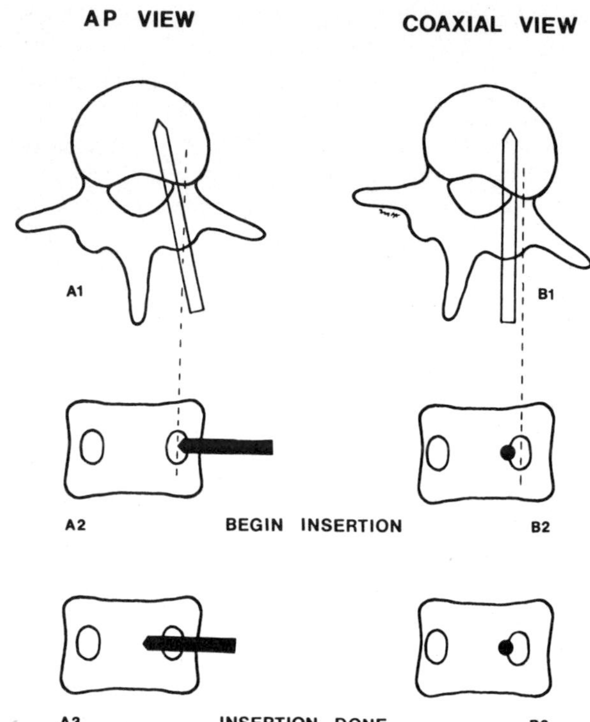

FIG 15–8.
AP vs. pedicle coaxial view for accuracy in visualizing breakout of the screw through the medial cortex of the pedicle. **A,** an AP view before the beginning of drill insertion **(A2)** shows the drill bit tip to appear centered over the pedicle. It is not apparent that breakout will occur. Even after drill insertion **(A3)** it is not apparent that breakout has occurred. **B,** with the pedicle coaxial view, breakout can be anticipated before the beginning of drill insertion **(B2).** After insertion **(B3),** breakout can be seen no less well. (Courtesy of C. Herndon, 1990.)

An alternative x-ray view for oblique screws, as emphasized previously,[95] is along the pedicle axis, i.e., along the intended screw path (Fig 15–8,B, "coaxial" view). A convenient method for using this view is as follows. First, a C-arm image intensifier is positioned so its central beam is along the pedicle axis. Next, the tip of the drill bit or probe is located over the center of the pedicle. Then the shaft of the drill bit or probe is rotated up to be oriented parallel to the x-ray beam so as to appear end-on as a spot (Fig 15–8,B and 15–9). Insertion can then follow with the foreknowledge that screw placement will be accurate.

Hole Preparation

A number of techniques have been described: drill bit,* curet,[39, 99] curved flat probe,[56, 146] and straight

*References 73, 86, 87, 95, 110–113, 132–136.

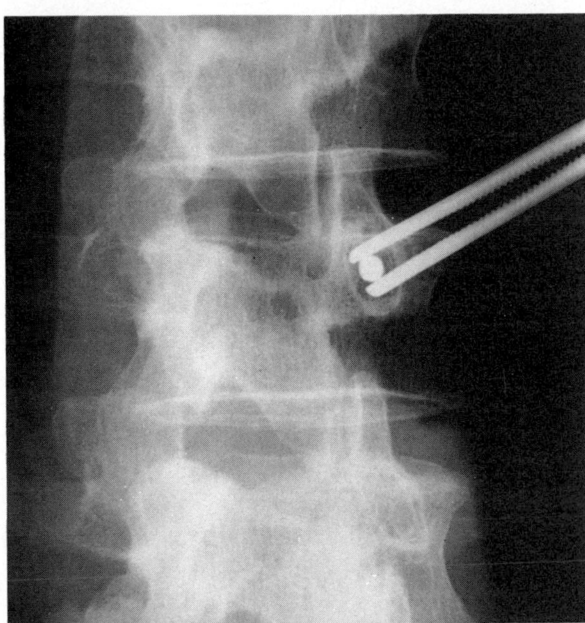

FIG 15–9.
Drill bit centered over the pedicle, with the image intensifier positioned for the "coaxial view." The jaws of a Kelly clamp are holding the dorsal end of the drill bit.

probe. However, only two comparative studies have been performed. Drill bit use was compared with a curved flat probe in a study by Moran et al.[120] that used screw pullout strength as an outcome measure. A reanalysis using the more appropriate two-tailed (rather than the one-tailed) *t* statistic[48, 88] of these data showed no difference between the drill bit and probe. The drill bit was compared with a conical-tipped straight probe in a study by George et al.[48] that also used pullout strength. Here, too, no difference was present.

Banta et al.[14] raise the concern that if too small a pilot hole is used, pedicle "blowout" (cortical breakage by expansion) may occur when the screw is inserted. Because a drill bit removes bone while a probe only compacts it, it may be that a "blowout" is more likely to be caused by screw placement into a probed hole than into a drilled hole. Because of the greater ease with which a dependably cylindrical hole can be formed by a drill bit and because the coaxial view precludes the need to "feel" one's way through the pedicle (possibly causing excessive trabecula damage), the author prefers the drill bit for hole preparation.

Depth of Insertion

Although some clinically based recommendations have been to insert the screw only part way into the vertebral body, biomechanical tests have shown that "deeper is stronger." The data of Lavaste,[100] when appropriately reanalyzed,[90] showed a significant strengthening effect of even a 5-mm increase in screw depth. Krag et al.[90] studied three screw insertion depths: 50%, 80%, and 100% of the distance from the posterior cortex to (but not through) the anterior cortex. There was a significant increase in strength with depth, and the relationship was approximately linear (Fig 15–10). The 100%-depth screws "to anterior cortex" are approximately twice as strong as the 50%-depth screws "just through the pedicle."

For sacral screws, it is often considered desirable to obtain a fairly deep insertion because the total loads at the sacrum are considered to be quite high and the available screw path length is not particularly long.[9, 35] On the other hand, there is considerable concern over the damage that anterior cortex penetration may produce, because of the narrow "safe zones" and the tight attachment of major neural and vascular structures to the anterior sacral cortex.[35, 43, 118] The author's impression is that many surgeons believe that anterior cortical penetration near the

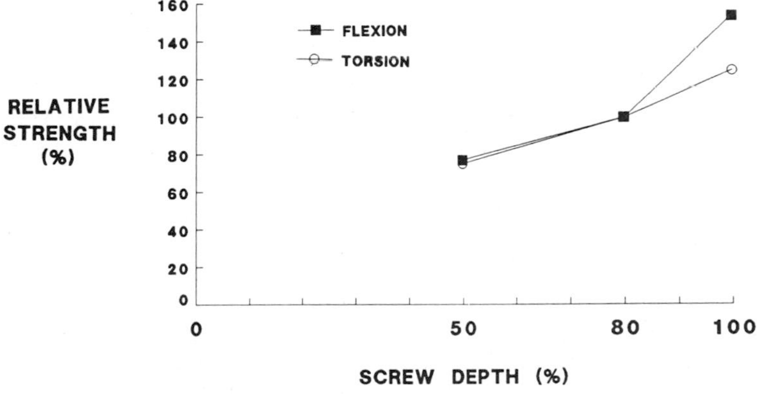

FIG 15–10.
Mean of the ratios between the strength of the 100%-depth screw and its contralateral 80%-depth screw for the flexion and for the torsion-loaded screw groups plotted against percent depth. Similar figures are given for the 50%- and 80%-depth screws.

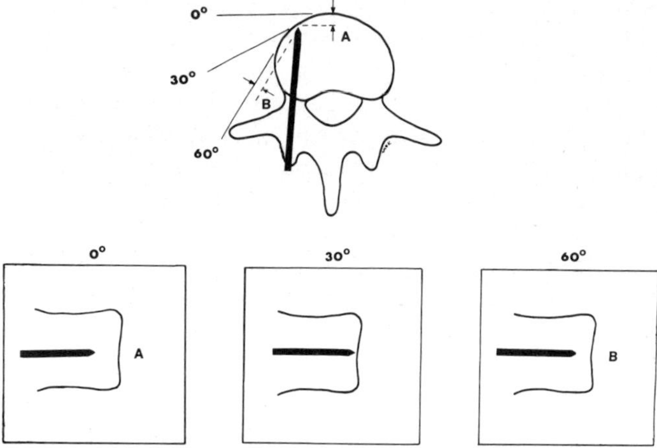

FIG 15–11.
"Near approach" x-ray view to decrease likelihood of anterior penetration. When the drill (or screw probe) tip is actually at the anterior cortex, the lateral view (0°) misleadingly shows the tip still to be some distance *(A)* away from the cortex. At too oblique an angle of view (60°), the tip again misleadingly appears to be some distance *(B)* away from the cortex. Only when the view is tangent to the point of penetration (30° in this case) does the tip appear most nearly to approach actual breakthrough. (From Krag MH: *Spine* 1991; 16:84–99. Used by permission.)

midline (by anteromedial screws) is less dangerous than that near the sacroiliac joint (by anterolateral screws).

Particularly with the deeper screw penetration, monitoring of the depth by one or more methods is desirable to avoid breaking through the anterior cortex. One method is the increased resistance to further drill bit or screw advancement that can sometimes be felt when the cortex is reached. Another method ("mallet method")[95] is to insert the drill bit or probe in the usual fashion partway to the anterior cortex and then complete the insertion by lightly tapping on it with a mallet; a distinct change in sound (rise in pitch) and increased vibration in the instrument shaft usually occur when the tip of the instrument contacts the anterior cortex. In osteopenic bone, however, caution must be used: neither method may be dependable.

A third method is to use radiographs to provide a direct assessment of the distance between the screw tip and the anterior cortex; however, the choice of x-ray view probably is important to avoid a misleading appearance. This same problem can occur during internal fixation of the hip[21, 101, 129, 144, 152, 154] and knee[42] and has been described in more detail elsewhere[95] for transpedicular screw placement. The lateral view may be very misleading and, as shown in Figure 15–11, gives a false sense of security[102, 112, 121]: if the screw tip penetrates the anterior cortex at a location away from the midline, the apparent distance from the screw tip to the cortex will be greater than the actual distance since the screw tip is "over the horizon." If, instead, the x-ray beam is directed obliquely (Fig 15–7,B) so that it is tangential to that point on the anterior cortex at which the screw would penetrate, the distance from the screw tip to the cortex is at a minimum (thus the name "near-approach view").[86, 95] Final screw advancement while imaging with this orientation will generally provide a more direct view of the relationship between the screw tip and the cortex than will a true lateral x-ray view.

Prevention or Repair of Screw Stripout

The use of polymethylmethacrylate (PMM) to prevent or repair stripout has been investigated in nonvertebral[78] and vertebral[164] applications and shown to provide a substantial increase in bone-screw interface strength. However, the problems associated with its use should be kept in mind: risk of its extrusion against cord or roots through cortical bone breaks, difficulty in its removal, or increased risk of infection. In an effort to avoid these problems, Pfeifer et al.[122] studied PMM use as well as two types of bone graft placed into the screw hole after screw pullout. The screw was reimplanted and then pullout tested again. Although the PMM repair was even stronger than the initial state, morselized bone graft was also fairly effective: it reconstituted 70% of the original strength. Whether the superior strength of the PMM is worth the potential complications remains to be established.

Linkage Between the Screw and Longitudinal Component

The major characteristics of this linkage from a biomechanical perspective are as follows.

1. *Positional adjustability.*—This affects how easily and to what extent the screws can be placed to "match the anatomy" instead of being forced by the implant into some suboptimal location. This also affects whether and how easily intervertebral realignment can be performed.

Plates with individual screw holes (e.g., Roy-Camille et al.,[136] Steffee et al.[146]) have the least adjustability; those with screw slots[108] have somewhat more. Fully articulated linkages (e.g., Dick et al.,[32] Kluger et al.,[80] Ölerud et al.,[121] or VSF[87, 89, 92]) have the most adjustability, as shown in Figure 15–12. This adjustability allows intervertebral realignment to be done by direct manipulation of the involved vertebra (using the transpedicle screws as "handles"). This may well provide better control and safety as well as a more thorough correction than any postural adjustment method.[105, 136]

2. *Positional control.*—Among currently available implants, those that have the least positional control between the screw and longitudinal element are those in which the screw passes through but is not mechanically locked to a plate.* With this arrangement, screw toggle

*References 19, 93, 108, 130–136, 149.

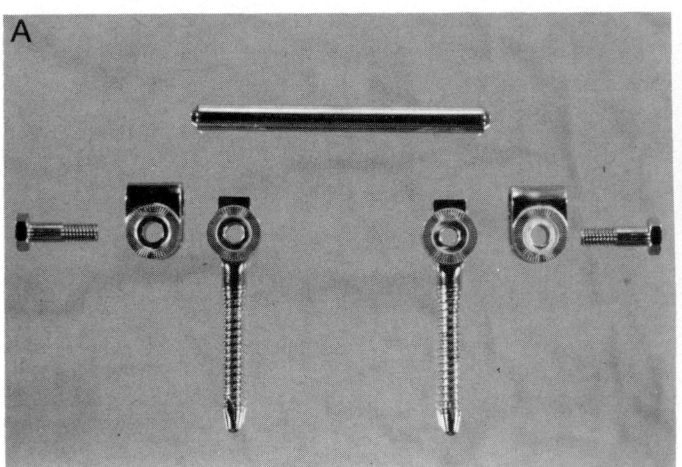

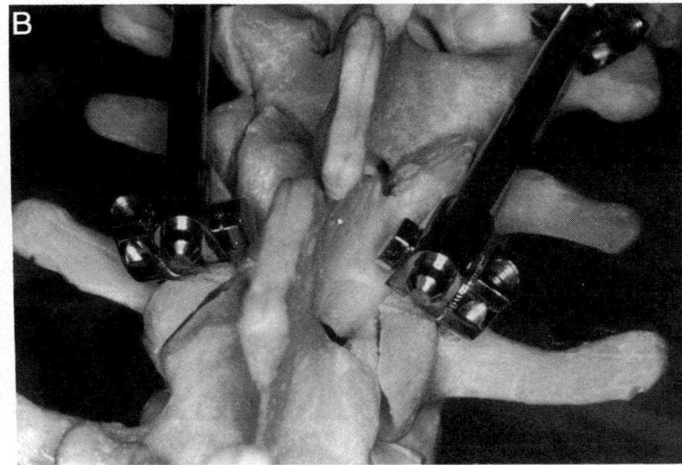

FIG 15–12.
A and **B,** fully articulated linkage between the Vermont Spinal Fixator screw and longitudinal rod. Flexion-extension occurs about the toothed interface, and axial rotation and distraction-compression occur between the clamp and rod. Tightening of the one bolt causes locking of both interfaces.

(up-down and medial-lateral) is controlled only by plate-bone interface forces over quite small contact surface areas (due to facet joint contours). Even a small amount of bone resorption probably leads to large reductions in plate-bone forces, which allows a kyphosis increase at the top and bottom screws. In addition, the screw toggle allows screw-bone interface forces to concentrate near the posterior cortex,[22] as shown in Figure 15–13, thereby reducing interface strength.

A small amount of toggle has been deliberately designed to be present in some implants.[38, 123] Although there is speculation that this is helpful to reduce peak stresses, it is by no means clear that this actually happens since within the toggle range there is little "braking action" or energy absorption. As a result, when the screw "fetches up" at the end of its toggle range, an abrupt peak in stress probably still occurs.

No toggle at all, but rather only a smooth elastic deflection is what occurs with implants in which each metal-metal interface is securely fastened. In this case there is no abrupt fetching up. A number of devices have used this type of linkage. Some of them require careful alignment of screws to match the longitudinal element,[141] some require bending of the screw or longitudinal element,[27, 67, 146] while others avoid either of these requirements by having sufficient adjustability in their linkage.[32, 80, 92, 121]

3. *Fatigue resistance.*—Little has been reported in this area, even though fatigue resistance is an important mechanical characteristic. Geiger et al.[47] tested various rods and plates by using cyclic loads to 24.1 Nm at 4 Hz: fatigue life ranged from 65,000 cycles for the Cotrel-Dubousset rod up to 220,000 cycles for the Harrington distraction rod. In the author's laboratory,[91] the assembled VSF was cycled at various load magnitudes up to 1×10^6 cycles. In no case did the articulating clamp loosen, although at high loads screw failure could eventually be obtained at the root of the first thread. This demonstrates that

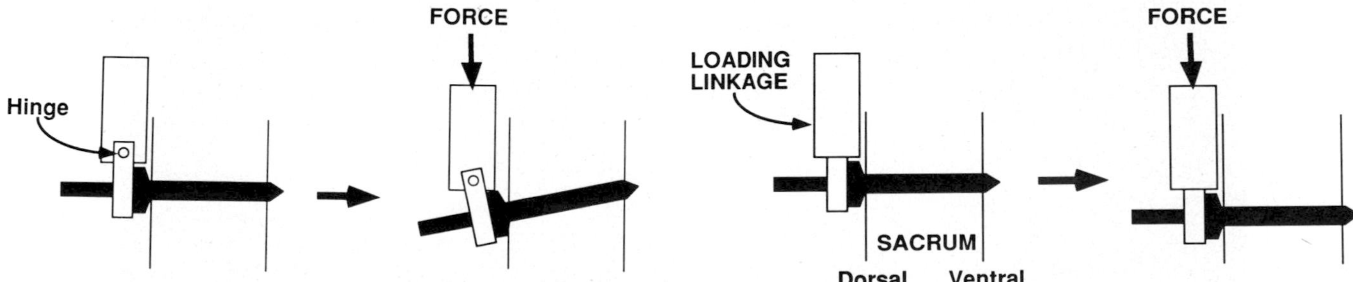

FIG 15–13.
A, semiconstrained linkage between screw and rod. A downward load on the screw causes stress concentration along the dorsal cortex. **B,** constrained linkage reduces the magnitude of stress concentration, distributes load more evenly along the screw length, and allows greater strength.

the articulation is not the "weak link" in the system. Similar testing of other systems is still needed.

4. *Other characteristics.*—The design used for linking the screw to the longitudinal component is one of the major determinants of the bulk and simplicity of the device and the ease of assembly. Although these aspects are not as readily quantified as are certain other mechanical characteristics (such as positional adjustability, stiffness, and fatigue strength), they nonetheless may be quite important. Bulky devices may encroach on adjacent facet joints, displace muscle tissue away from the normal position, produce increased dead space (possibly increasing the chance of infection), cause tenderness from adjacent tissue irritation, and occupy space otherwise available to the bone graft. Devices that are not simple and easy to assemble may be associated with longer operative times, increased risk of holes in sterile gloves, greater chance for incorrect implantation, and an overall greater "fiddle factor."

Longitudinal Component

The choice between plate and rod for this component is based upon many factors such as linkage design (the screw goes through vs. attaches to the side of the longitudinal component), ease of use intraoperatively, relative stiffness in different directions (i.e., flexion stiffness vs. lateral bend stiffness), and encroachment onto the graft bed. Although no comparative testing has been reported, certain observations seem worth noting. Rods may be bent as easily in one direction as another, while plates are much more resistant to lateral bending than they are to flexion. Plates that rest against the posterior cortex substantially obstruct the graft bed, while rods do so much less.

When more than two adjacent vertebrae are to be instrumented, two alternatives exist: (1) only the upper and lower vertebrae have screws (Fig 15–14,A), or (2) all the intermediate vertebrae also have screws (Fig 15–14,B). The choice between these alternatives should include the biomechanics involved.

Figure 15–15 compares a "short-span" implant with a "long-span" implant, which does not have screws in the intermediate vertebrae. In both of these cases, the bending moment *(M = Fd)* for the upper screws is the same, as is also true for the shear force *(F)*. For the rod, the peak stresses are higher for the long-span implant, but rod breakage has not been a problem with most implant systems.

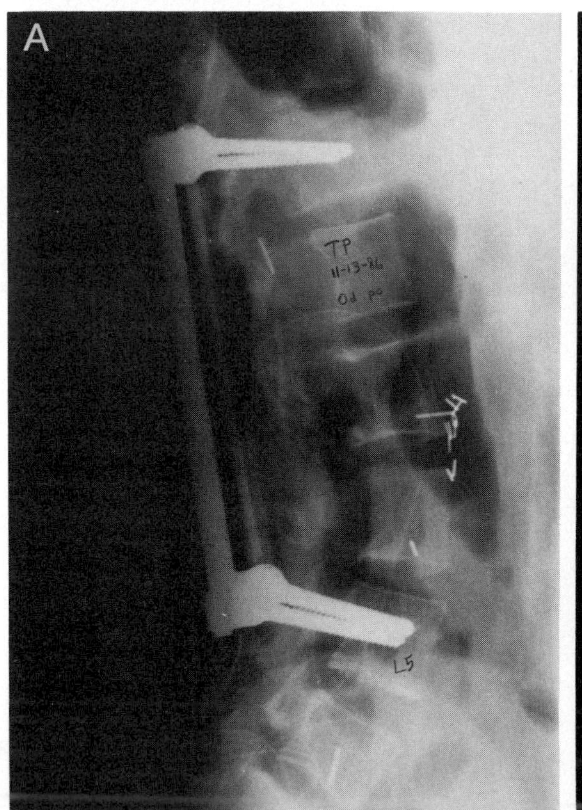

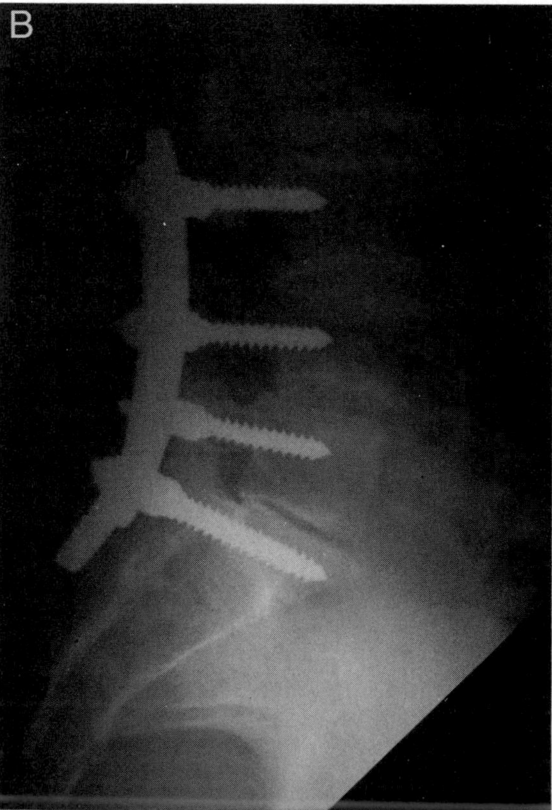

FIG 15–14.
Multiple vertebrae may be instrumented in two ways. **A,** screws placed into only the top and bottom vertebrae. The Vermont Spinal Fixator is shown. **B,** screws placed into each spanned vertebra. The Steffee Variable Spinal Plate is shown.

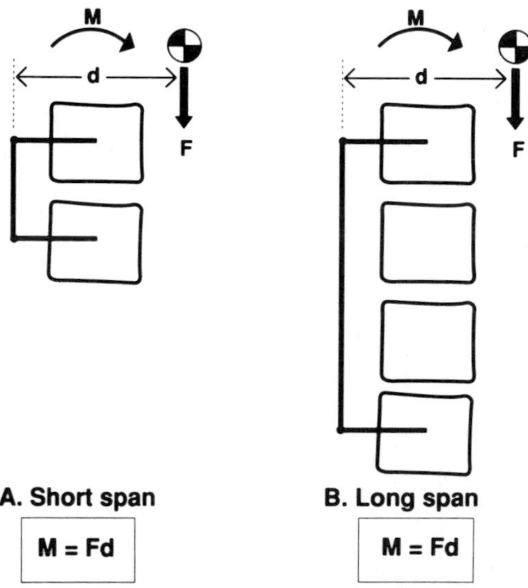

FIG 15–15.
Effect of implant length on the bending moment of the top screw. **A,** for a short-span implant, the bending moment is $M = Fd$. **B,** for a long-span implant, both F and d are unchanged; thus, M is also unchanged. (Courtesy of C. Herndon, 1990.)

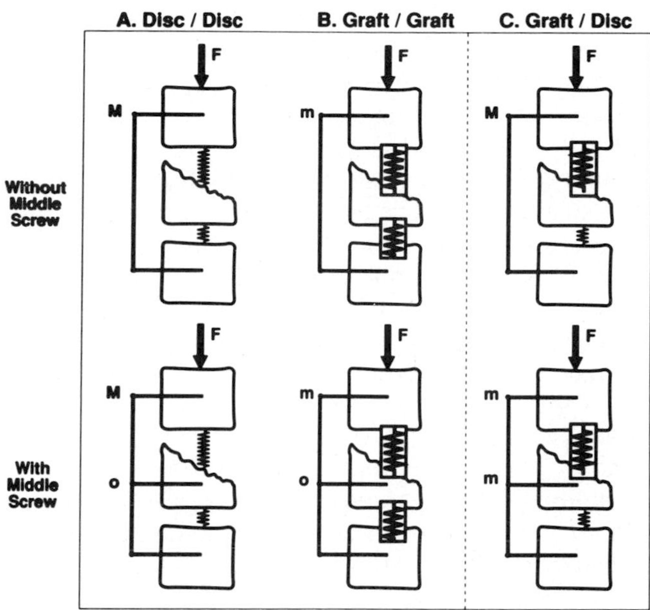

FIG 15–16.
Effect of the middle screw on the bending moment of the upper screw for three different constructs, each of which is exposed to load F. **A,** disc/disc with no interbody graft. The large bending moment *(M)* on the upper screw is not reduced by the addition of a middle screw since the latter carries very little of the load (bending moment = 0). **B,** graft/graft. Both interfaces are grafted. The upper screw bending moment is reduced to m by grafts, but the addition of the middle screw causes little further reduction. The middle screw itself carries very little load. **C,** graft/disc. Only the upper interspace is grafted, which does not reduce the bending moment of the upper screw very much because little load is transmitted from the middle to the lower vertebral body. Only for this rather unusual construct does the middle screw carry significant load *(m),* thereby reducing the bending moment of the upper screw from M to m. (Courtesy of C. Herndon, 1990.)

Figure 15–16 compares three-vertebrae instrumentation without a middle screw (upper row) with one with a middle screw (lower row). This is done for each of three situations. In the left column (Fig 15–16,A), only discs are present between vertebrae, shown by the flexible springs. In the middle column (Fig 15–16,B), an interbody graft is present at both the upper and lower levels, shown by the stiff springs. In the right column (Fig 15–16,C), an interbody graft is present only at the upper level. In each case, the same force, F, is applied. The resulting bending moment is shown for the upper screw and the middle screw (when present). The bending moment is either large *(M),* small *(m),* or negligible *(o).*

When no graft is present (Fig 15–16,A, upper) the bending moment on the upper screw is M. With the middle screw present (Fig 15–16,A, lower) this value is still M. Almost no decrease occurs in bending moment for the upper screw because the bending moment for the middle screw is almost 0 since it is attached to a nearly floating vertebra, which results in very little load sharing (assuming that the implant is much stiffer than the discs).

When both interbody grafts are present (Fig 15–16,B, upper), the bending moment on the upper screw is reduced to m. The addition of the middle screw (Fig 15–16,B, lower) again does not reduce the loads on the upper screw. This is because almost all loads transmitted by the upper graft to the middle vertebra is transmitted to the lower graft, but very little goes to the middle screw. Only in the rare situation in which there is a graft above and no graft below (Fig 15–16,C) does the middle screw share significantly in the load, thereby reducing the load on the upper screw.

By placing screws into only the top and bottom vertebrae, the number of screws is probably reduced to an absolute minimum. This correspondingly reduces the total risk associated with screw placement and decreases the overall operative time. These are the major benefits that result from using this construct, and it appears from the above analysis that no significant biomechanical price is paid by doing so. This is supported by clinical experience showing a very low screw breakage rate with devices using only four screws.[31–33, 80, 87, 121]

Performance of Intervertebral Realignment

Whether or not an implant allows realignment, and if so how easily, has to do with the interplay between screw, linkage, and longitudinal component. Realignment can be performed either before or after the transpedicle screws are inserted into the vertebra and attached to the longitudinal link (rod or plate). For systems in which the longitudinal link must be positioned before screw insertion,[105, 108, 136] reduction must be accomplished either by traction upon or positioning of the patient (described in further detail elsewhere)[105, 136] or by means of another temporarily implanted device such as Harrington distraction rods (although this may require additional dissection). If the longitudinal link can be applied after screw insertion, then it becomes possible to use the screw as a "handle" for controlling vertebral position and performing the reduction. In some cases, this may allow a successful reduction to be performed that otherwise might be attempted only by a separate anterior approach.[105]

Various instruments that attach to individual screws have been mentioned,[68, 80, 108] and the dorsally protruding shaft of a Schanz pin can be used in this fashion before it is cut off.[32, 113] Application of force to such screw extensions to produce realignment can be accomplished either manually or by means of an instrument. Whatever method is used, caution must be exercised so that excessive force is not placed upon any one screw, or else screw-vertebra loosening or screw bending can occur. To decrease the chance of this complication, our approach has been to develop a reduction frame that rigidly links together the right and left screws at each vertebral level, thereby producing balanced load sharing between the screws. The biomechanical relevance of this is indicated by the cadaveric testing performed by Kling et al.,[79] which shows that such cross-linked screws are more than twice as strong as a single screw alone ($P < .05$).

The use of this reduction frame (1) provides accurate control of position, (2) allows slower, more gradual reductions with less chance of excessive transient loads than might be feasible during manually performed reductions in difficult cases, (3) may be used to provide bridging between right and left screws for load equalization, (4) frees up surgical hands for other tasks, and (5) allows the implanted device to remain simple: the "tool" used for the reduction is not implanted in the patient but is returned to the "toolbox."

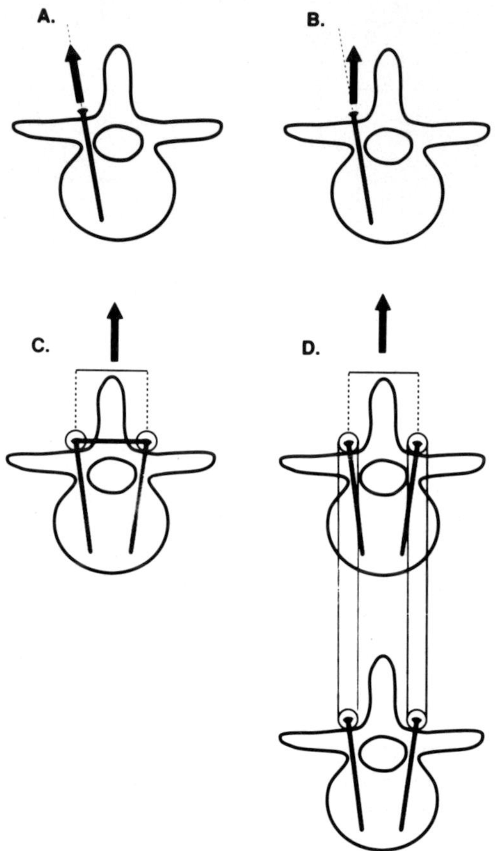

FIG 15–17.
Screw pullout test methods. **A,** pullout along the axis of the screw. This is probably not a load type commonly seen in vivo. **B,** pullout parallel to the sagittal plane more closely mimics loads produced by trunk flexion than does **A,** although the transverse connector effect of the lower vertebra (shown in **D**) is still not taken into account. **C,** transverse connector. The pullout load should be attached to the screws as shown, not to the middle of the connector, to duplicate the in vivo situation and to avoid bending the connector. The transverse connector effect of the lower vertebra (as shown in **D**), however, is missing here as well. **D,** transverse connector effect of the lower vertebra. The lower vertebra ties together the lower screws, which are attached by way of the longitudinal rods to the upper screws. The lower vertebra thereby strengthens the grip of the upper screw on the upper vertebra. This should be taken into account when measuring the effect of any implanted transverse connector. (Courtesy of C. Herndon, 1990.)

Transverse Connectors

Initially used for improving scoliosis deformity correction,[8] transverse connectors were later used for improving implant stiffness. For certain non–screw-based implants, some stiffness increase for some load types has resulted.[8, 10] For screw-based implants much remains to be learned, and some of the results so far are conflicting.

Wörsdörfer[162] compared the pullout strength of unilateral transpedicular Schanz screws with that of bilateral Schanz screws with a transverse connector. For the unilateral screw, whether the pullout was performed as shown in Figure 15–17,A or B is not clear. For the bilateral screws, the method was as shown in Figure 15–17,C. The bilateral, transversely connected screws were found to be just twice as strong as the unilateral screw, that is, there was a 0% strengthening effect per screw produced by the connector itself. This lack of strengthening was also found by Gurr and McAfee[55] for whole-implant stiffness of Cotrel-Dubousset implants for both torsion and axial compression.

Kling et al.[79] performed testing very similar to that of Wörsdörfer.[162] Here too, whether the unilateral pullout method was as shown in Figure 15–17,A or B is not clear. They found somewhat different results: the connector had a 31% strengthening effect for 4-mm Schanz screws and a 16% strengthening effect for 5-mm Schanz screws. However, intraspecimen controls and statistical analysis of significance were not reported.

Carson et al.[23] took a somewhat different approach and measured not the strength or stiffness of, but the strains on Steffee screws implanted into human cadaveric specimens in response to various loads applied to the vertebrae. They found little or no reduction in strains by the transverse connector when the screws were oriented 15 degrees or more away from the sagittal plane. That is, the connector was not carrying much load. Thus, as long as implant design or anatomic constraints do not prevent oblique screw placement, a benefit from the additional complexity and bulk of transverse connectors is not apparent.

The reason the connector did not carry much load is that the loads transmitted from the right to the left implant assembly were carried primarily by the instrumented vertebral bodies themselves. An example of this is shown in Figure 15–7. Here, resistance to lateral motion depends upon load transfer between the upper right and left screws by the upper vertebra itself and between the lower right and left screws by means of the lower vertebra. Except when the angles between pairs of screws are small, a transverse connector would add only little more resistance.

This same effect is present in response to pullout loads, as shown in Figure 15–17,D. Pulling away anteriorly of the upper vertebral body is resisted to an extent greater than twice the single-screw pullout strength (performed as shown in Figure 15–17,A or B). This additional resistance is provided by the two lower screws, which resist the tendency for the tips of the upper screws to separate during pull-away anteriorly of the upper vertebra. The lower screws are able to provide this additional resistance because they are linked together by the lower vertebra, which functions as a transverse connector, even without such a component being implanted. To understand the role of transverse connectors more fully, test results from the construct with an implanted transverse connector (shown in Figure 15–17,C) should really be compared with those from a construct without an implanted connector (Figure 15–17,D), but not to twice the value obtained from the constructs in Figure 15–17,A or B.

Whole-Implant Testing

Implant Stiffness

The stiffness level that is optimal remains to be established in terms of (1) facilitating the development of bony union, (2) preventing excessive stress shielding and related osteopenia, (3) preventing dangerous intervertebral deflections before bony union occurs, and (4) possible contribution toward an increased rate of degeneration of discs or facets at the ends of the fusion.

Optimal stiffness has not yet been established. The trade-off may well be between the likelihood of fusion and induced osteopenia, although the importance of the latter is not yet clear and presumably the latter will gradually remodel as longer-term resorption around the screws causes load shifting back to the bone graft mass. McAfee et al.[116, 117] showed a higher rate of fusion and some osteopenia with a stiffer implant. Johnston et al.[74] showed that graft stiffness varied inversely with rod stiffness. Goel and coworkers[50, 103] showed greater porosity around transpedicular screws that were less securely fixed by longitudinal plates.

Another biological issue besides fusion and osteopenia is that of whole-vertebra or vertebral-fragment motion: the stiffer the implant, the less such motion will occur. Certain limitations are imposed by the material properties: stiffer implants tend to tolerate fewer load cycles before failure (shorter fatigue life).

Finally, with regard to the increased rate of degeneration due to high implant stiffness, Hsu et al.[68, 69] have conjectured that such an effect may be present. This was based on a shorter time interval between surgery and the onset of clinically apparent degeneration in patients with Steffee plates as compared with those having bone graft alone. Alternative explanations are that the patients with Steffee plates had a greater amount of surgical dissection or actual impingement of the upper facet joint by the plates and screws, and that the stiffness of the plate itself contributed negligibly to this process.

Figure 15–18 illustrates a biomechanical argument to support this viewpoint. Along three motion segments of a normal spine (Fig 15–18,A), a specified overall amount of flexion is distributed approximately equally (33% at each motion segment). If a bone graft is added across the lower two motion segments and the same rotation is imposed (Fig 15–18,B), the bone graft will only allow a small motion to occur at the fused motion segment (perhaps 2% at each), and all the remaining motion (96%) occurs at the top motion segment. Motion at the top motion segment has thus been increased by 191% ([96%−33%]/33%).

If a flexible implant is added to the graft (Fig 15–18,C), the motion at the lower two motion segments will be further reduced, perhaps to half the previous value (down to 1% each). Although this concentrates 98% of the motion at the upper motion segment as compared with the situation in Figure 15–18,B, this represents an increase of only 2.1% ([98%−96%]/96%).

Even if a ten times stiffer implant is used (Fig 15–18,D) and the motion of the lower two motion segments is reduced to 0.1% as compared with the situation in Figure 15–18,B, the motion concentration is still increased by only 4.0% ([99.8%−96%]/96%). Since just the bone graft alone causes so much of the motion concentra-

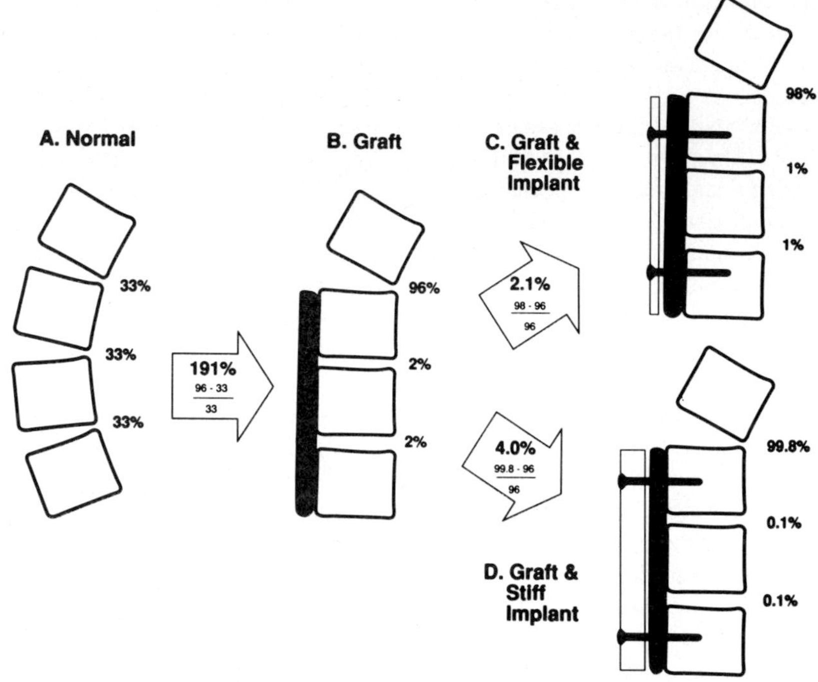

FIG 15–18.

Effect of a posterior bone graft and implant (flexible or stiff) on "motion concentration" at the motion segment immediately above the fusion. **A,** normal. Motion is evenly distributed across all three motion segments (33%, 33%, 33%). **B,** graft. For the same total motion, motion at the two lower motion segments is reduced to 2% each: 96% of the motion is "concentrated" at the upper motion segment. When compared with **A,** this is equivalent to a 191% increase at the upper motion segment. **C,** graft and flexible implant. Motion at the two lower motion segments is reduced to 1% each. Upper motion segment motion is increased to 98%. However, when compared with **B,** this is equivalent to only a 2.1% increase in motion concentration at the upper motion segment. **D,** graft and stiff implant. A very stiff implant reduces motion at the lower two motion segments to 0.1%. When compared with **B,** this still is equivalent to only a 4.0% increase in motion concentration. (Courtesy of C. Herndon, 1990.)

tion (which is closely related to stress concentration), it appears that the additional stiffness provided by the implant is not a major factor for increasing degeneration. This argument places all the more importance on avoiding damage to or implant contact with the upper facet joint during screw implantation.

Comparative Testing

A variety of vertebral levels, loading methods, performance parameters, and device comparisons have been used. These have been reviewed in detail elsewhere,[86] and thus the major findings alone will be described here.

For devices applied above the sacrum, the findings are as follows. Abumi et al.[1] found that an Ölerud external fixator, when compared with three other nonpedicle devices (Harrington compression rods, Luque rectangle, and Kaneda anterior screws and rods), was the "only device that provided sufficient stability . . . for all load types." Akbarnia et al.[4] rank-ordered the stiffness of various implants (Harrington rods without and with Edwards sleeves or wires, Luque rectangle, anterior Kaneda device without or with a cross-link, and Steffee plates) applied to calf spines. The overall greatest stiffness was from the Steffee plates. Ashman et al.[11] compared five different implants and found that all were approximately equally stiff but that higher strains were produced on screws that were securely attached to their longitudinal linking element vs. those for which some motion could occur at this junction. Ferguson et al.[45] found that a "one above–one below" VSF provided as much stiffness as "two above–two below" Jacobs rods or Harrington rods with circumlaminar wiring. In addition, they showed that the Roy-Camille plates were stiffer than the VSF rods and that both of these devices, unlike the rod-and-hook systems tested, were able to maintain lateral stability after cyclic loading. Gurr and McAfee[55] showed that a "one above–one below" Cotrel-Dubousset transpedicular implant with a rigid screw-rod connection applied to a highly unstable posterior instability model returned the overall construct stiffness back to normal. They also found that a "two above–two below" implant was even stronger than that in an intact state. Mann and coworkers[44, 114] reported that only when significant posterior disruption was present was supplementation with transfacet screws needed to bring the stiffness of the Syracuse "I" anterior plate construct up to that produced by the Dick internal fixator. Wörsdörfer[162] found that the Magerl external fixator provided greater overall positional control than any of the other nonpedicle implants studied.

Only two studies have been done that deal specifically with lumbosacral implantation of transpedicular screw-based devices. Asazuma et al.[7] used intact porcine L5, L6, L7, S1 specimens and compared Harrington distraction rods, Luque rods (Galveston technique), Steffee plates, the VSF and Zielke screws and rods without and with a Luque rectangle. They state that the VSF was "the most rigid construct overall," even though the screws were placed only into L5 and S1 (not into the intervening L6 and L7 vertebrae). Puno et al.[123] compared Luque rods (Galveston technique), the Luque rectangle, Steffee plates (without and with S2 screws), and three experimental screw-and-rod devices. Major findings included a troublesome bulkiness in the experimental articulated fixator and a substantially increased stiffness of the Steffee plate construct from the addition of a screw into the S2 lateral mass.

From these various tests, which involve a wide variety of devices, specimens, and methods, the following major conclusions may be drawn:

1. Transpedicle screw-based devices definitely convey better overall positional control than do other devices.
2. One component of this improved positional control is the improved security of the screw-pedicle/body interface vs. the hook-lamina or wire-lamina interface.
3. Devices that have secure screw-plate or screw-rod interface control can return normal stiffness to an injury model even if only one vertebra above and below the injury site is instrumented (rather than two or three above and below as with other devices).
4. When screw-vertebra interface failure occurs, it does not appear to threaten neural elements (i.e., the spinal canal and foramina remain intact).
5. The significance of different mechanical characteristics for the clinical situation needs to be kept in mind. Ultimate strength is an important measure since it may describe screw-bone failure, but stiffness is also important since the amount of deflection may affect bone or disc fragment motion.
6. The overall response of an implant to a variety of load types should be assessed since device response may be quite load type dependent and in vivo loads are likely quite varied.
7. Much remains to be learned concerning loads in vivo and the applicability of various experimental injury models to clinical situations.

REFERENCES

1. Abumi K, Panjabi MM, Duranceau J: Biomechanical evaluation of spinal fixation devices: Part III. Stability provided by six spinal fixation devices and interbody bone graft. *Spine* 1989; 14:1249–1255.
2. Aebi M, Etter C, Kehl T, et al: Stabilization of the lower thoracic and lumbar spine with the internal spinal skeletal fixation system: Indications, techniques, and first results of treatment. *Spine* 1987; 12:544–551.
3. Aebi M, Etter C, Kehl T, et al: The internal skeletal fixation system: A new treatment of thoracolumbar fractures and other spinal disorders. *Clin Orthop* 1988; 227:30–43.
4. Akbarnia BA, Merenda JT, Keppler L, et al: Surgical treatment of fractures and fracture dislocations of thoracolumbar and lumbar spine using pedicular screw and plate fixation. Presented at the 54th Annual Meeting of the American Academy of Orthopaedic Surgeons, San Francisco, 1987.
5. Ansell RH, Scales JT: A study of some factors which affect the strength of screws and their holding power in bone. *J Biomech* 1968; 1:279–302.
6. Armstrong GWD: Harrington instrumentation for spinal fractures. Presented at the Annual Meeting of the Scoliosis Research Society, Ottawa, Ontario, Canada, 1976.
7. Asazuma T, Stokes IAF, Moreland MS, et al: Intersegmental spinal flexibility with lumbosacral instrumentation: An in vitro biomechanical investigation. *Spine* 1990; 15:1153–1158.
8. Asher M, Carson W, Heinig C: A modular spinal rod linkage system to provide rotational stability. *Spine* 1988; 13:272–277.
9. Asher MA, Strippgen WE: Anthropometric studies of the human sacrum relating to dorsal transsacral implant designs. *Clin Orthop* 1986; 203:58–62.
10. Ashman RB, Birch JG, Bone LB, et al: Mechanical testing of spinal instrumentation. *Clin Orthop* 1988; 227:113–125.
11. Ashman RB, Galpin RD, Corin JD, et al: Biomechanical analysis of pedicle screw instrumentation systems in a corpectomy model. *Spine* 1989; 14:1398–1405.
12. Ashman RB, Johnson CE, Corin JD: Pedicle screw-plate function: Susceptibility to fatigue fracture. Presented at the 22nd Annual Meeting of the Scoliosis Research Society, Vancouver, 1987.
13. Baker LD, Hoyt WA: The use of interfacet Vitallium screws in the Hibbs fusion. *South Med J* 1948; 41:419–426.
14. Banta CJ, King AG, Dobezies EJ, et al: Measurement of effective pedicle diameter in the human spine. *Orthopedics* 1989; 12:939–942.
15. Bayley JC, Yuan HA, Fredrickson BE: The Syracuse I-plate. *Spine* 1991; 16(suppl):120–124.
16. Bechtol CO: Internal fixation with plates and screws, in Bechtol CO, Ferguson AB Jr, Laing PB (eds): *Metals and Engineering in Bone and Joint Surgery*. Baltimore, Williams & Wilkins, 1959, pp 152–171.
17. Berry JL, Moran JM, Berg WS, et al: A morphometric study of human lumbar and selected thoracic vertebrae. *Spine* 1987; 12:362–367.
18. Black RC, Gardner VO, Armstrong GWD, et al: A contoured anterior spinal fixation plate. *Clin Orthop* 1988; 227:135–142.
19. Blauth M, Tscherne H, Haas N: Therapeutic concept and results of operative treatment in acute trauma of the thoracic and lumbar spine: The Hannover experience. *J Orthop Trauma* 1987; 1:240–252.

20. Boucher HH: A method of spinal fusion. *J Bone Joint Surg [Br]* 1959; 41:248–259.
21. Brodsky JW, Barnes DA, Tullos HS: Unrecognized pin penetration of the hip joint. *Contemp Orthop* 1984; 9:13–20.
22. Carlson GD, Anderson DR, Abitbol JJ, et al: Screw fixation in the human sacrum: An in vitro study of the biomechanics of fixation. *Spine* 1992; 17(suppl):196–S203.
23. Carson WL, Duffield RC, Arendt M, et al: Internal forces and moments on transpedicular spine instrumentation. The effect of pedicle screw angle and transfixation: The 4R-4 bar linkage concept. Presented at the Annual Meeting of the Scoliosis Research Society, Amsterdam, 1989, pp 465–466.
24. Casey MP, Asher MA, Jacobs RR, et al: The effect of Harrington rod contouring on lumbar lordosis. *Spine* 1987; 12:750–753.
25. Chow D, Armstrong GWD, Feibel R, et al: The contoured anterior spinal plate: Design rationale and results of the first 25 cases. Proc Int Soc Study Lumbar Spine, Boston, 1990. *Orthop Trans* 1991; 15:308–309.
26. Coe JD, Warden KE, Herzig MA, et al: Influence of bone mineral density on the fixation of thoracolumbar implants: A comparative study of transpedicular screws, laminar hooks, and spinous process wires. *Spine* 1990; 15:902–908.
27. Cotrel Y, Dubousset J, Guillaumat M: New universal instrumentation in spinal surgery. *Clin Orthop* 1988; 227:10–23.
28. Daniels AU, Dunn HK: Anterior stabilization and implant system. Presented at the Annual Meeting of the Scoliosis Research Society, Seattle, 1980.
29. DeCoster T, Heetderks DB, Downey DJ, et al: Optimizing bone screw pullout force. *J Orthop Trauma* 1990; 4:169–174.
30. Denis F, Ruiz H, Searls K: Comparison between square-ended distraction rods and standard round-ended distraction rods in the treatment of thoracolumbar spinal injuries: A statistical analysis. *Clin Orthop* 1984; 189:162–167.
31. Dick W: *Innere Fixation von Brust- und Lendenwirbelfrakturen*. Bern, Switzerland, Hans Huber Verlag, 1984, pp 1–125.
32. Dick W: The "fixateur interne" as a versatile implant for spine surgery. *Spine* 1987; 12:882–900.
33. Dick W, Kluger P, Magerl F, et al: A new device for internal fixation of thoracolumbar and lumbar spine fractures: The "fixateur interne." *Paraplegia* 1985; 23:225–232.
34. Diehl K, Hanser U, Hort W, et al: Biomechanische Untersuchungen über die maximalen Vorspannkräfte der Knochenschrauben in verschiedenen Knochenabschnitten. *Acta Orthop Unfallchirurg* 1974; 80:89.
35. Dohring EJ, Krag MH, Johnson CC: Sacral screw fixation: A morphologic, anatomic and mechanical study. Presented at the Annual Meeting of the North American Spine Society, Monterey, Calif, 1990.
36. Drummond DW, Guadagni J, Keene JS, et al: Interspinous process segmental spinal instrumentation. *J Pediatr Orthop* 1984; 4:397–404.
37. Dunn HK, Daniels AU, McBride GG: Comparative assessment of the spine stability achieved with a new anterior spine fixation system. Presented at the 26th Annual Meeting of the Orthopaedic Research Society, Atlanta, 1980, p 192.
38. Edwards CC: Sacral fixation device: Design and preliminary results. Presented at the 19th Annual Meeting of the Scoliosis Research Society, Orlando, Fla, 1984.
39. Edwards CC: Spinal screw fixation of the lumbar and sacral spine: Early results treating the first 50 cases. Presented at the 21st Annual Meeting of the Scoliosis Research Society, Hamilton, Bermuda, 1986, p 99.
40. Edwards CC, Griffith P, Levine AM, et al: Early clinical results using the spinal rod sleeve method for treating thoracic and lumbar injuries. Presented at the Annual Meeting of the American Academy of Orthopaedic Surgeons, New Orleans, 1982.
41. Edwards CC, Levine AM: Early rod-sleeve stabilization of the injured thoracic and lumbar spine. *Orthop Clin North Am* 1986; 17:121–145.
42. El-Khoury GY, McWilliams FE: A simple radiological aid in the diagnosis of small avulsion fractures of the knee. *J Trauma* 1978; 18:275–277.
43. Esses SI, Botsford DJ, Huler RJ, et al: Surgical anatomy of the sacrum: A guide for rational screw fixation. *Spine* 1991; 16(suppl):283–288.
44. Falahee M, Mann K, Yuan H, et al: Biomechanical evaluation of augmented anterior and posterior short segment internal fixation for thoracolumbar burst fractures. Presented at the International Society for the Study of the Lumbar Spine, Miami, 1988.
45. Ferguson RL, Tencer AF, Woodard P, et al: Biomechanical comparisons of spinal fracture models and the stabilizing effects of posterior instrumentations. *Spine* 1988; 13:453–460.
46. Gardner ADH: Four years experience with an anterior spinal distraction device for the correction of kyphotic deformities, and its use as a permanent implant. Presented at the 17th Annual Meeting of the Scoliosis Research Society, Denver, 1982, p 122.
47. Geiger JM, Udovic NA, Berry JL: Bending and fatigue of spine plates and rods, and fatigue of pedicle screws. Presented at the Annual Meeting of the American Academy of Orthopaedic Surgeons, Las Vegas, 1989.
48. George DC, Krag MH, Johnson CC, et al: Hole preparation techniques (drill versus probe) for transpedicular screws: Effect upon pullout strength from human cadaveric vertebrae. *Spine* 1991; 16:181–184.
49. Gertzbein SD, MacMichael D, Tile M: Harrington instrumentation as a method of fixation in fractures of the spine: A critical analysis of deficiencies. *J Bone Joint Surg [Br]* 1982; 64:526–529.
50. Goel VJ, Lim TH, Gwon J, et al: Effects of rigidity of an internal fixation device: A comprehensive biomechanical investigation. *Spine* 1991; 16(suppl):155–161.

51. Goel VJ, Weinstein JN: *Biomechanics of the Spine: Clinical and Surgical Perspective*. Boca Raton, Fla, CRC Press, 1990, pp 1–295.
52. Grob D, Magerl F, McGowan D: Letter to the editor. *Spine* 1990; 15:3, 251.
53. Grobler LJ, Kempff PG, Gaines RW Jr: Comparing mersilene tape and stainless steel wire during segmental spinal instrumentation—evaluation of the macroscopical and microscopical tissue response in the baboon. Proc Scoliosis Res Soc Ann Mtg, Vancouver, BC, 1987. *Orthop Trans* 1988; 2:239.
54. Grobler LJ, Neale G, Wilder DG, et al: Anterior interbody stabilization with metal molds and cadaveric (allograft) bone: An experimental comparative investigation (6 month followup). Presented at the Annual Meeting of the American Academy of Orthopaedic Surgeons, New Orleans, 1990.
55. Gurr KR, McAfee PC: Cotrel-Dubousset instrumentation in adults: A preliminary report. *Spine* 1988; 13:510–520.
56. Guyer DW, Wiltse LL, Peek RD: The Wiltse pedicle screw fixation system. *Orthopedics* 1988; 11:1455–1460.
57. Haas N, Blauth M, Tscherne H: Anterior plating in thoracolumbar spine injuries: Indication, technique, and results. *Spine* 1991; 16(suppl):100–111.
58. Hadra BE: The classic: Wiring of the vertebrae as a means of immobilization in fractures and Potts' disease. *Clin Orthop* 1975; 112:4–8.
59. Hadra BE: Wiring of the spinous process in injury and Potts' disease. *Trans Am Orthop Assoc* 1891; 4:206.
60. Hall DJ, Webb JK: Anterior plate fixation in spine tumor surgery: Indications, technique, and results. *Spine* 1991; 16(suppl):80–83.
61. Hall JE: Dwyer instrumentation in anterior fusion of the spine: Current concepts review. *J Bone Joint Surg [Am]* 1981; 63:1188–1190.
62. Harrington PR: The history and development of Harrington instrumentation. *Clin Orthop* 1973; 93:110–112.
63. Harrington PR: Treatment of scoliosis: Correction and internal fixation by spine instrumentation. *J Bone Joint Surg [Am]* 1962; 44:591–610.
64. Harrington PR, Tullos HS: Reduction of severe spondylolisthesis in children. *South Med J* 1969; 62:1–7.
65. Heggeness MH, Esses SI: Translaminar facet joint screw fixation for lumbar and lumbosacral fusion: A clinical and biomechanical study. *Spine* 1991; 16(suppl):266–269.
66. Herrmann HD: Transarticular (transpedicular) metal plate fixation for stabilization of the lumbar and thoracic spine. *Acta Neurochirurg (Wien)* 1979; 48:101–110.
67. Horowitch A, Peek RD, Thomas JC, et al: The Wiltse pedicle screw fixation system: Early clinical results. *Spine* 1989; 14:461–467.
68. Hsu K, Zucherman JF, White AH, et al: Internal fixation with pedicle screws, in White AH, Rothman RH, Ray CD (eds): *Lumbar Spine Surgery: Techniques and Complications*. St Louis, Mosby–Year Book, 1987, pp 332–338.
69. Hsu KY, Zucherman J, White A, et al: Deterioration of motion segments adjacent to lumbar spine fusions. Presented at the Annual Meeting of the North American Spine Society, Colorado Springs, 1988.
70. Humphries AW, Hawk WA, Berndt AL: Anterior interbody fusion of lumbar vertebrae: A surgical technique. *Surg Clin North Am* 1961; 41:1685–1700.
71. Jacobs RR, Jauch EC, Jacobs CK, et al: Sacral and lumbar pedicle fixation: A biomechanical evaluation. Presented at the 33rd Annual Meeting of the Orthopaedic Research Society, San Francisco, 1987, p 382.
72. Jacobs RR, Nordwall A, Nachemson A: Stability and strength provided by internal fixation systems for dorsolumbar spinal injuries. *Clin Orthop* 1982; 171:300–308.
73. Jacobs RR, Schlaepfer F, Mathys R Jr, et al: A locking hook spinal rod system for stabilization of fracture dislocations and correction of deformities of the dorsolumbar spine: A biomechanic evaluation. *Clin Orthop* 1984; 189:168–177.
74. Johnston CE, Ashman RB, Baird AM, et al: Effect of spinal construct stiffness on early fusion mass incorporation: Experimental study. *Spine* 1990; 15:908–912.
75. Kaneda K, Abumi K, Fujiya M: Burst fractures with neurologic deficits of the thoracolumbar spine: Results of anterior decompression and stabilization with anterior instrumentation. *Spine* 1984; 9:788–795.
76. Kaneda K, Asano S, Hashimoto T, et al: Reconstruction of thoraco-lumbar spine with a bio-active ceramic vertebral spacer and the anterior spinal instrumentation. Proc Int Soc Study Lumbar Spine, Boston, 1990. *Orthop Trans* 1991; 15:308.
77. King D: Internal fixation for lumbosacral fusion. *Am J Surg* 1944; 66:357–361.
78. Kleeman BC, Gerhart TN, Hayes WC: Augmenting screw fixation in osteopenic trabecular bone. Presented at the Annual Meeting of the Society of Biomaterials, New York, 1987.
79. Kling TF Jr, Vanderby R Jr, Belloli DM, et al: Cross-linked pedicle screw fixation in the same vertebral body: A biomechanical study. Presented at the 21st Annual Meeting of the Scoliosis Research Society, Hamilton, Bermuda, 1986.
80. Kluger P, Gerner HJ: Das mechanische Prinzip des Fixateur Externe zur dorsalen Stabilisierung der Brust- und Lendenwirbelsäule. *Unfallchirurgie* 1986; 12:68–79.
81. Koranyi E, Bowman CE, Knecht CD, et al: Holding power of orthopaedic screws in bone. *Clin Orthop* 1970; 72:283–286.
82. Kostuik JP: Anterior fixation for burst fractures of the thoracic and lumbar spine with or without neurological involvement. *Spine* 1988; 13:286–293.
83. Kostuik JP: Anterior fixation for fractures of the thoracic and lumbar spine with or without neurologic involvement. *Clin Orthop* 1984; 189:103–115.
84. Kostuik JP: Anterior Kostuik-Harrington distractions systems for the treatment of kyphotic deformities. *Spine* 1991; 15:169–180.
85. Krag MH: Biomechanics of thoracolumbar spinal fixation: A review. *Spine* 1991; 16(suppl):84–99.

86. Krag MH: Biomechanics of transpedicle spinal fixation, in Weinstein JN, Wiesel S (eds): *The Lumbar Spine*. Philadelphia, WB Saunders, 1990, pp 916–940.
87. Krag MH: Lumbosacral fixation with the Vermont Spinal Fixator, in Lin PM, Gill K (eds): *Lumbar Interbody Fusion: Principles and Techniques of Spine Surgery*. Rockville, Md, Aspen Systems, 1988, pp 251–260.
88. Krag MH: Spine fusion: Overview of options and posterior internal fixation devices, in Frymoyer JW (ed): *The Adult Spine: Principles and Practice*. New York, Raven Press, 1991, pp 1919–1945.
89. Krag MH: The Vermont Spinal Fixator. *Spine State Art Rev* 1992; 6:121–145.
90. Krag MH, Beynnon BD, DeCoster TA, et al: Depth of insertion of transpedicular vertebral screws into human vertebrae: Effect upon screw-vertebra interface strength. *J Spinal Disorders* 1988; 1:287–294.
91. Krag MH, Beynnon BD, Frymoyer JW, et al: Fatigue testing of an internal fixator for posterior spinal stabilization. Presented at the 54th Annual Meeting of the American Academy of Orthopaedic Surgeons, San Francisco, 1987.
92. Krag MH, Beynnon BD, Pope MH, et al: An internal fixator for posterior application to short segments of the thoracic, lumbar, or lumbosacral spine: Design and testing. *Clin Orthop* 1986; 203:75–98.
93. Krag MH, Frymoyer JW, Beynnon BD, et al: An internal fixator for posterior application to short segments of the thoracic, lumbar, or lumbosacral spine: Design and testing, in White AH, Rothman RH, and Ray CD (eds): *Lumbar Spine Surgery: Techniques and Complications*. St Louis, Mosby–Year Book, 1987, pp 339–367.
94. Krag MH, Weaver DL, Beynnon BD, et al: Morphometry of the thoracic and lumbar spine related to transpedicular screw placement for surgical spinal fixation. *Spine* 1988; 13:27–32.
95. Krag MH, Van Hal ME, Beynnon BD: Placement of transpedicular vertebral screws close to anterior vertebral cortex: Description of methods. *Spine* 1989; 14: 879–883.
96. LaGrone MO: Loss of lumbar lordosis. A complication of spinal fusion for scoliosis. *Orthop Clin North Am* 1988; 19:383–393.
97. Lange F: Support for the spondylytic spine by means of buried steel bars attached to the vertebrae. *Am J Orthop Surg* 1910; 8:344–361.
98. Lange F: Support for the spondylytic spine by means of buried steel bars attached to the vertebrae (reprinted from the original). *Clin Orthop* 1986; 203:3–6.
99. Lavaste F: Biomechanique du rachis dorso-lombaire. *Deuxieme Journees d'Orthopedie de la Pitie* 1980; 2: 19–23.
100. Lavaste F: *Etude des Implants Rachidiens. Mémoire de Biomechanique* (thesis: "Ingeneur"). Ecole Nationale Supérieure des Arts et Metiers à Paris, 1977.
101. Lehman WB, Grant A, Rose D, et al: A method of evaluating possible pin penetration in slipped capital femoral epiphysis using a cannulated internal fixation device. *Clin Orthop* 1984; 186:65–70.
102. Levine AM, Edwards CC: Low lumbar burst fractures. *Orthopedics* 1988; 11:1427–1432.
103. Lim TH, Goel VJ, Park JB, et al: Quantification of the stress-induced bone porosity as a function of the rigidity of a fixation device—a canine study. International Society for the Study of the Lumbar Spine, Boston, 1990. *Orthop Trans* 1991; 15:309.
104. Liu YK, Njus GO, Bahr PA, et al: Fatigue life improvement of nitrogen-ion implanted pedicle screws. *Spine* 1990; 15:311–317.
105. Louis R: Fusion of the lumbar and sacral spine by internal fixation with screw plates. *Clin Orthop* 1986; 203:18–33.
106. Luque ER: Anatomic basis and development of segmental spinal instrumentation. *Spine* 1982; 7:256–259.
107. Luque ER, Cassis N, Ramirez-Wiella G: Segmental spinal instrumentation in the treatment of fractures of the thoracolumbar spine. *Spine* 1982; 7:312–317.
108. Luque ER, Rapp GF: A new semirigid method for interpedicular fixation of the spine. *Orthopedics* 1988; 11:1445–1450.
109. Lyon WF, Cochran JR, Smith L: Actual holding power of various screws in bone. *Ann Surg* 1941; 114:376–384.
110. Magerl F: Clinical application on the thoracolumbar junction and the lumbar spine, in Mears DC (ed): *External Skeletal Fixation*. Baltimore, Williams & Wilkins, 1983, pp 553–575.
111. Magerl F: External skeletal fixation of the lower thoracic and the lumbar spine, in Uhthoff HK, Stahl E (eds): *Current Concepts of External Fixation of Fractures*. New York, Springer-Verlag, 1982, pp 353–366.
112. Magerl F: External spinal skeletal fixation, in Weber BG, Magerl F (eds): *The External Fixator*. New York, Springer-Verlag, 1985, pp 290–365.
113. Magerl FP: Stabilization of the lower thoracic and lumbar spine with external skeletal fixation. *Clin Orthop* 1984; 189:125–141.
114. Mann KA, McGowan DP, Fredrickson BE, et al: Biomechanical investigation of short segment spinal fixation for burst fractures with varying degrees of posterior disruption. *Spine* 1990; 15:470–473.
115. Martin D, Cordey J, Rahn BA, et al: Bone screw displacement under lateral loading. Presented at the Second Meeting of the European Society of Biomechanics, Strasbourg, France, 1979.
116. McAfee PC, Farey ID, Sutterlin CE, et al: Device-related osteoporosis with spinal instrumentation. *Spine* 1989; 14:919–926.
117. McAfee PC, Farey ID, Sutterlin CE, et al: The effect of spinal implant rigidity on vertebral bone density: a canine model. *Spine* 1991; 16(suppl):190–197.
118. Mirkovic S, Abitbol JJ, Steinman J, et al: Anatomic consideration for sacral screw placement. *Spine* 1991; 16(suppl):289–294.
119. Moe JH, Denis F: The iatrogenic loss of lumbar lordosis. Proceedings of the Scoliosis Research Society 11th Annual Meeting. 1976. *Orthop Trans* 1977; 1:131.
120. Moran JM, Berg WS, Berry JL, et al: Transpedicular screw fixation. *J Orthop Res* 1989; 7:107–114.

121. Ölerud S, Karlström G, Sjöström L: Transpedicular fixation of thoracolumbar vertebral fractures. *Clin Orthop* 1988; 227:44–51.
122. Pfeifer BA, Krag MH, Johnson CC: Repair of failed pedicle screw fixation: A biomechanical study comparing polymethylmethacylate, morselized bone, and matchstick bone reconstruction. Presented to the American Academy of Orthopaedic Surgeons, Washington, D.C., 1992.
123. Puno RM, Bechtold JE, Byrd JE, et al: Biomechanical analysis of five techniques of fixation for the lumbosacral junction. Presented at the 33rd Annual Meeting of the Orthopaedic Research Society, San Francisco, 1987, p 366.
124. Rao SC, Mou ZS, Hu YZ, et al: The IVBF dual-blade plate and its applications. *Spine* 1991; 16(suppl):112–119.
125. Reimers C: Die dorsale Spannverstrebung von Wirbelsäulenabschnitten mittels innerer Schienung. *Chirurgie* 1956; 17:10–16.
126. Resina J, Alves AF: Technique of correction and internal fixation for scoliosis. *J Bone Joint Surg [Br]* 1977; 59:159–165.
127. Rezaian SM, Dombrowski ET, Ghista TDN, et al: Spinal fixator for surgical treatment of spinal injury. *Orthop Rev* 1983; 12:31–41.
128. Robbins S, Gertzbein S: Accuracy of pedicle screw placement in vivo. Presented at Annual Meeting of the Orthopaedic Trauma Association, Dallas, 1987, pp 27–28.
129. Rooks MD, Schmitt EW, Drvaric DM: Unrecognized pin penetration in slipped capital femoral epiphysis. *Clin Orthop* 1988; 234:82–89.
130. Roy-Camille R: Experience with Roy-Camille fixation for the thoracolumbar and lumbar spine. Acute spinal injuries: Current management techniques. University of Massachusetts Continuing Medical Education Course, Sturbridge, Mass, 1987.
131. Roy-Camille R, Demeulenaere C: Ostéosynthèse ju rachis dorsal, lombaire et lombo-sacré par plaque métalliques vissées dans les pédicules vertébraux et es apophyses articulaires. *Presse Med* 1970; 78:1447–1448.
132. Roy-Camille R, Saillant G, Berteaux D, et al: Early management of spinal injuries, in McKibbin B (ed): *Recent Advances in Orthopaedics*. New York, Churchill Livingstone, 1979.
133. Roy-Camille R, Saillant G, Berteaux D, et al: Osteosynthesis of thoraco-lumbar spine fractures with metal plates screwed through the vertebral pedicles. *Reconstr Surg Traumatol* 1976; 15:2–16.
134. Roy-Camille R, Saillant G, Berteaux D, et al: Vertebral osteosynthesis using metal plates. Its different uses. *Chirurgie* 1979; 105:597–603.
135. Roy-Camille R, Saillant G, Marie-Anne S, et al: Behandlung von Wirbelfrakturen und -luxation am thorakolumbalen Übergang. *Orthopaedie* 1980; 9:63–68.
136. Roy-Camille R, Saillant G, Mazel C: Internal fixation of the lumbar spine with pedicle screw plating. *Clin Orthop* 1986; 203:7–17.
137. Ryan MD, Taylor TKF, Sherwood AA: Bolt-plate fixation for anterior spinal fusion. *Clin Orthop* 1986; 203:196–202.
138. Ryan MD, Taylor TKF, Sherwood AA: New instrumentation for anterior lumbar and thoracolumbar interbody spinal fusion. Presented at the Scoliosis Research Society, Chicago, 1981.
139. Saillant G: Etude anatomique des pédicules vertébraux: Application chirurgicale. *Rev Chir Orthop* 1976; 62:151–160.
140. Schatzker J, Sanderson R, Murnaghan PJ: The holding power of orthopaedic screws in vivo. *Clin Orthop* 1975; 108:115–126.
141. Schreiber A, Suezawa Y, Jacob HAC: Preliminary report of 40 patients. Dorsal spinal fusion with a transpedicular distraction and compression system. *Orthop Rev* 1986; 15:93–96.
142. Scoles PV, Linton AE, Latimer B, et al: Vertebral body and posterior element morphology: The normal spine in middle life. *Spine* 1988; 14:1082.
143. Sell P, Collins M, Dove J: Pedicle screws: Axial pullout strength in the lumbar spine [briefly noted]. *Spine* 1988; 13:1075–1076.
144. Shaw JA: Preventing unrecognized pin penetration into hip joint. *Orthop Rev* 1984; 13:142–152.
145. Skinner R, Maybee J, Transfeldt E, et al: Experimental pullout testing and comparison of variables in transpedicular screw fixation: A biomechanical study. *Spine* 1990; 15:195–201.
146. Steffee AD, Biscup RS, Sitkowski DJ: Segmental spine plates with pedicle screw fixation: A new internal fixation device for disorders of lumbar and thoracolumbar spine. *Clin Orthop* 1986; 203:45–53.
147. Steffee AD, Sitkowski DJ: Posterior lumbar interbody fusion and plates. *Clin Orthop* 1988; 227:99–102.
148. Straub LR: Lumbosacral fusion by metallic fixation and grafts. *J Bone Joint Surg [Br]* 1949; 31:478.
149. Thalgott JS, LaRocca H, Aebi M, et al: Reconstruction of the lumbar spine using AO DCP plate internal fixation. *Spine* 1989; 14:91–95.
150. Thompson WAL, Ralston EL: Pseudarthrosis following spine fusion. *J Bone Joint Surg [Am]* 1949; 31:400–405.
151. Toumey JW: Internal fixation in fusion of the lumbo-sacral joints. *Lahey Clin Bull* 1943; 3:188–191.
152. Volz RG, Martin MD: Illusory biplane radiographic images. *Radiology* 1977; 122:695–697.
153. Waisbrod H, Gerbershagen HU: A pilot study of the value of ceramics for bone replacement. *Arch Orthop Trauma Surg* 1986; 105:298–301.
154. Walters R, Simon SR: Joint destruction: A sequel of unrecognized pin penetration in patients with slipped capital femoral epiphysis, in *Proceedings of the Eighth Open Scientific Meeting of the Hip Society*. St Louis, Mosby–Year Book, 1980.
155. Weinstein JN, Spratt KF, Spengler D, et al: Spinal pedicle fixation: Reliability and validity of roentgenogram-based assessment and surgical factors on successful screw placement. *Spine* 1988; 13:1012–1018.
156. Werlinich M: Anterior interbody fusion and stabilization with metal fixation. *Intern Surg* 1974; 59:269–273.
157. White AA III, Panjabi MM: *Clinical Biomechanics of the*

Spine, ed 2. Philadelphia, JB Lippincott, 1990, pp 1–722.
158. Whitecloud TS III, Butler JC, Cohen JL, et al: Complications with the Variable Spinal Plating system. *Spine* 1989; 14:472–476.
159. Williams EWM: Traumatic paraplegia, in Matthews DN (ed): *Recent Advances in Surgery of Trauma.* New York, Churchill Livingstone, 1963, pp 171–186.
160. Wilson PD, Straub LR: Lumbosacral fusion with metallic-plate fixation. *Instr Course Lect* 1952; 9:53–57.
161. Winter RB: Harrington instrumentation into the lumbar spine: Technique for preservation of normal lumbar lordosis. *Spine* 1986; 11:633–635.
162. Wörsdörfer O: *Operative Stabilisierung der thorakolumbalen und lumbalen Wirbelsäule: Vergleichende biomechanische Untersuchungen zur Stabilität und Steifigkeit verschiedener dorsaler Fixations-Systems* (thesis). Medizinisch-Naturwissenschaftliche Hochschule der Universität Ulm, 1981
163. Yuan HA, Mann KA, Found EM, et al: Early clinical experience with the Syracuse I-Plate: An anterior spinal fixation device. *Spine* 1988; 13:278–285.
164. Zindrick MR, Patwardhan A, Lorenz M: Effect of methylmethacrylate augmentation upon pedicle screw fixation in the spine. Presented at the International Society for the Study of the Lumbar Spine, Dallas, 1986.
165. Zindrick MR, Wiltse LL, Doornik A, et al: Analysis of the morphometric characteristics of the thoracic and lumbar pedicles. *Spine* 1987; 12:160–166.
166. Zindrick MR, Wiltse LL, Holland WR, et al: Biomechanical study of intrapedicular screw fixation in the lumbosacral spine. Presented at the Annual Meeting of the International Society for the Study of the Lumbar Spine, Sydney, Australia, 1985.
167. Zindrick MR, Wiltse LL, Widell EH, et al: Biomechanical study of interpedicular screw fixation in the lumbosacral spine. *Clin Orthop* 1986; 203:99–111.

16

Obtaining Spinal Stability

Charles C. Edwards, M.D., Thomas J. Kleeman, M.D.

Long-term spinal stability is most effectively achieved by directly opposing the forces of deformation to restore and maintain normal axial alignment. For the surgeon, this requires an understanding of the origins of instability and deformity, familiarity with stabilization techniques, and a set of biomechanical principles for planning an effective spinal reconstruction.

NORMAL SPINE MECHANICS

The forces of gravity and muscle contraction load the spine in all directions. In the normal spine, these loads are counterbalanced by opposing loads, spinal posture, and key anatomic structures in a delicate balance that provides a flexible, yet stable structural center for the human body. The two most troublesome forces that traverse the spine are anterior flexion and shear.

The body's center of gravity passes anterior to most regions of the spine. The center of rotation for most vertebrae is near the posterior cortex of the vertebral body.[52] The resulting flexion moment (rotational force) subjects the anterior column (vertebral bodies and discs) to compressive loading and the posterior ligaments to tensile loading. The extensor muscles, posterior ligaments, and anterior column work together to counterbalance the flexion moment and prevent kyphotic deformity.

Gravity and anterior muscle groups also act to translate individual vertebrae anteriorly. Facet joints serve as a buttress to limit both anterior and lateral translation at all levels of the spine except the upper cervical region, where translational forces are contained by the geometry of the occipital condyles at Oc–C1 and the odontoid process/transverse ligament complex at C1–2.

Whereas the anterior column, posterior ligaments, and facets provide fixed limits to the range of intervertebral motion, the paraspinal muscles serve to balance the normal forces crossing the spine. The effectiveness of these muscle groups is a function of posture. Postural curvatures such as lordosis and kyphosis increase the moment arm and hence the mechanical advantage of muscles on the concavity. Accordingly, lumbar lordosis makes it possible for the extensor muscles of the lower part of the spine to effectively counterbalance the flexion moment generated by the anteriorly displaced, upper-body center of gravity.

SPINE PATHOMECHANICS

Origins of Instability

Muscle Weakness

When the effectiveness of the counterbalancing muscles about the spine is compromised, spinal structures are subjected to greater loads. Paraspinous muscle effectiveness can be disrupted by postural deformity or muscle destruction. For example, if lumbar lordosis is lost, the extensor moment arm for the lumbar paraspinous muscles is greatly reduced, and they are less able to negate the large flexion forces traversing the spine. Sufficient kyphotic deformity can render the posterior stabilizing muscles essentially ineffective. Paraspinal muscle resection, radiation necrosis, ischemic necrosis from surgery, or dysfunction from denervation all reduce or eliminate the paraspinous counterbalance to flexion or other forces crossing the spine. As a result, the disc and facets are subjected to greater forward or lateral bending and shear forces. These abnormal forces can initiate or accelerate degenerative processes.

Axial Degeneration

Degenerative changes in the disc and facets lessen their stabilizing effectiveness. Disc degeneration is associated with a loss of proteoglycan and water, the two constituents primarily responsible for preservation of disc height and elasticity.[107] Without this elasticity, the anterior column is less able to resist compressive loading. Facet synovitis from overload or etiology destroys facet articular cartilage and may cause bony erosion to compromise the buttressing role of the facets. The result is an increased range of translational and axial motion across the affected vertebral motion segment. This abnormal motion leads to the "degenerative cascade" described by Kirkaldy-Willis and Farfan.[63] It may stimulate local nerves directly or through the emission of neural peptides to cause pain as discussed in Chapter 13.

Loss of Structures

Progression of instability from degenerative change is gradual and occurs over years. On the other hand, the onset of instability may be rapid, as in the case of trauma, infection, tumor destruction, or decompressive surgery. For example, flexion-compression injuries to the spine fracture the vertebral body and disrupt the posterior spinal ligaments to obliterate the two primary structures that limit the normal flexion forces working across the vertebral column. Likewise, metastatic disease and infection usually begin in the vertebral body and erode the structural integrity of the anterior column and its ability to resist flexion forces and their compressive effects. The facets are at the most risk from decompressive surgery. Adequate decompression of lateral recess stenosis mandates at least partial facetectomy. If the buttressing effectiveness of one or both facets is compromised at a time when segmental degenerative change has already created threshold instability, pain and listhesis are likely to follow.

Susceptible Zones

Certain regions of the spine are far more susceptible to instability than others. Susceptible zones often lie adjacent to structures such as the head, thorax, and pelvis, which are characterized by concentration of weight and relative rigidity. Their length becomes a moment arm (rotational lever arm) for the deforming forces, thus magnifying the effect of these forces on adjacent vertebral segments. Accordingly, degenerative change or trauma and resultant instability are most likely to occur in the upper part of the cervical spine (C1–2), the lower part of the cervical spine (C5–6), the thoracolumbar junction (T12–L2), or the lumbosacral junction (L4–S1). Long fusions can have a similar effect by concentrating forces that would normally be dissipated across several movable linkages at the first open joint on either side of the long fusion.

Origins of Deformity

Flexion Instability

As discussed above, loss of spinal musculature or facilitating posture can subject spinal structures to increased loads. Increased loads can accelerate degenerative change. Degeneration, gross trauma, tumor, infection, or surgical resection can destroy the stabilizing spinal structures. Without these protective structures, the *normal* forces acting across the spine become *deforming* forces. The *direction* of the deformity is determined by which structure(s) are compromised and the orientation of the spine at the level of instability.

The relationship between planes of instability, vertebral orientation, and resulting deformity can be seen in many common clinical scenarios. In the flexion-compression injury illustration, a vertebral body fracture allows the proximal part of the spine to rotate into flexion about its axis near the posterior body cortex. When the patient stands, the upper-body center of gravity is thus shifted anteriorly to produce a much greater flexion moment arm and, therefore, a much greater flexion force working against the fractured vertebra. Any initial kyphosis associated with the injury lessens the effectiveness of the posterior extensor muscles in counteracting this flexion moment. If the vertebral body fracturing is extensive and/or there is attenuation of the posterior ligamentous checkreins, progressive kyphosis is predictable.

Flexion instability can occur even without vertebral body fracture. Flexion-*distraction* forces may attenuate the posterior ligaments and tear the posterior portion of the anulus. Postinjury films may show little or no kyphosis. However, if the disruption occurs at the thoracolumbar junction where the spine is subjected to a considerable flexion moment, breakdown of the disc with a slight loss in anterior height may compound the flexion instability and allow anterior translation (listhesis) and kyphosis.

Rotational Instability

An asymmetrical load to the head, thorax, or pelvis can fracture a facet and disrupt the posterior ligaments and/or the annulus to leave residual instability in rotation. A common example is a unilateral facet fracture-subluxation in the neck. With loss of the facet buttress, the proximal part of the spine rotates anteriorly on the side of the fractured facet. This rotational instability often leads to foraminal narrowing and chronic pain.[88]

Anterior Shear Instability

Pars disruption in a lordotic portion of the spine allows anterior slippage of the proximal part of the spine. A pars defect cleaves the inferior facets from the rest of the vertebral body. The inferior facets hook over the superior facets of the vertebra below to block anterior translation. With erosive change of the facet joint or, worse yet, its removal or cleavage from the vertebral body in the case of a pars defect, the spine develops anterior translational instability.

Forward slippage after a hangman's fracture, degenerative L4–5 listhesis, or isthmic spondylolisthesis are all examples of deformity following the onset of anterior shear instability. C2 will slip forward on C3 after a C2 pars fracture (hangman's fracture) due to the flexion moment generated by the weight of the anteriorly displaced head. In the same manner, the lumbar spine will shift anteriorly on the sacrum when a pars defect occurs at L5 (isthmic spondylolisthesis). The potential slippage of the lower part of the lumbar spine is much greater because of the forward tilt of the lower lumbar vertebrae. Patients with a high degree of sacral lordosis therefore have spines more inclined to slip forward than do those with a relatively horizontal S1 end plate.

Lateral Instability

Facet erosion or resection renders the spine potentially unstable to lateral translation. When the base vertebral body is level and the lateral musculature is evenly balanced, lateral listhesis rarely occurs. However, if there is even a small degree of base vertebral obliquity (scoliosis), lateral listhesis with associated rotation is likely.

Posterior Listhesis

Retrolisthesis is usually the product of degenerative axial loss combined with compensatory lumbar lordosis. A combination of disc degeneration and facet erosion yields axial instability. Progressing inferiorly, most facets have an anterior-to-posterior inclination. Therefore, when the spine settles (axial shortening), it is directed slightly posteriorly by the orientation of the facets.

Significant retrolisthesis rarely occurs unless there is abnormal, usually compensatory, lordosis. For example, if a lumbosacral fusion leaves the lower part of the lumbar spine hypolordotic, the upper portion of the lumbar spine will hyperextend in an effort to maintain sagittal spine alignment (compensatory lordosis). This places the extension moment for the posterior spinal muscles at a mechanical advantage. The posterior pull of these muscles may be further accentuated by spasm. The combination of axial instability, the posteroinferior inclination of the facets, and an exaggerated posterior pull from the extensor muscles result in progressive retrolisthesis with foraminal impingement. Instrumented scoliosis fusions that extend across the lumbar lordosis to L4 or L5 and flatten the lumbar spine will also cause compensatory hyperlordosis and resulting painful retrolisthesis at the first open distal interspace. From an analysis of the data presented in papers on long scoliosis fusions, it appears that the degree of iatrogenic lumbar hypolordosis was a more important factor than fusion length in accelerating distal segment degeneration.[16, 54] In most cases studied, the instrumented hypolordosis was compensated by distal hyperlordosis to restore the near-normal overall lumbar lordosis required for sagittal balance.

A STRATEGY FOR RESTORING STABILITY

Stability implies freedom from abnormal spinal motion and its sequelae of chronic pain, neural compromise, or progressive deformity. To restore stability, we must therefore stop abnormal motion and prevent future loss of alignment. Instability and deformity usually result from the loss or compromise of stabilizing structures. Hence, most instabilities can be effectively treated either by replacing the stabilizing structures or by opposing the deforming forces. Surgical ethics requires that we select the approach that involves the least amount of surgery and risk for each case.

Replace Stabilizing Structures

Anterior Column Loss

The anterior column can be reconstructed with either bone grafts and/or reinforced methylmethacrylate. This will usually suffice if the posterior structures (ligaments, extensor muscles, and facets) are unimpaired. If there is equivocal posterior instability, supplemental anterior fixation is advisable. The simplest fixation option in the thoracic and lumbar spines is compression across the anterior graft or spacer by using a spinal rod attached to the adjacent vertebral bodies with spinal screws. In the cervical spine an anterior plate attached to adjacent vertebral bodies with screws provides effective fixation. With complete posterior ligamentous disruption, some surgeons will attempt anterior fixation with more complex fixators such as the Dunn[21] or Kaneda devices[61] for the thoracolumbar spine or a graft and plate for the cervical spine.[5] However, most spine trauma surgeons advise concurrent posterior fixation.

Posterior Spinal Ligamentous Disruption

The posterior ligaments function as a tension band or checkrein. This function is effectively replaced with posterior compression instrumentation. Short-segment compression rods are most effective. Low-profile L-shaped spinal hooks that will not project into the canal are placed over the lamina above the disruption and under the lamina below it. Normal interlaminar distance is restored by shortening (compressing) ratcheted rods between the hooks.[24, 29] When laminae are fractured, an effective tension band can be constructed by using pedicle screws connected by rods or plates.

Facet Loss

Replacement of facets can be more complicated. Magerl developed a facet plate for the cervical spine that relies on one point of distal screw fixation.[90] In the upper part of the cervical spine, the role of the odontoid can be restored after fracture with one or two screws placed in a superior direction from the base of the C2 body across the fracture into the proximal tip of the odontoid.[4, 43] In the lumbar spine, translational forces are high, and reconstruction of an effective buttress against translation usually requires two points of distal fixation.

Oppose Deforming Forces

For Anterior Column Loss

Loss of the anterior column leaves the spine unstable in flexion such that the normal flexion moment traversing the spine becomes a deforming force. Successful reconstruction requires either replacing the anterior column or directly opposing the deforming flexion force by providing an *extension* moment. An effective extension moment will counteract the instability and unload the anterior column. An extension moment requires three- or four-point loading. For example, the rod-sleeve and distraction-lordosis (D-L) constructs of the Edwards Modular Spinal System (EMSS) are designed to create an extension moment so as to unload the anterior column and negate flexion instability. In the rod-sleeve method, a polyethylene spacer is placed over the disrupted interspace and the facet joint to provide the fulcrum, while anatomic laminar hooks positioned 3 to 4 cm above and below the sleeves exert posteriorly directed force to generate an extension moment.[28, 33] The D-L construct for low lumbar fractures uses three pairs of screws for fixation.[31, 66] After distracting between the upper and lower screws with ratcheted universal rods, an adjustable connector is extended between the rods and midposition screws to provide the extension moment.

In order to *maintain* a dynamic extension force until union, both the rod-sleeve and D-L construct techniques generate sufficient three-point loading to bow the rod within its elastic range. Similar biomechanics are theoretically possible with a contoured plate or rod if two points of fixation are provided above and below the unstable segment to effect four-point loading. On the other hand, simply fixing the vertebrae above and below a burst fracture with a rigid plate or fixator does not generate a dynamic extension moment. Accordingly, these two-point fixation techniques consistently show greater loss of correction and late kyphosis.[22, 44, 50]

For Disruption of Posterior Ligaments

The instability from posterior ligamentous disruption can also be counteracted by creating an extension moment rather than replacing the posterior tension band. For example, when anterior surgery is performed and the facets are intact, focal extension can be effected by wedging an anterior interbody spacer between the affected vertebrae and fixing it in place with an anterior rod or plate. This will rotate the two vertebrae about the posterior annulus or facets into extension to unload the posterior ligaments.

For Facet Disruption

The rotational instability that follows *uni*lateral facet fracture-subluxation in the cervical spine can be reversed with the oblique wiring technique.[29, 35] A wire is passed through a hole in the subluxing inferior facet of the proximal vertebra, passed about the base of the spinous process of the adjacent distal vertebra, and tightened under image control to reduce the subluxation and provide a posteriorly directed rotational force to counteract rotational instability.

The translational instability that follows *bi*lateral facet destruction requires two-point distal fixation. In cases of thoracic and upper lumbar trauma, this is accomplished with segmental fixation. Examples include Luque sublaminar wires, bilaminar claws, and bridging sleeves. For low lumbar injuries and degenerative listhesis, two distal points of fixation are usually provided with screws attached to either spinal rods or plates.

Restore Alignment

To *maintain* long-term clinical stability, we must either replace the stabilizing structures or provide offsetting corrective forces, but we must also restore normal spine alignment. This does not mean that every portion of the spine must be straight, but it does mean that the spine must be left compensated in both the sagittal and coronal planes. Satisfactory overall alignment or compensation is indicated when the base of the neck (C7) or the skull (mastoid process and central sulcus of the posterior part of the neck) are positioned directly over the midline of the pelvis and hip joints. If the reconstructed spine is left decompensated, the likelihood of future clinical instability is high.

To maintain balance for ambulation and most other activities, a patient will do everything possible to keep his head directly over the center of the pelvis. If the fused spine is left relatively kyphotic, the patient will hyperextend any movable spinal segments above or below the fusion. This requires sustained effort by the extensor muscles, which may fatigue and become painful. Compensatory hyperlordosis also overloads open facet joints to accelerate degenerative change with pain, osteophyte formation, and lateral stenosis. Decompensation in the coronal plane has a similar sequela. If fused in lateral decompensation, the patient must maximally bend in the opposite direction to stand erect. Muscle fatigue combined with concave facet degeneration, osteophyte hypertrophy, and root irritation often follows.

Axial alignment also helps to maintain solid union and prevent progression of deformity. Once fused, the spine does not necessarily *remain* fused and motionless. Indeed, within the first year of fusion the bone is quite plastic and will remodel in response to the forces acting upon it. If regional forces are excessive, fatigue failure with microfractures, progressive slippage, and repair will occur. The result is progressive deformity in the face of a "solid" fusion.

Progressive kyphosis or scoliosis in a fused but decompensated spine is well known.[7, 26] However, the most frequent and dramatic examples we have personally observed are in patients with severe spondylolisthesis. In situ fusions for young patients with high slip angles (lumbosacral kyphosis) will usually leave the center of gravity anterior to the hip joints. Although the in situ fusion may be judged "solid" and the initial clinical course "successful," the abnormal flexion moment and anterior shear forces working against the fusion eventually cause progression of the deformity and late recurrence of pain or radiculopathy. Indeed, we see several young ladies each year who had "successful" in situ fusions of grade III or IV spondylolisthesis and then present in early adulthood with severe spondyloptosis.

Maximize Biocompatibility

In order to achieve lasting clinical spinal stability, careful attention must be directed toward preserving normal biomechanics for the *un*fused portions of the spine.

The importance of overall spinal alignment has already been discussed. For long-term biocompatibility, it is equally important to preserve the integrity of adjacent *unfused* facets so as to not overly stiffen the fused portion of the spine and thus preserve the cervical and low lumbar motion segments.

Protect Adjacent Facets

Some forms of pedicle screw fixation threaten the integrity of the adjacent proximal unfused facet joint. Partial resection of the facet or extensive disruption of its capsule damages the very joint that will be subjected to concentrated forces in the years ahead and can only accelerate degenerative change. In order to protect the adjacent proximal facet joint, screws should be inserted several millimeters distal and lateral to the center of the pedicle and directed in a mediosuperior position. Appropriate screw positioning can eliminate violation of the unfused lumbar facets. In the thoracic and upper portion of the lumbar spine where the small size of pedicles precludes significant screw angulation, laminar hooks provide secure attachment without risk to the adjacent unfused facets.

Do Not Overly Stiffen the Spine

Although data remain inconclusive, the long-term results will probably validate the admonition not to leave instrumentation in place that could overly stiffen fused portions of the spine. A lateral spinal fusion without instrumentation leaves approximately 1 to 2 degrees of motion across each interspace.[60] Instrumentation that permits an equivalent amount of motion should not affect the composite stiffness of the fused spine. However, implants with rigid connections that reduce this degree of motion alter the biomechanics of the instrumented portion of the spine. Animal studies demonstrate progressive osteopenia from stress shielding after fixation with rigid plates.[75, 95] More importantly, however, stiffening a fused segment transmits greater loads to the adjacent unfused segments that could accelerate future degenerative change. Hence, if the surgeon chooses to use very rigid implants, some consideration might be given to their future removal, particularly in the case of long fusions.

Preserve Motion Segments

Studies that attempt to correlate fusion length with acceleration of adjacent segment degeneration have been inconclusive.[16, 48, 54] Nevertheless, every additional vertebra fused removes a linkage and adds to the length and, hence, moment arm of the forces working through the fused segment and against the adjacent unfused segments. This phenomenon is magnified in the highly mobile cervical and lower lumbar vertebrae. The potential deleterious effect of a long fusion is compounded in the lower portion of the lumbar spine by the high loads at the base of the spine and the proximity of the pelvis with its long lever arms. Accordingly, it is important to restrict the length of low-lumbar fusions whenever possible to those vertebrae responsible for major pain, root impingement, or deformity.

THE SURGICAL ARMAMENTARIUM

Tools and materials are needed to stabilize the spine. Some are designed to provide immediate (short-term) stability, while others are intended to preserve that stability for many years.

Short-Term Stability

Brace, Cast, or Halo

Clinical stability, that is, freedom from abnormal motion and no pain, neural impingement, or deformity, is a relative term. Some conditions require only limited reduction in motion for several weeks until an inflammatory phenomenon subsides or a minor injury heals. A brace or cast will suffice for these conditions. A Philadelphia collar provides relative stability for the upper part of the cervical spine, while a Philadelphia collar with thoracic reinforcement (Yale brace) or a four poster will suffice for lower cervical conditions.[59] A Jewett brace counteracts the flexion moment working against the spine for disruptions between approximately T7 and L2.[81] A chair back brace or, preferably, a total-contact orthosis (TCO) will restrict motion between L1 and L5.[46, 70] Significant reduction in motion across the lumbosacral junction requires the addition of a thigh cuff.[46]

Material selection is important when fabricating braces. One-quarter-inch polypropylene has been the standard for fabricating total-contact braces and those with a thigh cuff addition. Recently, however, orthotists have begun using lighter-weight 3⁄16-in. polypropylene. To compare the effectiveness of these alternatives, we fabricated one brace in 3⁄16-in and another from ¼-in polypropylene from the same plaster mold. The lighter polypropylene brace permitted three times the range of motion on maximal effort between L4 and S1 (12 degrees) as compared with the ¼-in. brace (4 degrees).

When more stability is required than possible with bracing, plaster should be utilized. It is a crystalline material and, hence, much stiffer than plastics. Furthermore, more precise molding and three-point loading are possible.

All present brace and cast alternatives permit considerable motion in the upper part of the cervical spine. For relatively stable injuries such as most hangman's or Jefferson fractures, Philadelphia collar fixation is sufficient.[67] However, for unstable odontoid fractures and other unstable conditions without internal fixation, a halo vest is indicated. Although a halo vest is unable to maintain any sustained distraction, it is reasonably effective in preventing upper cervical angulation or translation.[59]

Implants

Internal fixation can provide far greater stability than braces, casts, or such external fixation devices as the halo vest. Implants used alone may eliminate spinal motion for some conditions. Examples include rigid variable spinal plates (VSP) (Steffee) plates (AcroMed Corp., Cleveland); most of the Cotrel-Dubousset (C-D) pedicle, screw, or multiple hook constructs (Stuart, Greensburg, Penn); and internal fixators such as the Vermont and Synthes Fixateur Interne (Synthes, Ontario). These implants have rigid articulations and deflect loads away from the spine to achieve stability.

Implants and Bone

Other implants work in conjunction with bone to provide stability. For example, the relatively flexible Wiltse Pedicle Screw System (Advanced Spine Fixation Systems, Stanton, Calif) and Luque plates (Zimmer, Warsaw, Ind) are not designed for significant reduction of deformity but rely on direct bone-to-bone contact in conjunction with the implant for achieving spinal stability. The compression construct (EMSS; Zimmer, Warsaw Ind) achieves rotational and translational stability by compressing across and thus locking the grafted facet joints. The anterior neutralization construct (EMSS) achieves stability in translation and rotation by compressing across an anterior bone graft or methacrylate spacer.

Implants and Ligaments

Some implants work in conjunction with spinal ligaments to stabilize the spine. The most common cervical example used is posterior tension band wiring. Tightening the interspinous wire rotates the vertebra into extension about the facets to tension the anterior longitudinal ligament. The rod-sleeve method functions in a similar way in the thoracic and upper part of the lumbar spine. Sleeves wedged over the facets at the disrupted level push anteriorly while proximal and distal hooks pull posteriorly to tension the anterior ligament. Taut anterior ligaments combined with compression across the unstable facets provide considerable stability in rotation and translation at the injured level with unsurpassed late maintenance of correction.[33, 53] In like manner, relatively flexible implants used in the treatment of kyphosis, scoliosis, or spondylolisthesis all achieve three-dimensional stability in part by tensioning formerly contracted ligaments.

In our opinion, implants that work in conjunction with bone or ligaments can achieve optimal stability without many of the drawbacks of more rigid implants when the requisite ligamentous and bony stock are present. When they are not, more rigid implants *or* anterior plus posterior fixation is certainly indicated.

Interbody Spacer Plus Ligaments

One-level segmental instability can be fixed with an interbody spacer in conjunction with the annulus and anterior and posterior spinal ligaments. Body spacers include iliac or fibular autologous grafts, cadaveric femoral or other bone, and carbon fiber spacers.[9] An interbody graft or spacer will enhance stability if it is shaped and positioned to both tension the annulus/anterior ligaments and maintain facet contact. This requires that the graft be (1) inserted in maximum distraction, (2) positioned in the anterior half of the interspace in front of the sagittal axis of rotation, and (3) wedge shaped to parallel the adjacent lordotic end plates. The resulting vertebral-graft friction and facet contact provide translational stability while the spacer itself provides axial stability. Without facet contact, only limited translational stability is achieved. Hence, interbody spacers are not adequate for patients with facet loss or erosion and significant translational instability without concomitant internal fixation.

Methylmethacrylate

Acrylic cement can provide immediate stability for the spine when used in conjunction with metal implants. Methacrylate will interdigitate with bone to stop motion for several days or weeks. It must be used with discretion, however, since it has many associated liabilities. Methacrylate alone is strong in compression but weak in tension and shear.[18] Fatigue failure at the bone-cement interface is likely after several weeks[74, 108] with resulting recurrence of clinical instability and possible cement dislodgement. Methacrylate is associated with a higher incidence of infection than are metallic implants.[74] In view of these liabilities, there is little or no present indication for the use of methacrylate on the posterior aspect of the spine. However, it can be useful as an anterior vertebral body spacer, particularly when combined with metal reinforcement for improved shear strength and bone fixation.

All surgical materials or devices used to obtain short-term stability are subjected to tension, bending, and shear forces. Depending on the surgical construct, either fatigue failure of the device causing breakage, fatigue failure at the bone-implant interface causing loosening, or fatigue failure of the material causing collapse is inevitable. Some of the fixation methods discussed above will suffice for several weeks, while others will maintain clinical stability for at least a year, but *all* will eventually fail without biological union.

Long-Term Stability

Permanent stability can only be achieved through the attainment of a solid bony fusion. In contrast with implants, a fusion can respond to the forces acting upon it with increased strength and repair of microfractures. Throughout the years, many materials have been used in an attempt to achieve a solid fusion. These include autologous bone, cadaveric allograft bone, artificially produced bone ceramic substitute, and osteoinductive proteins, both naturally and synthetically produced.

Autologous Bone

The "gold standard" since its initial use at the beginning of the century, autologous cancellous bone has the advantage of producing both osteoconduction and osteoinduction. Its large trabecular surface area allows for early remodeling by creeping substitution. In contrast with cancellous bone, cortical bone has the strength to withstand mechanical loading. However, it harbors fewer osteoinductive cells and has a low surface area-to-volume ratio. Hence, it requires vascular invasion to secure union, which makes it slower to both incorporate and remodel.

The advantages of autologous graft are offset to some extent by the added operative time, further blood loss, and occasional complications. These include the possibility of hemorrhage, most commonly from the superior gluteal artery, painful disruption of the sacroiliac joint, and cluneal nerve section with local hypoesthesia or dysesthesia. Some persisting discomfort at the donor site occurs in up to 15% of patients.[65] Infection is at least as common in the harvested site as in the actual back incision.[65, 110] Because of these various complications, attempts have been made to achieve fusion without extensive harvesting of bone. The most common substitute is cadaveric (allograft) bone.

Fresh Frozen Allograft

Freezing to −70°C allows for prolonged storage.[42] In the cervical spine, fresh frozen bone is said to be equal to autologous bone in obtaining *anterior* cervical fusion[11] and is satisfactory for posterior spinal fusion in pediatric and paralytic scoliosis populations.[1, 2, 76, 82] However, its use for *posterior* cervical fusions has caused a high rate of nonunion.[96]

Freeze-dried allograft has less immunogenicity and a longer shelf life than its fresh frozen counterpart.[47] Its disadvantage is a 50% reduction in mechanical strength.[83] Both fresh frozen and freeze-dried bone are osteoconductive but have minimal osteoinductive properties.[72, 93] Its use has been studied in the adult anterior cervical spine with results equal to the use of autograft.[93, 112]

Sterilization to eliminate transmission of the human immunodeficiency virus (HIV) and other viruses has been attempted with irradiation, autoclaving, and the use of ethylene oxide. Radiation is destructive to matrix proteins and greatly weakens the graft.[84] Autoclaving is also disruptive to matrix proteins and has been found to be detrimental to fusion attempts in animals.[12] Likewise, ethylene oxide causes a 70% decrease in bone induction with a high (76%) nonunion rate in adult thoracic and lumbar fusions with ethylene oxide–treated bone.[56] Hence at this time fresh frozen allograft is generally preferred despite the slight risk of viral transmission.

Results using fresh frozen or freeze-dried cadaveric bone vary according to the age of the patient and level of the spine. Most authors agree that either fresh frozen or freeze-dried allograft is effective for anterior cervical fusions in all age groups.[11, 73, 86, 93, 112] Fresh frozen allograft appears to be effective for adolescents in the treatment of thoracic scoliosis.[2] On the other hand, there is strong consensus that it is grossly inferior to autologous bone for adult thoracic and especially lumbar fusions. For example, Fernyhough and LaRocca, compared allograft with autograft in situ lumbar fusions performed by the same surgeon. The union rate for autograft was twice (53%) that of the allograft group (24%).[45] Similar results were reported by Gurr and associates.[51]

Decalcified bone matrix has received substantial interest in the last few years. Cadaver bone is soaked in hydrochloric acid, which reduces both its immunogenicity and mechanical strength.[104] However, both osteoinductive and conductive properties are retained. After implantation there is release of bioactive proteins within the bone matrix, most importantly, bone morphogenetic protein (BMP).[104] In one study of 40 adults, an 80% union rate was reported for posterolateral spine fusions when only decalcified bone matrix was used.[104]

Bone Morphogenetic Protein

BMP is produced by osteoblasts[79] and is found in high concentrations in dentin, bone, various sarcomas, and Paget disease.[106] It is found in decreased levels in patients with osteoporosis.[58] It acts on the mesenchymal cells in perivascular connective tissue to stimulate osteoblastic differentiation, migration, and proliferation.[106] In the protein family of growth factors, only BMP has been able to induce de novo endochondral ossification in extraskeletal sites.[100]

BMP can now be cloned by using recombinant DNA technology to provide sufficient quantities for clinical use.[49, 106] Since BMP is insoluble,[55, 80] it must be aggregated with such carriers as polylactic acid.[105] Animal studies using 100 mg of BMP aggregated with polylactic acid have shown significant accumulations of bone formation as early as 2 weeks and union by 12 weeks.[80] In spinal fusion studies on dogs, BMP in polylactic acid alone stimulated two to three times more bone than in controls with a 71% fusion rate.[69] Recently, BMP has been used clinically to augment autogenous bone grafts in patients with failed spinal fusions.[78] Very early results are favorable and without complications.[78]

Ceramic Bone Substitutes

Hydroxyapatite and tricalcium phosphate are both osteoconductive but remodel at different rates. Hydroxyapatite resorbs very slowly, if at all, while tricalcium phosphate usually resorbs within 6 weeks of implantation.[57] Hydroxyapatite can withstand compressive loading and is of value as a spacer for interbody fusions, whereas granular tricalcium phosphate is more useful in posterior spinal fusions.[57] The potential for combining the osteoinductive properties of BMP with the osteoconductive properties of a sterile artificial substitute such as tricalcium phosphate offers the potential for a successful autograft substitute in the future.

Instrumentation

It appears that successful union and, hence, long-term stability may be facilitated by the judicious use of instrumentation. Instrumentation serves to (1) reduce motion between vertebrae to a level conducive to union[85] and (2) promote axial loading across the facets and graft to stimulate callus maturation. There is growing evidence that appropriate instrumentation can enhance the rate of union for selected instabilities. When studies with similar patient populations and criteria for union are compared, greater union rates are typically reported for patients stabilized with instrumentation than when treated with in situ fusion alone in the case of both spondylolisthesis[26, 68] and lumbar pseudarthrosis.[40, 64, 97] Lorenz et al. recently reported fusion rates for various lumbar instabilities randomly treated with or without instrumentation by the same surgeons and found higher union rates for the instrumented groups.[68]

RECONSTRUCTING THE UNSTABLE SPINE

The early success of spine reconstructive surgery is largely determined by the degree to which the surgeon either reconstructs the stabilizing structures or opposes the forces of deformation. Long-term success is influenced by decisions made in regard to the length of instrumentation, the points and methods of fixation, the quality of alignment, and the use of anterior support, when indicated, and may be further influenced by the postoperative bracing regimen.

Corrective Forces

The first step in planning spine reconstructive surgery is to identify the planes of instability and the forces of deformation. The surgery should then be designed to repair the source of instability or directly oppose the forces of deformation. For example, if a fracture renders the spine unstable in flexion and compression, then distraction and extension forces are needed to reverse the deformity and maintain stability. If anterior shear forces are expected to dissuade union for spondylolisthesis, then a posteriorly directed force is needed to negate anterior shear instability. If a flexion-rotation injury to the neck produces unilateral facet fracture-subluxation with resultant rotational instability, then a rotational force in the opposite direction is needed to reduce the subluxation and maintain stability.

Length of Instrumentation

Once the corrective forces to be applied at surgery are selected, the next step is to determine the optimum length of instrumentation and fusion. In general, fusion should be limited to the painful pathology. For example, instrumentation and fusion for a grade II spondylolisthesis should be limited to the L5–S1 interspace. There is no justification for fusing to L4 unless the slip is severe with retrolisthesis and degenerative change at L4–5. Likewise, most thoracic and lumbar burst fractures can be fully reduced and stabilized with rod-sleeve instrumentation extending across just three interspaces for the midlumbar spine or four interspaces for thoracic injuries. It is difficult to justify longer instrumentation unless the lumbar arch is so disrupted that a bridging sleeve or double-claw construct is required.

Determining optimum instrumentation length is more difficult when treating degenerative lumbar scoliosis. Although vertebral deformity may extend from the sacrum to the thoracic spine, painful pathology is usually localized to the low lumbar vertebrae. Facet arthrosis and root impingement from lateral listhesis are common sources of pain. Although degenerative changes and/or proximal curves are often present, they are usually *not* the source of pain. Hence, instrumentation and fusion can sometimes be limited to the unstable low lumbar vertebrae.

Although it is desirable to limit instrumentation to the painful segments, it may be necessary to extend instrumentation in order to balance forces acting across the instrumentation so as to maintain fixation until fusion. When treating kyphosis, instrumentation length should be adjusted to provide for equal distances between the apex and the point of proximal and distal fixation. The standard in treating lumbar scoliosis is to instrument to stable (midline compensated) vertebrae both proximally and distally.[62] However, when treating degenerative lumbar scoliosis, it is possible to reconstruct only the unstable distal part of the lumbar spine with rods affixed to the sacrum. When using short distal instrumentation, the portion of rods fixed to the sacrum and inferior lumbar vertebrae for stability must approximate the length of the proximal portion of the rods used to correct the deformity. For example, if painful lateral angulation or listhesis occurs at the L4–5 interspace, distal fixation at L5 and S1 will be sufficient when instrumenting proximally to L3 but should be extended to S2 when instrumenting to L2.

Fixation Points

Determining the optimum length of instrumentation defines the proximal and distal points of fixation. The next step is to decide how many intervening points of fixation are needed to generate sufficient moment arms to provide the necessary corrective forces and to achieve adequate stability for successful union. At least two points of fixation distal to the point of instability are necessary to stabilize major translational deformities such as lateral listhesis or spondylolisthesis.[25] Either two pairs of hooks, two pairs of screws, or one pair of screws and an interbody spacer can provide the necessary two points of fixation.

How many points of fixation are necessary for optimum stability? Since thoracic vertebrae are intrinsically more stable than lumbar vertebrae, fewer fixation points are needed to achieve the same degree of ultimate stability. Likewise, since the application of posterior compression locks the facet joints, it is intrinsically far more stable in translation and rotation than a distraction construct, which *un*loads the facet joints. Accordingly, constructs fixed in compression require fewer fixation points than those left in distraction. The following recommendations are based on data from the Spinal Fixation Study Group series using the EMSS. For semirigid fixation in the *lumbar* spine, segmental fixation with hooks, screws, or sleeves is sufficient at every other vertebra left in compression and advisable for every vertebra left in distraction. In the *thoracic* spine and thoracolumbar junction, fixation at every third vertebra left in compression is sufficient and at every other vertebra left in distraction. Due to the high degree of cervical spine mobility, we recommend fixation at every cervical level instrumented in order to dispense with the need for postoperative halo vest protection.

Attachment Means

Once the vertebral fixation points are selected, we must decide on the optimum means of attachment for each site. In general, we recommend the means of attachment that affords secure fixation with the least amount of risk. Current fixation choices include wire and plates for the posterior portion of the cervical spine; hooks, screws, or sublaminar wires for the posterior aspect of the thoracic and lumbar spine; screws with rods or plates for vertebral bodies; and screws for the sacrum. For most posterior cervical reconstructions, wire provides secure fixation with the least risk.[17, 99, 103] Posterior cervical plate and screw fixation may be advantageous when major instability extends across multiple vertebra or across the occipital-cervical junction.[89, 90] For most situations, laminar hooks provide secure fixation with less time and risk than pedicle screws or multiple sublaminar wires in the thoracic and upper part of the lumbar spine.[32, 94] On the other hand, pedicle screw fixation is both safer and more effective than hook or wire fixation for the anterior aspect of the spine, sacrum, and fifth lumbar vertebra.[32]

Alignment

When reconstructing spinal deformity, it is essential that the spine be left fully compensated in both the sagittal and coronal planes. This will provide overall postural balance, limit the rate of deformity progression, and reduce the degree of required compensatory deformities with resultant muscle fatigue, degenerative change, and late pain. In order to restore or even maintain sagittal and coronal compensation when correcting deformities, the surgeon must obtain preoperative bending films and then calculate the amount of correction necessary to restore compensation, but not correct so much as to decompensate the patient in the opposite direction.

Correction of regional (i.e., lumbar) or even local (i.e., L5–S1) deformity may not be essential, but it is certainly advantageous to the patient. Any major deformity increases the moment arm for some muscle groups and reduces it for others. This imbalance promotes instability and gradual worsening of the deformity. For some deformities, particularly kyphosis, the greater the deformity, the further the center of gravity moves from the spine's axis of rotation, thus accentuating the deforming forces against the area of instability. Since both muscle and gravity forces cause increased motion, particularly tension and shear at the unstable level, the presence of the deformity superimposed on instability tends to aggravate pain and make union harder to achieve.

A little knowledge can be a dangerous thing when it comes to correcting long-standing deformity in the adult spine. For all their disadvantages, most chronic deformities present in a relatively stable position for that point in time. A well-intentioned attempt to provide *some* correction can unwittingly leave the spine in a less stable but still deformed position. This makes loss of fixation, recurrence of deformity, and nonunion likely occurrences. Hence, complete restoration of regional alignment to both correct deformity and leave the vertebrae to be fused in a stable position is our goal. If this goal cannot be accomplished, focal in situ fusion of a painful deformity is probably more advantageous than token reduction.

How much correction is necessary to maintain stable fixation until union? Numerous variables must be addressed to answer this question for a given case. A few general guidelines become apparent from the study of over 3,000 cases in the Spinal Fixation Study Group's (SFSG) documentation center. When treating kyphosis with posterior instrumentation and fusion alone, the spine must be left in no less than normal sagittal compensation. In addition, local deformity must be reduced enough to lower panthoracic kyphosis to under 45 degrees and residual thoracolumbar kyphosis to under 10 degrees, and lumbar kyphosis must be corrected to leave at least 20 degrees panlumbar *lordosis* with some net lordosis across any three vertebral segments.

The concept of reducing a spondylo-deformity into a "stable zone" was first published by Bradford.[8] He found that it was necessary to at least correct lumbosacral kyphosis as measured on a standing lateral radiograph to the extent that the L4 vertebral body fell within a zone created by projecting the anterior and posterior cortices of the sacral body. In addition, data from the SFSG series make it clear that translation should be reduced to the extent that the L5 body rests on the uppermost portion of the sacral dome for anterior support.

In the treatment of scoliosis, satisfactory alignment mandates compensation in the coronal plane. In addition, for a reconstruction to succeed, the forces acting on the instrumentation must be in balance. As previously discussed, this state is achieved when proximal and distal fixation is to stable (midline) vertebra or when the distal fixation of rods onto the sacrum or stable vertebra approximates the length of the proximal attachment to deformed and unstable vertebrae. In either case, equilibrium is signaled by vertical alignment of the rods on postoperative standing films.

Anterior Support

Although posterior surgery will suffice for reconstruction of most spinal instabilities, there are at least six specific indications for supplemental anterior graft support:

1. *Inadequate spinal alignment.*—When it is not possible to restore sagittal and coronal compensation or meet the minimum regional alignment criteria set forth in the preceding section, anterior surgery is indicated to improve correction and provide anterior column support.

2. *Excess vertebral body loss below L1.*—When normal alignment is restored, posterior instrumentation and fusion can completely unload the vertebral bodies and maintain stable alignment without anterior column support for most conditions between C2 and L2. We have shown that 80% of apparent vertebral body loss after burst fractures will be reconstituted following early restoration of anatomic alignment with posterior instrumentation alone.[38] However, the forces and potential range of motion in the lower part of the lumbar spine are sufficiently large that anterior grafting is sometimes indicated following acute trauma when more than 50% of vertebral body area is lost below L2. This degree of loss only occurs when more than half of the total vertebral body bone is crushed or has been displaced laterally beyond the normal circumference of the anterior column.

More anterior column support is needed in the case of degenerative conditions where the body has accommodated to chronic deformity than in the case of acute traumatic conditions where soft tissues remain in normal equilibrium. Upon review of SFSG cases to date, it appears that anterior grafting is indicated below L2 for degenerative deformities when more than 20% of vertebral body volume has been lost from erosion.

3. *After anterior disectomy or corpectomy.*—When anterior surgery is indicated to remove osteophytes, tumor, or an abscess pressing on the cord, anterior grafting is indicated to restore anterior column support, and posterior surgery is usually not necessary. Cervical spondylosis results in pain from local instability and/or foraminal encroachment. Anterior interbody fusion with a tricortical graft will provide foraminal distraction for decompression and sufficient stability for immediate pain relief with less surgery and risk than most posterior alternatives. In contrast, the results of anterior interbody grafts to indirectly decompress *lumbar* stenosis and provide sufficient fixation and graft surface for fusion have been less successful.[13, 101]

4. *To permit the use of or to facilitate posterior compression.*—Compression instrumentation appears to yield the highest union rates for lumbar instability and yet should not be used without intact facets to preserve foraminal height and provide rotational stability. The use of an interbody graft placed posterior to the midpoint of the vertebral body acts as a spacer to enable posterior compression in patients whose facets have been previously resected. Posterior compression across the interbody spacer tensions the anterior ligament for stability, while the graft spacer maintains foraminal height.

5. *To save low lumbar motion segments.*—Most degenerative and isthmic spondylolisthesis is characterized by instability in anterior translation and forward flexion. Two points of distal fixation are needed to generate the posterior translation and extension forces necessary to correct the deformity and oppose the deforming forces. For low-grade spondylolisthesis, providing a sufficient extension moment across the listhetic interspace will negate anterior translational instability enough to maintain stable fixation until fusion. In the treatment of L5–S1 isthmic spondylolisthesis, the two points of distal fixation are provided by screws at S1 and S2. In the treatment of degenerative listhesis at L4–5, the surgeon can use L5 screws for one point and either S1 screws or an L4–5 interbody spacer as the other. The interbody graft alternative is useful for those few patients who present with L4–5 spondylolisthesis and a rather normal L5–S1 motion segment. The graft serves to distract anteriorly, while the ratcheted rods or plates provide compression posteriorly.

6. *Recurrent Nonunions.*—Compression instrumentation with iliac grafting offers an 86% probability for successful repair of each pseudarthrosis.[39] In those few cases where meticulous iliac grafting combined with posterior compression instrumentation does not succeed, we practice anterior interbody fusion combined with repeat posterior compression instrumentation and fusion. The use of an anterior spacer positioned posterior to the midpoint of the vertebral body combined with preservation of some anterior longitudinal ligament and posterior compression instrumentation appears to provide ideal biomechanics for pseudarthrosis repair. The central anterior graft acts as a spacer to maintain disc space height, while the posterior compression instrumentation tensions the anterior ligament and locks the facets for great stability. The construct further directs all axial loading across the anterior and posterior grafts while blocking any disruptive tensile or translational forces. Early successful results with this tech-

nique for even recurrent pseudarthroses appear to exceed 95%.

Supplemental Anterior Fixation

Anterior interbody fusions obtain stability by tensioning surrounding ligaments; end-point translational and rotational stability is provided by the facets. When there is loss of the anterior ligament or probable disruption of the facets, supplemental anterior fixation is advisable. Since motion across each interspace is cumulative, the more interspaces an anterior graft traverses, the greater the vertebral-graft motion and the higher the probability of graft dislodgement or junctional nonunion. Therefore, anterior fixation should also be considered when an interbody graft is used to stabilize two or more motion segments following corpectomy.

Considerable stability can be obtained by compressing across anterior interbody or corpectomy grafts. The stability is provided by the potential friction generated between the vertebral bone and spacer (graft). The simplest method for generating anterior compression is with the anterior neutralization construct (EMSS). Spinal screws are placed across the vertebral bodies above and below the grafted segment. Height is restored by distracting with a ratcheted universal rod, the graft(s) is inserted with the spine held distracted, and then compression is applied to fix the graft in place. If additional stability is required, two rods may be placed side by side and cross-linked. Other alternatives that provide stable fixation in conjunction with an anterior graft for the low thoracic and lumbar vertebrae include the Kaneda device (AcroMed Corp., Cleveland)[61] and Yuan[111] and CASP-Armstrong plates (Surgical Dynamics, Alameda, Calif).[3] Low-profile cervical plates (Synthes, Paoli, La) provide the only current alternative for supplemental anterior cervical fixation.

Postoperative Bracing

Postoperative bracing serves four purposes: (1) an appropriate brace will oppose deforming forces working against the reconstruction to permit the use of less rigid instrumentation for long-term biocompatibility, (2) protecting the instrumentation from deforming forces will decrease the likelihood of fixation failure regardless of the instrumentation selected, (3) bracing will remind the patient to limit his activities, and (4) postoperative bracing appears to increase the probability of successful fusion. It is well established that a reduction in motion facilitates the early phases of bony union.[15] It is equally established that the later stages of bony union and graft consolidation are, in contrast, augmented by motion, particularly axial loading.[109] The ideal of a rigid to progressively flexible graft environment can be approached by combining semirigid fixation with postoperative bracing. The combination achieves sufficient reduction in motion to maximize early union. After several months, the brace can be modified or replaced to permit somewhat more loading across the graft and then removed to permit full physiologic loading and graft consolidation.

Data from the SFSG series demonstrates higher union rates when appropriate bracing is used in conjunction with semirigid posterior instrumentation and posterior grafting for long lumbosacral fusions, all lumbar distraction constructs, lumbosacral deformities, and lumbar pseudarthrosis.[91] Accordingly, bracing is indicated following these procedures to include a TCO with a thigh cuff for lumbosacral reconstructions and a ¼-in. polypropylene TCO alone for the more proximal surgeries. Cervical orthoses are indicated after anterior interbody fusions without internal fixation and after posterior cervical wiring procedures.

RECOMMENDED TECHNIQUES

The principles for obtaining spinal stability should remain relatively unchanged over time. The surgical techniques that best fulfill these principles are ever-changing. In the authors' opinion, the techniques outlined in this section offer the greatest chance for obtaining long-term clinical stability with the least amount of surgery and risk for 1992. The discussion will center on five types of instability: degenerative instability, cervical injury, thoracolumbar injury, chronic deformity, and vertebral body loss.

Degenerative Instability

Disc/Facet Degeneration

Motion segment degeneration gives rise to pain and/or root irritation. It is often difficult to decide whether the pain originates more from the annulus or facets. Fortunately, either anterior or posterior fusion will obliterate one side and unload the other. Hence, either anterior or posterior fusion provides acceptable treatment for degeneration without root impingement. When anterior surgery is selected, a large interbody graft will tension the anterior ligaments to provide sufficient stability for cases with early degenerative change but without gross instability or deformity. In contrast, posterior in situ fusion disrupts ligaments and reduces stability until fusion occurs. It is not surprising, therefore, that early reports suggest that union rates can be improved when posterior grafting is supplemented with instrumentation that effectively reduces intervertebral motion.[68]

Pseudarthrosis

Successful repair of pseudarthrosis seems to require greater stability than primary fusion. Maximum stability combined with axial loading through the facets and graft to stimulate bone formation is desirable. This appears to be most effectively accomplished with a compression construct.[40] Plate fixation can provide equal or greater stability but limits axial loading across the facets and fusion mass. As previously discussed, *recurrent* nonunions are best treated with anterior interbody fusion combined with posterior compression instrumentation and iliac grafting.

Cervical Injury

The great majority of cervical trauma requiring surgery results from flexion-distraction, rotation, compression, or translation injuries, and leaves the spine unstable in these positions.

Flexion-distraction ruptures posterior ligaments and one or both facet capsules to produce bilateral or unilateral facet dislocation. After facet reduction, a posterior tension band is required to restore the ligamentous checkrein and negate residual flexion instability. This is best accomplished with posterior interspinous wiring.[14] An effective tension band can be achieved with posterior cervical plates and screws[77] or Halifax clamps (Codman and Shurtleff, Inc., Randolph, Mass), but these devices limit bone area for fusion and certainly involve more complexity and risk than the highly effective and well-proven posterior wiring techniques.

Rotation of the head *without* distraction will fracture a facet and leave the spine unstable in rotation. Fixation with a halo vest[88] or interspinous wiring[19, 29, 35] is not particularly effective since they do not directly oppose the rotational instability. Rather, an oblique wiring technique from the proximal dislocating facet or lamina to the spinous process below will provide excellent maintenance of alignment and a nearly 100% union rate without the risk or complexity of cervical plates and screws.[35] If there is both rotational and flexion instability, oblique wiring can be combined with interspinous wiring. If there is vertebral body comminution as well, posterior plate fixation becomes indicated to address multiplanar instability.[20, 77, 90]

Compression injuries to the cervical spine cause vertebral-body burst fractures. Some injuries can be effectively treated with the application of posterior plates if they are contoured into lordosis, attached to the spine at two points distal to the unstable interspace, and applied with the cervical spine in longitudinal traction.[90] If a partial anterior corpectomy is necessary to decompress the cord, an anterior interbody fusion using tricortical iliac bone and stabilization with an anterior plate is recommended.[5, 98]

Fracture of the odontoid base leaves the upper part of the cervical spine unstable in *translation*. A Brooks[10] or Edwards[41] C1 or C2 bone block will provide adequate stability if the C1 arch is intact and postoperative halo vest protection is planned. If the C1 ring is fractured or deficient or if postoperative bracing is impractical, Bohler odontoid screw fixation will directly address translational instability.[4]

Thoracic and Lumbar Injury

The great majority of fractures to the thoracic and lumbar segments of the spine can be placed into three groups: those due to flexion-distraction, compression, or translational forces.

Flexion-distraction injuries usually cause tension failure of the posterior ligaments but may also cause tension failure of the posterior bony elements to produce a Chance fracture. Although both injury patterns can be treated with a hyperextension cast, patients are more comfortable and the end result superior after one-level compression instrumentation and fusion.[31]

Flexion-compression forces account for the great majority of unstable thoracic and lumbar fractures. They produce a continuum of injuries ranging from a classic burst fracture when compression predominates to a fracture-dislocation when flexion predominates.[34] In both cases, the anterior longitudinal ligament remains intact. If appropriate posterior reduction is performed within several days of the injury, indirect decompression of neural elements is accomplished in over 95% of cases.[33] We have found the simplest, safest, and most effective technique for these injuries to be the rod-sleeve method.[24, 33] If postoperative assessment discloses residual anterior neural impingement, we recommend secondary anterolateral decompression and grafting.[6, 34] If the surgeon chooses primary anterior decompression and fixation for selected severe burst fractures, then anterior fixation is obtained with a large tricortical iliac graft, two fibular sections, or an allograft femur packed with autologous cancellous bone,[24, 92] depending on the amount of anterior column loss. In each case, we recommend anterior fixation. The simplest and safest form of instrumentation is an anterior neutralization construct using one universal rod compressing across the graft in cases of mild instability and either two coupled rods, a plate,[111] or a Kaneda device (AcroMed Corp., Cleveland)[61] when there is a question of mild posterior ligamentous attenuation. In cases with known posterior disruption or facet fractures, supplemental posterior fixation is advised.

Translational or shear injuries occur when both the anterior longitudinal ligament and posterior ligaments and/or facets are disrupted. Shear injuries are diagnosed by vertebral displacement in both the sagittal and coronal planes without a loss of vertebral height.[34] Translational injuries with shear instability require fixation at two points distal to the injury. Two-point segmental fixation can be provided in descending order of stability with plates and pedicle screws, rods and pedicle screws, rods with clawed hooks proximally and distally, and rods affixed to the spine with sublaminar wires.

Chronic Deformity

Reduction of chronic deformity requires either the surgical release or stretching of contracted anterior ligaments.

The classic approach requires anterior surgery to section contractures and posterior surgery for reduction, fixation, and fusion.[71, 87] We have learned that equal or greater correction and stability can be achieved for most deformities when gradual posterior instrumented reduction is used to both stretch out the contracted tissues and hold the reduction until fusion. This method will usually save patients the added surgery and morbidity of a preliminary or combined anterior operation.

Post-traumatic kyphosis can be fully corrected even years after injury with the kyphoreduction construct (EMSS), unless an anterior bony bridge has formed.[37] Likewise, even severe L5–S1 spondylolisthesis can be fully corrected by using the spondylo-construct (EMSS) to provide gradual instrumented reduction.[23, 26] Indeed, it has not been necessary for us to approach the spine anteriorly in the treatment of our last 15 patients with spondyloptosis.

Degenerative spondylolisthesis is usually relatively flexible and can be treated with several different techniques. When we wish to indirectly decompress the canal by flattening the disc and opening the foramina and when the adjacent L5–S1 disc is also degenerated, we prefer the D-L construct (EMSS) to reduce an L4–5 degenerative listhesis.[36] It provides initial distraction to prevent "plowing" of the disc and then rotates L5 under L4 to correct the listhesis and restore lordosis. On the other hand, when the L5–S1 motion segment is relatively normal and asymptomatic, we suggest limiting instrumentation to the symptomatic level. This requires the use of a rigid one-level plate with or without an interbody graft or the use of a compression construct (EMSS) combined with an interbody graft.

Degenerative scoliosis with lateral listhesis can be reduced to a stable position by using gradual posterior instrumented reduction techniques. For lumbar deformities, we typically use screws for attachment to the sacrum and the low lumbar vertebrae and hooks in a bilaminar claw configuration for upper lumbar or low thoracic attachment. Correction of listhesis and upper lumbar scoliosis is accomplished with adjustable connectors between the ratcheted universal rods and either screws placed in selected lumbar pedicles or bilaminar claws. Low lumbar obliquity is addressed with either the same or separate rods distracting on the concavity and compressing on the convexity after partial convex-side facetectomies are performed. For very severe low lumbar scoliosis, a supplemental iliac strut rod is used to rotate the spine into a compensated position. Finally, the various rods are stabilized by cross-locking. Treatment of thoracic and thoracolumbar scoliotic deformities without listhesis can be accomplished by using various spinal systems (including the C-D, Texas Scottish Rite Hospital [Danek Medical, Inc., Memphis, Tenn], Isola [AcroMed Corp., Cleveland], or EMSS) combined with iliac fusion.

Vertebral Body Loss

In anterior collapse, one or more vertebral bodies can be destroyed or resected due to tumor or infection. Significant anterior column loss is associated with flexion instability and progressive kyphosis. If vertebral body loss from metastatic disease does not cause anterior cord pressure from tumor retropulsion, posterior instrumentation can correct the kyphotic deformity, negate flexion instability, and unload the anterior column without the need for anterior surgery.[28, 30] In the cervical spine, this can best be accomplished with posterior plates contoured into lordosis. In the thoracic spine, any of the hook-and-rod systems will suffice. Near the thoracolumbar junction, the standard or bridging rod-sleeve method provides the most effective extension moment with the least amount of instrumentation. If the surgeon wishes to avoid postoperative bracing and is willing to extend instrumentation over a greater distance, a bilaminar claw-to-bilaminar claw construct can be used with or without sleeves to maintain alignment. Either C-D, TSRH, Isola, or Edwards Instrumentation can be used for this purpose.

Corpectomy is required when there is neural impingement from retropulsion or when radiation combined with posterior instrumentation is unable to contain further anterior destruction or collapse. Anterior reconstruction following corpectomy is simplified by the fact that posterior structures usually remain. We recommend constructing an anterior spacer from a fresh frozen allograft femur packed with autogenous cancellous bone. If there is already kyphotic deformity, screws are placed medially to laterally across the adjacent vertebral bodies, and traction is applied with a universal rod and hook outrigger. After wedging the graft in place, compression is applied with the same rod to stabilize the construct. Additional cancellous bone is then packed anterior and lateral to the spacer.

For patients with limited life expectancy, the anterior reconstruction can be simplified by using a methacrylate spacer. To provide translational stability for this spacer, we use a threaded Harrington compression rod in the center of the methacrylate spacer that crosses the adjacent end plates. Nuts and cancellous washers are used to restore anterior column height before placing the methacrylate.[28] For intermediate life expectancies, we generally place rib or other graft material in front of the methacrylate spacer and find that it is usually incorporated.

In cases with vertebral infection, corpectomy is performed to eradicate the infection; thereafter, tricortical iliac grafts combined with the anterior neutralization construct (EMSS) will generally provide good fixation without recurrent infection. However, for virulent infections with local purulence, we use reinforced methacrylate combined with antibiotics to retard local infection. After several months, we add a short posterior compression construct and iliac fusion for long-term stability.

Vertebrectomy is performed to resect primary spinal tumors or circumferentially decompress the cord. Complete vertebrectomy leaves the spine highly unstable. However, its reconstruction is conceptually simple. It requires an anterior spacer (allograft femur with cancellous bone or reinforced methacrylate depending on the life expectancy) and a single-rod anterior neutralization construct combined with a short posterior compression construct from the first intact level above to the first intact level below the resection. Either a hook-to-hook or a screw-to-screw compression construct can be used depending on the anatomic level of the resection. For total vertebrectomy in the midlumbar area of the spine, we recommend extending the compression construct one additional level above and below the resected segment for both proximal and distal segmental fixation in order to enhance stability in translation and rotation. This can be accomplished by using plates and pedicle screws extending two levels above and below the resection or with any of the current segmental rod-hook systems.

When multiple vertebrectomies are performed, the surgeon might consider using an anterior prosthesis containing intramedullary extendable rods[28, 30] and should definitely apply four-point posterior fixation. Posterolateral grafting is worthwhile in cases where up to two full vertebrae have been resected. By using long corticocancellous strips of bone, we have observed successful union at postoperative exploration years later.

Total sacrectomy provides a notable reconstructive challenge. Successful fixation requires the use of screw attachment to both the sacrum and ilium with rods or struts affixing to the remaining lumbar spine at two or more points for each rod. Anterior column support requires grafting with cadaveric bone and anterior fixation to both ilia.[102] This approach contains many hazards. The prospects for graft incorporation are tenuous, and at least low-grade infection in the site of sacral tumor resection is common.

The second alternative following total sacrectomy is the biological sling concept.[27, 28, 30] We have found that the lumbar spine will gradually settle into the pelvis without interrupting remaining cauda equina function and reach a stable end point. Our longest survivor dispensed with his TCO brace after several years and now, after more than 10 years' follow-up, continues asymptomatic ambulation.

REFERENCES

1. Aprin H, Bowen JR, MacEwen GD, et al: Spine fusion in patients with spinal muscular atrophy. *J Bone Joint Surg [Am]* 1982; 64:1179–1187.
2. Aurori BF, Weierman RJ, Lowell HA, et al: Pseudarthrosis after spinal fusion for scoliosis. *Clin Orthop* 1985; 199:153–158.
3. Black RC, Gardner VO, Arnstrong GWD, et al: A contoured anterior spinal fixation plate. *Clin Orthop* 1988; 227:135–142.
4. Bohler J: Anterior stabilization for acute fractures and nonunions of the dens. *J Bone Joint Surg [Am]* 1982; 64:18–27.
5. Bohler J, Gaudernak T: Anterior plate stabilization for fracture-dislocations of the lower cervical spine. *J Trauma* 1980; 20:203–205.
6. Bohlman HH, Eismont FJ: Surgical techniques of anterial decompression and fusion for spinal cord injuries. *Clin Orthop* 1986; 154:57–67.
7. Boxall D, Bradford DS, Winter RB, et al: Management of severe spondylolisthesis in children and adolescents. *J Bone Joint Surg [Am]* 1979; 61:479–495.
8. Bradford DS: Closed reduction of spondylolisthesis: An experience in 22 patients. *Spine* 1988; 13:580–587.
9. Brantigan JW, Steffee AD, Geiger JM: A carbon fiber implant to aid interbody lumbar fusion. *Spine* 1991; 16:277–282.
10. Brooks AL, Jenkins EB: Atlanto-axial arthrodesis by the wedge compression method. *J Bone Joint Surg [Am]* 1978; 60:279–284.
11. Brown MD, Malinin TI, Davis PB: A roentgenographic evaluation of frozen allografts versus autografts in anterior cervical spine fusions. *Clin Orthop* 1976; 119:231–236.
12. Burwell RG: The fate of bone grafts, in Apley AG (ed): *Recent Advances in Orthopaedics*. London, Churchill, 1969, pp 115–207.
13. Calandruccio RA, Benton BF: Anterior lumbar fusion. *Clin Orthop* 1964; 35:63–68.
14. Capen DA, Garland DE, Waters RL: Surgical stabilization of the cervical spine. A comparative analysis of anterior and posterior spinal fusions. *Clin Orthop* 1985; 196:229–237.
15. Chao EYS: Biomechanics of external fixation, in Lane J (ed): *Fracture Healing*. New York, Churchill Livingstone, 1987, pp 105–122.
16. Cochran T, Irstam L, Nachemson A: Long term analysis and functional changes in patients with adolescent idiopathic scoliosis treated by Harrington rod fusion. *Spine* 1983; 8:576–584.
17. Coe JD, Warden KE, Sutterlin CE, et al: Biomechanical evaluation of cervical spinal stabilization methods in a human cadaveric model. *Spine* 1989; 14:1122–1131.
18. Crowninshield R, Pope MH, Hoaglund FT: A comparison of the tensile properties of bone and polymethylmethacrylate. *J Bone Joint Surg [Am]* 1974; 56:865.
19. Csongradi J, Whalen R, Pyka W, et al: Mechanical analysis of cervical spine stabilization techniques. *Orthop Trans* 1985; 9:348.
20. Domenella G, Berlanda P, Bassi G: Posterior approach osteosynthesis of the lower cervical spine. *Ital Traumatol* 1983; 9(suppl 1):107.
21. Dunn HK: Anterior stabilization of thoracolumbar injuries. *Clin Orthop* 1984; 189:116–124.

22. Ebelke DK, Asher MA, Neff J, et al: Survivorship analysis of VSP spine instrumentation in the treatment of thoracolumbar and lumbar burst fractures. *Spine* 1991; 16(suppl):428–432.
23. Edwards CC: Prospective evaluation of a new method for complete reduction of L5–S1 spondylolisthesis using corrective forces alone. *Orthop Trans* 1990; 14:549.
24. Edwards CC: Reconstruction of acute lumbar injury. *Op Tech Orthop* 1991; 1:106–122.
25. Edwards CC: Reduction of spondylolisthesis: Biomechanics and fixation. *Orthop Trans* 1986; 10:543–544.
26. Edwards CC: Reduction of spondylolisthesis, in Bridwell K, DeWald R (eds): *Textbook of Spinal Surgery*. Philadelphia, JB Lippincott, 1991, pp 605–634.
27. Edwards CC: Resection du rachis inferieur et du sacrum. *Rev Chir Orthop* 1987; 73:122–128.
28. Edwards CC: Spinal reconstruction in tumor management, in Uhthoff HK (ed): *Current Concepts of Diagnosis and Treatment of Bone and Soft Tissue Tumors*. New York, Springer-Verlag, 1984, pp 328–349.
29. Edwards CC: Spine stabilization: Analysis of surgical options, in Lane J (ed): *Fracture Healing*. New York, Churchill Livingstone, 1987, pp 215–257.
30. Edwards CC: The diagnosis and surgical management of spinal tumors using computed tomography, in Post JD (ed): *Computed Tomography of the Spine*. Baltimore, Williams & Wilkins, 1983, pp 704–737.
31. Edwards CC: Thoracolumbar trauma: Posterior reduction and fixation with the Modular Spinal System. *Semin Spine Surg* 1990; 2:8–18.
32. Edwards CC, Levine AM: Complications associated with posterior instrumentation in the treatment of thoracic and lumbar fractures, in Garfin S (ed): *Complications of Spine Surgery*. Baltimore, Williams & Wilkins, 1989, pp 164–199.
33. Edwards CC, Levine AM: Early rod-sleeve stabilization of the injured thoracic and lumbar spine. *Orthop Clin North Am* 1986; 17:121–145.
34. Edwards CC, Levine AM: Fractures of the lumbar spine, in Evarts CM (ed): *Surgery of the Musculoskeletal System*, ed 2. New York, Churchill Livingstone, 1990, pp 2237–2275.
35. Edwards CC, Matz SO, Levine AM: The oblique wiring technique for rotational injuries of the cervical spine. *Orthop Trans* 1985; 9:142.
36. Edwards CC, McConnell JR: The surgical reconstruction of degenerative lumbar stenosis and listhesis, in Andersson G, McNeill T (eds): *Spinal Stenosis*. St Louis, Mosby–Year Book, 1991.
37. Edwards CC, Rhyne A: Late treatment of post-traumatic kyphosis. *Semin Spine Surg* 1990; 2:63–69.
38. Edwards CC, Rhyne AL, Weigel MC, et al: 5–10 year results treating burst fractures with rod-sleeve instrumentation and fusion. *Orthop Trans* 1991; 15:728.
39. Edwards CC, Weigel MC: Treatment of 56 lumbosacral nonunions with compression instrumentation. Presented at the American Academy of Orthopaedic Surgeons Annual Meeting, Las Vegas, 1989.
40. Edwards CC, Weigel MC, Levine AM: Improved results treating lumbosacral nonunions with compression instrumentation. *Orthop Trans* 1988; 12:131.
41. Edwards CC, White JB, Levine AM: A new bone block construct for C1–2 fixation. *Orthop Trans* 1987; 11:5.
42. Ehrlich MG, Lorenz J, Tomford W, et al: Collagenase activity in banked bone. *Trans Orthop Res Soc* 1983; 8:166.
43. Esses SI, Bednar DA: Screw fixation of odontoid fractures and nonunions. *Spine* 1991; 16:483–485.
44. Fedder I: Use of the Olerud PSF device in treatment of thoracolumbar spine fractures. Unpublished manuscript, 1991.
45. Fernyhough JC, LaRocca SH: Lumbar spine fusions utilizing crushed freeze-dried cortico-cancellous allograft with cancellous autograft. North American Spine Society Exhibit, 1990.
46. Fidler MW, Plasmans MT: The effect of four types of support on the segmental mobility of the lumbosacral spine. *J Bone Joint Surg [Am]* 1983; 65:943–947.
47. Friedlaender GE: Immune responses to osteochondral allografts. *Clin Orthop* 1983; 174:58–68.
48. Frymoyer JW, Hanley EN, Howe J, et al: A comparison of radiographic findings in fusion and nonfusion patients ten or more years following lumbar disc surgery. *Spine* 1979; 4:435–440.
49. Gerhart TN, Kirker-Head CA, Kriz MJ, et al: Healing of large mid-femoral segmental defects in sheep using recombinant human bone morphogenetic protein (BMP2) *Trans Orthop Res Soc* 1991; 16:172.
50. Gertzbein SD, Robbins SE, Chow D, et al: The preliminary results of the AO internal fixator for spinal fractures. *Orthop Trans* 1989; 13:752–753.
51. Gurr KR, Barr S, Haddad R, et al: In vivo analysis of autograft versus allograft in posterior intertransverse fusions. Presented at the Scoliosis Research Society Minneapolis, Phoenix, Ariz, 1991, p 98.
52. Haher TR, Bergman M, O'Brien M, et al: The effect of the three columns of the spine on the instantaneous axis of rotation in flexion and extension. *Spine* 1991; 16(suppl):312–318.
53. Hanley EN, Starr JK: Junctional burst fractures. Presented at the American Academy of Orthopaedic Surgeons Annual Meeting, Anaheim, 1991.
54. Hayes MA, Tompkins SF, Herndon WA, et al: Clinical and radiological evaluation of lumbosacral motion below fusion levels in idiopathic scoliosis. *Spine* 1988; 13:1161–1167.
55. Heckman JD, Boyan BD, Aufdemorte TB, et al: The use of bone morphogenetic protein in the treatment of nonunion in a canine model. *J Bone Joint Surg [Am]* 1991; 73:750–764.
56. Herron LD, Newman MH: The failure of ethylene oxide gas-sterilized freeze-dried bone graft for thoracic and lumbar spinal fusion. *Spine* 1989; 14:496–500.
57. Jarcho M: Calcium phosphate ceramics as hard tissue prosthetics. *Clin Orthop* 1981; 157:260–277.
58. Johnson EE, Urist MR, Finerman GAM: Repair of segmental defects of the tibia with cancellous bone grafts augmented with human bone morphogenetic protein. *Clin Orthop* 1988; 236:249–257.

59. Johnson RH, Hart DL, Simmons EF, et al: Cervical orthoses. *J Bone Joint Surg [Am]* 1977; 59:332–339.
60. Johnsson R, Selvick G, Stromgvist B, et al: Mobility of the lower lumbar spine after posterolateral fusion determined by roentgen stereophotogrammetric analysis. *Acta Orthop Scand Suppl* 1988; 227:83.
61. Kanada K, Abumi K, Fujiya M: Burst fractures with neurologic deficits of the thoracolumbar-lumbar spine. *Spine* 1984; 9:788–795.
62. King HA, Moe JH, Bradford DS, et al: The selection of fusion levels in thoracic idiopathic scoliosis. *J Bone Joint Surg [Am]* 1983; 65:1302–1313.
63. Kirkaldy-Willis WH, Farfan HF: Instability of the lumbar spine. *Clin Orthop* 1982; 165:110–121.
64. Kornblatt MD, Casey MP, Jacobs RR: Internal fixation in lumbosacral spine fusion: A biomechanical and clinical study. *Clin Orthop* 1986; 203:141–150.
65. Kurz LT, Garfin SR, Booth RE: Harvesting autogenous iliac bone grafts: A review of complications and techniques. *Spine* 1989; 14:1324–1331.
66. Levine AM, Edwards CC: Low lumbar burst fractures: Reduction and stabilization using the modular spine fixation system. *Orthopedics* 1988; 11:1427–1432.
67. Levine AM, Edwards CC: Management of traumatic spondylolisthesis of the axis. *J Bone Joint Surg [Am]* 1985; 67:217–226.
68. Lorenz M, Zindrick M, Schwaegler P, et al: A comparison of single-level fusions with and without hardware. *Spine* 1991; 16:455–458.
69. Lovell TP, Dawson EG, Nilsson OS, et al: Augmentation of spinal fusion with bone morphogenetic protein in dogs. *Clin Orthop* 1989; 243:266–274.
70. Lumsden RM, Morris JM: An in vivo study of axial rotation and immobilization at the lumbosacral joint. *J Bone Joint Surg [Am]* 1968; 50:1591–1602.
71. Malcolm BW, Bradford DSA, Winter RB, et al: Posttraumatic kyphosis. *J Bone Joint Surg [Am]* 1981; 63:891–899.
72. Malinin TI, Brown MD: Bone allografts in spinal surgery. *Clin Orthop* 1981; 154:68–73.
73. Malinin TI, Rosomoff HL, Sutton CH: Human cadaver femoral head homografts for anterior cervical spine fusions. *Surg Neurol* 1977; 7:249–251.
74. McAfee PC, Bohlman HH, Ducker T, et al: Failure of stabilization of the spine with methacrylate. *J Bone Joint Surg [Am]* 1986; 68:1145–1157.
75. McAfee PC, Farey ID, Sutterlin CE, et al: Device-related osteoporosis with spinal instrumentation. *Spine* 1989; 14:919–926.
76. McCarthy RE, Peek RD, Morrissy RT, et al: Allograft bone in spinal fusion for paralytic scoliosis. *J Bone Joint Surg [Am]* 1986; 68:370–375.
77. Montesano PX, Juach EC, Anderson PA, et al: Biomechanics of cervical spine internal fixation. *Spine* 1991; 16:10–15.
78. Muschler GF, Lane JM, Dawson EG: The biology of spinal fusion, in Cotler JM, Cotler HB (eds): *Spinal Fusion*. New York, Springer-Verlag, 1990, pp 9–21.
79. Nakahara H, Takaoka K, Ono K: The effects of bone morphogenetic protein on periosteal osteogenic cells in vivo. *Trans Orthop Res Soc* 1989; 14:38.
80. Nilsson OS, Urist MR, Dawson EG, et al: Bone repair induced by bone morphogenetic protein in ulnar defects in dogs. *J Bone Joint Surg [Br]* 1986; 68:635–642.
81. Norton PL, Brown T: The immobilizing efficiency of back braces: Their effect on the posture and motion of the lumbosacral spine. *J Bone Joint Surg [Am]* 1957; 39:111–138.
82. Osebold WR, Mayfield JK, Winter RB, et al: Surgical treatment of paralytic scoliosis associated with myelomeningocele. *J Bone Joint Surg [Am]* 1982; 64:841–857.
83. Pelker RR, Friedlaender GE, Markham TC, et al: Effects of freezing and freeze-drying on the biomechanical properties of rat bone. *J Orthop Res* 1984; 1:405–411.
84. Pelker RR, Friedlaender GE, Panjabi MM, et al: Radiation-induced alterations of fracture healing biomechanics. *J Orthop Res* 1984; 2:90–96.
85. Perren SM, Cordey J, Gautier E: Rigid internal fixation using plates: Terminology, principles and early problems, in Lane J (ed): *Fracture Healing*. New York, Churchill-Livingstone, 1987, pp 139–151.
86. Rish BI, McFadden JTG, Penix JP: Anterior cervical spine fusion using homologous bone grafts. A comparative study. *Surg Neurol* 1976; 5:119–121.
87. Roberson JR, Whitesides TE: Surgical reconstruction of late post-traumatic thoracolumbar kyphosis. *Spine* 1985; 10:307–312.
88. Rorabeck CH, Bourne RB, Hawkins RJ, et al: Unilateral facet dislocations of the cervical spine: Diagnosis and results of treatment. *Orthop Trans* 1982; 6:471.
89. Roy-Camille R, Saillant G: Les traumatismes du rachis sans complication neurologique. *Int Orthop* 1984; 8:155–162.
90. Roy-Camille R, Saillant G, Mazel C: Internal fixation of the unstable cervical spine by a posterior osteosynthesis with plates and screws, in *The Cervical Spine*. Philadelphia, JB Lippincott, 1989, pp 390–421.
91. Schimandle J, Weigel MC, Edwards CC, et al: Indications for thigh cuff bracing following instrumented lumbosacral fusions. *Orthop Trans* 1992, in press.
92. Schlegel J, Yuan HA, Fredrickson B: Anterior interbody fixation devices, in Frymoyer JW (ed): *The Adult Spine*. New York, Raven Press, 1991, pp 1947–1959.
93. Schneider JR, Bright RW: Anterior cervical fusion using freeze-dried bone allografts. *Transplant Proc* 1976; 8:73.
94. Scoliosis Research Society: *Morbidity and Mortality Committee Report*. Scoliosis Research Society, 1987.
95. Smith KR, Hunt TR, Asher MA, et al: A study of bone stress shielding in the canine lumbar spine. *Orthop Trans* 1989; 13:97–98.
96. Stabler CL, Eismont FJ, Brown MD, et al: Failure of posterior cervical fusions using cadaveric bone graft in children. *J Bone Joint Surg [Am]* 1985; 67:370–375.
97. Stauffer RN, Coventry MB: Posterolateral lumbar spine fusion. *J Bone Joint Surg [Am]* 1972; 54:1195–1205.
98. Suh PB, Kostuik JP, Esses SI: Anterior cervical plate fixa-

tion with the titanium hollow screw plate system. *Spine* 1990; 15:1079–1081.

99. Sutterlin CE, McAfee PC, Warden KE, et al: A biomechanical evaluation of cervical spinal stabilization methods in a bovine model. *Spine* 1988; 13:795–802.
100. Tabas JA, Zasloff M, Wasmuth JJ, et al: Bone morphogenetic protein: Chromosomal localization of human genes for BMPI, BMP2A, and BMP3. *Trans Orthop Res Soc* 1991; 16:409.
101. Taylor TK: Anterior interbody fusion in the management of disorders of the lumbar spine. *J Bone Joint Surg [Br]* 1970; 52:784.
102. Tomita K, Tsuchiya H: Total sacrectomy and reconstruction for huge sacral tumors. *Spine* 1990; 15:1223–1227.
103. Ulrich C, Wörsdörfer O, Claes L, et al: Comparative study of the stability of anterior and posterior cervical spine fixation procedures. *Arch Orthop Trauma Surg* 1987; 106:226–231.
104. Urist MR, Dawson E: Intertransverse process fusion with the aid of chemosterilized autolyzed antigen-extracted allogeneic (AAA) bone. *Clin Orthop* 1981; 154:97–113.
105. Urist MR, Lietze A, Dawson E: Beta-tricalcium phosphate delivery system for bone morphogenetic protein. *Clin Orthop* 1984; 187:277–280.
106. Urist MR, Masiarz FR, Barr PJ, et al: Recombinant bone morphogenetic protein by a yeast expression system. *Trans Orthop Res Soc* 1990; 15:68.
107. Vasan NS, Gutteling EW, Lee CK, et al: A preliminary study of mechanically stress-induced changes in the extracellular matrix of the canine intervertebral disc. *Spine* 1991; 16:317–320.
108. Whitehill R, Barry JC: The evolution of stability in cervical spinal constructs using either autogenous bone graft or methacrylate cement. *Spine* 1985; 10:32–41.
109. Wolf JW, White AA, Panjabi MM, et al: Comparison of cyclic loading versus constant compression in the treatment of long bone fractures in rabbits. *J Bone Joint Surg [Am]* 1981; 63:805–810.
110. Younger EW, Chapman MW: Morbidity at bone graft donor sites. *Orthop Trans* 1987; 10:494.
111. Yuan HA, Mann KA, Found EM, et al: Early clinical experience with the Syracuse I-plate: An anterior spinal fixation device. *Spine* 1988; 13:278–285.
112. Zdeblick TA, Ducker TB: The use of freeze-dried allograft bone for anterior cervical fusions. *Spine* 1991; 16:726–729.

17

Spinal Orthoses

Gary A. Schneiderman, M.D., and Mark Hambly, M.D.

The use of orthotics in the treatment of spinal disorders dates back to antiquity. In 200 B.C. Galen attempted to correct scoliotic curves by wrapping bandages about the chest. Lumbosacral corsets, which were initially utilized as women's foundations, have been traced back 2,000 years to the Minoan period.[6] Tree bark corsets have been recovered from the dwellings of pre-Colombian Indians living in the southwestern United States circa 900 A.D.[2,45] And yet, the spinal orthotic remains a mainstay in the treatment of spinal disorders. The purpose of these devices is to limit motion, correct deformity, and reduce loads on the spine. A number of factors influence the ability of the orthotic to achieve these goals.

The patient's anatomy is of prime importance when considering a spinal orthosis. The first consideration is the spinal level involved. The usual subgroups of the spine—cervical, thoracic, and lumbar—can be further broken down to atlantoaxial (C1–2), midcervical (C3–T1), thoracic (T2–10), thoracolumbar (T11–L1), lumbar (L1–4), and lumbosacral (L4–S1). In general the cephalad and caudad extremes of the spine are more difficult to immobilize with an orthotic. Other anatomic factors include body habitus and skin condition. Orthotics require contact with the skin and are molded to the body's contours in order to achieve fixation. Patients who are overweight may be difficult to fit. Abnormalities of the skin such as the thin skin of a rheumatoid patient or the propensity for decubiti in a neurologically impaired individual may require modifications in the brace's design or fabrication material.

Biomechanical factors influencing the choice of an orthotic are the degree of instability, the degree of deformity, and the anticipated load on the spine. Understanding the plane of deformity or instability and anticipating the amount of load or force that is acting on the spine is essential in choosing the proper orthotic. No brace can provide absolute rigidity of fixation. Therefore, patients with significant instability or severe deformity or individuals in situations where large loads are possible may not be appropriate candidates for bracing.

Physiologic factors to consider include the quality of the bone, the neurologic status of the patient, and changes in function of the body's organ systems, including the respiratory, gastrointestinal, and renal systems. Despite the development of spinal implants that do not require external support, an orthotic might be considered in patients with internal spinal fixation who are osteoporotic or markedly unstable. On the other hand, bracing can have a detrimental effect on the patient's physiology. Changes in the vital capacity have been noted with thoracolumbosacral orthoses (TLSOs) in severe neuromuscular scoliotics.[33] The restrictive nature of a TLSO may be unbearable for the patient with chronic obstructive pulmonary disease. Abdominal distension associated with ileus makes casting and brace fabrication of the thoracolumbar spine difficult. Renal function has been noted to be altered in patients treated with braces for scoliosis.[1, 5] The negative effects of long-term orthosis use can be significant. Potential problems include atrophy; fibrosis; contractures of the paraspinal and anterior abdominal musculature, fascia, and ligaments; skin irritation; and psychological dependence.[3, 28, 32]

Cervical braces can be divided into cervical and cervicothoracic orthoses (Figs 17–1 to 17–4). With the exception of the halo apparatus, which allows for skeletal fixation to the skull, cervical orthoses support the neck by contact with the occiput and mandible cephalad and the shoulder girdle caudad. Cervicothoracic orthoses achieve further support by extending the brace inferiorly over the thorax. Another modification of the cervical orthosis is the head strap. In the Minerva type of brace this head strap is used for further immobilization. In the SOMI (skull, occiput, mandibular immobilizer) brace the head strap provides temporary support when the chin piece is removed to allow for mastication.

The degree of immobilization provided by the cervical braces varies with the level of injury and the brace design.[11, 12, 21] As has been reported by Johnson et al.,[11, 12] the soft collar provides little immobilization and may act solely as a reminder to the patient to limit motion. The remaining cervical and cervicothoracic orthoses provide variable amounts of immobilization. The degree of immobilization as described by Johnson et al. varies with the level of involvement, the brace design, and the plane of

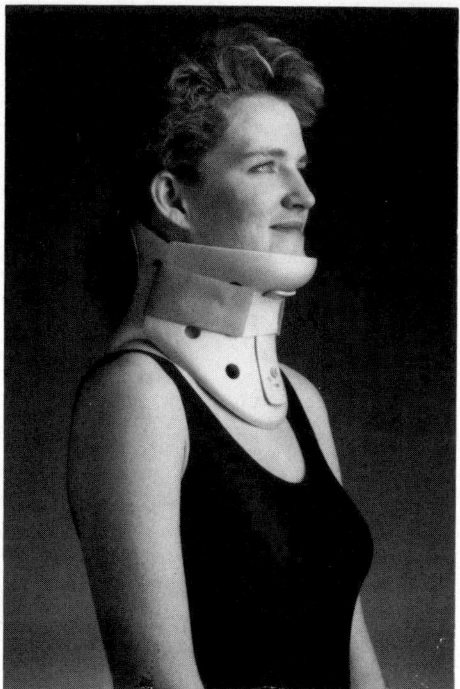

FIG 17–1.
Philadelphia collar, prefabricated.

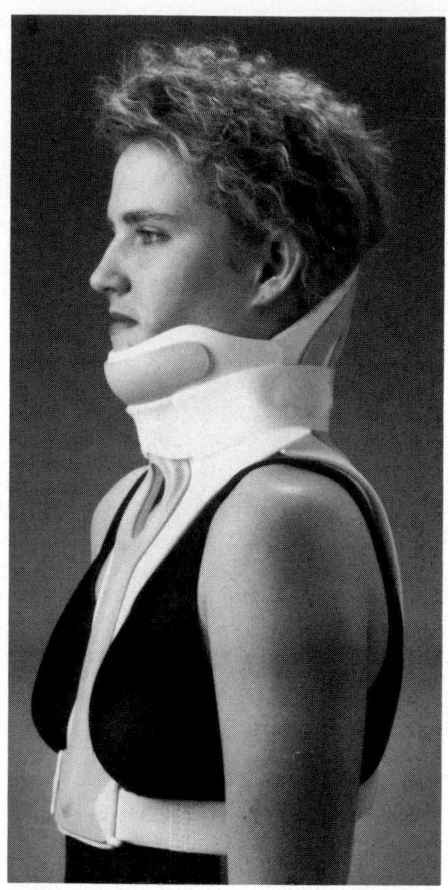

FIG 17–2.
Yale cervical orthosis. This brace represents a modification of the Philadelphia collar with further extension of support over the thorax.

instability.[11, 12] The orthotic choice is determined by the level and type of injury (Table 17–1).

The halo apparatus provides the greatest amount of immobilization in all planes of motion at every level of the cervical spine.[11, 12] First described by Perry and Nickel[37] in 1959, the halo uses pins to attach the cephalad ring of the brace to the skull. A series of upright bars connects the ring to the thoracic portion of the appliance. The thoracic portion may be either a cast, vest, or a series of contact pads. The cast has been shown to be more effective in limiting cervical motion, probably due to better contact conformation to the thoracic wall as compared with the vest.[48] The vests are generally "off the shelf" and are fitted by circumference rather than being custom-molded to the thorax (Fig 17–5). The use of longer vests to obtain greater trunk contact does not seem to improve immobilization.[40] The disadvantage of casting is that the application is more time-consuming and requires more patient positioning than does a vest. Skin hygiene under a cast may also be a problem, particularly in the neurologically impaired patient. Greater skull pin loosening has also been observed in patients treated in the halo cast vs. the vest.

Cervical motion still occurs in the halo.[11, 12, 15] The cervical spine is a mobile structure composed of multiple motion segments. In the halo, fixation points are at the end of this multisegmented structure rather than at each individual segment. Motion can occur between the fixation points, with flexion occurring at one segment while extension occurs at another. This "snaking" motion has been implicated as a mechanism for displacement of fractures and dislocations immobilized in a halo apparatus.

Loading and unloading of the cervical spine also occurs in the halo. Changes in load across the cervical spine have been noted with changes in patient position from supine to sitting. Shoulder shrugging pushes up on the shoulder straps of the vest or cast and can increase loads on the cervical spine.[15]

Recently, the thoracic portion of the halo has been redesigned in order to alleviate some of the problems with the halo vest and cast. Krag and Beynnon[16] have modified the brace by changing the vest to a system of pads that contact relatively immobile regions of the thoracic wall at the sternum, intrascapular area, and the lateral chest wall (Fig 17–6, A–C). No shoulder straps are necessary, and thus the problem of loading and unloading through them is negated. The pads can be easily adjusted to the contours of the body, and yet less skin area is contacted, which allows for better skin hygiene as compared with the halo cast or vest. Finally, the brace is easy to apply and adjust.

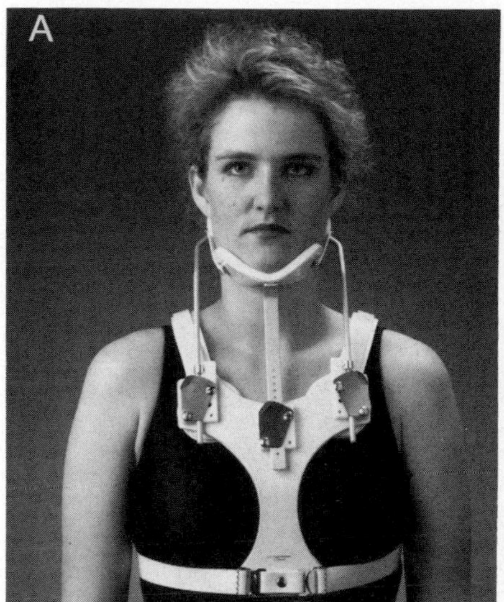

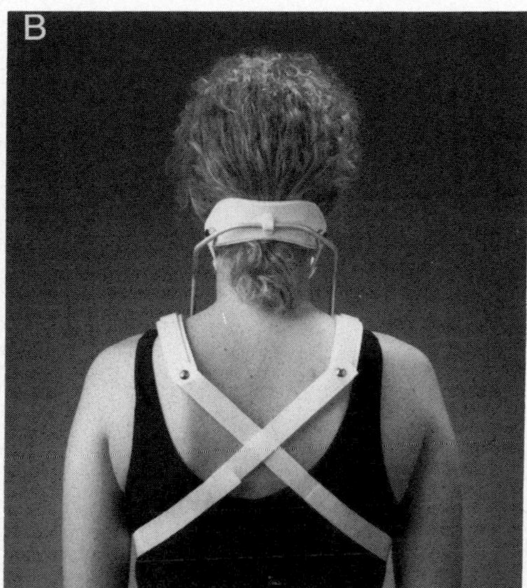

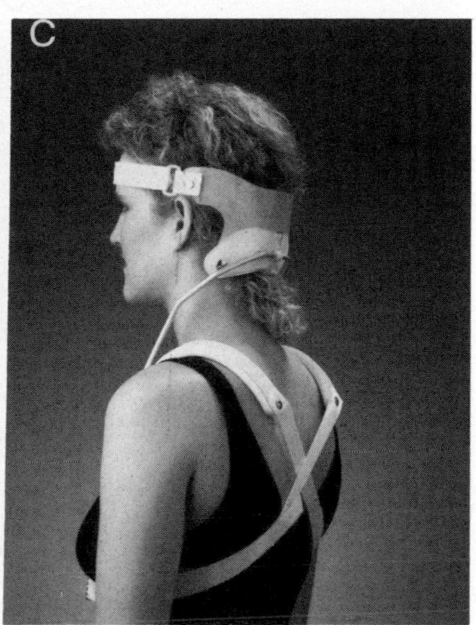

FIG 17-3.
A, SOMI frontal view demonstrating the mandibular support and anterior strap mechanism. **B,** SOMI posterior view showing the occipital support and crossed strap design. **C,** SOMI oblique view. Note the head strap applied with removal of the mandibular support. This addition to the appliance allows for mastication during meals. Restriction of motion is maintained by the brace despite removal of the mandibular support.

Use of the halo is not without complications. Pin loosening, infection, loss of reduction, skin decubiti, and skull perforation have all been described. Proper application of the brace and careful attention to the care of the pin sites is essential to prevent complications. Pins should be tightened initially to 6 to 8 ft-lb and retightened at 24 or 48 hours.[9] Pin care should be performed daily, including cleansing of the pin sites with peroxide or sterile saline and painting with an antiseptic solution such as povidone-iodine (Betadine). Ointment should not be used around the pins. If loosening occurs, the pins can be retightened as long as resistance is felt. Newer designs of pins and braces may be helpful in the future in the prevention of complications.

Research on the effectiveness of bracing in the thoracic spine has been primarily in the area of scoliosis. Use of the cervicothoracic lumbosacral orthosis (CTLSO) or

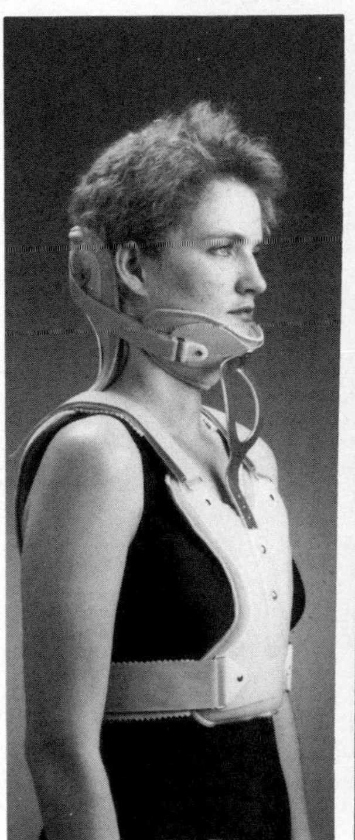

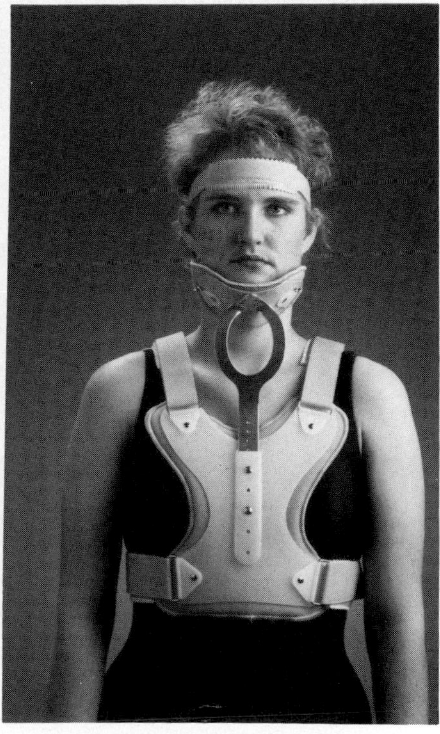

FIG 17-4.
Minerva-style cervical brace. **B,** frontal view, Minerva-style brace. Note the head strap used for additional support.

TABLE 17–1.
Selected Cervical Injuries and Orthoses Recommended*

Clinical Condition	Segmental Level	Plane of Instability	Recommended Orthoses
Ring C1 (Jefferson fracture)			
Stable	Occiput C1	All	Yale
Unstable	Occiput C2	All	Halo
Dens (odontoid types II and III)	C1–2	All	Halo
Atlantoaxial instability (rheumatoid)	C1–2	Flexion	SOMI
Neural arch C2 fracture (hangman's fracture)			
Stable	C2–3	Flexion	SOMI
Unstable	C2–3	All	Halo
Flexion injuries, midcervical C3–5	C3–5	Flexion	Yale, SOMI
Flexion injuries, lower cervical C5–T1	C5–T1	Flexion	Cervicothoracic
Extension injuries, midcervical C3–5	C3–5	Extension	Halo, cervicothoracic
Extension injuries, lower cervical C5–T1	C5–T1	Extension	Halo

*From Johnson RM, Owen JR, Hart DL, et al: *Clin Orthop* 1981; 154:34–45. Used by permission.

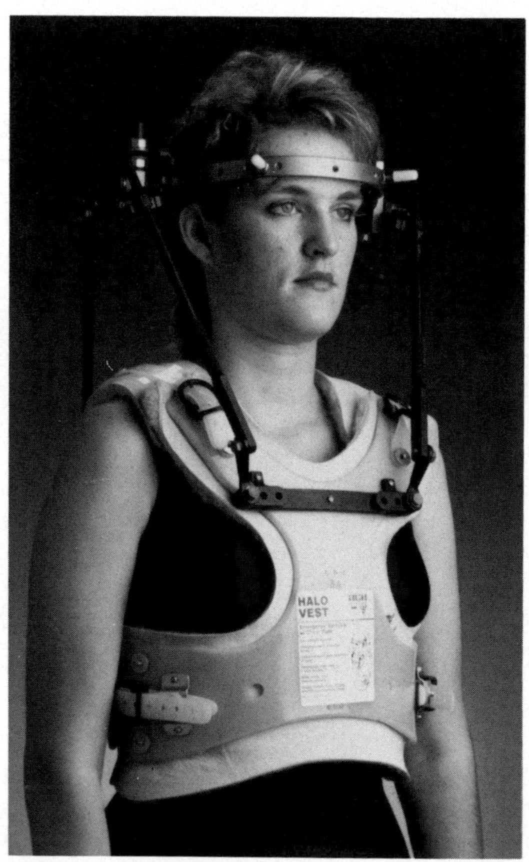

FIG 17–5.
Halo vest, Ace manufacturing design. Note the rigid shoulder straps and encompassing vest. Various vest sizes are available prefabricated. The halo ring, superstructure, and vest are magnetic resonance imaging (MRI) compatible.

the TLSO has been shown to reduce deformity and lessen loads on spinal implants in surgical patients stabilized with internal fixation.[32] Extrapolating this information to other pathologic entities in the thoracic spine such as fracture dislocations, infections, and tumors is difficult, and the data to date are limited (Fig 17–7, A and B). However, in the upper segment of the thoracic spine (T1–6), modifying a standard TLSO with a cervical extension (Fig 17–8) that provides for occipital mandibular contact has been recommended.[14] More rigid proximal fixation can be obtained with a halo applied to the TLSO. For the midthoracic spine (T7–11) a standard underarm TLSO is usually adequate. Significant instability may preclude the use of a brace in the absence of internal fixation.

The thoracolumbar junction (T11–L1) is the most frequent level of traumatic injury in the thoracic or lumbar spine. The effect of bracing at this level has been studied by Nagel et al.[31] Thoracolumbar injuries were inflicted on cadaveric preparations and stability assessed after the application of a Knight-Taylor brace, three-point hyperextension brace, and body cast. The three-point hyperextension brace was effective in reducing flexion by 27% but was ineffective at reducing extension. The Knight-Taylor brace reduced both flexion and extension by 20% but was poor in controlling lateral bending. Only the body cast controlled flexion, extension, and lateral bending.

Patwardhan has recently studied the thoracolumbar area by using finite analysis of cadaveric spines.[35] One- and two-level injuries were created with increasing levels of instability. A three-point hyperextension brace (Jewett brace) was used to stabilize the injury, and the brace's effectiveness at stabilizing the segment with increasing lev-

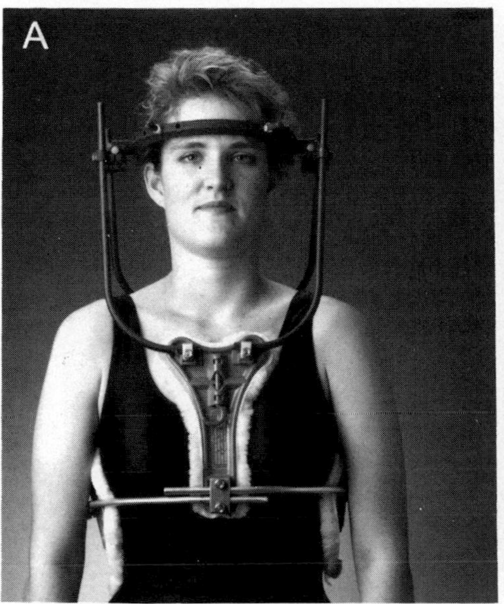

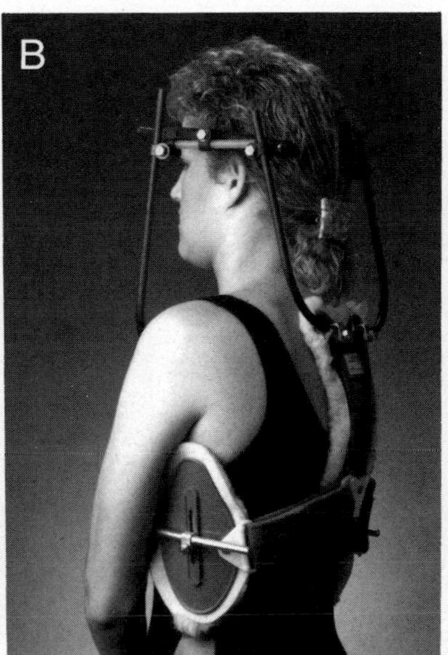

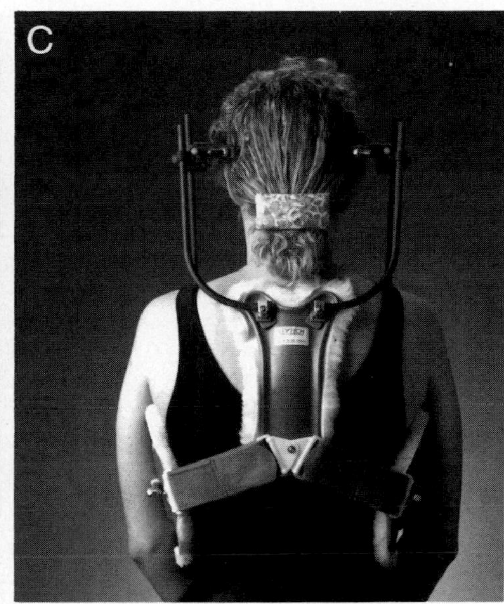

FIG 17–6.
Levtec halo vest designed by Krag and Beynnon. The anterior sternal pad attaches to the side pads and contact fixation obtained anteriorly and laterally. Note the absence of shoulder straps. **B,** lateral view of the pad system. **C,** posterior view demonstrating the limited contact of the posterior pad to the interscapular area.

els of instability was evaluated (Fig 17–9). If greater than 85% of the stiffness was lost in a single-level injury or 60% in two-level injuries, then the brace was ineffective at controlling flexion deformity. This would be the case in a severe three-column injury. Severe two-column injuries affecting one level could be controlled in the brace in low-level load situations.

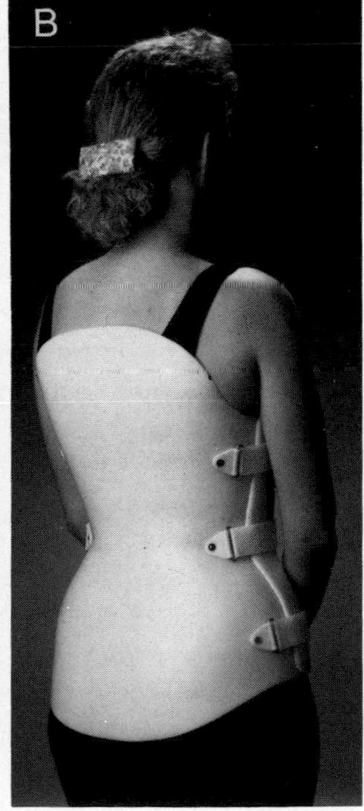

FIG 17–7.
A and **B,** standard underarm thoracolumbarsacral orthoses.

Bracing of the thoracolumbar spine has been found to be effective in the management of fractures.[13, 14, 39, 42] The argument against bracing as a primary treatment in the more severe injuries to this area is the risk of prolonged bed rest, concerns about spinal alignment and deformity, the importance of early immobilization and rehabilitation, and concerns about chronic pain and late neurologic deterioration due to stenosis or instability. However, the use of orthotics is well documented in the thoracolumbar spine, both as a primary method of treatment and as adjunctive support in the surgically stabilized patient.

In terms of primary treatment for acute thoracolumbar spine injuries, Jones et al. found satisfactory results in patients kept at bed rest for an average of 6 to 8 weeks followed by bracing an average of 16 weeks.[13] Reid et al., after following 21 neurologically intact patients with burst fractures, recommended bracing after 24 to 48 hours with a TLSO. Bracing was continued over 12 weeks with satisfactory results.[39] Weinstein retrospectively reviewed patients treated nonoperatively with thoracolumbar burst fractures over a 40-year period. The majority of patients were treated in a cast or brace and were neurologically intact. There were no complications related to the cast or brace. In general, nonoperative treatment resulted in a successful outcome with minimal pain, asymptomatic deformity, and only minimal risk of instability or stenosis. The neurologic outcome in patients with incomplete spinal cord injuries was comparable to patients treated surgically.[42]

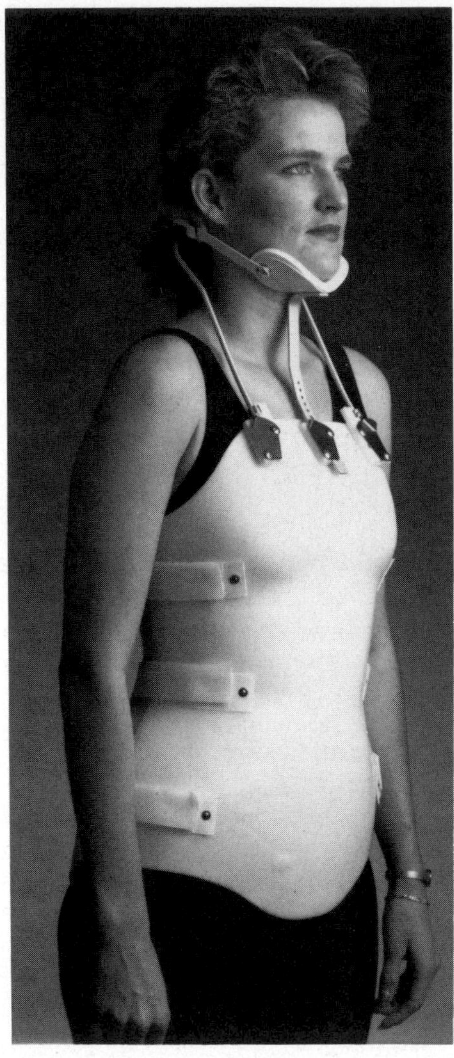

FIG 17–8.
Cervicothoracic lumbosacral orthosis. The addition of a SOMI appliance to the TLSO allows for improved immobilization in the lower cervical/upper thoracic vertebrae. Greater immobilization of the cervicothoracic junction is obtained with a halo rather than this design.

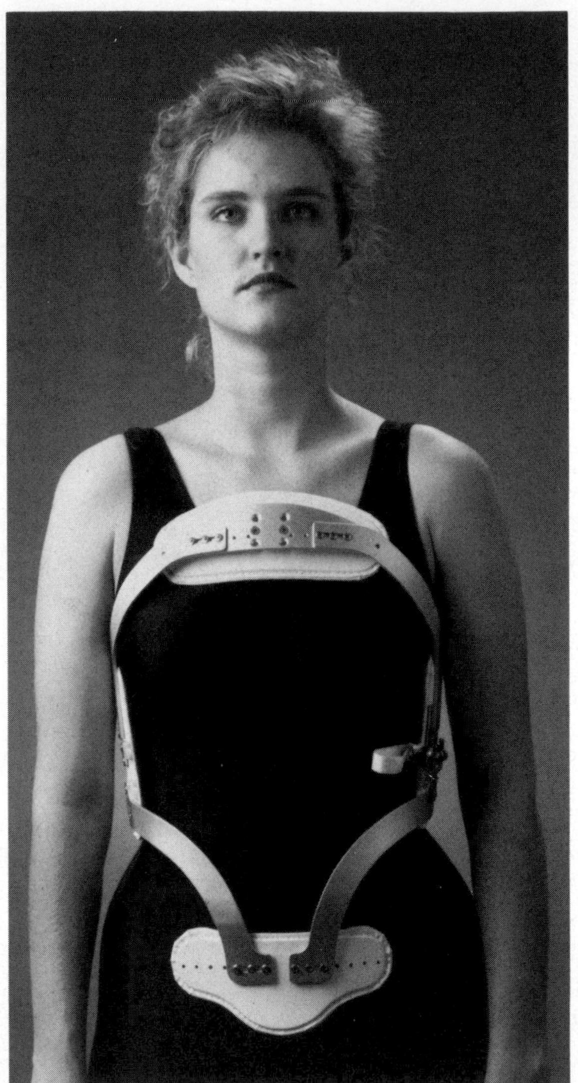

FIG 17–9.
Jewett hyperextension orthosis. A single pad is utilized posteriorly and two pads anteriorly to achieve "three-point" support.

In the lumbar spine, orthoses are utilized to exert either a corrective or supportive force in the spine. The first actual lumbosacral corset was made in 1530 for Catherine de Medici.[7] It was specifically designed to function as a lumbosacral corset. In 1863, Taylor designed a brace that utilized the principle of three-point fixation.[2] The Taylor brace was originally designed for the treatment of Pott's disease. While lumbosacral orthoses are still utilized in the treatment of infection, fractures, and deformity, they are probably most frequently used in the treatment of idiopathic low back pain.

Immobilization, stabilization, maintenance or correction of deformity, and decreased joint loading are all biomechanical goals of external immobilization of the spine. Immobilization of the trunk, increased intra-abdominal pressure, and modification of trunk muscle function have all been implicated as mechanisms by which lumbosacral orthoses function.[28]

The degree of immobilization of the lumbar spine varies of course with the brace's design. The more rigid orthoses utilize three-point fixation to limit flexion and extension. Three-point fixation is created by applying forces proximally and distally to the segment to be immobilized. A third oppositely directed counterforce between the proximal and distal forces is used to achieve three-point fixation. If the counterforce is placed anteriorly to the spine and the proximal and distal forces posteriorly, then a flexion movement is created. Examples of this are the Williams brace or Raney jacket. Conversely, if the counterforce is placed posteriorly and the proximal and distal forces are anterior to the spine, then an extension movement is created as in the Jewett hyperextension brace.

A lumbosacral orthosis relies upon two-point fixation proximally and distally and the inherent rigidity of the brace to control axial rotation. Axial rotation of the lumbosacral joint averages 6 degrees while standing during maximal rotation and 1.5 degrees while walking. However, Lumsden and Morris found that during normal level walking an orthosis did not appear to decrease lumbosacral rotation and in some subjects it actually increased rotation.[20]

Lateral bending is limited by the addition of longitudinal lateral supports that provide two-point fixation. The rigidity of the support and the quality of the interface at the thorax and pelvis determine to what degree lateral bending is limited. A lumbosacral corset, chairback brace, and molded TLSO have all been shown to restrict lateral bending by 29%, 45%, and 49%, respectively.[17]

The degree of immobilization of intersegmental motion depends upon the type of orthosis utilized. Fidler and Plasmans compared the canvas jacket, Raney jacket, body jacket cast, and pantaloon-type cast.[8] Each respective orthosis was studied by using roentgenographic measurements. Motion was reduced at each level by approximately 30%. Midlumbar motion was reduced approximately 66% by both the Raney jacket and body jacket cast. Neither of these orthoses were more effective than a corset in immobilizing the proximal part of the lumbar spine. Intersegmental motion at the L4–5 and the L5–S1 levels was reduced by 92% by the pantaloon cast. The effect of a molded TLSO, chairback brace, and lumbosacral corset on gross body motion was studied by Lantz and Schultz.[18] An orthosis limited motion by up to 20% in flexion and 45% in extension.

Intra-abdominal pressure is increased with almost all lumbar braces.[10] The reduction of load on the lumbar spine by an orthosis may be due to this increase. However, this effect is not well understood. While the load on the lumbar spine has been shown to decrease with an increase in the intra-abdominal pressure,[49] other studies have demonstrated increased load.[50]

Decreases in trunk muscle activity have been considered as a mechanism whereby a lumbar brace reduces load on the spine. However, myoelectric studies have demonstrated that orthoses such as a chairback brace or molded TLSO inconsistently reduce the myoelectric activity of the erector spinae and abdominal musculature.[18, 30, 41] The true mechanism by which an orthotic reduces pain in the lumbar spine remains unknown.

Fixation of an orthosis to the body is difficult in that the soft tissues interface between the brace and the body's bony prominences. This relatively loose layer of tissue forces the brace to rely on friction for fixation. Fixation proximally is not as problematic as it is distally at the pelvis. The thorax has a greater surface area upon which the orthosis can act than does the pelvis. More complete fixation of the lumbosacral joint (92%) can be obtained if the hip joint is immoblized with a single spica thigh extension added to the brace. Unfortunately, this may render the patient more disabled or uncomfortable. A droplock hinge between the TLSO and the spica extension can be used to allow the hip joint to be mobilized when necessary (Fig 17–10). This allows for ease of brace application and improves comfort.

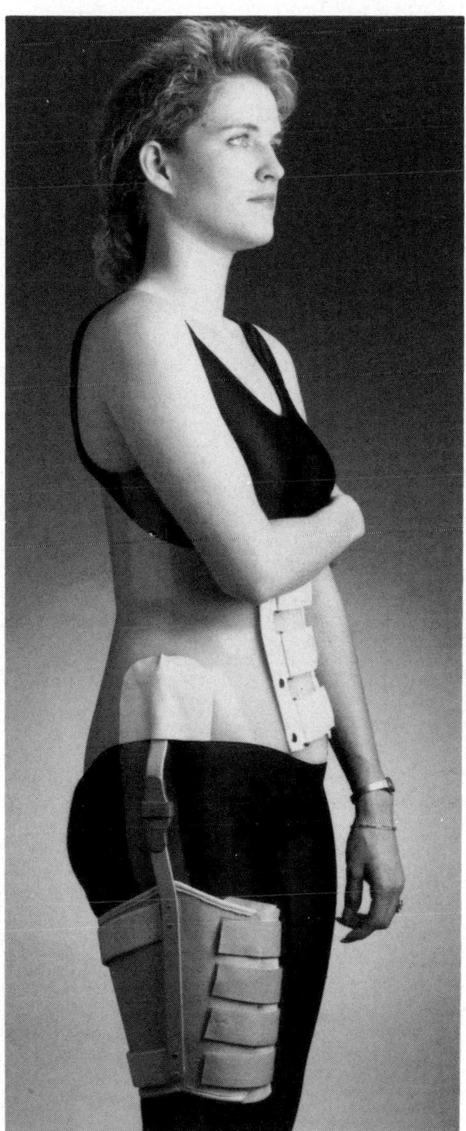

FIG 17–10.
Boston overlap brace with the addition of a single thigh spica. This particular design incorporates the use of a droplock hinge that attaches the Boston overlap brace to the thigh gaiter. The droplock is raised to allow for flexion of the hip, which allows for easier application of the brace. The droplock is then set and the thigh fixed to the torso via the brace, thus providing additional restriction of motion at L4–5 and L5–S1.

The orthosis prescribed should be as comfortable as possible while both standing and sitting. Compliance becomes a significant problem if the orthosis is unduly cumbersome.

Lumbar spine orthoses have been commonly prescribed and reported as effective in clinical use. However, very few well-controlled studies exist.[2, 25] Patient populations with low back pain of unknown etiology treated with an orthosis have yielded inconclusive results.[2, 24, 25] Reliable reproducible results have been obtained in patients with discrete pathologic conditions such as spondylolysis or spondylolisthesis.[19, 23, 45] Idiopathic low back pain is probably the most common indication for spinal bracing. This would include acute lumbosacral strain, internal disc disruption, and myofascial syndrome. Accurate diagnosis allows the specific biomechanical needs of the patient to be addressed.

The lumbosacral corset is the orthosis most commonly prescribed for the lumbosacral strain.[36] A corset can be fabricated with or without stays. The material and its configuration determine its ultimate rigidity. Controversy exists as to whether lordosis or kyphosis is effective. Inflatable bladders have also been added to increase intra-abdominal pressure in a uniform manner. Angular movements have been shown to be decreased by approximately 66% of normal with a canvas corset.[8] Axial rotation was not well controlled, however. A significant placebo effect along with a massaging effect has been associated with the use of an orthosis.[10, 28]

Internal disc disruption has been treated with any number of orthoses. The relative unloading of the disc by posteriorly displacing axial forces, postural modification, and limitation of gross motion is the goal. Restoration of the lumbar lordosis with bracing has been shown to reduce pain.[22]

Spondylolysis and spondylolisthesis in the adolescent have been successfully treated in patients with a rigid flexion brace (Boston) (Fig 17–11, A and B). The spondylolytic defect healed in 16% of this group.[23] A canvas corset can also be used effectively.[46] In adults with documented 25% to 50% spondylolisthetic slip, a rigid thermoplastic flexion brace provided complete pain relief in 87% and some relief in the remaining 13%.[45]

Some success has been achieved in the treatment of spinal stenosis with bracing.[23, 45, 47] A flexed posture may provide relief from neurogenic claudication and back pain. Consequently, the orthosis should maintain flexed posture and provide adequate stabilization. Unfortunately, rigid braces are not generally tolerated by elderly patients. Severe symptomatic spinal stenosis is poorly treated with an orthotic.

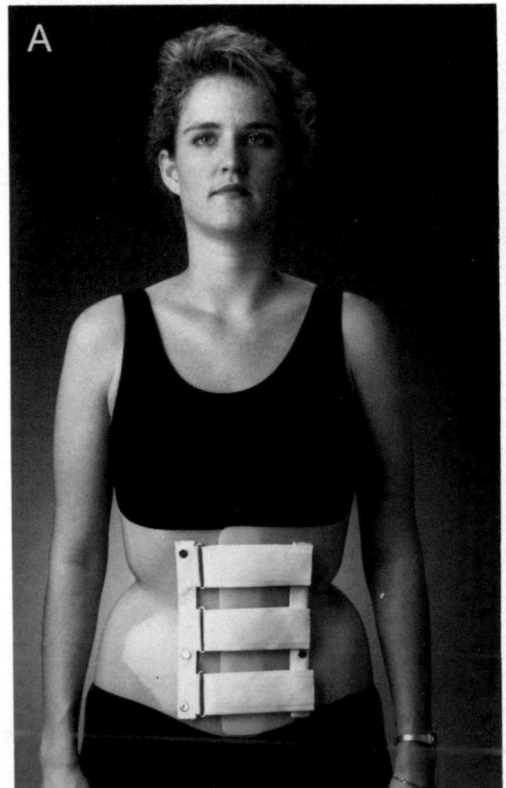

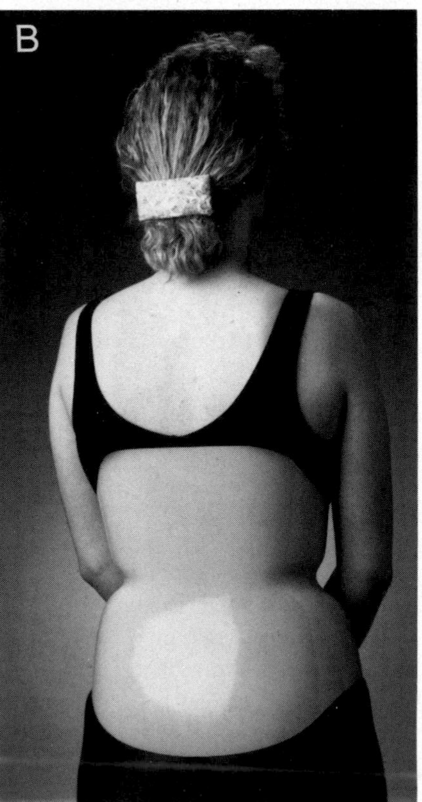

FIG 17–11.
Boston overlap brace. Note that this brace has an anterior closure. It is available prefabricated in a number of sizes.

Degenerative instability such as degenerative spondylolisthesis can be treated with bracing. Significant postdecompression instability is more difficult to treat orthotically.

Lumbar spondylitis requires control of segmental motion at the involved levels. During the acute phase a TLSO, pantaloon cast, or body jacket are effective in conjunction with appropriate medical treatment. Once the acute pain and spasm have subsided, an orthosis that is less rigid is adequate.

In summary, use of external support in spinal disorders remains an effective method of treatment with careful selection of the appliance. A successful result in terms of relief of pain, stabilization of instability, and reduction of deformity can be achieved.

REFERENCES

1. Aaro S, Berg U: The immediate effect of the Boston brace on renal function in patients with idiopathic scoliosis. *Clin Orthop* 1982; 170:243–247.
2. Ahlgren SA, Hansen T: The use of lumbosacral corsets prescribed for low back pain. *Prosthet Orthot Int* 1978; 2:101–104.
3. American Academy of Orthopaedic Surgeons: *Atlas of Orthotics: Biomechanical Principles and Application*. St. Louis, Mosby–Year Book, 1975, pp 312–360.
4. American Academy of Orthopaedic Surgeons: *Orthopaedic Appliances Atlas*. Ann Arbor, Mich, Edwards, 1952, pp 180–187.
5. Berg U, Aaro S: The long term effect of Boston brace treatment on renal function in patients with idiopathic scoliosis. *Clin Orthop* 1983; 180:169–172.
6. Evans A: *The Palace of Minos at Knossos*, vol 1. London, MacMillan, 1921, p 503.
7. Ewing E: *Fashion in Underwear*. Batsford, 1971, p 13.
8. Fidler MW, Plasmans CMT: The effect of four types of support on the segmental mobility of the lumbosacral spine. *J Bone Joint Surg [Am]* 1983; 65:943–947.
9. Garfin SR, Botte MJ, Waters RL, et al: Complications in the use of the halo fixation device. *J Bone Joint Surg [Am]* 1986; 68:320–325.
10. Grew ND, Deane G: The physical effect of lumbar spine supports. *Prosthet Orthot Int* 1982; 6:79–87.
11. Johnson RM, Hart DL, Simmons EF, et al: Cervical orthoses. *J Bone Joint Surg [Am]* 1977; 59:332–339.
12. Johnson RM, Owen JR, Hart DL, et al: Cervical orthoses, a guide to their selection and use. *Clin Orthop* 1981; 154:34–45.
13. Jones RF, Snowdon E, Coan J, et al: Bracing of thoracic and lumbar spine fractures. *Paraplegia* 1987; 25:386–393.
14. Keefer B, Levine AM: Total contact orthoses for immobilization of thoracolumbar fractures. *Orthop Nurs* 1985; 6:36–54.
15. Koch RA, Nickel VL: The halo vest, an evaluation of motion and forces across the neck. *Spine* 1978; 3:103–107.
16. Krag MH, Beynnon BD: A new halo-vest: Rationale, design and biomechanical comparison to standard halo-vest designs. *Spine* 1988; 13:228–235.
17. Lantz SA, Schultz AB: Lumbar spine orthosis wearing. 1. Restriction of gross body motions. *Spine* 1986; 11:834–837.
18. Lantz SA, Schultz AB: Lumbar spine orthosis wearing. 2. Effect on trunk muscle myoelectric activity. *Spine* 1986; 11:838–842.
19. Larsson U, Choler U, Lidstrom A, et al: Autotraction for treatment of lumbagosciatica: A multicentre controlled investigation. *Acta Orthop Scand* 1980; 51:791–798.
20. Lumsden RM, Morris JM: An in vivo study of axial rotation and immobilization at the lumbosacral joint. *J Bone Joint Surg [Am]* 1968; 50:1591–1602.
21. McCabe JB, Nolan DJ: Comparison of the effectiveness of different cervical immobilization collars. *Ann Emerg Med* 1986; 15:50–53.
22. McKenzie RA: Prophylaxis in recurrent low back pain. *NZ Med J* 1979; 89:22–23.
23. Micheli LJ, Hall JE, Miller ME: Use of modified Boston brace for back injuries in athletes. *Am J Sports Med* 1980; 8:351–356.
24. Million R, Hall W, Nilsen KH, et al: Assessment of the progress of the back-pain patient. *Spine* 1982; 7:204–211.
25. Million R, Nilsen KH, Jayson MIV, et al: Evaluation of low back pain and assessment of lumbar corsets with and without back supports. *Ann Rheum Dis* 1981; 40:449–454.
26. Deleted in proofs.
27. Deleted in proofs.
28. Nachemson A: Orthotic treatment for injuries and diseases of the spinal column. *Phys Med Rehabil* 1987; 1:11–24.
29. Deleted in proofs.
30. Nachemson A, Schultz AB, Anderson GBJ: Mechanical effectiveness studies of lumbar spine orthoses. *Scan J Rehabil Med Suppl* 1983; 9:139.
31. Nagel DA, Koogle TA, Piziali RL, et al: Stability of the upper lumbar spine following progressive disruptions and the application of individual internal and external fixation devices. *J Bone Joint Surg [Am]* 1981; 63:62–70.
32. Nash CL: Current concepts review. Scoliosis bracing. *J Bone Joint Surg [Am]* 1980; 62:848–852.
33. Noble-Jamieson CM, Heckmatt JZ, Dabowitz V, et al: Effects of posture and spinal bracing on respiratory function in neuromuscular disease. *Arch Dis Child* 1986; 61:178–181.
34. Norton PL, Brown T: The immobilizing efficiency of back braces. Their effect on the posture and motion of the lumbosacral spine. *J Bone Joint Surg [Am]* 1957; 39:111–138.
35. Patwardhan AG, Li S, Gavin T, et al: Orthotic stabilization of thoracolumbar injuries, a biomechanical analysis of the Jewett hyperextension orthoses. *Spine* 1990; 15:654–661.
36. Perry J: The use of external support in the treatment of low back pain. Report of the Subcommittee on Orthotics of the Committee on Prosthetic-Orthotic Education. National Academy of Sciences, National Research Council. *J Bone Joint Surg [Am]* 1970; 52:1440–1442.
37. Perry J, Nickel VL: Total cervical spine fusion for neck paralysis. *J Bone Joint Surg [Am]* 1959; 50:1400–1409.
38. Deleted in proofs.

39. Reid DC, Ha R, Davis LA, et al: The nonoperative treatment of burst fractures of the thoracolumbar junction. *J Trauma* 1988; 28:1188–1194.
40. Wang GJ, Moskal JT, Albert T, et al: The effect of halo-vest length on stability of the cervical spine. A study in normal subjects. *J Bone Joint Surg [Am]* 1988; 70:357–360.
41. Waters RL, Morris JM: Effects of spinal supports on the electrical activity of muscles of the trunk. *J Bone Joint Surg [Am]* 1970; 52:51–60.
42. Weinstein JN, Collato P, Lehman TR: Long term follow-up of nonoperatively treated thoracolumbar spine fractures. *J Orthop Trauma* 1987; 1:152–159.
43. Deleted in proofs.
44. Whitehill R, Richman JA, Glaser JA: Failure of immobilization of the cervical spine by the halo vest. *J Bone Joint Surg [Am]* 1986; 68:326–332.
45. Willner S: Effect of a rigid brace on back pain. *Acta Orthop Scand* 1985; 56:40–42.
46. Wiltse LL: Personal communication, 1990.
47. Deleted in proofs.
48. Wolf JW, Jones HC: Comparison of immobilization of the cervical spine by halo casts versus plastic jackets. Presented at the Cervical Spine Research Society Annual Meeting, Palm Beach, Fla, 1980.
49. Gracovetsky S, Farfan H, Helleur C: The abdominal mechanism. *Spine* 1985; 10:317–324.
50. Nachemson AL, Andersson GB, Schultz AB: Valsalva maneuver biomechanics: Effects on trunk loads of elevated intraabdominal pressures. *Spine* 1986; 11:476–479.

PART V

BASIC SCIENCE OF SPINE-ASSOCIATED FEATURES

18

*Bone**

W. Thomas Edwards, Ph.D., and Hansen A. Yuan, M.D.

Bone is an adaptive tissue. It is the ability of bone to remodel and, when required, to heal that distinguishes this tissue from other structural, load-bearing materials. Bone is continually undergoing the process of remodeling, with bone formation and resorption proceeding through life. This adaptation of bone is known to depend on metabolic factors,[110] age,[94, 137, 140] race, gender,[18, 46] nutrition, disease, pharmacologic agents,[1, 3, 10, 57] and mechanical stimulation.[108] These factors have been extensively reviewed through studies of osteoporosis and metabolic disorders of bone.[1, 8, 30, 57, 87–89] The mechanical and biological parameters that control remodeling and adaptation play an important role in spine rehabilitation.

NORMAL BONE

Bone is most commonly regarded for its role as the main structural component of the skeleton. In this function, normal mineralized bone maintains the structural integrity of the skeleton within the constraints of physiologic morphology and anatomy. However, bone also serves an equally important function as the primary reservoir for calcium in the maintenance of calcium balance in the body. In these competing roles, bone strength will be sacrificed to provide calcium when required.

The microscopic structure of bone can be divided into three main categories: primary, secondary, and woven bone. Primary bone is new bone that occupies a space where bone has not existed before. Secondary bone is the result of bone remodeling and is the result of bone resorption and bone deposition.[78] The distinction between primary and secondary bone is important because it is believed that different processes control the apposition of bone in each case. Both the strength and stiffness are greater for primary bone in comparison to secondary bone.[78] Both primary and secondary bone are lamellar. The microstructure of woven bone is random, not lamellar. In adults, woven bone is associated with pathologic conditions and response to trauma. In rehabilitation, secondary bone modified through bone remodeling is of principal concern.

Three structural forms of bone tissue may be found in the spine. Trabecular and cortical bone are most common and form the vertebrae, and following injury (fracture of the vertebra) woven bone may occur. In the vertebral body, trabecular bone constitutes over 99% of the volume of bone. The cortical shell of the vertebral body is generally less than 1 mm thick, in the range of 0.4 to 1.3 mm. The density of the trabecular bone depends on age, level of activity, and general health (Fig 18–1). In healthy individuals the apparent density of trabecular bone (the mass of bone mineral per unit volume) in the vertebral body is greater than 150 mg/mL. In osteoporosis or conditions of extreme osteopenia, the risk of atraumatic fracture of the vertebrae become significant for densities below 65 mg/mL.

Bone and the Requirement for Calcium Regulation

The structural function of bone is secondary in many respects to the body's regulation of calcium. The amount of free calcium is tightly controlled. Under physiologic conditions, the total plasma calcium is about 10 mg/dL with part bound to protein and part diffusible. About 47% of the total plasma calcium is ionized Ca^{2+}. Calcium deficiency affects clotting and other systems and in extreme cases may result in hypocalcemic tetany.[42]

Both systemic and local factors regulate the calcium balance through the rate of bone turnover.[109] Systemic control of bone remodeling is required for the regulation of calcium balance. Ninety-nine percent of the body's calcium is stored in bone. Therefore, in this capacity bone represents the primary reservoir for calcium in the body. Local regulation of bone mass must meet the potential systemic demands for calcium while sustaining the strength of the bone in the active mechanical environment. The strength of the bone in the spine is dependent on the bone density, bone quality, and bone morphology.[50, 51, 82, 95] There is evidence that the relative percentage of calcium in comparison to other constituents of bone varies with age and metabolic condition.[25] The failure of either the sys-

*Support for contributing research was provided in part by grants from the AcroMed Corporation, NIH grant AR-33066, and the AO/ASIF Research Foundation. Additional resources were provided by the Department of Orthopedic Surgery, SUNY Health Science Center, Syracuse.

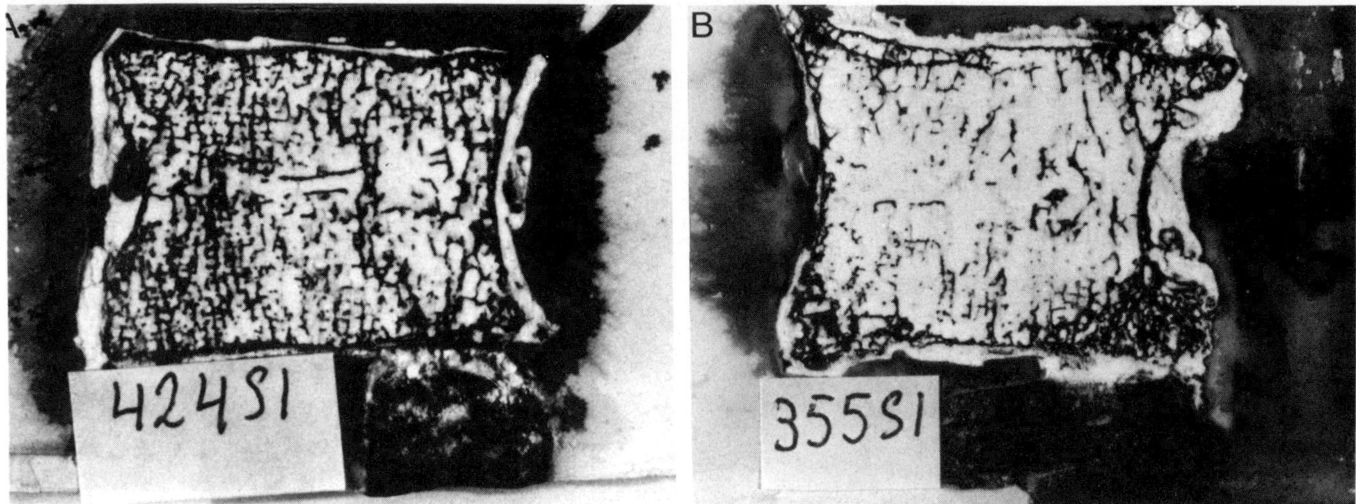

FIG 18–1.
Specimens used for bone density assessment of the distribution of trabecular bone in the midsagittal plane. Specimens were sectioned and then dyed to enhance the bone contrast. Bone is shown in black (India ink); the interspaces are shown in white (confectioner's sugar). **A,** normal bone density. **B,** osteoporotic specimen.

temic or local regulatory processes will result in significant calcium imbalance or localized weakness of bone with increased risk of fracture.

Systemic Regulation of Calcium

In the regulation of calcium, bone remodeling is controlled through the interaction of hormones produced by several organ systems (Fig 18–2). Three main hormones are involved in the systemic regulation of calcium: 1,25-dihydroxyvitamin D_3, (1,25[OH]$_2$ D_3), parathyroid hormone (PTH), and calcitonin. The endocrine systems involved in this process interactively control the release of calcium from bone through the effect of these hormones.[110, 112]

In the systemic regulation of calcium, the hormone 1,25(OH)$_2$$D_3$ is recognized as the principal mediator of bone metabolism. Reichel et al.[112] provide an excellent description of these systemic interactions in their review of the role of vitamin D in the regulation of bone and mineral metabolism.

Multiple forms of vitamin D_3 occur between synthesis and the final active state 1,25[OH]$_2$$D_3$. Vitamin D_3 is synthesized in the skin in the presence of ultraviolet light,[53] and taken into the bloodstream from the intestine. In the liver, hydroxylation of vitamin D_3 occurs to yield 25-hydroxyvitamin D_3 (25[OH]D_3), which circulates freely in the bloodstream. Finally, in the kidney 25(OH)D_3 is transformed to 1,25(OH)$_2$$D_3$ through a two-step process and released to the blood.[112] Ionic factors (PO_4^-, Ca^{2+}, and H^+) and endocrine factors (estrogen, calcitonin, growth hormone, prolactin, insulin, and glucocorticoids) modulate the transformation of vitamin D_3 in the kidney.

Factors known to influence the production of 1,25 (OH)$_2$$D_3$ include PTH, phosphate, and serum calcium. A high intake of phosphate results in decreased serum levels of 1,25(OH)$_2$$D_3$.[105] The principal regulators of 1,25(OH)$_2$$D_3$ production are PTH and 1,25(OH)$_2$$D_3$ itself.[112]

Calcitonin decreases bone resorption.[7, 76] It has been used in the treatment of conditions characterized by high bone turnover rates such as Paget disease[55] and conditions that result in hypercalcemia.[56] Calcitonin may also be effective in limiting bone loss in high-turnover osteoporosis.[15] Estrogen, androgens, insulin, and other factors act systemically to stimulate osteoblasts and bone formation. Interleukin-1 (IL-1), prostaglandin E_2 (PGE_2), 1,25(OH)$_2$$D_3$, epidermal growth factor, and others factors are known stimulators of bone resorption.

Local Regulation of Bone

Bone remodeling at the cellular level is an interactive process involving groups of cells organized in units called basic multicellular units (BMUs) by Frost.[39] BMUs are functional units that include osteoblasts (bone-forming cells) and osteoclasts (bone-resorbing cells). At this local level the BMU must interpret systemic and local stimuli and, when appropriate, initiate bone remodeling. Stimuli include systemic and local chemical signals, mechanical stresses and strains, and electrical signals.

The normal sequence of bone remodeling is a cyclic process with four main steps: activation, resorption, reversal, and formation (ARRF) (Fig 18–3).[109] In this sequence activation occurs first. Lining cells, presumably of osteoblastic linage,[109] cover the inactive bone surface. Osteoblasts possess receptors for 1,25(OH)$_2$$D_3$.[112] Stimula-

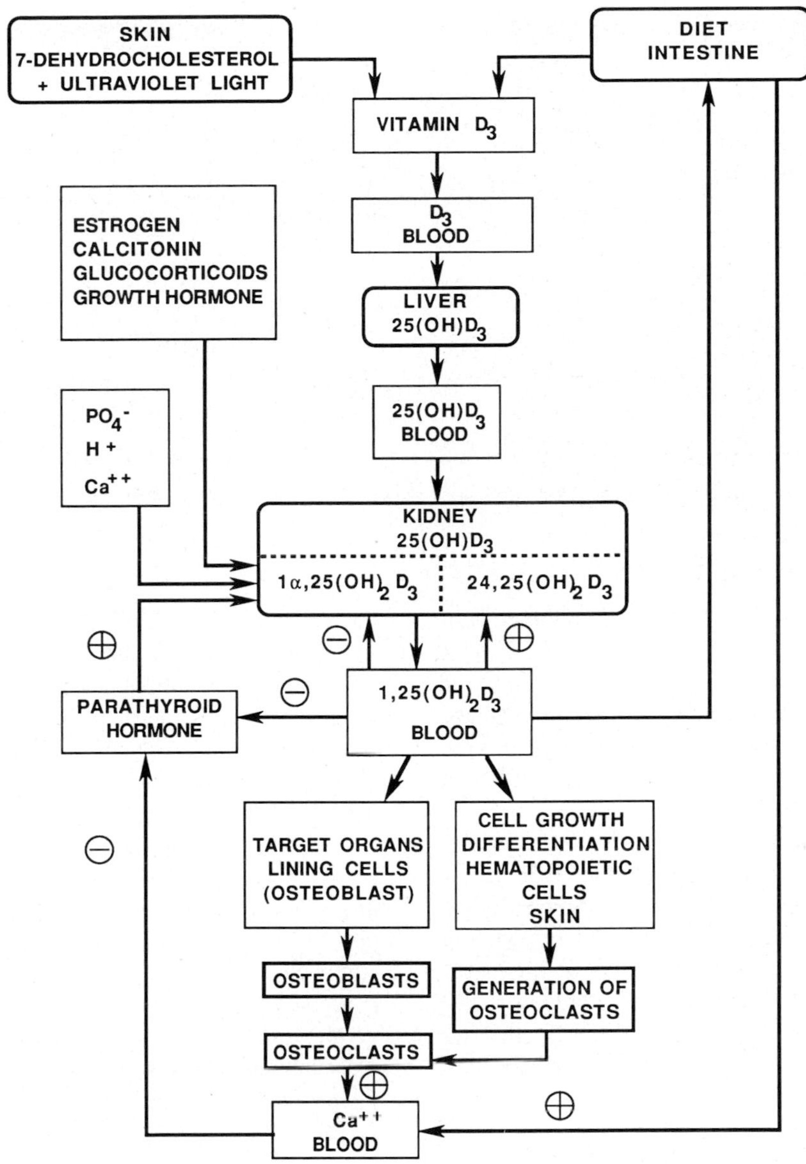

FIG 18–2.
Systemic regulation of bone remodeling and calcium balance.[110, 113]

tion by $1,25(OH)_2D_3$ increases alkaline phosphatase production[70] and the synthesis of osteocalcin by the osteoblast.[100] These cells respond to $1,25(OH)_2D_3$ and other factors. During activation the lining cells contract, expose the bone surface, and provide access by the osteoclasts. Bone resorption is then initiated through the maturation and attachment of osteoclasts to the bone surface. Following the resorption of bone mineral and matrix the reversal phase occurs. Raisz indicates that macrophages may appear on the bone surface at this phase and suggests that they may produce factors to initiate bone formation.[109] During bone formation osteoblasts produce unmineralized bone matrix (osteoid). This osteoid is mineralized following a lag, the mineralization lag time, of about 10 days.[78] The mineralized bone is mostly a complex salt, hydroxyapatite $Ca_{10}(PO_4)_6(OH)_2$.[41]

It is not surprising that mediators must signal the initiation and completion of each stage of the process in view of the coordinated interaction of the cells of the BMU throughout the remodeling processes. Many potential mediators that may serve this function have been identified and were reviewed by Raisz.[109] Osteoblasts and lining cells possess receptors for PTH and $1,25(OH)_2D_3$. Osteoclasts do not respond to these systemic factors. PGE_2 causes a transient inhibition of osteoclastic activity.[72] In bone cell cultures, mechanical stress results in increased

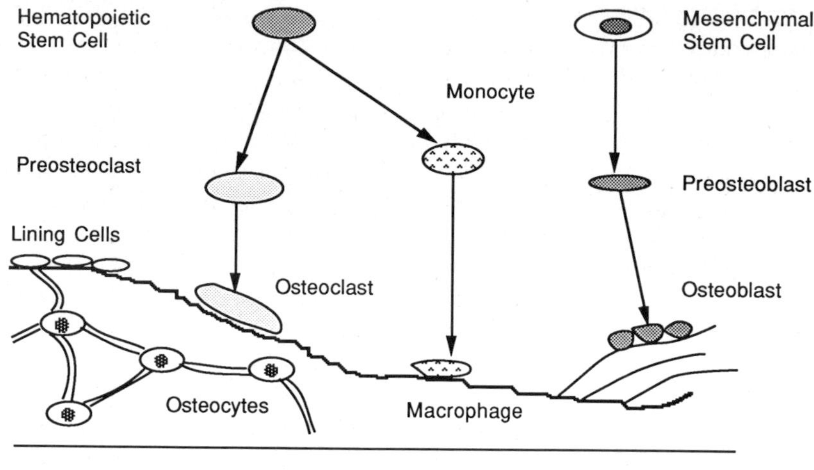

FIG 18–3.
Local remodeling of bone.[79, 110]

PGE_2 production.[126] The administration of indomethacin can reverse bone loss due to immobilization.[132] IL-1α is a stimulator of bone resorption. Low concentrations of IL-1α can interact with PTH and cytokines to increase bone resorption.[23] Locally produced insulin-like growth factor (IGF-1) can produce cell replication and collagen synthesis.

However, current pharmacologic interventions are designed to modify the remodeling cycle of the BMU to either add or reduce local bone mass. This is accomplished by attempting to decouple the ARRF steps of remodeling and alter the balance between bone formation and bone resorption. Unfortunately, the local process is only partially understood, and much work remains to quantify the dynamics of this process.

Structural Features of Bone

There are two major forms of bone within the axial skeleton, cortical and trabecular bone. Cortical bone (compact bone) forms the surface of the vertebrae and is thickest in the region of the lamina and the facets. The density of the cortical bone is about 2 g/mL. Trabecular bone (also called spongy or cancellous bone) is most plentiful within the vertebral body and to a lesser extent in the center portion of the pedicles and the posterior elements. The density of trabecular bone varies significantly with age and other factors but ranges from 0.05 g/mL to 0.3 g/mL. Morphologic analysis of the cancellous bone within the vertebral body has demonstrated that the structure of the trabeculae resembles plates and rods oriented primarily in the superoinferior direction.

Trabecular Morphology and Density Distribution Within the Vertebrae

The density of the bone and the trabecular architecture is not uniform within the vertebra but varies throughout. In the vertebral body three regions of trabeculae can be distinguished in the horizontal plane: two sections of higher-density bone near the superior and inferior end plates that consists of plates of trabeculae and a central section consisting of rods of trabeculae.[5] The biomechanical effects of altered morphology are dependent on both bone density and trabecular architecture.

In the spine the density of the vertebrae can be assessed with high-resolution, noninvasive skeletal imaging procedures such as computed tomography and digital radiography.[8, 42, 82] The accuracy of noninvasive density measurements from the lumbar vertebrae with quantitative computed tomography (QCT) was demonstrated by Genant et al.[42] and others. Other methods for the noninvasive measurement of bone density in the spine include dual-photon absorptiometry (DPA) and dual-energy x-ray absorptiometry (DEXA).[77, 80, 119]

The accuracy and precision of these density measurement techniques have continued to improve with each generation of equipment.[77, 79] At present the DEXA or DPA methods are accepted for patient screening and treatment monitoring. QCT, however, remains the only available technique for independently assessing the spatial distribution of the density of the trabecular bone within the vertebrae. QCT requires higher x-ray exposure in comparison to DEXA and DPA.[77] These techniques have been used to quantify the variation of density within the vertebrae. QCT measurements of bone density in the horizontal plane have shown that the highest density and strength is found at the posterolateral portion of the vertebral body adjacent to the region of the pedicles.[26, 27, 33] With the assumption that bone strength is proportional to density squared, measurements indicate that the strength of the posterior portion of the centrum is greater than the anterior region.[33, 63]

The architecture of trabecular bone may further be

quantified by specifying the bone thickness, the area fraction of bone, the orientation of the trabeculae, and the number in the horizontal and vertical directions. These parameters are generally assessed from measurements of plane sections of trabecular bone by using stereologic techniques.[140, 147, 148] Keller et al. in their stereologic examination of the cross-sectional distribution of bone density (measured by bone area fraction) obtained similar findings.[63] Their measurements demonstrated variations in bone density over the cross section, with the higher densities in the posterolateral position of the body. Wu et al measured the variation of bone density and strength in the midsagittal plane of the vertebral body (Table 18–1). From our area fraction measurements of cancellous bone in 17 L1 midsagittal regions, the highest densities were observed adjacent to the end plates (area fractions, >0.29). Regions of lowest density were found in the central portions of the vertebral bodies, above the midline of the body (area fractions, <0.20).[153]

The structural architecture of trabecular bone has been examined during the process of bone loss. Studies by Arnold[5] and Parfitt[101] indicate that as bone density decreases, there are increasing perforations of trabecular plates, that leave rods of vertically oriented trabeculae. It was reported that the thickness of the horizontal trabeculae decreases while some vertical trabeculae increase in thickness as compensation.[5, 6, 13] It has been suggested that horizontal vertebral trabeculae may be lost preferentially with compensatory thickening of the vertical trabeculae.[109] However, there is disagreement about whether the loss of bone density in the vertebrae is accompanied by generalized trabecular thinning or by a specific loss of lateral struts and compensatory trabecular thickening. It has been reported that the thickness of the horizontal trabeculae decreases more rapidly than that of the vertical trabeculae as bone density decreases.[102] Merz and Schenk observed decreased trabecular thickness with decreased density and ascribed the scatter in data at low densities to hypertrophy of the remaining trabeculae.[90] Eder measured the thickness of the horizontal and vertical trabeculae directly and found that both decreased with loss of density.[30a]

This relationship of trabecular architecture to the strength of the bone within the vertebral body was again studied by using stereologic measurements. Snyder et al. found that as the relative density of the trabecular bone increased, the change in the number of horizontal and vertical trabeculae occurred at equal rates (Fig 18–4).[34, 124] At higher densities the spacing between horizontal and vertical trabeculae was almost identical, but at lower densities the differences in spacing between horizontal and vertical trabeculae become progressively greater.[34, 124] From a biomechanical perspective, the vertical trabeculae represent columns supporting compressive loads, and the horizontal trabeculae act as cross struts stabilizing these columns. A change in the spacing between trabeculae represents a change in the effective length of the members. As the spacing between horizontal trabeculae increases, the effective length of the vertical trabeculae increases. This results in a decrease in stability of the vertical trabeculae under compressive loads. The study indicates that the number of vertical trabeculae in a vertebral body is greater than the number of horizontal trabeculae at all densities. The reduction in horizontal and vertical trabeculae occurs at equal rates as bone density decreases in osteoporosis. Similar results would be anticipated with disuse. These changes in bone density and architecture produce a reduction in bone strength that is greater than that predicted from density alone and correlates better to density raised to a power.

Relation Between Bone Density and Strength

Many have investigated the relationship between the density and strength of bone. It is widely accepted that density is the primary determinant of trabecular strength and that cancellous bone is made up of compact bone.[12] However, with increasing age a decrease in water content, age-related changes in the matrix, and reduced numbers of osteocytes contribute to a reduction in strength. Dickenson measured the tensile strength of strips of femoral cortical

TABLE 18–1.

Mean Percent Area Fractions for 20 Regions Within the Midsagittal Vertebral Slice for L1*

		Post			ANT	Mean	SD
	SUP	33.2	29.3	29.8	31.7	31.0	1.8
		24.2	19.8	19.8	24.0	22.0	2.5
L1		24.2	21.1	23.2	26.6	23.8	2.2
		29.5	21.5	24.2	23.7	24.7	3.4
	INF	37.8	31.6	29.1	32.7	32.8	3.6
	Mean	29.8	24.7	25.2	27.7		
	SD	5.9	5.4	4.2	4.2		

*Enclosed in the box are the percent area fractions for the 20 regions of interest. The mean percent area fractions and standard deviations for the rows are calculated to the right of the box, and the mean percent area fractions and standard deviations for each column are listed below the box.

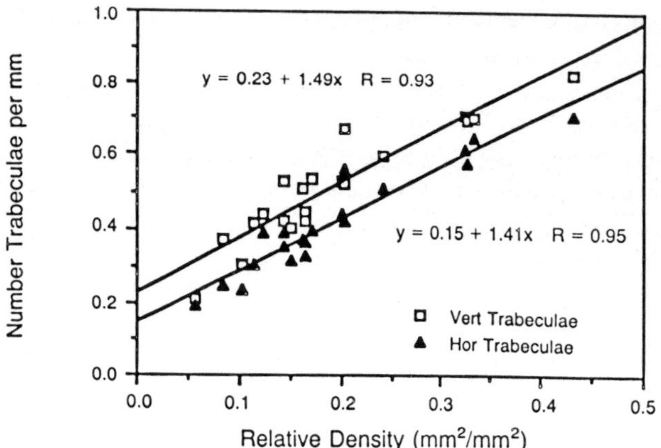

FIG 18–4.
Number of vertical *(vert)* and horizontal trabeculae in relation to relative bone density (area fraction of bone). The slopes of the regression lines were not statistically different ($t = 0.70$, $P > .05$); however, the y-intercepts were statistically different ($t = 3.49$, $P < .05$).

bone and found that osteoporotic bone showed less strength and stiffness than normal bone due to higher porosity.[25] They also found that osteoporotic bone had a higher mineral content than normal bone. Galante et al. found that the density of the bone in trabeculae ranged from 1400 to 2000 kg/m^3.[40] The changes in the properties of cancellous bone with age clearly warrant further study.

The relative strength of cancellous bone is dependent not only on the density and strength of the mineralized bone tissue but also on the architecture of the trabeculae. The cells formed by trabecular bone can be examined by distinguishing between open and closed structures. A network of trabecular rods produces open cells, and a network of trabecular plates provides closed cells.[5, 43] Gibson analyzed the relationship between the strength and the density of cancellous bone with the assumption of open and closed cell models.[43] Gibson found that bone failed by buckling or by plastic yield. The yield condition was dependent on the density of bone per volume (the apparent or relative density) raised to a power. The magnitude of the exponent ranged from 3/2 for the plastic yield of the open-cell model to a power of 3 for the closed-cell buckling model. These values are consistent with experimental data.

From experimental data the strength of cancellous bone is proportional to the apparent density squared ($S \alpha \rho^2$).[16] Carter and Hayes measured the strength of human and bovine bone and found the strength dependent on apparent density (ρ^2) and strain rate ($\dot{\epsilon}$),

$$S = 68\ \dot{\epsilon}^{0.06}\ \rho^2,$$

with S in megapascals and density in kilograms per cubic centimeter.[11, 12] The elastic modulus was measured and found to depend on the apparent density cubed:

$$S = 3{,}790\dot{\epsilon}^{\ 0.06}\ \rho^3.$$

Lang et al. found that the modulus of vertebral trabecular bone would best be represented by density squared rather than density cubed.[71] The cubic form of these equations was confirmed by additional studies by others.[16] These differences may in part be explained by the types of the trabecular architecture analyzed by Gibson[43] and the possible changes in the trabecular structure with bone loss and aging.

The compressive load supported by the spinal column is distributed between the anterior and posterior vertebral components and further divided in the vertebral body between the cortex and the trabecular centrum. In studies of the compressive response of the spine, it was found that 75% to 80% of the force is supported by the vertebral body and the remainder is supported by the facets and the posterior components.[65] Direct measure of the facet contact pressure demonstrated that the vertical component of facet load is transmitted by bony contact of the tip of the inferior facet with the lamina of the vertebrae below.[35] The anterior load is supported by the vertebral body and the intervertebral disc.[145]

The relative contribution of the vertebral cortex to the strength of the vertebral body has been measured in compression. In an early study Rockoff et al. found that the vertebral cortex accounts for 40% to 75% of the strength of the vertebra.[114] McBroom et al. removed the cortex from ten L1 vertebral bodies and compared the strength of these with paired L3 vertebrae.[82] We observed a reduction of only about 10% in the strength of the specimens with no cortex in comparison to the intact pairs. These studies indicate that for compressive loads, the trabecular bone within the vertebral centrum may account for up to 72% of the vertebral strength.

Mechanics of Bone Remodeling

Changes in the density and structure of bone reflect the sacrifice of bone to maintain the calcium and the adaptive response of bone to mechanical and other stimuli. The adaptive response of the BMU is called bone remodeling. Remodeling in general may include bone repair and the formation of new bone but requires the local cellular interactions of the BMU.

Trabecular bone is metabolically more active than cortical bone and undergoes specific histologic and morphologic changes with bone loss. For the central portion of the vertebral body, Arnold presented a sequence of five events for bone loss in osteoporosis: (1) a normal honeycomb structure of young adults that is composed of solid plates of bone without perforations, (2) the appearance of numerous small perforations in the plates, (3) expansion of the perforations and conversion of plates to rods, (4) progressive narrowing and loss of horizontal trabecular elements, and (5) atrophy of vertical rods and compensatory hypertrophy of residual plates.[5] Observations by others support this course. Merz and Schenk found a decreasing trabecular thickness with decreasing density.[90]

Historic Origin of the Theory of Bone Remodeling

Several reviews have traced the history of the concepts of the biomechanics of bone remodeling.[78, 115] The formal expression of the relationship between the architectural features of bone (cancellous bone) and the mechanical environment was first presented in the early 19th century by Bourgery.[9] The general concepts were refined and made more specific by the collaborative work of the anatomist Meyer and the engineer Culmann.[91] This work focused attention on the similarity of the trajectories of structural members in the Culmann crane to the orientation of trabecular bone in the femoral head. Between 1869 and 1892 these concepts were further developed and published by Wolff.[150, 151] Roux attempted to explain the trajectories studied by Wolff through a new principle of functional adaptation.[116] Debate on these biomechanical aspects of bone remodeling appeared immediately and has continued unresolved to the present.[158]

Mechanoreceptors in Bone

The adaptation of bone in response to mechanical stimuli (or the lack of stimuli) implies that these mechanical inputs must be "received" and interpreted by the cells in the BMU. Early studies have shown that a network of canaliculi join the osteocytes within bone and the lining cells on the bone surface.[78] Martin and Burr[78] indicate that Weidenreich first suggested that the canaliculi join the lacunae of adjacent osteons,[141] and that this was demonstrated later by Curtis et al. in their study of human long bones.[19] The network of cell processes connects by gap junctions and therefore can rapidly exchange ions.[54] These interconnections constitute a means of intercellular transduction of mechanical input. The details of these cellular interactions that sense mechanical load are not well understood.[17]

Theories appear in the literature for the remodeling and adaptation of bone that are based either on stress (dependent on the loads over an area of bone) or on strain (dependent on the deformation of bone).[52] In a so-called linear-elastic material, the stress is proportional to strain, and the stress and strain (or changes in stress and strain) are perfectly correlated. Consequently, in this ideal case there is no effective difference in the use of either stress or strain for the interpretation of the biomechanical response of bone during the application of loading over time, to quantify the remodeling process.

Unfortunately, bone is not a static material but is dynamic. Therefore the adaptive response and the properties of bone differ from the ideal linear-elastic case. The current shortcoming of current remodeling theories is that they are each controlled by only a single remodeling parameter. No adaptive model of bone has been presented that relates the biomechanical stimuli (modulated by strain and stress) to the local and systemic metabolic processes. Models based on a single remodeling parameter cannot describe both the systemic and local interactions of the calcium balance and bone mechanics. Specific biomechanical parameters that could initiate bone remodeling and possible thresholds are currently debated.

HYPERTROPHIC CONDITIONS

The heterotopic formation of bone is associated with the degenerative cascade of the spine with aging and may occur following injury. The degenerative cascade is a sequence of conditions in the spine that is characterized by changes in the mobility of the spinal motion segment in the formation of bone at the perimeter of the disc and at the facets. Aging with associated changes in the biochemistry of the disc and factors that alter the biomechanics of the spine motion segments are underlying primary causes.

Biomechanically the distribution of load between anterior and posterior components is a contributing factor in bone formation. It has been observed in degenerated motion segments that there is an increase in the surface area of the vertebral end plates with the formation of osteophytes. In the facet joints there is also an increase in surface area with a change in facet geometry and additional bone formation.[143]

Through this process the mechanics of the intervertebral disc, the vertebral body, and the facets are closely linked. One hypothesis is that the degeneration of the intervertebral disc may initiate the degenerative cascade (Fig 18–5).[155] In this sequence, as the intervertebral disc degenerates, a cascade of biomechanical events occurs. With the loss of central pressure from the nucleus pulposus due to degeneration or injury, the anterior portion of the compressive load supported by the spine is redistributed to the annulus fibrosus.[113] There is a loss in overall height of the

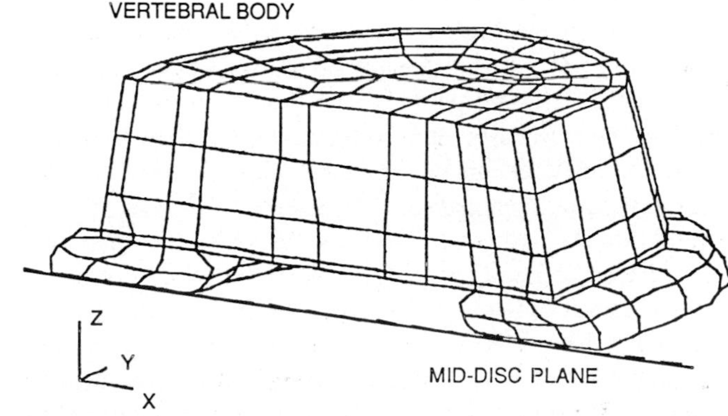

FIG 18–5.
Three-dimensional finite-element model of the vertebral disc with disc pressure reduced to zero (nucleus removed). The model demonstrates a loss in the disc height and a change in the fiber orientation of the annulus around the perimeter of the disc.[156]

disc and a redistribution of the stresses within the fibers of the annulus fibrosus, with the load shifting to the perimeter of the intervertebral disc. The new alignment of the fibers is consistent with the formation of osteophytes around the perimeter of the end plate, an increase in the bone density adjacent to the cortex of the vertebral body, and a decrease in the trabecular bone density in the centrum. With the loss in height of the intervertebral disc, the stiffness of the motion segment is decreased, and translations of the motion segment in the anterior, posterior, and lateral directions increase. Translation in excess of about 2 to 3 mm in the sagittal plane has been associated with the threshold of clinical instability.[106] With this hypermobility the loading and motion of the facets increase. These changes are consistent with the degeneration of the facets that leads to stenotic conditions of the intervertebral foramina[60, 154]; however, further research is needed to examine this and other possible hypotheses. At this time it is difficult to separate the biochemical and biomechanical factors in this cascade.

Restoration of normal canal size can occur through limited manipulation and bone remodeling without progressive degeneration. This has been documented in several series.[38] Fredrickson et al. observed the remodeling of bone within the canal over a period of 18 months and found a significant reduction in canal impingement (Fig 18–6).[38] The process was dependent on age but may occur to varying degrees in all age groups.

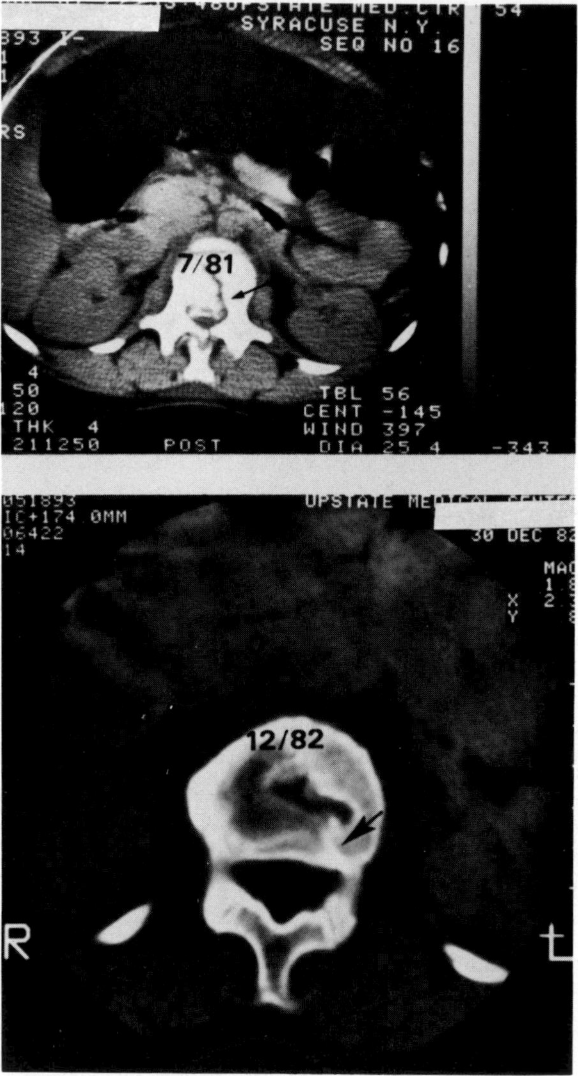

FIG 18–6.
A, significant canal compromise of 50% or greater can resolve over time. The process is age dependent but has been observed in all age groups. **B,** marked reconstitution of the canal over a period of 18 months.[39]

OSTEOPENIA

Research on bone and metabolic conditions of bone has increased as the health care emphasis swings to address the problems of an aging population in the United States. Studies have provided data on bone that should be considered in the rehabilitation of spinal disorders and corrective procedures.

Loss of Bone Strength With Age

The biomechanical strength of the vertebral body depends not only on the density of the trabecular bone but also on the vertebral geometry and the structural arrangement of the trabeculae. It is well known that significant loss of bone mineral occurs beyond the age of 30 years, particularly following menopause.[18, 68] Studies by Mosekilde and Mosekilde showed that in addition the cross-sectional area of a vertebra increases with age.[96] In our previous investigation of the effects of both density and vertebral area, we found that the product of area and trabecular density squared correlates better with vertebral strength than does density alone.[82] However, these measures have not identified changes in the trabecular architecture as bone density decreases. The capabilities of noninvasive methods such as QCT and DPA were demonstrated for the measurement of vertebral density, although few studies have correlated these measurements to the morphologic changes of the trabeculae with progressive idiopathic bone loss.[63, 124]

Metabolic and Disease-Related Causes

Changes in bone density, particularly the loss of bone strength, has been identified for conditions that affect the metabolism of bone and in disease processes. Patients with rheumatoid arthritis (RA) require special consideration due to the effect of this disorder and treatments for RA on bone. Systemic rheumatic diseases initially can have predominantly hand signs.[121] However, multiple sites are affected, including the cervical spine, lungs, airway, bone, and bone marrow, and attention must be given to organs that may be affected by the systemic involvement that occurs with rheumatoid disease. An overall assessment of the status of the patient's arthritis, general health and preparedness for the procedure, and the rehabilitation that follows is necessary.[121] Intraoperatively and postoperatively rheumatoid patients may require supplementary corticosteroids and an adjustment of the dose of their antirheumatic medications. These medications may affect bone healing and the density of bone.[109]

Skeletal demineralization in patients with chronic alcoholism has been reported. A radiographic survey was made by Spencer et al. of 96 fully ambulatory male patients admitted to a rehabilitation center for patients with chronic alcoholism.[127] The age of these patients ranged from 24 to 62 years. They found that 45 of the 96 male patients, 47% of this group, showed radiographic evidence of extensive bone loss. Thirty-one percent of these 45 patients with bone loss were relatively young (aged 31 to 45 years), and half of that group of 14 patients were less than 40 years old. The difficulty with such studies is control for nutrition, activity, and other potentially confounding factors. However, excessive use of alcohol is clearly a contributing factor to reduced bone density.

Nonsteroidal anti-inflammatory drugs (NSAIDs) are also known to inhibit bone healing, in addition to recognized beneficial effects. NSAIDs and other analgesics are frequently used in the conservative treatment of low back pain. NSAIDs as a group of drugs have numerous biological and clinical effects attributed to them. The earliest known biological effect of NSAIDs was their effect on cellular energy metabolism.[122, 145, 146] With the discovery that most of the NSAIDs inhibit prostaglandin production from arachidonic acid, much of the recent efforts have explored this mechanism as the basis for their clinical and biochemical effects.[137, 138] Unfortunately, causal and other interrelationship between the observed biological effects attributed to NSAIDs are not well known. The inhibition of prostaglandin formation has been frequently attributed to the anti-inflammatory properties of NSAIDs, but this relationship is not as clear as has been assumed. By inhibiting cyclo-oxygenase, not only proinflammatory prostaglandin (e.g., E, A, and B types) but also anti-inflammatory prostaglandin (e.g., $F_{2\alpha}$) production is diminished.[123, 137, 138] These contradictory effects and the lack of direct prostaglandin antagonists makes identifying the exact role of present NSAIDs in the relationship between prostaglandin inhibition and their anti-inflammatory properties difficult. Also, other inflammation-modulating properties such as stabilization of lysosomal membrane[1, 2] and prevention of superoxide release from polymorphonuclear leukocytes may not be dependent on prostaglandin inhibition.[1, 2]

Reported effects of PGE_2 on bone metabolism are contradictory,[28, 109, 110] and it may be concentration dependent and lead to either bone resorption or formation. The exact biochemical modulation of bone repair by prostaglandins is not known, but they may affect bone formation by stimulation of the replication as well as differentiation of osteoblasts from primitive mesenchymal cell lines.[94, 111] PGE_2 appears to have a preventive action on the cortisol-induced decrease in DNA content in osteoblast culture.[111] However, after 24 hours of treatment, no demonstrable effect on collagen synthesis was noted.[111] Another site of modulation in bone repair may be in bone remodeling since PGE_2 was shown to be a strong promoter of osteoclast differentiation from stem cells, most likely through a cyclic adenosine monophosphate (cAMP)-mediated mechanism.[94] This is further substantiated by the fact that indomethacin was shown to inhibit haversian canal remodeling in rabbits.[128, 130] Release of prostaglandins E and F from the rabbit tibia and surrounding muscles after fracture has been reported.[21] Since prostaglandin is an important modulation of inflammation, it would be expected to play an important role in early fracture healing. It has been theorized that PGE_1 and PGE_2 may play a role in bone resorption in the early phase of fracture repair as well as improve local oxygenation by increasing vasodilation.

The inhibitory effect on bone formation by ibuprofen and indomethacin has been utilized clinically to inhibit heterotopic bone formation in total-hip replacement patients with documented successes.[36, 64, 120] Through investigation of these inhibitory effects in experimental bone-healing and fracture models a number of investigators have shown that use of these agents may lead to delayed bone healing as well as increased nonunion of fractures.*

Disuse

Mechanical loading and physical activity are needed to maintain and possibly enhance bone density in the spine. Sustained immobilization or disuse results in a loss of bone mass with several stages of bone remodeling. This process of bone loss due to reduced bone strain was studied in animal immobilization models, following spinal cord injury, as a result of bed rest, and due to space weightlessness.[133]

Allison and Brooks, in one of the earliest studies of disuse, examined the effects of reduced strain in the forelimbs of mongrel dogs for three disuse conditions: (1) excision of the proximal end of the humerus, (2) resection of the brachial plexus, and (3) plaster casting of the dogs' forelimbs.[4] Bone tissue specimens were examined directly over a period of 1½ to 45 weeks. Three phases of bone remodeling were observed. During weeks 1 to 4, loss of trabecular bone was found, in weeks 4 to 14, bone was resorbed from the periosteal and endosteal surfaces of the cortical bone; and from weeks 14 to 45, intracortical resorption of bone occurred. Similar patterns of trabecular

*References 3, 62, 73, 113, 129, 134, 135.

and cortical bone remodeling were observed in studies of rabbits[44] and monkeys[61] and in humans.

The effects of immobilization in patients with spinal cord injuries was observed by Minaire et al.[92] The trabecular bone volume and the thickness of the cortical bone of iliac biopsy samples were compared with controls. They found that the trabecular bone volume decreased for 25 weeks following immobilization and then bone loss leveled off at an average value of 12.1% trabecular bone volume. Meade observed that this value was above the threshold at which risk of vertebral collapse occurs.[86]

The change in bone mass of the os calcis following chronic bed rest has also been measured. Donaldson et al. observed three subjects for 30 to 36 weeks.[29] Over this period, the net calcium loss increased. However, they found that bone loss due to bed rest was reversible, with os calcis bone mineral increasing beyond the pre-experiment values after 18 to 36 weeks of reambulation.

These studies indicate that activity, which provides bone strain, is needed to maintain bone mass, but it is still uncertain to what extent exercise can be used to enhance bone mass, particularly in the elderly.[37] Krolner et al. found that aerobic exercise over a period of 8 months maintained lumbar spine bone mineral density in elderly women.[69] Lumbar bone mineral density was also improved in a study by Dalshy et al.[20] that combined walking, jogging, and stair climbing. Higher bone mineral density due to higher loading has been observed by several research groups in studies of weight lifters.[46a] Pruitt found in a study of postmenopausal women near the age of 54 years that weight training maintained lumbar bone mineral density but had no significant effect on the bone density of the wrist or femoral neck.[107]

Consequence of Reduced Bone Density

Variations in the density and strength of bone within the vertebral body may contribute to differences in segment stiffness and to the strength of spinal instrumentation. Researchers have examined the variation of the density of the trabecular bone within the vertebral body. Regions of higher-density bone are found adjacent to the vertebral end plates[125] and in the posterolateral portions of the vertebral body.[33, 83, 84]

Studies such as that of Halvorson et al[49] have shown that the density of bone in the vertebra has a strong influence on the pullout strength of transpedicular screws. It is clear that the strength and stiffness of transpedicular screws are dependent not only on the depth of screw insertion and screw design but also on the distribution and strength of the bone within the vertebral body. Although the loads supported along the length of pedicle screws are not exactly known,[66] screws placed in regions of higher-density bone and in contact with the cortex provide more secure fixation.

Variations in screw orientation and depths of insertion have been advocated.[24, 75, 117, 118] Krag et al. studied the morphology of vertebrae and the effects of depth of penetration on screw strength.[67] Their data showed that 80% depth of penetration produces an approximately 30% stronger purchase for the pedicle screw as compared with only 50% depth of penetration. Zindrick et al. studied screws implanted to various depths with controlled displacements of the dorsal end of the screw in either a mediolateral or a cephalocaudal direction.[157] Their data showed greater strength for implants to the cortex vs. screws to a 50% depth for both the mediolateral and the cephalocaudal displacements. Zindrick et al. also compared the length of the screw path at different medial-lateral approach angles and showed that a slightly longer path length results from insertion along the pedicle axis rather than parallel to the sagittal midline of the body.[156]

STABILIZATION IN SPINE FUSION AND FRACTURE HEALING

Indications for surgery vs. conservative treatment now depend primarily upon the assessment of the relative stability of the fractured region. Internal fixation is less needed in the case of a stable fracture and may increase the period of hospitalization. The benefit of internal fixation becomes apparent for the patient with an unstable fracture of the vertebral column. In this case, conservative treatment has almost no advantage except the avoided risk of an operation. Operative management is timesaving, may reduce the rehabilitation cost, and provides the necessary correction and stabilization of the fracture. Several factors are key to the biomechanical interpretation and optimization of spine stabilization, including (1) the magnitude of the observed forces and moments and (2) the clinical parameters believed to correlate with successful fusion, in particular, bone strain.

Internal Control of Strain and Bone Healing

Posterior lumbar fusions have been performed since the early 1900s. The initial fusions were done posteriorly and involved bone grafting in the area of the spinous process. A significant nonunion rate was encountered, and subsequent clinical experience showed that posterolateral fusions over the transverse process and facet area have a higher success rate. Various explanations have been given for this phenomenon, including (1) that the surrounding musculature provides better vascularity for the graft and (2) that the transverse processes are located closer to the center of rotation and therefore the fusion mass is subjected to less strain.

The concept of interfragmentary strain was initially presented by Perren and Cordey[103, 104] Their work was in long-bone fracture healing.[103, 104] They emphasized that developing callus goes through numerous stages from the earliest granulation tissue to eventual reconstitution of normal bony architecture. They postulated that in the early phases of healing the tissues are of low strength but can tolerate significant elongation and strain without difficulty. As the tissues mature, they have the ability to increase in strength and rigidity. The amount of elongation that tissues tolerate without developing a nonunion varies depending upon the stage of callus. Perren and Cordey postulated that if at any time during this continuum of healing the strain is greater than the tissues can tolerate, then this leads to nonunion.

It is generally accepted that following injury the spine must be stabilized to promote healing. The assessment of the relative stability of the motion segment has been based on stiffness, the load-displacement response, overall segment motion, and the motion along the affected region. Of these parameters, measurement of the apparent strain (the motion over the affected region divided by the length of the region) best reflects the mechanical environment of the bone graft or fixed segment.

Nagel et al. noted a significant difference in the rate of fusion of bone grafts in sheep with respect to the strain between the lamina.[97] Using small cancellous and corticocancellous bone grafts across the decorticated lamina of the lumbar spine and the sacrum, they observed that the interlumbar areas always healed but the lumbosacral joint rarely fused. They found that the mean strain at the lumbosacral joint was 36% while the strain was only 10% at the L5–6 joint (where fusion always occurred).

Earlier work by Thomas in conjunction with Kirkaldy-Willis in the early 1970s supported the work of Nagel.[131] They performed experimental spinal fusions on guinea pigs and dogs and were predominantly interested in the effect of the spinal fusion and the development of possible spinal stenosis.[131] They did, however, report the same relatively high nonunion rate at the lumbar sacral junction and postulated, again, that this was secondary to increased motion or strain in the area.

Optimal Strain Condition in Spine Healing

Although numerous studies have been done to define the stiffness of various constructs involving these fixation devices, to date the ideal mechanical environment for the fusion mass to be exposed to has not been resolved.[31, 32, 47, 48, 59, 152] The mechanical strain measured across the region of injury or fusion has been successfully employed to characterize the degree of spinal immobilization in response to combinations of applied loads and can be measured for all types of instrumentation. Adequate control of strain during the healing process may optimize the biomechanical conditions for the best rate of healing and surgical outcome.

Purcell et al. provide one of the earliest in vitro comparative studies of the biomechanics of strain after internal fixation.[108] Compression-flexion loads were applied to the thoracolumbar spine segments. The posterior elements between T12 and L1 were disrupted and then stabilized by using various Harrington rod constructs. Distraction (motion) across the T12–L1 defect was used to monitor stability. The effective strain allowed for each construct may be calculated from an analysis of the geometry of their experimental system. For all constructs that were considered adequate, the strain was between 2% and 10% for loading up to about 35 nm. These adequate Harrington constructs were clinically acceptable at that time.

Recent laboratory studies have shown a higher rate of fusion and improved strength of the fusion mass with more rigid fixation devices. Studies suggest that by limiting motion between the adjacent vertebrae of a grafted region, on the basis of overall strain a nonunion is less likely to occur, and fusion will result. Others have shown that for small strains it may be possible to excessively shield the fusion region from strain, which could lead to osteopenia.

This hypothesis was tested in an animal model by McAfee et al.[81] In this study, anterior and posterior disruptions were created in 42 dogs at the L5–6 level. Measurements were made of the stiffness of the construct after the instrumentation was removed, the anterior strain between the vertebral bodies, the density of the vertebral bodies, and the bone formation rate. Comparison was made of five sets of instrumentation constructs in torsion, compression, and flexion. One group was destabilized with no fusion (A/P TRANS), a second group had posterior lateral fusion (PLF), the next had Luque rod plus fusion (LI+PLF), the fourth group had Harrington instrumentation plus fusion (HI+PLF), and the fifth had CD pedicular screws with fusion (CDI+PLF).[81] The animals were followed for a period of 6 months, and all of the 42 dogs survived to the conclusion of the study.

From the data of McAfee et al.,[81] comparisons can be made of success of fusion and the effect of strain on the vertebral body density (Fig 18–7). A comparison of vertebral body density vs. the percent fusion demonstrated that as the rigidity of the construct increased, the rate of percent fusion increased and the density of the bone within the vertebral body decreased (Fig 18–7,A). With respect to strain between the vertebral bodies, as the construct and the fusion mass became more rigid, the axial strain anteriorly decreased, and the rate of fusion increased (Fig 18–7,B). Finally, the reduction in axial strain also resulted in a reduction of the bone density of the vertebral body (Fig 18–7,C). These results indicate that in this animal model an increase in graft stiffness provides a reduction in axial strain and a loss of bone in the region of reduced strain (here the vertebral body).

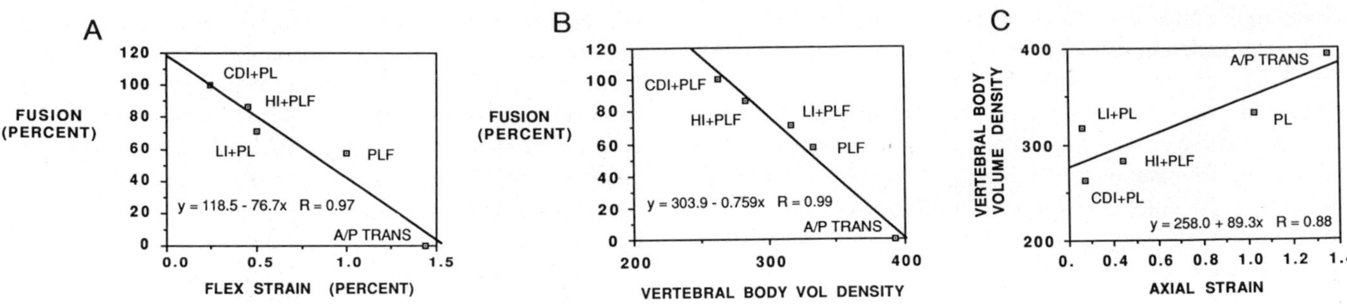

FIG 18–7.
A, the percent rate of fusion increases with decreased strain and increasing implant rigidity. See the text for a designation of instrumentation and constructs. **B,** vertebral body density was lower for constructs with high rigidity and a higher percent rate of fusion. **C,** vertebral body density was reduced for constructs that provided low axial strain. (Data from McAfee PC, Farey ID, Sutterlin CE, et al: *Spine* 1989; 14:919–926.)

The limitation of strain across the spine motion segment may vary between conservative and surgical techniques. Wendsche et al. reviewed the results of 19 patients with unstable injuries of the thoracolumbar spine.[142] Poor late results were recorded from 11 of them who had undergone conservative or inadequate surgical treatment. Axial malposition of severe clinical disorders were among the findings.

Johnsson et al. directly monitored patients to determine the influence of the duration and amount of postoperative lumbar immobilization on the consolidation of posterolateral lumbosacral fusions.[58] In their study the trunk was immobilized with a molded rigid lumbar orthosis after surgery. They found that the rate of fusion healing was higher for patients immobilized for 5 months in comparison to patients immobilized for only 3 months. By using roentgen stereophotogrammetric analysis, motion across the fusion region was measured in vivo. In patients with fusion, sagittal translations decreased beginning at 3 to 6 months from 2.4 mm to less than 0.7 mm. In patients with poor fusions, motion was initially higher, 5.8 at 2 months, and decreased to 4.4 mm at 1 year. It was concluded that maintenance of reduced motion (strain) for up to 5 months significantly improved the fusion rate.

Therefore, these studies suggest that by limiting motion between the adjacent vertebrae of a grafted region a nonunion is less likely to occur, and fusion will result. Increasing segment stiffness by modification of instrumentation, a construct, or the use of external bracing reduces strain across the region of healing. On the basis of overall strain, defined by the change in length per unit reference length between the laminae, spinal levels with more than 36% distraction should result in nonunion, and levels with less than 10% should fuse satisfactorily.[97, 98] On the other hand, for small strains with less than approximately 2% distraction it may be possible to excessively shield the fusion region from strain, which could lead to osteopenia.

Mechanics of Internal Fixation—Variable-Stiffness Fixation

These studies indicate the importance of strain in the healing process. The concept of a window of optimal strain during healing of a spine fusion implies an upper and a lower bound. Excessively low strains are associated with disuse or stress shielding and result in osteopenia; high strains contribute to the formation of nonunion. The optimal levels of the strains needed for control of bone strength and the possible effect of a variation in the strain over time are currently unknown.

General concepts can guide treatment. Load is redistributed anteroposteriorly in the stabilization of the spine during the fusion process (Fig 18–8). Three load-bearing paths or regions provide mechanical support across the motion segment: an anterior region (the vertebral body); a posterior region that includes both vertebral components

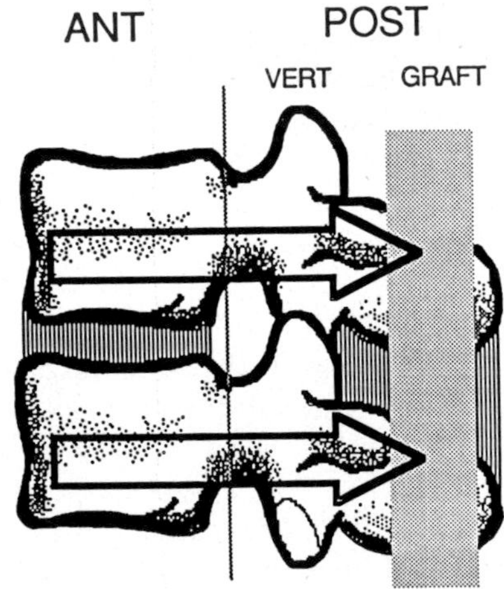

FIG 18–8.
Compressive load is redistributed from the anterior portion of the motion segment to the posterior graft during the fusion process. Three load-bearing paths provide mechanical support across the motion segment: an anterior *(ant)* region (the vertebral body), a posterior *(post)* region that includes vertebral *(vert)* components and graft material, and the implant.

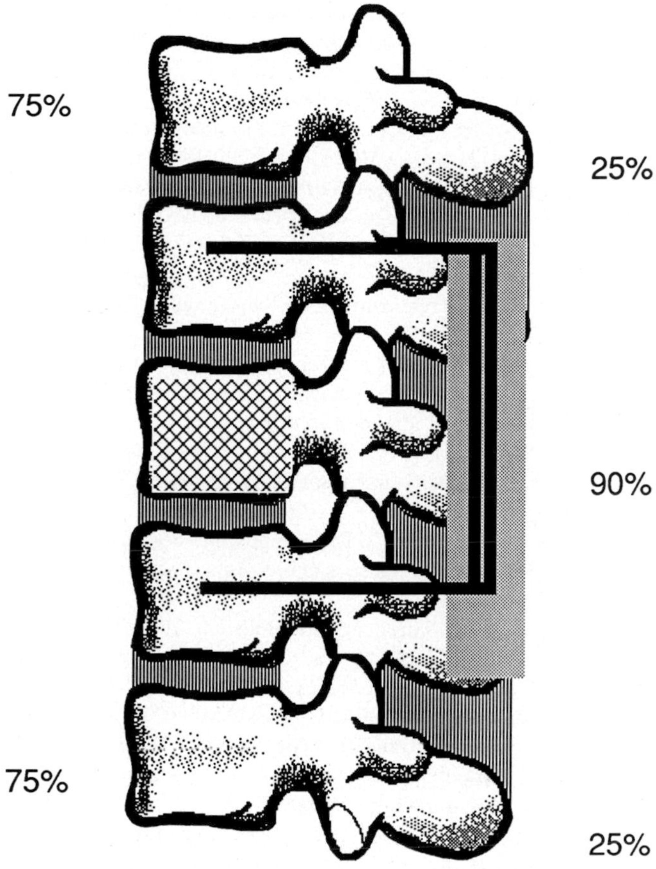

FIG 18–9.
The load follows the region or path of highest stiffness. Normally the vertebral body supports about 75% to 80% of the compressive load in the spine with the posterior elements supporting the remaining 25% to 20%.

and the graft material; and if an implant is applied, the implant itself constitutes the third region. These regions reflect the three columns considered in spinal injury.[22] With the placement of a graft or construct, the load is shifted from the body posteriorly toward the graft or the implant (Fig 18–9). Normally the vertebral body supports about 75% to 80% of the compressive load in the spine, with the posterior elements supporting the remaining 25% to 20%.[65] The load follows the region or path of highest stiffness. The vertebrae below the level of instrumentation have a more physiologic distribution of load. Support across an anterior fracture of a spine segment with posterior stabilization would shift the load posteriorly and distribute it between the vertebra and the posterior construct (Fig 18–10). The relative distribution depends entirely upon the relative stiffness of these three load paths.

The effect of this redistribution of load has been examined by Lipscomb et al.[74] They found that there were changes in bone density in the adjacent vertebra following fusion. In 26 patients followed with a mean age of 35 years, they observed that bone loss of about 15% to 16% in the adjacent vertebra above or below the fusion occurred sometime between 3 to 12 months. At 12 months' follow-up 23% of the subjects in this investigation continued to have a low bone density level. Sixty-one percent recovered, and in that group some of them actually had a higher density than the baseline values.

Goel et al. investigated the effect of reducing the stiffness of an internal fixation device over time.[45] The study used in vitro experimental tests and an analysis of the structural stiffness of the canine spine to guide a subse-

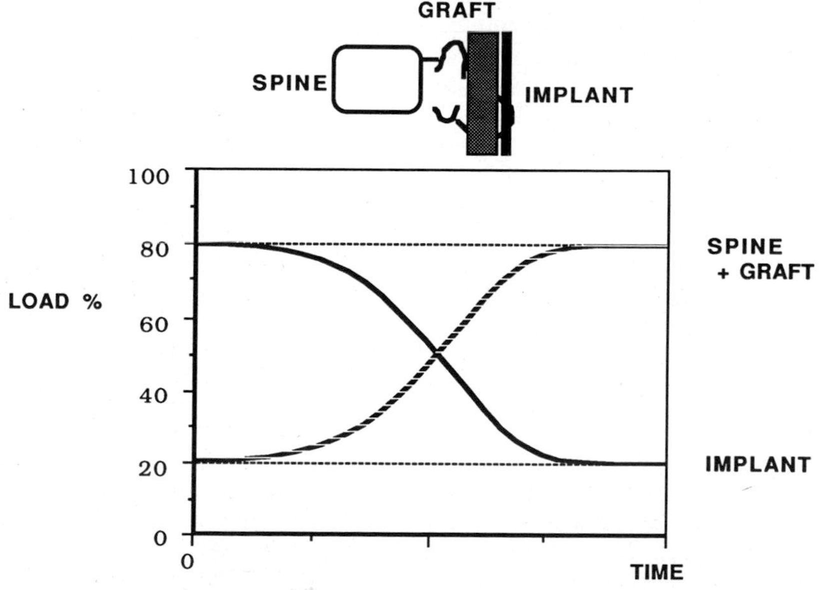

FIG 18–10.
Initially, an implant assumes most of the load across the area to be stabilized while the spine and the graft are shielded from strain. Over time, this distribution of load and strain changes as the graft becomes stronger or as the spine heals.

quent in vivo study. The quality of bone within the stabilized segment was assessed 6 months following surgery. Stabilization was obtained by using posterior VSP (Steffee) plates and modified VSP plates. The modified instrumentation had polymer washers between the plate and the integral nut. They found that the use of polymer washers increased bone growth around the screws and that the porosity of the bone was improved in comparison to the more rigid configuration.

SPINAL BONE DENSITY DURING REHABILITATION

Although the optimal conditions for fusion and fracture healing in the spine have not been quantified, it is clear that this process is not static. The fusion mass is initially flexible and increases in stiffness as the bone mineralizes. Initially, an implant assumes most of the load across the area to be stabilized, while the spine and the graft are shielded from strain. Studies suggest that strain between approximately 2% and 10% may provide an optimal window of initial conditions for healing in the spine. The amount of strain across a region of healing bone in the spine should provide an early indication of the success of fusion or the stability of a healing fracture.[58] Over time, this distribution of load and strain changes as the graft becomes stronger or as the spine heals.

The mechanical and biological parameters that control remodeling and adaptation processes are now only partially understood. Each of these factors and the regulation of bone metabolism play an important role in spine rehabilitation. In most rehabilitative situations it is not feasible to maintain bone at densities in the normal range throughout the spine. The end result reflects a balance of the maintenance of bone density, calcium regulation, and strength. The current challenge is the identification of the time course of strain and metabolic factors during the healing process that could promote the development of devices or orthoses that optimize these conditions over time.

REFERENCES

1. Abramson S, Korchak H, Ludewig R, et al: Modes of action of aspirin-like drugs. *Proc Natl Acad Sci USA* 1985; 82:7227–7231.
2. Abramson S, Weismann G: The mechanism of action of nonsteroidal anti-inflammatory drugs. *Arthritis Rheum* 1989; 32:1–9.
3. Allen HL, Wase A, Bear WT: Indomethacin and aspirin: Effect of nonsteroidal anti-inflammatory agents on the rate of fracture repair in the rat. *Acta Orthop Scand* 1980; 51:595–600.
4. Allison N, Brooks B: An experimental study of the changes in bone which result from nonuse. *Surg Gynecol Obstet* 1921; 33:250.
5. Arnold JS: Trabecular pattern and shapes in aging and osteoporosis. *Metab Bone Dis Suppl* 1980; 2:297–308.
6. Atkinson PJ: Variation in trabecular structure of the vertebrae with age. *Calcif Tissue Res* 1967; 1:24–32.
7. Austin LA, Heath H: Calcitonin. Physiology and pathophysiology. *N Engl J Med* 1981; 304:269–278.
8. Biggemann M, Hilweg D, Brinckmann P: Prediction of the compressive strength of vertebral bodies of the lumbar spine by quantitative computed tomography. *Skeletal Radiol* 1988; 17:264–269.
9. Bourgery JM: Trate complet de l'anatomie de l'homme. I *Osteologie* 1832.
10. Brandt KD: Effects of nonsteroidal anti-inflammatory drugs on chrondrocyte metabolism in vitro and in vivo. *Am J Med* 1987; 83(suppl 5A):29–34.
11. Carter DR, Hayes WC: Bone compressive strength: The influence of density and strain rate. *Science* 1976; 194:1174–1176.
12. Carter DR, Hayes WC: The compressive behavior of bone as a two-phase porous structure. *J Bone Joint Surg [Am]* 1977; 49:954–962.
13. Cassucio C: An introduction to the study of osteoporosis (biochemical and biophysical research in bone aging). *Proc R Soc Med* 1962; 55:663–668.
14. Cheal EJ, Mansmann KA, DiGioia AMI, et al: Role of interfragmentary strain in fracture healing: Ovine model of a healing osteotomy. *J Orthop Res* 1991; 9:131–142.
15. Civitelli R, Gonnelli S, Zacchei F, et al: Bone turnover in postmenopausal osteoporosis: Effect of cacitonin treatment. *J Clin Invest* 1988; 82:1268–1274.
16. Cowin SC: *Bone Mechanics*. Boca Raton, Fla, CRC Press, 1989.
17. Cowin SC, Moss-Salentijn L, Moss ML: Candidates for the mechanosensory system in bone. *J Biomech Eng* 1991; 113:191–197.
18. Cummings S, Kesley J, Nevitt M, et al: Epidemiology of osteoporosis and osteoporotic fractures. *Epidemiol Rev* 1985; 7:178–208.
19. Curtis T, Ashraft S, Weber D: Canalicular communication in the cortices of human long bones. *Anat Rec* 1985; 212:336–344.
20. Dalsky D, Stocke K, Ehsani A, et al: weight-bearing exercise training and lumbar bone mineral content in postmenopausal women. *Ann Intern Med* 1988; 108:824–828.
21. Dekel S, Lenthal G, Francis MJO: Release of prostaglandin from bone and muscle after tibial fracture. *J Bone Joint Surg [Br]* 1981; 63:185–189.
22. Denis F: Spinal instability as defined by the three-column spine concept in acute spinal trauma. *Clin Orthop* 1984; 189:65–76.
23. Dewhirst F, Ago J, Peros W, et al: Synergism between parathyroid hormone and interleukin-1 in stimulating bone resorption in organ culture. *J Bone Miner Res* 1987; 2:127–134.
24. Dick W, Kluger P, Magerl F, et al: A new device for internal fixation of thoracolumbar and lumbar spine fractures: The "fixateur intern." *Paraplegia* 1985; 23:225–232.

25. Dickenson RP, Hutton WC, Stott JRR: The mechanical properties of bone in osteoporosis. *J Bone Joint Surg [Br]* 1981; 63:233–238.
26. Dickie DL, Goldstein SA, Flynn MJ, et al: Regional vertebral bone density distribution measurements and their correlation to whole bone strength. Presented to the Orthopaedic Research Society, San Francisco, 1987.
27. Dickie DL, Goldstein SA, Flynn MJ, et al: Vertebral rBMD distribution and fracture characteristics: In vitro and in vivo results. Presented to the Orthopaedic Research Society, Atlanta, 1988.
28. Dietrich JW, Raisz LG: Prostaglandin in calcium and bone metabolism. *Clin Orthop* 1975; 111:228–236.
29. Donaldson C, Hulley S, Vogel J, et al: Effect of prolonged bed rest on bone mineral. *Metabolism* 1970; 19:1071.
30. Eastell R, Wahner H, O'Fallon W, et al: Unequal decrease in bone density of lumbar spine and ultradistal radius in Colles' and vertebral fracture syndromes. *J Clin Invest* 1989; 83:168–174.
30a. Eder M: Der Strukfurumbau der Wirbelspogiosia. *Virch Arch Pathol Anat* 1960; 333:509–522.
31. Edwards WT: Biomechanics of the spine—spine stabilization. How much is enough? Presented to the North American Spine Society. Monterey, Calif, 1990.
32. Edwards WT, Hayes WC, White AA III, et al: Variation of lumbar spine stiffness with load. *J Biomech Eng* 1987; 109:35–42.
33. Edwards WT, McBroom RC, Hayes WC, et al: Variation of density in the vertebral body measured by quantitative computed tomography. *Trans Orthop Res Soc* 1986; 11:205.
34. Edwards WT, Snyder BD, Van der Linde JM, et al: Correlation of computed tomography measurement with trabecular morphology of human vertebrae. Presented to the Orthopaedic Research Society, Las Vegas, 1989.
35. El-Bohy A, Yang K-H, King A: Experimental verification of facet load transmission by direct measurement of facet lamina contact pressure. *J Biomech* 1989; 22:931–941.
36. Elmstedt E, Lindholm TS, Nilson OS, et al: Effect of ibuprofen on heterotopic ossification after hip replacement. *Acta Orthop Scand* 1985; 56:25–27.
37. Fiatarone MA, Marks EC, Ryan ND, et al: High-intensity strength training in nonagenarians. *JAMA* 1990; 263:3029–3034.
38. Fredrickson BE, Yuan HA, Bayley JC: The nonoperative treatment of thoracolumbar injuries. *Semin Spine Surg* 1990; 2:70–78.
39. Frost HM: *Bone and Remodelling Dynamics*. Springfield, Ill, Charles C Thomas, 1963.
40. Galante J, Rostoker W, Ray RD: Physical properties of trabecular bone. *Calcif Tissue Res* 1970; 5:236–246.
41. Ganong WF: *Review of Medical Physiology*. Los Altos, Calif, Lange Medical, 1977.
42. Genant HK, Turski PA, Moss AA: Advances in CT assessment of metabolic and endocrine disorders. *Adv Intern Med* 1983; 28:409–447.
43. Gibson LJ: The mechanical behavior of cancellous bone. *J Biomech* 1985; 18:317–328.
44. Gieser M, Treuta J: Muscle rarification and bone formation. *J Bone Joint Surg [Am]* 1958; 40:282.
45. Goel VK, Kim T, Gwon J, et al: Biomechanical effects of rigidity of an internal fixation device: A comprehensive investigation. Presented to the International Society of the Lumbar Spine, Heidelberg, Germany, 1991.
46. Goldsmith NF, Johnston JO: Bone mineral: Effects of oral contraceptives, pregnancy, and lactations. *J Bone Joint Surg [Am]* 1975; 57:657–668.
46a. Granhed H, Jonson R, Hansson T: The loads on the lumbar spine during extreme weight lifting. *Spine* 1987; 12:146–149.
47. Gurr K, McAfee P, Shih C-H: Biomechanical analysis of anterior and posterior instrumentation systems after corpectomy. *J Bone Joint Surg [Am]* 1988; 70:1182–1191.
48. Gurr K, McAfee P, Warden K, et al: Roentenographic and biomechanical analysis of lumbar fusions: A canine model. *J Orthop Res* 1989; 7:838–848.
49. Halvorson TL, Kelly LA, Thomas KA, et al: Effects of bone mineral density on pedicle screw fixation. Presented to the North American Spine Society, Keystone, Colorado, 1991.
50. Hansson T, Roos B, Nachemson A: The bone mineral content and ultimate compressive strength of lumbar vertebrae. *Spine* 1980; 5:46–55.
51. Hansson T, Keller T, Stengler D: Mechanical behavior of the human lumbar spine II. Fatigue strength during dynamic compressive loading. *J Orthop Res* 1987; 5:479–487.
52. Hart R, Davy D: Theories of bone remodeling and remodeling, in Cowin S (ed): *Bone Mechanics*. Boca Raton, Fla, 1989, CRC Press, pp 253–277.
53. Holick M: The cutaneous photosynthesis of previtamin D_3: A unique photoendocrine system. *J Invest Dermatol* 1981; 76:51–58.
54. Holtrop M, Weinger J: Ultrastructural evidence for a transport system in bone, in Talmage R, Munson P (eds): *Calcium Parathyroid Hormone and Calcitonins*. Amsterdam, Excerpta Medica, 1972.
55. Hosking DJ: Calcitonin and diphosphate in the treatment of Paget's disease of bone. *Metab Bone Dis* 1981; 4:317–326.
56. Hosking DJ, Bijvoet OLM: Therapeutic use of calcitonin, in Parsons JA (ed): *Endocrinology of Calcium Metabolism*. New York, 1982, Raven Press, pp 485–535.
57. Johnson BE, Lucasey B, Robinson RG, et al: Contributing diagnoses in osteoporosis: The value of a complete medical evaluation. *Arch Intern Med* 1989; 149:1069–1072.
58. Johnsson R, Stromqvist B, Axelsson P, et al: Influence of spinal immobilization on consolidation of posterolateral lumbosacral fusion: A roentgen stereophotogrammetric and radiographic analysis. *Spine* 1992; 17:16–21.
59. Johnston CEI, Ashman RB, Baird AM, et al: Effect of

spinal construct stiffness on early fusion mass incorporation. Experimental study. *Spine* 1990; 15:908–912.
60. Kao HC, Fay LA, Yuan P, et al: The effect of lumbar distraction and decompression in reducing intervertebral canal stenosis. Presented to the International Society of the Lumbar Spine, Chicago, 1992.
61. Kazarian LE, Von Gierke H: Bone loss as a result of immobilization and chelation: Preliminary results in *Maccaca mulatta*. *Clin Orthop* 1969; 65:67.
62. Keller J, Bunger C, Anderassen TT, et al: Bone repair inhibited by indomethacin. *Acta Orthop Scand* 1987; 58:379–383.
63. Keller T, Moeljanto E, Main J, et al: Distribution and orientation of bone in the human lumbar vertebral centrum. *J Spinal Disorders* 1992; 5:60–74.
64. Kjaersgaard-Andersen P, Schmidt SA: Indomethacin for prevention of ectopic ossification after hip arthroplasty. *Acta Orthop Scand* 1986; 57:12–14.
65. Kou YF, Edwards WT, Hayes WC, et al: Time dependent load distribution in the lumbar intervertebral joint. Presented to the Orthopaedic Research Society, Las Vegas, 1986.
66. Krag M, Pope M, Wilder D: Mechanisms of spine trauma and features of spinal fixation methods. Part 1: Mechanisms of injury, in Ghista D (ed): *Spinal Cord Injury Medical Engineering*. Springfield, Ill, Charles C Thomas, 1986, pp 133–157.
67. Krag MH, Beynnon BD, Pope MH, et al: Depth of insertion of tranpedicular screws into the human vertebrae: Effect upon screw-vertebra interface strength. *J Spinal Dis* 1989; 1:287–294.
68. Krolner B, Nielsen SP: Bone mineral content of the lumbar spine in normal and osteoporotic women: Cross-sectional longitudinal studies. *Clin Sci* 1982; 62:329–336.
69. Krolner B, Toft B, Nielson SP, et al: Physical exercise as a prophylaxis against involutional bone loss: A controlled trial. *Clin Sci* 1983; 64:541–546.
70. Kurihara N, Ishizuka S, Kiyoki M, et al: Effects of 1,25-dihydroxyvitamin D_3 in osteoblastic MC3T3-E1 cells. *Endocrinology* 1986; 118:940–947.
71. Lang S, Moyle D, Berg E, et al: Correlation of mechanical properties of vertebral trabecular bone with equivalent mineral density as measured by computed tomography. *J Bone Joint Surg [Am]* 1988; 70:1531–1538.
72. Lerner UH, Ransjo M, Ljunggren O: Prostaglandin E_2 causes a transient inhibition of mineral mobilization, matrix degradation, and lysosomal enzyme release from mouse calvarial bones in vitro. *Calcif Tissue Int* 1987; 40:323–331.
73. Lindholm TS, Tornkvist H: Inhibitory effect on bone formation and calcification exerted by the anti-inflammatory drug ibuprofen. *Scand J Rheumatol* 1981; 10:38–42.
74. Lipscomb H, Grubb S, Talmage R: Spinal bone density following spinal fusion. Presented to the Orthopaedic Research Society, Las Vegas, 1987.
75. Magerl FP: Stabilization of the lower thoracic and lumbar spine with external skeletal fixation. *Clin Orthop* 1984; 189:125–141.
76. Marie PJ, Caulin F: Mechanisms underlying the effects of phosphate and cacitonin in bone histology in postmenopausal osteoporosis. *Bone* 1986; 7:17–22.
77. Markel M, Wikenheiser M, Morin R, et al: A comparison of four noninvasive techniques to measure bone healing: QCT, MRI, SPA, and DEXA. Presented to the Orthopaedic Research Society, New Orleans, 1990.
78. Martin RB, Burr DB: *Structure, Function and Adaptation of Compact Bone*. New York, Raven Press, 1989.
79. Mazess RB, Cameron JR, O'Connor R, et al: Accuracy of bone mineral measurement. *Science* 1964; 145:388–389.
80. Mazess RB, Trempe JA, Bisek JP, et al: Calibration of dual-energy x-ray absorptiometry for bone density. *J Bone Miner Res* 1991; 6:799–806.
81. McAfee PC, Farey ID, Sutterlin CE, et al: Device-related osteoporosis with spinal instrumentation. *Spine* 1989; 14:919–926.
82. McBroom R, Hayes W, Edwards W, et al: Prediction of vertebral body compressive fracture using quantitative computed tomography. *J Bone Joint Surg [Am]* 1985; 67:1206–1214.
83. McBroom RJ, Hayes WC, Edwards WT, et al: Non-invasive prediction of vertebral fracture risk. Presented to the Orthopaedic Research Society, Atlanta, 1984.
84. McCubbery D, Cody D, Kuhn J, et al: Static and fatigue failure properties of thoracic and lumbar vertebral bodies and their relation to regional density. Presented to the Orthopaedic Research Society, New Orleans, 1990.
85. McGill SM, Norman RW: Partitioning of the L4-L5 dynamic moment into disc, ligamentous, and muscular components during lifting. *Spine* 1986; 11:666–678.
86. Meade J: The adaptation of bone to mechanical stress: Experimental and current concepts, in Cowin S (ed): *Bone Mechanics*. Boca Raton, Fla, CRC Press, 1989, pp 211–251.
87. Melton LJ III, Eddy DM, Johnston CC Jr: Screening for osteoporosis. *Ann Intern Med* 1990; 112:516–528.
88. Melton LJ III, Riggs BL: Epidemiology of age-related fractures, in Avioli LV (ed): *The Osteoporotic Syndrome: Detection, Prevention, and Treatment*. New York, Grune & Stratton, 1983, pp 45–72.
89. Melton LJ III, Riggs BL: Risk factors for injury after a fall. Symposium on falls in the elderly: Biological and behavioral aspects. *Clin Geriatr Med* 1985; 1:1–15.
90. Merz WA, Schenk RK: Quantitative structural analysis of human cancellous bone. *Acta Anat (Basel)* 1970; 75:54–66.
91. Meyer GH: Die architektur der spongiosa. *Arch Anat Physiol Wiss Med* 1867; 34:615–628.
92. Minaire P, Meuneir P, Edouard C, et al: Quantitative histological data on disuse osteoporosis: Comparison with biological data. *Calcif Tissue Res* 1974; 17:57.
93. Mongiorgi R, Romagnoli R, Olmi R, et al: Mineral alterations in senile osteoporosis. *Biomaterials* 1983; 4:192–196.
94. Morita I, Toriyama K, Murota S: Effects of prostaglandin E_2 on phenotype of osteoblast-like cells. *Adv Prostaglandin Thromboxane Leukotriene Res* 1989; 19:419–422.

95. Mosekilde L: Age-related changes in vertebral trabecular bone architecture-assisted by a new method. *Bone* 1988; 9:247–250.
96. Mosekilde L, Mosekilde L: Normal vertebral body size and compressive strength: Relations to age and to vertebral and iliac trabecular bone compression strength. *Bone* 1986; 7:207–212.
97. Nagel DA, Edwards WT, Schneider E: Biomechanics of spinal fixation and fusion. *Spine* 1991; 16(suppl 3):151–154.
98. Nagel DA, Kramers PC, Rahn BA, et al: Experimental model of lumbo-sacral nonunion. Presented to the International Society of Orthopaedic Surgery and Trauma, Munich, 1987.
99. Nilsson B, Westlin N: Bone density in athletes. *Clin Endocrinol* 1971; 77:179–182.
100. Pan L, Price P: The effect of transcriptional inhibitors on the bone–carboxyglutamic acid protein response to 1,25-dihydroxyvitamin D_3 in osteosarcoma cells. *J Biochem* 1984; 259:5844–5847.
101. Parfitt AM: Age-related structural changes in trabecular and cortical bone: Cellular mechanisms and biomechanical sequences. *Calcif Tissue Int* 1984; 36:123–128.
102. Parfitt AM, et al: Relationship between surface, volume, and thickness of iliac trabecular bone in aging and in osteoporosis. *J Clin Invest* 1983; 72:1396–1409.
103. Perren SM: Physical and biological aspects of fracture healing with special reference to internal fixation. *Clin Orthop* 1979; 138:175–190.
104. Perren SM, Cordey J: The concept of interfragmentary strain, in *Current Concepts of Internal Fixation of Fractures*. New York, Springer-Verlag, 1980, pp 63–77.
105. Portale A, Halloran B, Murphy M, et al: Oral intake of phosphorus can determine the serum concentrate of 1,25-dihydroxyvitamin D by determining its production rate in humans. *J Clin Invest* 1986; 77:7–12.
106. Posner I, White AA III, Edwards WT, et al: A biomechanical analysis of the clinical stability of the lumbar and lumbosacral spine. *Spine* 1982; 7:374–389.
107. Pruitt LA, Jackson RD, Bartels RL, et al: Weight-training effects on bone mineral density in early postmenopausal women. *J Bone Miner Res* 1992; 7:179–185.
108. Purcell G, Markolf K, Dawson E: Twelfth thoracic–first lumbar vertebral mechanical stability of fractures after Harrington-rod instrumentation. *J Bone Joint Surg [Am]* 1981; 63:71–78.
109. Raisz LG: Local and systemic factors in the pathogenesis of osteoporosis. *N Engl J Med* 1988; 318:818–828.
110. Raisz LG, Koolemans-Beynen AR: Inhibition of bone collagen synthesis by prostaglandin E_2 in organ culture. *Prostaglandin* 1974; 8:377–385.
111. Raisz LG, Kream BE: Regulation of bone formation. *N Engl J Med* 1983; 309:2935.
112. Reichel H, Koeffer HP, Norman AW: The role of the vitamin D endocrine system in health and disease. *N Engl J Med* 1989; 320:980–991.
113. Ro J, Sudmann E, Marton PF: Effect of indomethacin on fracture healing in rats. *Acta Orthop Scand* 1976; 47:588–599.
114. Rockoff SD, Sweet E, Bluestein J: The relative contribution of trabecular and cortical bone to the strength of human lumbar vertebrae. *Calcif Tissue Res* 1975; 3:163–175.
115. Roesler H: The history of some fundamental concepts in bone biomechanics. *J Biomech* 1987; 20:1025–1034.
116. Roux W: Der züchtende Kampf der Teile, oder die "Teilauslese" im Organismus, in Engelman W (ed): *Theorie der "Funktionellen Anpassung."* Leipzig, Germany, 1881.
117. Roy-Camille R, Saillant G, et al: *Posterior Spinal Fixation with Transpedicular Screws and Plates*. Paris, Boulevard de Hopital, 1983.
118. Roy-Camille R, Saillant G, Mazel C: Internal fixation of the lumbar spine with pedicle screw plating. *Clin Orthop* 1986; 203:7.
119. Sambrook P, Bartlett C, Evans R, et al: Measurement of lumbar spine bone mineral: A comparison of dual photon absortiometry and computed tomography. *Br J Radiol* 1985; 58:621–624.
120. Schmidt SA, Kjaersgaard-Andersen P, Pendersen NW, et al: The use of indormethacin to prevent the formation of heterotopic bone after total hip replacement. *J Bone Joint Surg [Am]* 1988; 70:834–838.
121. Schneller S: Medical considerations and perioperative care for rheumatoid surgery. *Hand Clin* 1989; 5:115–126.
122. Smith MJH, Dawkins PD: Salicylates and enzymes. *J Pharm Pharmacol* 1971; 23:729–744.
123. Smith RJ: Modulation of phagocytosis by and lysosomal secretion from guinea-pig neutrophils: Effect of nonsteroid anti-inflammatory agents and prostaglandins. *J Pharmacol Exp Ther* 1977; 200:647–657.
124. Snyder BD, Edwards WT, Hayes WC: Trabecular changes with vertebral osteoporosis (letter). *N Engl J Med* 1988; 319:793–794.
125. Snyder BD, Edwards WT, Van der Linde JM, et al: Stereological assessment of trabecular structure on the lumbar vertebral body: Biomechanical implications. Presented to the Orthopaedic Research Society, Las Vegas, 1989.
126. Somjen D, Binderman I, Berger E, et al: Bone remodelling induced by a physical stress is prostaglandin E_2 mediated. *Biochim Biophys Acta* 1980; 627:91–100.
127. Spencer H, Rubio N, Rubio E, et al: Chronic alcoholism: Frequently overlooked cause of osteoporosis in men. *Am J Med* 1986; 80:393–397.
128. Sudmann E, Bang G: Indomethacin-induced inhibition of haversian remodeling in rabbits. *Acta Orthop Scand* 1979; 50:621–627.
129. Sudmann E, Hagen T: Indomethacin-induced delayed fracture healing. *Arch Orthop Unfallchir* 1974; 85:151–154.
130. Sudmann E, Tveita T, Hald JJ: Lack of effect of indomethacin on ordered growth of the femur in rats. *Acta Orthop Scand* 1982; 53:43–49.
131. Thomas I, Kirkaldy-Willis WH, Singh S, et al: Experimental spinal fusion in guinea pigs and dogs: The effect of immobilization. *Clin Orthop* 1975; 112:363–375.

132. Thomson P, Rodan GA: Immobilization produces increased bone resorption and decreased formation in rats (abstract). *J Bone Miner Res* 1986; 1(suppl 1):23.
133. Tilton F, Degioanni J, Schieder V: Longterm follow-up of Skylab bone demineralization. *Aviat Space Environ Med* 1980; 51:1209.
134. Tornkvist H, Lindholm TS: Effect of ibuprofen on mass and composition of fracture callus and bone. *Scand J Rheumatol* 1980; 9:167–171.
135. Tornkvist H, Lindholm TS, Netz P, et al: Effect of ibuprofen and indomethacin on bone metabolism reflected in bone strength. *Clin Orthop* 1984; 187:255–259.
136. Tsai K-S, Heath H III, Kumar R, et al: Impaired vitamin D metabolism with aging women: Possible role in pathogenesis of senile osteoporosis. *J Clin Invest* 1984; 73:1668–1672.
137. Vane JR: Inhibition of prostaglandin synthesis as a mechanism of action for aspirin-like drugs. *Nature* 1971; 231:232–235.
138. Vane JR: Mode of action of aspirin and similar compounds, in Robinson HJ, Vane JR (eds): *Prostaglandin Synthesis,* New York, Raven Press, 1974.
139. Vose G, Stover B, Mack P: Quantitative bone strength measurements in senile osteoporosis. *J Gerontol* 1961; 16:120–124.
140. Weibel H: Stereological techniques for microscopic morphometry. *Princip Electron Microsc* 1979; 3:261–271.
141. Weidenreich F: Uber sehnenverknocherunger und faktoren dew knochenbildung. *Z Anat Entwichlegeschichte* 1923; 69:558–597.
142. Wendsche P, Michek J, Unger C: Treatment of unstable thoracolumbar spinal injuries—determination of its present status and a preliminary report on transpedicular stabilization. *Zentralbl Chir* 1988; 113:520–529.
143. White AH, Rothman RH, Ray CD: *Lumbar Spine Surgery: Techniques and Complications*. St Louis, Mosby–Year Book, 1987.
144. White AA III, Panjabi MM: *Clinical Biomechanics of the Spine*. Philadelphia. JB Lippincott, 1978.
145. Whitehouse MW: Some biochemical and pharmacological properties of anti-inflammatory drugs. *Prog Drug Res* 1965; 8:321–429.
146. Whitehouse MW: The molecular pharmacology of anti-inflammatory drugs: Some possible mechanisms of action at the biochemical level. *Biochem Pharmacol (Suppl)* 1968; 17:293–307.
147. Whitehouse WJ: A stereological method for calculating internal surface areas in structures which have become anistropic as the result of linear expansions or contractions. *J Microsc* 1974; 101:169–176.
148. Whitehouse WJ: Cancellous bone in the anterior part of the iliac crest. *Calcif Tissue Res* 1977; 23:67–76.
149. William TJ, Peck MJ: Role of prostaglandin-mediated vasodilation in inflammation. *Nature* 1977; 270:530–532.
150. Wolff J: *Das Gesetz der Transformation der Knochen*. Berlin, Hirchwald, 1892.
151. Wolff J: Uber die Bedeutung der Architektur der Spongiosa. *Zentrabl Med Wiss VI Jahrgang* 1869; 223–234.
152. Wu J, Shry JS, Chao E, et al: Comparison of osteotomy healing under external fixation devices with different stiffness characteristics. *J Bone Joint Surg [Am]* 1984; 66:1258–1264.
153. Wu SS, Edwards WT, Zou D, et al: Transpedicular vertebral screws in human vertebrae: Effect on screw-vertebra interface stiffness. *Trans Orthop Res Soc* 1992; 17:459.
154. Yoo J, Zou D, Edwards WT, et al: Alteration of neuroforaminal size secondary to cervical motion. Presented to the American Orthopaedic Association, Palm Beach, Fla, 1991.
155. Zhang CY, Edwards WT: Refined analysis of deformations and stress within the human intervertebral disc following discectomy. Presented to the International Society of the Lumbar Spine, Chicago, 1992.
156. Zindrick MR, Wiltse LL, Doornik A, et al: Analysis of the morphometric characteristics of the thoracic and lumbar pedicles. *Spine* 1987; 12:160–166.
157. Zindrick MR, Wiltse LL, Widell EH, et al: A biomechanical study of intrapedicular screw fixation on the lumbosacral spine. *Clin Orthop* 1986; 203:99–122.
158. Zschokke E: *Weiter Untersuchenger uber das Verhaltnis der Knochenbildung zur Statik und Mechanik des Vertebraten-skelettes*. Zurich, Art Institute Orell Fussli. 1892.

19

Ligament

Rocky S. Tuan, Ph.D.

Ligaments of the spine represent the connective structures between adjacent vertebrae. The principal function of the spinal ligaments is to restrain the extremes of motions, either in multiple or single segments.[13] An example of the first category is the ligamentum nuchae, a dense and fibrous posterior midline band running from the external occipital protuberance to the spinous process of C7. Ligaments of the second category include those of the lower and upper halves of the cervical spine, e.g., the anterior longitudinal ligament, posterior longitudinal ligament, ligamentum flavum, alar ligaments, etc.

The function of the spinal ligaments as motion-restraining structures necessarily involve a great deal of tensile load and large mechanical strain, as high as 25% in the supraspinous and interspinous ligaments for 30 newton-meters (Nm) of flexion with no preload.[38] In addition to intrinsic degenerations of the ligaments as part of the aging process, primary degenerations of the intervertebral discs can often lead to secondary structural changes in the ligaments as a result of acute or repetitive load shifts from the discs.[23] Repair of such mechanical damages is often slow owing to the acellular nature and poor vascularization of the ligaments.[43]

This chapter reviews the anatomy, histology, morphology, cell biology, and biochemical composition of ligaments, as well as changes in these properties as a function of development, age, injury and mechanical perturbations.

LOCATION AND APPEARANCE

In the cervical spine, two sets of ligaments provide support and security as well as allow movement of the head: the external craniocervical ligaments, which lie outside the vertebral canal, and the internal craniocervical ligaments, which lie within the vertebral canal.[13, 32] The former include (1) the ligamentum nuchae, which extends from the external occipital protuberance to the posterior tubercle of the atlas and all other spinous processes of the cervical vertebrae; (2) the ligamentum flavum, present between the arch of the atlas and the lamina of the axis; (3) various membranous, fibroelastic bands (anterior and posterior atlanto-occipital membranes and anterior and posterior atlantoaxial membranes); and (4) capsular ligaments surrounding the joints between the occipital condyles of the skull band and the superior surface of the atlantal facets and all around the atlantoaxial facet articulations. On the other hand, the internal craniocervical ligaments include (1) the tectorial membrane, a cranial prolongation of the posterior longitudinal ligament that extends from the posterior surface of the body of the axis to the anterior edge of the foramen magnum and blends with the cranial dura mater; (2) the atlas cruciform ligament, which attaches transversely to the tubercles on thc inner side of each lateral mass of the atlas and emanates at the midpoint of the transverse ligament to attach vertically to the basilar part of the occipital bone and to the posterior surface of the body of the axis; (3) the apical ligament, which connects the odontoid apex to the anterior midpoint of the foramen magnum; (4) the alar ligaments, which stretch obliquely upward and outward from the superolateral aspects of the odontoid process to the inner sides of the occipital condyles; and (5) accessory ligaments extending from the anterior longitudinal ligament and running from the base of the odontoid to the lateral mass of the atlas.

In the thoracolumbosacral spine, an extensive array of motion segment ligaments are functional.[13, 19, 32] The common ones include the supraspinous and interspinous ligaments, ligamentum flavum, intertransverse ligaments, and posterior and anterior longitudinal ligaments. In the thoracic spine, each motion segment also has costovertebral and costotransverse articulations. In the lumbosacral and sacroiliac articulations, a larger number of additional, strong ligaments provide the necessary stability.

In general, ligaments are fibroelastic bands. Among the ligaments of the spine, the ligamentum flavum is unique because of its composition (see below) and yellow appearance.[13, 19] Structurally, the ligaments, like the capsule, consist of a proximal bone insertion, the substance of the ligament, and the distal bone insertion (Fig 19–1).[9] Discrete changes in matrix composition and cellular histology accompany the ligament insertion into bone and are discussed in detail below.

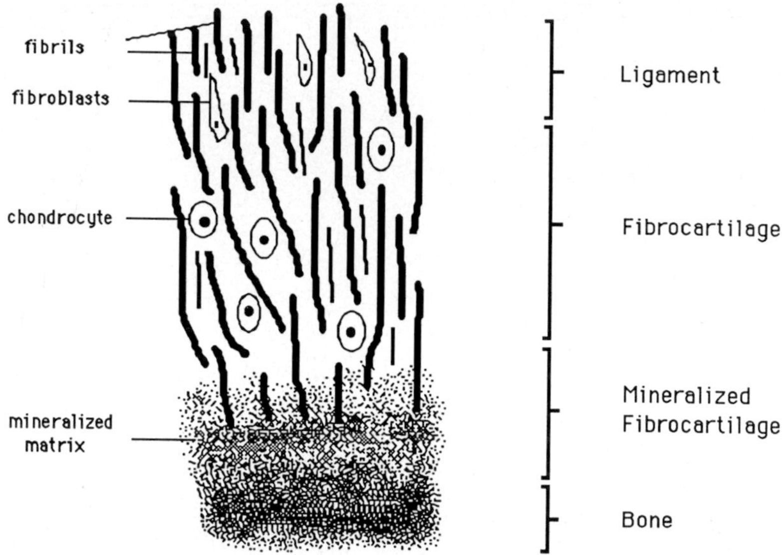

FIG 19-1.
Schematic structure of ligament attachment to chondro-osseous tissue. The ligament proper, consisting of collagen and elastin fibrils, is interphased to fibrocartilage and mineralized fibrocartilage, which are assimilated into the mineralized matrix of bone.

HISTOLOGY, MORPHOLOGY, AND CELL BIOLOGY

A hallmark of the histology of ligaments is their relatively high acellularity and the abundance of extracellular matrix. Ultrastructurally, ligaments consist primarily of highly oriented, densely packed collagen fibrils that often form layered sheets or lamellae (Fig 19–2). Yahia et al.[44] recently reported on the ultrastructure of human interspinous ligament and ligamentum flavum. Elastic and elaunin fibers with interspersed small-diameter collagen fibrils make up the ligamentum flavum. On the other hand, the interspinous ligament is constituted predominantly of collagen fibrils, and elastic fibers are seen in the most ventral part of the ligament. The cylindrical elastic fibers, which consist of elastin and other protein components (see below), generally lie parallel to the collagen fibrils. Cells that are found are principally fibroblast-like, and chondrocytes are found only near the attachment sites. Proteoglycans are also detected and appear to form a regular interfibrillar linking.

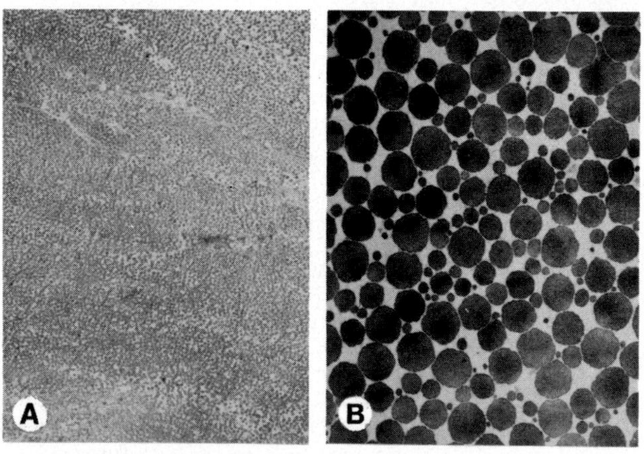

FIG 19-2.
Ultrastructure of collagen fibrils in a transverse section of a ligament. **A,** low magnification showing the abundance of fibrils. **B,** high magnification showing the different populations of fibrils of varying diameters. (Adapted from Gibson MA, Kumaratilake JS, Cleary EG: *J Biol Chem* 1989; 264:4590–4598.)

The structural transition seen in ligament attachment to bone is similar to that observed for tendons, i.e., a transition from the elastic ligament to the rigid bone (see Fig 19–1). This is accomplished by the tissue assuming different zones of stiffness—ligament, fibrocartilage, mineralized fibrocartilage, and bone.[9] Insertions may vary in the obliquity of the angle between the collagen fibrils of the ligament and the bone such that the site of insertion may be either periosteal or intraosteal; these differences are likely to affect the response of the insertion to loading and immobilization.[25, 28]

The ligamentum flavum may undergo symptomatic calcification to give rise to calcified nodules. A recent study[24] reports the presence of extracellular matrix vesicles and, in some areas of the ligament, thick wall-bound matrix giant bodies with or without mineral deposits. These calcified vesicles are also present in the wide mineralized areas among the collagen and elastic fibers in the ligament. It is thus conceivable that abnormal calcification of the ligament involves a mechanism similar to that normally responsible for growth plate mineralization, i.e., with the involvement of matrix vesicles, extracellular membrane-bound structures that have been postulated as nucleating centers of matrix mineralization.[7] Interestingly, another recent study[22] described cases of cervical radiculomyelopathy caused by calcium pyrophosphate dihydrate crystal deposition disease (CPPDcdd) that were accompanied by nodular calcifications in the cervical ligamentum flavum. Light and electron microscopy and x-ray diffraction and microanalysis showed the association of hydroxyapatite with calcium pyrophosphate dihydrate in these nodules. The investigators suggest that CPPDcdd and "calcification of the ligamentum flavum" are the same disease and that the hydroxyapatite in the calcification nodules is transformed from calcium phosphate dihydrate.

The most distinctive aspect of the ligaments is their extracellular matrix, which like other skeletal connective tissues, determines the mechanical properties of the ligaments. The predominant component is collagen type I (see below), which is organized ultrastructurally into parallel, densely packed fibrils of varying sizes aligned along a given axis of the ligament (Fig 19–2). Occasionally, the lamellae of collagen fibrils may be found aligned obliquely to each other, e.g., in the central portion of the transverse ligament, the collagen fibers cross each other at an angle of approximately 30 degrees.[34] This type of fibrillar arrangement of the ligaments resembles that found in tendons and is grossly different from that of other skeletal connective tissues such as cartilage and bone. For example, in cartilage a loose collagenous network is found, whereas in bone, obliquely aligned, densely packed, and mineralized collagen fibrils are observed (Fig 19–3).[5] In general, aging of the ligaments is usually accompanied by an increase in the volume of the extracellular matrix.

The principal cell type found embedded in the dense matrix of the ligament is the fibroblast.[5] Other cells found occasionally in the ligament include endothelial and nerve cells. However, a recent study[11] reported the localization of substance P–like immunoreactive and neurofilament protein immunoreactive fibers in the supraspinous ligament of the rabbit, which indicates that the tissue is in fact richly innervated, a fact that may contribute to the etiology of low back pain.

Recently, the technique of magnetic resonance imaging (MRI) has begun to be applied for the examination of spinal cord trauma[21] and spinal ligaments.[18] For example, the latter study reported that the ligamentum flavum may be analyzed as a structure with intermediate signal intensity on images obtained with short and long repetition times (Fig 19–4). Sagittal images with short repetition times appear to be effective for evaluating relationships between the ligamentum flavum, spinal canal, and nerve roots. Changes in the shape or thickness of the ligaments on MRI are seen to correlate with degenerative changes. However, calcification and fat infiltration, both well depicted on anatomic sections, are not visualized on MRI.

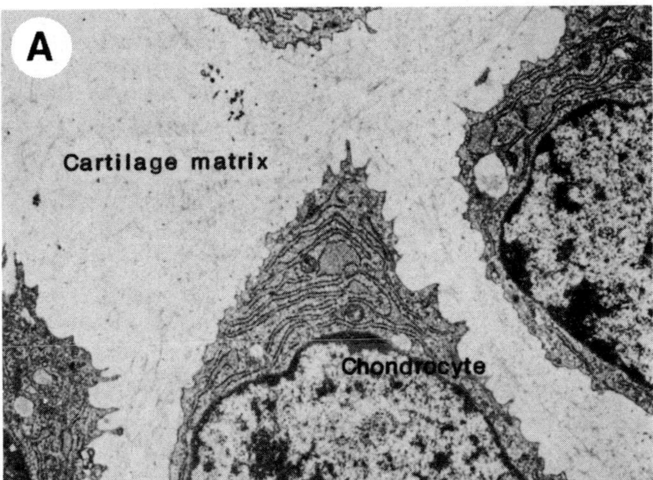

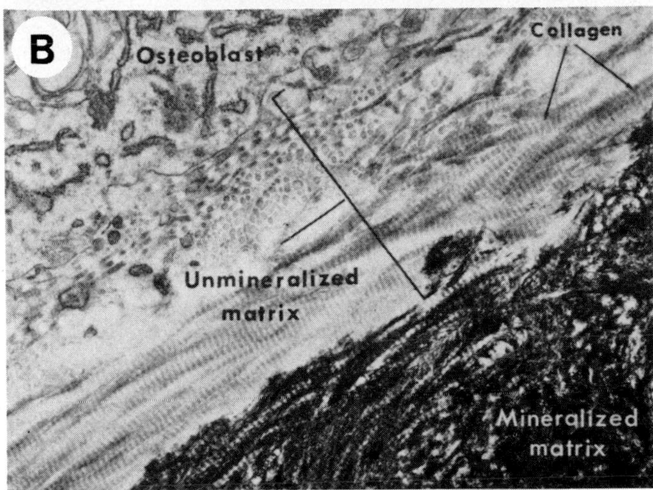

FIG 19–3.
Ultrastructure of collagenous matrix in cartilage **(A)** and bone **(B).** In cartilage, chondrocytes are surrounded by a matrix consisting of a fibrous meshwork of collagen interspersed with proteoglycans. In bone, highly structured collagen fibrils are found in the matrix, which undergoes extensive mineralization. (Adapted from Bloom W, Fawcett DW: *A Textbook of Histology*, Philadelphia, WB Saunders, 1975.)

In addition to MRI, other methods have also been used to examine the structure of ligaments. For example, both polarized light microscopy and x-ray diffraction have been applied,[4] both techniques taking advantage of the highly ordered nature of the matrix of parallel collagen fibrils and elastic fibers.

As described above, cells of the ligament are embedded in a prodigious matrix and must therefore exhibit unique adhesive properties with respect to the matrix components. In general, cells utilize a number of mechanisms in their interactions with the extracellular matrix. Most of these involve cell surface matrix receptors known as integrins,[4] which operate by recognizing and binding to spe-

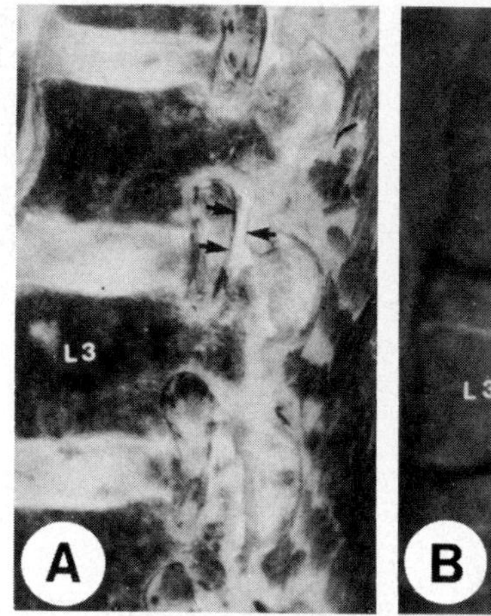

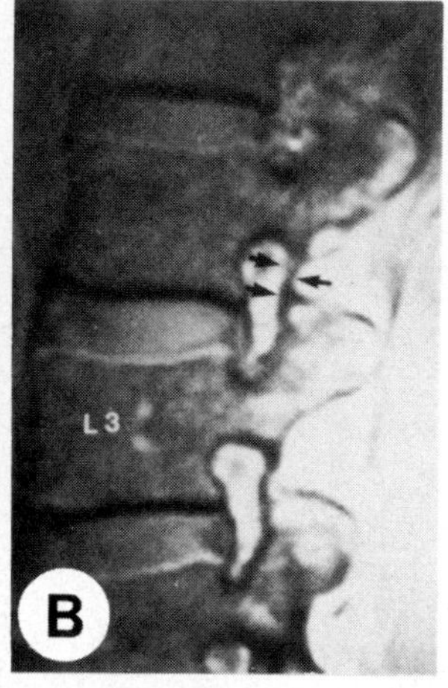

FIG 19–4.
Imaging of ligamentum flavum by MRI. Parasagittal cryomicrotomic sections were examined by conventional light microscopy (**A**) or MRI (**B**). The sections were through the lateral border of facet joint and pedicle. The ligamentum flavum appeared as a yellowish stripe under light microscopy (*arrows* in **A**) and showed low signal intensity on MRI (*arrows* in **B**). (From Ho PS, Yu SW, Sether LA, et al: *Radiology* 1988; 168:468–472. Used by permission.)

cific amino acid sequences in a number of matrix proteins, including fibronectin, collagen, etc. (Fig 19–5). Sauk et al. have characterized the ability of ligament cells to spread on a number of bone and skeletal matrix proteins and the relationship of the spreading to stress tolerance of these cells.[37] Interestingly, cells that persistently spread on type I collagen and bone sialoprotein-I are found to be clearly more resistant to heat stress than other cells. These results appear to indicate that specific spreading of the ligament cells to the surrounding matrix is a prerequisite for

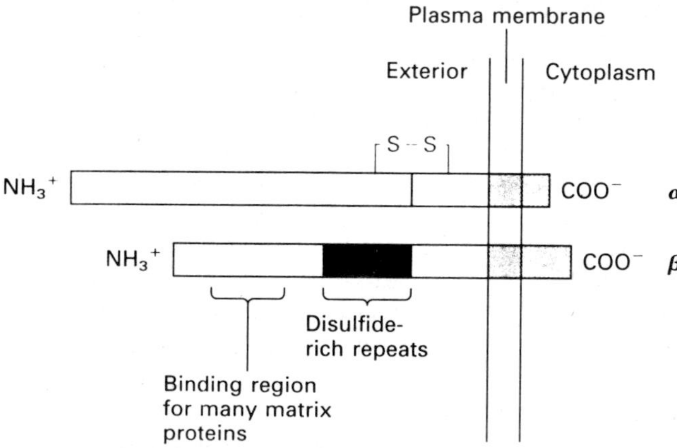

FIG 19–5.
The structure of the integrin class of cell-surface receptors. Two transmembrane polypeptides, α and β, whose molecular weight varies from about 100 to 140 kDa make up an integrin receptor. The amino terminal of the β-chain, which is exposed to the extracellular milieu, is responsible for the binding to extracellular matrix macromolecules, including collagen types, fibronectin, proteoglycans, etc.

stress tolerance. It remains to be established whether tolerance to mechanical stress, a functional requirement for ligament cells, also operates via such cell-spreading mechanisms.

BIOCHEMICAL COMPOSITION

Collagen

As mentioned above, the principal biochemical component of ligaments is collagen, specifically, type I. Collagen is the most abundant single protein in most vertebrate animals.[12, 26] The basic unit of collagen is the tropocollagen molecule, a triple helix of three polypeptide chains, each about 1000 amino acid residues in length (Fig 19–6). This threefold, left-hand helical structure of the polypeptide, which consists of 3.3 residues per turn, is unique to the collagen molecule. Three of these polypeptide chains wrap around one another in a right-hand manner, with hydrogen bonds extending between the chains. Every third of the amino acid residues along any given chain is glycine, whose limited side-chain structure is absolutely essential for the compactness of the triple helical conformation. Formation of the individual helices also dictates that the preceding amino acid residue be proline or hydroxyproline. Thus, a repetitive theme in the sequence is glycine-X-proline or glycine-X-hydroxyproline, where X is some other amino acid. Another unusual feature of

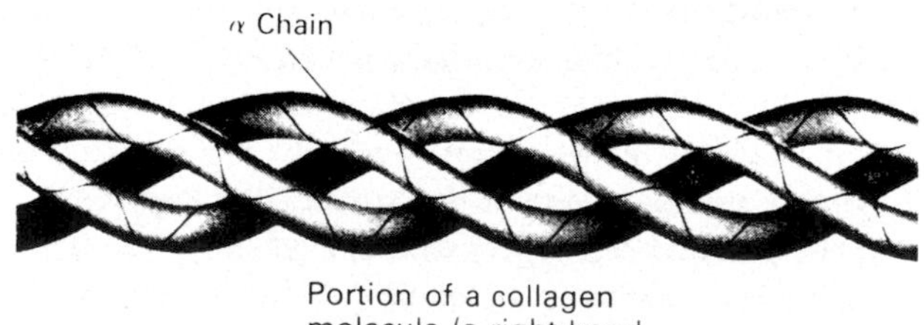

13
-Gly-Pro-Met-Gly-Pro-Ser-Gly-Pro-Arg-
22
-Gly-Leu-Hyp-Gly-Pro-Hyp-Gly-Ala-Hyp-
31
-Gly-Pro-Gln-Gly-Phe-Gln-Gly-Pro-Hyp-
40
-Gly-Glu-Hyp-Gly-Glu-Hyp-Gly-Ala-Ser-
49
-Gly-Pro-Met-Gly-Pro-Arg-Gly-Pro-Hyp-
58
-Gly-Pro-Hyp-Gly-Lys-Asn-Gly-Asp-Asp-

FIG 19–6.
The structure of collagen consists of three polypeptide chains denoted as α-chains wrapped around one another in a right-hand triple helix. The amino acid sequence of collagen as exemplified by the α_1-chain of type II collagen (residues 13 to 66) shows every third residue to be glycine (Gly) and the abundance of proline (Pro) and hydroxyproline (Hyp).

collagen is the extensive modification of proline to hydroxyproline and, to a lesser extent, lysine to hydroxyllysine. These hydroxylation reactions involve ascorbic acid, vitamin C, as a cofactor. This explains the disease of scurvy as a result of vitamin C deficiency, which is caused by weakening of the collagen fibers due to insufficient production of hydroxyproline. The individual tropocollagen molecules pack together in a collagen fiber in a unique fashion: each is about 300 nm long, and each overlaps its neighbor by about 64 nm, thus resulting in a characteristic banded appearance of the fibers. Such organization of the collagen fibers results in their mechanical strength. Finally, part of the mechanical properties of collagen may be attributed to the high degree of cross-linking of the individual molecule to one another via lysine side chains (Fig 19–7). Many lysine residues are oxidized to aldehyde derivatives, which can then react with either another lysine residue or one another to produce an aldol cross-link. This process continues through life, and the accumulation of cross-links renders the collagen increasingly less elastic and more brittle. Many incidents involving the skeletal tissues that are associated with aging, such as fractures or rupture of ligaments and tendons, are probably a result of this biochemical reaction.

Type I collagen, the principal collagen type of ligament, is a heterotrimer of tropocollagen polypeptides that consists of two α1 chains and one α2 chain. The α1 and α2 polypeptides are each derived from separate genes. At least 14 distinct types of collagen encoded by 25 different genes have been identified[20]; in fact, type XII collagen has been detected in ligaments by immunohistochemistry.[39] A number of recent studies have revealed that collagen gene mutations are associated with and perhaps are directly responsible for several skeletal anomalies, including osteogenesis imperfecta[31] and some forms of osteoarthritis.[3] It is not known, however, whether such mutations affect ligament functions.

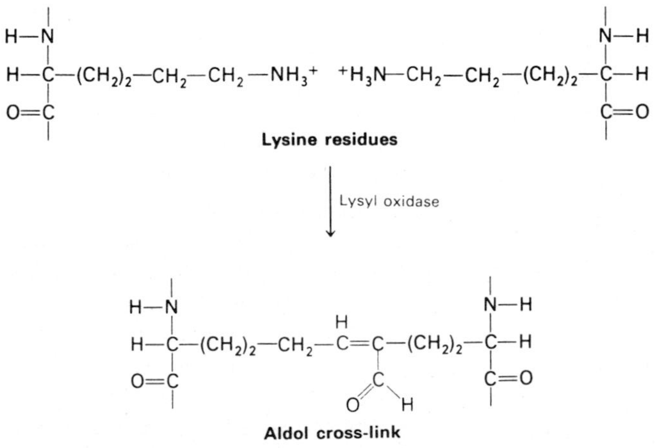

Lysine residues

Lysyl oxidase

Aldol cross-link

FIG 19–7.
Formation of an aldol cross-link from two lysine side chains in collagen. The reaction is catalyzed by the enzyme lysyl oxidase, which requires vitamin C as a cofactor.

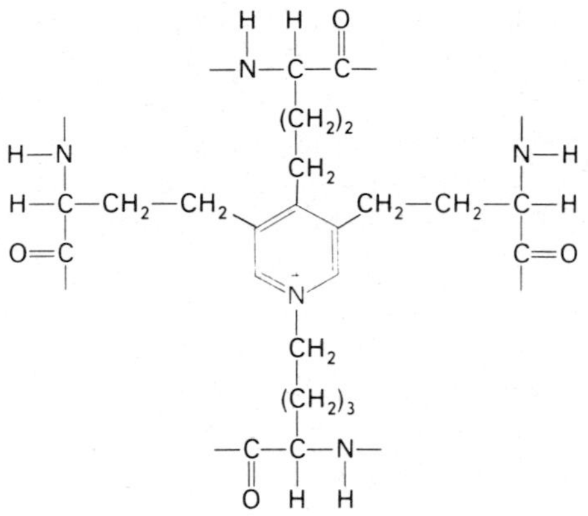

FIG 19–8.
Structure of the cross-link product desmosine, which is formed from four lysine residues in elastin.

Elastin

Elastic fibrils are found predominatly in the extracellular matrix of ligaments.[44] The principal component, over 90%, of the microfibrils is elastin.[5] Among the spinal ligaments, the ligamentum flavum has a uniquely high elastic content (80%) vs. the collagen content (20%), which gives the ligament a yellow appearance.[13] The polypeptide chain of elastin is rich in glycine and alanine and is very flexible and easily extended.[36] Proline residues are also abundant, although little hydroxyproline is present. Lysine residues are also present in elastin and are often involved in cross-links (Fig 19–8). Mechanically, it is these chemical cross-links that prevent the elastin fibers from extending indefinitely and allow them to "snap back" upon removal of tension. The lysine-derived chemical cross-links in elastin are different structurally from those in collagen; specifically, four lysine residues combine to form a desmosine or isodesmosine cross-link. This tight aggregation of four lysine residues ensures that a highly stretchable, interconnected network is formed readily in elastin.

Proteoglycans

The major function of proteoglycans, which are highly negatively charged macromolecules, is to permit the tissue to hydrate as a result of the water shell around the charged anionic sites and thereby maintain the viscoelastic properties of the tissue.[16] Although the chemical composition of the proteoglycans of ligaments is not well understood, it is most likely structurally analogous to those found in cartilage, perhaps differing in the proportion of the various glycosaminoglycan chains.[17] The major components of a proteoglycan molecule are glycosaminoglycans (Fig 19–9), which are polysaccharide chains made up of repeating disaccharide units, usually a derivative of glucosamine or galactosamine, at least one of the sugars in the disaccharide bearing a negatively charged carboxylate or sulfate group. Some of the most common glycosaminoglycans are hyaluronic acid, chondroitin sulfate, keratin sulfate, heparan sulfate, and heparin. In the proteoglycan from cartilage (Fig 19–9), keratin sulfate and chondroitin sulfate chains are covalently attached to a polypeptide backbone called the core protein via a link protein. The entire proteoglycan complex is very large, with a molecular mass of 2×10^6 Da and a dimension of several microns. Cartilage proteoglycans are also usually associated with hyaluronic acid

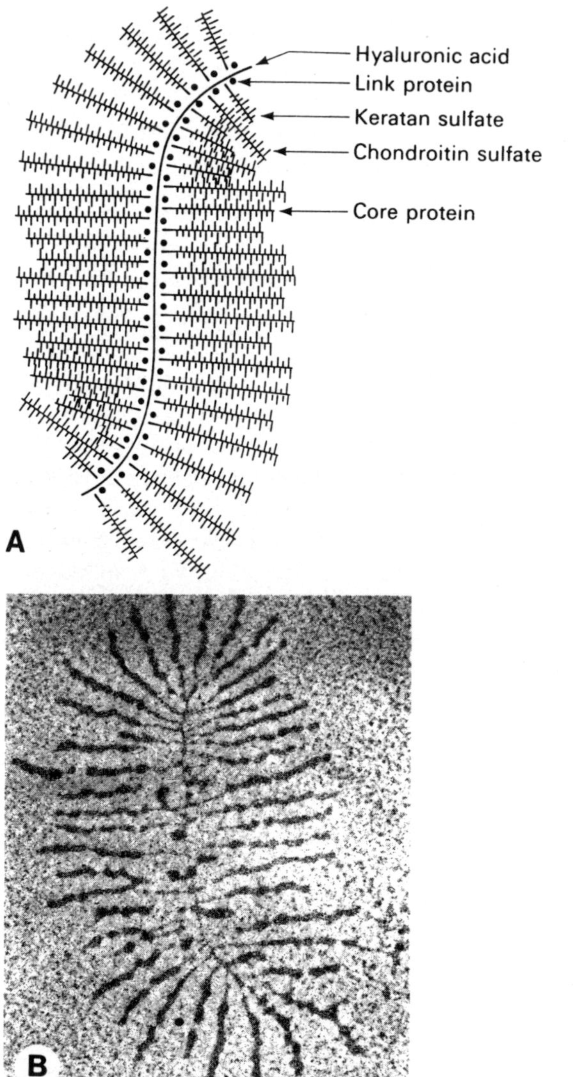

FIG 19–9.
Structure of a cartilage proteoglycan aggregate **(A),** which consists of glycosaminoglycans (keratin sulfate, chondroitin sulfate) covalently attached to core protein and bound via the link protein to a hyaluronic acid chain. **B,** electron micrograph showing the dimension of the aggregate (magnification, 6,000×).

to form supramacromolecular complexes with a molecular mass of over 20×10^6 Da. The presence of such large molecular complexes explains the unique viscoelastic characteristics of hyaline cartilage. The proteoglycans of ligaments have been described as interspersed between the collagen fibers[13, 44] and most likely serve a similar function. Histologically, proteoglycans may be conveniently detected by cationic histochemical stains such as alcian blue[35] because of their anionic nature.

As indicated above, the water content of a fibrous connective tissue such as a ligament defines its viscoelastic properties. Therefore, under situations where proteoglycans are lost, for example, during immobilization of a joint, water loss is also observed and is accompanied by ligamentous weakening as measured by energy absorption to failure.[23]

Other Extracellular Matrix Components

Recent biochemical analysis[15] has revealed the presence of other components in ligaments, in particular those in the elastin-associated microfibrils. Gel electrophoresis has identified five major components of molecular weights 340, 78, 70, 31, and 25 kDa. The 31-kDa species has been named microfibril-associated glycoprotein (MAGP).[14] All of the protein components are rich in acidic amino acids and cystine. It is postulated that the 78-kDa species and MAGP are both constituents of the 340-kDa species, which in turn is the subunit of which the 12-nm microfibrils are composed. The identity and relationship to microfibrils of the 70- and 25-kDa proteins are presently unknown.

STRUCTURAL CHANGES AS A FUNCTION OF DEVELOPMENT, AGE, MECHANICAL STRESS, AND DISEASE

The formation and attachment of ligaments to bone occur during prenatal development via regional specialization of cells at the attachment site. For example, for insertion into a metaphysis or diaphysis, the most distal region consists of germinal and resting cells, and the most proximal region consists of cells capable of bone formation, whereas the intermediate region contains maturing cells synthesizing extracellular matrix.[42] It should be noted that for the most part ligaments do not directly insert into the completely osseous region of the bone; instead, the insertion site is often localized to the overlying fibrous and fibrocartilaginous regions. This type of attachment mechanism allows active integrated growth of the chondro-osseous tissue. Furthermore, since similar tensile-responsive components, i.e., ligaments and fibrocartilage, interact, a progressive gradation of elasticity is accomplished. With skeletal maturation, the nature of such attachments is gradually altered, so the tendency toward soft-tissue, i.e. ligament, disruptions is increased as a function of age.

Aging is a principal cause of structural changes in ligaments such as fraying, partial ruptures, necrosis, and cyst formation.[8] In general, the tensile properties of the ligaments become reduced.[10, 27, 29] An age-related reduction in the amount of elastin to collagen has been reported and is possibly the consequence of elevated elastase activity.[5, 13] Mechanical stresses can also favorably or adversely alter the structural integrity of ligaments.[1, 2, 6, 43] For example, joint immobilization has been observed to result in (1) disorganized cellular and fibrillar alignment, (2) increased collagen degradation, (3) reduced collagen cross-linking, and (4) loss of proteoglycans and the associated water. The end point is characterized by weakening of the ligaments.

Finally, a number of diseases have been found to be manifested as changes in ligament functions and structure. Examples include Baastrup's disease,[8] spinal stenosis,[40] and symptomatic calcification as described above,[22, 24] all of which disrupt the normal structure of the ligaments.

REMARKS AND PROSPECTS

When compared with other skeletal tissues, the biology of spinal ligaments is relatively poorly understood. Some of the outstanding issues include the following. What are the cellular and molecular mechanisms underlying the formation of the spinal ligaments during embryonic development? How is ligament morphogenesis correlated temporally and spatially with vertebral morphogenesis, which is a highly patterned process involving resegmentation of somites and the migration and condensation of sclerotomal cells? How are the microfibrils assembled in concert with the selective gene expression of elastin isoforms?[30] What other minor collagen types are involved in the structuring of collagen fibers and what are their functions? What cellular and biochemical interactions mediate the attachment and abnormal detachment of ligaments from osteochondral tissue sites? What is the extent and functional involvement of innervation in spinal ligaments? What processes other than selective proteolytic degradation are responsible for the age- and immobilization-associated alterations in ligament structure? How do all of the above processes integrate into the biomechanical characteristics of ligaments? Are there valid experimental animal models for diseases involving spinal ligaments such as those being used for osteopetrosis, rheumatoid arthritis, etc.?[33] Can ligament biology and cellular functions be reproduced in a valid manner by in vitro methodologies such as those used in the study of cartilage and chondrogenesis?[41] These issues clearly should be addressed by future research on spinal ligaments.

Acknowledgment

The author's research is supported in part by grants from the National Institutes of Health, the March of Dimes Birth Defects Foundation, the United States Department of Agriculture, and the Orthopaedic Research and Education Foundation.

REFERENCES

1. Akeson WH, Amiel D, LaViolette D: The connective tissue response to immobility. *Clin Orthop* 1967; 51:183–197.
2. Akeson WH, Amiel D, Woo SL: Immobility effects on synovial joints. *Biorheology* 1980; 17:95–110.
3. Ala-Kokko L, Baldwin CT, Moskowitz RW, et al: Single base mutation in the type II procollagen gene (COL2A1) as a cause of primary osteoarthritis associated with a mild chondrodysplasia. *Proc Natl Acad Sci USA* 1990; 87:6565–6568.
4. Albelda SM, Buck CA: Integrins and other cell adhesion molecules. *FASEB J* 1990; 4:2868–2880.
5. Allbright JA, Brand RA: *The Scientific Basis of Orthopaedics*, ed 2. East Norwalk, Conn, Appleton & Lange, 1987.
6. Amiel D, Woo SL, Harwood FL, et al: The effect of immobilization on collagen turnover in connective tissue. *Acta Orthop Scand* 1982; 53:325–332.
7. Anderson HC: Vesicles associated with calcification in the matrix of epiphyseal cartilage. *J Cell Biol* 1969; 41:59–74.
8. Bywaters EGL: The pathological anatomy of idiopathic low back pain, in White AA III, Gordon SL (eds): *American Academy of Orthopaedic Surgeons Symposium on Idiopathic Low Back Pain*. St Louis, Mosby–Year Book, 1982, pp 144–177.
9. Cooper RR, Misol S: Tendon and ligament insertion. *J Bone Joint Surg [Am]* 1970; 52:1–21.
10. Dumas GA, Beaudoin L, Drouin G: In situ mechanical behavior of posterior spinal ligaments in the lumbar region: An in vitro study. *J Biomech* 1987; 20:301–310.
11. el-Bohy A, Cavanaugh JM, Getchell ML, et al: Localization of substance P and neurofilament immunoreactive fibers in the lumbar facet joint capsule and supraspinous ligament of the rabbit. *Brain Res* 1988; 460:379–382.
12. Eyre DR: Collagen: Molecular diversity in the body's protein scaffold. *Science* 1980; 207:1315–1322.
13. Frymoyer JW, Ducker TB, Hadler NM, et al (eds): *The Adult Spine: Principles and Practice*. New York, Raven Press, 1991.
14. Gibson MA, Hughes JL, Fanning JC, et al: The major antigen of elastin-associated microfibrils is a 31-kDa glycoprotein. *J Biol Chem* 1986; 261:11429–11436.
15. Gibson MA, Kumaratilake JS, Cleary EG: The protein components of the 12-nanometer microfibrils of elastic and nonelastic tissues. *J Biol Chem* 1989; 264:4590–4598.
16. Hassel JR, Kimura JH, Hascall VC: Proteoglycan core protein families. *Annu Rev Biochem* 1986; 55:539–567.
17. Hey NJ, Handley CJ, Ng CK, et al: Characterization and synthesis of macromolecules by adult collateral ligament. *Biochim Biophys Acta* 1990; 1034:73–80.
18. Ho PS, Yu SW, Sether LA, et al: Ligamentum flavum: Appearance on sagittal and coronal MR images. *Radiology* 1988; 168:468–472.

19. Hukins DW, Kirby MC, Sikoryn TA, et al: Comparison of structure, mechanical properties, and functions of lumbar spinal ligaments. *Spine* 1990; 15:787–795.
20. Jacenko O, Olsen BR, LuValle P: Organization and regulation of collagen genes. *CRC Crit Rev Eukary Gene Express* 1991; 1:327–353.
21. Kalfas I, Wilberger J, Goldberg A, et al: Magnetic resonance imaging in acute spinal cord trauma. *Neurosurgery* 1988; 23:295–299.
22. Kawano N, Matsuno T, Miyazawa S, et al: Calcium pyrophosphate dihydrate crystal deposition disease in the cervical ligamentum flavum. *J Neurosurg* 1988; 68:613–620.
23. Kim YE: *An Analytical Investigation of the Ligamentous Lumbar Spine Mechanics* (dissertation). Iowa City, University of Iowa, 1989.
24. Kubota T, Kawano H, Yamshima T, et al: Ultrastructure study of calcification process in the ligamentum flavum of the cervical spine. *Spine* 1987; 12:317–323.
25. Laros GS, Tipton CM, Cooper RR: Influence of physical activity on ligament insertions in the knees of dogs. *J Bone Joint Surg [Am]* 1971; 53:275–286.
26. Miller EJ, Gay S: The collagens: An overview and update. *Methods Enzymol* 1987; 144:3–41.
27. Nachemson AL, Evans JH: Some mechanical properties of the third human lumbar interlaminar ligament (ligamentum flavum). *J Biomech* 1968; 1:211–220.
28. Noyes FR, Torvik PJ, Hyde WB, et al: Biomechanics of ligament failure. *J Bone Joint Surg [Am]* 1974; 56:1406–1418.
29. Panjabi MM, Goel VK, Takata K: Volvo Award in biomechanics: Physiologic strains in the lumbar spinal ligaments. An in vitro biomechanical study. *Spine* 1982; 7:192–203.
30. Paulovich RP, Anwar RA: Developmental regulation of the mRNAs for elastins a, b, and c in foetal calf nuchal ligament and aorta. *Biochem J* 1989; 261:227–232.
31. Prockop DJ, Kivirikko KI: Heritable diseases of collagen. *N Engl J Med* 1984; 311:376–386.
32. Reckling FW, Reckling JAB, Mohn MP: *Orthopaedic Anatomy and Surgical Approaches*. St Louis, Mosby–Year Book, 1990.
33. Rojkind M: *Connective Tissue in Health and Disease*. Boca Raton, Fla, CRC Press, 1990.
34. Saldinger P, Dvorak J, Rahn B, et al: Histology of the alar and transverse ligaments. *Spine* 1990; 15:257–261.
35. San Antonio JD, Tuan RS: Chondrogenesis of limb bud mesenchyme in vitro: Stimulation by cations. *Dev Biol* 1986; 115:313–324.
36. Sandberg LB, Soskel NT, Leslie JG: Elastin structure, biosynthesis, and relation to disease state. *N Engl J Med* 1981; 304:556–579.
37. Sauk JJ, Van Kampen CL, Norris K, et al: Persistent spreading of ligament cells on osteopontin/bone sialoprotein-I or collagen enhances tolerance to heat shock. *Exp Cell Res* 1990; 188:105–110.
38. Shirazi-Adl A, Drouin G: Load-bearing role of facets in a lumbar segment under sagittal plane loadings. *J Biomech* 1987; 20:601–613.
39. Sugrue SP, Gordon MK, Seyer J, et al: Immunoidentification of type XII collagen in embryonic tissues. *J Cell Biol* 1989; 109:939–945.
40. Tsuyama N: Ossification of the posterior longitudinal ligament of the spine. *Clin Orthop* 1984; 184:71–84.
41. Tuan RS: Ionic regulation of chondrogenesis, in Hall BK, Newman S (eds): *Cartilage: Molecular Aspects*. Boca Raton, Fla, CRC Press, 1991, pp 153–178.
42. Videman T: *An Experimental Study of the Effects of Growth on the Relationship of Tendons and Ligaments to Bone at the Site of Diaphyseal Insertion* (dissertation). University of Helsinki, 1970.
43. Woo SL-Y, Buckwalter JA: *Injury and Repair of the Musculoskeletal Soft Tissues*. Park Ridge, Ill, American Academy of Orthopaedic Surgeons, 1988.
44. Yahia LH, Garzon S, Strykowski H, et al: Ultrastructure of the human interspinous ligament and ligamentum flavum. *Spine* 1990; 15:262–268.

20

Disc

Casey K. Lee, M.D.

The intervertebral disc is the most important stabilizer of the three-joint complex of a spinal motion segment. The disc is made of three component structures: the nucleus pulposus, the annulus fibrosus, and the vertebral end plates. All three components are structured in such a way that the disc allows angular motions in six planes about three axes, stability against horizontal displacement, and effective load transmission capability.

The structures and functions of the disc and its components are changing constantly throughout life from birth to death. Three common causes for changes are the natural aging process (maturation and involution), disruption and degradation by various pathologic conditions, and secondary biological responses to the above two.

THE VERTEBRAL END PLATE

The vertebral end plate is made of a thin plate of bone and a thin layer of cartilage, which form an interface between the vertebral bone and the disc. The central area of the end plate is the opposing area to the nucleus pulposus, and the peripheral ring is over the annulus fibrosus. The vertebral end plate transforms from a flat or less concave plate during the early age into a concave plate when the upright posture is assumed.[24] The vertebral end plates go through significant changes throughout life by aging.[5, 24] These changes include gradual disappearance of the cartilage plate on the bone and gradual calcification of the cartilage plate. In advanced age, bone may come in direct contact with the nucleus pulposus, especially in individuals with Schmorl's nodes.

Two important functions of the vertebral end plates are even and effective stress distribution to the disc from the bone and diffusion across the plate between the vertebral body and the disc.[13, 21] The vertebral end plate is the weakest structure of the disc under axial compressive load. In the normal lumbar disc, stress distribution in the vertebral end plate is even throughout the entire cross-sectional area under axial and under bending compression.[13] This is probably due to the fluidlike action of nucleus pulposus. In a degenerated disc uneven distribution of the axial stress was observed in the peripheral ring area of the disc over the annulus fibrosus.[13] With advancing age, permeability of the end plates decreases.[24] This may have adverse effects on the nutritional and biomechanical status of the disc.

Failure of the vertebral end plates is most commonly due to excessive axial compression.[3, 6] The pathologic findings of end plate failure vary from subtle changes to a complete burst fracture.[14, 20] Subtle and minor failure of the end plate may not be detectable on routine roentgeographic examination. These changes can, however, be detected by discographic examination.[4, 14] Schmorl's nodes are a noticeable form of end plate failure with migration of nuclear material into the bone. The vertebral end plate and the vascular structure in it are observed to have unmyelinated nerve fibers that may be capable of nociception.[15] The nociceptive mechanism may be either by biochemical by-products from degradation of the disc that may come in contact with these nerve endings or by mechanical disturbances of the end plates.[4]

THE NUCLEUS PULPOSUS

The nucleus pulposus is made of collagen fibrils embedded in mucoprotein gel substance and occupies about 40% to 60% of the cross-sectional area of the disc. It contains a large amount of water (70% to 80% by weight) and is incompressible. The functions of the nucleus pulposus are unclear, but it is postulated that (1) it distributes stress evenly from the vertebral body to other components of the disc, (2) it transforms axial compressive force into tangenitial stress in the annulus (hoop stress), (3) it acts like a ball bearing during bending movements, and (4) it maintains disc height by hydrostatic and osmotic pressure actions.

In children and young adults, the nucleus pulposus has no vascular or neural structures; however, it comes in contact with vascular structures from the vertebral end plates in the later part of adult life. The natural aging process of the nucleus pulposus was well studied by Ritchie and Fahrni and others[2, 12, 24]: it loses water content and becomes more fibrotic and less mucoid. The nuclear cavity enlarges as age advances. The chemical composition of the nucleus pulposus also changes: Chondroitin sulfate, which constitutes 80% of the total acid mucopolysaccharides in newborn infants, decreases with age while keratosulfate increases. The size of the proteoglycan aggregates also become smaller with aging.

Since the normal nucleus pulposus is an incompressible, gel-like mobile substance, isolated traumatic injury to the nucleus pulposus is not likely to occur. Pathologic conditions that mainly involve the nucleus pulposus are rare. The loss of nucleus pulposus may occur in certain pathologic conditions such as in infections and autoimmune diseases. However, the more common cause for the loss of nucleus pulposus is surgical removal or degradation by chemonucleolysis. Does the removal of the nucleus pulposus significantly alter the function of the disc? Markoff and Morris found that the removal of the nucleus pulposus did not cause significant changes in the compressive load-deflexion characteristics of the disc in their experimental studies on fresh human cadaveric spines.[19] They postulated that there appeared to be a "self-sealing mechanism" of the annular hole. Brinkman and Horst measured increased loss of disc height (1.53 mm) and increased radial bulge of the disc (0.37 mm) after partial discectomy in their experiment.[3] Spencer et al. found that chemonucleolysis of the canine lumbar disc caused a significant increase in flexibility (10%), especially in flexion and torsion.[26] Wakano et al. found from an in vivo canine study that chymopapain injection into the canine intervertebral disc caused significant reduction of disc height and compressive stiffness in the disc 3 weeks postinjection, but these were returning toward normal in discs 3 months postinjection.[27] The long-term effects of nuclectomy on a disc with no other significant abnormality appear to be minimal. Bradford et al. observed reconstitution of disc height on a follow-up evaluation after chymopapain injection in dog spines.[2] It appeared that the nucleus pulposus was regenerated. The nuclear regeneration after chemonucleolysis has been occasionally observed in young adult subjects, but the frequency and the extent of regeneration is not well understood.

Although these experimental studies show measurable amounts of changes in the biomechanical characteristics of the disc after nuclectomy, their clinical significance is not well understood.

THE ANNULUS FIBROSUS

The annulus fibrosus is made of concentric lamellae (12 to 20 layers) of collagen fibers embedded in proteoglycan ground substance. The collagen fibers run obliquely (30 degrees) between the vertebral end plates.[9] The annulus fibrosus contains chondrocytes and has nerve endings in the outer half of the thickness, which may have significant roles for nociceptive function.[28, 29] The annulus fibrosus is the most important stabilizing structure of the disc in all planes—axial compression, torsion, bending, and horizontal translation.[7]

In normal discs, the anterior portion of the annulus fibrosus is thicker than the posterior part. The number of lamellae are the same, but the lamellae in the posterior portion of the disc are packed closer together. With the advancement of age, the arrangement of the annulus changes.[24] The anterior rim of the annulus bulges inward toward the nuclear cavity, especially the anterolateral parts, and the posterolateral parts bulge outward. This rearrangement of the annulus with aging transforms the nucleus pulposus into a triangular or cloverleaf form in the horizontal plane. At the same time, there is a gradual loss of proteoglycan content in the annulus and an increase in the number of circumferential clefts between lamellae as age advances. In late adult life, it is common to find many circumferential and radial tears. It is probable that these age-related changes may be the results of "wear and tear" due to normal physiologic loading conditions. A degenerated annulus fibrosus is more susceptible to injury as it loses its extensibility.

The annulus fibrosus is similar to ligamentous structures of a joint. The stability, mobility, and maximum strength of the annulus depends on the biomechanical characteristics of the annulus. An excessive force beyond the maximum strength or an excessive motion beyond the physiologic range will probably cause an injury to the structure. Changes in material characteristics as in degeneration by aging may have significant effects on the maximum strength, stiffness, and the range of motion.

Injury Mechanisms

A normal disc has a very high axial compressive modulus. The biomechanical behaviors of the annulus fibrosus have been extensively studied.[1, 3, 7, 8, 11, 18] The maximum axial compressive force to failure of the annulus fibrosus is estimated to be 7,000 newtons, while the maximum compressive force of the vertebral end plate is only about 2,500 newtons.[3, 7] A normal disc has a very small amount of displacement and radial bulge under axial compression. According to the biomechanical study of Brinkman et al., a normal disc only loses 0.6 mm of disc height and demonstrates a 0.34-mm radial bulge of the posterior of the disc under 1,700 newtons of axial compressive force.[3] The annulus fibrosus is also the main stabilizer against torsional and horizontal displacements. The normal range of horizontal displacement of the normal disc is 8% of the anteroposterior diameter of the disc, and the maximum torsional range is 5% to 10%. The annulus will fail beyond these limits. The range of motion in flexion-extension of a lumbar motion segment varies at different levels. It ranges from 8 to 9 degrees at the upper lumbar disc to 17 to 18 degrees at L5–S1.[8] The maximum tensile strength of the annulus fibrosus is about 16 newton-meters. The collagen fibers in the annulus are likely to fail when they are elongated more than 4% of their resting length.[11]

The most common injury mechanism of the annulus fibrosus is trauma. The annulus fibrosus is a lamellated fiber–ground substance, composite structure. Unphysiologic external forces applied on the disc can produce abnormal stress and strain in the annulus fibrosus, and they may cause delamination (circumferential tear), fiber rupture (radial tear), or ground substance degradation. Three common injury mechanisms of the annulus fibrosus are compression, torsion, and bending.[1, 6, 7, 11] Since the annulus fibrosus has a very high compressive modulus under axial compression, it is not likely injured by excessive axial compressive loading. In such a case, the vertebral end plates will fail first. An excessive compressive load, however, may result in radial tears of the annulus in a degenerated disc and may even cause disc herniation. An excessive torsional load is likely to produce circumferential tears of the annulus fibrosus, especially in the posterolateral areas of the disc where the stress level is higher due to the oval shape of the disc and the reentrant concavity of the posterior disc wall. Excessive forward bending is also considered by Hickey and Hukins to be an injury mechanism of the annulus fibrosus.[11] However, the oval shape of the disc with its posterior reentrant concavity produces a stress-shielding effect on the posterior of the annulus fibrosus. Rupture of the posterior part of the annulus with central disc herniation is more common at the disc levels where the posterior reentrant concavity is less, as in the L5–S1 level. Excessive strain or sprain may also cause ground substance degradation. The mechanism for ground substance degradation by trauma is not well established. Chondrocytes in a traumatized annulus fibrosus may release proteolytic enzymes to degrade proteoglycan ground substance.[17] Beside trauma, other pathologic conditions such as infection or autoimmune disease may cause progressive ground substance degradation. Exposed fibers in the area with depleted ground substance are predisposed to traumatic rupture or delamination.

Failure of the annulus fibrosus may be either in the form of predominantly fiber failure, predominantly ground substance failure, or various combinations of these two depending on the mode of injury and host reactions.

The type of injury of the annulus also depends on the magnitude and mode of the applied force, geometry of the disc, and the inherent strength of the structure.[7] A physiologic load to a normal annulus fibrosus may become an excessive traumatic force to a degenerated annulus fibrosus. A degenerated annulus fibrosus loses its extensibility and is predisposed to failure under less than the normal maximum strength.

Pathologic Conditions

Kirkaldy-Willis et al. described the degenerative process of the disc: Circumferential tear to radial tear to disc disruption and disc resorption to instability to stenosis.[16] Radial tears of the annulus fibrosus may be associated with disc herniation. However, Crock described disc resorption to be a separate entity.[4] In the natural aging process, annular disruption may follow the general sequence described by Kirkaldy-Willis et al.[16] In a traumatic injury, either radial or circumferential tears may occur as an isolated initial injury depending on the mode of application of the traumatic force. On observation of discographic evaluation of patients with low back pain, one can find various patterns of annular tears and varying degrees of involvement of the cross-sectional area. A confluent tear pattern involving a quadrant of the disc in a young adult may be the result of one severe traumatic injury or the result of repeated multiple injuries. "Internal disc disruption" may be an inclusive term to describe all types of *mechanical* disruption of the annulus fibrosus (circumferential, radial, or combined tear and internal multiple disruption), while "disc resorption" may include biochemical degradation of the disc.

Disc Resorption

There appears to be at least two different types of disc resorption: primary and secondary disc resorption. In primary disc resorption, the proteoglycan ground substance is first selectively degraded, and the collagen fibers are preserved. This type of disc resorption is seen in the early stages of disc space infection or after chymopapain injection. Autoimmune disorders may also cause primary disc resorption. Secondary disc resorption is a gradual enzymatic degradation of the disc secondary to internal disc disruption. Not all discs with internal disc disruption will have disc space collapse after disc resorption. Determining factors for secondary disc resorption are not known. Pain and/or neurocompressive symptoms are common clinical presentations of these pathologic conditions of the annulus fibrosus. Pathophysiologic nociceptive mechanisms of disc lesions are not clearly understood. There are three possible areas of the disc where nociceptive endings may be located: the outer half of the annulus, which contains nerve endings; the outermost layer and the peridiscal soft tissue, which are richly innervated from the sinu-vertebral nerves and autonomic nerve branches; and the sub–end plate's vertebral body, which has direct communication and contact with the nucleus pulposus in adult life. Noxious stimuli to the nociceptive structures in these areas may be mechanical, biochemical, or a combination of the two. Abnormal internal stress and strain in the area of an annular tear could be the mechanical irritation to the nociceptive endings in the annulus. The abnormal radial bulge could cause abnormal stretching of the peridiscal structures or nerves and cause a nociceptive response. A localized large disc bulge, for example, could cause nerve root compression symptoms. Other possible mechanical causes of nociception are disc herniation and instability. The biochemical nature of the nociceptive mechanism is less well understood. Injured chondrocytes in the annulus fibrosus may release various proteolytic enzymes and other chemical substances. Some of these chemical by-products of injured tissue may be capable of directly stimulating the nociceptive endings, or they may act on the nociceptive ending to lower the threshold level. Some may come in contact with vascular structures in the peridiscal area or the sub–end plate's vertebral body and produce inflammatory reactions and nociceptive irritation. Symptoms produced by disc herniation are typical examples of the combination of these two nociceptive mechanisms: the mechanical and biochemical nature. The acute phase of symptoms of disc herniation is probably due to a combination of the biochemical and mechanical nociceptive mechanisms. During the chronic phase of disc herniation, the characteristics of pain change from acute severe pain to dull paresthesia. This change in the characteristics of pain symptoms, which occurs usually 2 to 4 weeks after the onset without any noticeable change in the size of disc herniation, strongly suggests the biochemical-inflammatory nature of the nociceptive mechanism of disc herniation during the acute phase. Crock postulated that the sub–end plate's vascular structure in the vertebral body may play an important role in the nociceptive mechanism of some disc diseases.[4] In "isolated disc disruption," biochemical by-products of degenerating discs may come in contact with these vascular structures and produce inflammatory nociceptive responses.

THE BIOLOGIC HEALING PROCESSES OF THE DISC INJURY AND DEGENERATION

An injury to the disc often initiates both the degenerative and reparative processes at the same time. These two processes progress in parallel, but the speed and extent of each process is not the same. The reparative process in the injured disc takes several forms: Early and delayed cellular responses in the middle substances of the annulus, scarring at the very peripheral area of the annulus fibrosus, and osteophyte formation. During the early phase after an injury to the annulus, cells in the annulus demonstrate reparative responses and produce proteoglycan to seal the tear.[17, 23] This reparative process, however, is apparently very limited, and the progressive degenerative process follows. A cut or tear of the most peripheral layer of the annulus heals well with scar tissue, but a deficit in the deeper layer is not repaired by scarring.[10, 22, 25] A radial tear on the annulus in experimental animal studies shows repairing at the periphery by scarring, but the deeper tear shows progressive degeneration without healing. Osteophyte formation about the vertebral end plates is probably a reparative response to the altered mechanical stress by injury and/or degeneration. The location, size, and shape of osteophyte formation is probably governed by the status of stress changes. Marginal osteophytes add to the cross-sectional area of the disc, especially at the strategic peripheral areas to effectively resist bending and torsional moments. This is a very effective means of restabilizing the injured disc and protecting the weakened disc from further injuries.

DIAGNOSTIC AND THERAPEUTIC CONSIDERATIONS

The successful outcome of treatment (nonoperative or operative) for low back disorders depends on understanding the injury mechanisms, pathophysiology, pathologic anatomy, and the natural course of various disc disorders, as well as an accurate diagnosis of the pathologic conditions. In spite of recent advancements in understanding disc biomechanics and the availability of diagnostic techniques, an accurate diagnosis of various pathologic conditions remains very difficult. Some important reasons are (1) a poor understanding of nociceptive mechanisms; (2) the inability to differentiate painful pathologic conditions from nonpainful aging (degenerative) conditions, both having the same appearances; and (3) a poor understanding of the clinical significance of the results of various diagnostic techniques. Because of the difficulty of arriving at an accurate diagnosis and because of poor understanding of the natural course of various disc pathologic conditions, the predictable outcome of various treatment modalities has not been established for most pathologic conditions of the disc.

ANNULAR TEARS

Traumatic injury to the disc may produce annular tears or vertebral end-plate injuries causing painful symptoms. The probable nociceptive mechanisms may be mechanical, i.e., local changes in stress/strain patterns, biochemical, or both. A diagnosis of these pathologic conditions is difficult to establish in clinical practice, but the injury history, physical findings (pain-provocative maneuvers), magnetic resonance imaging (MRI), and occasionally pain-provocative/relieving tests (such as discography) may be useful. It has been thought that most of these injuries become asymptomatic with nonoperative treatment of rest and protection from further injury.

However, the mechanism for pain relief from these injuries is not well understood. Since the healing of an annular tear and the reparative mechanisms of chondrocytes in the annulus are very limited, the mechanism for pain relief in these injuries may be by other biological compensatory mechanisms. Can the injured disc ever retain the preinjury biomechanical characteristics? Does the injured disc always have less than normal biomechanical strength? Do repeated injuries have an accumulative effect? When does an injured disc reach the state in which the biological compensatory mechanisms are insufficient to cope with daily activities and the painful symptoms persist?

No satisfactory answers to these questions are yet available. Answers to these questions will help guide clinicians in establishing various treatment plans: activity guidance, exercises, job counseling, and indications for surgical treatment.

DISC HERNIATION

The pathologic condition of disc herniation causing low back pain and radicular irritation symptoms has been extensively studied for diagnosis, natural history, and treatment responses.

INSTABILITY

Instability causing pain, neurologic problems, and/or deformity due to various disc disorders is another poorly understood topic. This is mainly due to the lack of correlation between the structural defects, biomechanical changes, and nociceptive mechanisms. Other reasons are an inability to adequately assess the balance between the degenerative and reparative processes and the inability to evaluate the injured or degenerated disc's capacity to tolerate external loads without causing nociceptive irritation or neurologic problems.

REFERENCES

1. Adams MA, Hutton WE: The relevance of torsion to the mechanical derangement of the lumbar spine. *Spine* 1981; 6:241–248.
2. Bradford DS, Cooper KM, Oegema TR: Chymopapain chemonucleolysis and nucleus pulposus regeneration. *J Bone Joint Surg [Am]* 1983; 65:1220–1231.
3. Brinkman P, Horst M: The influence of vertebral body fracture, intradiscal injection, and partial discectomy on the radial bulge and height of human lumbar discs. *Spine* 1985; 9:138–145.
4. Crock HV: Internal disc disruption, a challenge to prolapse fifty years on. *Spine* 1986; 11:650–653.
5. Edelson JG, Nathan H: Stages in the natural history of the vertebral end-plates. *Spine* 1988; 13:21–26.
6. Farfan HF: *Mechanical Disorders of the Low Back*. Philadelphia, Lea & Febiger, 1973, pp 134–143, 200–206.
7. Farfan HF, Cossette JW, Robertson GH, et al: The effects of torsion on the lumbar intervertebral joints: The role of torsion in the production of disc degeneration. *J Bone Joint Surg [Am]* 1970; 52:468–497.
8. Froning EC, Frohman B: Motion of the lumbosacral spine after laminectomy and spine fusion correlation of motion with the results. *J Bone Joint Surg [Am]* 1968; 50:897.
9. Fung YB: Biomechanics, its scope, history and some problems of centenuum mechanics in physiology. *Appl Mech Rev* 1968; 21:1–20.
10. Hampton D, Laros G, McCarron R, et al: Healing potential of the annulus fibrosus. *Spine* 1989; 14:398–401.
11. Hickey DS, Hukins DW: Relation between the structure of the annulus fibrosus and function and failure of the intervertebral disc. *Spine* 1980; 5:106–116.
12. Hirsch C, Paulson S, Sylven B, et al: Biophysical and physiological investigation on cartilage and other mesenchymal tissues. VI. Characteristics of human nuclei pulposi during aging. *Acta Orthop Scand* 1952; 22:179.
13. Horst M, Brinkman P: Measurement of the distraction of axial stress on the end-plate of the vertebral body. *Spine* 1981; 6:217–232.
14. Hsu KY, Zuckerman JF, Derby R, et al: Painful lumbar end-plate disruptions: A significant discographic finding. *Spine* 1988; 13:76–78.
15. Jackson HC, Winkelman RK, Bickel WH: Nerve endings in the human lumbar spinal column and related structures. *J Bone Joint Surg [Am]* 1966; 48:1272–1281.
16. Kirkaldy-Willis WH, Wedge JH, Young-Hing K, et al: Pathology and pathogenesis of lumbar spondylosis and stenosis. *Spine* 1978; 3:319–328.
17. Lipson SJ, Muir H: Proteoglycans in experimental intervertebral disc degeneration. *Spine* 1981; 6:194–210.
18. Markoff KL: Deformation of the thoracolumbar intervertebral joints in response to external loads. A biomechanical study using autopsy material. *J Bone Joint Surg [Am]* 1972; 54:511–532.
19. Markoff KL, Morris JM: The structural components of the intervertebral disc. A study of their contributions to the ability of the disc to withstand compressive forces. *J Bone Joint Surg [Am]* 1985; 56:675–687.
20. McFaden KD, Taylor JR: End-plate lesions of the lumbar spine. *Spine* 1981; 14:867–869.
21. Ogata K, Whiteside LA: Nutritional pathways of the intervertebral disc: An experimental study using hydrogen washout technique. *Spine* 1981; 6:211–216.
22. Osti OL, Vernon-Roberts B, Fraser RD: Annulus tears and intervertebral disc degeneration. An experimental study using an animal model. *Spine* 1990; 15:762–767.
23. Pedrini-Mille A, Weinstein JN, Found EM, et al: Stimulation of dorsal root ganglia and degeneration of rabbit annulus fibrosus. *Spine* 1990; 15:1252–1256.
24. Ritchie JH, Fahrni WH: Experimental surgery, age changes in lumbar intervertebral discs. *Can J Surg* 1970; 13:65–71.
25. Smith JW, Walmsley R: Experimental incision of the intervertebral disc. *J Bone Joint Surg [Br]* 1951; 33:612–625.
26. Spencer DL, Miller JAA, Schultz AB: The effects of chemonucleolysis on the mechanical properties of the canine lumbar disc. *Spine* 1985; 6:555–561.
27. Wakano K, Kasman R, Chao EY, et al: Biomechanical analysis of canine intervertebral discs after chymopapain injection. A preliminary report. *Spine* 1983; 8:59–68.
28. Weinstein J, Claverie W, Gibson S: The pain of discography. *Spine* 1988; 13:1344–1348.
29. Yoshizawa H, Obrien JP, Smith WT, et al: The neuropathology of the intervertebral discs removed for low back pain. *J Pathol* 1980; 132:95–104.

21

Cartilage

Heikki Vanharanta, M.D.

A major goal in rehabilitating patients with chronic low back pain is to restore the load-bearing capacity of the spine. This function depends greatly on the unique role of cartilaginous tissues, discs, and facet joints. The traditional methods of physical medicine and rehabilitation have been strongly rooted in physical mechanics as well as muscle and pain physiology. However, critical evaluation of these methods has not verified their value in treating back pain,; however, an injury may have altered the normal mechanics of the spine and is frequently associated with painful muscle spasm. In addition, many studies do not support the theory that pain originates in the muscles, but rather in the cartilaginous tissues, which are also involved in the mechanical properties of the spine.[39] Thus when treating patients with back pain, rehabilitation of cartilaginous tissue is essential. This tissue has great healing potential, and its natural healing process needs to be nurtured. In this chapter the reactions of cartilage tissues to common treatment methods such as unloading, loading, immobilization, and remobilization will be discussed.

The effects of various physical and even pharmacologic treatments on cartilage are not very well understood. However, histologic and biochemical research in recent years has resulted in a greater knowledge of both the pathogenesis of degenerative diseases and the effects of conservative rehabilitation methods on cartilage tissues. Unfortunately, most of this research has been performed in animals and in diarthrodial joints, so there may be reservations concerning how well results from these models relate to the human spine. However, the similarity of the living cells in the cartilaginous structures in these models justifies cautious application of the results in practical rehabilitation medicine. The advances seen recently in the rehabilitation of patients with back pain comply well with the results of the animal research, and it appears that the theoretical knowledge based on these studies has some potential to also be the basis for the prevention of low back pain.

STRUCTURE OF CARTILAGE

Cartilaginous tissues in the back, as elsewhere in the body, allow loaded motion between bones with low frictional resistance. In lumbar motion segments we have cartilage-type tissues in the discs, their end plates, and the apophyseal joints. The annular and nuclear tissues of the disc in many ways resemble normal hyaline cartilage despite their structural and metabolic differences. All these structures are hydrated, fiber-reinforced composites, with collagen fibers embedded in a gel of proteoglycans providing architectural framework and strength. The mechanical needs of different types of cartilaginous tissues are reflected in the composition of these structures. For example, the disc annulus has more type I collagen fibers than do the nucleus, end plates, or facet joints. Type I collagen gives more tensile strength than type II collagen, which predominates in cartilaginous tissues exposed to compressive loads.

The strength variance of these structures among individuals depends on the quality of collagen and proteoglycans produced by the fibrocytes and chondrocytes living within the matrix. Contrary to general belief, the cells in the cartilage tissues are active throughout life in producing the matrix substances; however, the level of activity decreases with age. Genetic factors as well as environmental factors such as nutrition, hormones, and stimulation or irritation of the cells will affect the quality of the matrix produced.

Collagen fibers form the primary structure in cartilage and discs, thus making the integrity of the collagen network crucial. The other main proteins of the matrix synthesized by the chondrocytes are proteoglycans entrapped in the collagen network in a volume of only 20% of their maximum molecular domain in dilute solution.[2] Proteoglycans are composed of glycosaminoglycan chains linked with a protein core. The glycosaminoglycans are polyanions, and so their counterions exert an osmotic pressure of several atmospheres that is resisted by the collagen network. Due to this osmotic pressure cartilage is exceptionally hydrated.

The physical properties of cartilage are affected by the relationship of collagen, proteoglycans, and water. The tensile strength of cartilage is correlated with its collagen content and modified by prestressed tension due to the osmotic pressure related to the proteoglycan content. The compressive stiffness of cartilaginous tissue is therefore directly proportional to its proteoglycan content.[12]

DEGENERATION OF CARTILAGE

Degeneration of cartilaginous tissues is generally a very slow phenomenon caused by multiple etiologies. Due in part to this and to the failure of imaging methods to visualize the early stages of degeneration, initial painful lesions cannot yet be recognized in clinical practice. However, in recent years some progress has been made in identifying a clear relationship between low back pain and disc deterioration,[41] and also the degeneration of posterior joints has been found to be a very likely source of low back pain.[17]

In the early stages, osteoarthritic cartilage shows considerable potential for repair.[18] But at the same time, the catabolic activity is also elevated, and treatment providers need to know what effect their recommendations have on the balance between biosynthetic and degradative activities. Many pharmacologic and physical treatment procedures either accelerate or decelerate the degenerative process. In degenerative diseases there may often be many painful lesions in the same individual as well as the potential for many new painful lesions if the tissues are irritated or the degenerative process is accelerated. For example, the internal risk factors for degenerative disc disease are the same for every disc within an individual.

The water content of cartilage increases during the early phases of human cartilage degeneration. This hydration occurs very early before the histologic appearance of the cartilage changes.[14] This change will influence the biomechanical properties of the joint and also alters the microenvironment of the cartilage cells. It is speculated that the fibrillar network of collagen will somehow become weak, perhaps by collagenolytic enzymes, and allow increased cartilage hydration. There is no significant difference in collagen content between osteoarthritic and normal cartilage.[11] However, there is an increased rate of collagen synthesis in osteoarthritic joints.

Both proteoglycan synthesis and the number of cells producing proteoglycans are increased in osteoarthritic joints. However, the increased synthesis is not enough to counteract the rapidly decreasing proteoglycan content. Metabolic activity of the chondrocytes varies with their location on the joint surface. The areas frequently exposed to heavy loading produce much matrix, thus indicating mechanic stimulation of the synthesis rate. The thickness of cartilage is approximately inversely proportional to the cell density. The amount of cartilage matrix maintained by one cell reflects the total load transmitted by the joint.[33] Newly synthesized proteoglycans of osteoarthritic joints have some structural differences when compared with normal proteoglycans, but there is no difference in their catabolism. When a minimal degradation of proteoglycans in cartilage starts, degradation of proteoglycans will rapidly diffuse throughout the cartilage.[18]

CONTROLLING THE RISK FACTORS OF DEGENERATION

In designing a rehabilitation program it is important to recognize the multietiologic nature of disc and cartilage degeneration and the potential risk factors in each patient. However, most of the epidemiologically identified risk factors are very difficult to eliminate. For example, only a few of the known risk factors of sciatica can be eliminated, including smoking, obesity, excessive driving, vibration, and continuous sitting; even occupation may to some extent be changed. Other risk factors that cannot be altered are genetic factors, inborn skeletal abnormalities, height, age, and sex. These are the strongest risk factors for degeneration.[3] However, in the treatment process we have several potential ways to control some risk factors for cartilage degeneration. The usual treatment methods such as unloading, immobilization, and remobilization all have both beneficial and harmful effects on cartilage. Properly controlling these treatment methods offers much potential in controlling the degradation of cartilaginous tissues.

Unloading of Cartilage

Early studies by Retterer in 1908 found that the thickness of humeral head cartilage was reduced in guinea pigs after amputation of a forelimb; the normal orientation of the cells was also disturbed, but the chondrocytes survived the prolonged non–load bearing.[28] This type of cartilage could not resist heavy loads but would demonstrate osteoarthritic changes. Later Oláh and Kostenszky reported marked losses of glycosaminoglycans in an unloaded joint.[19] From these and other studies it is evident that long-term unloading is not beneficial to cartilaginous tissue.

Unloading of cartilaginous tissues is often achieved in the back by bed rest. The disc pressure is very low when the subject is lying supine. Rest is still a widely used method in treating patients with low back pain. In acute situations it has been found to be beneficial.[45] Correspondingly, in a rabbit study, free mobilization immediately after a disc injury was found to deteriorate the discs much more than resting in a cage.[1] Currently, prolonged bed rest is widely criticized and justly so based on the animal studies mentioned above. The atrophying effect of prolonged rest on cartilage needs to be explained to patients with chronic back pain because patients generally think just the opposite. The belief that joints will wear out with use is very common among the general public and even among some medical practitioners.

Immobilization and Static Loading

Rigid immobilization quickly atrophies cartilaginous tissue in discs and joints and is often used to induce experimental osteoarthritis in diarthrodial joints.[9] Early osteoarthritic changes can be observed in a period of days and even macroscopic changes within 3 weeks. In the spine, within 3 months after spinal fusion in dogs, the rate of transport of oxygen, glucose, and sulfate into the discs of fused segments had decreased, metabolic rates were affected, and the discs had lost matrix.[4]

For less stable immobilization, braces are often used for treating patients with various types of low back pain problems and also as a postoperative treatment. Braces provide less rigid immobilization, so extrapolating from results seen in experiments with fused vertebrae or splinted diarthrodial joints may lead to exaggerations. However, when the effects on cartilaginous tissue are considered, immobilization combined with static loading is generally negative. Many studies support the view that even nonrigid splinting of a joint has a potentially degenerative effect and seems to lead to cartilage atrophy. In a canine study, the proteoglycan synthesis rate of chondrocytes decreased by 41% after 6 days of immobilization, and after 3 weeks proteoglycan aggregation was no longer demonstrated.[21]

The in vitro works that found the static loading of chondrocyte culture to decrease the proteoglycan synthesis of chondrocytes[22] correspond well with the recent autopsy study by Videman et al.[43] in which sedentary workers were found to have more disc degeneration than those engaged in more active occupations. The adverse effect of static loading of discs is a potential side effect of workplace ergonomic design focused on reducing or changing the loading mechanisms of the spine.

Immobilization has been widely used after joint surgery, but today surgeons use more continuous passive movement due to the side effects of immobilization. In experimental works by Salter et al. the effect of immobilization after trauma to cartilage was destructive.[31] In treating patients with back pain, immobilization with a brace is still used frequently after spinal fusion surgery. Disc degeneration with stenosis and osteophytes above the fusion is often seen years after the surgery was performed. An explanation for this overuse is often mentioned because of elimination of movement elsewhere in the spine. The overuse of a disc or cartilage tissue is always relative, however. Immediate postoperative immobilization of the disc will evidently reduce its load-bearing ability, and with mobilization the disc becomes more sensitive to degenerative trauma or even painful disc rupture if the mobilization is rapid.

However, immobilization has been found to have a positive effect if only used for short periods of time. Palmoski and Brandt reported that immobilization of the knee for 12 weeks after anterior cruciate ligament transection prevented the development of osteoarthrosis of the knee joint, although articular cartilage atrophy ensued.[23] Also, other experimental studies support the concept that a brief period of immobilization after an injury will protect the joints against further damage but that long-term immobilization is harmful. These experimental studies give some support to the use of postoperative immobilization after back surgery; however, possible atrophy of cartilaginous tissues needs to be addressed in the postoperative rehabilitation program.

Remobilization

Remobilization of patients with back pain is one of the most common rehabilitation activities. In early works made by Moll it was observed that degenerative changes associated with immobilization of rabbit knees generally developed after the immobilization had ceased, i.e., during the remobilization period.[16] In a later study contradicting these results, Sood observed that immobilization-induced regressive changes were reversible by remobilization.[32] Palmoski and Brand found that the ability to reverse osteoarthritic changes was dependent on the aggressiveness of the remobilizing activities.[20] Canine knee cartilage that had been exposed to vigorous running for 3 weeks after being immobilized for 3 weeks showed continuing decreases in cartilage thickness and uronic acid content, although net proteoglycan synthesis increased. In the control group, which ambulated freely for 3 weeks, the cartilage thickness, uronic acid content, and net proteoglycan synthesis were normalized. Similar results have been reported by Tammi and coworkers.[34]

These studies correspond with the clinical observations that if remobilization is performed quickly and vigorously, the result in back motion is worse than if remobilization is introduced over a longer period of time. For this reason, many chronic back pain programs include a preconditioning program lasting a few weeks before starting aggressive work hardening.

While both immobilization and mobilization may hasten the degenerative process in cartilage, it seems that their repeated combination hastens it even more. Michelson and Riska found that daily motion exercises of otherwise immobilized joints increased degeneration and decreased function.[15] Correspondingly, Videman found that experimental osteoarthritis is more severe in periodic immobilization of a joint than in continuous immobilization when the total immobilization time is the same.[42] Thus the side effects of immobilization cannot be reduced by periodic mobilization. Cartilage very slowly adapts to motion, and this gradual adaptation needs to be considered when designing rehabilitation programs.

Loading of Cartilaginous Tissue

Epidemiologic studies demonstrate a very clear association between heavy work and degenerative diseases in both the spine and joints. However, there is increasing evidence that this association might be more closely related to injuries rather than to joint loading in the workplace.[29] Discs of physically active people, either in work or in sports, have been found to withstand more load before rupturing than do discs of less physically active people.[25] In the joints of former athletes, even in international champions, no increased incidence of osteoarthritis has been identified.[26]

The majority of experimental animal works indicate that loading makes cartilaginous tissue strong. In early animal studies by Retterer, one forelimb was amputated, and so an increased load was forced onto the remaining forelimb.[28] Cartilage thickness was increased, and superficial cartilage cells were hypertrophied in the load-bearing joints. Correspondingly, Saaf found enlarged cells and increased basophilia in the intercellular matrix of guinea pigs after exercising on a motor-driven treadmill.[30] Lanier found that daily, forced exercise for 12.5 months prevented the degenerative changes seen in control mice.[10] More recent studies have found that increased load bearing will result in increased hexosamine, glucosamine, and glycoprotein levels in cartilage.[7] The fact that cartilage responds directly to mechanical stress was verified by applying cyclic or static compressive stresses to articular cartilage in vitro. Proteoglycan synthesis was increased by cyclic stress but reduced by static stress.[22]

Studies by Salter and coworkers clearly demonstrated the effect of motion.[31] The application of continuous passive motion is currently a standard in the postoperative treatment of large joints; however, there are no devices to provide this treatment to patients with back pain. Studies by Palmoski et al. have shown that not only is movement necessary to maintain a joint's integrity, but loading is also needed.[24]

Tammi and coworkers demonstrated that moderate physical training of normal joints activates the chondrocytes, which respond by augmented matrix proteoglycan content in the intermediate or deep zone of cartilage and improve the biomechanical properties of articular cartilage.[34] Three months of vigorous training increased the nutrient supply to the discs of dogs, increased the rate of glycolysis, and decreased the amount of lactate in the disc nucleus.[5, 6] However, physical training may also have adverse effects on cartilaginous tissue. Krause was the first to report a strenuous running program resulting in decreased cartilage matrix.[8] There have been other studies verifying his findings. In the works by Tammi et al., strenuous training reversed the benefit of moderate training on the proteoglycan concentration and biomechanical properties of cartilage.[34] Immediate loading through running on an injured rabbit disc deteriorated the disc more than staying relatively inactive in a small cage.[1]

Repetitive impact loading was found to induce osteoarthritic changes.[27] Prior to this, microfractures with healing and stiffening of the subchondral bone were observed. This study demonstrated the important role of subchondral bone in the development of osteoarthrosis, and this may also have a role in disc degeneration.

STIMULATION OF CHONDROCYTES

Cyclic loading seems to be a mechanical stimulus for a chondrocyte to produce more matrix macromolecules as glycosaminoglycans.[27] Decreased compression or static compression decreases the cellular activity. Vibration has also been found to reduce the synthesis rate.[40] One of the mediators of synthesis activity appears to be cyclic adenosine monophosphate (cAMP). High levels of cAMP in the chondrocytes are associated with a greater synthesis of matrix macromolecules. Pressure seems to increase both the penetration of calcium ions into the cells and intracellular cAMP levels. Different mechanisms of chondrocyte activity have been speculated to be voltage-dependent channels, the inositol system, and the action of adenyl cyclase.[33] Loading and unloading greatly influence the pH level of tissue, thus controlling the synthesis rate of new matrix. The loading of a disc will pump water with H^+ ions out of the tissue, and during unloading "fresh" water is drawn back into the tissue.

HEATING AND TRACTION OF JOINTS

Hot packs, deep heating modalities, and traction are still widely used in treating patients with low back pain. This approach is based on a very mechanical concept of low back pain. There have been many clinical studies attempting to demonstrate the effectiveness of these treatments, but none have been very convincing. Generally the effectiveness of these treatments is the same as spontaneous healing. Warming and massaging back muscles will certainly relax them. In experimental works, heating a joint has generally affected capsular tissues[35, 37, 38] and did not increase but rather decreased joint mobility.

Traction of the spine will not pull a protruded tissue back into the disc as has been speculated. Also, traction has not been found to decrease the osteoarthritic process of immobilized or remobilized joints.[42]

MEDICATION DURING REHABILITATION

In developing the new anti-inflammatory drugs much attention has been focused on the effect of the drug on the production of glycosaminoglycans by the chondrocytes. In laboratory studies some anti-inflammatory drugs were found to be safer for cartilage than others. Although anti-inflammatory drugs seem to be important even in the rehabilitation phase of low back pain, it is evident that new drugs for rehabilitation patients will be introduced in the near future. For example, in experimental studies the effect of glycosaminoglycan polysulfate has been very effective in slowing the osteoarthritic process both in diarthrodial joints and in discs.[1, 36] Clinical evidence in patients is still lacking, however.

SUMMARY

The biological knowledge of cartilage tissue degeneration has greatly increased in recent years, and this has resulted in rehabilitation medicine gaining a firmer pathophysiologic basis for treating degenerative diseases of cartilaginous tissues. In the past, pain was the main guide in rehabilitation, which gave the patient control of his treatment program. Today the target of back rehabilitation is to restore the loading ability of the spine guided by the physiology of cartilaginous tissues. Basically the principles are the same as Wolff's law of "form follows function" originally described for bones. In applying the physiologic knowledge of cartilaginous tissues in the rehabilitation of patients with back pain, we can achieve better results despite the multilateral medicopsychosocial problems of patients with chronic back pain as has been demonstrated in several successful rehabilitation programs.[13]

REFERENCES

1. Gill K, Videman T, Shimizu T, et al: Experimental intervertebral disc degeneration (abstract). Presented at the International Society for the Study of the Lumbar Spine, Rome, 1987.
2. Hascall VC, Hascall GK: Proteoglycans, in Hay EO (ed): *Cell Biology of Extracellular Matrix*. New York, Plenum, 1981, pp 39–63.
3. Heliovaara M: *Epidemiology of Sciatica and Herniated Lumbar Intervertebral Disc*. Helsinki, Social Insurance Institution, 1988, p 76.
4. Holm S, Nachemson A: Nutritional changes in the canine intervertebral disc after spinal fusion. *Clin Orthop* 1982; 169:243–258.
5. Holm S, Nachemson A: Variations in the nutrition of the canine intervertebral disc induced by motion. *Spine* 1983; 8:866–874.
6. Holm S, Rosenqvist A-L: Morphological and nutritional changes in the intervertebral disc after spinal motion (abstract). *Scand J Rheumatol Suppl* 1986;60:117.
7. Kostenszky KS, Oláh EH: Functional adaptation of the articular cartilage. *Acta Biol Hung* 1975; 26:157–164.
8. Krause W-D: *Mikroskopische Untersuchungen am Gelenkknorpe lextrem, funktionell belasteter Mäuse* (thesis). Cologne, Germany, Gouder & Hansen, 1969.
9. Langenskjold A, Michelsson J-E, Videman T: Osteoarthritis of the knee in rabbits produced by immobilization. Attempts to achieve a reproducible model for studies on pathogenesis and therapy. *Acta Orthop Scand* 1979; 50:1–14.
10. Lanier R: The effects of exercise on the knee-joints of inbred mice. *Anat Rec* 1946; 94:311–321.
11. Mankin HJ, Lippiello L: Biochemical and metabolic abnormalities in articular cartilage from osteoarthritic human hips. *J Bone Joint Surg [Am]* 1970; 52:424–434.
12. Maroudas A: Physiochemical properties of articular cartilage, in Freeman MAR (ed): *Adult Articular Cartilage*. Tunbridge Wells, England, Pitman Medical, 1979, pp 215–290.
13. Mayer TG, Gatchel RJ, Mayer H, et al: A prospective two-year study of functional restoration in industrial low back injury: An objective assessment procedure. *JAMA* 1987; 258:1763–1767.
14. McDevitt CA, Gilbertson E, Muir H: An experimental model of osteoarthritis: Early morphological and biochemical changes. *J Bone Joint Surg Br* 1977; 59:24–35.
15. Michelson J-E, Riska EB: The effect of temporary exercising of a joint during an immobilization period: An experimental study on rabbits. *Clin Orthop* 1979; 144:321–325.
16. Moll A: Experimentelle Untersuchungen über den anatomischen Zustand der Gelenke bei andauernder Immobilisation derselben. *Virchows Arch* 1886; 105:466–485.
17. Mooney V, Robertson J: The facet syndrome. *Clin Orthop* 1976; 115:149–156.
18. Muir H, Carney SL: Pathological and biomechanical changes in cartilage and other tissues of canine knee resulting from induced joint instability, in Helminen HJ, et al (eds): *Joint Loading*. Bristol, England, Wright, 1987, pp 47–63.
19. Oláh EH, Kostenszky KS: Effect of altered functional demand on the glycosaminoglycan content of the articular cartilage of dogs. *Acta Biol Hung* 1972; 23:195–200.
20. Palmoski M, Brandt KD: Running inhibits the reversal of atrophic changes in canine knee cartilage after removal of a leg cast. *Arthritis Rheum* 1981; 24:1329–1337.
21. Palmoski M, Perricone E, Brandt KD: Development and reversal of a proteoglycan aggregation defect in normal canine knee after immobilization. *Arthritis Rheum* 1979; 22:508–517.
22. Palmoski MJ, Brandt KD: Effects of static and cyclic compressive loading on articular cartilage plugs in vitro. *Arthritis Rheum* 1984; 27:675–681.
23. Palmoski MJ, Brandt KD: Immobilization of the knee prevents osteoarthritis after anterior cruciate ligament transection. *Arthritis Rheum* 1982; 25:1201–1208.
24. Palmoski MJ, Coyler RA, Brandt KD: Joint motion in the absence of normal loading does not maintain normal articular cartilage. *Arthritis Rheum* 1980; 23:325–334.
25. Porter RW, Adams MA, Hutton WC: Physical activity and the strength of the lumbar spine. *Spine* 1989; 14:201–203.
26. Puranen J, Alaketola L, Peltokallio P, et al: Running and primary osteoarthritis of the hip. *Br Med J* 1975; 276:424–425.
27. Radin EL, Martin RB, Burr DB, et al: Effects of mechanical loading on the tissues of the rabbit knee. *J Orthop Res* 1984; 2:221–234.
28. Retterer E: De l'influence de la suractivité fonctionelle sur

la structure du cartilage diarthrodial. *C R Soc Biol (Paris)* 1908; 64:117–120.

29. Riihimaki H: Back pain and heavy physical work: A comparative study of concrete reinforcement workers and maintenance house painters. *Br J Indust Med* 1985; 42:226–232.
30. Saaf J: Effects of exercise on adult articular cartilage. *Acta Orthop Scand Suppl* 1950; 7:1–86.
31. Salter RB, Simmonds DF, Malcolm BW, et al: The biological effect of continuous passive motion on the healing of full-thickness defects in articular cartilage. *J Bone Joint Surg [Am]* 1980; 62:1232–1251.
32. Sood SC: A study of the effects of experimental immobilization on rabbit articular cartilage. *J Anat* 1971; 108:497–507.
33. Stockwell RA: Structure and function of the chondrocyte under mechanical stress, in Helminen HJ, et al (eds): *Joint Loading*. Bristol, England, Wright, 1987, pp 126–148.
34. Tammi M, Paukkonen K, Kiviranta I, et al: Joint loading-induced alterations in articular cartilage, in Helminen HJ, et al (eds): *Joint Loading*. Bristol, England, Wright, 1987, pp 64–88.
35. Vanharanta H: Effect of short-wave diathermy on mobility and radiological stage of the knee in the development of experimental osteoarthritis. *Am J Phys Med* 1982; 61:59–65.
36. Vanharanta H: Glycosaminoglycan polysulphate treatment in experimental osteoarthritis in rabbits. *Scand J Rheumatol* 1983; 12:225–230.
37. Vanharanta H, Eronen I, Videman T: Effect of ultrasound on glycosaminoglycan metabolism in the rabbit knee. *Am J Phys Med* 1982; 61:221–228.
38. Vanharanta H, Eronen I, Videman T: Shortwave diathermy effects on ^{35}S-sulfate uptake glycosaminoglycan concentration in rabbit knee tissue. *Arch Phys Med Rehabil* 1982; 63:25–28.
39. Vanharanta H, Guyer RD, Ohnmeiss DD, et al: Disc deterioration in low-lack syndromes: A prospective, multi-center CT/discography study. *Spine* 1988; 13:1349–1351.
40. Vanharanta H, Nykanen M, Eronen I, et al: Experimental study on the effect of vibration on rabbit joints. *J Orthop Rheumatol* 1988; 1:109–112.
41. Vanharanta H, Sachs BL, Spivey MA, et al: The relationship of pain provocation to lumbar disc deterioration as seen by CT/discography. *Spine* 1987; 3:295–298.
42. Videman T: Experimental osteoarthritis in the rabbit. Comparison of different periods of repeated immobilization. *Acta Orthop Scand* 1982; 53:339–347.
43. Videman T, Nurminen M, Troup JDG: Lumbar spine pathology in cadaveric material in relation to history of back pain, occupation, and physical loading. *Spine* 1990; 15:728–740.
44. Videman T, Vanharanta H: Daily repeated traction in developing osteoarthritis. An experimental study in rabbits. *Ann Chir Gynaecol* 1983; 72:200–206.
45. Wiesel SW, Cuckler JM, DeLuca F, et al: Acute low back pain: An objective analysis of conservative therapy. *Spine* 1980; 5:324–330.

22

*Muscle**

Michael L. Pollock, Ph.D., James E. Graves, Ph.D., David M. Carpenter, M.S., Daniel Foster, M.S., Scott H. Leggett, M.S., and Michael N. Fulton, M.D.

Low back pain (LBP) is one of the most common and costly medical problems in western society.[2, 36, 39] The problem afflicts both the young and the old and often well-conditioned athletes. The etiology of LBP is diverse, and many factors have been associated with its incidence. Soft-tissue weakness in the area surrounding the lumbar spine is often mentioned as a primary risk factor for LBP.[2, 11, 59, 65, 68] Likewise, strengthening the lower back musculature has long been recognized as an important component in the rehabilitation of LBP.[2, 43, 54, 55] Thus it is important to study the physiologic principles associated with improving lumbar muscle strength and endurance. Training for muscular strength is also associated with the strengthening of connective tissue.[11, 84]

New technology, e.g., methods for standardizing testing procedures and computerized dynamometers, have improved evaluation techniques for determining the muscular strength and endurance of the lumbar extensor muscles. For example, the measurement of lumbar extension strength is complicated by the involvement of the stronger gluteal and hamstring muscles. Mayer and Greenberg[52] noted that the lumbar-pelvic rhythm, i.e., a compound movement that involves pelvic rotation plus lumbar extension, during lumbar testing contributed to the lumbar extension strength measurement. New technology has now made it possible to isolate the lumbar muscles by pelvic stabilization so that the lumbar musculature can be more effectively measured and trained.[38, 77]

This chapter will summarize the basic physiologic principles associated with muscular strength evaluation, as well as the development and maintenance of muscular strength through exercise training. Within this framework, much of our research experience with testing and training the isolated lumbar extensor muscles will be synthesized and reviewed. Normative data for both men and women and strength curve interpretation will be provided. Other important factors will be discussed with regard to evaluating and conditioning the lumbar extensor musculature, e.g., static and dynamic testing techniques, muscle fiber fatigue characteristics, the effect of counterweighting to account for the weight of the head and torso mass, the concept of stored energy (total torque and net muscular torque [NMT]), lumbar muscle strength curves, and the trainability of the isolated lumbar extensor muscles.

BASIC MUSCLE PHYSIOLOGY AND PRINCIPLES OF RESISTANCE TRAINING

Muscular strength refers to the maximum amount of force or tension that a muscle or muscle group can generate. Muscular endurance pertains to the ability of a muscle to sustain repeated contractions of a submaximal nature. Each plays an important role in the treatment and prevention of LBP and injury.[45] Moreover, muscular strength and endurance may be improved through a program of resistance training.[20] For this reason, clinicians should be familiar with the basic principles of resistance training. While the theory behind resistance training is simple; strengthen a muscle by making it work harder (the overload principle), the physiologic process by which a muscle becomes stronger is complex and involves neural, morphologic, and biochemical adaptations.[58]

Physiologic responses to resistance training include improvements in muscular strength and endurance and increases in muscle mass,[81] bone mass,[79] and connective tissue thickness.[79] Additional responses include alterations in stored levels of intramuscular aerobic and anaerobic metabolites and enzymes[14] and enhanced motor unit recruitment.[75] Increases in muscle mass occur primarily due to the hypertrophy of individual muscle fibers. This process is related to an accelerated synthesis of the contractile proteins within the muscle cell. The key factor initiating muscular hypertrophy is an increase in the tension or force that the muscle must generate. It is this increase in muscular tension that also causes the proliferation of associated bone and connective tissue cells.[79]

*Research funded by the MedX Corp., Ocala, Fla. The Center for Exercise Science is a multidisciplinary research laboratory and educational facility of the Departments of Medicine, Exercise and Sport Sciences, and Physiology at the University of Florida and the Geriatric, Research, Education, and Clinical Center (GRECC) of the VA Medical Center, Gainesville, Fla. Since September 1987 we have completed extensive research with specialized equipment designed to evaluate and rehabilitate the spine.

In addition to an increase in muscle mass, neural adaptations contribute greatly to improved levels of muscular strength and endurance. With regular exercise, the neural control of muscular contraction is enhanced. This occurs primarily as a result of greater motor unit recruitment and an increase in the frequency of motor unit firing.[75] Resistance training may also cause the abatement of protective sensory mechanisms (such as the Golgi tendon reflex) that normally inhibit muscular contraction and the expression of strength.[37] The relative contributions of hypertrophy and neural adaptation differ along the time course of strength development. During the initial stages of a resistance training program (the first 3 to 4 weeks) gains in strength are primarily due to neural changes. Beyond this point, hypertrophy becomes the major factor accounting for further gains in strength.[61] This has important implications concerning the duration of resistance training programs in which hypertrophy is a primary consideration.

The fiber-type composition of a muscle is another important consideration in the development of strength and endurance. Most skeletal muscles consist of a heterogeneous mixture of several fiber types. The performance or functional characteristics of a muscle are dependent on the relative distribution of these fiber types within the muscle. Although there is a broad spectrum of fiber types, generally three basic types are described. A muscle consisting mainly of slow-twitch (type I) fibers will demonstrate a limited potential for force production and an enhanced capacity for muscular endurance. A muscle consisting mainly of fast-twitch (type IIa and IIb) fibers will demonstrate an enhanced potential for force production and a limited capacity for muscular endurance. Type I fibers are associated with a high oxidative (aerobic) capacity and type IIb fibers with a high glycolytic (anaerobic) capacity. The type IIa fibers appear to adapt toward a more oxidative or glycolytic characteristic depending on how they are stimulated, i.e., trained for strength or trained for endurance.[78] A muscle consisting of an even mixture of type I and type II fibers will display moderate capacities for both strength and endurance.

The fiber-type composition of a muscle has a bearing on the degree to which the overall functional capacity of the muscle may be altered or improved through resistance training. A predominantly fast-twitch muscle possesses greater potential for improvements in strength and hypertrophy than a predominantly slow-twitch muscle does. The opposite would be true for the development of muscular endurance.

Resistance training is associated with specific alterations in the metabolic characteristics of a muscle.[12, 14, 81–83] High-intensity resistance training is associated with increases in the concentration of phosphogenic and glycolytic substrates and an increase in the activities of enzymes reflecting an anaerobic-glycolytic metabolism.[12] Long-term high-intensity strength training is also associated with the attenuation of certain aerobic-oxidative enzymes.[82] These changes reflect an overall reduction in the aerobic capacity of muscle and, as mentioned above, are associated with the transformation of the characteristics of the type IIa fiber to the type IIb fiber. Moderate to low-intensity resistance training has been shown to promote increases in the activity of enzymes associated with aerobic metabolism.[14]

Another consideration in the response of a muscle to resistance training is the order of fiber-type recruitment. Motor units are generally recruited in order of their size, with the largest-strongest motor units being recruited last.[75] When the demands of exercise require little force production from a muscle, as in lifting a light weight very slowly, motor units of slow-twitch fibers are recruited. As the weight load or speed of movement increases and greater force becomes necessary, motor units of fast-twitch fibers are also recruited. This pattern of recruitment ensures that slow-twitch fibers are recruited during the performance of low-intensity and long-duration (aerobic) activities. Fast-twitch fibers are only recruited during high-intensity (anaerobic) activities.

The components of the prescription for resistance exercise training include frequency, intensity, volume, duration, and mode of activity. Depending on the goals of the training program, these components may be manipulated in such a way as to elicit a specific training response.

The frequency of resistance training refers to the number of training sessions completed per week. Although there are relatively few studies reporting the effects of various training frequencies on the development of muscular strength, it is generally felt that a minimum of three workouts per week per muscle group is required to produce optimal improvements.[20] However, recent research has shown that training one time per week is sufficient to produce maximal improvements in the strength of the isolated lumbar extensor muscles.[26] This response to training one time per week appears to be unique to the lumbar extensors and will be discussed later in this chapter under "training responses."

The requirements for resistance exercise training frequency vary on an individual basis. Several factors determine an individual's optimal training frequency. The foremost of these is the ability to recover. This refers to the amount of rest required between training sessions. It has been demonstrated that three training sessions per week performed on alternate days (one day of rest between) allows adequate recovery, especially for the novice exerciser.[1] Several sources suggest that as one advances and is better able to tolerate resistance exercises, training frequency may be increased.[5, 20, 80] Recovery ability is therefore partially dependent on the training status of the muscle.

Recovery ability is also affected by the intensity of training. Generally, a more intense training session necessitates a longer rest period. This is likely related to the degree of "damage" inflicted on the exercising muscle. Several sources suggest using the degree of residual muscle soreness as a parameter to determine the adequacy of recovery following a training session.[20] If soreness or fatigue are still present to a great degree at the onset of subsequent training sessions, this is probably an indication of incomplete recovery. Under these circumstances, the frequency, intensity, or volume of training may have to be reduced to prevent more serious muscular injury and symptoms of overtraining.

The intensity of training refers to the degree of overload that a muscle encounters during exercise. The required intensity of resistance training differs depending on the specific goals of a program. High-intensity exercises employ a high level of resistance and a low number of repetitions. Low-intensity exercises employ a low resistance and a high number of repetitions. High-intensity exercises stimulate maximal improvements in muscular strength, whereas low-intensity exercises are best suited for developing muscular endurance. According to Fleck and Kraemer,[20] repetition maximum (RM) loads of 6 or less have the greatest effect on strength development, while RM loads of 20 or more have the greatest effect on the development of muscular endurance. RM loads ranging between 6 and 20 would stimulate improvements in both strength and endurance, although the magnitude of improvement would not be as great for either. This is why most experts recommend 8 to 12 repetitions of exercise for general fitness and strength endurance development.[73, 88] It should be noted that an increase in muscular strength is associated with an increase in muscular endurance. As maximal strength increases, the percentage of strength needed to lift a given weight load decreases.

Training volume refers to the total amount of exercise performed during a single training session. This is usually expressed in terms of the total number of sets completed per exercise session, along with the total number of repetitions completed per set. The total time under load is another way to express training volume. The general consensus in the literature is that two to five sets of exercise are required to stimulate maximal gains in strength.[20] However, substantial improvements in strength result from completing a single set of exercises performed to volitional fatigue (maximum effort).[6] There is much controversy concerning the number of sets required to develop maximal strength. This controversy exists due to the fact that training intensity varies among sets used in multiple-set training studies, i.e., volitional fatigue may not have been required for all sets. As will be discussed later in this chapter under "training responses," a recent study that compared the effect of one vs. two sets of exercise (8 to 12 RM) found one set to be equally as effective for the development of isolated lumbar extension strength.[24]

The duration of training refers to the length of a resistance training program. This is usually expressed in terms of the number of weeks or months of training. As mentioned previously, neural adaptation is primarily responsible for improvements in muscular strength during the early stages of a resistance training program, after which hypertrophy accounts for most of the strength gain. Significant increases in muscle mass have been observed within 2 months following the onset of resistance training.[81] Near-maximum improvements in strength are known to occur following as little as 12 weeks of resistance training.[12] However, peak improvements in strength and hypertrophy typically require a much longer duration of training.[20] An atrophied or weak muscle possesses a greater potential for hypertrophy and strength gain than does a trained muscle.[13, 33] Moreover, an atrophied or weak muscle will also demonstrate a faster rate of growth and strength gain than a trained muscle. However, since an atrophied muscle is further away from achieving its maximum potential for growth and strength development, it will most likely require a longer duration of training.

The mode of activity refers to the type of exercise employed during a resistance training program. Muscular strength and/or endurance may be developed through the use of either isometric (IM) or dynamic exercise. IM exercise stimulates improved levels of strength, but only at or near the specific joint angle trained.[42] With IM exercise, multiple contractions at different joint angles are required in order to stimulate improvements in strength throughout a full range of motion (ROM). Full-range improvements in strength are achieved through the use of dynamic exercise, provided that they are performed slowly throughout a full ROM.[29] Dynamic exercises that require both concentric and eccentric contractions of the exercising muscle have been shown to produce superior gains in strength vs. the same exercise requiring either concentric or eccentric contractions only.[31]

The mode of activity is related to the type of resistance training equipment used during training. The various types of resistance training equipment differ according to the nature of the resistance they provide, with most equipment providing one of three types of resistance: (1) constant load, (2) variable resistance, or (3) isokinetic (accommodating) resistance.

Constant-load devices provide a consistent, unchanging weight load throughout all points of a given ROM. This is not to be confused with constant resistance, which requires that the resistance be continually applied perpendicular to the moving limb or body segment. The most widely used form of constant-load devices are free weights or barbells. Free weights are extremely popular because of their affordability, diversity, and overall ease of use. However, strength is known to vary throughout a range of joint motion. With free weights exercise is limited by the weakest position in the ROM. In other words, one may lift only as much weight as possible at the weakest joint angle. Thus, the muscle is never required to contract maximally in its stronger positions. This compromises the potential effectiveness of these devices from the standpoint of stimulating maximal improvements in strength through a full ROM. An additional disadvantage of free weight exercise is that a partner or "spotter" is often required to safely perform certain lifts. The lower part of the back is especially vulnerable to injury if proper technique is not used in lifting and lowering the weight from the floor.

Variable-resistance devices attempt to provide a resistance curve that matches the ideal strength curve of the exercising muscle. Resistance is varied with cams and pulleys, which ultimately provides the exerciser with a mechanical advantage at certain points through the ROM. The intended effect is to allow a variable resistance through the ROM to provide a maximal overload throughout. Theoretically, this would provide a more effective stimulus to the exercising muscle and result in a greater full-range effect.

For both constant- and variable-resistance exercise devices, performing repetitions with a slow controlled movement is recommended. Rapid movements under load are associated with the development of momentum that minimizes potential training effects. In addition, rapid movements may be associated with dangerously high impact forces and an increased risk of injury.

Isokinetic resistance machines are designed for exercise at a preselected constant velocity of movement. Once a constant velocity is achieved, resistance is supposed to be supplied to the exercising muscle equal to the amount of force produced at all points through a given ROM. In theory, this allows the exercising muscle to contract maximally at all points through its ROM. Moreover, this could be accomplished at speeds of movement that simulate those used in the performance of certain athletic or functional activities.

A major limitation of isokinetic exercise machines is that it is impossible to move at a constant velocity through a full ROM. Acceleration and deceleration occur at the beginning and end of isokinetic exercises.[63] Acceleration occurs as the exercising body segment "catches up" to the machine's movement arm, and deceleration occurs as the limb nears its limits of joint movement. Since the exercising limb is not moving at the preset speed of movement, maximal resistance is not provided at these positions. Acceleration and deceleration of a different nature occur as the dynamometer attempts to control the speed of movement. When the exercising limb accelerates beyond the preset speed of movement, it is immediately slowed by a sudden and partial braking and releasing of the machine's movement arm. This leads to the development of potentially harmful impact forces. Greater speeds of movement result in progressively greater impact forces.[63] These impact forces are referred to as "torque overshoot" and represent an artifact of isokinetic testing. In addition to increasing the variability associated with estimating the true isokinetic torque, impact forces may result in injury to the exercising muscle or its associated joint structures. Finally, with the exception of some recent models, isokinetic resistance devices fail to provide resistance during the eccentric phase of muscular contraction. The major limitation of variable-resistance machines is that they fail to account for individual differences in the shapes of strength curves. The resistance curve provided by a particular machine may be appropriate for one individual and inappropriate for another.

A program of resistance training must be progressive in order to continue to produce gains in muscular strength and endurance. To ensure continued gains in strength, the intensity of training must be increased or maintained. In order to ensure maximal improvements in muscular endurance, the volume of training must be steadily progressed. In either case, the rate of progression should be gradual. A typical convention is to increase the resistance by 5% when the exerciser is able to complete the prescribed number of repetitions per set for a given exercise. This will minimize the risk of muscular and/or orthopaedic injury. Finally, any improvements in muscular strength and/or endurance brought about by a training program are of limited value if training is not continued. With detraining, a large part of the improvement in muscular strength and endurance will eventually be lost. Therefore, it is recommended that training be carried on systematically throughout one's lifetime. However, once a new level of conditioning is attained, maintenance of muscular strength and endurance may be achieved through a program of reduced training. This usually involves a decrease in the frequency of training. A recent study that investigated the effects of reduced training on the maintenance of isolated knee extension strength found that the improvements in strength achieved during an initial 18-week training period at a frequency of three times per week were maintained following a 12-week program of reduced training at frequencies of one or two times per week.[28] The key component in the maintenance of muscular strength appears to be the intensity of training.

If the intensity of training is maintained, improved levels of strength are not lost. Even though the long-term (greater than 12 weeks) effects of reduced resistance training have yet to be established, it appears that it takes less to maintain than it does to attain strength and endurance. It is important to recognize that missing a workout once in a while should have no significant effect on maintaining strength and endurance. The main point is not to stop training altogether.

REQUIREMENTS FOR ACCURATE EVALUATION OF LUMBAR EXTENSION FUNCTION

The primary function of skeletal muscle is to generate force. In most instances, forces generated by skeletal muscles are used for anatomic stabilization or to produce movement. The accurate quantification of the force-generating capacity of the lumbar extensor muscles requires isolation of the lumbar extensors via pelvic stabilization, compensation for the influence of gravity on upper body mass, testing through a full ROM, and a safe and reliable method of testing.

Pelvic Stabilization

As mentioned in the beginning of this chapter, only a small portion of the total trunk extension movement is due to lumbar extension. Under normal circumstances, the lumbar extensors work in conjunction with the larger, more powerful gluteus and hamstring muscles (which rotate the pelvis) to extend the trunk. This compound movement, consisting of pelvic rotation and lumbar extension, is often referred to as lumbar-pelvic rhythm and encompasses approximately 180 degrees of movement. The lumbar extensor muscles are capable of approximately 72 degrees of trunk extension.[18, 38]

To isolate the lumbar extensors from the muscles that rotate the pelvis, pelvic stabilization is required.[27, 70, 77] One method of stabilizing the pelvis when testing lumbar extension strength in the seated position is to restrict pelvic rotation by applying a restraining force to the lower extremities (Fig 22–1). When the legs are adequately restrained, backward rotation of the pelvis is minimized. Smidt et al.[77] have documented the effectiveness of this strategy for stabilizing the pelvis and have shown that a considerable error in lumbar extension strength measurement occurs when the pelvis is not adequately stabilized. Further evidence of the importance of pelvic stabilization to isolate the lumbar extensors comes from the results of lumbar extension exercise training with and without pelvic stabilization. Graves et al.[30] showed that isolated lumbar extension strength was not affected by training on "low back" exercise machines that did not stabilize the pelvis. This study will be covered in more detail later in this chapter.

Gravity Compensation

When evaluating muscular function in the sagittal plane, gravitational force will act upon the mass of the involved body parts and influence the observed torque measurements.[19, 32, 66, 89] Head, arms, and torso mass detract from lumbar extension torque measurements when the trunk is in flexed positions and adds to the measurements made in extended positions of the ROM (See Fig 22–2). Winter et al.[89] have reported that when gravitational forces are not considered during muscular strength testing, measurement errors may exceed 500%. The magnitude of error associated with a lack of gravity compensation for body

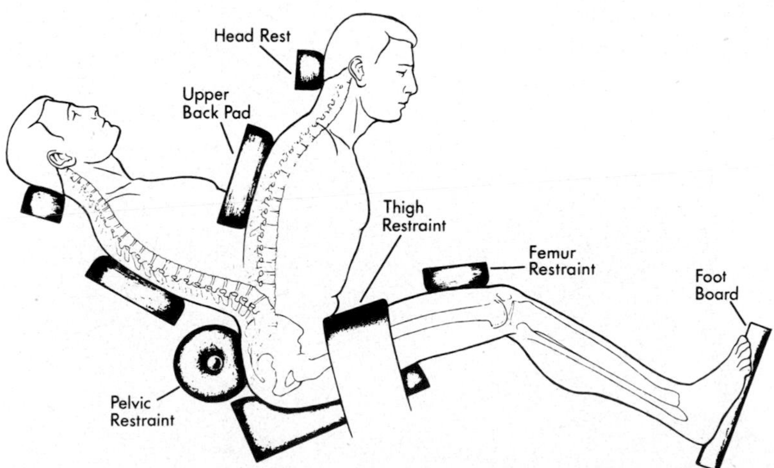

FIG 22–1.
Restraining mechanisms for isolating the lumbar extensor muscles. A force that is imposed against the bottom of the feet is transmitted by the lower parts of the legs to the femurs at an angle of approximately 45 degrees. The knee and thigh restraints limit upward movement of the knees, upper aspect of the thighs, and pelvis. The pelvic restraint prevents movement of the pelvis in the direction of extension.

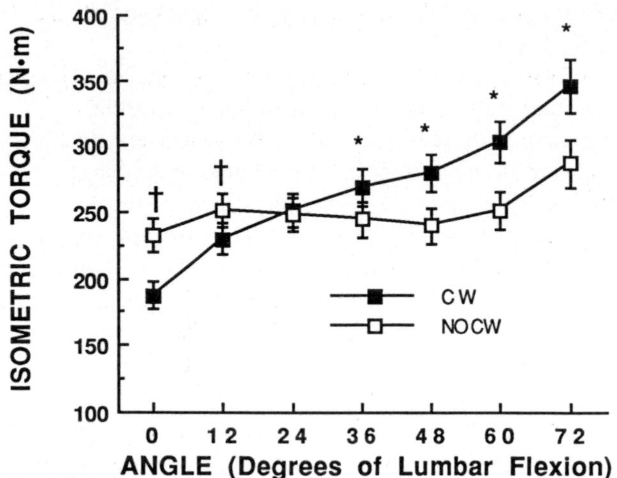

FIG 22–2.
The influence of upper-body mass during lumbar extension torque evaluation in the seated position. A group of 34 subjects was tested for isolated lumbar extension strength with a counterweight *(CW)* and again without a counterweight *(NOCW)*. *The CW trial was significantly higher than the NOCW trial ($P \leq .05$). †The NOCW trial was significantly higher than the CW trial ($P \leq .05$). (Data from Fulton M, Pollock M, Leggett S, et al: Effect of upper body mass on the measurement of isometric lumbar extension strength. Presented at the Orthopaedic Rehabilitation Association Conference, San Antonio, Tex, 1990.)

mass when evaluating lumbar extension function has been described by Fulton et al.[22] and represents as much as 25% of the mean torque values (Fig 22–2).

Some dynamometers have employed correction algorithms and/or mechanical devices to compensate for the effects of gravitational force on muscular torque measurements. However, there has been little research to validate the accuracy of these procedures. Recently, Pollock et al.[71] studied the accuracy of a counterweight procedure designed to compensate for the effect of gravity acting upon upper body mass during IM lumbar extension torque testing. The authors used a prototype lumbar extension machine (MedX; Ocala, Fla) that allowed testing in the sagittal plane while using the counterweight procedure. The machine could also be rotated 90 degrees to enable testing in the transverse plane without the need for a counterweight because gravity no longer influences upper body mass in the direction of lumbar extension (Fig 22–3). Seventy-four subjects were tested isometrically through a 72-degree ROM in both planes. The resulting torque curves indicated no significant difference between the two conditions from 72 to 12 degrees of extension (Fig 22–4). The difference observed at 0 degrees (15 newton-meters) was small, and the correlation between tests was $r = 0.91$. These data validate the effectiveness of the counterweight procedure to compensate for upper body mass during IM lumbar extension strength testing in the seated position.

Importance of Testing Through a Full Range of Motion

The normal IM lumbar extension torque curve is linear, descends from flexion to extension, and encompasses a ROM of approximately 72 degrees.[25] Patients with LBP and individuals who are predisposed for LBP due to existing pathologies often exhibit a limited ROM[21, 74] and abnormally shaped IM lumbar extension torque curves that are characterized by weakness at certain positions in the ROM (Fig 22–5) but not necessarily through the entire ROM.[21] Testing at a single position or through a limited

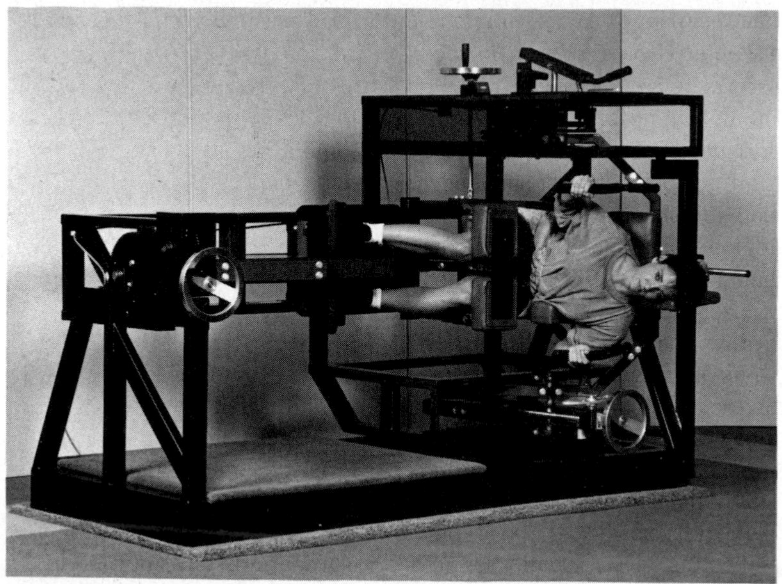

FIG 22–3.
Lateral lumbar extension machine (MedX Corp., Ocala, Fla). This machine was used for data collected in Figure 22–4.

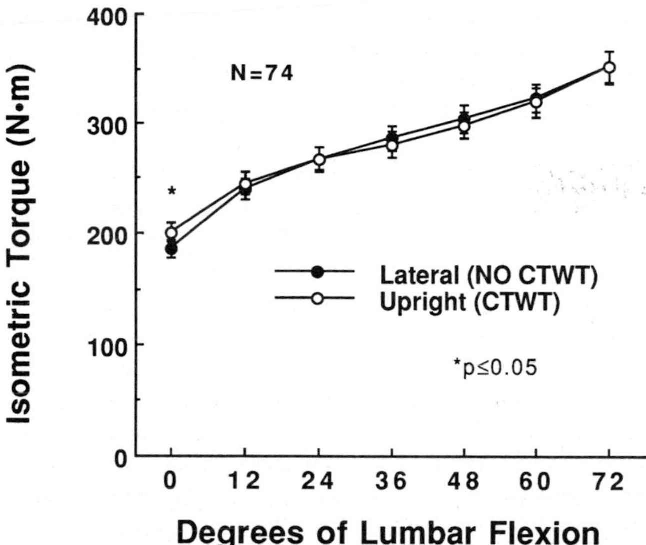

FIG 22–4.
Isometric torque values for lumbar extension strength testing in the sagittal plane with upper body mass counterweighted *(CTWT)* and in the transverse plane without the need for counterweighting *(NO CTWT)*. (From Pollock M, Graves J, Leggett S, et al: *Med Sci Sports Exerc* 1991; 23(suppl):66. Used by permission.)

ROM may not identify potentially significant abnormalities. Also, exercise training programs for prevention and rehabilitation may have a varied influence throughout the ROM.[27, 29] Testing through a full ROM is important to provide a complete profile of strength for the purposes of patient screening and evaluation. Patients undergoing treatment for LBP often improve their ROM during the healing process, and full-ROM strength testing is important to monitor this progress as their condition improves.

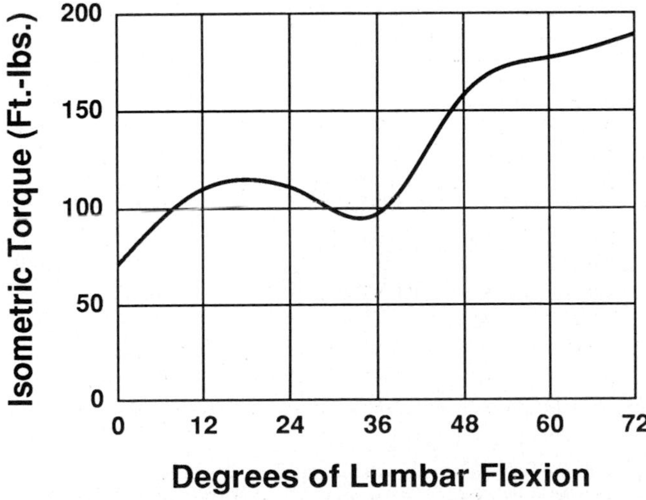

FIG 22–5.
Example of an abnormal isometric lumbar extension strength curve. Note the weakness at 36 degrees of lumbar flexion that is causing a deviation from the normal linear torque curve by angle relationship.

The importance of full-ROM evaluation is further illustrated by athletes involved in unique training programs. Waterskiing, for example, overloads the lumbar extensors in the extended portion of the ROM as the skier leans back to resist the pull of the tow boat. As a result of this overload and the principle of specificity of training, water-skiers are unusually strong in the extended portion of the ROM but not in flexion (Fig 22–6).[46] Full-ROM lumbar extension strength training generally produces the greatest effect in the extended portion of the ROM (to be discussed later in "training responses"). A case study involving 10 weeks of lumbar extension strength training at a frequency of once every 2 weeks (five training sessions) by a competitive slalom skier, however, showed a 60% increase in strength in full flexion (72 degrees of lumbar flexion) and a 22% improvement in strength at 20 degrees of lumbar flexion, which was the initial position of peak strength.[38] The specific adaptations to waterskiing and to full-ROM lumbar extension strength training in a previously untrained water-skier could only be observed by accurate full-ROM evaluation.

Dynamic exercise tests do not have the ability to assess strength through a full ROM. Isotonic tests are limited to the quantification of strength at the weakest position in a ROM. Isokinetic tests are associated with a period of acceleration at the beginning of the ROM and a period of deceleration at the end of the ROM. The acceleration and deceleration phases of the test are responsible for producing a bell-shaped curve that is characteristic of all isokinetic exercise tests, regardless of the muscle group being evaluated. The amount of information lost during an isokinetic

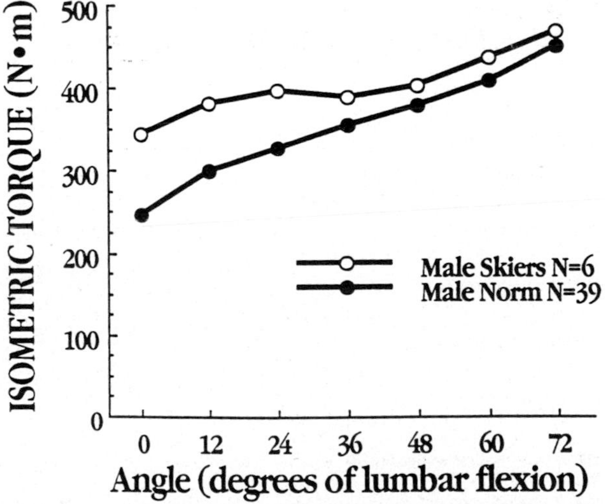

FIG 22–6.
Isometric lumbar extension torque curves for elite professional male water-skiers and normal (untrained) males. (Data from Leggett SH, Pollock ML, Graves JE, et al: Physiological evaluation of elite professional water-skiers. Presented at the International Congress on Sports Medicine and Human Performance, Vancouver, Canada, 1990.)

test depends on the speed of movement and can consist of as much as 50% of the ROM during lumbar extension strength testing.[53]

Due to the limitations of assessing strength through a ROM with dynamic exercise tests, IM measures are often used to describe strength through a ROM.[44] IM strength of compound lumbar-pelvic function has been evaluated.[52] A multi-joint angle IM exercise test has been described that can accurately assess isolated lumbar extension torque through a full ROM.[25] Advantages of this test include a high degree of reliability and low variability in addition to providing a full ROM profile for lumbar extension torque. The accuracy of isokinetic measures of muscular strength have been questioned due to the need for mathematical interpretation of the oscillations in observed torque (impact forces) caused by constant braking and releasing of the servomechanism that controls movement velocity.[4, 62, 63, 76] Because IM exercise tests involve no movement, impact forces are not found when the generation of muscular tension is slow and controlled.

While IM measures of muscular torque have the advantage of reliability, accuracy, and provision of a full-ROM profile, multi–joint-angle IM tests can be limited by fatigue associated with the testing procedure. Graves et al.[29] showed that the shape of the IM lumbar extension torque curve is influenced by the order of testing, i.e., IM lumbar extension torque measurements are affected by the previously performed IM contractions. This order effect is not influenced by exercise training. Therefore, as long as the order of testing is standardized, a multi–joint-angle test can be used to quantify changes in strength through a full ROM. When it is imperative to obtain maximal IM torque measurements at multiple positions through a ROM, a sufficient amount of time between contractions must be allowed to ensure adequate recovery.

Reliability of Isometric Testing

In order for test results to be meaningful, they must be reliable. Otherwise, it is impossible to determine whether deviations from normative data or changes resulting from intervention programs represent true differences or whether they are a reflection of the unreliability of the test. Graves et al.[25] evaluated the reliability and variability associated with measuring IM lumbar extension strength through a 72-degree ROM. One hundred thirty-six men and women completed IM lumbar extension strength tests on 3 separate days. On days 1 and 2, subjects completed two tests separated by a 20- to 30-minute rest interval. For each test, IM lumbar extension torque was measured at 72, 60, 48, 36, 24, 12, and 0 degrees of lumbar flexion. The mean IM torque values, within day reliability coefficients and test variability over the seven positions measured, improved from day 1 to day 2. Mean strength values and reliability statistics showed no further improvements from day 2 to day 3. Values for single test variability ranged from 20.3 to 24.3 newton-meters (Nm), which represented 6.7% to 11.0% of the mean torque value (see Table 22–1). Because of the improvement noticed from day 1 to day 2, a practice test is recommended to obtain the most reliable results for the lumbar extension muscles. Using the most reliable data observed, Graves et al.[25] reported normative IM lumbar extension torque for men and

TABLE 22–1.

Reliability of Multiple–Joint Angle Isometric Strength Tests

Study	Correlation Coefficient	Joint Angle 1	2	3	4	5	6	7	8
Knee extension*	*r*†	0.98	0.98	0.98	0.98	0.94	0.95	0.93	0.90
	SEE/$\sqrt{2}$%‡	4.8	4.9	5.0	4.7	7.1	6.6	8.3	10.3
Lumbar extension§	*r*	0.97	0.94	0.95	0.96	0.94	0.92	0.81	
	SEE/$\sqrt{2}$%	7.2	6.7	8.2	7.9	9.9	11.1	11.6	
Cervical extension¶	*r*	0.96	0.95	0.94	0.96	0.94	0.96	0.92	0.90
	SEE/$\sqrt{2}$%	9.8	8.8	8.0	7.4	8.4	8.4	8.6	10.2
Cervical rotation‖	*r*	0.97	0.96	0.97	0.97	0.97	0.94	0.91	
	SEE/$\sqrt{2}$%	7.9	8.4	7.3	6.8	6.4	8.9	15.1	
Torso rotation**	*r*	0.97	0.95	0.96	0.93	0.91	0.87	0.85	
	SEE/$\sqrt{2}$%	5.8	7.2	6.2	8.3	9.3	11.1	16.7	

*Knee extension joint angles are 70, 85, 100, 115, 130, 145, 160, and 171 degrees of knee extension. Data from Graves JE, Pollock ML, Jones AE, et al: *Med Sci Sports Exerc* 1989; 21:84–89.

†Pearson product-moment correlation coefficient describing test-retest reliability.

‡Single test variability described by dividing the standard error of the estimate (SEE) by $\sqrt{2}$ and expressed relative to the mean torque values at each angle.

§Lumbar extension angles are 72, 60, 48, 35, 24, 12, and 0 degrees of lumbar flexion. Data from Graves JE, Pollock ML, Carpenter DM, et al: *Spine* 1990; 15:289–294.

¶Cervical extension angles are 126, 108, 90, 72, 54, 36, 18, and 0 degrees of cervical flexion. Data from Leggett SH, et al: *Am J Sports Med,* 1991; 19:653–659.

‖Cervical rotation angles are 72, 48, 24, 0, −24, −48, and −72 degrees of cervical rotation. Data from Trinkle JP: *Quantitative assessment of isometric cervical rotation strength* (thesis). University of Florida, 1990.

**Torso rotation angles are 54, 36, 18, 0, −18, −36, and −54 degrees of torso rotation. Data from Carpenter DM, et al: *Int J Sports Med* 1991; 2:246.

women. The normal curves are linear and descend from flexion to extension (Fig 22–7).

The variability of muscular strength measures made on humans under the most carefully standardized conditions is generally 5% to 10%.[87] This variability is considered to be normal human biovariation and is caused by the fact that there are a variety of factors that can influence human strength on a day-to-day basis. Some important factors that can influence human strength measurements include but are not limited to the amount of sleep, the time of day, the time since the last meal, recent physical activity, physiologic stress, and motivation. It is prudent to standardize as many of the factors as possible to obtain the most reliable test results.

Research from our laboratory on the reliability of multiple–joint-angle IM strength testing has also been evaluated for the knee extensors, cervical extensors, and the muscles that rotate the torso and neck (MedX). Results from these studies are summarized in Table 22–1. The data show a high degree of repeatability and low variability for all muscle groups studied through a full ROM. The only exception is variability associated with the measurement of torso rotation torque in the fully contracted position (22%).

Safety

An additional advantage of IM testing is that it is a relatively safe method to evaluate muscular strength. Momentum developed during dynamic modes of exercise often results in impact forces when this momentum is suddenly halted. This occurs during isokinetic exercise when

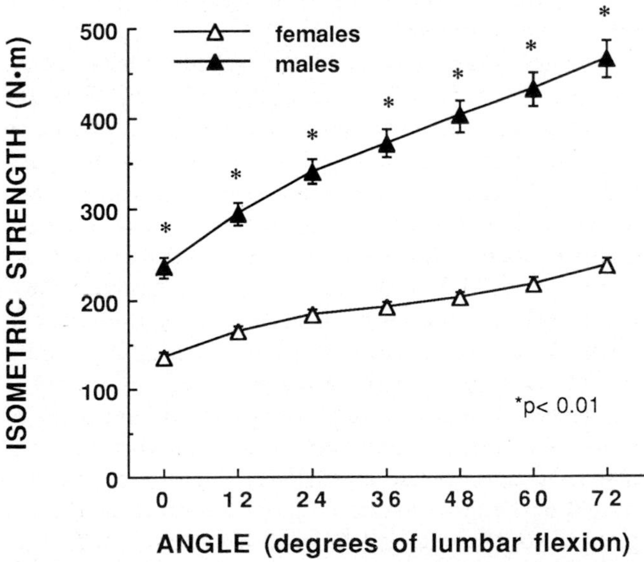

FIG 22–7.
Isometric lumbar extension torque values for normal men and women. (Data from Graves JE, Pollock ML, Carpenter DM, et al: *Spine* 1990; 15:289–294.)

the acceleration of the involved body part is halted by the movement arm of the device as it attempts to maintain preset velocity.[62, 63, 76] The impact forces resulting from this situation represent a testing artifact (described as torque overshoot) and are potentially dangerous, especially in patients with LBP.[57, 67] Research[51, 56] has shown that isokinetic trunk extension torque production can increase with increasing movement speed. This is in violation of the force-velocity relationship for muscular contraction (i.e., maximal force production decreases as movement velocity increases).[35] These data cannot be explained physiologically and probably result from the inability to accurately interpret the impact forces associated with isokinetic exercise testing, i.e., the greater the speed of movement, the greater the impact forces generated.

Testing for Lumbar Extension Net Muscular Torque

The mechanical properties of skeletal muscle have elastic and contractile components.[10] Elastic and strain (compression) energy may also be stored in connective tissue and bone. Measured torque resulting from voluntary muscular contraction is a combination of torque generated by the stored energy of the stretched (or contracted) muscle and its associated joint structures and force generated by the excitation-coupling process. Although both the elastic and contractile properties of muscle have been studied in vitro and in vivo, there has been no attempt to separate and quantify these two components in vivo by using computerized dynomometry.

The total torque generated during lumbar extension testing in the seated position consists of voluntary and involuntary components. Involuntary torque has been observed in the flexed positions of the ROM when subjects have been instructed to relax prior to voluntary contraction. Presumably this involuntary or "stored energy" torque represents the sum of the elastic energy of the fully stretched lumbar extensor muscles: the upward force on the torso caused by compression of the abdomen and the downward force of gravity acting upon the torso (if no counterweight is used to compensate for torso mass).

To quantify the involuntary and contractile components of measured torque during lumbar extension, an experiment was conducted in which subjects were secured in a lumbar extension machine with the addition of a harness that was designed to hold the torso against the movement arm of the machine.[8] The movement arm was positioned and locked at the first test angle (72 degrees of lumbar flexion), and the subjects were instructed to relax. The subjects' involuntary torque (stored energy) was displayed on a computer monitor (Fig 22–8) and recorded.

After the involuntary torque was recorded by the computer, the subjects were requested to perform a maximal IM contraction. The maximal or total torque value ob-

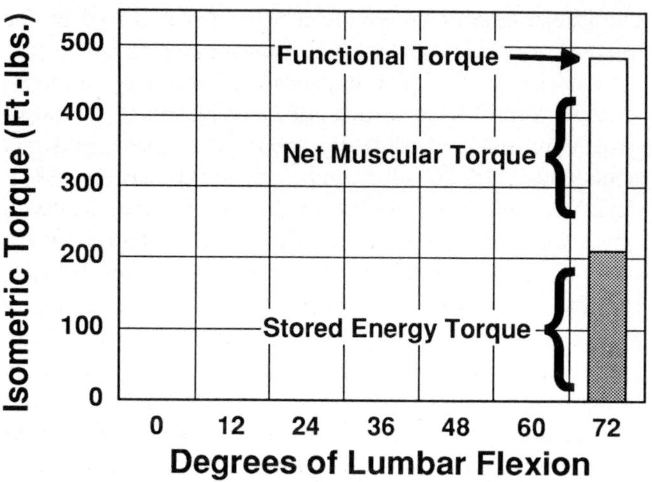

FIG 22–8.
Resting involuntary torque is first recorded by the computer. The subject then performs a maximal isometric contraction, and the total torque is recorded. The difference between the total torque and the torque due to involuntary factors represents the net muscular torque.

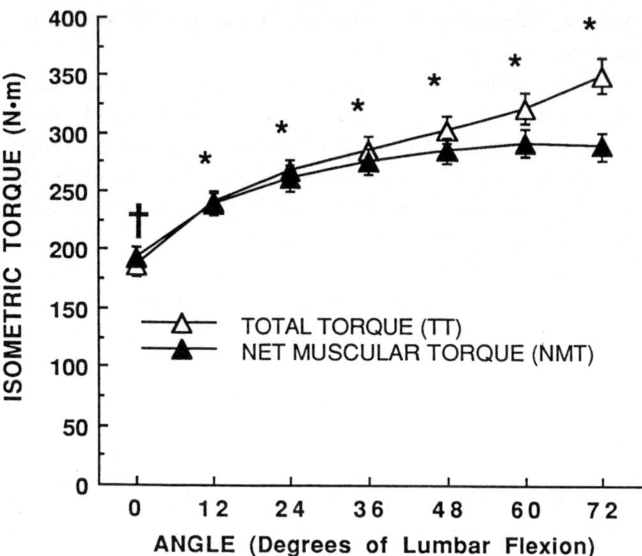

FIG 22–9.
Total torque and net muscular torque through 72 degrees of lumbar motion. (Data from Carpenter DM, Leggett S, Pollock M, et al: *Med Sci Sports Exerc* 1991; 23(suppl):65.)

served represents the torque generated by muscular contraction plus the torque due to the previously described involuntary factors. Subtracting the involuntary torque from the total torque measurement yields a measure of NMT. The NMT measure is the torque generated by volitional muscular contraction.

This procedure was then repeated at six additional test positions through the 72-degree ROM. Following the test, total-torque and NMT curves were compared. The area between these two curves represents the involuntary torque that was generated throughout the lumbar extensor ROM. As illustrated in Figure 22–9, involuntary factors can dramatically affect total functional torque. At 72 degrees of lumbar flexion, involuntary factors accounted for over 20% of the total torque value.

The concept of NMT is unique because it describes the force due to volitional contraction with the exclusion of other variables that can influence muscular torque measurements. Because of the limitations associated with dynamic torque measurements NMT can only be obtained during IM strength testing. The ability to quantify NMT will improve the ability to interpret and monitor measurements of lumbar function.

Fatigue Characteristics of the Lumbar Extensors

The fatigue characteristics of skeletal muscle have been studied and described in detail.[16] As previously described in this chapter, the fatigue characteristics of skeletal muscle are to a large extent related to the fiber-type composition of the muscle. The most common methodology used to investigate muscle fiber–type composition has been the histochemical treatment of muscle biopsies. This technique is invasive, requires sophisticated biochemical laboratory equipment and highly trained personnel, and obviously cannot be applied practically by the average health care professional interested in muscle fatigue characteristics. In addition, the technique is limited in its inability to differentiate along a continuum of fiber types and produces highly variable results in humans due to the inability to obtain sufficient quantities of muscle for evaluation. More importantly, while histochemical analysis of muscle biopsies may qualitatively describe muscle fiber–type composition, it does not provide a measure of muscular performance.

Fatigue characteristics of the isolated lumbar extensors may be evaluated by using the following three-part testing procedure.[38] This procedure has been referred to as a fatigue response test (FRT). Subjects are first positioned and secured in the lumbar extension machine so that the pelvis is stabilized as previously described. Then the multi–joint-angle IM lumbar extension test described earlier is performed through a full ROM. Immediately following the IM test, subjects complete a dynamic exercise with a preselected weight load. We have successfully used a weight load equal to 50% of the peak torque generated at 72 degrees of lumbar flexion during the IM lumbar extension torque test. Subjects perform as many dynamic variable-resistance lumbar extensions as possible until the weight load can no longer be lifted through a full 72 degrees of ROM (volitional fatigue). To ensure standardization of the procedure, subjects/patients are instructed to maintain an exercise cadence of 2 seconds for the concentric phase of the contraction (lifting the weight), a 1-second pause in the extended position, and 4 seconds for the eccentric phase of the contraction (lowering the weight). Finally, within 60 seconds following the final dynamic repetition, subjects complete a second, seven-angle, maximal-effort IM test. A subject's "fresh" IM torque curve and the IM torque curve generated immediately following the dynamic exercise are compared for analysis. The area separating the two curves represent the fatigue associated with performing the dynamic exercise.

The fatigue response of subjects completing the three-part FRT is a continuum. Figure 22–10 illustrates the results of two subjects who demonstrate dramatically different responses to the FRT. The two bottom test results (at 72 degrees) represent a subject whose fresh IM strength was increased by 8% following six dynamic lumbar extensions with a moderate level of resistance. The top two test results (at 72 degrees) represent a subject who lost 45% of his fresh IM strength following only six dynamic lumbar extensions, also to moderate fatigue. Both subjects exercised with the same work load (200 lb). These two varied responses are likely due to differences in fiber-type composition. The relationship between muscle fiber–type composition and the fatigue characteristics of skeletal muscle is well documented.[16, 20]

Current pre-employment strength testing procedures often use peak torque as a predictor of how well suited an individual may be for job-related tasks requiring a frequent amount of lifting.[40] The basis for this rationale is that stronger individuals are less likely to suffer a low back injury when placed in situations requiring repetitive or heavy lifting. There is evidence to suggest, however, that in certain situations it is the stronger worker who is at a greater risk for injury.[3] This may be due to the fact that stronger individuals often fatigue rapidly. It cannot be overlooked, however, that stronger individuals may be more likely to be placed into high-risk jobs.

The FRT may be a better predictor of an individual's risk for back injury than peak torque is. Those individuals who demonstrate a large decrement in strength with only a few repetitions of exercise may not be suited for jobs requiring repetitive lifting despite their ability to generate high levels of peak torque. Thus, the FRT may provide a useful method of evaluating the risk of low back dysfunction in an industrial setting. In addition, fatigue response characteristics are important to consider for the most appropriate prescription of resistance training exercises for the development and maintenance of muscular strength.

Most individuals (approximately 70%) show a 10% to 25% decrease in strength following the FRT. Approximately 10% are fatigue resistant and show less than a 10% reduction in strength. Another 20% show a high degree of fatigue (>25% decrease in strength). Individuals with greater than 25% fatigue responses tend to be either very strong individuals or patients with LBP. Patients/subjects who show extreme fatigability during the FRT should train less frequently and with fewer repetitions (6 to 8 repetitions) of exercise. Those who show little or no fatigue can train more frequently and with a greater number of repetitions (15 to 20 repetitions). Continued research is warranted to clarify the relationship between muscular endurance of the lumbar spine, risk of LBP, and the prescription of low back exercise.

EXERCISE TRAINING RESPONSES OF THE LUMBAR SPINE

Lumbar Extension Exercise Training in Subjects Without Low Back Pain

This section will deal with our 5 years' experience in exercise training of the isolated lumbar extensor muscles. Where appropriate, comparisons with other training studies from the literature will be made and recommendations

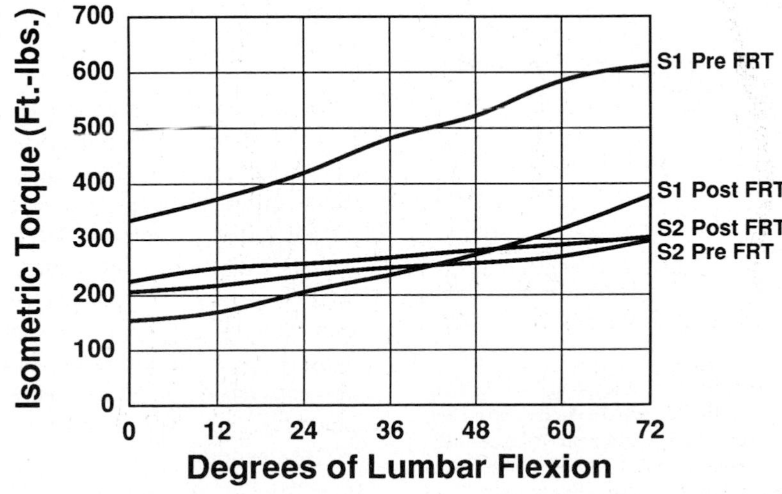

FIG 22–10.
Isometric torque values prior to and following an acute bout of dynamic lumbar extension exercise (fatigue response test *[FRT]*).

for exercise prescription inferred. The MedX lumbar extension machine (Ocala, Fla) was used for all investigations.

One of our first training studies was conducted on 25 healthy volunteers: 18 men (aged 33 ± 11 years) and 7 women (22 ± 1 years).[72] Fifteen of these subjects were assigned to an exercise group that trained 1 day per week for 10 weeks. Ten were assigned to a nonexercising control group. Training consisted of one set of full-ROM, variable-resistance lumbar extension exercises with a weight load that allowed 6 to 15 repetitions to volitional fatigue (maximal effort). Both groups were tested before and after training by using the multiple-joint, seven-angle IM testing protocol mentioned earlier.

The results showed that the exercise group significantly improved their isolated IM lumbar extension strength through a full 72 degrees of ROM while the controls did not change (Fig 22–11). A unique finding of this study was the magnitude of the training response of the isolated lumbar extensor muscles. The 42% increase at 72 degrees (full flexion) to a 102% increase at 0 degrees (full extension) is much higher than what is normally found following training of other muscle groups. A review by Fleck and Kraemer[20] showed that the average increase in strength for most studies using IM or isotonic testing and training of a variety of different muscle groups was between 20% and 30%. It has been shown that participants who are untrained and who are low in strength with respect to their potential for strength gain have a greater capacity to acquire strength than do those who are highly trained or who are already close to their maximum strength potential.[13, 33] de Vries[13] and Fleck and Kraemer,[20] in recent reviews of exercise prescription for resistance training, alluded to the importance of this concept when evaluating the effectiveness of training programs. Thus, the magnitude of the training response observed for the isolated lumbar extensor muscles shows that they were initially very weak. Another significant factor was that 10 of the 15 subjects in the exercise group had been training regularly on the Nautilus low back machine (Nautilus Sports Medical Industries, Inc., Independence, Va). If the lumbar extensor muscles had been trained, further increases in strength would not have been expected.

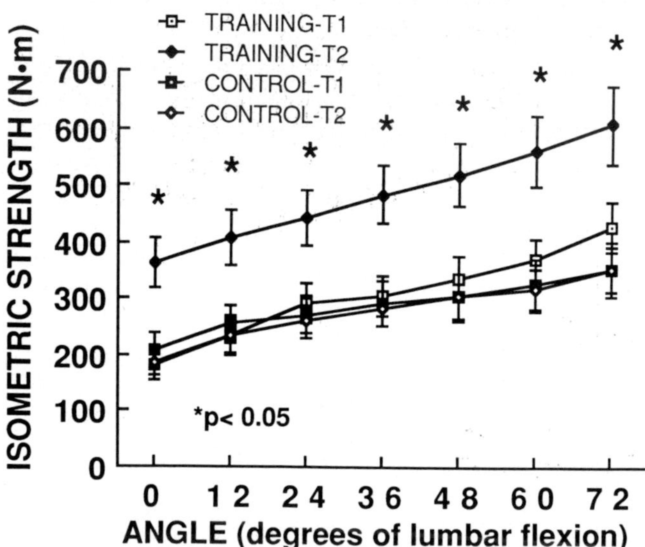

FIG 22–11.
Torque (newton-meters) measurements for isometric strength of the lumbar exterior muscles at 0, 12, 24, 36, 48, 60, and 72 degrees of lumbar flexion. T1 and T2 show measurements before and after 10-week training, respectively. Data represent means ± SEM. (From Pollock ML, Leggett SH, Graves JE, et al: *Am J Sports Med* 1989; 17:624–629. Used by permission.)

How can these unusually large increases in strength of the lumbar extensors, in particular, the latter half of the ROM, be explained? A reasonable explanation is that the strength of these muscles is not normally developed or maintained with existing exercise methods. These machines do not isolate the lumbar extensor muscles through pelvic stabilization. As mentioned earlier in this chapter, without proper stabilization of the pelvis, the larger, stronger gluteus and hamstring muscles do most of the exercise in back extension. This situation may be equivalent to that of a muscle that has been placed into a cast; it is in a state of chronic disuse, atrophies quickly, and loses its size and strength.[15–17, 47, 49, 64, 85] Thus, it appears that the lumbar extensor muscles never develop strength to their full potential and become atrophied from chronic disuse. This has important implications for primary prevention and rehabilitation of LBP since the lumbar extensor muscles seem to be the weak "link" in the "muscle chain" that protects the lower part of the back.

Whether the magnitude of strength gain found in this study was attributable to hypertrophy related to specific biochemical or histochemical adaptations to training or neural factors was not studied. But based on the time course of strength improvement discussed earlier by Moritani and de Vries,[61] most likely some of the early changes in strength could be attributable to neural factors, with hypertrophy being predominant thereafter. Some have suggested that a learning factor may have influenced the magnitude of strength gain. As mentioned in the evaluation and reliability section of this chapter, the learning associated with the testing procedure takes place during the initial test.[25] Since the subjects in this study had multiple tests initially and since the control group showed no increase in strength during the course of the study, learning was not considered an attributable factor in the results of this study.

As mentioned earlier, frequency of training is an important component of the exercise prescription for resistance training. Most experts recommend three training sessions per week for optimal results.[20, 73, 88] Although the strength increase from our initial training study was considered unusually large, only 1 day per week of training was used. Would a lesser or greater frequency of training elicit a different response? To answer this question 72 healthy men (31 ± 9 years old) and 42 women (28 ± 10 years old) volunteered to train for 12 weeks and were randomly assigned to training frequencies of one time every 2 weeks, one time per week, two times per week, or three times per week or to a nonexercising control group.[26] Each training session consisted of one set of full-ROM dynamic, variable-resistance exercise with a work load that allowed 8 to 12 repetitions to volitional fatigue. Figure 22–12 shows the adjusted post-training IM torque values for the various groups. When compared with the control group all exercise training groups improved their strength through a full ROM. Although there was a trend for the once-every-2-week group to show a smaller strength increase with training, the increases in torque found post-training were not statistically significant among groups.

Whether the groups exercising twice or three times per week would improve to a greater extent if they were allowed a longer time period to adapt to training was investigated in a follow-up study. Eighty-five of the subjects from the previously mentioned 12-week training study continued to exercise in the same manner for an additional 8 weeks for a total of 20 weeks of training. Increases in IM torque found at 20 weeks of training for the various exercise groups again showed no significant difference among groups.[7] Since the group training once every 2 weeks increased their dynamic training weight to a lesser extent than did the other exercise groups and because there were no differences among the groups training once, twice, or three times per week, 1 day per week of lumbar extension training is recommended for normal use.

The aforementioned studies of Pollock et al.,[72] Graves et al.,[26] and Carpenter et al.[7] all showed unusually large increases in isolated lumbar extension strength, with a greater magnitude of gain shown in the latter half of the ROM. Since most training studies in the literature have been conducted for 10- to 12-week durations, little evidence is available concerning further increases in strength beyond 12 weeks.[20] Also, most studies have only reported peak strength; thus inference as to whether strength increases are proportional through the full ROM is not well documented.

Carpenter et al.[7] evaluated the shape of the IM torque curve following 12 and 20 weeks of isolated lumbar extension training. The data from Figure 22–13 show that most of the increase in strength associated with lumbar extension exercise occurred during the first 12 weeks of training. Training up to 20 weeks showed no change in peak strength (72 degrees of lumbar flexion) from the 12-week testing period, but significant increases were found from 48 to 0 degrees of lumbar flexion. The time-by-angle interaction statistic showed that there was a change in the shape

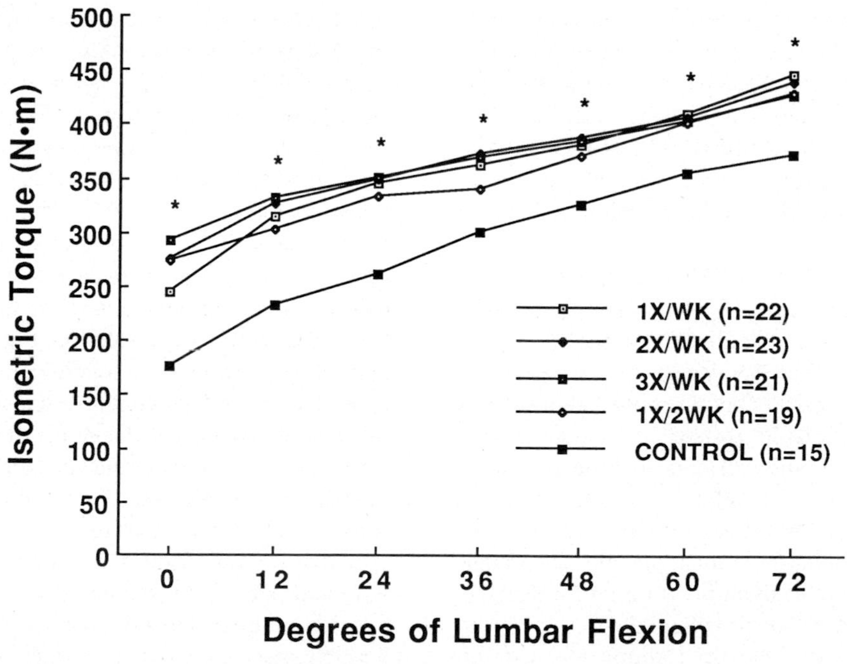

FIG 22–12.

Adjusted post-training isometric torques for the control group and the groups that trained dynamically every other week (1×/2WK), once per week (1×/WK), twice per week (2×/WK), and three times per week (3×/WK). *Control is less than 1×/2WK, 1×/WK, 2×/WK, 3×/WK ($P \leq .05$). (From Graves JE, Pollock ML, Foster D, et al: *Spine* 1990; 15:504–509. Used by permission.)

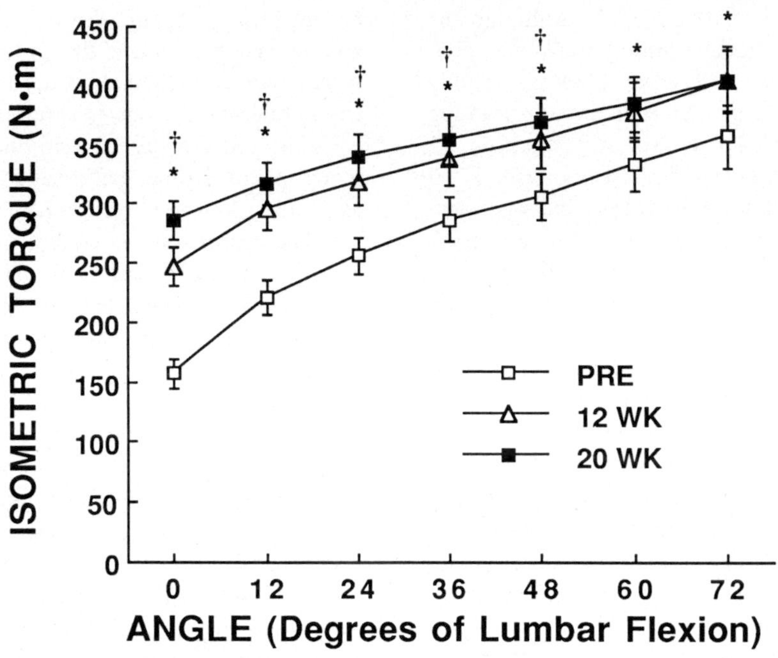

FIG 22–13.
Initial *(PRE)*, 12-week, and 20-week isometric torque values for the combined group. *PRE is less than 12-week and 20-week torques ($P \leq .01$). †Twelve-week is less than 20 week ($P \leq .05$). Values represent means ± SEM. (From Carpenter DM, Graves JE, Pollock ML, et al: *Phys Ther* 1991; 71:580–588. Used by permission.)

of the lumbar extension IM strength curve. The ratio of torque from 72 to 0 degrees of lumbar flexion was reduced from 2.3:1 prior to training to 1.6:1 at 12 weeks and 1.4:1 at 20 weeks. The flattening of the torque curve in the extended positions following training supports the contention that the lumbar extensor muscles are disproportionately weak in the mid to extended parts of the ROM. One of the more important points that can be surmised from this study is the importance of full-ROM testing and training, for if only peak torque were measured, inferences made from the results would have been different and limited.

To evaluate the specificity of IM training for developing lumbar extension strength, 14 volunteers trained with IM exercise at the same seven angles that are used for testing.[26] They trained one time per week for 12 weeks and were compared with a group that exercised dynamically once per week with variable resistance. Figure 22–14 shows that both the IM and variable-resistance training groups made significant and similar improvements in IM torque through the full ROM when compared with the control group. Thus, the results show that multiple–joint-angle IM training is as effective as dynamic training for developing full-ROM IM lumbar extension strength.

The full-range effect of the IM training was not surprising since it has been shown that both IM and dynamic training at specific joint angles results in a strength effect on either side of trained areas.[23, 27, 41, 48] The dynamic exercise was performed in a slow controlled manner that simulated the multiple IM efforts.[69] This plus the variable-resistance cam were effective in ensuring a full-ROM training response. Thus, either IM or dynamic variable-resistance training can be recommended for developing lumbar extension strength. Also, improvements in strength from periodic IM testing can be expected to stimulate improvement in some patients or research subjects.

To evaluate the effects of volume of training on lumbar extension strength, 110 volunteers exercised one time per week for 12 weeks with either one (n = 42) or two (n = 53) sets with 8 to 12 repetitions per set to volitional fatigue.[24] The results showed significant and similar full-ROM strength improvements for both exercise groups as compared with the controls (see Fig 22–15). Although the multiple-set (volume of training) issue is controversial, it appears that with the lumbar extensor muscles an added set of exercise has no advantage for most subjects.[20] Whether three sets of lumbar extension training would be superior to one set is not known, but based on the magnitude of results already found with one set plus the added time and cost that would result from a program of three sets per day, it would not be recommended.

To evaluate the effect of pelvic stabilization during variable-resistance lumbar extension training on isolated IM lumbar extension strength, 72 healthy men and women (aged 31.8 ± 10 years) trained 1 day per week for 12 weeks.[30] Subjects were randomly assigned to one of four

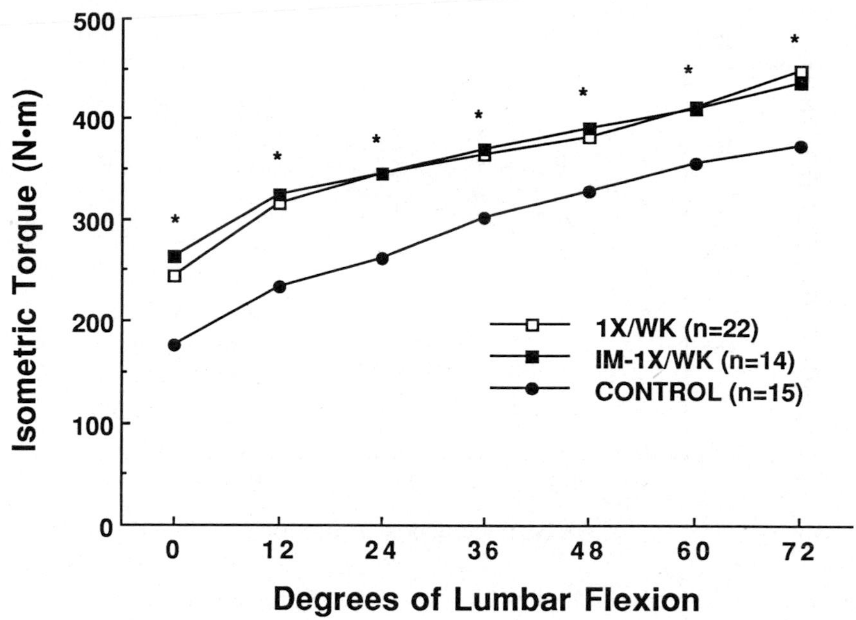

FIG 22–14.
Adjusted post-training isometric torques for the control and the groups that trained isometrically one time per week (IM-1×/WK) and dynamically one time per week (1×/WK). *Control is less than IM 1×/WK, 1×/WK ($P \leq .05$). (From Graves JE, Pollock ML, Foster D, et al: *Spine* 1990; 15:504–509. Used by permission.)

groups: Eagle (n = 19; Cybex, Ronkonkoma, NY); Nautilus (n = 19; Nautilus Sports Medical Industries, Independence, Va); MedX (n = 19; Ocala, Fla); and a control (n = 15). Only the MedX lumbar extension machine isolated the lumbar extensor muscles through pelvic stabilization. All training groups improved significantly in the dynamic training weight used for each specific apparatus (Eagle, 19.8 kg; Nautilus, 18.8 kg; and MedX, 23.8 kg). Adjusted post-training isolated IM torques, however, increased significantly only in the MedX group (see Fig 22–16). These data showed that pelvic stabilization is required to effectively condition the lumbar extensor muscles. Improve-

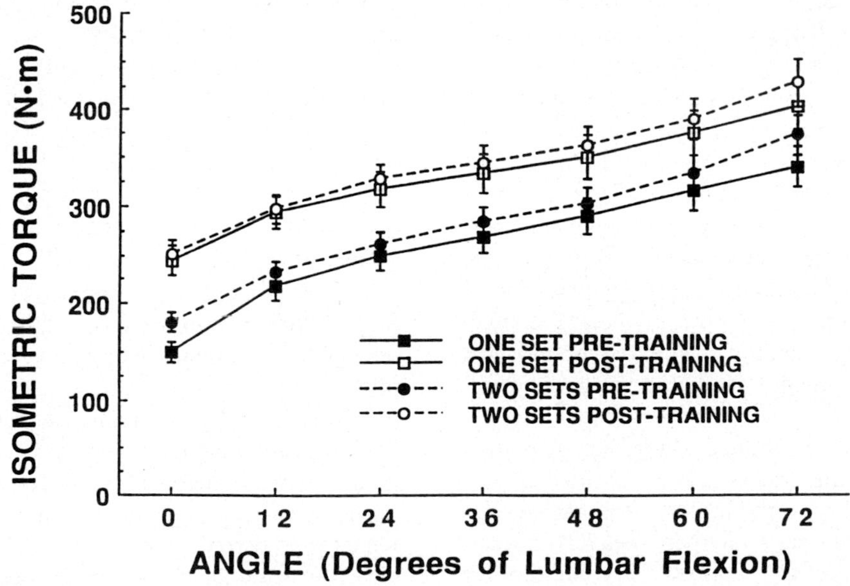

FIG 22–15.
Torque (newton-meters) measurements for isometric strength of the lumbar extensor muscles at 0 to 72 degrees of lumbar flexion. Data show pre-training and post-training results of groups that trained by doing either one set or two sets of exercises. (Data from Graves JE, Holmes BL, Leggett SH, et al: Single versus multiple set dynamic and isometric lumbar extension training. Presented at the World Confederation for Physical Therapy 11th International Congress, London 1991, pp 1340–1342.)

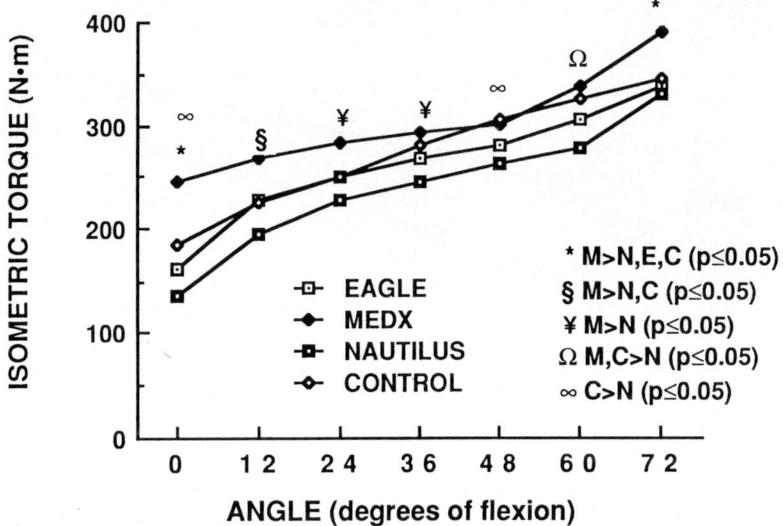

FIG 22–16.
Adjusted post-training isometric torque for the control group and the groups that trained by using Nautilus, MedX, or Eagle equipment. (From Graves JE, Webb D, Pollock ML, et al: *Int J Sports Med* 1991; 10:43. Used by permission.)

ments in the dynamic training weight noted for those groups that exercised without pelvic stabilization were likely due to strength increases in the gluteus and hamstring muscles.

An important question concerning both the primary prevention and rehabilitative settings is how much exercise training is necessary to maintain strength once it has been attained? It is generally known for both aerobic endurance and strength training exercise that it takes less to maintain fitness than it does to attain it.[28, 34] The key factor is not to stop altogether (detrain). It appears that frequency and duration of training can be greatly reduced, and as long as intensity of effort is maintained, a significant reduction in fitness will not occur. For example, Graves et al.[28] trained 50 healthy volunteers aged 25 ± 5 years two to three times per week for up to 18 weeks. Training consisted of one set of seven to ten repetitions of bilateral knee extension exercise to fatigue. Subjects were then placed into groups who stopped or reduced their training to 2 or 1 day/week for 12 weeks. The detraining group lost 68% of the IM strength that they gained during training, while the groups that completed at least one quality workout per week maintained their strength.

Although the above-mentioned study has important implications for long-term fitness and rehabilitation programs, how might it relate to the lumbar extensor muscles that need to be exercised only 1 day per week? To investigate this question Tucci et al.[86] trained 50 volunteers for 10 to 12 weeks with isolated lumbar extension exercise. After this training period, subjects were randomized into a group that detrained and into two groups that reduced their training to once every 2 weeks or once every 4 weeks for 12 weeks. Training consisted of one set of 8 to 12 repetitions of dynamic variable-resistance exercise to fatigue. The detraining group lost strength significantly through the full ROM (Fig 22–17). Both reduced training groups were able to maintain their lumbar extension strength with only a nonsignificant trend for the group training once every 4 weeks to decrease in strength from 0 to 24 degrees of ROM (see Figs 22–18 and 22–19). The important finding of this study is that once a participant/patient reaches a certain strength level in a preventive/rehabilitative program, he can maintain most if not all of his strength by returning to the clinic just one time per month. This would be considered cost-effective for long-term management of LBP and feasible for patients who have busy schedules or who live in an outlying area to the clinic.

The importance of accurate full-range testing was evident in the reduced-training study because if only peak torque were known, interpretation of the results would have been limited. For example, the detraining group lost 89% of their previous gains in their strongest position but were able to maintain approximately 60% at their weakest point.

Because reduced training frequency has important implications for long-term preventive and rehabilitative programs, more research is necessary to evaluate lesser frequencies of training and to conduct experiments over a longer time period. Even so, because of the trend for a decrease in strength in the last 24 degrees of ROM for the group training once every 4 weeks, it can probably be considered the minimal threshold of training necessary for full-ROM strength maintenance of the lumbar muscles (Fig 22–19).

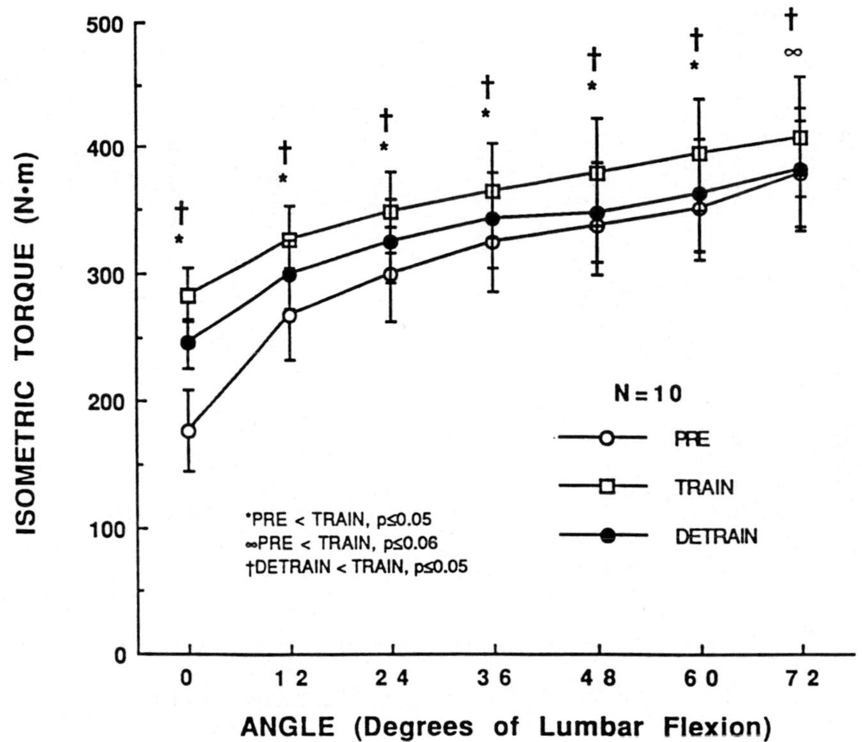

FIG 22–17.
Isometric torque (newton-meters) following 12 weeks of training *(TRAIN)* and 12 weeks of detraining *(DETRAIN)*. *PRE* = pretraining results. (From Tucci JT, Carpenter DM, Pollock ML, et al: *Spine,* in press. Used by permission.)

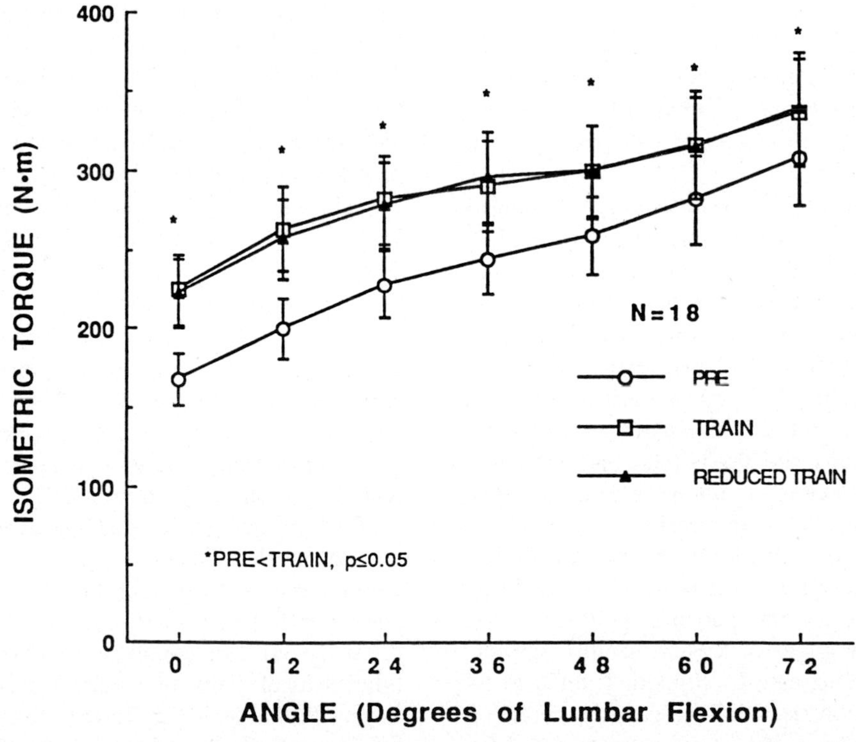

FIG 22–18.
Isometric torque (newton-meters) following 12 weeks of training *(TRAIN)* and 12 weeks of reduced training one time every 2 weeks. *PRE* = pretraining results. (From Tucci JT, Carpenter DM, Pollock ML, et al: *Spine,* in press. Used by permission.)

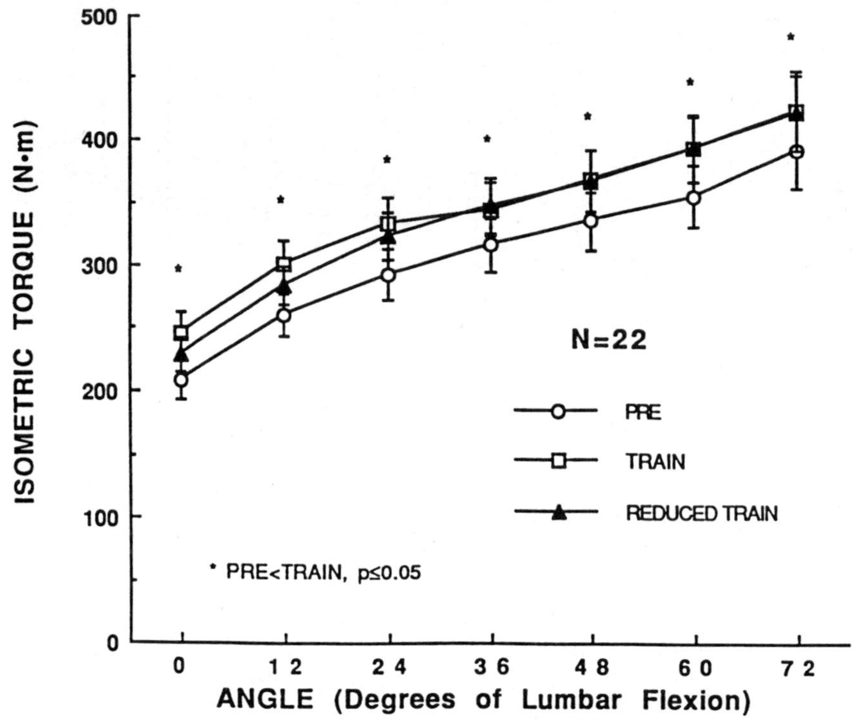

FIG 22–19.
Isometric torque (newton-meters) following 12 weeks of training *(TRAIN)* and 12 weeks of reduced training one time every 4 weeks. *PRE* = pretraining results. (From Tucci JT, Carpenter DM, Pollock ML, et al: *Spine*, in press. Used by permission.)

Exercise Training for Patients With Chronic Low Back Pain

Most of the preceeding information on exercise training has been with healthy subjects without LBP. This section will describe our training studies with patients with chronic LBP.

Our first group experience with chronic LBP included 12 subjects (aged 41 ± 3 years) who had mild chronic LBP for at least 2 years.[50] The purpose of the study was to determine the effects of variable-resistance training of the isolated lumbar extension muscles on the development of muscular strength and reduction of symptoms of chronic LBP. The evaluation included the seven-angle IM isolated lumbar extension test, a clinical examination, and the assessment of symptoms by the Prolo pain and Oswestry LBP disability questionnaires. Training consisted of one set of 10 to 15 repetitions of variable-resistance lumbar extension exercise 1 day per week for 12 weeks. Post-training adjusted values showed that IM torque increased significantly at all angles for the patients with LBP (Fig 22–20). A comparison group of normal healthy subjects made a slightly higher increase in strength from 0 to 24 degrees of lumbar flexion than did the patients. Training weights increased from 60 to 101 kg for patients with LBP and 68 to 110 kg for the subjects with no LBP.

The important finding of this study was the fact that LBP decreased significantly with training in patients with chronic LBP: 10 of 12 patients reported reduced functional status initially and 5 of 12 post-training (Prolo score), and the average Oswestry disability rating was 8% initially and 1% post-training. Thus, patients with mild chronic LBP may not present with lower-than-normal lumbar extension strength and appear to respond to resistance training in a similar fashion as normal subjects. More importantly, symptoms of LBP were decreased with specific training of the lumbar extensor muscles.

Even though the above-mentioned study showed promising results for relief of symptoms in patients with LBP, the study included a small sample and lacked the sophistication of having a randomized control group. Thus, a randomized clinical trial was designed and implemented with 55 patients with chronic LBP.[74] Patients ranged from 22 to 65 years of age, and the average duration of pain was 65 months. Forty-six percent of the sample were not working due to LBP, and 35% reported workmen's compensation as their primary income. Prior to participation in the study, patients completed the West Haven–Yale Multidimensional Pain Inventory (WHYMPI) and Sickness Impact Profile and were tested for isolated IM lumbar extension strength. Subjects were than randomly assigned to a 10-week exercise group (n = 31) or a wait-list control

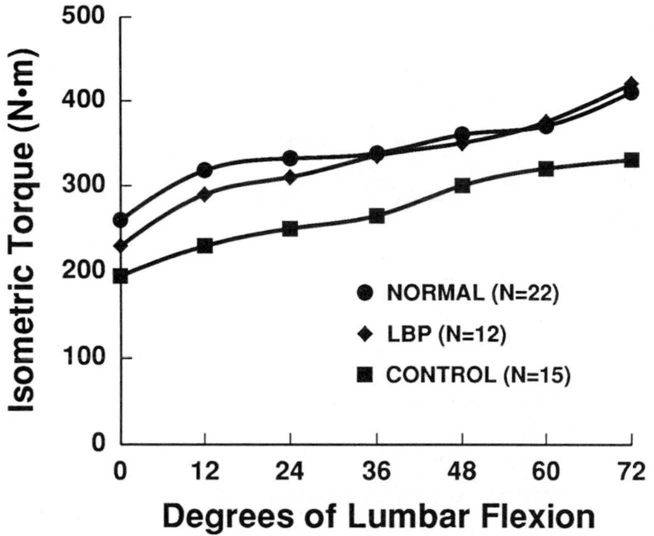

FIG 22–20.
Adjusted post-training isometric torques for the control group, normal group, and group with chronic low back pain *(LBP)*. Training was once per week for 12 weeks. Control is less than normal and patients with LBP at all angles tested ($P \leq .05$). (Data from MacMillan M, Pollock ML, Graves JE, et al: Effect of lumbar extensor resistance training on symptomatology and strength of patients with mild chronic low back pain (unpublished data). Department of Orthopaedics and the Center for Exercise Science, University of Florida, 1988.

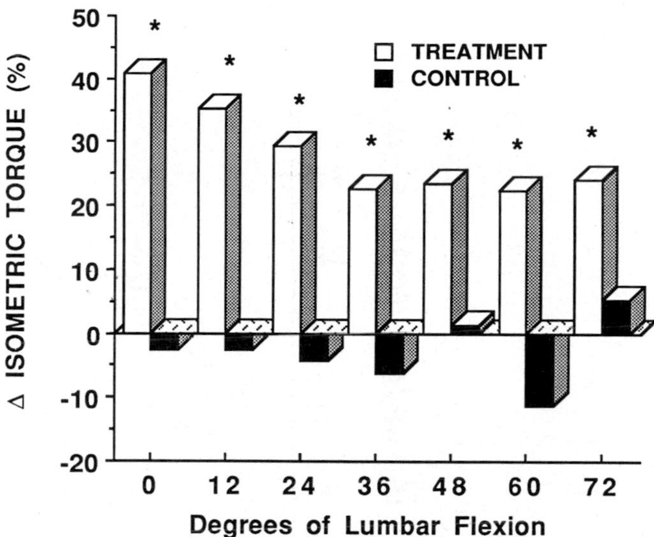

FIG 22–21.
Data show the percent change in isometric torque for a control and treatment group from 0 to 72 degrees of lumbar flexion. The treatment group performed lumbar extensor exercise once per week for 12 weeks. (Data from Risch SV, Norvell NK, Pollock ML, et al: *Spine,* in press.)

group (n = 23). The exercise group trained with variable-resistance dynamic exercise two times per week for 4 weeks followed by one time per week for 6 weeks for a total of 10 weeks. The control group did not train and were instructed not to change their life-style.

There were no pretreatment differences between groups on measures of strength, prior medical history, self-reported pain, psychological distress, stress, or activity levels. Post-treatment results showed that the exercise group increased IM strength through a full ROM while the control group did not change (Fig 22–21). Self-reported pain was measured by a subscale of WHYMPI that ranged from 0 for no pain to 6 for severe pain. The exercise group reported a significant decrease in pain as compared with the control group as well as decreases in scores on the physical and psychosocial subscale of the Sickness Impact Profile. Thus, the findings from this randomized clinical trial support the results from our earlier study, i.e., increased full-range strength and decreased symptoms in the exercise group, as well as an increase in physical and psychosocial function in the exercise group.

Since progressive resistance exercise training has been shown to be so effective in increasing isolated lumbar extension strength in both primary and rehabilitative programs and because many patients with LBP have limited range of lumbar motion, there was a need to evaluate the influence of limited-ROM exercise training on the development of full-ROM lumbar extension strength. Therefore, 58 healthy men and women (aged 30 ± 11 years) were randomly assigned to one of three training groups or to a control group that did not train.[29] Training was conducted one time per week for 12 weeks and consisted of one set of 8 to 12 repetitions of variable-resistance lumbar extension exercise to volitional fatigue. One group trained from 72 to 36 degrees of lumbar flexion (A), one from 36 to 0 degrees of lumbar flexion (B), and one at full ROM from 72 to 0 degrees of lumbar flexion (AB). The seven-angle isolated IM lumbar extension test described earlier was used to evaluate the training response. Post-training adjusted scores showed that all training groups increased in lumbar extension torque at all angles measured vs. the controls (Fig 22–22). Also, the greatest increases in torque were found for groups A and B in their respective ranges of training. These results are in agreement with research concerning the specificity of exercise and its effect on improvement of muscular strength.[27, 38, 58] For example, the data presented earlier on elite water-skiers showed a disproportionate strength curve in the latter half of the ROM (see Fig 22–6).[46] This was produced by specific limited-range heavy work near full extension.

The above findings also indicated that limited ROM lumbar extension training through a 36-degree ROM was effective for developing strength in an adjacent range of lumbar extension. These findings are in agreement with other investigators who have shown an extension of the training effect in an adjacent untrained area.[23, 27, 41, 48]

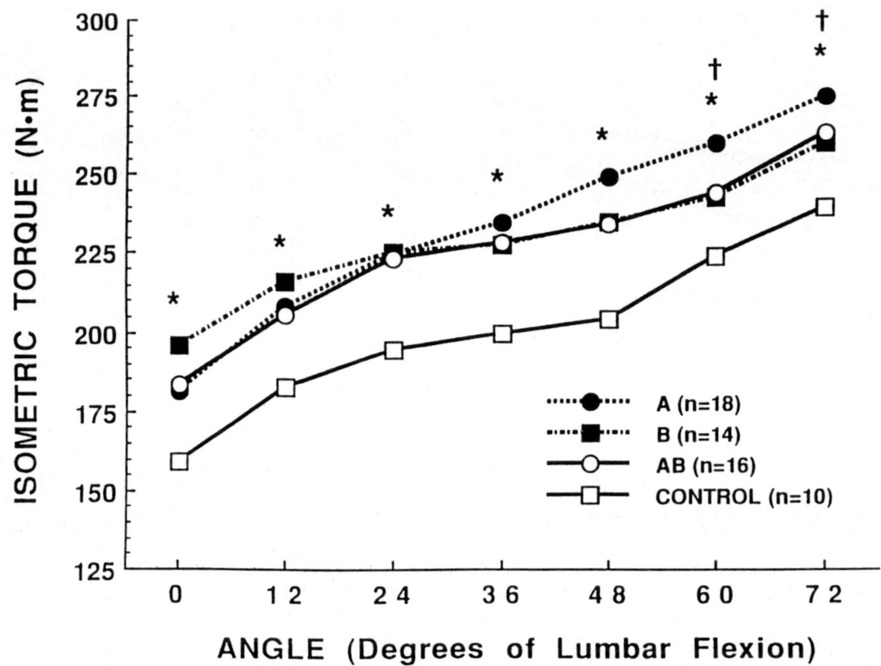

FIG 22–22.
Adjusted post-training isometric torque values (newton-meters) for the limited-ROM training *(A* and *B),* full-ROM training *(AB),* and control groups. Group A trained through a ROM limited between 72 and 36 degrees of lumbar flexion. Group *B* trained through a ROM limited between 36 and 0 degrees of lumbar flexion. Group *AB* trained through a 72-degree range of lumbar motion. *Control is less than *A, B, AB* ($P \leq .05$). †*A* is greater than *B* ($P \leq .05$). (From Graves J, Pollock M, Leggett S, et al: *Med Sci Sports Exerc* 1992; 24:128–133. Used by permission.)

Since many patients with LBP have limited ROM in the lumbar spine, the above findings have important implications for rehabilitation programs. Patients who are limited in ROM due to muscle weakness may benefit beyond their range of training and increase ROM. Thus, conservative progression in ROM will not compromise strength gain in the adjacent ROM not exercised.

REFERENCES

1. Atha J: Strengthening muscle. *Exerc Sport Sci Rev* 1981; 9:1–73.
2. *Back Injuries: Cost, Causes, Cases, and Prevention*. Washington DC, Bureau of National Affairs, 1988.
3. Battie M, Bigos S, Fisher L, et al: Isometric lifting strength as a predictor of industrial back pain reports. *Spine* 1989; 14:851–856.
4. Bemben M, Grump K, Massey B: Assessment of technical accuracy of the Cybex II isokinetic dynamometer and analog recording system. *J Orthop Sports Phys Ther* 1988; 10:12–17.
5. Berger RA: Application of research findings in progressive resistance exercise to physical therapy. *J Assoc Phys Ment Rehabil* 1965; 19:200–203.
6. Braith RW, Graves JE, Pollock ML, et al: Comparison of two versus three days per week of variable resistance training during 10 and 18 week programs. *Int J Sports Med* 1989; 10:450–459.
7. Carpenter DM, Graves JE, Pollock ML, et al: Effect of 12 and 20 weeks of resistance training on lumbar extension torque production. *Phys Ther* 1991; 71:580–588.
8. Carpenter D, Leggett S, Pollock M, et al: Quantitative assessment of isometric lumbar extension net muscular torque. *Med Sci Sports Exerc* 1991; 23(suppl):65.
9. Chaffin DB, Herrin GD, Keyserling WM: Preemployment strength testing. *J Occup Med* 1978; 67:403–408.
10. Chapman AE: The mechanical properties of human muscle. *Exerc Sport Sci Rev* 1985; 13:443–501.
11. Colletti LA, Edwards J, Gordon L, et al: The effects of muscle building exercise on bone mineral density of the radius, spine, and hip in young men. *Calcif Tissue Int* 1989; 45:12–14.
12. Costill DL, Coyle EF, Fink WF, et al: Adaptations in skeletal muscle following strength training. *J Appl Physiol* 1979; 46:96–99.
13. deVries HA: *Physiology of Exercise for Physical Education and Athletics,* ed 4. Dubuque, Iowa, WC Brown, 1986, p 14.
14. Dudley GA: Metabolic consequences of resistive-type exercise. *Med Sci Sports Exerc* 1988; 20(suppl):158–161.
15. Edstrom L: Selective atrophy of red muscle fibers in the quadriceps in long-standing knee joint dysfunction. Injuries to the anterior cruciate ligament. *J Neurol Sci* 1970; 11:551–558.
16. Edwards R: Human muscle function and fatigue, in Porter R, Whelan J (eds): *Human Muscle Function and Fatigue: Physiological Mechanisms*. London, Pitman Medical, 1981.
17. Edwards RHT, Jones DA: Diseases of skeletal muscle, in

Peachey LD (ed): *Handbook of Physiology,* section 10, *Skeletal Muscle.* Bethesda, Md, American Physiological Society, 1983, pp 633–672.
18. Farfan H: Muscular mechanism of the lumbar spine and the position of power and efficiency. *Orthop Clin North Am* 1975; 6:135–144.
19. Fillyaw M, Bevins T, Fernandez L: Importance of correcting isokinetic peak torque for the effect of gravity when calculating knee flexor to extensor muscle ratios. *Phys Ther* 1986; 66:23–31.
20. Fleck SJ, Kraemer WJ: *Designing Resistance Training Programs.* Champaign, Ill, Human Kinetics Books, 1987.
21. Fulton M, Jones G, Pollock M, et al: Rehabilitation and testing . . . conservative treatment for lower-back and cervical problems. *Rehabil Management* 1990; 3:2–40.
22. Fulton M, Pollock M, Leggett S, et al: Effect of upper body mass on the measurement of isometric lumbar extension strength. Presented at the Orthopaedic Rehabilitation Association Conference, San Antonio, Tex, 1990.
23. Gardner GW: Specificity of strength changes of the exercised and nonexercised limb following isometric training. *Res Q* 1963; 34:98–101.
24. Graves JE, Holmes BL, Leggett SH, et al: Single versus multiple set dynamic and isometric lumbar extension training. Presented at the World Confederation for Physical Therapy 11th International Congress, London, 1991, pp 1340–1342.
25. Graves JE, Pollock ML, Carpenter DM, et al: Quantitative assessment of full range-of-motion isometric lumbar extension strength. *Spine* 1990; 15:289–294.
26. Graves JE, Pollock ML, Foster D, et al: Effect of training frequency and specificity on isometric lumbar extension strength. *Spine* 1990; 15:504–509.
27. Graves JE, Pollock ML, Jones AE, et al: Specificity of limited range of motion variable resistance training. *Med Sci Sports Exerc* 1989; 21:84–89.
28. Graves JE, Pollock ML, Leggett SH, et al: Effect of reduced training frequency on muscular strength. *Int J Sports Med* 1988; 5:316–319.
29. Graves J, Pollock M, Leggett S, et al: Limited range-of-motion lumbar extension strength training. *Med Sci Sports Exerc* 1992; 24:128–133.
30. Graves JE, Webb D, Pollock ML, et al: Effect of training with pelvic stabilization on lumbar extension strength (abstract). *Int J Sports Med* 1991; 10:403.
31. Hakkinen K, Komi PV: Effect of different combined concentric and eccentric muscle work regimens on maximal strength development. *J Hum Move Studies* 1981; 7:33–44.
32. Herzog W: The relation between the resultant moments at a joint and the moments measured by an isokinetic dynamometer. *J Biomech* 1988; 21:5–12.
33. Hettinger T: *Physiology of Strength.* Springfield, Ill, Charles C Thomas, 1961.
34. Hickson RC, Foster C, Pollock ML, et al: Reduced training intensities and loss of aerobic power, endurance and cardiac growth. *J Appl Physiol* 1985; 58:492–499.
35. Hill A: The heat of shortening and the dynamic constants of muscle. Presented at the Royal Society of London, 1938, pp 136–195.
36. Holbrook TL, Grazier K, Kelsey JL, et al: *The Frequency of Occurrence, Impact and Cost of Selected Musculoskeletal Conditions in the United States.* Chicago, American Academy of Orthopaedic Surgeons, 1984.
37. Ikai M, Steinhaus AH: Some factors modifying the expression of human strength. *J Appl Physiol* 1961; 16:157–163.
38. Jones A, Pollock M, Graves J, et al: *The Lumbar Spine.* Santa Barbara, Calif, Sequoia Communications, 1988.
39. Kelsey JL, White AA, Pastides H, et al: The impact of musculoskeletal disorders on the populations of the U.S. *J Bone Joint Surg [Am]* 1979; 61:959–964.
40. Kishino N, Mayer T, Gatchel J, et al: Quantification of lumbar function. Part 4: Isometric and isokinetic lifting simulation in normal subjects and low-back dysfunction patients. *Spine* 1985; 10:921–927.
41. Knapik JJ, Mawdsley RH, Rammos NV: Angular specificity and test mode specificity of isometric and isokinetic strength training. *J Orthop Sports Phys Ther* 1983; 5:58–65.
42. Knapik JJ, Wright JE, Mawdsley RH, et al: Isometric, isotonic, and isokinetic torque variations in four muscle groups through a range of joint motion. *Phys Ther* 1983; 63:938–947.
43. Kraus H, Nagler W: Evaluation of an exercise program for back pain. *Am Fam Physician* 1983; 28:153–158.
44. Kulig K, Andrews J, Hay J: Human strength curves. *Exerc Sport Sci Rev* 1984; 12:417–466.
45. Lee C: The use of exercise and muscle testing in the rehabilitation of spinal disorders. *Clin Sports Med* 1986; 5:271–276.
46. Leggett SH, Pollock ML, Graves JE, et al: Physiological evaluation of elite professional waterskiers. Presented at the International Congress on Sports Medicine and Human Performance, Vancouver, Canada, 1990.
47. Lindboe CF, Platou CS: Disuse atrophy of human skeletal muscle. *Acta Neuropathol* 1982; 56:241–244.
48. Lindh M: Increase in muscle strength from isometric quadriceps exercises at different knee angles. *Scand J Med* 1979; 11:33–36.
49. MacDougall JD, Elder GCB, Sale DG, et al: Effects of strength training and immobilization on human muscle fibers. *Eur J Appl Physiol* 1980; 43:25–34.
50. MacMillan M, Pollock ML, Graves JE, et al: Effect of lumbar extensor resistance training on symptomatology and strength of patients with mild chronic low back pain (unpublished data). Department of Orthopaedics and the Center for Exercise Science, University of Florida, Gainesville, 1988.
51. Marras J, King A, Joynt R: Measurements of loads on the lumbar spine under isometric and isokinetic conditions. *Spine* 1984; 9:176–188.
52. Mayer L, Greenberg B: Measurement of the strength of trunk muscles. *J Bone Joint Surg* 1942; 4:842–856.
53. Mayer T, Gatchel R: *Functional Restoration for Spinal Disorders.* Philadelphia, Lea & Febiger, 1988.
54. Mayer T, Gatchel R, Kishino N, et al: Objective assess-

ment of spine function following industrial injury. A prospective study with comparison group and one-year follow-up. *Spine* 1985; 10:482–493.
55. Mayer T, Smith S, Keeley J, et al: Quantification of lumbar function. Part 2: Sagittal plane trunk strength in chronic low-back pain subjects. *Spine* 1985; 10:765–772.
56. Mayer TG, Gatchel RJ, Mayer H, et al: A prospective two-year study of functional restoration in industrial low back injury. *JAMA* 1987; 258:1763–1767.
57. Mayhew T, Rothstein J: Measurement of muscle performance with instruments, in Rothstein J (ed): *Measurement in Physical Therapy*. New York, Churchill Livingstone, 1985, pp 57–102.
58. McArdle W, Katch F, Katch V: *Exercise Physiology: Energy, Nutrition, and Human Performance,* ed 3. Philadelphia, Lea & Febiger, 1991.
59. McNeill T, Warwick D, Anderson GBJ, et al: Trunk strengths in attempted flexion, extension and lateral bending in healthy subjects and patients with low back disorders. *Spine* 1980; 5:529–538.
60. Meuller EA, Rohmert W: Die geschwindigkeit der muskelkraftzunahme bei isometrischem training. *Arbeitsphysiologie* 1963; 19:403–419.
61. Moritani T, deVries HA: Neural factors versus hypertrophy in the time course of muscle strength gain. *Am J Phys Med* 1979; 58:115–130.
62. Murray D: Optimal filtering of constant velocity torque data. *Med Sci Sports Exerc* 1986; 18:603–611.
63. Murray DA, Harrison E: Constant velocity dynamometer: An appraisal using mechanical loading. *Med Sci Sports Exerc* 1986; 18:612–624.
64. Musacchia XJ, Steffen JM, Fell RD: Disuse atrophy of skeletal muscle, animal models. *Exerc Sport Sci Rev* 1988; 16:61–87.
65. Nachemson AL, Lindh M: Measurement of abdominal and back muscle strength with and without low back pain. *Scand J Rehabil Med* 1969; 1:60–69.
66. Nelson S, Duncan P: Correction of isokinetic torque recordings for the effect of gravity. *Phys Ther* 1983; 63:674–676.
67. Nisell R, Ericson M, Nemeth G: Tibiofemoral joint forces during isokinetic knee extension. *Am J Sports Med* 1989; 17:49–54.
68. Nordgren B, Scheile R, Linroth K: Evaluation and prediction of back pain during military field service. *Scand J Rehabil Med* 1980; 12:1–7.
69. Osternig LR, Bates BT, James SL: Isokinetic and isometric force relationships. *Arch Phys Med Rehabil* 1977; 58:254–257.
70. Peterson C, Amundsen L, Schendel M: Comparison of the effectiveness of two pelvic stabilization systems on pelvic movement during maximal isometric trunk extension and flexion muscle contractions. *Phys Ther* 1987; 67:534–539.
71. Pollock M, Graves J, Leggett S, et al: Accuracy of counterweighting to account for upper body mass in testing lumbar extension strength. *Med Sci Sports Exerc* 1991; 23(suppl):66.
72. Pollock ML, Leggett SH, Graves JE, et al: Effect of resistance training on lumbar extension strength. *Am J Sports Med* 1989; 17:624–629.
73. Pollock ML, Wilmore JH: *Exercise in Health and Disease: Evaluation and Prescription for Prevention and Rehabilitation,* ed 2. Philadelphia, WB Saunders, 1990.
74. Risch SV, Norvell NK, Pollock ML, et al: Lumbar strengthening in chronic low back pain: Physiological and psychological benefits. *Spine,* in press.
75. Sale DG: Neural adaptation to resistance training. *Med Sci Sports Exerc* 1988; 20(suppl):135–145.
76. Sapega A, Nicholas J, Sokolow D, et al: The nature of torque "overshoot" in Cybex isokinetic dynamometry. *Med Sci Sports Exerc* 1982; 14:368–375.
77. Smidt G, Herring T, Amundsen L, et al: Assessment of abdominal and back extensor function: Quantitative approach and results for chronic low-back patients. *Spine* 1983; 8:211–219.
78. Staron RS, Hikida RS, Hagerman FC: Reevaluation of human muscle fast-twitch subtypes evidence for a continuum. *Histochemistry* 1981; 78:33–39.
79. Stone M: Implications for connective tissue and bone alterations resulting from resistance exercise training. *Med Sci Sports Exerc* 1988; 20(suppl):162–168.
80. Stone M, O'Bryant H: *Weight Training: A Scientific Approach*. Minneapolis, Bellweather Press, 1987.
81. Tesch PA: Skeletal muscle adaptations consequent to long-term heavy resistance exercise. *Med Sci Sports Exerc* 1988; 20(suppl):132–134.
82. Tesch PA, Komi PV, Hakkinen K: Enzymatic adaptations consequent to long-term strength training. *Int J Sports Med* 1987; 8(suppl):66–69.
83. Tesch PA, Thorsson A, Kaiser P: Muscle capillary supply and fiber type characteristics in weight and power lifters. *J Appl Physiol* 1984; 56:35–38.
84. Tipton CM, James SL, Mergner W, et al: Influence of exercise on the strength of the medial collateral knee ligaments of dogs. *Am J Physiol* 1970; 218:894–901.
85. Tomanek RJ, Cooper RR: Ultrastructural changes in tenotomized fast- and slow-twitch muscle fibers. *J Anat* 1972; 113:409–424.
86. Tucci JT, Carpenter DM, Pollock ML, et al: Effect of reduced training frequency and detraining on lumbar extension strength. *Spine,* in press.
87. Wakim K, Gersten J, Elkins E, et al: Objective recording of muscle strength. *Arch Phys Med* 1950; 31:90–100.
88. Wescott W: *Strength Fitness: Physiological Principles and Training Techniques*. ed 3. Dubuque, Iowa, WC Brown, 1991.
89. Winter D, Wells R, Orr G: Errors in the use of isokinetic dynamometers. *Eur J Appl Physiol* 1981; 46:397–408.

23

Neural Tissue: Spinal Cord, Conus Medullaris, Cauda Equina Nerve Root

Eric J. Wall, M.D., and Steven R. Garfin, M.D.

Spine neural tissue has little mechanical function in comparison to the surrounding bones, ligaments, discs, and muscles. However, the spinal cord and nerve roots do undergo biomechanical stresses during normal human activity. The spinal cord stretches with spine flexion and relaxes with spine extension. In addition, upper- and lower-extremity motion can transmit tension to the spinal nerve roots. More severe neural stress is involved in spinal column trauma, disc protrusion, and the tethered cord syndrome.

Many investigators have studied the pathophysiology of spinal tissue injury. Ischemia, edema, hemorrhage, and axon/myelin degeneration are involved in the injury cascade.[2] Relatively little is known, however, about the biomechanics of neural tissue during injury or repair. The following is a summary of current knowledge on the biomechanics of the neural elements of the spine with regard to normal and pathologic stresses.

SPINAL CORD

The major structural component of the spinal cord is its dural envelope. The dura is fixed to the surrounding spinal canal at the occiput and sacrum and, segmentally, at the intervertebral foramen. Strong fibrous connections exist between the ventral thecal sac and the vertebral bodies.[25] Twenty-one pairs of dentate ligaments anchor the spinal cord to the surrounding dura from just cephalad to the first cervical roots down to the last thoracic or first lumbar roots.[1] Cerebrospinal fluid surrounds the spinal cord. A layer of epidural fat and veins encase the dura within the bony spinal column.

Brieg and Marions reported that spinal cord tension increases with spine flexion and relaxes with extension.[5, 6] They believed that neurologic symptoms could be altered through a change in spinal neural tension. and described a "thrust effect" in which any spinal canal encroachment becomes more significant as the longitudinal neural tissue tension increases. Tencer and colleagues showed that axial distraction of the spinal column by as little as 5.2 mm significantly increased the contact pressure between the spinal cord dura and bone in the canal.[32] In vivo studies using enhanced computer tomographic and magnetic resonance scans have confirmed structural changes in the spinal cord with spine motion. Stevens et al. noted a change in cervical spinal cord length with flexion and extension on human enhanced computed tomographic scans and myelograms.[27] The cervical spinal cord cross-sectional area decreased from 80.3 to 70.5 mm^2 between scans in extension and scans in flexion, thus indicating that the cord narrows as it stretches during flexion. Condon and Hadley quantified cervical spinal cord deformation by using dynamic magnetic resonance scanning.[9] Curve-fitting computer programs allowed for in vivo measurement of cord deformation, angulation, and width.

The biomechanics of acute spinal cord injury are relatively unexplored. Autopsy findings in 48 patients with cervical spine trauma indicated that only 3 patients had total cord tissue disruption and many of the patients with clinical evidence of total cord lesions had incomplete contusion and parenchymal hemorrhages.[4] Spinal cord injury usually involves a transient contusion of the spinal cord at the time of injury, which triggers a cascade of progressive damage.[15] Persistent disc or bone fragments in the canal can add to the original injury. Using an experimental spinal cord injury model in which weights were dropped onto an exposed spinal cord, Hung and associates demonstrated a pressure wave in the cerebrospinal fluid that propagated above and below the site of impact.[13] When the spinal fluid was released from the dural sac prior to impact, deformation of the spinal cord was found to increase, which suggests a protective role for the cerebrospinal fluid. Closed methods of spinal cord injury (with an intact spinal column) required more than 20 times the amount of momentum to produce cord injury equivalent to the open weight-drop methods.[7]

A pseudo–Young's modulus for in vivo animal spinal cords tested under tension is reported to be 22 newtons/cm^2.[7] This modulus varied with the history of loading and deformation characteristics, which suggests a viscoelastic behavior of spinal cord tissue. Motor function recovery was seen after transient spinal cord elongations of up to 50%.

The failure tensile stress of the dura was found to be essentially uniform along the cord at about 28 newtons/cm^2, as were failure strain (34%) and dural thickness (0.27 mm).[31] This elastic behavior of the dura was felt to be important, given that cervical flexion can increase dural strain up to 20%. When the dura reaches its circumferential elastic limit, it may confine a swollen post-traumatic spinal cord and lead to the equivalent of a spinal cord compartment syndrome.[1] Scarff reported on the intraoperative appearance of the spinal cord in a patient with an acute spinal cord injury.[21] He stated that "the dura was opened and there was an instantaneous and violent rupture of the cord and extrusion of it through the dural incision." In another patient, "fully 2 in. of the cord was thus 'blown out' within a few seconds" after opening the dura. In contrast, Shapiro et al. found that tissue pressure adjacent to a spinal cord weight-drop impact site was less than 10 mm Hg above resting levels within the first 24 hours after injury.[23] Despite the latter study, however, most authors feel that the dura acts as a restricting membrane, which may become significant during spinal cord edema.

CONUS MEDULLARIS

The conus medullaris is the tapering end of the spinal cord and is located at the thoracolumbar junction of the spinal column. The lower portion of the spinal cord is fixed by the lowest pair of dentate ligaments, and the filum terminale connects the tip of the conus to the fascia over the dorsum of the coccyx. The roots of the conus medullaris are held in a fixed relation to one another by a thin web of arachnoid tissue that probably has very little mechanical strength.[33]

Little biomechanical data exist regarding the conus despite the high number of traumatic injuries to this area. Animal experiments on the tethered spinal cord syndrome have shown that the filum terminale possesses far greater extensibility than any spinal cord segments.[30] It may function as a buffer in preventing the cord from overstretching. The lumbar, sacral, and coccygeal segments elongate under traction only below the attachment of the lowest pair of dentate ligaments. When the dentate ligaments are sectioned, the spinal cord at the involved level shows greater elongation.

CAUDA EQUINA/NERVE ROOTS

The cauda equina consists of the intrathecal nerve roots below the conus medullaris and extends from approximately the L1–2 intervertebral level to the sacrum. These roots are held together by invaginations of pia and arachnoid into an organized pattern and are bathed in a column of cerebrospinal fluid. As each lumbar nerve root exits the spinal canal, it hooks around the inferior margin of the subjacent pedicle and enters the intervertebral foramen[8] (Fig 23–1). The dura ensheathes the exiting root and fuses with it at the level of the dorsal root ganglion to become a tough fibrous capsule.[18]

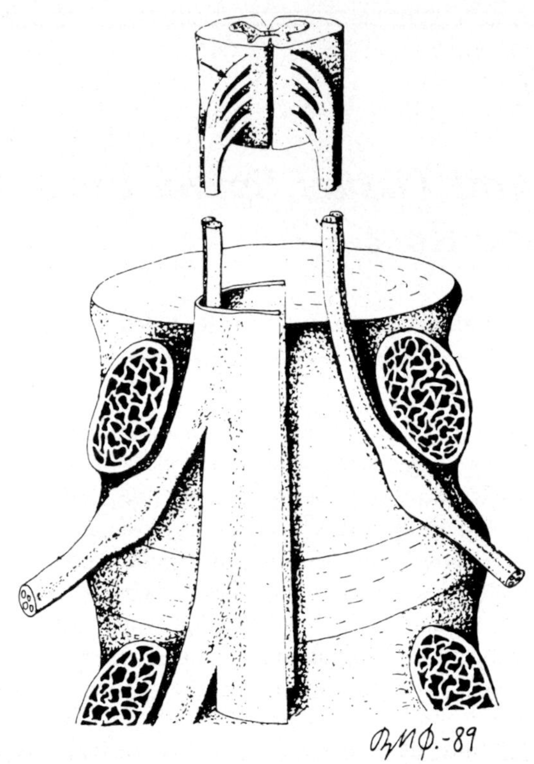

FIG 23–1.
Posterior view of nerve roots exiting the thecal sac. Each nerve root hooks around the subjacent pedicle. The dura ensheathes each root and fuses with it at the level of the dorsal root ganglion.

The cauda equina roots occupy approximately 50% of the thecal sac cross-sectional area, which allows for significant canal compromise before neural impingement occurs. Schönström and Hansson observed that cerebrospinal fluid pressure did not begin to rise until the human cauda equina was constricted to 45% of its normal cross-sectional area.[22] This pressure increased to 50 mm Hg with narrowing down to 37% of the normal area and increased to 100 mm Hg with constriction to 33% of the normal area. Delamarter and associates[10] studied spinal stenosis in an animal model and found significant nerve dysfunction at constriction greater than 50% of cauda equina cross-sectional area. More damage was observed in the extradural nerve roots than the intradural nerve roots, which suggests a protective role of the thecal sac for the cauda equina nerve roots.

Olmarker reported that direct compression of cauda equina nerve roots with pressures of 50 to 100 mm Hg leads to changes in intraneural blood flow, vascular permeability, axonal transport, and nerve conduction.[18] Rydevik and colleagues feel that one mechanism for nerve compression injury is related to the pressure gradient that develops between the compressed and noncompressed parts of the nerve, the so-called edge effect[19] (Fig 23–2). Tissue displacement is largest at the edges of the compressed nerve segment and leads to pronounced injury of nerve fibers and intraneural vessels at that location. Sharpless demonstrated that spinal nerve roots exiting the thecal sac proper acquire a structural feature that protects them from compression effects before they enter the intervertebral foramen, but the dural sheath did not appear to play an important role.[24]

Brieg and Marions showed that the cauda equina nerve roots elongate with flexion of the cervical spine and relax into a wavy pattern with neck extension.[6] They reported that neural tissue does not slide in the canal during spinal motion but rather adapts to length changes by passive deformation. Inman and Saunders measured the total change in length of the spinal canal from full flexion to complete extension at 7 cm, thus suggesting that the neural elements must undergo considerable in vivo motion.[14]

As the nerve root exits the thecal sac proper, a layer of dura envelops the nerve root before it enters the intervertebral foramen. Inman and Saunders felt that the spinal nerve in the intervertebral foramen was relatively free, being attached to the surrounding skeletal structures only by fine areolar tissue.[14] Consequently, they noted a pistoning of the nerve root within the foramen of up to 2 to 5 mm with spine flexion and extension that was most pronounced at the upper lumbar levels. Tension on the sciatic nerve produced up to 7 mm of root motion within the foramen of the L4 through S2 nerve roots.

Other authors disagree and find substantial fibrous connections between the root sleeves and the intervertebral foramina.[17] The nerve root sheaths adhere to their respective intervertebral foramina, which serve as segmental fixation points of the spinal cord and meninges.[25] Most of the motion in the peripheral nerves is not transmitted to the spinal nerve roots because of the dampening effect of this dural fixation at the intervertebral foramen. de Peretti et al. concluded that the intervertebral foramen acts as an "almost insuperable barrier" to movements imposed from outside nerves.[11] With heavy tension on the distal spinal nerve (≥1.5 kg) they described minimal root sleeve motion, with no tension transmitted to the nerve roots enclosed within the thecal sac. Spencer and coworkers studied the fixation of lumbosacral nerve roots and found that in addition to the previously described sites of dural fixation at the occiput, the filum terminale, and the nerve root foramen, there were ventral dural attachments to the anterior wall of the spinal canal.[25] They reported that traction on the spinal nerve produced slight distal migration of the nerve in the foramen by slightly everting the tissue on the outer face of the foramen.

The pathomechanics of disc protrusion involves primarily nerve root tension forces rather than compression forces.[6] At the common site of disc protrusion, the nerve root is free to become displaced posteriorly and does not become compressed between the disc and the posterior spinal canal wall unless the herniation is large. Usually the protruding disc increases tension on the nerve root, just as the bridge on a guitar increases tension on the guitar string. Spencer et al. performed a static free-body analysis of a disc protruding on a nerve root and reported that tension on the nerve root develops to counteract the force of the protruding disc.[26] They measured contact pressures of 0.5 to 5 newtons during simulated lumbar disc protrusions.[4] They similarly measured nerve root contact pressure and found that it could be reduced with simulated disc space narrowing, thereby relieving tension in the nerve root.[26] As an aside, these researchers suggested that this could possibly be the mechanism of pain relief from chemonucleolysis.

Beel and colleagues observed that when a lumbar nerve root was pulled away from the spinal cord in an animal experiment, failure occurred at the cord-root junc-

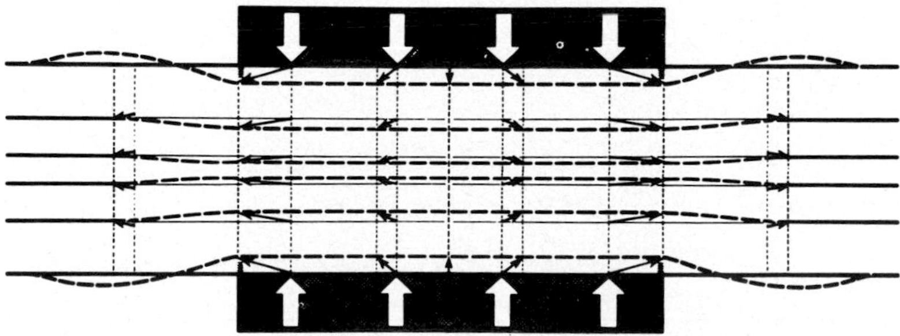

FIG 23–2.
Schematic demonstrating nerve tissue deformation secondary to circumferentially applied pressure. The pressure application leads to a bidirectional displacement of nerve tissue from the compressed nerve segment toward the noncompressed parts of the nerve. The *interrupted lines* show the positions of different tissue layers during compression. The *arrows* are vectors that indicate the displacement of nerve tissue components as a result of the applied pressure. Note that the displacement is maximal at the edges of the compressed segment.

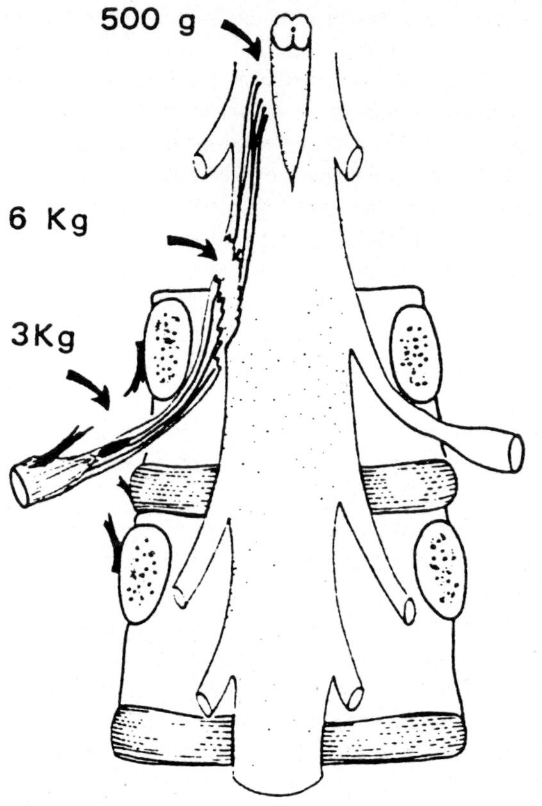

FIG 23–3.
The sites of fixation of human lumbar nerve roots and their ultimate tension before failure. Nerve roots avulse from the conus with 0.5 kg of tension, fail at the nerve root takeoff from the thecal sac with 6.0 kg of tension, and rupture at the periphery of the neural foramen with 3.0 kg of tension.

tion.[3] Cadaver studies performed by de Peretti and associates demonstrated that lumbar spinal roots avulsed from the conus with only 0.5 kg of tension. Rupture at the nerve root takeoff site from the thecal sac required 6.0 kg, and failure at the periphery of the neural foramen required 3.0 kg[11] (Fig 23–3). Kwan and colleagues compared the tensile strength of human intrathecal nerve roots with the more distal part of the foraminal nerve root with its associated dural sheath.[16] They found that the unsheathed intrathecal nerve roots failed at one fifth the load of the corresponding foraminal nerve roots. Additionally, both portions of the nerve roots were shown to have a nonlinear stress-strain curve (Fig 23–4). Little tension develops in the nerve root during the initial lengthening as shown by the large "toe region" of the curve. However, with increased lengthening of the nerve root, tension begins to develop rapidly. The large toe region probably protects the nerve root from excessive tension during the normal physiologic motion of the spine and limbs.

Spinal nerve viscoelasticity has not been quantified systematically but may be involved in a nerve root's ability to decrease tension or encroachment pressure over time. Creep is the lowering of contact pressure in a tissue after a fixed protrusion, and stress relaxation is the lowering of tension after a fixed stretch. Spencer and associates, in a model of fixed disc protrusion on a nerve root, showed a 27% lowering of contact force between the first and third trials of the experiment and a 17% decrease in contact force after 150 seconds.[26] This finding demonstrates the viscoelastic nature of neural tissue.

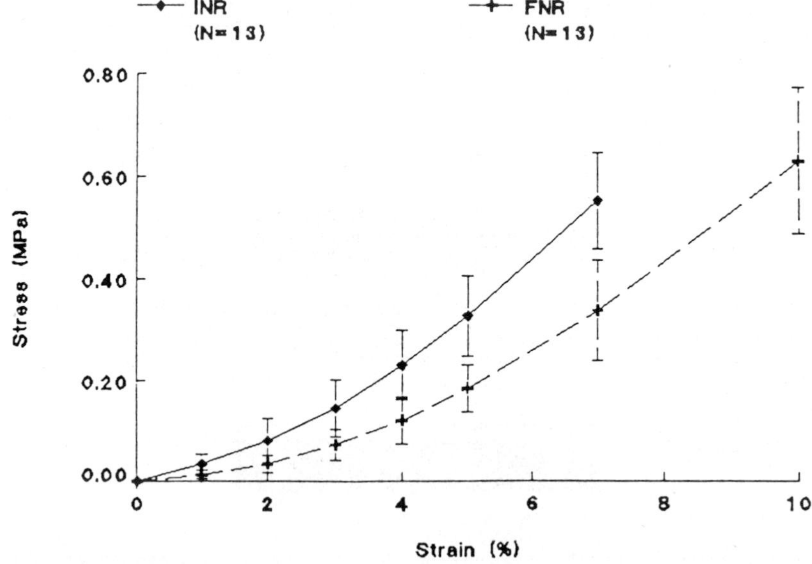

FIG 23–4.
The nonlinear stress/strain behavior of the human lumbar intrathecal *(INR)* and foraminal nerve roots *(FNR)*. Note the "toe region" where increased strain causes little increased stress.

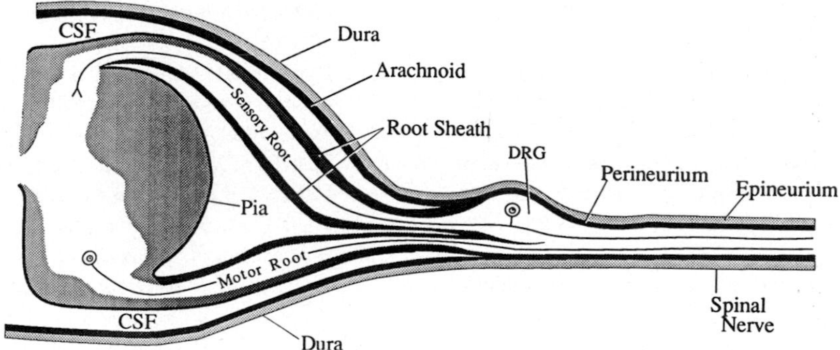

FIG 23–5.
Cross section of spinal cord with a nerve root. Thecal sac dura ensheathes the exiting nerve root and fuses with it at the level of the dorsal root ganglion *(DRG)*. Beyond the dorsal root ganglion begins the spinal nerve.

DORSAL ROOT GANGLION

The dorsal root ganglion (containing the sensory nerve cell bodies) lies in the intervertebral foramen and is enclosed by a strong capsule of dura. Rydevik et al. showed a significant elevation of endoneurial tissue pressure in the dorsal root ganglia of rats after transient mechanical compression.[20] Therefore, a "mini–compartment syndrome" may play a role in the biomechanics of dorsal root ganglia injury. Increased dorsal root ganglia tissue pressure has also been implicated in the pathogenesis of spinal stenosis neural injury and symptoms.[10]

SPINAL NERVE AND PERIPHERAL NERVES

More biomechanical information is available on the peripheral nerve than the spinal nerve root. The peripheral nerve is more amenable to study because it is longer and easier to dissect out than the spinal nerve root. The data available on the peripheral nerve have often been assumed to relate to the spinal nerve root; however, there are significant anatomic differences that probably make that assumption invalid.

The intrathecal spinal nerve roots lack a contiguous sleeve of strong connective tissue and hence float virtually naked in a bath of cerebrospinal fluid. The axons of the spinal nerve roots are enclosed in endoneurial tissue that is similar to the endoneurium of the peripheral nerves.[12] However, nerve roots contain only one fifth the collagen of the peripheral nerve.[28] Sunderland and Bradley believe that the endoneurium is the primary tissue resisting elongation of the spinal nerve root.[29] Coating the nerve roots within the cerebrospinal fluid is a thin layer of connective tissue called the "root sheath." This thin filmy layer is analogous to the pia mater that covers the spinal cord and probably has little mechanical function. As each nerve root sequentially exits the thecal sac proper, it becomes surrounded by a tough dural membrane. At the level of the dorsal root ganglion the spinal nerve root ends and becomes the spinal nerve.[18] More distally, the dura surrounding the spinal nerve slowly changes in composition to become the epineurium and perineurium of the peripheral nerve (Fig 23–5).

Animal studies reveal that peripheral nerves are ten times stronger than the spinal nerve roots under tensile loading.[3] Sunderland and Bradley mechanically tested human sacral nerve roots and found that they failed at lower loads than did peripheral nerves.[29] They attributed this to the lack of a perineurium in the roots, which provides most of the tensile strength of a peripheral nerve. Peripheral nerve axons have a triple layer of connective tissue protection: a fibrous epineurium surrounds the entire nerve, the fascicles are bound circumferentially and individually by perineurium, and the axons are covered by endoneurium. Vascular and connective tissue bundles also course throughout the epineural boundaries of a peripheral nerve to provide additional strength. In contrast, protection of the spinal nerve roots resides in the cerebrospinal fluid, the thecal sac, and the surrounding bony spinal column. Elastic limit, failure strain, viscoelasticty, nonlinear stress-strain behavior, and conduction changes with tension have been studied in the peripheral nerve, but their relevance to the spinal nerve roots and spinal nerve is unknown.

This chapter has shown that biomechanical forces are involved in normal spine motion and in many pathologic neural tissue states of the spine. More research is needed before a clear understanding of spinal cord and root injury can be appreciated. A complete biomechanical profile of the spine neural tissue will aid in the development of techniques to prevent, treat, and rehabilitate spinal injuries.

REFERENCES

1. Albin MS, White RJ: Epidemiology, physiopathology, and experimental therapeutics of acute spinal cord injury. *Crit Care Clin* 1987; 3:441–452.
2. Banik NL, Hogan EL, Hsu CY: The multimolecular cas-

cade of spinal cord injury. *Neurochem Pathol* 1987; 7:57–77.

3. Beel JA, Stodieck LS, Luttges MW: Structural properties of spinal nerve roots: Biomechanics. *Exp Neurol* 1986; 91:30–40.
4. Bohlman HH: Acute fractures and dislocations of the cervical spine: An analysis of 300 hospitalized patients and review of the literature. *J Bone Joint Surg [Am]* 1979; 61:1119–1142.
5. Breig A: Overstretching of and circumscribed pathological tension in the spinal cord—a basic cause of symptoms in cord disorders. *J Biomech* 1970; 3:7–9.
6. Breig A, Marions O: Biomechanics of the lumbosacral nerve roots. *Acta Radiol* 1962; 1:1141–1160.
7. Bunegin L, Hung T-K, Chang GL: Biomechanics of spinal cord injury. *Crit Care Clin* 1987; 3:453–470.
8. Cohen MS, Wall EJ, Brown RB, et al: Cauda equina anatomy: Extrathecal nerve root and dorsal root ganglion. *Spine* 1990; 15:1248–1251.
9. Condon BR, Hadley DM: Quantification of cord deformation and dynamics during flexion and extension of the cervical spine using MR imaging. *J Comput Assist Tomogr* 1988; 12:947–955.
10. Delamarter RB, Bohlman HH, Dodge LD, et al: Experimental lumbar spinal stenosis. *J Bone Joint Surg [Am]* 1990; 72:110–120.
11. de Peretti F, Micalef JP, Bourgeon A, et al: Biomechanics of the lumbar spinal nerve roots and the first sacral root within the intervertebral foramina. *Surg Radiol Anat* 1989; 11:221–225.
12. Gamble HJ: Comparative electron-microscopic observations on the connective tissues of a peripheral nerve and a spinal nerve root. *J Anat* 1964; 98:17–25.
13. Hung T-K, Albin MS, Brown MS, et al. Biomechanical responses to open experimental spinal cord injury. *Surg Neurol* 1975; 4:271–276.
14. Inman VT, Saunders JB: The clinico-anatomical aspects of the lumbosacral region. *Radiology* 1942; 38:669–678.
15. Janssen L, Hansebout RR: Pathogenesis of spinal cord injury and newer treatments. *Spine* 1989; 14:23–32.
16. Kwan MK, Rydevik B, Myers RR, et al: Biomechanical and histological assessment of human lumbosacral spinal nerve roots. *Trans Orthop Res Soc* 1989; 13:348.
17. Murphy RW: Nerve roots and spinal nerves in degenerative disk disease. *Clin Orthop* 1977; 129:46–60.
18. Olmarker K: *Spinal Nerve Root Compression* (thesis). University of Göteborg, Sweden, 1990.
19. Rydevik B, Brown MD, Lundborg G: Pathoanatomy and pathophysiology of nerve root compression. *Spine* 1984; 9:7–15.
20. Rydevik BJ, Myers RR, Powell HC: Pressure increase in the dorsal root ganglion following mechanical compression. *Spine* 1989; 14:574–576.
21. Scarff JE: Injuries of the vertebral column and spinal cord, in Brock S (ed): *Injuries of the Brain and Spinal Cord and Their Coverings*. New York, Springer, 1960, pp 530–589.
22. Schönström N, Hansson T: Pressure changes within the cauda equina following constriction of the cauda equina. *Spine* 1988; 13:385–388.
23. Shapiro K, Shulman K, Marmarou A, et al: Tissue pressure gradients in spinal cord injury. *Surg Neurol* 1977; 7:275–279.
24. Sharpless SK: Susceptibility of spinal roots to compression block. NIH Workshop, Feb 2–4, 1975, in Goldstein M (ed): NINCDS Monograph No 15, 1975, pp 155–161.
25. Spencer DL, Irwin GS, Miller JAA: Anatomy and significance of fixation of the lumbosacral nerve roots in sciatica. *Spine* 1983; 8:672–679.
26. Spencer DL, Miller JAA, Bertolini JE: The effect of intervertebral disc space narrowing on the contact force between the nerve root and a simulated disc protrusion. *Spine* 1984; 9:422–426.
27. Stevens JM, O'Driscoll DM, Yu YL, et al: Some dynamic factors in compressive deformity of the cervical spinal cord. *Neuroradiology* 1987; 29:136–142.
28. Stodieck LS, Beel JA, Luttges MW: Structural properties of spinal nerve roots: Protein composition. *Exp Neurol* 1986; 91:41–51.
29. Sunderland SL, Bradley KC: Stress-strain phenomena in human spinal nerve roots. *Brain* 1961; 84:120–124.
30. Tani S, Yamada S, Knighton RS: Extensibility of the lumbar and sacral cord. Pathophysiology of the tethered spinal cord in cats. *J Neurosurg* 1987; 66:116–123.
31. Tencer AF, Allen BL, Ferguson RL: A biomechanical study of thoracolumbar spine fractures with bone in the canal. Part III. Mechanical properties of the dura and its tethering ligaments. *Spine* 1985; 10:741–747.
32. Tencer AF, Ferguson RL, Allen BL: A biomechanical study of thoracolumbar spinal fractures with bone in the canal. Part II. The effect of flexion angulation, distraction, and shortening of the motion segment. *Spine* 1985; 10:587–589.
33. Wall EJ, Cohen MS, Abitbol JJ, et al: Intrathecal nerve root organization at the level of the conus medullaris. *J Bone Joint Surg [Am]* 1990; 72:1495–1499.

PART VI

TRAUMA

24

Regional Spinal Cord Injury Centers

David F. Apple, M.D.

HISTORY

A spinal cord injury center was first developed in the United States in Boston by Dr. Donald Munro in the late 1940s and early 1950s at the University Hospital. About the same time, Drs. Ernst Bor, Estin Comar, and Herbert Talbert were developing spinal cord injury treatment centers within the Veterans Administration system. In 1964, the staff at Rancho Los Amigos Hospital set up a spinal cord injury unit that was modeled after the concepts that had been developed by Sir Ludwig Guttmann at Stoke Mandeville Hospital in England during the mid 1940s. In 1968, a group of physicians treating spinal cord injury wrote to Congress about the needs of spinal cord injury victims and the poor coordination of care. As an outgrowth of these talks, Congress, through the Rehabilitation Service Administration, funded the first model spinal cord injury care system at Good Samaritan Hospital in Phoenix, Arizona.

DEFINITION

In engineering terms, a system is defined as an assemblage of components operating within a prescribed boundary and united by some form of interaction or interdependence to form a coherent or integrated whole. This definition is applicable to the system that was set up in Arizona with the Good Samaritan Hospital cooperating with the Barrow Neurologic Institute to form the spinal cord injury center.

Defining the state of Arizona as the boundaries, the system of care developed had five components. The first component was easy access for the injured patient to the center via a good emergency evacuation system managed by well-trained emergency service personnel. The second ingredient was a traumatology service to provide the expertise necessary to manage not only the spinal cord injury but multiple trauma. The third prerequisite was a rehabilitation program utilizing the multidisciplinary team approach to ensure that the injured patient received maximal benefit consistent with the neurologic deficits. The spinal cord injury rehabilitation center had to be able to furnish the fourth component, which was psychosocial and vocational services that prepared the patient to return to an altered, meaningful life permitting effective community reintegration. The final component was a comprehensive follow-up program that ensured the patient continuing medical, vocational, and other support services as required.

DEVELOPING A SPINAL CORD INJURY CENTER

The development of a spinal cord injury center initially hinges around two critical ingredients. One, there must be a sufficient patient population to support the center. The minimum number of dedicated beds it takes to operate a center efficiently is 12, with 16 being more appropriate. These figures are derived from the critical staffing elements. A single therapist can manage 6 to 8 patients, and if an aide is added, the number can be expanded to 10. However, because of vacation time, sickness, and ongoing education requirements, at least an additional half-time and preferably another full-time therapist is necessary. By this reasoning, the number of 12 to 16 patients is ascertained.

With an average length of stay for all patients in a good center being approximately 90 days, or a patient turnover of 4 per bed per year, there would need to be 48 to 56 new spinal cord injury admissions per year in order to sustain a center. It would take a population of approximately 1½ million based on the current incidence rate of 30 new injuries per million of population in order to sustain a center.

The second critical ingredient is a physician knowledgeable in the management of spinal cord injury patients who will make the time commitment necessary to develop a center. It is the physician's responsibility, along with cooperation from the hospital administration, to develop the necessary interhospital agreements and to mold the paraprofessional staff into a functional unit capable of managing the patients efficiently.

Once the population base and physician have been identified, it is necessary to establish a dedicated area in which to manage the spinal cord–injured patients. Next, a team of paraprofessionals with either spinal cord injury experience or an educational exposure in spinal rehabilitation beyond the general rehabilitation training must be recruited. The team that is developed needs to include at least the following: nursing, physical therapy, occupational therapy, social work, and therapeutic recreation—a multidisciplinary team. Available on a consultative basis should be experts in psychology, speech therapy, vocational counseling, and nutrition. This group must meet on a weekly basis to assess the patient's progress and to continue development and modification of each patient's program.

From a medical standpoint, the team needs to have available, at least on a consultation basis, the following medical subspecialties: orthopedics, neurosurgery, internal medicine, respiratory medicine, cardiology, gastroenterology, urology, neurology, physical medicine, psychiatry, and dentistry. Occasionally, hematology-oncology and endocrinology services are utilized.

In the classic sense, this team functions as a multidisciplinary team. There is a trend at this time to have the team function on an interdisciplinary level. This means that each patient's rehabilitation issues, rather than being discipline oriented, that is occupational therapy, physical therapy, etc., become goal oriented, that is, dressing, feeding, wheelchair skills, etc. Superimposed on the team function is the patient education that must take place. In a minimal-size center, this process is fragmented among the various disciplines, but in a larger center, an educational person becomes a valuable member of the team.

Once the core has been developed, the external components of the center must be addressed. On the front or acute injury end, transfer agreements with the referring hospitals within the catchment area should be developed. The agreement encourages an early transfer of recently injured patients to the center. At the very least the agreement would mandate involvement of the center's physician in the early care of the patient on a consultative basis until such a time as the patient could be transferred for intensive spinal cord care.

On the back end or discharge, there are two elements that need to be addressed. One, community reintegration, can be accomplished by identifying the appropriate agencies within the catchment area that will provide educational, vocational, and quality-of-life needs, including recreation activities, leisure time activities, and counseling on personal, financial, and marital issues. The final element that needs to be addressed is follow-up care. This may be provided by the physician in the center or by returning the patient to the referring physician. If the latter is to occur, the physician must be provided with a summary of the patient's capabilities, general medical situation, and medications.

When all these pieces are in place, a center has been developed that will provide the patient with the benefits to be discussed subsequently. As a simple measure of center program expectations, an average paraplegic patient should be managed from the time of injury to completion of rehabilitation in 80 to 90 days and the average quadriplegic in 95 to 105 days.

CASE STUDY: PART 1

In order to help clarify center functions, following a patient through a programmatic outline will demonstrate a center's activities.

The patient, a 25-year-old man, was riding his motorcycle home after having had "several beers," lost control, and was thrown from the cycle. Emergency medical service was summoned to the accident scene. Their initial evaluation indicated that the patient was unable to move his legs and was complaining of shoulder pain. With appropriate cervical control, he was positioned in anatomic alignment and a cervical collar applied. He was placed on a spine board for transportation to the ambulance and thus to the closest hospital.

Following arrival in the emergency room, the treating physician obtained no history of loss of consciousness, and there was good memory of the event. The past history included being involved in a motorcycle accident at the age of 15 years in which he fractured both upper extremities and both lower extremities. Physical examination revealed that the pupils were equal and reactive. There was no blood in the external auditory canals. Sensory examination was normal to the elbows with no movement in the upper extremities. There was no respiratory distress. There was crepitus and tenderness around the right shoulder. The remainder of the examination was unremarkable. Radiographs were ordered of the entire spine, the chest, the right shoulder, and the skull. Skull radiographic findings were negative. Chest radiographs demonstrated fracture of the midportion of the clavicle on the right side. The shoulder x-ray studies demonstrated the fractured clavicle. The only abnormal findings in the spine radiographs was a small chip fracture from the inferior body of C6 with no malalignment.

Treatment in the emergency room consisted of starting an intravenous catheter, inserting a Foley catheter, and continuing immobilization in the cervical collar. Methylprednisolone in a dosage of 30 mg/kg was administered intravenously per the recommended protocol at the time of the accident. The emergency room physician contacted the spinal cord injury center 60 miles away, and arrangements were made for transfer by helicopter.

The receiving physician, an orthopaedist at the spinal cord injury center, met the patient in the emergency room about 2½ hours after the injury. The history obtained at that time corroborated the history of drinking and history of the previous motorcycle accident. The patient had full memory of the event and admitted to smoking a pack of cigarettes a day for the past 10 years. Examination revealed puffiness around both orbits. There was previously noted crepitus around the right shoulder. Motor and sensory examinations revealed sensation down the anterolateral aspect of the forearm to just below the elbow bilaterally at the C4 dermatome. Motor examination revealed the deltoids to be functioning at grade IV and biceps functioning at grade III. There was no motor function below, thus indicating a C5 motor level. A bulbocavernosus reflex was present, and a diagnosis of C5 Frankel A quadriplegia was established. Review of the x-ray films accompanying the patient demonstrated no abnormalities in the lumbar-thoracic spine. There was a fracture of the inferior lip of the body of C6 with soft-tissue swelling anterior to the body of C3 and no malalignment.

The patient was placed in cervical traction by using Gardner-Wells tongs. The methylprednisolone protocol of 5.4 mg/kg was instituted every hour for 23 hours. The patient was transferred to the computed tomographic (CT) scanner for imaging the abdomen, cervical spine, and skull. CT of the skull indicated fractures of both orbits that were essentially nondisplaced. CT of the abdomen was negative. CT of the cervical spine demonstrated lamina fractures at C4 and C5 and a body fracture of C6. The spinal canal showed no encroachment and was not stenotic. The patient was transported to the spinal intensive care unit for ongoing care.

Consultation was obtained from plastic surgery for evaluation of the orbital fractures. The urologist was consulted regarding bladder management. Respiratory medicine was asked to assess anticipated pulmonary problems with a long history of smoking. Preventive ulcer management was also instituted to cover the high dose of steroids plus the stress phenomenon of the injury. The fractured clavicle was managed effectively by positioning in bed until such time as the patient would be able to get up.

On the first day following the injury, the patient was evaluated by physical therapy, occupational therapy, and the social work department. The nursing service was involved with skin management. Appropriate turning while in traction was instituted, and appropriate padding of the bony prominences was begun. The nursing service also began early bowel and bladder management. The purpose of instituting these services early was to prevent potential complications of skin sores, to prevent joint contractures, and to prevent deconditioning of muscles that were partially or fully innervated.

The orthopaedist determined that appropriate management in this case was a halo jacket because any posterior procedure would involve long internal fixation that would need to extend from C3 to C7. If approached anteriorly, plating of at least C4 to C7 and probably a halo for additional immobilization would be required. A halo was applied on the third postinjury day, and the patient was allowed out of bed that same day. On the fifth day, the patient had progressed from sitting in the wheelchair at bedside for 2 to 3 hours to going to the therapy gym for 4 hours of involvement in both individual and group therapy programs.

During the course of the 90-day rehabilitation period, the patient was involved in the team effort. The team met on a weekly basis to initially set long-term goals and establish short-term goals for the coming week. These goals would be altered as the patient made progress by this weekly monitoring system. Additionally during the 90-day rehabilitation period, the patient would be involved in at least four family sessions. The initial session would be largely devoted to the medical aspect of the spinal cord problem in relation to intact nervous system functions and what alterations occur with a spinal cord injury. Additionally, the patient would be given a general outline of the rehabilitation course. A second involvement of the family would take place prior to the patient being allowed to go out on a pass to be sure that significant others were trained in the patient's requirements for assistance. Additional meetings with the family and patient would be scheduled to further update the patient's programs and any alterations in family involvement. A final review with the patient and family would take place just prior to discharge to be sure that everyone was comfortable with the patient's programs and the amount of help required.

The Rehabilitation Team

A brief review of the members of the rehabilitation team and their functions will help in indicating how the team functions.

Nursing

Nursing care is significant during the early postinjury period when the patient is still sick from the injury. During this time the nurse provides the traditional services but also becomes increasingly involved with skin as well as bowel and bladder management. The patient needs to know appropriate relief measures such as padding bony prominences, being turned at night, and performing weight shifts during the day. Regarding bladder management, the patient needs to progress from an indwelling Foley catheter to definitive bladder management, which in most institutions is intermittent catheterization. The patient, whether or not able to do this himself, needs to understand how it is done and at what times. All patients require a bowel program; this is most effectively done by using the dilatation procedure on an every-other-day schedule, preferably at night when the patient will have more time to perform this activity, which may require an hour.

Physical Therapy

The physical therapist is responsible for developing mobility skills for the patient. This includes getting in and out of bed whether by a Hoyer lift, by sliding board transfers, or by unassisted transfers. In addition to getting in and out of bed, the patient will need to know how to get from the wheelchair to the toilet seat, to the tub, to the car, and in the appropriate instances, to and from the floor.

Additionally, it is ideal that the patient understand the maintenance of his wheelchair. In the case of a patient who would be able to ambulate with braces, gaiting activities with or without the use of functional electrical stimulation are the responsibility of the physical therapist.

Occupational Therapy

The occupational therapist is primarily concerned with activities of daily living. These include feeding, shaving, brushing teeth, grooming, bathing, dressing, and undressing, as well as communication skills. The occupational therapist must work conjointly with the physical therapist, particularly in the area of wheelchair skills and especially with the high-level quadriplegic when adaptive equipment is required to manage the wheelchair. Various power control options such as the arm, the head, chin blink, or eyebrow switches may be needed. Additionally, these two therapists need to cooperate with patients who are capable of driving and need mobility skills to get in and out of the vehicle but require hand controls for shifting and braking and wheel adaptations for steering.

Social Work

Social work is involved to help the patient with coping with the injury emotionally, vocationally, and financially. The social worker should address with the patient those areas regarding family functioning without the services of the injured individual. How the patient is going to cope with either working at an altered job level or not being able to work at all and how the patient will deal with differences encountered in his altered world are social work concerns. The social worker should also help with insurance problems and funding of necessary durable medical equipment and be sure that all resources that are available to the patient from any public areas are fully utilized.

Psychology

The psychologist takes a more in-depth approach to the ramifications of the injury and how it affects the individual dynamics. In order to do this, testing is helpful for determining how the patient handles life situations in order to better ascertain what help is needed to cope with the spinal cord injury problem. Additionally, there are concerns regarding sexuality and sexual functioning that need to be addressed, and the psychologist is instrumental in this.

Therapeutic Recreation

With a spinal cord injury, most patients are going to have more leisure time than they had prior to the injury. Thus identifying recreational activities preinjury and either adapting this interest or shifting to a similar interest that the patient can do is important. If the patient can be shown that he can participate and enjoy a sport or leisure activity, he may be more likely to develop a positive approach and return to work.

Education

An educational specialist is helpful in evaluating how a patient learns. Once the learning style is determined, it is easier to effectively teach the patient about his spinal cord injury, the altered body systems, and how they will function postinjury. This is particularly important in teaching the patient skin management, bowel programs, and bladder programs. If the patient is an auditory learner, most of this can be done through a lecture. If the patient is a visual learner, audiovisual equipment will help. If the patient is an active learner, demonstration of techniques will be the most effective teaching method. Knowing all this conserves patient and staff time in the overall rehabilitation program.

Nutrition

Involving a nutritionist early in the patient's injury allows early intervention to prevent weight and protein loss and to reduce complications due to malnutrition such as increased urinary and respiratory infections. Proper diet and nutrition will enhance the patient's ability to participate in therapy programs.

Vocational Counseling

At the appropriate time, usually about midway through the rehabilitation course, a vocational counselor can become active in evaluating the patient's potential for returning to a previous job. If this is not possible, identifying areas of skill and interest directs the patient in career planning postdischarge.

Meeting on a regular basis, this team of professionals can develop a patient's program in a coordinated way. Once the team becomes goal oriented rather than discipline oriented, the process moves along more quickly and with less problems so that at the time of discharge there are no loose ends that have been missed.

The final job of the rehabilitation team is to arrange for community reintegration. This means that the team has identified the appropriate resources in the patient's locale for obtaining the necessary services. This may mean supplies such as catheters and medications. It means identifying people to do the necessary work to be sure that the dwelling place is altered to accept a wheelchair and the bathroom and kitchen are accessible. It means being sure that the patient has identified a physician within the community who can handle general medical needs and, it is hoped, the more simple spinal cord injury needs. Arrangements should be made for the patient to return on a periodic basis to the spinal cord injury center for evaluation of the neurologic status as well as follow-up on the various programs and skills learned while an inpatient.

CASE STUDY: PART 2

Regarding the patient in the case study, his rehabilitation program from the time of injury to discharge was 91 days. He regained functional strength and developed grade III wrist extensors, which made him a functional C6 quadriplegic. He was independent in skin management, being able to observe posterior skin with a mirror. He was independent with his bowel program and used a dilatation stick. He was independent with his bladder program after having been taught to do intermittent catheterization with the use of a hand brace. He was in a wheelchair with "quad pegs," and because he was planning to go to school, a power wheelchair with a hand control was ordered. He was independent in all of his transfers without the use of a sliding board. Regarding activities of daily living, he required minimal assistance in meal preparation only. He was able to dress his upper extremities independently but required assistance with socks and shoes. He was able to do all his grooming. He could use a toilet with an elevated toilet seat. He could bathe himself, but required assistance in getting in and out of the bathtub. He was totally independent in all communication skills. He had been taught to drive a van by using hand controls. He had not obtained his own van at the time of discharge, but it had been ordered. Appropriate prescriptions had been given for modifications for getting in and out of the van and for driving.

His family had prepared a sketch of the house, and modifications suggested by the physical therapist and occupational therapist had been made. The school he was attending had been contacted, and the campus was wheelchair accessible. Arrangements were made for him to have a room on the first floor of the dormitory, with the school assisting in recruiting attendant help that he needed at bedtime and on arising in the morning. The psychologist had discussed sexuality and sexual functioning with him. The vocational rehabilitation counselor was assisting in helping to fund the modifications on his van and any modifications that needed to be done in the school setting. The patient understood all his programs and was capable of teaching his needs to an aide. His parents learned all his programs and were comfortable with assisting and providing what he needed. Copies of his records were sent to his physician in his hometown as well as to the student health center at the college he would be attending. Arrangements were made for him to return to the spinal center in 2 months for evaluation.

BENEFITS OF REGIONAL SPINAL CORD INJURY CENTERS

Regional spinal cord injury centers have been in existence since 1972. One of the primary functions of regional centers has been a centralized data base, which was first maintained in Phoenix, Arizona, at the Good Samaritan Hospital under the direction of Dr. John Young. Subsequently, these efforts were transferred to the University of Alabama at Birmingham under the direction of Dr. Sam Stover. During these 18 years, over 15,000 patients have been entered into the data system, which allows extensive analysis. The benefits of regional spinal cord injury centers can be identified in five different areas. They would be general benefits, primarily statistical; patient benefits; economic benefits; research benefits; and educational benefits.

General Benefits

The large statistical base at the National Spinal Cord Injury Statistical Center indicates that the male-to-female ratio is 4:1. The highest reported incidence is among persons between 15 and 20 years of age. The annual incidence has dropped from an early estimation of as high as 50 new injuries per million of population per year down to 30 per million per year. The etiology of this large group is depicted in Table 24–1. As regards the time of injury, the peak is in July with 11.5%, followed by August at 10.7%, June at 9%, and May and September at approximately 8.7%. The largest percentage (18.6% each day) occurs on Saturday and Sunday, with the remaining days of the week being approximately equal. Over the years of data collection, the percentage of quadriplegics vs. paraplegics has remained approximately the same, with slightly more than half being quadriplegic. However, there has been a gradual increase in the number of incomplete injuries from 38% in 1973 to 53.8% in 1984. These statistics, while not of significance to the individual, do have overall implications for programmatic decisions and thus are invaluable to the industry.

Patient Benefits

Benefits to the patient can be viewed in three areas: (1) neurologic function, (2) secondary complications, and (3) life expectancy. With the increase in the number of incompletely injured patients over the years, the eventual neurologic function has improved. Even of those who initially were graded as complete or Frankel A, almost 7% improved at least one Frankel grade by the time of discharge. Of those admitted as Frankel B, that is, sensory sparing only, 10% became worse, and 28% improved at least one Frankel grade. In those admitted as Frankel C, 56% became Frankel D, and 1.5% fully recovered. In those admitted as Frankel D, that is, useful motor function

TABLE 24–1.
Etiology and Incidence of Spinal Cord Injury

Motor vehicle accidents	47.7%
Falls	20.8%
Sports	14.2%
Acts of violence	14.6%
Others	2.7%

TABLE 24–2.
Effect of Admission Time on Complication Rate

Complication	Early Admission (Day 1) (%)	Delayed Admission (Days 2–60) (%)	*P* Value
Contractures	3.3	5.3	.03
Heterotopic ossification	3.3	6.1	.004
Gastrointestinal hemorrhage	3.4	4.1	.45
Atelectasis	19.7	25.5	.002
Pneumonia	16.5	19.7	.06
Deep-vein thrombosis	16.3	13.3	.06
Pulmonary embolus	4.0	5.5	.06
Cardiac arrest	4.0	6.5	.02
Chills and fever (urosepsis)	23.7	27.3	.07
Abnormal renal function	0.2	1.4	.004
Pressure sore (any grade)	35.2	46.0	.0001
Pressure sore (grade 2, 3, or 4)	21.7	25.9	.02

distal to the level of injury, 4% obtained full recovery, and 2% worsened.

Another area of patient benefit is a reduction in the number of secondary complications due to spinal cord injury. Table 24–2 indicates the difference when the patient is admitted within 24 hours of injury and when admission is delayed up to 60 days postinjury. All of these secondary complications are important. However, the one that creates the most immediate economic problem as well as increases the length of stay is the presence of pressure sores. A 1988 estimate revealed that the average cost of a pressure sore was about $58,000 for hospital stay expenses. Therefore, reduction in this area alone has had significant benefit.

Analysis of Table 24–2 indicates that patients admitted to a regional spinal cord injury center should have a lower incidence of contractures, cardiac arrest, atelectasis, heterotopic ossification, renal dysfunction, and significant pressure sores. The remainder of the areas are statistically not significant, but all tended to be lower in the early admission group. The overall 12-year survival rate for all spinal cord–injured patients in the system was 88.2% of the normal rate. This, however, varied by age, neurologic level, and extent of the lesion. The 12-year survival rates range from 95% for young persons with neurologically incomplete lesions to a low of 18.1% for older persons with complete quadriplegia. A comparison of 5-year survival rates for patients treated in a model spinal cord injury center vs. a similar group of northern California residents is demonstrated in Table 24–3.

TABLE 24–3.
Spinal Injury Center Patients

Neurologic Classification	Model System Survival Rates (%)	Northern Calif. Residents (%)
All persons	87	84
C1–3 complete injury	75	34
C4–T1 complete injury	78	70
T2–L3 complete injury	95	84

Economic Benefits

The economic benefit, mainly determined by the length of the hospital stay, is influenced by many factors, the most important one being the number of secondary complications. If one compares the group of patients admitted to regional spinal cord injury centers within 24 hours of injury with those admitted 2 to 60 days postinjury, acute hospitalization is shorter by 13 days, and the rehabilitation stay is decreased by 3 days. The average total hospitalization is 113 days vs. 136 days in those admitted later. In comparing the length of stay in a regional spinal cord injury center with those of non–center-treated spinal cord–injured patients in the uniform data system group, the hospital days were decreased by 18 for center-treated patients.

Rehospitalization following the initial rehabilitation program is also an important aspect of the economics. Forty percent of the patients are rehospitalized an average of 12 days during the second year after injury. By the 12th year, this is decreased to 25% of patients for 8 hospital days. There are presently no data available to compare with non–center-treated patients. The direct cost incurred in the treatment of spinal cord–injured patients ranges from $72,000 for persons with neurologically incomplete paraplegia to $153,000 for persons with neurologically complete quadriplegia (Table 24–4).

If regional spinal cord injury center charges are adjusted to 1989 dollars, the charges show an increase from approximately $73,000 in 1974 to $80,000 in 1988 for an increase of only 9.5%. This relatively small rise over 14 years was possible because of a reduction in the length of stay over the same interval. The fact that there was any rise at all is explained by the increase in the number of ventilator-dependent quadriplegic patients who survived and thus incurred a higher rehabilitation charge. Finally, in the economic analysis, there has been a reduction in the number of patients being discharged to a nursing home from 4% to 2.6%. Additionally, the number of persons returning to employment increases from an immediate postinjury return of 17% to a peak of 38%. Again, there are no data available regarding non–regional center patients in this economic parameter. However, there seems to be sufficient indication that regional spinal cord injury centers show a definite economic benefit to the patient and to society.

RESEARCH

The regional spinal cord injury centers have provided a good opportunity for collaborative research. Many of the

TABLE 24–4.
Costs of Spinal Cord Injury Care per Person by Neurologic Level and Extent of Lesion

Cost Period	Incomplete Paraplegia ($)	Complete Paraplegia ($)	Incomplete Quadriplegia ($)	Complete Quadriplegia ($)
Acute care and rehabilitation, 1988–89 model system patients	71,980	83,649	88,210	153,312
Total first postinjury year	72,859	87,868	134,957	173,131
Second postinjury year	4962	9213	8682	12,276
Each subsequent year	9009	14,032	24,886	43,663
Present value of lifetime direct costs	210,379	274,939	461,957	571,854
Present value of lifetime foregone earnings	151,253	200,164	188,150	308,054

items that need to be addressed require a population that is not available to any one regional center, and thus collective research has been necessary and possible. Over the years of regional spinal cord injury center designation, there are currently 13 centers and 6 former centers that have produced over 500 research papers. Almost three quarters, or 73%, were devoted to three major topic areas: medical complications including associated injuries and their treatment, 33%; rehabilitation including functional prognosis, cost, and outcome, 28%; and surgery of any type, 12%. The bibliography of these papers has been compiled as Appendix A in the publication, *Spinal Cord Injury—The Model.*

EDUCATION AND TRAINING BENEFITS

Educational activities undertaken by the majority of the regional spinal cord injury centers included individual lectures as a part of the courses. There were center-sponsored activities such as conferences, courses, workshops, panel discussions, demonstrations, and exhibits. There were staff presentations in the area of research and teaching at scientific meetings as well as poster presentations. The regional centers developed material for professional education, resident education, and patient and family education. Materials utilized have been videotapes, slide tape programs, slide series, films, books, posters, manuals, information packets, and public service announcements. The target audiences for these activities have been medical students, residents, fellows, emergency medical technicians, nurses, physical therapists, occupational therapists, speech pathologists, social workers, psychologists, vocational counselors, consumers, third-party payers, community organizations, and patients. In these educational activities, all potential areas have been addressed, that is, acute care, medical complications, rehabilitation management, prevention, research, costs, program evaluation, and cure of spinal cord injury.

Because of the benefits of a regional spinal cord injury center, it is hoped that more will develop in the future. This may occur with federal funding such as received by the 13 regional model spinal cord injury systems, with state funding such as the Florida Spinal Cord Injury System, or probably more feasibly, similar to the voluntary uniform data system group in upstate New York. These centers need to develop in areas where there is the required 1½ million population base to effectively develop and maintain a viable spinal cord injury center.

SUGGESTED READING

1. American Spinal Injury Association: *Standard for Neurologic Classification of Spinal Injury Patients.* April 1989.
2. Donovan WH, Bedbrook G: *Spinal Cord Injuries: Comprehensive Management and Research,* ed 2. Oxford, Blackwell, 1976.
3. Hardy AG, Rossier PB: *Spinal Cord Injuries.* Stuttgart, Germany, Georg Thieme, 1972.
4. Guttmann L: *Spinal Cord Injuries, Comprehensive Management and Research,* ed 2. Oxford, Blackwell, 1976.
5. Proceedings of the National Consensus Conference on Catastrophic Illness and Injury: *Spinal Cord Injuries.* Sheppard Spinal Center for Treatment of Spinal Injuries, 1990.
6. Sutton NG: *Injuries of the Spinal Cord: The Management of Paraplegia and Tetraplegia.* London, Butterworths, 1973.
7. University of Alabama at Birmingham: *Spinal Cord Injury: The Facts and Figures.* 1986.
8. Yashon D: *Spinal Injury.* New York, Appleton-Century-Crofts, 1978.

25

Traumatic Spinal Injuries—Cervical, Thoracic, Lumbar

William H. Donovan, M.D., and Howard B. Cotler, M.D.

Spinal cord injury (SCI) is a malady that affects approximately 7000 to 10,000 individuals per year in the United States. Its prevalence is about 900 per million, or approximately 175,000 to 200,000 cases. Its incidence is also quoted as being between 20 and 40 per million population. It affects males four times more frequently than females, and although it is found to occur in all age groups, the mean age is 29 years, the median age is 25, and the mode age is 19. Etiologies of this condition vary from country to country, but in the developed countries the distribution is generally as follows: motor vehicle, 48%; falls, 21%; sports, 14%; acts of violence, 15%; and other, 3%.[78]

In recent years, considerable emphasis has been given to two important concepts concerning the delivery of health care to spinal cord–injured persons. One involves the regionalization of care for catastrophic disabilities such as head injury, spinal injury, and severe burns. While the incidence of these conditions is relatively low, the extent of impairment is extremely high. It is also extremely costly, not only because required hospitalization, including rehabilitation, is long but also because adequate care cannot be delivered unless providers make a commitment to ensuring that adequate numbers of trained personnel, facilities, and equipment are available. Cost-effectiveness under these conditions cannot be readily achieved unless the above elements are concentrated in regional centers and all spinal cord–injured patients are sent there. The elements that should be available in such centers have been presented by the American Spinal Injury Association (ASIA)[35] and have subsequently been adapted as standards by the Commission on Accreditation of Rehabilitation Facilities.[11] The other important concept, which flows directly from this, is the programmatic approach toward the care of catastrophic disabilities both during the acute and rehabilitation phases. Spinal cord–injured patients in this scheme are to be treated in designated areas within the hospital or hospital complex. That is, disabilities are not mixed but are segregated according to their unique needs and differences. This permits a concentration of trained staff to allow an economy of effort with respect to patient care and family/patient education.

The federal government has supported these concepts in several ways. One way was the development and designation of regional model centers that could provide systems of care for spinal cord–injured patients all the way from rescue, emergency care, acute care, and rehabilitation to long-term care and community reintegration. The rest of this chapter will focus on some of these aspects and the information that is needed in order to provide comprehensive care.

DIAGNOSIS

When a newly injured person with an SCI arrives at the emergency room, the neurologic examination should be performed after one has established that the circulatory and respiratory systems have been truly stabilized. Following that, attention can be turned to the neurologic examination, which will disclose the neurologic level,[76] the degree of incompleteness as measured by the Frankel grade,[31] and the motor index score.[53, 76]

The establishment of a sensory level depends upon one's knowledge of the typical sensory dermatome maps.[21, 76] The sensory level is designated as the lowest level in which all sensory modalities, i.e., sharp/dull, pain/temperature, proprioception, vibration, light touch, and deep pressure, are perceived as normal. In patients with complete injuries, some of these modalities will also be felt one to three dermatomes below the last normal one. This partial sparing of some neurologic function is referred to as the zone of partial preservation. In incomplete lesions, some or all of the sensory modalities may be felt in a diminished or normal fashion for some distance below the level of injury. However, in order for a sensory impairment to be designated as incomplete, this preservation of sensation must extend as far as the lowest sacral segments.[76]

To determine the motor level, a knowledge of the "key muscles" (Table 25–1) as well as their innervation is crucial. It is important to remember that most muscles have a dual and sometimes triple innervation. That is, usually two segments (via their corresponding nerve roots) provide innervation to each muscle. Because of this, a muscle cannot

TABLE 25–1.
Spinal Cord Injury Motor Index Score*

Suggested Spinal Cord Injury Motor Index Score†			
Grade on Right	Muscle	Grade on Left	Key Muscles for Motor Level Classification‡
5	C5	5	C4 Diaphragm C5 Deltoid and/or biceps
5	C6	5	C6 Wrist extensors
5	C7	5	C7 Triceps C8 Flexor profundus
5	C8	5	T1 Hand intrinsics
5	T1	5	
5	L2	5	T2–L1 Use sensory level, abdominal reflexes, and Beevor's sign to help localize the lowest normal neurologic segment
5	L3	5	
5	L4	5	L2 Iliopsoas L3 Quadriceps
5	L5	5	L4 Tibialis anterior L5 Extensor hallucis longus
5	S1	5	S1 Gastrocnemius
50		50	S2–5 Use sensory level

Total Score 100

Motor grading system:

0—Absent (total paralysis)
1—Trace (palpable or visible contraction)
2—Poor (active movement through ROM§ with gravity eliminated)
3—Fair (active movement through ROM against gravity)
4—Good (active movement through ROM against resistance)
5—Normal

*The key muscles, shown on the right, are tested according to the muscle grading system located on the lower left. A perfect score is illustrated on the upper left.

†This motor index score, when used accurately, provides a numerical grading system to document improvement or deterioration of motor function. (Motor index score adapted from a scoring system by Lucas JT, Ducker TB: *Ann Surg* 1979; 45:151–158.)

‡This motor neurologic level is considered the lowest intact segment when the muscle grade is fair (grade 3) or greater. Most of these key muscles have dual innervation. By assigning a single level to each muscle as shown above, it is understood that this is a simplification. The key muscles above the chosen level must all test as normal (grade 5) while the chosen level tests to at least grade 3.

§ROM = range of motion.

perform at normal strength unless it has both segments contributing to its innervation. The biceps, for example, is a C5–6 muscle. If all of its C5 but none of its C6 innervation were functioning, the muscle would not test as normal. It would likely have enough strength to give a grade 3 or possibly a grade 4 level of performance but not a 5. Conventional muscle grading is described as follows: 0, no movement; 1, trace, i.e., perceptible contraction with or without some movement; 2, poor, i.e., contraction sufficient to provide movement through a full range, gravity eliminated; 3, fair, i.e., movement through full range, against gravity; 4, good, i.e., the ability to provide some resistance to movement; and 5, normal strength.[76] Therefore, the motor level is determined by knowing the lowest key muscle that gives a normal grade, the next lower key muscle that gives a fair grade, and finally the next lower key muscle that gives a 0 grade. The lowest normal myotome (i.e., the lower motor neurons in that spinal segment and the muscles they innervate) is the key muscle in this sequence that gives a fair grade.[21, 76] The zone of injury may be reflected in the motor as well as the sensory examination by the finding of grade 1 to 4 strength in muscles below the lowest normal myotome. But as with the sensory examination, this must be found in more than three myotomes below the last normal one before the lesion can be classified as motor incomplete.

The Frankel grade is next determined. In 1969, Frankel et al. described a functional grading system for incomplete lesions of the spinal cord.[31] The letter "A" was designated to describe a complete lesion; "B" described a lesion with only the preservation of sensation, regardless of whether it was perceived normally or in a diminished manner; "C" described a lesion with preservation of some sensation and

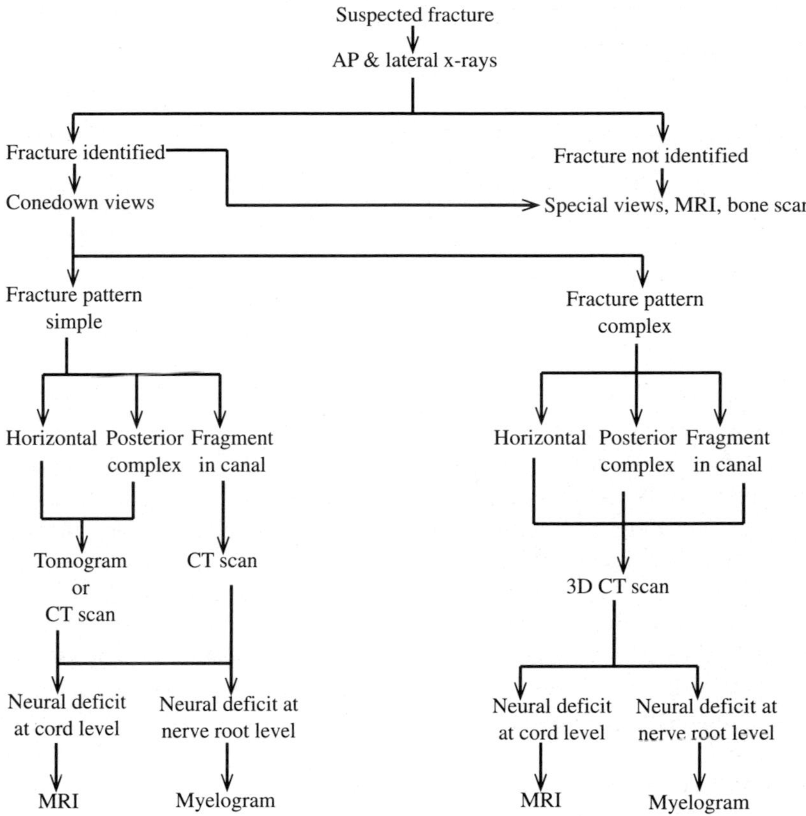

FIG 25–1.
Algorithm for investigating spinal fractures. (From Young W: *Cent Nerv Syst Trauma* 1985; 2:109–114. Used by permission.)

some motor function, but the motor function was insufficient for functional activities such as ambulation; and "D" described an injury where the degree of motor function was useful. A patient with a cervical lesion in which ambulation is possible, even though it requires braces and crutches, would be classified as having a "D" lesion. "E" described a lesion that was marked by complete recovery, although the persistence of hyperreflexia did not preclude an "E" grade. The ASIA has recently modified Frankel's classification.[76] A, B, and E remained the same, but C and D were changed as follows: if the majority of the key muscles below the level of injury test as less than grade 3, the lesion was considered a C lesion. Otherwise, if the majority key muscles are grade 3 or better, the lesion was classified as D. Finally, the motor index score is determined by testing the strength of all the key muscles according to the muscle scale given above. Five muscles in each extremity are examined. A perfect score is 100 if each muscle receives a grade of 5 (Table 25–1).

The sensory and motor levels localize the lesion within the longitudinal axis of the spinal cord. The Frankel grade and the motor index score describe the degree of incompleteness or conduction of action potentials through the area of injury. From this information, reasonable functional expectations can be predicted and reasonable comparisons made between patient groups (see the section on functional expectations).

In the high-level quadriplegic it is also important to determine the precise extent of diaphragmatic function. The latter should be evaluated directly by fluoroscopic examination and indirectly by using parameters such as the vital capacity and negative inspiratory force. As in all patients, a Frankel grade must never be assigned without examination of the sacral segments (anus and genitalia) for sensory and motor sparing. In addition, since patients with cervical spine injury may also sustain a head injury, careful documentation of the mental status should be carried out as well as the Glasgow coma scale, if applicable.

SPINAL IMAGING

The physical neurologic examinations as well as the mechanism of injury deduced from plain films may offer the most significant information regarding the vertebral column injury and its potential for instability. Although routine radiology is essential, the introduction of newer radiologic techniques can provide more information about

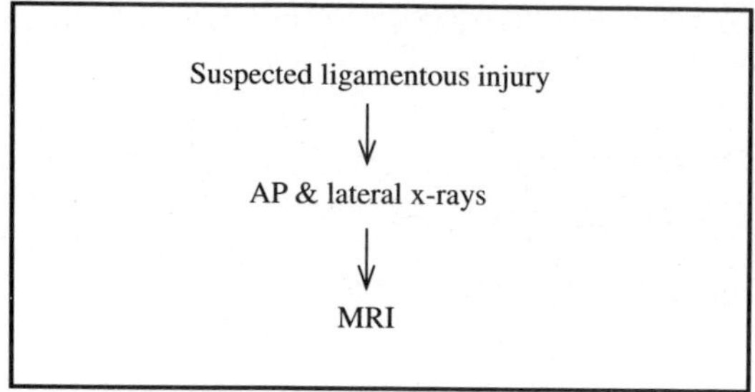

FIG 25–2.
Soft-tissue delineation.

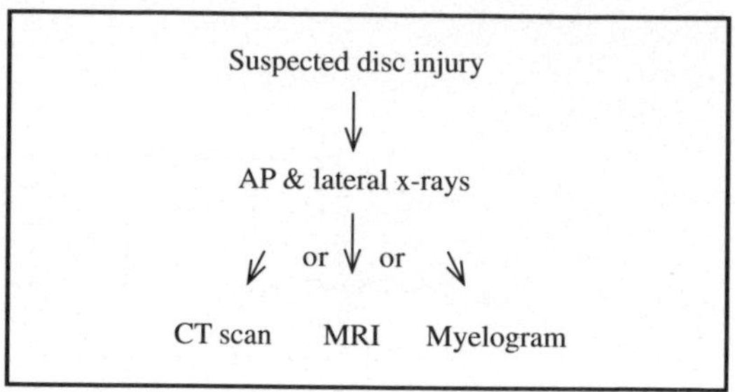

FIG 25–3.
Disc injury.

the extent of soft-tissue trauma, the patterns of fracture, and the concurrent neurologic injury (Figs 25–1 to 25–3).

Through a radiologic assessment, the definitive diagnosis of the type of spinal column trauma may be accurately obtained. Lateral (Fig 25–4,A) and anteroposterior (AP) (Fig 25–4,B) or biplane roentgenograms of any area suspected of injury should be performed. A total-spine series of biplane roentgenograms should be performed on any patient with a major spinal injury because there is approximately a 5% incidence of another fracture, either contiguous or at a distant site,[9] that may be masked by the anesthesia below the spinal cord injury.

The extent of gross deformity, i.e., vertebral displacement, loss of vertebral height, or kyphosis, is usually determined by plain roentgenograms. In evaluating the cervical spine, the cross-table lateral view is the most helpful (Fig 25–5). All seven cervical vertebrae must be visualized. A lateral radiograph revealing less than seven cervical vertebrae (Fig 25–6,A) requires either a cross-table lateral view with traction applied to the arms or a "swimmer's view" (Fig 25–6,B). The three views of the cervical spine that are included in the initial series of plain radiographs are (1) cross-table lateral and/or "swimmer's view," (2) AP, and (3) open mouth (Fig 25–7). The addition of Weir pillar views to this initial series allows one to identify an unstable injury in greater than 99% of the patients even if changes in

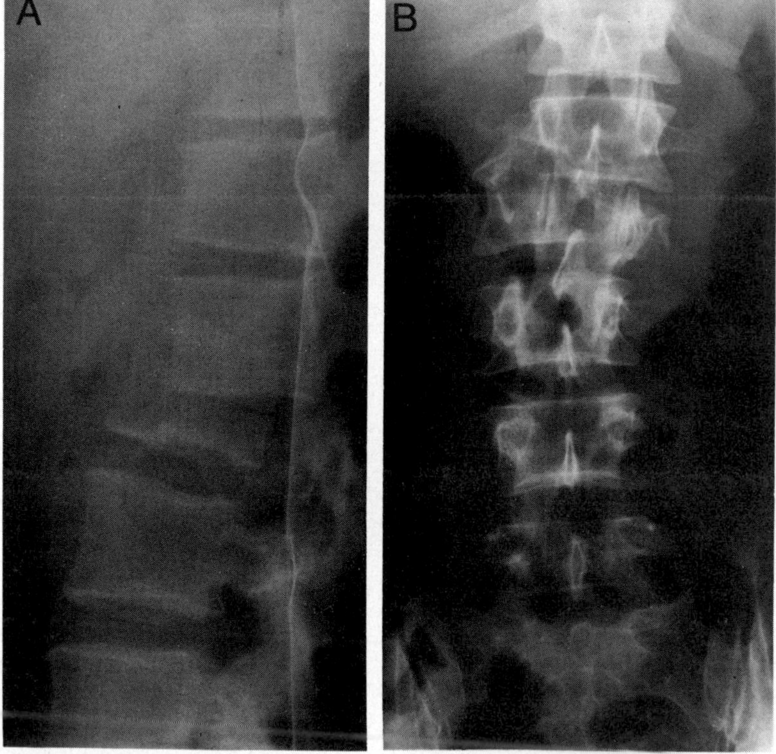

FIG 25–4.
A, lateral roentgenogram of an L1–2 fracture dislocation. **B,** AP roentgenogram of an L1–2 fracture-dislocation. Note the amount of translation that was not evident on the lateral view **(A).**

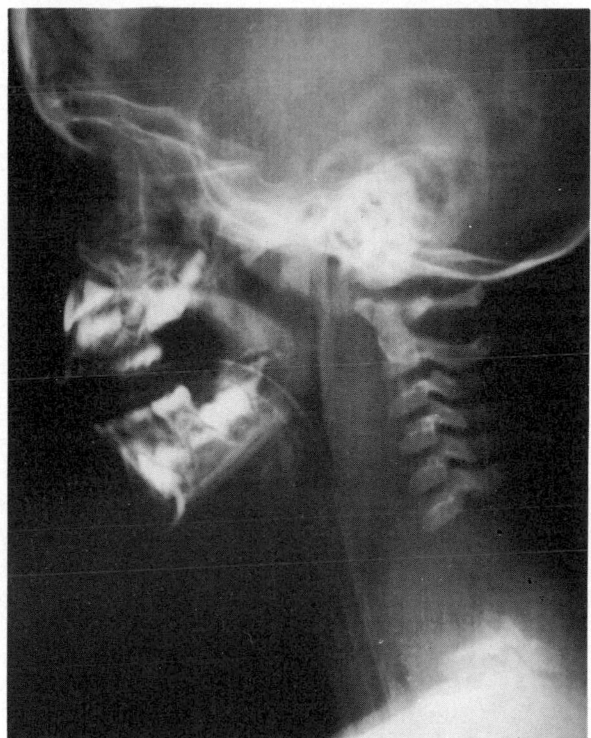

FIG 25–5.
Lateral radiograph of a pediatric C6–7 distraction injury.

mentation are present.[48] Lateral flexion and extension roentgenograms of the cervical spine are obtained during the initial assessment when there is no obvious bony injury in a patient who is alert with minimal or no neurologic deficit and when there is minimal hazard of producing a neurologic deficit. Thoracic, lumbar, and sacral injuries are also initially evaluated by cross-table lateral and AP views.

Fracture detail that is difficult to visualize on plain roentgenograms may be better assessed by biplane (AP and lateral) tomography. Tomography (Fig 25–8) is useful for studying the posterior joints, neural arches, and transverse fractures.

Metrizamide myelography or metrizamide-enhanced computerized axial tomographic (CAT) scanning has previously been indicated in the following circumstances.[58]

1. Neurologic deterioration in the incomplete or intact spine-injured patient
2. Preoperative evaluation of an incomplete lesion in a patient undergoing a spine stabilization procedure
3. Lack of anatomic correlation of a vertebral column injury with a neurologic deficit
4. Electrical studies (somatosensory evoked potentials) that do not correlate with the neurologic deficit
5. A recovering neurologic injury that stabilizes or plateaus early.

Myelography may be of benefit in the diagnosis of extradural lesions (i.e., disc herniation or hematoma) or for intramedullary pathology, i.e., a post-traumatic syrinx.

A CAT scan (Fig 25–9) provides excellent assessment of the spinal canal and horizontal definition of a fracture and bony encroachment of neural elements. Three-dimensional CAT scanning (Fig 25–10,A and B) may

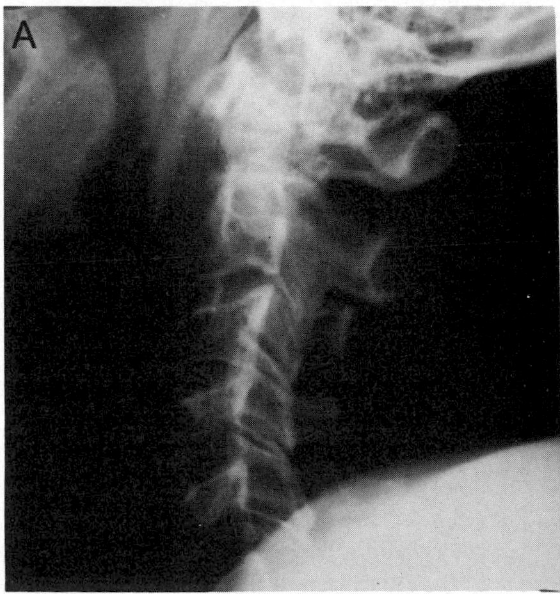

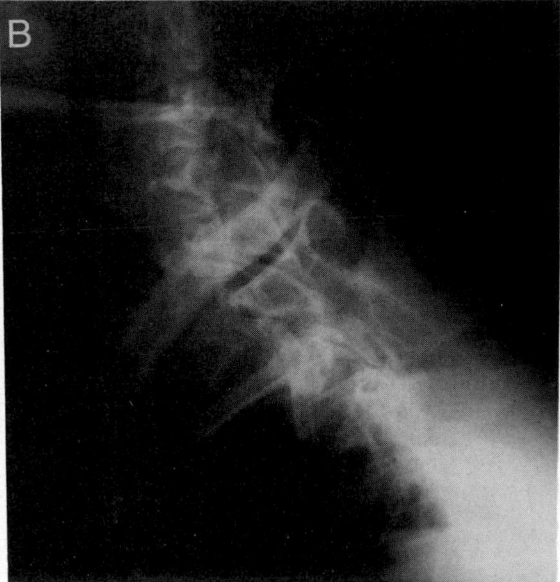

FIG 25–6.
A, lateral radiograph showing only six cervical vertebrae. **B,** the swimmer's view displays a C6–7 malalignment that was secondary to bilateral C7 facet fractures.

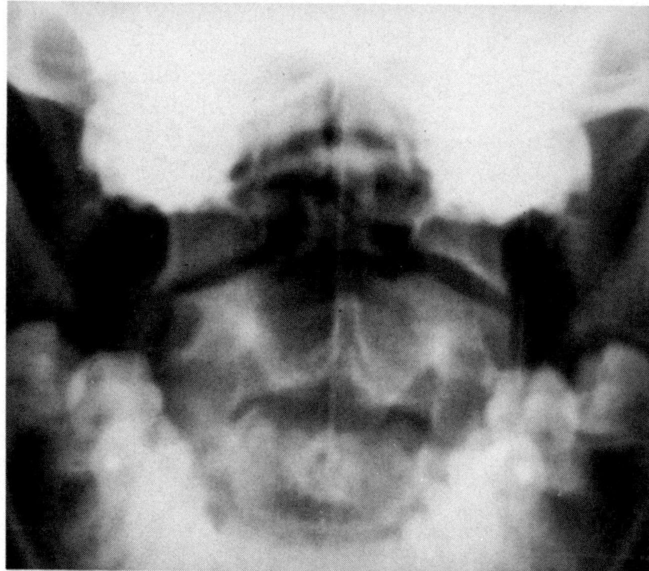

FIG 25–7.
Open mouth view of a type II odontoid fracture.

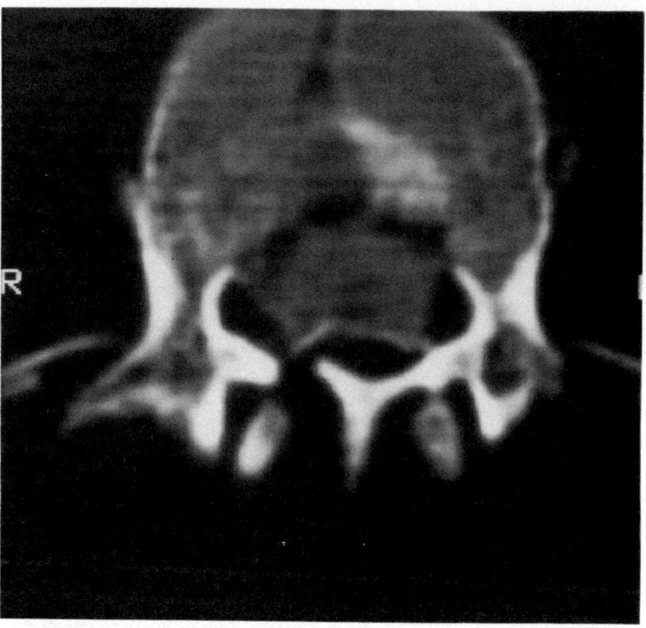

FIG 25–9.
Axial CAT scan of a lumbar-level burst fracture with approximately 90% canal compromise. Note the right-sided laminar fracture that was associated with dural laceration and entrapped nerve roots.

delineate the degree of kyphotic angulation and the extent of injury, better define retropulsed intraspinal fragments, and aid in surgical planning by providing a better image of the injury.[49]

Magnetic resonance imaging (MRI) (Fig 25–11) is increasingly becoming recognized as a diagnostic imaging modality. MRI may be useful in staging or determining the exact structures injured in order to determine stability. Also, MRI has shown promise in detecting and characterizing cord injuries in patients with acute paralysis and predicting the potential for neurologic recovery.[4]

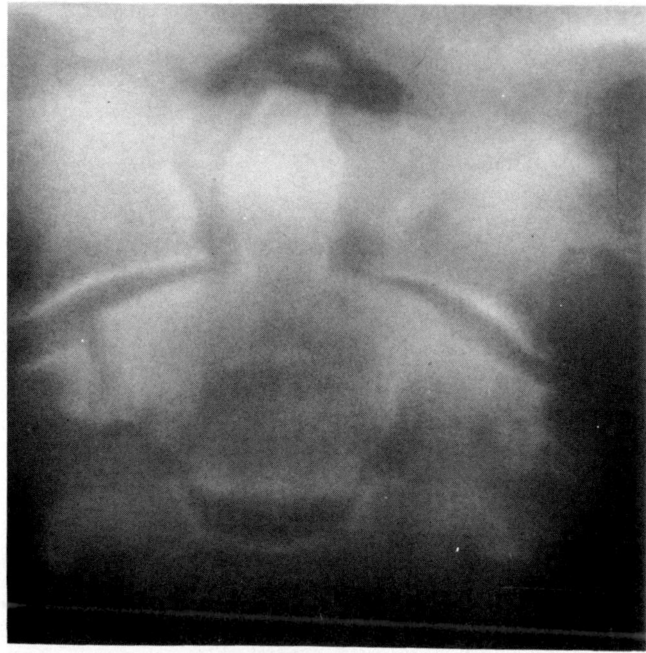

FIG 25–8.
An AP tomogram of C2 displays a C2 lateral mass fracture and a type I odontoid fracture.

It must be emphasized in obtaining these special views that are afforded by computed tomography (CT) and MRI that the patient has to be placed in a confined area for an extended period of time. Therefore, anyone who is experiencing medical instability, particularly of the cardiovascular or respiratory systems, must be watched extremely closely, and one must be prepared to delay the diagnostic procedure or remove the individual if the patient's distress becomes extreme. Also, the importance of pressure relief must not be ignored during this time.

As techniques for imaging acute traumatic spinal injuries improve, the exact anatomic structure that has failed may be determined. Identification of the number of failed anatomic structures plays a direct role in the determination of spinal instability and may give insight into the force vectors of injury that may need to be reversed by manipulation, traction, or surgery for deformity correction.

PATHOLOGY

The structural and ultrastructural changes that occur after damage to the spinal cord have been studied in both laboratory animals and postmortem human subjects. Laboratory experiments have been carried out primarily on the cat. In experimentally induced SCI, these animals are seen to develop scattered petechial hemorrhages in the central

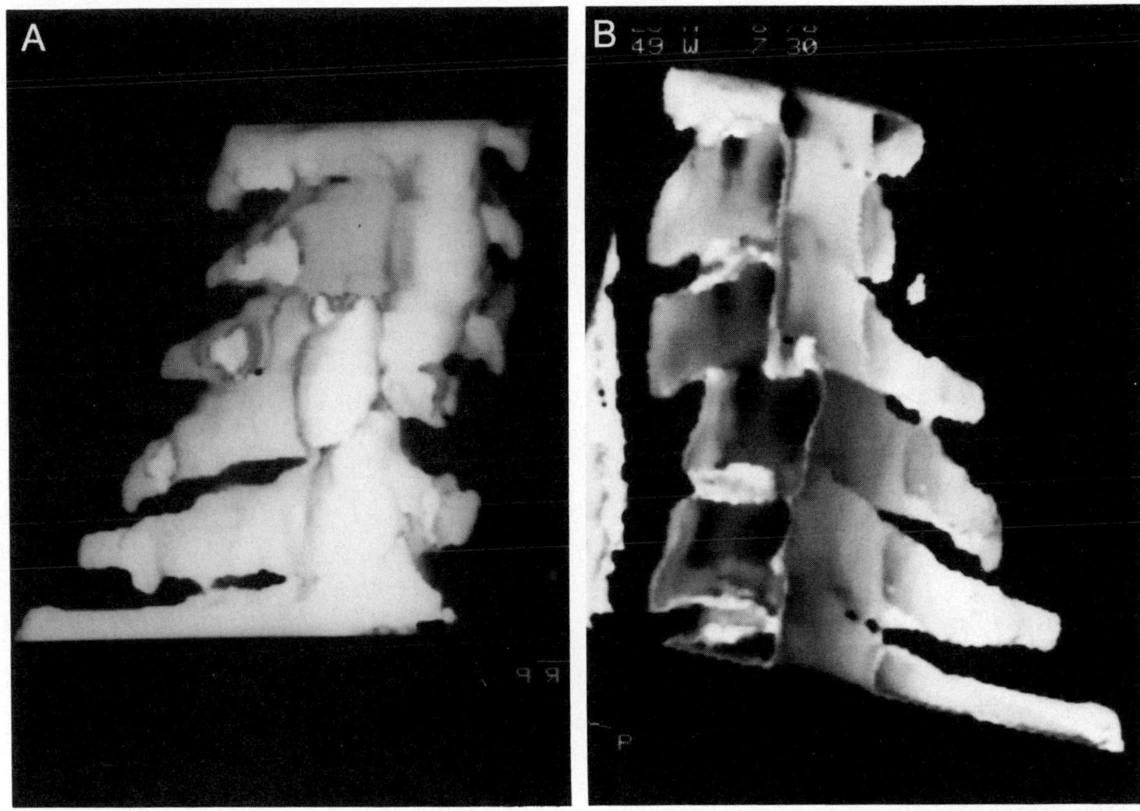

FIG 25–10.
Three-dimensional CAT scan of a C4–5 bilateral facet dislocation. **A,** the lateral view shows one of the facet dislocations. **B,** the midsagittal view displays the canal compromise.

gray matter within the first 15 minutes, and these enlarge and coalesce by 1 hour.[10, 82] The extrusion of blood into the gray matter generally reaches a maximum in 3 to 4 hours, and by 24 to 36 hours the gray matter has undergone hemorrhagic necrosis. The white matter begins to show petechial hemorrhages at 3 to 4 hours. Myelinated fibers show enlargement of the periaxonal space and fraying of the myelin. By 24 to 36 hours, long tracts show extensive structural degeneration.[47]

Kakulas has studied hundreds of severely traumatized spinal cord specimens obtained from people who were dead on arrival at a medical facility.[44] He found that despite its delicate semifluid nature, the cord may appear normal to the naked eye after trauma despite significant damage to the adjacent bony structure, ligaments, and muscles. This is particularly true in patients who died instantly upon impact. In others, the spinal cord showed petechial hemorrhages, edema, and disruption of the parenchyma. In many specimens, some continuity of long tracts appeared to be preserved. Complete dehiscence of the spinal cord was a rare finding from closed trauma. In patients who survived for a period of 12 to 24 hours, vascular changes became prominent, and hemorrhages in the white and gray matter were noted to be similar to those described in the cat.

Animal experimentation has yielded information concerning blood flow to the spinal cord following injury, and vasospasm and constriction of the arterial supply have been a constant observation. The cause of the vasoconstriction has not been fully defined and serotonin, catecholamines, and prostaglandins have each been implicated as causal agents.[64] In addition to being potent vasoconstrictors, norepinephrine and serotonin potentiate platelet aggregation. The decreased cord perfusion after injury may therefore occur from platelet aggregation coupled with chemically mediated large-vessel vasoconstriction and thrombosis.[60] The presence of intracellular calcium after disruption of neuron cell membranes also appears to be a major factor in causing cell dysfunction and death.[90]

In his study of patients with SCI who died weeks to months after their injury, Kakulas described macrophage activity removing debris and establishment of the process of gliosis.[44] Macrophages were seen to be actively engaging in ingestion of necrotic spinal cord tissues mainly in the central areas of the cord and the adjacent posterior columns. A glial meshwork was seen to begin to demarcate

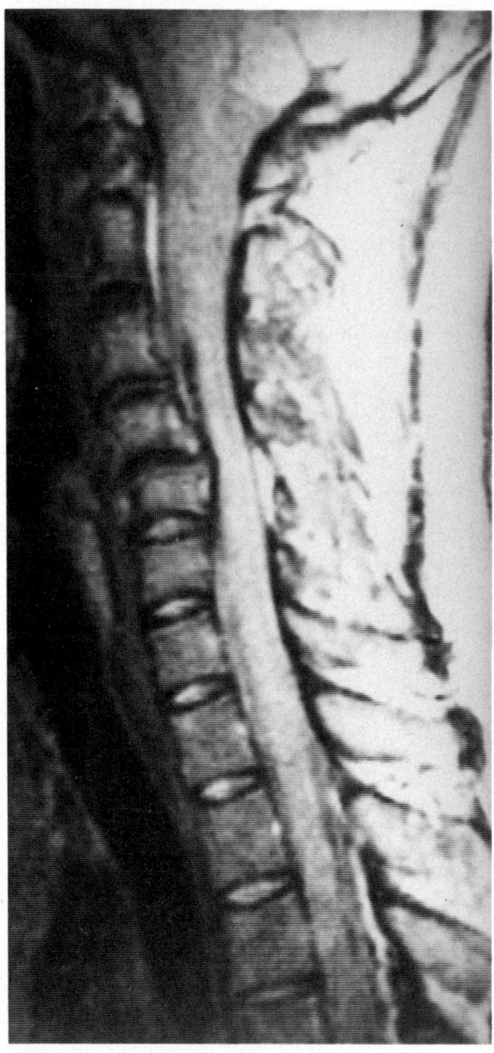

FIG 25–11.
A sagittal T1-weighted image of the cervical spine with a large C4–5 disc herniation and spinal cord compression.

the lesion from the tracts.[44] One could infer that concomitant biochemical changes must be occurring in the cord's various neuropeptides and other neurotransmitters, but information of this nature is only beginning to become available.[41]

Studying the material found in patients who died months to years after their injuries affords the ability to learn of chronic changes after spinal cord injury. This stage is characterized by the presence of multilocular cysts with thick glial walls, sensory nerve root regeneration, and a residuum of descending and ascending central nervous system fibers at the level of the lesion. Often the subarachnoid space is obliterated by fibrous tissues, which may also enter and mix with the glial network. These glial scars may also be the source of abnormal neuropeptide release. Regenerating nerve roots, which are a feature of the chronic stage, rarely enlarge sufficiently to form a neuroma with compression of the cord remnant.[44]

It is known that months to years after an SCI a small percentage of patients may develop a condition known as post-traumatic cystic myelopathy, which may cause clinical deterioration with involvement of higher (and lower) spinal cord segments. For reasons not entirely known, the cysts that occur in most patients enlarge in this small subgroup sufficiently to cause symptoms of neurologic compromise. This can become extremely critical in the cervical region where the loss of one segment adds significant impairment, particularly when the C3 and C4 areas become involved. In patients whose injuries occur in the cauda equina, some demonstrate a continuing active fibrosis of the nerve roots that may persist after many years.

At the present state of the art, medical science can do little to try to reverse the vascular and cellular reactions that occur after trauma to the spinal cord. However, Bracken and colleagues[5] have recently presented evidence that methylprednisolone administered in large doses within 8 hours of injury can reduce the ultimate neurologic impairment. Despite any advantage that methylprednisolone may give, it is important to eliminate the possibility of further injury that may be caused by improper handling of an unstable spinal column during the rescue and retrieval. Further, it is necessary to reduce aggravating factors such as hypotension and hypoxia that will add to the neurologic deficits if they are allowed to develop.

In essence, the extent of the destruction of neural tissue and the potential for recovery depend primarily upon the magnitude of force that has been impacted on that neural tissue within the spinal cord at the moment of injury. Now it appears that this can be modified by methylprednisolone. However, it is generally true that whether the trauma be minor or major, the spinal cord immediately loses its ability to conduct action potentials. Only time will reveal how much neurotrauma actually occurred, for if the injury was indeed very minor, recovery will occur quickly and totally. If it was major, it will never recover at all. However, between these two extremes there are significant gradations that may result in incomplete SCIs. In general, the sooner recovery occurs, the more that will occur, and the later it is noted, the less it will occur.

While regeneration of the spinal cord still appears a long way off for humans, progress has been made in this area. Aguago and colleagues[1] have recently accomplished the feat of getting central nervous system axons to grow through a peripheral nerve bridge and then synapse with cells on the other side of the bridge in the optic nerve of the rat. It is hoped that this accomplishment will be followed by similar accomplishments in other locations and in other species, particularly with the aid of oligodendrocyte-inhibiting techniques as developed by Schwab.[73]

Incomplete lesions to the spinal cord may take the form of several syndromes based upon the anatomic relationships of the neural tracts and gray matter. These syndromes of incompleteness include the following.[21]

1. The central cord syndrome.—In this lesion, the central gray matter is damaged far more than the peripheral white matter. It occurs primarily in the cervical region, and one sees a pattern of paralysis in the upper extremities due to destruction of the anterior horn cells that serve this region of the body. There is often sparing of some or all of the more peripheral white matter that allows these tracts to conduct past the area of injury. They are thus able to energize the motor neurons in the lumbar and sacral areas. Therefore, depending upon the magnitude of the injury and the involvement of the white matter, the individual will be left with impairment of the upper extremities, less impairment of the lower extremities, and very possibly, preservation of bowel, bladder, and sexual function.

2. Anterior cord syndrome.—This syndrome displays a neurologic picture that reflects the destruction of the anterior two thirds of the cord. This includes the central gray and the white matter in the anterior and lateral columns of the cord. Thus, dorsal column function is preserved, and the individual has position and vibratory sense below the level of the lesion but lacks pain, temperature, and motor function.

3. Brown-Sequard syndrome.—This reflects the presence of function in only half of the spinal cord. This syndrome is manifested by ipsilateral loss of motor function, vibration, and position sense. The unique feature here is the loss of pain and temperature on the contralateral side of the body. Therefore, the injured person retains the feelings of pain and temperature on the paralyzed side.

4. The posterior column syndrome.—This consists of the loss of position and vibratory sense only, with preservation of the other motor and sensory modalities. This is rarely seen as a result of trauma.

It is important to remember that these syndromes are rarely "pure." That is, closed trauma rarely causes an exact manifestation of any one of the above syndromes. For example, someone will usually not manifest a Brown-Sequard syndrome in the pure form but rather will manifest an impairment of both sides of the spinal cord with one being more involved than the other.

BIOMECHANICS OF SPINAL TRAUMA

Clinical biomechanics has been defined by White and Panjabi[85] as "that body of knowledge that employs mechanical facts, concepts, principles, terms, methodologies, and mathematics to interpret and analyze normal and abnormal human anatomy and physiology." The analysis of spinal trauma by using biomechanical modeling gives important insight into the mechanism of injury, failure of anatomic structures, and forces required for deformity correction.

The basic unit of spinal anatomy is one motion segment, which has been identified as the functional spinal unit (FSU). The FSU is composed of two adjacent vertebrae, the intervening disc, the facet joints, and the connecting ligamentous structures. When an FSU is unable to resist or withstand physiologic forces or when excessive loading results in failure of the FSU with the potential for neurologic injury, the condition of spinal instability exists. White and Panjabi[85] further defined clinical spinal instability as "the loss of the ability of the spine under physiologic loads to maintain its pattern of displacement so that there is no initial or additional neurological deficit, no major deformity, and no incapacitating pain."

Vertebral column instability is based on radiologic imaging of acute spinal injuries to identify and analyze deformities and pathologic load conditions, which when coupled with neurologic involvement serve as good predictors of instability. White and Panjabi[85] have provided detailed checklists of radiologic and clinical factors affecting stability.

Spinal instability was described by Holdsworth[39, 40] on the basis of the fracture pattern seen on plain roentgenograms; he classified simple wedge fractures, burst fractures, and extension injuries as stable and classified dislocations, rotational fracture-dislocations, and shear fractures as unstable. Kelly and Whitesides[45] proposed a two-column model with an anterior weight-bearing (compression) column of vertebral bodies and a posterior (tension-resisting) column of neural arches. The three-column model, which was independently postulated by Denis[17, 18] and McAfee[55] by using CAT scans, brought attention to the middle vertebral structures. The three-column model proposes (1) the anterior column, including the anterior two thirds of the vertebral body and disc; (2) the middle column composing the posterior third of the vertebral body, the annulus fibrosus, and the posterior longitudinal ligament; and (3) the posterior column, which included the remaining posterior structures. Column failure is based upon application of pathologic loads where (1) the anterior vertebral body complex fails with compression loads, (2) the middle column fails with extreme axial loads, and (3) the posterior column fails after excessive flexion (or tension) loads. With excessive extension forces, rupture of the anterior longitudinal ligament and intervertebral disc can occur. Translational, subluxation, and/or dislocation injuries can often affect all three columns.

CLASSIFICATION OF SPINAL INJURIES

Of the numerous spinal injury classification systems proposed, few have gained the recognition required for widespread acceptance. In general, the classification of spinal injuries is based upon morphologic injury patterns that reflect the pathomechanics of the injury. Although there may be a multitude of force vectors acting upon the spine to create a fracture pattern, the primary mechanisms are compression, distraction, and torsion.[33] The compression mechanism may result in impaction, splitting, or burst fractures. The distraction mechanism may include posterior disruption, including the arch; posterior disruption, which is purely ligamentous; or anterior disruption, which results from hyperextension. Torsion results in the most unstable injury because it adds a component of force along the z (long) axis.

INITIAL TREATMENT

Regardless of the position in which one finds the injured person, every effort must be made to stabilize the spine. This can be done with a backboard or neck brace and strapping the patient to the board while he is extricated, e.g., from the car or construction site.

If the respiratory status is extremely impaired and emergency tracheostomy or cricothyroidotomy becomes necessary, it may not be possible to apply a cervical collar. The same may be true if extensive bleeding is present in the cervical area. In such an instance, the head must be stabilized with sandbags applied laterally. It must be remembered that when the spinal cord has been damaged, the patient is vulnerable to the development of pressure ulcers because of impaired sensation. Therefore, the patient must be turned at regular intervals, preferably every 2 hours, *regardless* of the fact that his spine may be unstable and must be immobilized. Turning is also necessary to facilitate drainage of the bronchial tree. When turning is performed, the patient must be log-rolled, and the chin, sternum, and symphysis pubis kept in a straight line at all times. When supine, the cervical and lumbar lordoses should be supported by towels or pillows. The backboard or splint of hard material must be removed as soon as the patient arrives at a hospital where definitive care can be given.

It is generally agreed among experts in the field that patients with SCI should be taken to a trauma center that has the services of a neurosurgeon, orthopedic surgeon, or preferably both. In addition, only lifesaving and emergency measures should be applied before the patient is taken to such a center. A trauma center that is attached or closely affiliated with an SCI center is the most preferable place for a spinal cord–injured person's initial care.

The patient should be transported in an ambulance or helicopter if at all possible and should only be given narcotics and other analgesics if the patient is actually complaining of severe pain since many individuals do not complain of pain as long as they are stabilized and handled with care.

Upon arrival at a trauma center, an intravenous line should be established if not already present, and the circulatory and respiratory systems must be stabilized. An indwelling urethral catheter and, usually, a nasogastric tube should be placed. The neurologic and radiographic examinations described earlier should then be carried out.

In the case of cervical injuries, efforts at stabilization will usually center around the application of external support such as a cervical brace of one form or another or the application of cervical traction by calipers or tongs such as the Gardner-Wells tongs. It is extremely important when dealing with a high-level cervical injury, such as those that may impair respiratory function, that the amount of traction be applied very cautiously since it is possible to easily overdistract an injury in the upper part of the cervical spine. Thus, frequent spine radiographs should be taken if the amount of traction is increased.

In the past, most patients with high-level cervical injuries either were neurologically intact or died. In recent times due to the rapid advances in life support systems and the wider availability of such services, many patients who would have died are now saved and are placed on artificial ventilation. Thus, it is possible for someone to survive who not only is paralyzed in the arms and legs but is also unable to breathe at all or unable to breathe adequately. Therefore, every effort must be made to foster conditions that will also favor the survival of as many nerve cells as possible in the zone of injury within the spinal cord. In addition to careful rescue and immobilization referred to earlier, it is important to avoid complications that are known to affect neural tissue adversely such as hypoxia and hypotension. Therefore, the respiratory and circulatory systems must be carefully supported.

MANAGEMENT OF SPINAL INJURIES

The management of spinal column and spinal cord injuries is controversial, and most of the discussion has focused on the concept of stability.* Historically, nonoperative management was popular for patients referred to spinal centers in Europe and Australia. In the United States, when patients arrived at spinal cord centers weeks or months after the injury, postural reduction was often the only option prior to the beginning of a rehabilitation program.† This approach in some cases resulted in spinal deformity, pain, and a relatively long hospitalization.‡ To-

*References 3, 13, 14, 16, 18, 22, 24, 27, 28, 30, 31, 36, 37, 40, 43, 49, 51, 67, 77, 81, 84, 87.

†References 2, 3, 8, 31, 36, 37, 51, 79, 89.

‡References 25, 34, 52, 54, 56, 61, 63, 68, 72.

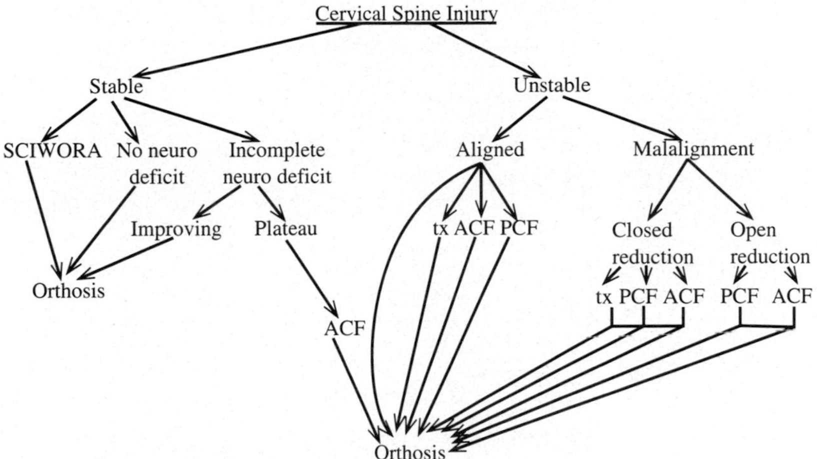

FIG 25–12.
Algorithm for the treatment of cervical spinal injuries. *SCIWORA* = spinal cord injury without radiologic abnormalities; *tx* = traction; *ACF* = anterior cervical fusion; *PCF* = posterior cervical fusion.

day, when operative intervention in competent hands can be performed safely, hospitalization time may be shortened, spinal deformity may be prevented, neurologic recovery may be maintained or enhanced, and mobilization may be started earlier with resulting psychological and physiologic benefit to the patient.§

The prompt reduction of acute spinal injuries with spinal deformity is a basic principle that has been widely accepted for quite some time. The spinal deformity should be reduced as promptly as possible.[15] Some believe that this will also relieve the bony pressure upon the injured spinal cord. The question as to which method is the safest and most efficient has stirred controversy. Postural reduction and manipulation vs. operative reduction are both techniques that may be equally effective and safe in skilled hands. The real controversy centers around how to achieve stabilization of the reduced spine so that the spinal cord may reside in an area safe from reinjury and the patient may be mobilized into a rehabilitation program for societal reentry (Figs 25–12 and 25–13). These concerns then bear direct relevance to the concept of spinal stability. The restoration of spinal stability to an injured spine may come either from a direct surgical repair of the injured spinal column by employing bone grafting and usually some form of metallic instrumentation or from a natural healing or "autofusion" of injured bony tissues while an orthosis is employed. Another area of key concern is healing of the injured tissues. Will they be able to sustain the forces of daily living while maintaining continued spinal cord protection?

Most stable spinal injuries are treated nonoperatively. Generally, fractures are designated as relatively stable if there is less than 25% to 30% loss of vertebral body height, only one of three columns is injured, there is less than 30 degrees of kyphosis, and there is less than 10 degrees of scoliosis.[59] These patients are immobilized in bed until the pain has decreased and then mobilized in an appropriate orthosis for a period of 6 to 12 weeks. The majority of patients will have no neurologic deficits, but oc-

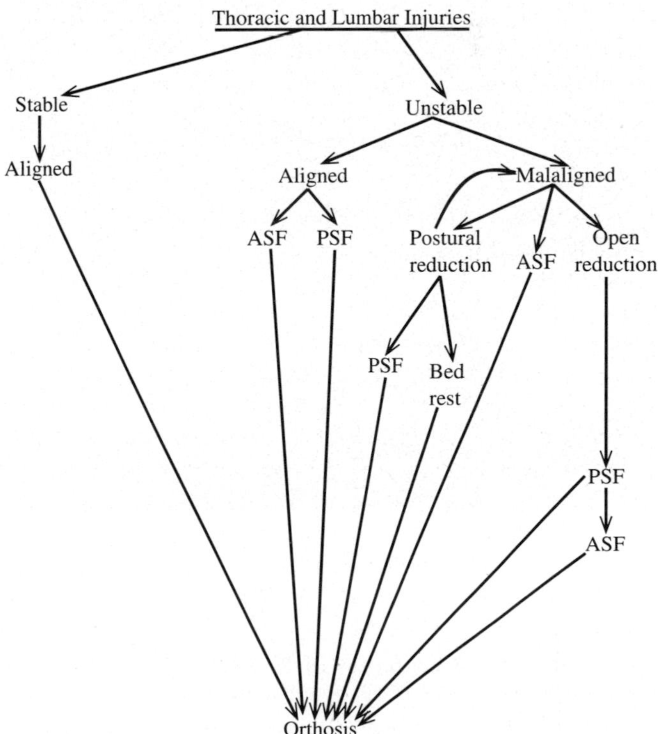

FIG 25–13.
Algorithm for the treatment of thoracic and lumbar spinal injuries. *ASF* = anterior spinal fusion; *PSF* = posterior spinal fusion.

§References 19, 26, 29, 38, 42, 52, 56, 81, 83.

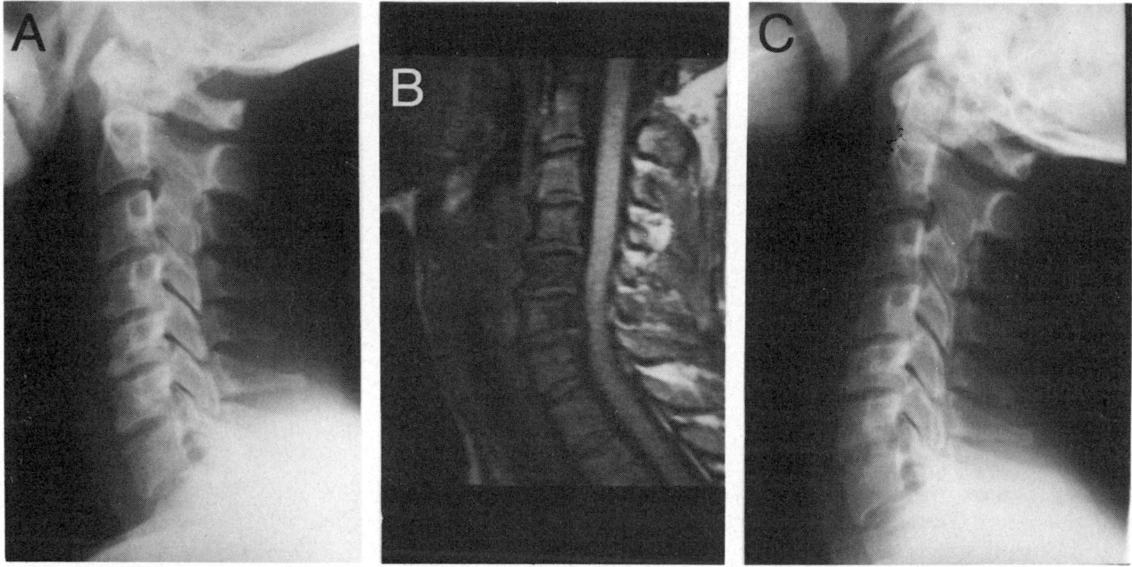

FIG 25–14.
A, lateral radiograph after a motor vehicle accident in a patient with radiculopathy. **B,** MRI shows a C6–7 herniated disc and spinal cord compression. **C,** lateral radiograph after anterior discectomy and fusion with an iliac crest bone graft.

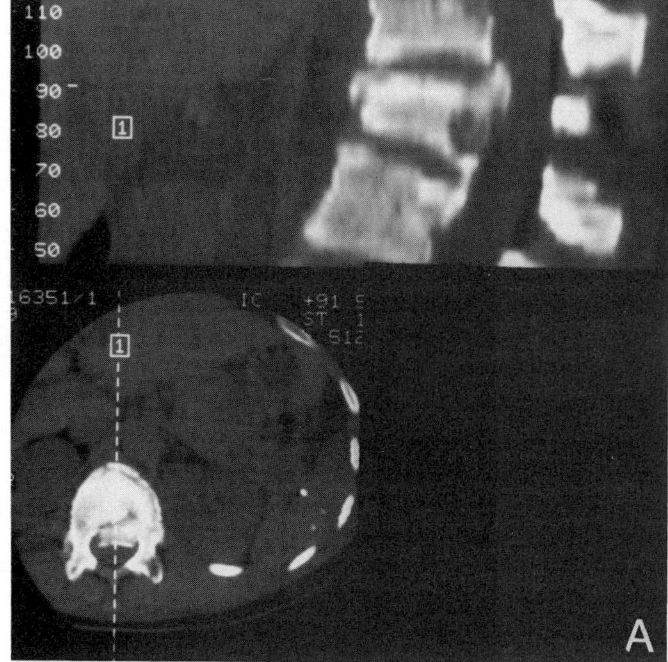

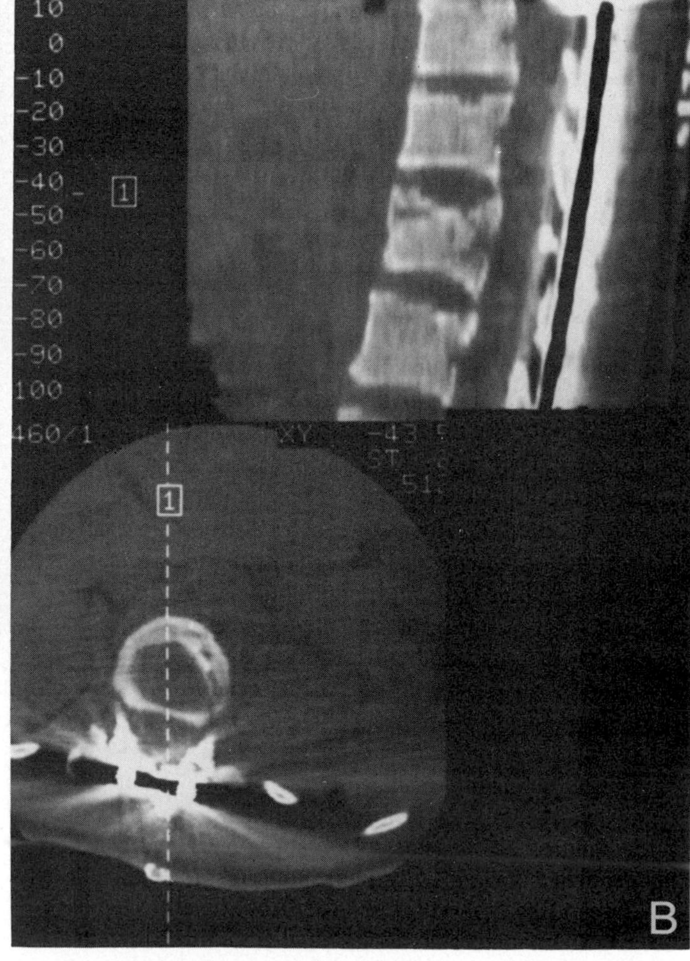

FIG 25–15.
Preoperative **(A)** and postoperative **(B)** axial and sagittal CAT scans after treatment of an L1 burst fracture with Harrington rods.

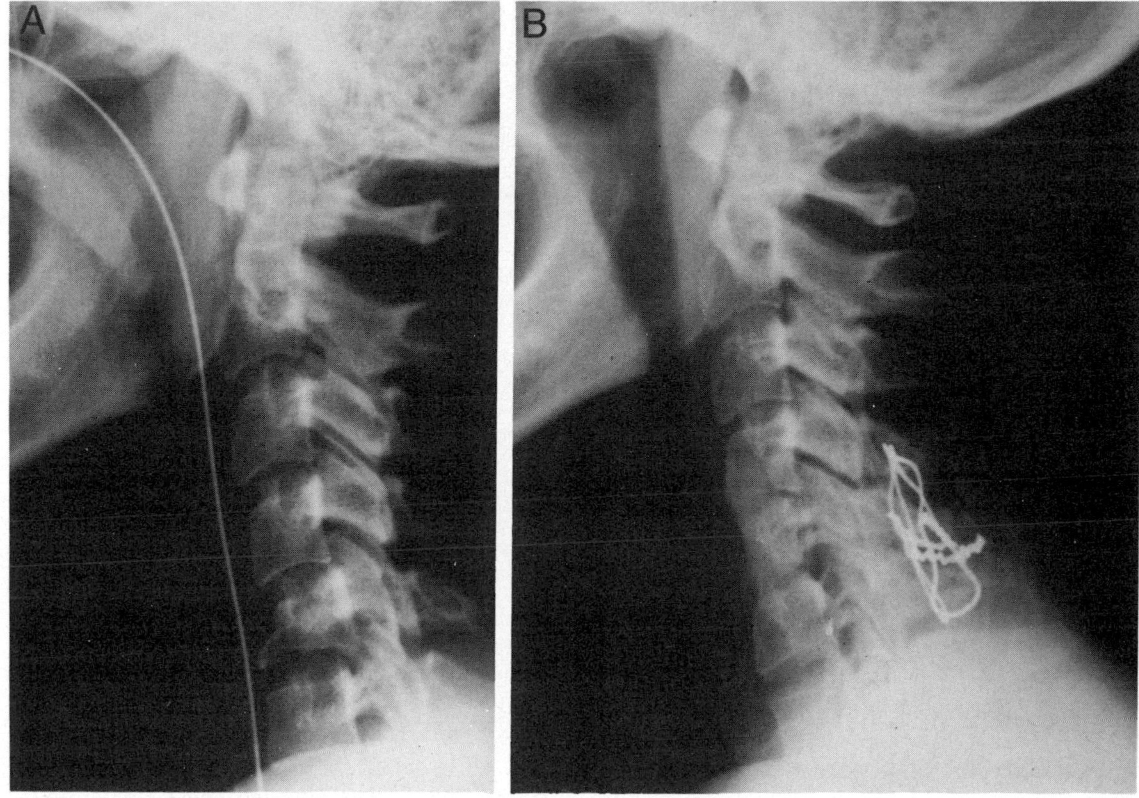

FIG 25–16.
A, lateral radiograph of a C5 compression (teardrop) fracture in a patient with incomplete quadriplegia. **B,** postoperative lateral radiograph after anterior C5 vertebrectomy and fusion and posterior fusion with wire internal fixation.

casionally an SCI without radiologic abnormalities (SCIWORA)[65, 71] or varied neurologic deficits are associated with stable injuries. Should a progressive significant deformity develop, as diagnosed by regular radiographic examinations, then operative intervention will be necessary.

An unstable spinal injury requires restoration of vertebral column alignment while consideration is given to maintaining the balance between mobility and stability.[6] Many institutions generally recommend surgical stabilization for unstable spinal injuries. Unstable injuries may be stabilized by either anterior and/or posterior procedures, but the anterior procedure is generally reserved for those patients requiring decompression of the spinal cord or more bony support for the anterior column (Fig 25–14, A–C). Unstable compression injuries are usually managed by a posterior procedure (Fig 25–15,A and B), with the noted exception of when there is a deficient anterior column. In cases where there is a deficient anterior column, then stability needs to be restored by an anterior bone graft and internal fixation or an anterior decompression and fusion and a posterior fixation procedure (Fig 25–16,A and B). The noted exceptions to these generalizations are at the C1–2 levels and fractures of the upper part of the thoracic spine. At the level of C1 and C2, most injuries are treated nonoperatively by traction techniques and then halo immobilization for 6 to 12 weeks (Fig 25–17). Unless there are multiple rib fractures or dislocations, the upper part of the thoracic spine (T1–9) is usually also amenable to nonoperative care due to the inherent stability that the thoracic cage with rib attachments imparts. There are a multitude of new instrumentations available for stabilization of acute unstable spinal injuries, and each one has advantages and disadvantages that must be considered prior to usage (Table 25–2).

Decompression of the spinal canal and its contents is indicated for any patient with an incomplete neurologic injury who worsens neurologically. Some authors also include those who fail to recover, and who continue with a significant neurologic deficit. The best decompression of neural tissue is often a reduction or realignment of the spine, and then if there is any residual compression, that specific area can be approached (Fig 25–18,A and B). The major disadvantage of the anterior approach is the magnitude of the surgery itself. Laminectomy alone is virtually never indicated today for traumatic spinal injuries.

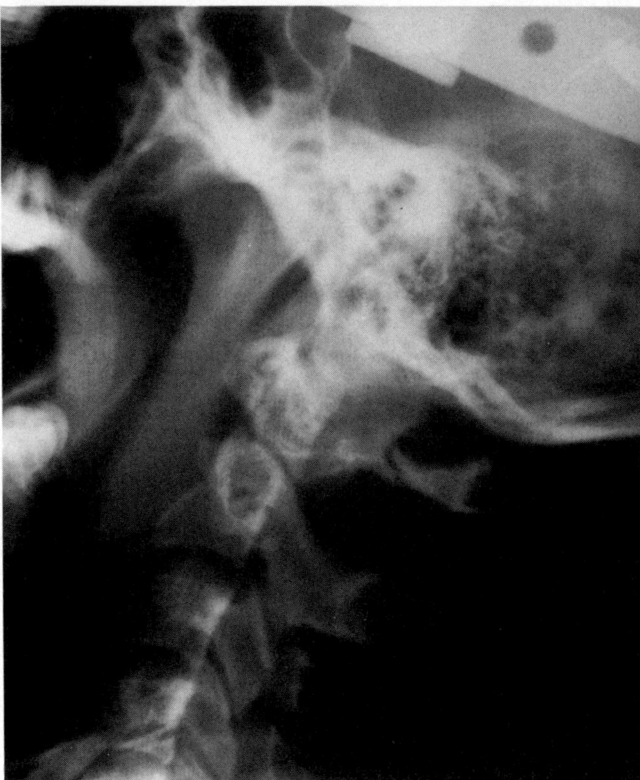

FIG 25–17.
C1 (Jefferson) and type II odontoid fractures that were treated nonoperatively with a halo vest.

TABLE 25–2.
Devices for Stabilization of Spinal Injuries

Cervical spine
Roy-Camille plates
Louis plates
Halifax clamp
Orosco plates
Caspar plates
Thoracic and lumbar spine
Rod and hook devices
Harrington rods
Edwards modular spinal system
Jacob distraction rods
Segmented devices
Luque rods and sublaminar wires
Cotrel-Dubousset system
Pedicle screw devices
Fixateur interne (AO internal fixator)
Fixateur externe (AO external fixator)
Steffee plates
Luque plates
AO plates
Olerud spinal fixator
Vermont spinal fixator
Harms device

FUNCTIONAL EXPECTATIONS

When it comes to predicting functional outcomes or functional expectations, the spinal cord readily lends itself to such predictions since each neurologic level (or segment) controls specific muscles and transmits sensory information from its dermatome. The distribution is similar but not exactly the same among all individuals. When considering functional expectations, it is useful to group several levels together. While it is understood that the lower levels within each group will perform better than the higher levels, the expectations for each group are nearly the same. The expectations given below are for musculoskeletal as well as for bowel, bladder, and sexual function.

Levels Below S2

Below S2, only bowel, bladder, and sexual function are affected. Patients in this group have acontractile bladders and lax sphincters, and males are generally impotent. Intermittent catheterization is often used unless patients are easily able to overcome sphincter resistance by strain and the Credé method. Some urinary and fecal incontinence may occur with a Valsalva maneuver. For this reason, it is preferred that stool softeners be avoided and the stool consistency be firm. Males and females may need to wear incontinence pads if dribbling is a problem. Artificial sphincters may be appropriate for some in this group. They require the patient to inflate and deflate the artificial sphincter by squeezing hydraulic fluid through tubes and valves implanted under the skin. There are usually no motor deficits except perhaps to the foot intrinsics, which could lead to hammertoe deformities.

Levels L4, L5, S1, and S2

In the L4–S2 group, indwelling catheters are rarely needed, while intermittent catheterization is often used. These patients also generally have lax sphincters and areflexic, acontractile detrusors. Therefore, elimination may also be accomplished by increasing abdominal pressure, and postvoid residual urine volumes close to zero are often achievable. However, incontinence may also occur, particularly with a Valsalva maneuver. If dribbling is significant, males may use an external collecting system consisting of a condom, a tube, and a collecting bag, and females may wear absorbent pads. Artificial sphincters may also be surgically implanted. Bowel elimination is usually accomplished by strain, Credé's maneuver, and often manual removal from the rectal vault. As with the first group, suppositories may be tried but are often ineffective due to the inability to induce reflex emptying. Since the anal sphincters may also be lax, some fecal soiling may occur when straining; therefore, patients generally prefer a more firm stool.

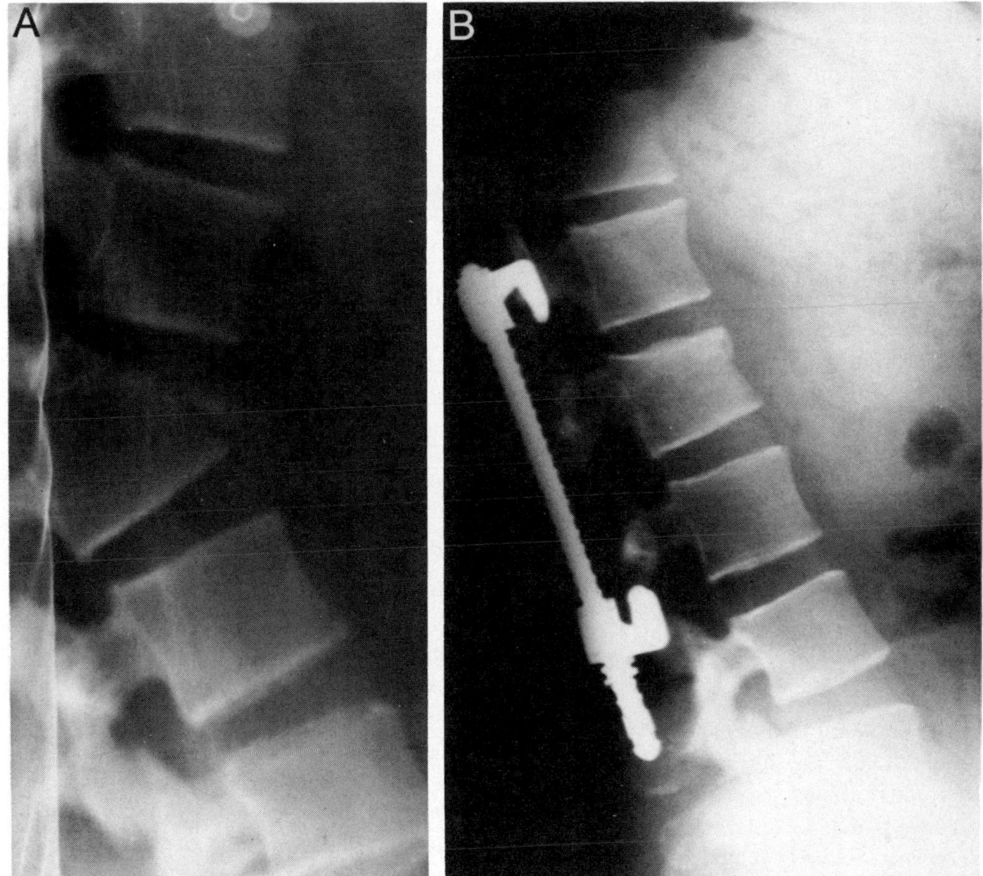

FIG 25–18.
A, lateral radiograph of an L1 distraction injury in a patient with incomplete paraplegia. **B,** a postoperative lateral radiograph shows anatomic alignment and stabilization with Edwards instrumentation and a bone graft. The patient had a complete neurologic recovery.

In both of these groups, in order to circumvent the male patient's inability or difficulty in obtaining an erection, a penile prosthesis consisting of semirigid silicone or one with an inflatable mechanism[74] can be surgically implanted. The patient's erectile ability can also be influenced by the injection of papaverine and/or phentolamine into one of the corpora cavernosa.[7] More recently, prostaglandin E has been used successfully in this regard.[50] Condom-type devices employing a vacuum principle have also been successful in some patients. Competent sexual counseling should be offered before any such procedures or devices are recommended so that the patients and their partners can assess their expectations and feelings toward each other.

Transfers, eating, dressing, and personal hygiene pose no problem. The patient's ambulation is often quite good even without orthoses, although L5 lesions will benefit from the ankle stability provided by two ankle-foot orthoses (AFOs) that essentially "lock" the ankle joint, i.e., prevent both dorsiflexion and plantar flexion. Two canes or crutches are required by some when the hip abductors and extensors are weak, although at the lower levels one cane may be sufficient, even for long distances. Wheelchairs are not needed in most cases. At the lower levels in this group, driving without special hand controls can be achieved, although hand controls may be preferred by some patients. No attendant care is necessary.

Levels L1, L2, and L3

At these levels, urethral and anal sphincters are inclined to be hyperreflexic, and involuntary tone will keep them in the closed position. Bladder elimination may still be accomplished by abdominal pressure if the sphincteric pressures are not too great. If they are, it may be necessary to use a procedure called anal stretch,[46] which consists of manually dilating the anal sphincter and thereby relaxing the urethral sphincter to permit bladder emptying by the Valsalva maneuver. Alternately, intermittent catheterization may be used by this group also. External collecting systems for the male and absorbent pads for the female are less necessary since it is usually possible for the bladder to store enough urine so the patient will remain dry between catheterizations or voidings. Anticholinergics may be needed if the bladder is too hyperreflexic to store sufficient volumes to allow catheterizations every 4 hours. Anticholinergics will usually improve bladder capacity. Bowel leakage is less of an issue, although should diarrhea occur, incontinence would still be a problem. The use of reflex stimulation of peristalsis to enhance bowel emptying is more successful. Timing, i.e., after a meal (taking advantage of the gastrocolic reflex), use of a suppository, and digital stimulation are more effective than in patients with lower lesions. Transfers, eating, dressing, and personal hygiene are independent after training.

Bipedal ambulation will usually require knee-ankle-foot orthoses (KAFOs) and two crutches or perhaps even a walker. The gait pattern used may be either the four-point, "swing-through," or "swing-to" type, depending on the ability of the hip flexors (L2, L3) to advance the limb. Wheelchairs at these levels are usually not discarded, particularly not at the higher levels because they will be needed for long distances. Automobile driving requires the use of hand controls. No attendant is necessary.

Levels T7–12

Bladder and bowel function is similar to the more rostral lumbar levels. However, the bladder may be more hyperreflexic. Males and females may be managed with intermittent catheterization but will often require anticholinergics for this to be workable. If the male desires to stop catheterizing and void, a sphincterotomy may be necessary to allow him to void with acceptable pressures and residual volumes if the sphincter is too hypertonic. External collecting devices are then needed and are now practical since newer materials cause less skin irritation.

The higher the level between T7 and T12, the greater the loss of control over the abdominal and back musculature. Since these muscles are used for coughing, the higher the lesion, the less effective the cough. Therefore, these patients are at greater risk for developing respiratory infections, particularly the smokers among them.

Transfers, eating, dressing, and personal hygiene are easily achieved through training. Bipedal ambulation with KAFOs and crutches at these levels is less and less functional the higher the level and is used mostly for exercise. The wheelchair is the main mode of propulsion. Therefore, use of public buildings, public toilets, etc., is restricted to those that are wheelchair accessible. Hand controls are required for automobile driving.

Levels T1–6

Bladder elimination is essentially as described for T7–12. Control of leakage usually requires anticholinergics and the maintenance of sterile urine. Males may avoid this and wear external collecting systems all the time, providing that voiding pressures and volumes are acceptable. Females may find that leakage is not controlled sufficiently regardless of anticholinergics and sterile urine and choose a catheter with drainage to a leg bag. Bowel function control is as above. Transfers, eating, dressing, and personal hygiene, while achievable, require much training.

Bipedal ambulation is no longer practical for many in this group, even for exercise, because of poor trunk control, although some patients might choose to attempt it. The wheelchair is the main mode of locomotion or mobilization. Hand controls and sometimes external trunk support are required for automobile driving. Usually no attendant is necessary, although a roommate could be helpful.

Levels C7 and C8

At these levels, the hands are involved. Training now takes longer because special adaptive equipment is needed and manual manipulative techniques need to be learned.

Wearing an external collector is preferred by many men. Providing that voiding pressures and residual volumes are acceptable, bladder elimination can be accomplished by stimulating the micturition reflex. Sphincterotomies may be required to lower the voiding pressure to an acceptable range (under 80 cm H_2O). As with all groups with contractile bladders, this will be helpful only if the detrusor has sufficient contractibility to expel the urine once the resistance has been reduced. Intermittent catheterization is difficult although not impossible, particularly for the C8 lesion. Many females will use a continuous indwelling Foley catheter. Autonomic dysreflexia may be a significant problem, particularly if the catheter becomes obstructed. Bowel function, particularly the insertion of suppositories and the use of digital stimulation of the anus, becomes more difficult for the patient to perform himself but can be achieved with a finger splint or can be performed by an attendant.

Due to grip weakness, modifications of the wheelchair to make propulsion easier may be required, such as applying friction tape, tubing, or projections on the handwheel rims. Some will require power wheelchairs. Transfers usually require a sliding board, and electric beds are usually necessary. Clothing modifications such as the use of snaps or Velcro will circumvent the difficulty these patients have with buttons. Dressing and personal hygiene may require partial use of an attendant for donning pants and total-body bathing. Special adaptations of bathroom systems are required. Hand controls and sometimes steering wheel attachments are necessary for automobile driving. The C7 level is the most rostral level compatible with needing no attendant whatsoever, although many will not achieve this goal.

Level C6

Bladder and bowel function is the same as for the C7/C8 levels, but intermittent catheterization is not practical for most patients since they usually cannot do it themselves and it must be done by an attendant. Most females and many males will require an indwelling catheter, either urethral or suprapubic.

The only remaining hand and wrist function at this level is extension or dorsiflexion of the wrist. Triceps function is lost; therefore the patient cannot forcibly extend his elbow. Elevating the trunk from the sitting surface is more difficult since only the shoulder depressors can be used, and then only if the elbows are free of flexion contractures and can be placed in full extension. Therefore, preservation of full range of elbow motion is essential. Eating skills are achieved by using adaptive equipment applied to the hands such as a wrist-driven flexor hinge (tenodesis) splint that creates opposition of the thumb to the second and third fingers by dorsiflexing the wrist. A cuff worn over the hand with a slot for a spoon or fork (universal cuff) may also be used.

Ambulation in a manually operated wheelchair with modifications of the wheel rims as above is still possible on level, smooth surfaces. However, electric wheelchairs are also needed for more difficult terrain. The completion of total dressing and personal hygiene usually requires an attendant. Some patients can achieve this independently with the aid of loops sewn onto the clothes into which they can hook a finger, but this is often too time-consuming. Pull-over garments for the upper part of the torso are usually preferable to buttoned shirts because of the difficulty of manipulation of buttons, snaps, and the like. If the arms are long enough, a sliding board is used for transfers. Transfers in and out of bed and on and off a toilet can be achieved, and car transfers can also be achieved by certain patients without assistance. The use of a van with a lift makes car travel and driving easier and more practical. An attendant or at least a helpful roommate is usually required to assist with dressing, personal hygiene, and in some cases, transfers. Some of the bladder care, e.g., application of the external collector, and bowel care, e.g., suppository insertion and cleanup, also require assistance. Such patients are rarely able to live alone.

Level C5

At this level the patient has shoulder and elbow flexion function but no wrist and hand function. Bladder management is essentially as for C6. Male patients cannot apply an external collector independently. For bowel function, an attendant must provide a suppository, digital stimulation, and cleanup functions. Eating, except perhaps for cutting, can be developed with everything set up (i.e., food already cut, cartons opened, and straws inserted), but transfers, dressing, and personal hygiene are usually totally dependent on an attendant.

Ambulation is by electric wheelchair that the patient controls by placing his hand on a stick mounted on the control box of the wheelchair on the same side as the stronger arm. Automobile driving capability depends upon residual shoulder motion, but a van is absolutely necessary. A full-time attendant is necessary to assist with most functions but need not be at the patient's side at all times. With appropriate seat cushions, these patients can sit for 8 to 10 hours a day with perhaps some pressure relief provided by the attendant or by intermittently reclining the seat back by power controls.

Other adaptive equipment used by some patients with lesions at C5 include battery-powered and cable-operated wrist-driven flexor hinge splints. Ball bearing feeders (mobile arm supports) anchored to the wheelchair that allow the patient to feed himself and do some facial grooming can be used by weak C5 patients and C4 patients. To operate the mobile arm supports, the patient places the arms in special troughs attached to movable hinged bars. By using the shoulder muscles, the patient can make the troughs swivel to bring his arms toward the body and move them out again and also to tip the troughs downward at the elbow to raise the hands (Fig 25–19).

Levels C1, C2, C3, and C4

Acutely, the C4 level is the last compatible with life, unless at the time of the accident assisted respiration was provided by someone in the vicinity. C1, C2, and many C3 patients invariably require permanent assisted ventilation, as do some of the C4 patients. A battery-powered portable respirator can, for most, be fitted to the wheelchair. The C1–3 patients usually require a permanent tra-

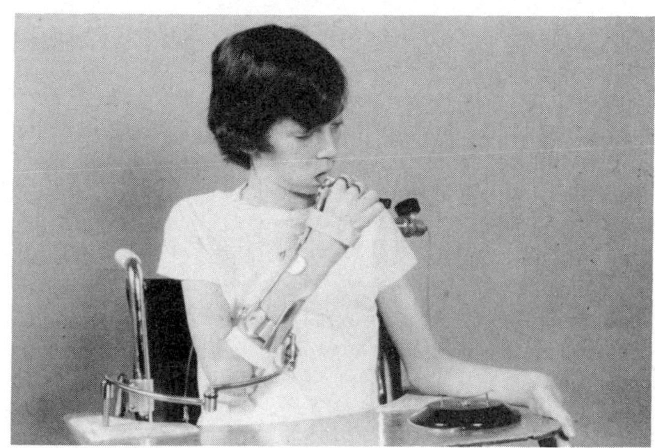

FIG 25–19.
Demonstration of the use of a mobile arm support, also known as a ball bearing feeder.

cheostomy and special techniques to control lung and throat secretions. Some will be helped by phrenic nerve stimulators providing that the nerve is viable, and this will reduce reliance on the ventilator. Others will gain some time off the ventilator with a pneumobelt.

C1–4 patients can use a chin, mouth, or breath control device and perhaps a voice-controlled device to operate electric wheelchairs. They may have greater control of their environment through so-called environmental control systems. In these systems, the patient can control a telephone, radio, television, lights, buzzer, and the like from one place. Selection of one of these options is made by using breath, tongue, sound, or residual muscle power to activate the system. A full-time trained attendant is required for the patient and should always be available.

PREVENTION OF COMPLICATIONS

The importance of alterations of function of the respiratory, cardiovascular, digestive, urinary, and integumentary systems following SCI has been recognized for many years.[88]

These complications are usually preventable if the patient is cared for by doctors, nurses, and other personnel who are experienced with the spinal cord–injured patient's unique problems. In a regional system of care, patients with SCI are referred quickly to an SCI center (just as burn patients are referred to a burn center), where the staff expertise, facilities, and equipment are available to meet their needs. Such a system permits this extraordinary care to be available on a cost-effective basis[21] because the incidence of SCI is too low even when using the highest incidence figures (5 to 6 per 100,000 population)[32] to financially justify every community hospital providing these services. When complications are prevented, resources are not squandered on their treatment. By avoiding them and remaining healthy, the patient can progress faster in his rehabilitation.

Respiratory System

Coincident trauma to the chest will obviously focus the surgeon's attention on the respiratory management of patients with SCI. Rib fractures, for example, are not infrequent and occur in approximately 25% of all thoracic spine injuries.[88]

However, medical complications may also compromise respiratory function, and the surgeon must be aware that most can be prevented. Information from the National Spinal Cord Injury Data Research Center indicated that the most common respiratory complications were pneumonia and atelectasis, 8% and 11%, respectively, in paraplegics and 17% and 19%, respectively, in quadriplegics. The incidence of pulmonary emboli was 4% in paraplegics and 5% in quadriplegics.[88]

Factors that increase the risk of atelectasis and pneumonia include (1) a neurologic level above T10, which impairs the effectiveness of cough; (2) a history of smoking beyond five to ten pack-years, which is often associated with a hypersecretory state due to long-standing chronic bronchitis; (3) obesity; and (4) a recent history of general anesthesia. If a patient's ability to cough is compromised because of either paralysis of the abdominal and thoracic musculature or pain due to rib fractures or the spinal trauma itself, secretions can pool in the respiratory tree and occlude the patient's airways. These atelectatic segments collapse and become no longer ventilated. If they still remain perfused, however, unoxygenated blood returns to the left heart, mixes with the oxygenated blood, and is circulated throughout the body, thereby lowering the oxygen content of the arterial blood. The resulting hypoxemia impairs the function of all body organs and further impairs the ability of the unaffected parts of the lungs to exchange gases effectively.[69] If this remains uncorrected, a condition requiring ventilatory support and tracheotomy can quickly arise.

Atelectasis, pneumonia, and respiratory insufficiency from muscle fatigue are preventable if the primary physician anticipates them. It is most helpful to assess all patients initially, particularly the quadriplegics and high-level paraplegics, for vital capacity and negative inspiratory force on a daily basis. This provides the physician with important information as to the patient's respiratory reserve. Under resting conditions with no increased metabolic demand, e.g., from fever, a tidal volume of 500 mL is needed to provide adequate gas exchange. If a patient's vital capacity falls below 1500 mL, respiratory fatigue may ensue because the patient is using one third or more of his maximum effort just to provide the necessary ventilation. If the vital capacity drops below 1000 mL, a potentially serious problem of respiratory insufficiency may be imminent due to fatigue of the diaphragm. The diaphragm is a muscle of inspiration only. In a quadriplegic, expiration occurs passively. More importantly, without the thoracic and abdominal muscles, he cannot cough and therefore cannot move secretions.

Even in the absence of space-occupying conditions, e.g., hemothorax, the vital capacity may be compromised by increasing atelectasis and/or increased secretion production. Therefore, every effort must be made to assist the patient in raising these secretions. Since the cough mechanism is absent in quadriplegics and impaired in most paraplegics, the nursing or respiratory therapy staff must be available and knowledgeable in the techniques of chest physiotherapy, including assisted coughing. Even if the patient has been tracheotomized and ventilatory support has been instituted, chest physiotherapy and assisted coughing should be performed even though the latter may be less effective with the tracheostomy. In neurologically intact patients, suctioning alone through an endotracheal catheter does nothing directly to raise secretions from the periphery of the lungs. It only does so secondarily by stimulating a cough. However, if the patient's cough is absent or weak, the secretions may never be moved from the periphery, where they are liable to occlude the smaller bronchioles. Further, vigorous suctioning in quadriplegics can cause sinus arrest due to excessive unopposed vagal tone triggered by the carinal reflex. It must be remembered that quadriplegia is a condition of sympathetic blockade. Only assisted coughing plus chest physiotherapy (in the patient with an SCI above T10) can bring secretions from the periphery.

Deep Venous Thrombosis and Pulmonary Embolus

Clinically obvious deep venous thrombosis occurs in 15% of paraplegics and 4% of quadriplegics.[88] The incidence is, in fact, probably much higher if it is actively searched for, particularly through radionuclide scanning. Thigh and calf measurements should be monitored daily, and if a discrepancy of more than 2 cm appears and increases, venography should be performed. The authors prefer radionuclide venography because it not only provides information as to the presence or absence of deep venous thrombosis but can also supply some information as to the age of the clot. In the authors' experience, it also gives better imaging of the pelvic veins. Treatment of this condition, once diagnosed, includes heparin by continuous infusion and maintenance of the activated partial thromboplastin time (APPT) between 1.5 and 2.0 times control. The patient may be switched to warfarin (Coumadin) therapy after 3 to 5 days of heparin treatment with the goal of achieving the same control range.

Much debate still exists over the efficacy of prophylactic doses (minidoses) of heparin. It has been reported[66, 70] that minidose heparin, i.e., 5000 units of heparin administered every 8 or 12 hours, decreases the incidence of deep venous thrombosis and pulmonary emboli. Information available to date indicates that heparin probably does decrease but not eliminate the incidence of deep venous thrombosis and pulmonary emboli. Ideally, it should be started within the first 48 hours post-trauma. Merli and colleagues have reported augmentation of the prophylaxis from heparin with the use of functional electrical stimulation (FES).[57]

Urinary System

Complications involving the urinary tract following SCI are more numerous than those of any other system. The most frequent complication of these is urinary tract infection (UTI). The National Spinal Cord Injury Data Research Center reported an incidence of UTI of 66% in paraplegics and 70% in quadriplegics.[88] This includes both symptomatic and asymptomatic bacteriuria. In fact, the figure would probably approach 100% if colonization of the bladder were recorded in all cases.

The clinician must recall that spinal shock manifests itself initially by total flaccidity, regardless of whether the lesion is in the cord or the cauda equina. This applies to the bowel and the bladder as well as the skeletal muscles. If the lesion is suprasacral, i.e., within the cord but above the conus medullaris, eventually the bladder should regain reflex activity. There are instances of suprasacral lesions, however, when the bladder may remain flaccid for an extended period of time, even well after reflex activity has returned to the skeletal muscles. Regardless of the location of the lesion, however, the bladder must be catheterized as part of the initial treatment.

While it is true that intermittent catheterization has been a significant advance in the management of paraplegic and quadriplegic patients and its use avoids many of the complications of the indwelling catheter, it seems pointless to the authors to begin intermittent catheterization immediately. The risk of overdistension of the bladder (because of the administration of too much fluid for the bladder to store in a 4-hour period) is too great at a time when frequently more than one intravenous line is running. In addition, it may be necessary to monitor the urinary output on an hourly basis, and intermittent catheterization more frequently than every 4 hours becomes increasingly impractical to perform. Therefore, it is the authors' policy to place an indwelling Foley catheter, using a closed system, and change this catheter once weekly. The patient is treated by continuous drainage until all intravenous fluids have been removed and oral fluids can be limited on an average to 200 mL every 2 hours. This should ensure a volume of no more than 400 mL of urine every 4 hours. Intermittent catheterization should be continued throughout the acute phase, with one exception. If pyelonephritis or sepsis develops, particularly when intravenous catheters are required, a closed-system indwelling catheter should be reinserted and fluids forced.

Treatment of "asymptomatic bacteriuria" during the acute period postinjury is still a matter of debate. The issue is somewhat clarified when one defines what is meant by asymptomatic bacteriuria. In the minds of many urologists, it simply means that there is no fever. Colonization of the urinary bladder by bacteria in significant numbers (i.e., greater than 100,000 colonies per milliliter) may produce symptoms other than fever. These include lethargy, nausea, incontinence between catheterizations, and an increase in spasticity (after reflexes to the skeletal muscles have returned), and consequently, the rehabilitation effort may become impaired. It is the authors' opinion, therefore, that during the acute phase postinjury, colonization of the urinary tract in significant numbers should be treated by an appropriate antibiotic even in the absence of fever. Frequently, if the bacteriuria is not treated properly, fever, septicemia, and symptoms of pyelonephritis will develop. If they do, the patient will require intravenous antibiotics and bed rest for a period of 7 to 10 days and his nutritional status will likely suffer due to the loss of appetite during the illness. If the patient has been exposed to the risks and benefits of an internal stabilization procedure to allow early mobilization, he will be unable to take advantage of those benefits while febrile. No one knows ahead of time whether or not bacteriuria will progress to septicemia. Thus, it is best to keep the urinary tract free of bacteriuria while monitoring urine cultures once or twice per week. If fever should develop, it will be reassuring to know that the urinary tract is not the source because the urine is sterile.[21] Later, after the catabolic effects of the trauma and surgery have been reversed and the patient's resistance is normalized, bacteriuria, if it is truly asymptomatic, may be treated expectantly.

Integumentary System

It cannot be emphasized strongly enough that not only is the complication of a decubitus ulcer (pressure necrosis) the most unnecessary and the most reprehensible of complications to beset the spinal cord–injured patient, but it is also the most costly. Statistics from the National Spinal Cord Injury Data Research Center indicate that if a spinal cord–injured patient develops even one decubitus ulcer serious enough to require plastic surgery, it increases the cost of hospitalization fivefold. That same study revealed that 20% of paraplegics and 26% of quadriplegics cared for within the model systems developed pressure ulcers. Subsequent studies[23, 62] disclosed that the likelihood of the development of pressure necrosis increased significantly the longer a patient was cared for in a community hospital prior to referral to an SCI center. In one study, patients whose referral to an SCI center was delayed more than 6 weeks showed a 35% incidence of pressure sores. These ulcers can be prevented only by a meticulous and alert nursing staff who are aware of the need for turning the patient every 2 hours coupled with careful inspection of the skin over the bony prominences each time the patient is turned. Redness that fails to fade after 15 minutes necessitates an alteration of the turning schedule to avoid worsening of the condition. Turning accomplishes more than simple pressure relief; it also facilitates pulmonary drainage. Whether the patient is turned manually or by a rotating bed, careful attention to other nursing needs must be carried out.

Each time a patient is turned, not only is his skin inspected, but the perineum is checked for soilage, the catheter is checked for proper drainage, the intravenous lines are inspected, the need for suctioning is determined, and the patient is questioned in regard to his general comfort. Mechanical beds do not do any of these things, and they alone do not prevent sores. They can reduce the need for strength on the part of the personnel caring for the patient.

Digestive System

There is no need to begin a bowel program until bowel sounds have returned. If the initial examination discloses a large amount of hard stool in the rectal ampulla, this may be gently removed and is all that is required on the first day. Occasionally, the period of ileus will last longer than the usual 3 to 5 days, and intra-abdominal pathologic findings such as infection or abscess should be ruled out. Following a thoracolumbar fracture it is not uncommon for a large retroperitoneal hematoma to occur. This may be responsible for prolongation of the ileus also. However, once bowel sounds have returned and the patient is begun on oral or nasogastric feedings, most patients with SCI (except those mentioned earlier) require a stool softener to allow the passage of stool by peristalsis more easily since abdominal muscles may be weak and the patient may be unable to bear down effectively. A suppository and digital stimulation of the rectal mucosa to initiate defecation are also required. The authors prefer that bowel programs be performed once daily during the acute period to avoid the problems of constipation.

Since steroids are used routinely,[5] it would seem reasonable to use an H_2 blocker to prevent acid production by the parietal cells of the gastric fundus.

Musculoskeletal System

The tendency to develop contractures in paralyzed limbs of the spinal cord–injured patient is somewhat different from that of the head-injured patient. The latter frequently demonstrates an increase in tone postinjury, while the former is always flaccid until the period of spinal shock has passed. As long as range of motion is performed on a daily or twice-daily basis, it is unlikely that fixed contractures will develop during the acute phase; therefore, the wearing of resting splints while in bed becomes unnecessary. The one joint that is perhaps an exception to the above is the shoulder. The capsule of the shoulder is so redundant that it easily loses this redundancy unless the joint is passed through full range of motion. In addition, the authors have found that the problem of adhesive capsulitis, which is so common in quadriplegics and patients with brachial plexus lesions, can be significantly reduced if the arms are placed in a 90-degree abducted position while the individual is supine.[75]

Psychological System

Information regarding the proper methods of treatment of the psyche of the spinal cord–injured person exists. Not all patients appear to need to pass through the classic phases of recovery from trauma, namely, shock, denial, anger, depression, and gradual elevation of spirits.[80] These manifestations will vary considerably with one's neurologic deficit, one's family support, and the confidence that the patient and family have in the facility and its staff. In the acute phase postinjury, the authors have found that it is most important that the family be kept apprised of the medical status of the injured person in a timely fashion. It is also their confirmed opinion that blunt perfunctory statements regarding the prognosis for recovery during the first few weeks postinjury are neither valuable, necessary, nor helpful in any way. The authors believe that "a hope for the best, but prepare for the worst" attitude is the best one to convey to the patient and his family during this time.

Mobility

The authors have chosen to emphasize complications and medical management of the spinal cord–injured patient during the foregoing paragraphs. From the spinal cord physician's point of view, complications that may be acquired by the patient with SCI cannot be simply ascribed to bed rest. It is the neglected patient at bed rest who develops complications, not the patient simply at bed rest per se. Surgery that is necessary to correct significant spinal deformity is not questioned. However, overenthusiasm directed at getting the patient "out of bed" based simply on the naive belief that he will be better off both mentally and physically and operating on the spine for this reason only are to be discouraged. Decisions regarding the issue of early mobilization should be based carefully on factors such as concomitant injuries, general medical condition, absence of medical complications, and the reliability of the allied health personnel to care for the patient competently, as well as on concerns such as ensuring spinal stability and the early mobilization that internal fixation will allow. It is true that in patients with thoracolumbar injuries early mobilization does reduce the length of hospitalization as well, all other factors being equal.[16] The paraplegic patient generally does not experience respiratory difficulties as severe as those of the quadriplegic, nor does he usually have the accompanying circulatory insufficiency, namely, orthostatic hypotension. In addition, the full use of the upper extremities and innervation of the trunk do allow the performance of mobilization activities earlier if internal stabilization is performed. On the other hand, the period of bed rest necessary to ensure proper healing of a thoracolumbar or lumbar fracture without surgery is approximately 10 to 12 weeks as compared with only 6 weeks for a cervical fracture.

Therefore, since the paraplegic patient has more things to do when out of bed and less pathophysiologic changes to adjust to than does a quadriplegic patient, the rationale for internal stabilization and fusion for purposes of early mobilization is on a sounder footing than the rationale for those with neck injuries. Internal stabilization of cervical fractures has been shown to shorten the acute care hospital stay[12] but does not significantly shorten the total hospitalization (acute care and rehabilitation) and does achieve better alignment of the cervical spine.[20]

REFERENCES

1. Aguago A: Regrowth and connectivity of regenerating axons from the adult mammalian CNS. Presented at the Annual Neurotrauma Symposium, Phoenix. October 1989.
2. Bedbrook GM, Sir: Fracture dislocations of the spine with and without paralysis. A case for conservatism and against operative techniques, in Leach RE, Hoaglund FT, Riseborough EJ (eds): *Controversies in Orthopaedic Surgery*. Philadelphia, WB Saunders, 1982, pp 423–455.
3. Bedbrook GM, Sir: Treatment of thoracolumbar dislocation and fractures with paraplegia. *Clin Orthop* 1975; 112:27.
4. Bondurant FJ, Cotler HB, Kulkarni MV, et al: Acute spinal cord injury: A study using physical examination and magnetic resonance imaging. *Spine* 1990; 15:161–168.
5. Bracken MB, Shephard MJ, Callus WF: A randomized, controlled trial of methylprednisolone or naloxone in the treatment of acute spinal cord injury. *N Engl J Med* 1990; 322:1405–1411.
6. Bradford DS, Thompson RC: Fractures and dislocations of the spine. Indications for surgical intervention. *Minn Med* 1976; 7:711.
7. Brindley GS: Cavernosal alpha-blockade: A new technique for investigating and treating erectile impotence. *Br J Psychiatry* 1983; 143:322.
8. Burke DC, Murray DD: The management of thoracic and thoraco-lumbar injuries of the spine with neurological involvement. *J Bone Joint Surg [Br]* 1976; 58:72.
9. Calenoff L, Chessare JW, Rogers LF, et al: Multiple level spinal injuries: The importance of early recognition. *Am J Radiol* 1978; 130:665.
10. Campbell JB, DeCrescito V, Tomasula JJ, et al: Effects of antifibrinolytic and steroid therapy on the contused spinal cord of cats. *J Neurosurg* 1974; 40:726–733.
11. Commission on Accreditation of Rehabilitation Facilities: *Standards Manual for Organizations Serving People With Disabilities*. Tucson, 1989.
12. Cotler HB, Cotler JM, Alden ME, et al: The medical and economic impact of closed cervical spine dislocations. *Spine* 1990; 15:448.
13. Cotler HB, Cotler JM, Stoloff A, et al: The use of autografts for vertebral body replacement of the thoracic and lumbar spine. *Spine* 1985; 10:748.
14. Cotler HB, Miller LS, DeLucia FA, et al: Closed reduction of cervical spine dislocations. *Clin Orthop* 1987; 214:185.
15. Cotler HB, Scott AC: Unstable cervical spine dislocations: Recognition, assessment, management. *J Musculoskel Med* 1989; 6:29.
16. Davies WE, Morris JH, Hill V: An analysis of conservative (non-surgical) management of thoraco-lumbar fractures and

fracture-dislocations with neurological damage. *J Bone Joint Surg [Am]* 1980; 62:1324.
17. Denis F: Spinal instability as defined by the three-column spine concept in acute spinal trauma. *Clin Orthop* 1984; 198:65.
18. Denis F: The three-column spine and its significance in the classification of acute thoraco-lumbar spinal injuries. *Spine* 1983; 8:817.
19. Dickson JH, Harrington TR, Erwin WD: Results of reduction and stabilization of the severely fractured thoracic and lumbar spine. *J Bone Joint Surg [Am]* 1978; 60:799.
20. Donovan WH, Cifu DX, Shotte DE: Neurological and skeletal outcomes in 113 patients with closed injuries to the cervical spinal cord. *Paraplegia* 1992; 30:533.
21. Donovan WH, Bedbrook GM: Comprehensive management of spinal cord injury. *Clin Symp* 1982; 34:1–36.
22. Donovan WH, Carter RE, Bedbrook GM, et al: Incidence of medical complications in spinal cord injury: Patients in specialized, compared with non-specialized centers. *Paraplegia* 1984; 22:282–290.
23. Donovan WH, Dwyer AP: An update on the early management of traumatic paraplegia (nonoperative and operative management). *Clin Orthop* 1984; 189:12.
24. Doppman JL, Girton M: Angiographic study of the effect of laminectomy in the presence of acute anterior epidural masses. *J Neurosurg* 1976; 45:487.
25. Dorr LD, Harvey JP Jr, Nickel VL: Clinical review of the early stability of spine injuries. *Spine* 1982; 7:545.
26. Edwards CC, Levine AM: Early rod-sleeve stabilization of the injured thoracic and lumbar spine. *Orthop Clin North Am* 1986; 17:121.
27. Evans DK: Anterior cervical subluxation. *J Bone Joint Surg [Br]* 1976; 58:318.
28. Ferguson RL, Allen BL Jr: A mechanistic classification of thoracolumbar spine fractures. *Clin Orthop* 1984; 189:77.
29. Flesch JR, Leider LL, Erickson DL, et al: Harrington instrumentation and spine fusion for unstable fracture and fracture-dislocations of the thoracic and lumbar spine. *J Bone Joint Surg [Am]* 1977; 59:143.
30. Fountain SS: Transverse fractures of the sacrum: A report of six cases. *J Bone Joint Surg [Am]* 1977; 59:486.
31. Frankel HL, Hancock DO, Hyslop G, et al: The value of postural reduction in the initial management of closed injuries of the spine with paraplegia and tetraplegia. *Paraplegia* 1969; 7:179–192.
32. Frankowski RF: Comprehensive center for CNS trauma, in *Galveston-Houston Health Services Area Progress Report Year II*. Houston, 1982, p 27.
33. Gertzbein S: A new classification of spinal injuries. Personal communication, 1990.
34. Gertzbein SD: Assessment of cervical spine instability, in Tator CH (ed): *Early Management of Spinal Cord Injury*. New York, Raven Press, 1982, pp 41–52.
35. *Guidelines for Facility Categorization and Standards of Care: Spinal Care Injury*. Chicago, American Spinal Injury Association, 1981.
36. Guttman L, Sir: Surgical aspects of the treatment of traumatic paraplegia. *J Bone Joint Surg [Br]* 1949; 31:399.
37. Guttman L, Sir: Surgical aspects of the treatment of traumatic paraplegics and tetraplegics following surgical procedures. *Paraplegia* 1969; 7:38.
38. Hannon K: Harrington instrumentation in fractures and dislocations of the thoracic and lumbar spine. *South Med J* 1976; 69:1269.
39. Holdsworth F, Sir: Fractures, dislocations and fracture-dislocations of the spine. *J Bone Joint Surg [Br]* 1963; 45:6.
40. Holdsworth F, Sir: Fractures, dislocations and fracture-dislocations of the spine. Review article. *J Bone Joint Surg [Am]* 1970; 52:1534.
41. Hughes JT: The new neuroanatomy of the spinal cord. *Paraplegia* 1989; 27:90.
42. Jacobs RR, Asher MA, Snider RK: Thoracolumbar spinal injuries. A comparative study of recumbent and operative treatment in 100 patients. *Spine* 1980; 5:463.
43. Jacobs RR, Nordwall A, Nachemson A: Reduction, stability, and strength provided by internal fixation for thoracolumbar spinal injuries. *Clin Orthop* 1982; 171:300.
44. Kakulas BA: Pathology of spinal injuries. *Cent Nerv Syst Trauma* 1984; 1:117–129.
45. Kelly RP, Whitesides TE: Treatment of lumbo-dorsal fracture-dislocations. *Ann Surg* 1968; 167:705.
46. Kiviat MD, Zimmerman TA, Donovan WH: Sphincter stretch: A new technique resulting in continence and complete voiding in paraplegics. *J Urol* 1975; 114:895.
47. Koenig C, Dohrman GJ: Histopathologic variability in "standardized" spinal cord trauma. *J Neurol Neurosurg Psychiatry* 1977; 40:1203.
48. Kreipke DL, Gillespie KR, McCarty MC, et al: Reliability of indication for cervical spine films in trauma patients. *J Trauma* 1989; 29:1438–1439.
49. Kricun ME: *Imaging Modalities in Spinal Disorders*. Philadelphia, WB Saunders, 1988.
50. Lee LM, Stevenson RWD, Szasz G: Prostaglandin E versus phentolamine/papaverine for the treatment of erectile impotence: A double blind comparison. *J Urol* 1989; 141:549.
51. Leidholt JD, Young JJ, Hahn DR, et al: Evaluations of late spinal deformities and fracture-dislocations of the dorsal and lumbar spine in paraplegics. *Paraplegia* 1969; 7:16.
52. Lewis J, Kibben B: The treatment of unstable fracture-dislocations of the thoracolumbar spine accompanied by paraplegia. *J Bone Joint Surg [Br]* 1974; 56:603.
53. Lucas JT, Ducker TB: Motor classification of spinal cord injuries with mobility, morbidity and recovery indices. *Ann Surg* 1979; 45:151–158.
54. Luque ER, Cassis M, Ramirez-Wiella G: Segmental spinal instrumentation in the treatment of fractures of the thoracolumbar spine. *Spine* 1982; 7:312.
55. McAfee PC, Yuan HA, Fredrickson BE, et al: The value of computed tomography in thoracolumbar fractures. An analysis of 100 consecutive cases and a new classification. *J Bone Joint Surg [Am]* 1983; 65:461.
56. McSweeney T: Deformities of the spine following injuries to the cord. *Hand Neurol* 1976; 26:159.
57. Merli GJ, Rensman B, Doyle L, et al: Prophylaxis for deep vein thrombosis in acute spinal cord injury comparing two

doses of low molecular weight heparinoid (org 10172) in combination with either external pneumatic compression or electrical stimulation. Presented to the American Spinal Injury Association, Orlando, Fla, May 1990.

58. Meyer PR Jr: *Surgery of Spine Trauma*. New York, Churchill Livingstone, 1988.
59. Meyer PR Jr, Cotler HB: Fusion technologies in traumatic injuries, in Cotler JM, Cotler HB (eds): *Spinal Fusion: Science and Technique*. New York, Springer-Verlag, 1990, pp 189–246.
60. Naftchi NE, Demeny M, DeCrescito V, et al: Biogenic amine concentrations in traumatized spinal cords of cats. Effects of drug therapy. *J Neurosurg* 1974; 40:52–57.
61. Nicoll EA: Fractures of the dorso-lumbar spine. *J Bone Joint Surg [Br]* 1949; 31:376.
62. Oakes DD, Wilmot CB, Hall KM, et al: Benefits of early admission to a comprehensive trauma center for patients with spinal cord injury. *Arch Phys Med Rehabil* 1990; 71:637.
63. Osebod WE, Weinstein SL, Sprague BL: Thoracolumbar spine fractures: Results and treatment. *Spine* 1981; 6:13.
64. Osterholm JL: Noradrenergic mediation of traumatic spinal cord autodestruction. *Life Sci* 1974; 14:1363–1384.
65. Pang D, Wilberger JE: Spinal cord injury without radiographic abnormalities in children. *J Neurosurg* 1982; 57:114–129.
66. Perkash A: Experience with management of deep vein thrombosis in patients with spinal cord injury. *Paraplegia* 1980; 18:2.
67. Pierce DS, Barr JS Jr: Fractures and dislocations at the base of the skull and upper cervical spine, in *The Cervical Spine*. Philadelphia, JB Lippincott, 1983, pp 196–206.
68. Roberts JB, Curtis PH: Stability of the thoracic and lumbar spine in traumatic paraplegia following fracture or fracture-dislocation. *J Bone Joint Surg [Am]* 1970; 52:115.
69. Robin ED: Dysoxia. *Sci Am* 1983; 14:1–10.
70. Ruckley CV, Thurston C: Pulmonary embolism in surgical patients: 1959–1979. *Br Med J* 1982; 284:1100.
71. Ruge JR, Sinson GP, McLane DG, et al: Pediatric spinal injury: The very young. *J Neurosurg* 1988; 68:25–30.
72. Sareff J: *Assessment of the Late Results of Traumatic Compression Fractures of the Thoracolumbar Vertebral Bodies*. Stockholm, Karalinska Hospital, 1977, pp 1–88.
73. Schwab ME: Regeneration of nerve fibers in the lesioned rat spinal cord following neutralization of neurite growth inhibitors. Presented at Spinal Cord Injury in the 90s: Future Trends in Medical Management and Treatment, Dallas, November 1990.
74. Scott FB, Bradley WE, Timm GW: Management of erectile impotence. *Urology* 1973; 2:80–82.
75. Scott JA, Donovan WH: The prevention of shoulder pain and contracture in the acute tetraplegia patient. *Paraplegia* 1981; 19:313.
76. *Standards for Neurological Classification of Spinal Injury Patients*. Chicago, American Spinal Injury Association, 1988.
77. Stauffer ES: Open reduction and internal fixation of unstable thoracolumbar fractures and dislocations, in Leach RE, Hoaglund FT, Riseborough EJ (eds): *Controversies in Orthopaedic Surgery*. Philadelphia, WB Saunders, 1982, pp 446–454.
78. Stover SL, Fine PR (eds): *Spinal Cord Injury—The Facts and Figures*. Birmingham, The University of Alabama at Birmingham, 1986, pp 13–15.
79. Stranger JK: Fracture-dislocations of the thoraco-lumbar spine with special references to reduction by open and closed operations. *J Bone Joint Surg* 1947; 29:107.
80. Trieschmann RB: *The Psychological, Social and Vocational Adjustment in Spinal Cord Injury: A Strategy for Future Research*. Los Angeles, Easter Seal Society, 1978, pp 21–71.
81. Watson-Jones R, Sir: Injuries of the spine, in Wilson JN (ed): *Fractures and Joint Injuries,* ed 5. Edinburgh, Churchill Livingstone, 1976, pp 798–849.
82. Weirich SD, Cotler HB, Marayana PA, et al: Histopathologic correlation of magnetic resonance imaging signal patterns in a spinal cord injury model. *Spine* 1990; 15:630–638.
83. Wharton GW: Stabilization of spinal injuries for early mobilization. *Orthop Clin North Am* 1978; 9:271.
84. White AA, Panjabi MM: *Clinical Biomechanics of the Spine*. Philadelphia, JB Lippincott, 1978.
85. White AA, Panjabi MM: *Clinical Biomechanics of the Spine,* ed 2. Philadelphia, JB Lippincott, 1990.
86. Whitesides TE: Traumatic kyphosis of the thoracolumbar spine. *Clin Orthop* 1977; 128:78.
87. Yosipovitch Z, Robin GC, Makin M: Open reduction of unstable thoracolumbar spinal injuries and fixation with Harrington rods. *J Bone Joint Surg [Am]* 1977; 59:1003.
88. Young JS, Burns PE, Bowen AM, et al: *Experience of the Regional Spinal Cord Injury System*. Phoenix, Good Samaritan Medical Center, 1982, p 32.
89. Young JS, Dexter WR: Neurological recovery distal to the zone of injury in 172 cases of closed traumatic spinal cord injury. *Paraplegia* 1978; 16:39.
90. Young W: The role of calcium in spinal cord injury. *Cent Nerv Syst Trauma* 1985; 2:109–114.

26

Rehabilitation of Acute Spinal Cord Injury

Jack E. Zigler, M.D.

Traumatic spinal cord injury (SCI) is often an instantaneous devastating occurrence that immediately shifts the focus of a young individual's life. Once the urgent initial decisions regarding stabilization of the spine and management of concurrent medical difficulties are resolved, rehabilitation becomes the single most important concern to the young paraplegic or quadriplegic. The skills that are taught to this individual in the next 4 to 6 months will have a significant impact on the quality of life that that person may enjoy. The rehabilitation team's "best shot" at successful primary teaching will occur during this post-traumatic window, and the opportunity must not be lost.

In a formalized rehabilitation program, goals are established following a comprehensive team assessment in collaboration with the patient. These goals must be realistic and meaningful to the patient and address his present physical status. The thrust of treatment should be toward maximizing the patient's potential, not on dwelling upon the lost functions. Strengthening a single wrist extensor muscle may superficially appear to be a trivial accomplishment, but in the C6 quadriplegic it may allow the patient to grasp a utensil and, with the appropriate setup, to feed himself. This small act may reaffirm some measure of independence in an individual who has watched himself lose the abilities of self-care.

In the early phase of treatment, the patient may be encouraged to depend on others. As they advance in therapy, patients must philosophically shift from a sick role to become informed consumers of medical care. These individuals must evolve from dwelling upon the physical limitations of their injury, the highly structured schedule of the spinal injury center, the regimentation of any inpatient care facility, and the taken-for-granted provisions of all basic needs to break through the "exemption from normal social role responsibilities"[6] and reenter the community as an active member of society.

Rehabilitation philosophies differ from institution to institution. The treatment team at each particular facility needs to agree on a uniform approach so that patients may be instructed in an unconfused manner. At Rancho Los Amigos Medical Center (Rancho), the philosophy is to direct treatment toward long-term functional outcomes. These outcomes, or goals, are set through collaboration among the treatment team, the patient, and significant others. These goals not only address the functional skills each person requires but also incorporate the long-term costs to the musculoskeletal system. Patients with postpolio syndrome have demonstrated the adverse effects of overtaxing weak muscles. Many individuals who were encouraged to reach their highest level of functioning with little regard for the long-term effects on their musculoskeletal structures suffered irreversible damage over the years. In the spinal-injured population, this concern is often manifested in the selection of equipment. For example, an electric rather than manual wheelchair is recommended for a patient with a weak shoulder girdle who is planning to return to school. Although the patient might be able to propel the manual wheelchair initially, the long-term effect of overuse of the shoulder muscles would be negative. Rehabilitation must be considered from a long-term perspective.

Another important aspect of successful rehabilitation is providing the patient with positive role models. Other spinal cord patients or staff members serve in this role and in so doing enable the patient to benefit from their experiences, to identify with them, and to see a positive future. This role modeling is achieved through roommates, groupmates in group treatment, and individual peer counselors.

Following completion of the inpatient rehabilitation of the patient with SCI, a highly specialized health care team is required to meet the patient's ongoing needs. At Rancho, lifelong follow-up is provided by a spinal injury primary-care clinic in which a primary nurse screens patients, who are then referred to the appropriate health care provider.

The philosophy of a team approach to rehabilitation was popularized by Rancho in the care of polio patients and has been adapted to the care and management of SCI. These patients require daily maintenance of all health care problems both related and unrelated to the primary neurologic injury.

Nursing staff and allied health and psychological services are essential to the care and treatment of the cord-injured adult. Speech therapy, sexual counseling, and recreational therapy are also essential. Finally, social work often provides aid to the achievement of the final goal—discharge to the outside world.

A staff of highly skilled and well-trained nurses and nursing assistants is needed to ensure a smooth transition to the rehabilitation hospital. Successful rehabilitation is dependent upon care and treatment of the many problems that occur in the quadriplegic and paraplegic patient, and complications of poor treatment can impede the achievement of rehabilitation goals.

Complications of poor skin care can be extremely expensive and require the use of special types of support beds and/or plastic surgical flap procedures. Complications can be prevented by nursing team vigilance, by pressure relief, and by proper instruction in bed and wheelchair pressure raises. Monitoring patient education in this area is a vital part of the rehabilitation nursing process. Avoidance of repeat hospitalizations for pressure sore management is a nursing-directed goal. The average extension of hospitalization when a pressure sore occurs in the acute rehabilitation phase is 7 to 10 days. Prophylaxis begins with the nursing staff education program.

Bowel programs are instituted on admission after an accurate neurologic diagnosis has been established. Manual evacuation and suppository programs are provided and taught to the patient. Dietary guidance is also a vital part of the bowel program education process.

Bladder evacuation programs are supervised by the urology service at Rancho, but the intermittent catheterization programs are often observed and taught by nursing services. Due to the size of the Rancho Rehabilitation Service, an independent "catheterization team" is utilized, but the daily nursing contact and care can be involved in this program as well.

Autonomic functions such as blood pressure and pulse rate may also be altered following SCI. Average values in a quadriplegic are a heart rate of 60 and a blood pressure of 100/60 mm. High-level thoracic paraplegics may experience similar changes but to a lesser degree. Patients who have been on prolonged bed rest may experience limited compensatory vasoconstriction and reduced sympathetic activity with resulting orthostatic hypotension. Nursing treatment for this condition includes the use of an abdominal binding or corset, snug-fitting support hose, or elastic wraps on the lower extremities. Patients should practice sitting up in bed, slowly raising the head of the bed 10 to 20 degrees at a time, and stopping frequently if dizziness occurs. Patients who are sitting in a wheelchair and experience dizziness may be treated by reclining the wheelchair or elevating the lower extremities.

Autonomic dysreflexia is caused by stimulation of the sympathetic and parasympathetic systems, which causes a reflex rise in blood pressure that cannot be relieved by normal compensatory mechanisms due to the SCI. If not controlled, the precipitous rise in blood pressure may lead to a cerebral vascular accident or other vascular injury. Symptoms of autonomic dysreflexia include a pounding headache, sweating above the level of injury, facial flushing, urticaria or "goose bumps" above the level of injury, and/or nasal congestion. Common causes of dysreflexia include bladder distension, kidney stones, bladder infection, spasms, too rapid emptying of the bladder, or blocked catheter tubing. Colonic distension can also cause dysreflexia secondary to hard stools, excessive gas, stretching the rectum, or rough digital removal of stool from the rectum. Skin may also be irritated from sunburn or frostbite, pressure sores, or even an excessively tightened leg bag.

The occurrence of autonomic dysreflexia demands immediate action. Nursing intervention includes sitting the patient up in an attempt to positionally lower the blood pressure. Blood pressure should be monitored immediately. Any tight clothing should be loosened. Catheter tubing should be checked to be sure that there is no kink or other drainage problem, and the patient's catheter bag should be emptied. The catheter should be gently irrigated with 30 mL of irrigating solution, and if there are no results, the catheter should be quickly changed. Only 500 mL of urine should be removed following recatheterization. After several minutes, additional urine can be drained from the bladder. Rapid bladder drainage may lead to bladder spasm, which could once again elevate the blood pressure. If a patient voids reflexively, the bladder should be stimulated to empty by tapping in the suprapubic region, pulling the pubic hair, or stroking the inside of the thigh.

Most of these potential complications are unique to the spinal cord–injured patient. For this reason, nursing care of these patients has become extremely specialized.

Other consulting services required for the acute spinal cord rehabilitation team include urology; medicine; surgery; ear, nose and throat; plastic surgery; and dental services. Other subspecialty areas are often required as well, depending upon the patient's preinjury status or the severity of trauma.

It is necessary to screen for admission to the rehabilitation service if these services are not readily available. Some patients require a more extensive primary hospital stay so that consulting services can institute management at an earlier stage. Prolongation of rehabilitation can actually result from an inappropriate early transfer to the rehabilitation facility.

An ancillary service that is managed by the physical therapists at Rancho is the seating clinic. In the clinic, appropriate wheelchair positioning and pressure relief are designed and fabricated for maintenance of skin integrity.

Outpatient and inpatient consultation is available to prevent the need for surgical flap coverage. Since the 1982 average length of stay cost of readmission for a single pressure sore was $70,000, these preventive services are essential.

The catastrophe of an SCI has a dramatic emotional impact on the individual as well as his family. Psychological intervention plays an important role in addressing the various issues related to this often complicated process of recovery and adjustment. The role of the psychologist can vary from the traditional to the more informal consultant.

SCI results in multiple changes in the individual's life that he is forced to deal with. There are changes in his social status as he instantly becomes a member of a minority that generally has a socially devalued role and one in which he is seen as less desirable and less capable. His socioeconomic status and interpersonal relationships may be dramatically altered. The inability to perform certain functions affects the individual's vocational, social, and familial roles. Being unable to carry out job-related tasks may result in economic dependence and places pressure on other family members to alter their role. Friendships and family relationships often suffer from the stress and may deteriorate or completely dissolve.

The area of sexual function/dysfunction is of prime concern to this patient population. The psychologist plays an important role in addressing the area of sexuality. Sex function is managed in the same fashion as other areas of functioning of the individual in an attempt to establish a pattern of life as close to that of premorbid functioning as possible. A formal sex function program has two components: an educational group series designed to address the issues on a general level and an individual sex function evaluation designed to address individual specific sex function issues with a physician and the psychologist present. The program provides an opportunity to address the areas of sexual dysfunction, alternative behaviors, precautions, and other areas related to sexual counseling.

PHYSICAL THERAPY IN SPINAL CORD INJURY

Prior to initiating treatment, the physical therapist must first complete a comprehensive evaluation to ascertain the patient's functional level of neurologic injury, establish long-term goals, and devise a treatment plan that allows the patient to meet these goals.

The evaluation consists of eight major areas of emphasis: (1) sensory testing, (2) motor control, (3) respiratory function, (4) joint range of motion, (5) muscle tone, (6) skin integrity, (7) bulbar function (for respirator-dependent or head-injured patients), and (8) functional level.

A spinal cord–injured patient is usually described by level of injury. In the literature, the term *level* may be bony, neurologic, or functional. For purposes of this discussion, the term "functional level" will be used. Functional level is determined by the lowest level at which sensation is bilaterally intact and muscles innervated at that segment have a manual muscle test grade of fair-plus (3+) or better. This level is used by the entire team when establishing a diagnosis and prognosis for the patient's functional outcome. Since muscles receive innervation from multiple neural levels, it is felt that the fair-plus grade indicates complete innervation by the primary neurologic source.

The patients are further described as having complete or incomplete injuries. The patients described in this chapter are labeled incompletely injured only if sacral sparing is present. To be considered to have sacral sparing, the patient may only have perianal sensation or the ability to flex his great toe. This indicates that some communication still exists between the motor cortex and the most distal portion of the spinal cord. As a prognostic indicator, it gives more hope that the patient will have some return of function below the level of injury, although it is impossible to predict the degree of return. Sacral sparing cannot be determined if the patient is in spinal shock.[2]

A patient with a complete injury has no voluntary muscle control or sensation lower than several nerve root levels below the functional level of injury. Incomplete injuries have better recovery potential. Generally, the greater the initial sparing and the faster the neurologic recovery, the better the prognosis.[7]

When the initial evaluation has been completed, the physical therapist is ready to set the functional goals that the patient is expected to reach. The initial discussion will deal with the patient with a complete injury. Goal setting for the incompletely injured patient and the respirator-dependent patient will follow.

The goals that the physical therapist believes the patient will achieve are based on the function each innervated muscle provides. The goals presented here are reasonable, provided that no interfering factors exist. Factors that may limit functional outcome include significant spasticity, inadequate fixed range of motion at key joints, lack of patient acceptance of the injury, poor social support systems, or a less-than-optimal living situation to which the patient will be returned. Keeping this information in mind, the therapist is able to identify functional capabilities associated with key muscles at each segmental level.

Each spinal nerve level that remains intact is of critical importance when setting functional goals for the quadriplegic patient. For example, a patient with a C5 injury will be able to flex and abduct his shoulders and flex his elbows. However, all these movements will be weak given their dual innervation by C5 and C6 nerves. These patients may be able to propel a manual wheelchair with adapted handwheels, but because of their muscle weakness and limited endurance, a power wheelchair with hand controls would be the most functional. The person with a C5 injury will require assistance for all transfer and bed mobility activities.

If the C6 level is intact, the patient's function improves greatly. In addition to normal shoulder girdle strength, the C6 level provides some function to the clavicular portion of the pectoralis major, the serratus anterior, and the extensor carpi radialis longus. A patient with this level of injury will have much better wheelchair propulsion endurance and may be able to perform sliding board transfers, roll from supine to prone to provide pressure relief when in bed, and perform independent forward-bending pressure relief while in his wheelchair.

At the C7 level, the patient has full innervation to the clavicular portion of the pectoralis major, the serratus anterior, and the extensor carpi radialis brevis and longus muscles. In addition, the sternal pectoralis major, triceps, and latissimus dorsi are partially innervated. The presence of this additional nerve level greatly increases the patient's functional abilities. Most patients will be able to perform independent transfers to multiple surfaces and perform depression-type raises. The presence of the serratus anterior and latissimus dorsi provides the essential components of the force couple for shoulder girdle stability. This additional shoulder girdle stability will enable him to propel his wheelchair easily on a variety of surfaces and on inclines.

FUNCTIONAL SKILLS FOR THE QUADRIPLEGIC PATIENT

Transfers

The ability to move from one surface to another is called a transfer. Being able to perform this activity independently greatly increases a person's independence. There are two basic types of active transfers that can be performed: sliding board transfers and depression transfers.

The sliding board transfer is performed by placing a polished wooden or plastic (commercially available) board under the patient to bridge the gap between the patient and the surface he will be transferring to. The patient then utilizes the decreased friction of the board (in comparison to the friction of bed sheets or upholstery) to slide from one surface to another. Assistance to perform this transfer can range from the total assistance required by a C4 quadriplegic to the independent type that a C6 quadriplegic could perform provided that he is able to place the board and have sufficient trunk balance to perform the maneuver safely.

The second type is a depression transfer. To perform this type of transfer, the person must be able to lift his buttocks off one surface and bridge the gap to the second surface. All paraplegics utilize this type of transfer; so do those quadriplegics who are able to use the muscles of the shoulder girdle in conjunction with locked elbows to achieve the lift needed.

If a person has sufficient upper-extremity strength and good trunk balance, transferring down to and up from widely varying heights allows even greater independence. This ability will allow such individuals to transfer out of their wheelchairs down to the ground and to get to the bottom of the bathtub. This decreases the need for equipment such as a bath bench.

Wheelchair Skills

The spinal injury population achieving the best reintegration into society includes those who attain the highest level of functional independence. Wheelchair skills are an integral part of this learning process. Being able to propel a wheelchair on the hospital ward does not indicate that a person will be able to function outside the hospital. Rehabilitation is not complete until a patient has achieved higher-level wheelchair skills, if these are physically possible. These include the ability to transfer from the wheelchair to the ground, propel the wheelchair on uneven surfaces such as grass and dirt, propel up and down at least 10-degree slopes, handle curb cutouts, and perform wheelies to enable them to go over small obstacles and up and down curbs without cutouts.

All paraplegics should be able to achieve independence in these skills with the exception of those with severe spasticity or those with higher-level injuries (T2–5) who are unable to achieve adequate balance. Low-level quadriplegics (C6–8) are sometimes able to achieve a fair amount of proficiency in these advanced skills. The most difficult are transferring out of the chair to the ground and wheelies.

EQUIPMENT

Wheelchair Prescription

The prescription of a wheelchair is necessary for all spinal injury patients for whom full-time walking is not a goal. Wheelchairs have undergone a radical change in the recent past, and selecting the most appropriate chair requires some study. The price of wheelchairs can vary from about $750 for an "economy model" to greater than $15,000 for a high-tech chair. In this era of third-party payment, the therapist must be able to justify the need for an expensive wheelchair. The following is a brief introduction to the various types of wheelchairs available on the market today.

A manual wheelchair requires the patient to provide the motive power by pushing on the rims of the wheels. If a good grip is not present, the rims can be modified by coating them with plastic to increase the friction and substitute for the patient's inadequate grip. The type of wheelchair found in most hospitals is inappropriate for the spinal injury population for a number of reasons. Of primary importance to this population is a chair that is lightweight, has a low center of gravity and high maneuverability, and folds or disassembles easily for transporting in a vehicle. A standard hospital wheelchair weighs about 50 to 75 lb, while the ultralight models can weigh as little as 17 lb. The increase in price to obtain a lightweight chair can be easily justified when trauma to the shoulder joint from repeated lifting of the wheelchair is considered. In addition, the low center of gravity and high maneuverability of these chairs allows the spinal-injured person to handle most architectural barriers with a much lower expenditure of energy than that required in a standard-weight chair.

Power wheelchairs can vary from a manual wheelchair with an add-on motor to a computer-operated chair controlled by voice or breath. Due to the frequency of breakdown of parts, the prescription should contain only necessary components. These can range from power-reclining systems that enable the person to provide ischial pressure relief independently to custom-made seating systems to maintain proper posture. The most elaborate and expensive wheelchairs are used by the ventilator-dependent patients who also require sophisticated power-activation controls such as head or tongue control switches.

The philosophy at Rancho is that all patients who are unable to perform an independent pressure relief maneuver receive a power wheelchair with a power recliner. Patients able to perform independent pressure relief but who have limited ability to propel a manual wheelchair receive a lightweight wheelchair with an add-on motor. The patients who receive power wheelchairs with recliners also receive a manual wheelchair as a backup. Having the second manual wheelchair enables patients to have continued mobility while the power chair is being repaired.

Weight is also a factor to be considered. Power wheelchairs weigh at least 350 lb and cannot be transported easily without a van. Manual chairs can weigh as little as 18 to 20 lb and are very easily transported.

The most important consideration in wheelchair prescription is the functional capability the chair provides. Having a power wheelchair may enable a higher-level quadriplegic (C1–4) to return to the work force. When prescribing a wheelchair all the factors listed previously (injury level, physical requirements, and transportability) must be weighed to provide the patient with the most useful wheelchair.

Wheelchair Cushions

Of equal importance to the wheelchair is the wheelchair cushion the patient sits on. Skin breakdown over the ischial tuberosities is a frequent cause of rehospitalization in the spine-injured population. Having the proper cushion goes a long way toward preventing this totally unnecessary and costly complication. A large variety of cushions are available on the market. Prices vary from about $70.00 to $250.00. Component material also varies. The cushions may be made of foam that can be cut out on a custom basis to provide ischial pressure relief. Other cushions contain air or gel.

Capillary occlusion and tissue necrosis result from 13 to 34 mm of unrelieved pressure. The cushion should serve to prevent the person from bearing excessive weight on the ischial tuberosities through one of two means: total relief over bony prominences or total contact with the buttocks and lower extremities to disperse the pressure over a wider area. At Rancho we believe that proper seating is important enough to merit an outpatient clinic. The clinic, held twice each week to service the large spinal-injured population, provides custom cushion modifications and replacement of worn or "bottomed-out" cushions. In addition, a seating center is in operation daily to deal with difficult seating problems and prescription of seating systems for severely involved patients of all diagnoses.

Bathroom Equipment

Prior to prescribing equipment for the bathroom, the therapist should make a visit to the patient's home. If this is not possible, a detailed drawing should be made by the patient's family that demonstrates placement of the tub, sink, and commode and the width of the door and all the distance measurements between the fixtures. Without this information, it will be impossible to obtain equipment that will be useful.

The first and most important bathroom accessory is the commode. If the patient is unable to assist in any aspect of the bowel program, a commode chair should be considered. Many of the models available commercially can be wheeled directly over the toilet. While the bowel program can be carried out in bed, the upright position allows gravity to aid elimination and is more aesthetically acceptable to the patient and family.

If the patient can transfer to the toilet, a raised toilet seat with a slide cutout that allows access to the rectum for suppository insertion, digital stimulation, and hygiene is desirable. The addition of armrests may provide the patient with enough stability to enable him to carry out his toileting independently.

There are a variety of bath benches available that provide varied support for patient bathing. Depending on the patient's level of transfer skills and balance, the bench can range from a small seat inside the tub that is the same height as the tub rim to an elaborate bench that extends outside the tub and provides a cushioned surface for the patient to slide along. Because some of this equipment is bulky, it is wise to wait until the patient achieves good balance and transfer ability before trying out the various types. The greater the patient's skills, the smaller and simpler the equipment will need to be.

Grab bars are a good addition in most bathrooms near the commode or in the tub. These range from 12 to 18 in. and provide the patient with a sturdy hand hold if some additional balance assistance is required.

OCCUPATIONAL THERAPY WITH SPINAL CORD-INJURED PATIENTS

Philosophy

The occupational therapist's role is to guide the patient with SCI toward his optimal level of function and toward attaining the greatest degree of self-sufficiency and independence in activities of daily living (ADL). To meet these goals the therapist evaluates new ways to accomplish tasks and provides the patient with guidance in achieving skills in a safe and supportive environment. Facilitating successful performance empowers the patient and allows him to risk attempting the challenge of new tasks. The therapist and patient collaboratively formulate goals. In a continuous dialogue, the therapist serves to outline realistic attainable goals, and the patient selects those goals that are most meaningful to him.

The functioning of patients with SCI and especially of quadriplegics is significantly enhanced by the use of equipment. The therapist aids the patient in selecting the most appropriate device and in training him to use it. In order to best meet patients' equipment needs, careful consideration must be given to the discharge environment and to the patient's ability to maintain the equipment in good repair. To simplify patients' daily routines, it is important to select essential equipment only and to avoid overloading the patient with unnecessary devices. In choosing upper-extremity functional orthoses, one versatile device should be chosen over several devices. This allows the patient to avoid having to change orthoses for different activities.

The Evaluation Process

The evaluation process includes interviews and physical testing. The purpose of the interviews is to establish rapport with the patient and to gather data regarding the patient's preinjury occupational behavior—the patient's daily routines, vocational roles, and leisure pursuits. Other needed information is gathered, such as prior living situation, driving status, and the physical layout of the patient's home. Additionally, the occupational therapist describes to the patient his professional role. The physical assessment includes joint range of motion, motor strength and control, muscle tone sensation, functional evaluation, prevocational evaluation, and driving evaluation.

Goal Setting

As with the evaluation process, goal setting involves a continuous process of reexamination for the purpose of meeting an individual patient's needs. To meet these needs, long-term goals are established. These goals are functional in nature and describe the expected level of functioning upon discharge from the hospital. The functional level established by the team during the evaluation process serves as a useful guideline in forming long-term goals. It assists in guiding patients toward realistic, attainable goals, thus minimizing failure. Many extenuating factors may necessitate the reformulation of these goals. Factors such as age, height, weight, physical endurance, and life-style may all contribute to a unique goal formulation. In the case of a patient with a C6 functional level, for example, the guideline suggests that he can learn to dress the upper part of his body independently. However, if the patient experiences severe upper-torso spasms, this goal may be unrealistic, and he may be able to achieve this goal with assistance only.

In order to achieve long-term goals, the therapist analyzes each goal and breaks it down into its basic sequential components. Short-term goals are weekly objectives that form the building blocks toward attaining independence.

Typical Considerations in the Treatment of C5 Quadriplegics

Quadriplegics functioning at the C5 level may be able to independently don and doff their orthoses. Following assistance in setup, they are able to feed, brush their teeth, wash their face, apply makeup, shave, and comb their hair. In addition, they are expected to be able to write, type, and execute more complex desk, vocational, and leisure activities. C5 quadriplegics may also be able to drive a specially equipped van independently.

To reach these goals, upper-extremity management must first be addressed. As with high-level quadriplegics, upper-extremity deformity, edema, and pain must be prevented and managed. Functional joint range is maintained through bed and wheelchair positioning, daily ranging, and educating the patient and care givers. While the patient is lying in bed, emphasis is placed on avoiding direct pressure on the glenohumeral joint. C5 quadriplegics may develop elbow flexion and forearm supination contractures due to unopposed biceps activity. To avoid such deformities, the elbow must be maintained in extension and the forearm in full pronation. If limitations develop, serial casting with long-arm casts is most effective.

As with high-level quadriplegics, in order to maintain the functional position of the hand, the hand and forearm are initially placed in a prefabricated temporary splint to be later replaced with a custom-made wrist-hand orthosis (WHO).

Strengthening of the upper extremities begins as soon as the patient's neck is stabilized. Strict precautions are taken in order to protect the spine from further damage.

For the first 4 weeks following neck stabilization with a halo vest, shoulder and elbow exercises are only performed bilaterally with minimum resistance.

With these precautions in mind, it is recommended that strengthening begin as soon after the injury as possible. With the aid of an overhead frame, springs, and slings, the patient can begin upper-extremity active assistive exercises while still in bed. Neuromuscular electric stimulation (NMES), an electric current that brings about muscle excitation and induces motor response, provides for additional muscle activation when the patient is down in bed.[7] In the wheelchair, strengthening is achieved through the use of orthotic devices and weights as well as through therapeutic and functional activities.

Mobile arm supports are often used during the initial period following bed rest in order to support the arms and enhance proximal shoulder movement (Fig 26–1). Mobile arm supports assist patients whose deltoid strength is poor (grade 2) or, better, in achieving shoulder flexion, thus enabling them to increase their strength and endurance through repetitive motion. Additionally, it allows them to perform functional activities involving the head, such as feeding, hygiene, and grooming. When the deltoids and biceps develop fair-plus (grade 3+) or better strength and when endurance improves, the mobile arm support is no longer needed.

Strengthening is also achieved by a program of progressive exercises through the use of mobile arm supports and skateboards. Next, active exercises are performed against gravity. To further resist muscles, mechanical resistance is applied through the use of weights and through exercise machines specially developed to meet the needs of the quadriplegic. For further details regarding upper-extremity strengthening, Hill's chapter on this subject in the book *Spinal Cord Injury* is highly recommended.[5]

Because the C5 quadriplegic does not have either wrist or finger musculature, adaptive equipment is necessary for hand function. At Rancho, most C5 quadriplegics achieve hand function through the use of the ratchet WHOs mentioned previously. This orthosis eliminates the need for a variety of adaptive devices. With the ratchet WHO, the individual is trained to pick up, hold, manipulate, and release objects.

To achieve optimal functioning with the ratchet WHO, the patient must fully understand the purpose and function of the orthosis. Once the patient learns the operation of the ratchet, a graded therapeutic activity program is initiated. Training may begin with picking up and releasing soft, medium-sized objects such as sponge cubes. Next, repetitive functional activities such as holding a spoon and feeding may be practiced. More difficult activities requiring fine-motor coordination such as writing and donning and doffing the orthosis are initiated only when less complex tasks have been mastered. The grading of activities from simple to complex is designed to provide the patient with successful experiences, thereby enhancing motivation, confidence, and self-esteem.[1]

Since many rehabilitation centers do not provide their patients with orthotic devices, other methods for holding objects are used. The universal cuff, also known as the utensil holder, is the most common device used for feeding. This cuff fits around the palm of the hand and has a

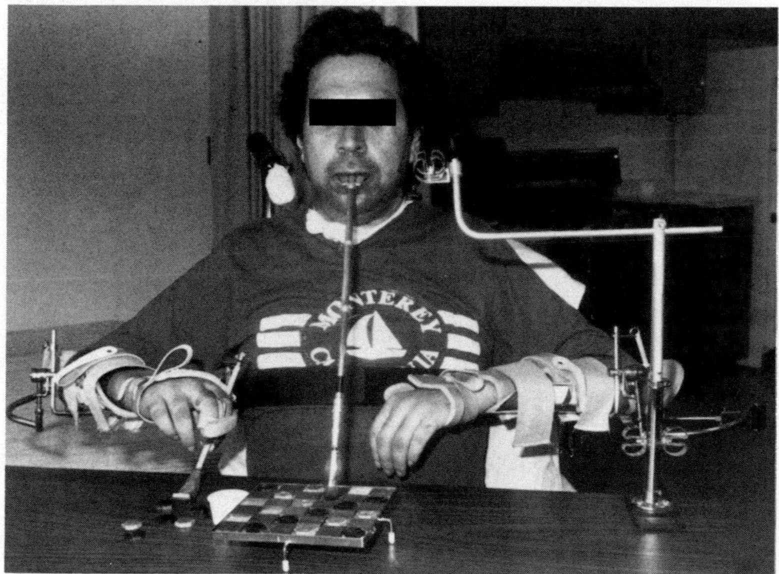

FIG 26–1.
A patient participating in occupational therapy using mobile arm supports, upper-extremity orthotics, and a mouth stick.

pocket for inserting utensils. To change the activity, the patient or an aide must change the tool inserted into the pocket. Other activities that can be achieved with a universal cuff include brushing the teeth and performing some light recreational activities. Other common adaptive devices are made for writing, typing, feeding, and performing hygiene and grooming activities.

As with high-level quadriplegics, a critical element in the rehabilitation process of the C5 quadriplegic involves enhancing independence through the effective use of attendants and community resources. A home visit is carried out in order to ensure a barrier-free and safe home environment. Additionally, training in the community is carried out, and group discussions regarding attendant management, child care, transportation, and returning to school or work are held.

The situation of the C5 quadriplegic with some C6 root escape of the wrist extensors is significantly different from that of other C5 quadriplegics because he can achieve a greater degree of independence. This is due to the very important role of wrist extensors in hand function through tenodesis (the functional finger closure of the hand when the wrist is extended and the opening of the fingers when the wrist is flexed). This motion, which is caused by tendon tightness, is used by the quadriplegic patient to grasp, release, and manipulate light objects.

In order to enhance functional tenodesis, maintenance of correct hand position and range as well as strengthening of the wrist are of critical importance. In order to maintain the functional finger tightness necessary for optimal tenodesis action, care must be taken to maintain a correct relationship between the fingers and wrist at all times to avoid stretching the finger flexors and losing the tenodesis action. While ranging or pursuing functional activities, the wrist is maintained in extension when the fingers are flexed. When the fingers are extended, the wrist is flexed. Occasionally, spasticity may interfere with functional tenodesis. When medications and splinting do not improve hand function, percutaneous phenol blocks to motor points administered by the physician may decrease spasticity and thereby improve hand opening and closure.[3] To increase wrist strength, the static WHO, used to maintain a functional hand position for C1–4 quadriplegics, is replaced by a dynamic orthosis called the wrist-action wrist-hand orthosis (WAWHO). This orthosis allows for active-assistive wrist extension with the aid of a rubber band attached to a post above the wrist.

For prehension and for maintaining tenodesis, the C5 quadriplegic with wrist extension motor return of at least fair-plus (3+) or above uses the wrist-driven wrist-hand orthosis (WDWHO), also called the wrist-driven flexor hinge hand splint. To achieve closure the patient extends his wrist, thereby transferring mechanical force to the fingers. To open the hand, gravity assists in wrist flexion and causes finger extension. To assist weak fair-plus (3+) wrist extensors, a vertical post with rubber bands is added. With the WDWHO, the patient learns to perform most activities. These include self-care skills such as feeding, brushing the teeth, and grooming, as well as community skills such as shopping and banking (Fig 26–2).

Prevocational training involves exploring with the patient his interests as well as his vocational aptitudes. Exploring work skills, the therapist provides the patient with a simulated work setting in which the patient can become aware of his capabilities and limitations. As in the case of high-level quadriplegics, gathered prevocational data are given both to the patient and to an appropriate vocational counselor.

Driving training is performed in a specially adapted van. Steering wheel and other sensitized controls are fitted to meet individual needs, and driving demands are gradually increased as the patient gains proficiency and confidence in driving. Special attention must be placed on safety considerations. Factors that may interfere with safe driving such as spasticity, spasms, and medications' side

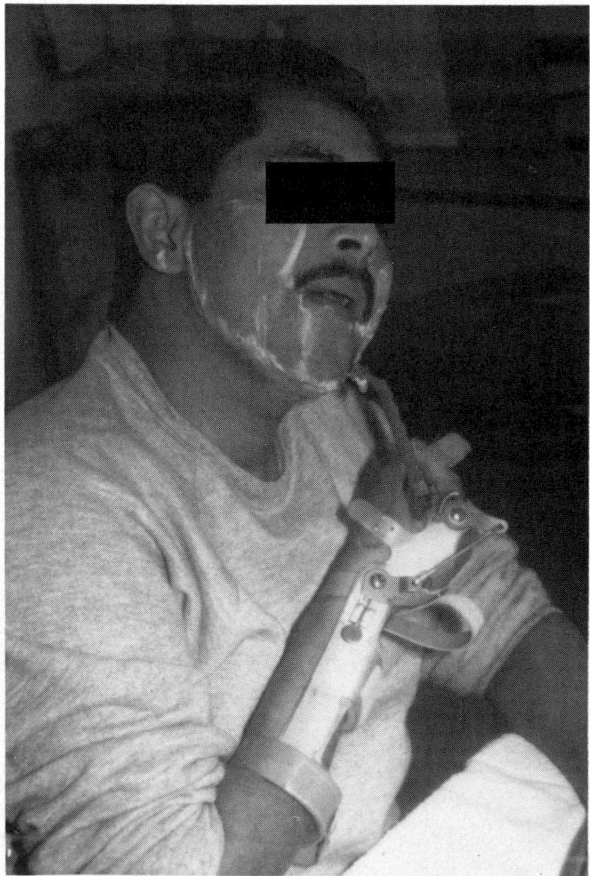

FIG 26–2.
A patient shaving with a wrist-driven wrist-hand orthosis.

effects must be addressed before the patient is allowed to drive independently.[4]

Treatment of the Paraplegic Patient

The functional goals in the rehabilitation of the paraplegic patient are complete independence in all self-care, home, and community skills. This independence is possible because the paraplegic patient has intact upper extremities and can therefore perform all activities with compensatory techniques.

Upper-extremity strengthening is frequently necessary following a long period of immobility. The progressive resistive program may begin in bed by using wrist weights and barbells and continues with modified universal gym equipment in physical therapy.

A prerequisite for any functional activity is good wheelchair balance. It is optimal for the patient to be able to use both upper extremities without having to support himself. In general, a high-level thoracic injury (T1–8) leaves the patient with intact upper extremities so that he can carry out all his transfers, wheelchair activities, and self-care independently. These patients do have significantly reduced trunk control as compared with the lower-level thoracic injuries (T9–12). The patient with an injury at T9–12 level has sufficient trunk stability to allow him to perform high-level wheelchair skills. Examples of these skills are wheelies and transfers out of the chair to the ground. The ability to transfer to the floor means that the patient will need less equipment at the completion of rehabilitation, such as a tub bench.

When the level of injury is in the lumbar region, ambulation becomes a feasible goal. Patients with injuries at the L1–3 level may be able to ambulate at the household level with knee-ankle-foot orthoses (KAFOs) because their hip flexors and adductors are innervated. At the L4 level the quadriceps become innervated. A manual muscle grade of fair-plus (3+) may enable the patient to ambulate in ankle-foot orthoses (AFOs). The gluteus medius and tensor facia lata receive partial innervation at L5. These muscles provide adequate hip stability to allow all patients to walk with AFOs (Fig 26–3). At the sacral level, ambulation may be possible without the use of orthoses.

Table 26–1 illustrates the functional goals that a spinal cord–injured patient can be expected to achieve at the time of discharge from therapy. Again, it must be stressed that these goals are merely guidelines.

Incomplete Paraplegia

The patient with an incomplete injury may be unable to achieve goals higher than a patient with a complete injury of the same level. It is with these patients that the manual muscle test grade of "fair-plus" (3+) becomes most critical. Muscles that are graded below F+/3+ have insufficient strength to take on any significant tasks. The

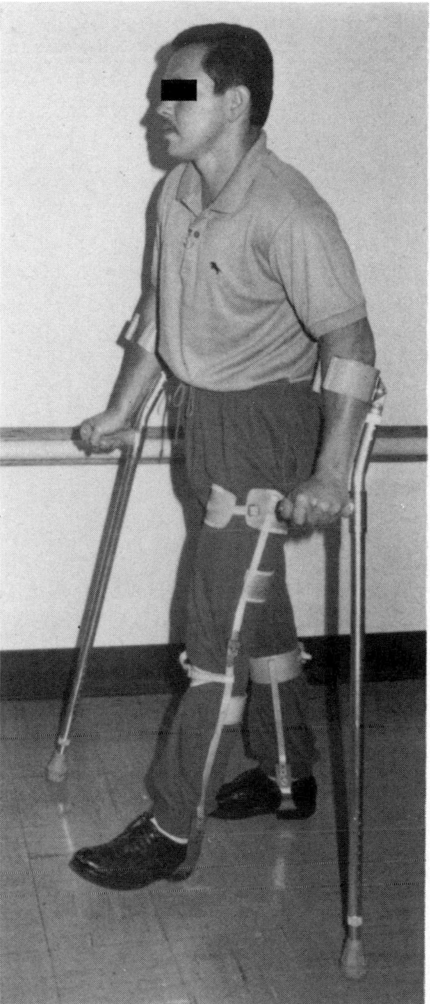

FIG 26–3.
A patient ambulating in a KAFO/AFO combination. When quadriceps strength is fair-plus or better, the knee joint of the KAFO can usually be unlocked.

patient should be made aware of the strength needed for many functional activities. This will allow him to be more realistic about his future without taking away all hope. Patients with trace and poor muscle grades in their trunk and lower extremities are frequently resistant to participating in therapy that stresses basic body handling skills. They frequently feel that all effort should be placed on ambulation and strengthening of the leg muscles. The best recommendation is that the patient be told that walking is very difficult and that all the skills he must learn first will contribute to his ultimate functional capabilities through a total-body approach to muscle strengthening.

Functionally, light self-care skills such as grooming and hygiene pose no difficulty for the paraplegic individual. However, self-care skills that involve the lower part of the body and demand adequate body-handling skills require the therapist's intervention. Lower-body dressing

TABLE 26–1.

Functional Goals for Patients With Complete Spinal Cord Injury (Consider Age, Sex, Weight, Body Type, and Motivation)

	Quadriplegics*				Paraplegics*			
Goal*	C1–4: Neck, Upper Trapezoids	C5: Deltoids, Biceps	C6: Wrist Extensors	C7–8: Triceps, Weak Hand	T1–8: Chest Extension	T9–12: Trunk Extension	L1–2 Hip Extensors	L3–5 Knee Extensors
Relief of skin pressure								
(I) With electric recliner	X	X						
(I) Forward loop or lean		*	*	*				
(I) Depression raises			X	X	X	X	X	X
Wheelchair propulsion								
Electric	X	X	*	*				
Manual with projection rims		*	*					
Manual with friction rims			X	*				
Manual with standard rims			*	X	X	X	X	X
Bed transfers								
Mechanical/manual lift	X	*						
(A) Sliding board	*	X	*					
(I) Sliding board			X	*				
(I) Depression			*	X	X	X	X	X
Car transfers								
Mechanical lift/dependent	X	X	*					
(A) Sliding board		*	*					
(I) Sliding board			X	*	*			
(I) Depression			*	X	X	X	X	X
Toilet transfers								
Mechanical lift to commode	X	X						
(A) Sliding board to commode		*	*					
(I) Sliding board to raised seat			X	*				
(I) Depression to raised seat			*	X	X	X	X	X
Tub transfers								
(A) Sliding board to tub bench		*	*					
(I) Sliding board to tub bench			X	*				
(I) Depression to tub bench			*	X	X	X	X	X
(I) To bottom of tub						*	*	*
Cough								
Dependent manual	X	X						
Self manual		*	X	*	*			
Independent			*	X	X	X	X	X
Curb management								
(I) 2 in. curbs			*	X				
(I) 4 and 6 in. curbs				*	X	X	X	X
Wheelchair into car								
(A) Dependent/unable			*					
(I) With loop on wheelchair			*					
Independent			X	X	X	X	X	X
Ambulation								
Physiologic				*	*	*	X	
Household							X	
Limited community							*	X
Community							*	X

*I = independent; A = assisted; X = most patients; * = some patients.

should begin when the hip flexion range is 0 to 110 degrees to avoid stretching the low back muscles in long sitting. Optimally, the patient should also be able to come to a sitting position from a supine one, maintain his balance in a long sitting position, and roll from side to side. Since these skills take time and much practice to develop, it is often necessary to begin training with compensatory techniques. Initially, these techniques may involve bringing up the back of the hospital bed to maintain long sitting and using assistive devices such as a dressing stick to reach the feet. When dressing in bed is mastered, the patient is trained to dress in the wheelchair.

To ensure success, the patient's thorough understanding of the purpose and procedure used to accomplish the task is critical. Audiovisual aids that show a paraplegic dressing in bed and in the wheelchair are helpful additions to the therapist's instruction.

Safety precautions must be of special consideration in showering and bathing training. Slippery surfaces make it difficult to maintain balance, especially when the arms are engaged in washing the body. The patient must be taught to prepare all needed supplies nearby to avoid precarious reaching. Patients must also learn to test the water temperature with their hands before entering the water to avoid burns. Simulating bathing conditions to resemble those at the patient's home makes training more relevant and valuable to the individual.

Once the paraplegic has learned to perform all self-care skills, treatment must focus on preparing the patient to meet the challenges of home life. Most home skills such as meal preparation, housekeeping, and laundry remain realistic and require only minimal instruction to be performed from a wheelchair. Training must emphasize planning skills, energy conservation, and safety precautions. Knowledge of the patient's home floor plan assists in making instruction specific to the architectural barriers the patient will encounter. The final goal in home skills training is to enable the patient to apply his knowledge to any situation that may arise. The patient must develop the ability to plan ahead, to organize efficiently, and to problem-solve effectively.

Day passes and overnight passes provide an excellent opportunity for the patient to test the skills learned in the hospital at home. Detailed discussions of information gathered on passes allow the patient to practice problem solving with the help of the occupational therapist. Group discussions in which patients are encouraged to provide their own solutions to problems are very helpful.

To complete the transition from the hospital to the community, community living skills training is essential. Community outings provide an opportunity to enable the patient to begin finding ways to manage in the community from the wheelchair. These outings may include taking a bus, shopping, and dining out. As with home skills, emphasis is placed on thorough planning prior to the activity. Group discussions serve to educate patients about community resources and their rights to services.

Another crucial element in obtaining independence is engaging in meaningful work. Following an in-depth evaluation of the patient's vocational interests, aptitude, and physical abilities, the patient is encouraged to try out different vocational activities in a simulated work environment. Work site evaluation may help prepare the patient to return to a previous job. Prevocational and vocational counselors assist in the process of vocational evaluation and continue training the patient after discharge from the hospital.

As with other ADL, driving training with the paraplegic patient requires less instruction than with the quadriplegic patient. Driving training must include behind-the-wheel practice sessions with hand controls and instruction in transferring the wheelchair in and out of the car. As with other activities, safety is of primary concern. Spasm patterns and spasticity are evaluated, and the patient is alerted to special considerations that he must attend to while driving.

Discharge Planning and Follow-Up

A critical goal for the rehabilitation team is to facilitate the patient's smooth transition from the hospital to his home and community. To accomplish this goal discharge planning must begin early in the rehabilitation process. The involvement of the patient's significant others must be encouraged early, especially with patients who will require assistance in ADL. Family members are encouraged to observe therapy, ask questions, and learn to perform the routine care that they may need to engage in at home such as ranging the patient.

An early visit to the patient's home will facilitate a successful transition from the hospital to the community. During this visit the patient, the physical therapist, and the occupational therapist meet with the patient's family at home to prepare for the patient's homecoming. Discussion is focused on the removal of architectural barriers that interfere with the patient's ability to perform daily routines independently and achieve maximal wheelchair accessibility and safety. To many families and patients, the home visit is a startling confrontation with the reality of disability. To reduce anxiety often aroused during the visit, skills learned in rehabilitation must be practiced and utilized in the home setting. Unfortunately, many patients do not have a clear discharge destination until the end of their rehabilitation stay. With these patients, home visits are conducted at discharge.

Day passes and overnight passes are extremely useful in preparing the patient for community reentry. During

TABLE 26–2.
Equipment That May Be Ordered for Patients With Complete Spinal Injury

	Injury Level*								
Equipment	C2–3	C4	C5: Shoulder Biceps	C6 Wrist Extensors	C7–8: Hand	T1–10: Chest	T11–12: Trunk	L1–3: Hip Flexors	L4–5: Knee Extensors
Lightweight W/C	X	X	X	X	X	*	*	*	*
Standard-weight W/C						X	X	X	X
Electric W/C with hand control		–	X	*					
Electric W/C with tongue control	X								
Electric W/C with chin control	X	X							
Custom cushion	X	X	X	X	X	X	X	X	*
Hill holders				X	X				
W/C trunk supports	X	X	X	–					
Sliding board	–	X	X	X	X	X			
Swivel bar			–	–					
Ramp	X	X	X	X	X	X	X	X	
Lumbar-sacral orthosis (corset)	X	X	X	X	X	–			
Elastic hose	X	X	X	X	X	X	X	–	–
Knee-ankle-foot orthosis (KAFO)						–	–	X	
Ankle-foot orthosis (AFO)								X	X
Forearm crutches						–	–	X	X
Pickup walker								–	–
Raised toilet seat				–	X	X			
Commode chair			–	–	–	–			
Bathtub seat			–	X	X	X			
Grab bars				–	X	X			
Lucite lapboard	X	X	X	–	–				
Mobile arm supports, radial or standard		X	X	–					
Suspension slings	X	X	–	–					
Basic long opponens wrist-hand orthosis	X	X	X						
Hand orthosis with lumbar bar					X	–			
Ratchet wrist-hand orthosis		–	X	–					
Wrist-driven flexor wrist-hand orthosis			–	X	X				
Plaster wrist-hand orthosis	X	X	X	–					
Plastazote wrist-hand orthosis	X	X	X	–					
Mouth stick	–	X	X						
Pincher mouth stick	–	X	X						
Adapted grooming equipment		X	X	X	X				
Adapted feeding equipment		X	X	X	X				
Driving cuff			–	X	X				
Hi-low hospital bed (manual)	X	X	X	X	–				
Bed rails	X	X	X	X	–				
Lift and sling	X	X	X	–	–				
Tub attachment for lift	–	–	–	–					
Scifoam mattress (Polyfloat)	–	–	–	–	–	–	–		
Firm mattress for bed in home	–	–	–	–	–	X	X	–	–
Suppository instructions									
Urinal bag clamp	X	X	X	X	X	–			

*X = usually ordered; – = occasionally ordered; * = optional these passes the patient is encouraged to try out new skills learned in therapy. Following passes the patient and the therapist attempt to solve those problems that the patient encountered and could not independently solve. On these passes, trial use of adaptive equipment is important in identifying the patient's specific needs.

In order to ensure that needed adaptive equipment and orthoses do not end up in the closet, the patient must have a good understanding of the function and routine maintenance of these devices. Supplementing discussion with written instructions on the care of equipment aids in ensuring its proper functioning. The patient must also have tried alternative ways to achieve goals that are attained with equipment and fully appreciate their pros and cons. This will allow him to continue to independently assess the use of his equipment. Prior to discharge, the patient must also have a clear understanding of how to obtain repairs when equipment malfunctions. He must also be instructed and well practiced in a routine home strengthening program in order to maintain and increase his functional ability.

Lifelong follow-up by a SCI health care team provides the spinal cord–injured patient with specialized care to meet his evolving problems and needs. If the patient and therapist identify new functional goals, further treatment is planned by the outpatient team to achieve these goals. Patients who are unable to come to the hospital's outpatient clinic are referred to other health care providers.

Patients who either are homebound or require more extensive follow-up at home are referred to the Visiting Nurse Association (VNA).

Equipment needs are evaluated at the time of discharge by the appropriate therapists. The patient's level of goal achievement is moderated by realistic functional expectations and the social situation in determining what adaptive devices, equipment, and functional aids are necessary. These decisions are made on a case-by-case basis. Typical equipment prescriptions according to the level of injury are illustrated in Table 26–2.

Acknowledgments

Acknowledgments are made to coauthors and contributors on the staff at Rancho: Michal Atkins, M.A., O.T.R.; Cheryl Resnik, M.S., P.T.; Daniel Capen, M.D.; Melinda Wallace, R.N.; and Gary Bresee, Ph.D.

REFERENCES

1. Baumgarten JM: Upper extremity adaptations for the person with quadriplegia, in Adkins HV (ed): *Spinal Cord Injury Clinics in Physical Therapy,* vol 6. New York, Churchill Livingstone, 1985.
2. Daniels L, Worthingham C: *Muscle Testing: Techniques of Manual Examination.* Philadelphia, WB Saunders, 1946.
3. Garland DE, Lilling M, Keenan MA: Percutaneous phenol blocks to motor points or spastic forearm muscles in head-injured adults. *Arch Phys Med Rehabil* 1984; 68:243–245.
4. Gowland C, Simoes N: *A Driver Training Program for Persons With Physical Disabilities,* ed 2. Rancho, NM, PSA, 1984.
5. Hill JP: *Spinal Cord Injury: A Guide to Functional Outcome in Occupational Therapy.* Rockville, Md, Aspen Systems, 1986.
6. Parsons T: *The Social System.* Glencoe, Ill, Free Press, 1951.
7. Reiser T, Mudiyam R, Waters R: Orthopaedic evaluation of spinal cord injury and management of vertebral fractures, in Adkins HV (ed): New York, Churchill Livingstone, 1985.

27

Rehabilitation of Chronic Spinal Cord Injury

Robert R. Menter, M.D.

The focus of attention in spinal cord injury (SCI) care is shifting from issues of acute care and early rehabilitation to issues of long-term care. While a solid volume of literature has been developed on the issues of acute care, very little has been established that relates to the issues of long-term care.

To understand long-term care, one must have a grasp of the influence of aging on both the able-bodied person and the individual with a disability. Aging presents three lifelong developmental processes all overlapping but distinctively different:

1. Physiologic changes of the body
2. Societal changes
3. Issues of self-realization

Because these are three very broad overlapping areas, the subject of aging can be approached from many different perspectives. Loss of muscle mass with the resultant decreased strength, decreasing range of motion and osteoarthritis leading to pain and decreased function, and increasing urologic and bowel problems may all be considered under physiologic change. Under the topic of societal changes, one thinks of growth and development as a child, leaving the home, marriage and parenting, loss of one's parents, and loss of a spouse. Within the category of self-realization are issues of growth and development to young adulthood, development of ethics and morality, spiritual discovery, and finding meaning in life.

Perhaps one of the most distinctive features of aging in both the able-bodied and in people with disabilities is the increasing uniqueness and differentiation of each individual within the aging process. An examination of 100 C6 quadriplegics 20 years old would reveal 100 people with a very similar profile of functional abilities, health impairment, and organ system reserves. A look at this same group 30 years later would show tremendous variations in weight, range of motion, cardiac reserve, strength, and functional ability.

RESEARCH ON SPINAL CORD INJURY AGING

Little is known about the effects of aging in SCI. At this time, most information is anecdotal and limited to each individual's perspective. Survival with SCI appears to have evolved through a series of steps. Those who survived SCI sustained in the 1940s and 1950s have low-level and mid-level paraplegia. It was not until the 1960s and 1970s that those with low-level quadriplegia (C7 and C8 levels) and then finally mid-level quadriplegia (C5 and C6 levels) survived in significant numbers. Only since the 1980s, with its vastly improved emergency medical care, has the survival of persons with high-level quadriplegia (C1 through C4) been possible.[22]

In studying problems associated with aging in SCI it must be remembered that those with paraplegia are now approaching 30 to 40 years' cumulative aging. Those individuals with low-level quadriplegia are reaching the 20-year postinjury milestone, and people with high-level quadriplegia, as a group, are now only 10 years postinjury.

Equally difficult to understand is the problem of differing rehabilitation goals that prevailed during the different decades of injury. In the 1950s rehabilitation was defined as survival, and goals were merely to get home to a sedentary existence. Sedentary life-styles have their own set of complications such as obesity, increased cardiovascular disease, and increased smoking. In contrast, during the 1970s and 1980s, rehabilitation goals called for very active life-styles with involvement in the community and as much independence as possible. These goals may have contributed to entirely different patterns of aging, including overuse syndromes, the wearing out of joints and muscles, and the effects of increased stress that result from trying to compete in the community. Clearly, because of the differing goals of rehabilitation, the individuals injured in the 1950s and 1960s may have very different patterns of aging from those injured in the 1970s and 1980s.

Recently, a clear difference in aging patterns depending upon the age of onset of SCI has become apparent. Traditionally, onset in youth has been the common factor of most spine injuries. However, as the aging of America continues, more and more people are living into their 60s, 70s, and 80s and are developing degenerative changes of the cervical spine with associated spinal stenosis. Significant numbers of these individuals with narrowed spinal canals are experiencing elderly-onset SCI rather than the usual youth-onset SCI. Initial studies indicate that these older individuals have quite different clinical courses after SCI than do their younger counterparts.[4, 17, 23, 24, 38]

PRELIMINARY FINDINGS

In 1982 Craig Hospital asked Dr. George Hohmann, Ph.D., to speak on issues of aging in SCI. Dr. Hohmann had incurred an SCI in World War II and had lived with paraplegia for 40 years. He identified six categories of problems experienced by fellow WW II SCI survivors.[16]

1. Orthopedic problems
2. Neurologic complications
3. Medical infections
4. Obesity
5. Family problems
6. Psychosocial problems

Orthopedic problems included increasing pain and restricted range of motion, particularly in the arms, shoulders, and neck. Many were thought to be overuse syndromes as a result of chronic use of the arms and shoulders to perform tasks they were not designed to perform. Equally significant was the increasing incidence of fractures of osteoporotic lower extremities. Less understood but a more frightening problem was the collapse of the spine at or below the level of injury as a result of developing Charcot joint changes below the level of paralysis.

Neurologic complications included the development of a significantly higher incidence of carpal tunnel syndrome and ulnar nerve atrophy than in the normal population. The former may be related to the trauma that the palms and wrists sustain secondary to using crutches and wheelchairs. The latter is related to the pressure on the elbows received from wheelchair armrests or other support surfaces. Other individuals suffered from mysterious loss of neurologic function above the level of their injury, which now is understood to be post-traumatic cystic myelopathy.

Obesity, a secondary complication of sedentary lives, became a significant problem when it prevented spouses from providing safe, necessary assistance for bowel care, transfers, and other activites of daily living. In many cases individuals were forced to move to nursing homes to obtain adequate care in the face of their obesity.

Family problems were reflected by the cumulative long-term effects on spouses who provided continuous care in addition to all their other responsibilities. With age, the demands on spouses became greater while their own increasing age made them less able to provide that care. Another problem noted was that the individuals with spinal injuries had to adopt aging-related life-style changes earlier than their able-bodied family members who had yet to feel the onset of aging.

Psychosocial problems were manifested by withdrawal from life in the absence of overt depression. Such withdrawal reflected a sense of helplessness and loss of control over life. Accompanying this was a loss of interest in sexuality and loss of self-esteem and hope.

Roberta Trieschmann, Ph.D., and Barry Corbet, filmmaker and author, have continued to explore the issues of SCI aging. Dr. Trieschmann published *Aging With a Disability* in 1987, which uses both personal stories and literature reviews to expand our knowledge on aging with disability. Barry Corbet published a series of interviews with aging SCI survivors in the "Options Group Revisited: Perspectives on Aging" (1987) and produced a movie, *Survivors 1989,* which explores the feelings and adaptive processes of aging with a disability. In England others have raised similar concerns, such as Rodney Coe, a quadriplegic of 22 years who reported significant changes in function and quality of life, and Silver, Zarb, and others, who published results of aging spinal cord injury survivors in England.[7, 8, 28, 32]

THE AGING PROCESS

Aging is multifactorial in its origin. The following are major components determining the aging process:

1. Genetic factors
2. Trauma
3. Life-style
4. Stress adaptation
5. Sociological role

Of these major determinants, genetic characteristics are the only ones over which there is no control. How we choose to live our life determines trauma risk factors, life-style, how we adapt to stress, and our sociological role. Since four of the five major determinants of aging are under our control, it follows that many of the consequences of aging are preventable or postponable.[3, 34, 35]

Modifiers of the Aging Process

Studies of longevity have shown the following determinants to be significant:

1. Diet
2. Exercise
3. Smoking

4. Retirement and work
5. Marital status
6. Social activities

In each area there is an optimal balance that lends itself to good health.

An important factor in the aging process is the cumulative effect of life-style circumstances such as smoking, exercise, nutrition, and economic support. The cumulative negative or positive effects of each of these may substantially alter system reserves and functional abilities.

How stress is managed is a significant factor in aging. Unmanaged stress may lead to such diverse problems as hypertension, heart disease, obesity, peptic ulcer disease, and respiratory disease. Each of these medical conditions can interfere with an individual's life-style. Good health requires effective stress management to prevent the focus of stress on any target organ by dissipating it in a more constructive manner.

Wellness is the concept that best encompasses the principles of controlling the consequences of aging and achieving longevity with as high a quality of life as possible. Wellness is defined as a life-style to achieve the best health possible. Key components of wellness programs involve nutrition, physical awareness, stress reduction, and self-responsibility. While most information relating to wellness has been developed in the able-bodied population, there is every reason to believe that these same principles hold true for people with disabilities such as SCI.[29]

Examples of Normal Aging

Physiologic aging is the steady erosion of the reserve built into each organ system of the body. As the reserve is gradually diminished, disruption of normal function of that system increases. The following are examples of normal changes of aging by system in several organ systems of able-bodied persons and some of the concerns these changes create in spinal cord–injured people.[2, 3, 26]

In the normal skeletal system, aging is reflected in osteoarthritis, with associated decreased range of motion and increased pain. Another normal aging change is osteoporosis and its associated increased risk of fractures. These normal aging changes—when imposed on an individual with SCI who already has decreased range of motion, pain, and osteoporosis—may produce an accelerated aging pattern with consequences noted at a much earlier age than in the able-bodied population.

The normal muscular system reflects aging with decreases in strength. This additional aging-induced loss of strength may significantly change the ability of individuals with SCI to be independent and care for themselves.

The normal gastrointestinal system manifests aging with decreased volumes of saliva, acid, bile, and pancreatic juice. In addition, there is decreased peristalsis leading to constipation. These normal changes, when superimposed on pre-existing problems of decreased peristalsis and concomitant constipation found in SCI, may produce accelerated refractory bowel dysfunction.

The normal skin ages with a thinning of the skin and dermis and a loss of subcutaneous fat. When combined with neurotropic skin, loss of protective sensation, and decreased muscle tone (as in SCI), there may be increased difficulty in maintaining sitting time and tolerance.

THE SPINAL CORD INJURY AGING MODEL

Research has identified what are typical aging patterns in all systems of the body. In any given individual, however, the particular pattern of aging will vary. In an individual with severe asthma, the pulmonary reserves may be exhausted at an early age, which then has an impact on overall bodily function. In a person with rheumatoid arthritis, the pattern of aging may be expressed by decreasing range of motion and increasing pain, both of which lead to decreased overall function. In an individual with SCI, there may be dramatic changes in many systems, such as skin sensitivity, bladder function, and bowel function. All may interfere with the overall mobility and health of the system. Nonetheless, because there is a tremendous amount of reserve built into each organ system and because of the complex system of adaptation offered by rehabilitation, most people do continue to function, even if at a reduced capacity.

Over the years, a conceptual model of how aging may affect or have an impact on the total function of the spinal-injured individual has been developed. Conceptually, there are three phases following the onset of a spinal injury: phase 1, acute restoration; phase 2, maintenance; and phase 3, decline (Fig 27–1).

Acute restoration is the process by which an individual moves from having virtually no function immediately following a spinal injury to regaining the maximum amount of function that is consistent with this level of neurologic injury. Thus, an individual with paraplegia could become independent but would still require a wheelchair or braces. An individual with C5 quadriplegia would be unable to do many of the things that someone with paraplegia could but might still reach a maximum function consistent with the injury level. Usually, the acute rehabilitation phase is completed within 2 years following the injury.

The maintenance phase is an indefinite but very lengthy phase during which time the person maintains the level of functioning that was established following the injury and successful rehabilitation.

The last phase, decline, occurs with the gradual onset of the physiologic aging process. Function may decline as a result of decreased muscle strength, decreased joint

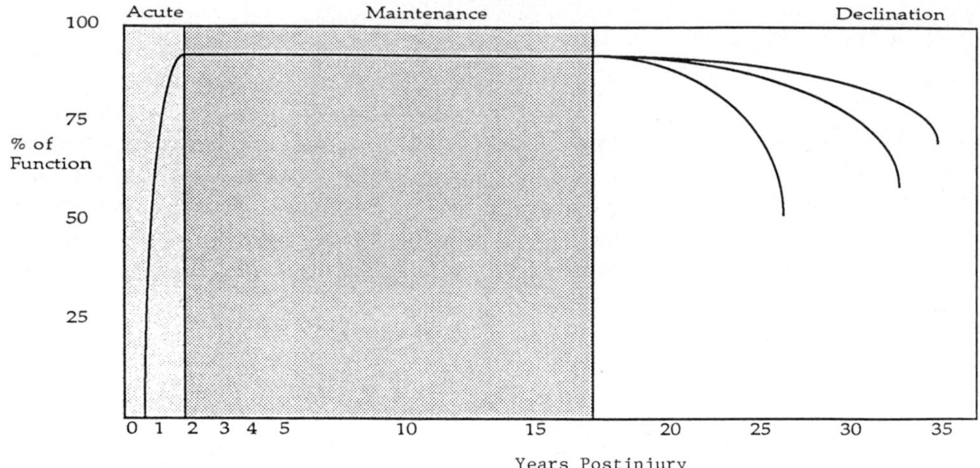

FIG 27–1.
Model of aging and physical disability.

range of motion, decreased respiratory or cardiovascular capacity, and increased frequency of skin breakdown. All, either individually or together, cause a steady erosion of organ reserve and an overall decrease in function. Very little is known about this phase. There may or may not be specific patterns of decline among individuals. Regardless, the goal is to understand the process so that individuals may take action to control or prevent their consequences.

This model of aging can be applied to other disability groups as well as individuals. Generally, the populations of head injury and SCI and polio survivors each reflect the characteristics of a different phase.

Working backward, postpolio survivors typify the last or decline phase of aging. Now approaching 40 years postonset, in the 1980s this group began exhibiting aging-related concerns for which they were totally unprepared. They were equally unprepared for the life-style alterations they were forced to make. Changes like increasing pain, weakness, and fatigue all exceeded what was expected for their age, and new behaviors were demanded. More physical aids were required, physical activity had to be limited, and survivors were forced to consider ways to preserve as much function and activity for the future as possible.

The second or maintenance phase is best illustrated by the majority of the SCI population. Members of this group, as a rule, are continuing at the level of function they attained following their injury. For the most part few new problems or needs are arising.

Finally, the first or acute restoration phase is best illustrated by the traumatic head injury population. Within this population the optimal treatment programs to restore function are still evolving.

Although the SCI and traumatic head injury groups are still in the early stages of the model, it can be predicted that each will move through the successive stages and have its own patterns of decline.

By utilizing this model as well as the previously discussed overlapping developmental spheres of the aging process, it is possible to understand how each individual will have his own unique pattern of aging based upon physiologic age, societal interaction, self-realization, anatomic or neurologic level of injury, and the length of time postinjury.

LONG-TERM MANAGEMENT OF SPINAL CORD INJURY

The key to long-term SCI management is a change in philosophical orientation of the rehabilitation team. In the acute care and early rehabilitation phase, the physician and rehabilitation team are the experts, and the patients are very unknowledgeable. Patient goals and outcomes are very similar at each level of injury. However, once patients have returned to the community, they become the experts and are increasingly knowledgeable of their problems, their resources, and their limitations. Moreover, in the community, the problems and needs become increasingly diverse. During the maintenance phase, the rehabilitation team and physician need to change roles and become resources for individuals as they solve problems they encounter in their communities and living situations. Quite different skills will be needed as special information and knowledge are developed to address issues not identified in the early rehabilitation care. The following are examples from the orthopedic and neurologic areas that were identified in current long-term follow-up programs. Also provided are some suggestions on how to work with them.

1. *Posture problems in the wheelchair.*—The problems of paretic muscles, decreasing range of motion, and spasticity increase with time and lead to increasing problems of posture in the wheelchair. Frequently, the patient's first complaint in the clinic is discomfort in the lower part

of the back. In addition to adequate urologic evaluation to rule out renal disease and/or bladder disease and after baseline x-ray films of the spine, a referral should be made to physical and occupational therapists with special interest and background in SCI posture problems. Many times, the discomfort in the back will be alleviated by a better seat cushion and/or back support system. In particular, the restoration of lumbar lordosis while sitting in the wheelchair will frequently give relief to low back discomfort. Underlying musculoskeletal pathology such as contractures at the hips, knees, ankles, and feet may have to be corrected to ensure a more appropriate sitting platform and distribution of weight. Heterotopic ossification contributing to contractures should be addressed very carefully. Surgery should be performed only if the process is proved to be inactive on a three-phase bone scan. Consultation with physicians having previous experience in heterotopic ossification surgery is desirable. Antibiotic coverage of the urinary bacteria during the perioperative period is crucial to prevent secondary infection. The use of etidronate disodium before and after heterotopic ossification surgery is mandatory. Radiation and nonsteroidal anti-inflammatory medications may play support roles in controlling the recurrence of heterotopic ossification.[31]

2. *Spasticity*.—One of the most frequent causes of increasing disability is spasticity interfering with function and/or causing increased pain. The causation needs to be thoroughly evaluated with attention to bladder, bowel, decubiti, fractures, cystic myelopathy, and contractures, all of which can cause an increase in the severity of spasms. Spasms have both positive and negative features. Positive features include better circulation and more frequent weight shifts, thus minimizing skin breakdown. Negative features include interfering with positioning and functional activities and/or causing pain. Goals of treatment are to control, not eliminate the spasms that interfere with function and/or cause pain. The initial treatment of choice is oral medication, usually baclofen. If baclofen is inadequate in controlling spasm and/or creates too many undesirable side effects, consideration may be given to procedures such as percutaneous thermorhizotomy or intrathecal baclofen pumps.[10, 15, 19, 20, 25, 39]

3. *Progressive neurologic loss of sensation and/or motor function above the base level of paralysis established at the original injury*.—This problem may be due to either progressive post-traumatic cystic myelopathy and/or the myelomalacic degenerative changes secondary to tethering of the spinal cord at the SCI injury site. Documentation of progressive motor sensory deterioration is necessary before surgical intervention can be justified. Diagnostic studies using magnetic resonance imaging (MRI) can frequently identify, track, and document the myelopathic process. Surgical intervention can be justified to prevent further neurologic deterioration but should be referred to neurosurgeons with specific experience in these areas.[33]

4. *Impaired shoulder function relating to rotator cuff disease and/or tendonitis*.—Poor body mechanics and incorrect transfer techniques are significant factors contributing to this frequent problem. Obesity is a contributing factor and should be addressed through increased attention to nutrition and appropriate exercise. All individuals with recurrent tendonitis and/or bursitis of the upper extremities require evaluation by experienced therapists to evaluate body handling techniques. Other ways of decreasing the stress on the joints is to use more adaptive equipment in place of strenuous transfers. Finally, nonsteroidal anti-inflammatories along with other symptomatic treatments commonly used in musculoskeletal disease should be undertaken.[1, 27, 37]

5. *Peripheral nerve entrapment problems*.—Carpal tunnel and ulnar nerve entrapment pathology have been identified in as many as 86% of patients with SCI over 15 years postinjury. Workup involves standard nerve conduction studies. Once diagnosed, symptoms may be controlled by conservative measures such as education about causes and use of night splints for the wrists and elbow pads at the elbows. Individuals with symptoms not responding to conservative treatment and individuals with progressive symptoms are candidates for standard surgical decompression. Each individual deserves an evaluation by an experienced therapist who can review all body-use activities to identify and correct any patterns that may be creating the pathology.[9, 13]

6. *Pain*.—This is one of the most common problems interfering with the quality of life. Pain can be musculoskeletal in origin, or it may be central (spinal cord) in origin. Overall, pain appears to increase with time. Factors influencing pain are poor posture, no leisure time interest or social activities, and inadequate social and financial support systems. All pain workups require a complete psychosocial assessment in addition to physiologic and therapy evaluations.[12, 14]

7. *Fractures due to the combination of osteoporosis, secondary paralysis, osteoporosis of aging, insensitive extremities, spasticity, and contractures*.—These processes all lead to increased fractures of the lower extremities. The most common fractures are in the supracondylar femur and proximal tibial metaphysis region, but fractures do occur at all locations. Most fractures are treated conservatively in pillow splints with good results. If surgical procedures are considered, they must take into account severe osteoporosis, severe spasticity, and neurotropic skin. Early range of motion needs to be initiated to prevent joint contractures.[11, 18]

8. *Fatigue*.—Fatigue is one of the most common problems affecting life-style and the quality of life. It is probably due to the gradual decrease in strength of the re-

maining functioning muscles. With increased weakness, greater effort is necessary to accomplish the same activities previously accomplished without fatigue. Many times, fatigue can be lessened by using more assistive equipment, setting lower levels of expectations, and breaking up the day with rest periods.

9. *Charcot spine.*—A small number of cases have developed Charcot joints at the thoracolumbar spine junction either a few years or many years postinjury. These are usually asymptomatic in terms of discomfort but do create progressive postural problems and, in some cases, audible crepitation as the joint moves. Surgery on a Charcot spine is fraught with many problems. Both anterior and posterior stabilization is necessary. Diagnostic workups should include conventional films with flexion-extension stresses, computerized axial tomography (CAT) studies, MRI to rule out osteomyelitis, and in some cases aspiration of fluid in the Charcot joint to rule out infection.[30, 36]

An overview of other nonorthopedic or non-neurologic changes secondary to aging includes the following[5]:

1. Urologic problems: pyelonephritis, renal calculi, prostatic hypertrophy with obstruction, recurrent infection
2. Nutrition disorders: obesity
3. Bowel dysfunction: constipation, gallbladder disease, esophageal reflux
4. Skin breakdown: decubiti, edema with stasis ulcers
5. Peripheral vascular disease
6. Respiratory problems: pneumonia, bronchitis
7. System infections of various etiologies

NONMEDICAL AGING ISSUES

Equally important but less frequently addressed are the societal, familial, and environmental changes each person encounters. How these changes are identified and handled frequently creates the stresses leading to the many medical issues previously identified.[6]

All too often the rehabilitation team fails to identify and work on these issues because they are less amenable to treatment with medications, therapy, equipment, or surgery. These areas require the commitment of the entire rehabilitation team, with particular focus on follow-through and follow-up in the community.

LONG-TERM FOLLOW-UP PROGRAM

After acute rehabilitation, annual follow-up with complete reassessment by the physician and rehabilitation team is indicated for 2 to 5 years. After the first few years, individuals seem to fall into three groups. One group is composed of those able to self-direct their care and follow-up. They need contact every 2 to 3 years as necessary. A second group includes those requiring very closely supervised, structured follow-up every 6 to 12 months. The last group of individuals consists of those who switch back and forth between structured and unstructured follow-up depending on stress and how they are handling it. In all individuals with SCI, a comprehensive physiologic and psychosocial baseline should be established every 5 years. More frequent follow-up will be necessary for many individuals depending on their clinical course. These comprehensive evaluations need to be completed at established SCI treatment centers with comparative data bases and previous comparative records of the patient to identify any changes.

FUTURE

The understanding of patient needs and program resources for long-term care of spinal-injured patients is very incomplete at this point. Studies are under way to try to develop a data base of normal aging processes that will lend itself to the development of new programs to help both the patients and the medical treating teams understand what to expect and what resources will be necessary to meet those needs.[20, 21]

REFERENCES

1. Bayley JC, Cocran TP, Sledge CB: The weight-bearing shoulder. *J Bone Joint Surg [Am]* 1987; 69:676–678.
2. Birren JE: *Handbook of Aging*. In Finch CE, Schneider EL (eds): *Handbook of the Biology of Aging,* vol 1. Birren JE, Schaie KW (eds): *Handbook of the Psychology of Aging,* vol 2. Binstock RH, Shanas E (eds): *Handbook of Aging and the Social Sciences,* vol 3. New York, van Nostrand Reinhold.
3. Bortz W: Disuse and aging. *JAMA* 1982; 248:1203–1208.
4. Brady S: Implications of aging in spinal cord injury. *Spinal Cord Injury Nurs* 1988; 3:4344.
5. Brenes G, LaPorte RE, Collins E: High density lipoprotein cholesterol concentrations in physically active and sedentary spinal cord injured patients. *Arch Phys Med Rehabil* 1986; 67:445–450.
6. Callahan D: Families as caregivers: The limits of morality. *Arch Phys Med Rehabil* 1988; 69:323–328.
7. Coe RG: 22 years a tetraplegic. *Lancet* 1982; 1:789–790.
8. Corbet B: *The Options Group: Perspectives on Aging With Spinal Cord Injury*. New York, North American Reinsurance Corp, March 1987.
9. Davidoff G, Werner R, Waring W: Compressive mononeuropathies in chronic paraplegia. *Paraplegia* 1991; 29:17–24.
10. Donovan WH, Carter E, et al: Clonidine effect on spasticity: A clinical trial. *Arch Phys Med Rehabil* 1988; 69:193–194.
11. Freehafer AA, Hazel CM, Becker CL: Lower Extremity Fractures in Patients with SCI. *Paraplegia* 1981; 19:367–372.

12. Frisbie JH, Aquilera EJ: Chronic pain after SCI: An expedient diagnostic approach. *Paraplegia* 1990; 28:460–465.
13. Gellman H, Chandler DR, et al: Carpal tunnel syndrome in paraplegic patients. *J Bone Joint Surg [Am]* 1988; 70:517–519.
14. Green B, Edgar R: Pain: Spinal injury, in *Current Therapy in Neurological Surgery,* vol 2. Toronto, BC Decker, 1989; pp 294–297.
15. Herz DA, Parsons KC, Pearl L: Percutaneous radiofrequency foraminal rhizotomies. *Spine* 1983; 8:729–732.
16. Hohmann G: Aging in SCI Survivors. WWII Craig Hospital 5th Annual John S. Young Lectureship, May 1982.
17. Hooker EZ: Problems of veterans spinal cord injured after age 55: Nursing implication. *J Neurosci Nurs* 1986; 18:188–195.
18. Ingram RR, Suman RK, Freeman PA: Lower limb fractures in chronic spinal injured patients. *Paraplegia* 1989; 27:133–139.
19. Kasdon DL, Lathi ES: A prospective study of radiofrequency rhizotomy in the treatment of post traumatic spasticity. *Neurosurgery* 1984; 15:526–529.
20. Katz RT: Management of spasticity. *Am J Phys Med Rehabil* 1988; 67:108–116.
21. Mather JH: A philosophy of caring for the elderly. *Paraplegia News*, 1986, pp 18–22.
22. Menter RR: Aging and spinal cord injury: Implication for existing model systems and future federal, state and local health care policy. Spinal cord injury: The model 72-80. Presented at the National Consensus Conference, Atlanta, December 1990.
23. Menter RR, Whiteneck G, Charlifue S, et al: Impairment, disability handicap and medical expenses of persons aging with SCI. *Paraplegia* 1991; 29:613–619.
24. Ohry A, Shemesh Y, Rozin R: Are chronic spinal cord injured patients (SCIP) prone to premature aging? *Med Hypotheses* 1983; 11:467–469.
25. Penn RD, et al: Intrathecal baclofen for severe spinal spasticity. *N Engl J Med* 1989; 320:1517–1521.
26. Shock NW: *Normal Human Aging: The Baltimore Longitudinal Study of Aging*. US Department of Health and Human Services, NIH Publication 84-2450, 1984.
27. Silfverskiold JP, Waters RL: Shoulder pain and functional disability in SCI patients. *Clin Orthop* 1991; 272:141–145.
28. Silver J, Creek G, Moore M, et al: *Personal and Social Implications of SCI. A Retrospective Study*. London, Thames Polytechnic, 1987.
29. Smith EL, Serafass RC: *Exercise and Aging. The Scientific Basis*. Hillside, NJ, Enslow, 1981, pp 45–57, 167–178.
30. Sobel JW, Bohlman HH, Freehafer AA: Charcot's arthropathy of the spine following SCI. *J Bone Joint Surg [Am]* 1985; 6:771–776.
31. Stover SL, Tulloss JR, Niemann KM: Experiences with resection of heterotopic ossification in SCI. *Clin Orthop* 1991; 263:71–77.
32. Trieschmann RB: *Aging with a Disability*. New York, Demos, 1987.
33. Williams B: Post traumatic syringomyelia: An update. *Paraplegia* 1990; 28:296–313.
34. Williams ME: Clinical implications of aging physiology. *Am J Med* 1984; 76:1049–1054.
35. Williams TF: *Rehabilitation in the Aging: Philosophy and Approaches*. New York, Raven Press, 1984.
36. Wirth CR, Jacobs RL, Rolander SD: Neuropathic spinal arthropathy: A review of the charcot spine. *Spine* 1980; 5:558–567.
37. Wylie EJ, Chakera TMH: Degenerative joint abnormalities with paraplegia of duration greater than 20 years. *Paraplegia* 1988; 26:101–106.
38. Yarkony GM, et al: SCI rehabilitation outcome: The impact of aging. *J Clin Epidemiol* 1988; 41:173–177.
39. Young RR, Delwaide PJ: Spasticity drug therapy. *N Engl J Med* 1981; 304:28–33, 96–99.

28

*Role of the Physical Therapist in the Management of Patients With Acute Spinal Cord Injury**

Michelle Lazarski, P.T., and Mary Sinnott, L.P.T., M.Ed.

Successful rehabilitation of the patient with acute spinal cord injury (SCI) begins, ideally, within 24 hours after the injury and involves the skilled and coordinated services of the entire rehabilitation team. Comprehensive rehabilitative care is established through teamwork involving physiatrics, nursing, physical therapy, occupational therapy, speech therapy, social work, and psychology. With SCI, not only is the neurologic system affected, but many other systems such as the cardiovascular, gastrointestinal, urologic, respiratory, and musculoskeletal systems are affected as well. In the initial phase of rehabilitative care (i.e., from the time of injury to the time of admission to a rehabilitation unit) it is important for the physical therapist to be knowledgeable about the multisystem involvement associated with SCI so that appropriate intervention can be provided and prevent complications that can result from SCI. It is the prevention of these complications that will allow for full and uninterrupted participation in later phases of a rehabilitation program eventually leading to a greater level of functional independence.

With advances in emergency medical care, more people are surviving spinal injuries than in the past. However, the severity of the incurred trauma often leads to medical and/or surgical instability that in the past would have delayed the start of rehabilitative care. Given the advancements made in our understanding of the healing process and recovery, rehabilitation professionals can begin intervention upon patient admission, if necessary, to establish an interdisciplinary plan of care. This helps to ensure the outcome from the initial acute phase of care in preparation for a more intensive and/or aggressive program once medical/surgical stability has been achieved.

In addressing the role of the physical therapist, it is the intention of this chapter to address only those systems that have an impact on mobility. For each system, the dysfunction, measurement, and implications will be discussed.

*Supported in part by awards from the National Institute on Disability and Rehabilitation Research to the Regional Spinal Cord Injury Center of Delaware Valley (H133N00027) and the National Rehabilitation Research and Training Center in Spinal Cord Injury (H133B80017).

CLASSIFICATION OF SPINAL CORD INJURY

Level of Injury

SCI can be classified by the bony level of injury or neurologic level of injury. In order to provide consistency of care, it is preferable to use the American Spinal Injury Association (ASIA) standards for classification in which the neurologic level of injury is used to describe the level of SCI.[1] As described by ASIA, the neurologic level of injury is the lowest neurologic segment with *both* motor and sensory function preserved. The criteria for determining the lowest intact neurologic segment are bilateral muscle grades of at least 3/5 (or fair) and all sensory modalities intact at that level bilaterally.

Severity of the Lesion

The severity of functional impairment after SCI is determined by the neurologic level of injury and the degree of tissue trauma to the cord at that level.

A complete injury is one in which there is total destruction of neural tissue resulting in the loss of all motor or sensory function below the zone of injury. The zone of injury is considered to be within three neurologic levels below the point of trauma to the spinal cord when muscle grades are less than 3/5 and partial sensory function exists. Remember that the zone of injury does not change the definition of the neurologic level of injury.

Incomplete injuries indicate that the spinal cord is only partially damaged at that level. An incomplete injury is one in which any motor and/or sensory function is preserved below the zone of injury. Incomplete injuries can present very differently depending on the area affected within the spinal cord. Therefore, incomplete injuries are further classified into syndromes.[1]

SPINAL CORD INJURY SYNDROMES

1. *Central cord.*—The pathophysiologic process is primarily limited to the central portions of the gray and

white matter. Because of the neurologic configuration of the corticospinal tract, upper-extremity weakness is often more profound than lower-extremity weakness.

2. *Brown-Sequard syndrome.*—This injury is typically the result of a penetrating wound that severs half of the spinal cord. The clinical presentation is ipsilateral paralysis and loss of proprioception, deep touch, vibration, and contralateral sensory loss of pain, temperature, and pressure.

3. *Anterior cord syndrome.*—Here the pathophysiologic process is limited to the gray and white matter of the anterior portion of the spinal cord, primarily affects the major corticospinal tracts (motor), and spares posterior column (sensory) function. The clinical presentation is motor paralysis with preservation of proprioception, deep touch, and vibration.

4. *Posterior cord syndrome.*—The opposite of an anterior cord syndrome, the motor tracts in the anterior section of the spinal cord are spared, and therefore, motor function is preserved. However, there is severe impairment of posterior column function with loss of proprioception, deep touch, and vibration.

In order to clarify the classification of spinal injuries, ASIA recommends the use of the Frankel grading system as defined below[1]:

FRANKEL SPINAL CORD INJURY GRADING SYSTEM

- Frankel A.—*Complete:* No preservation of motor or sensory function below the zone of injury
- Frankel B.—*Incomplete:* Sensory intact, that is, preservation of sensation below the zone of injury except for phantom sensation
- Frankel C.—*Incomplete preserved motor:* Nonfunctional grades (i.e., less than 3/5); preserved motor function without useful purpose; sensory function may or may not be preserved
- Frankel D.—*Incomplete preserved motor/functional:* Preserved voluntary motor function that is functionally useful (i.e., greater than 3/5)
- Frankel E.—*Complete recovery:* Complete return of all motor and sensory function but may still have abnormal reflexes

NEUROLOGIC IMPAIRMENT

Dysfunction

Muscle Paralysis/Paresis

A complete SCI affecting the cervical spine will result in quadriplegia, whereas an incomplete lesion in the cervical spine will result in quadriparesis. Likewise, an injury sustained at the thoracic or lumbar level will result in paraplegia or paraparesis, depending on the extent of injury to the spinal cord.

The spinal cord terminates distally at the conus medullaris. This is usually at the L1 vertebral level since the spinal cord is shorter than the spinal canal, although considerable anatomic variation does exist.[21] Spinal cord injuries above the L1 vertebral level will result in an upper motor neuron lesion since neurons contained in the central nervous system (CNS) are affected. Upper motor neuron lesions result in spastic paralysis due to sparing of the lower motor neuron reflex arc. Injuries below the L1 vertebra may result in a lower motor neuron lesion. Below the L1 level the canal contains the peripheral lumbar and sacral nerve roots that form the cauda equina. These peripheral nerves continue to descend through the remainder of the spinal canal to exit from the respective lumbar and sacral foramina.[17] Cauda equina injuries are considered to be peripheral nerve injuries and have the potential to regenerate as peripheral nerves elsewhere in the body.[21] Table 28–1 lists the muscles affected in SCI by neurologic level.

Sensory Loss

The degree and characteristics of sensory impairment will be dependent on the area of the spinal cord affected as well as the neurologic level of injury. The neurologic level of injury (and the syndrome if it is an incomplete injury) can be determined by evaluating sensory dermatome stimulation. The most frequently tested modalities of sensation are light touch, pain discrimination, and proprioception.

Muscle Tone

In addition to the neurologic impairments of muscle and sensation, abnormal tone is another consequence of SCI. During the period of spinal shock, usually lasting 24 to 48 hours postinjury, the patient with an SCI will present with flaccid paralysis and areflexia. The end of spinal

TABLE 28–1.
Key Muscles Affected in Spinal Cord Injury*

Level	Muscle	Function
C4	Diaphragm, upper trapezius	Shoulder shrug
C5	Deltoid and biceps	Elbow flexion
C6	Extensor carpi radialis, longus and brevis	Wrist extension
C7	Triceps	Elbow extension
C8	Flexor digitorum profundus	Finger flexion
T1	Hand intrinsics, interossi	Finger abduction, adduction
L2	Iliopsoas	Hip flexion
L3	Quadriceps	Knee extension
L4	Tibialis anterior	Ankle dorsiflexion
L5	Extensor hallucis longus	Great toe extension
S1	Gastrocnemius and soleus	Ankle plantar flexion

*Adapted from American Spinal Cord Injury Association: *Standards for Neurologic Classification of Spinal Cord Injury Patients* (revised). Chicago, April 3–17, 1990.

shock is marked by the return of sacral and deep tendon reflexes. If there is an upper motor neuron lesion, flaccidity will be replaced by spasticity. If there is a lower motor lesion, flaccidity will remain.

Measurement

Manual Muscle Test

In order to assess neurologic impairment one of the most frequently performed evaluations by the physical therapist is the manual muscle test (MMT). In order to provide objective measurements of strength and document changes in neurologic function it is crucial to perform daily MMTs on key muscle groups for the acute spinal cord–injured patient. The grading system used for MMT is based on a score of 0 to 5 or zero to normal as per Daniels and Worthingham.[4] ASIA recommends the use of the numeric grading system (Table 28–2). Plus (+) and minus (−) are commonly used in conjunction with this scoring system to further refine the evaluation. For instance, if less than half the range is actively completed by the patient, the lower grade with a plus is given. If greater than half the range is actively achieved, then the higher score with a minus sign is given.[4] This scoring system is helpful in noting strength changes, especially when progress is slow and minimal functional gains are seen. This scoring system varies slightly from the motor index scoring system, a part of the ASIA classification that numerically indicates the severity of the SCI. A score of 100 would indicate no motor deficits; likewise, a low score would indicate a more severe lesion. The score is calculated by adding the muscle grades from the bilateral upper and lower extremities; however, minus signs are not used, but plus signs are accepted.

MMT is a key examination used in classifying the neurologic level of injury. However, objectivity and reliability are sometimes difficult to achieve in the patient with acute injury due to positioning limitations, poor compliance due to medical status, pain, and medications. Particularly with the SCI population the validity of the examination is dependent on careful positioning, observation, palpation, and stabilization to prevent muscle substitution. Examples of muscle substitution often seen that should be prevented are in the hand, where tenodesis is often mistaken for finger flexion, and at the shoulder, where extension, external rotation, and forearm supination are used to simulate triceps motion. There is controversy regarding the use of MMT to assess strength in the presence of abnormal increases in muscle tone.

Tone

The presence or absence of abnormal tone should be included in an SCI evaluation. Tone needs to be evaluated for the presence of flaccidity, flexor or extensor spasticity, clonus, and/or associated reactions. The degree of spasticity can vary from mild to moderate to severe. The quality of motor control must not be overlooked because spasticity and/or spasms can mask true motor strength as well as affect the patient's ability to perform smooth, isolated movements. Thus, spasticity and/or spasms should not be mistaken for voluntary control.

Sensation

Sensory tracts can carry more than one modality. Therefore, when evaluating sensation a dermatome chart should be followed, and one modality is evaluated for each tract. The following is a list of the appropriate tract and its associated evaluative modality:

- Lateral spinothalamic tract: sharp/dull discrimination
- Anterior spinothalamic tract: light touch
- Dorsal columns: proprioception

It is important to accurately assess the sensory impairment since it will have an impact on prognosticating functional outcomes and recovery.[3]

Implications

Functional Implications Based on Neurologic Impairment

Although there are many factors involved in projecting functional outcome, with an SCI a major predictor of function is the neurologic level of injury and the presence of certain key muscle functions. The following chart summarizes the anticipated functional goals for a patient with *complete* uncomplicated SCI involving C3–4 to L3–S3 (Table 28–3).

TABLE 28–2.
Muscle Testing Grading System

Score	Action
5/5 (normal) and 4/5 (good)	Full motion *against gravity* and tolerating maximum (to moderate) resistance with a break test
3/5 (fair)	Full motion *against gravity* without tolerating manual resistance
2/5 (poor)	Full motion, *gravity eliminated,* without manual resistance
1/5 (trace):	Only a visible or palpable contraction elicited
0/5 (zero)	Absence of palpable or visible muscle contraction

TABLE 28–3.

Anticipated Functional Levels in Spinal Cord Injury From Magee Rehabilitation and Thomas Jefferson University Hospitals*

	Pulmonary Hygiene	A.M. Care	Feeding	Grooming	Dressing	Bathing	Bowel and Bladder Routine
C3–4	Totally assisted cough	Total dependence	Unable to feed self. Drink with long straw after set up	Total dependence	Total dependence	Total dependence	Total dependence
C5	Assisted cough	Independent with specially adapted devices with set up	Independent with specially adapted equipment for feeding after set up	Independent with specially adapted equipment for grooming after set up	Total dependence	Total dependence	Total dependence
C6	Some assistance required in supine positions. Independent in sitting position	Independent with equipment	Independent with equipment. Drink from glass	Independent with equipment	Independent upper dressing. Assistance with lower dressing	Independent uppers and lowers with equipment	Independent for bowel routine. Assistance with bladder routine
C7	As above	Independent	Independent	Independent with equipment	Potential for independence in upper and lower dressing	Independent with equipment	Independent
C8–T1	As above	Independent	Independent	Independent	Independent	Independent	Independent
T2–10	T2–6 as above. T6–10 independent	Independent	Independent	Independent	Independent	Independent	Independent
T11–L2	Not applicable	Independent	Independent	Independent	Independent	Independent	Independent
L3–S3	Not applicable	Independent	Independent	Independent	Independent	Independent	Independent

*From Staas W, et al: Rehabilitation of the SCI patient, in Delisa JA (ed): *Rehabilitation Medicine: Principles and Practice*. Philadelphia, JB Lippincott, 1988, pp 646–647. Used with permission.

Bed Mobility	Pressure Relief	Transfers	Wheelchair Propulsion	Ambulation	Orthotic Devices	Transportation	Communications
Total dependence	Independent in powered recliner wheelchair. Dependent in bed or manual wheelchair	Total dependence	Independent in pneumatic or chin control–driven power wheelchair with powered reclining feature	Not applicable	Upper extremity. Outside powered orthosis. Dorsal cockup splint	Dependent on others in accessible van with lift	Read with specially adapted equipment. Specially adapted phone. Unable to write. Type with special adaptions
Assisted by other and equipment	Most require assistance	Assistance of one person with or without transfer board	Independent in powered chair indoors and outdoors. Short distances in manual wheelchair with lugs, indoors	Not applicable	As above	As above	Same as above
Independent with equipment	Independent	Potentially independent with transfer board	Independent manual wheelchair with plastic rims or lugs indoors. Assistance outdoors and with elevators	Not applicable	Wrist-driven orthosis	Independent driving with specially adapted van.	Independent phone. Write with equipment. Type with equipment. Independent turning pages
Independent	Independent	Independent with/without transfer board except to/from floor with assistance	Independent manual wheelchair indoors and outdoors except curbs	Not applicable	None	Independent driving car with hand controls or specially adapted van. Independent wheelchair into car placement	Independent with equipment for phone, typing, and writing. Independent turning pages
Independent	Independent	Independent including to/from floor	Independent manual wheelchair indoors and out	Not applicable	None	As above	Independent
Independent	Independent	Independent	Independent	Exercise only (not functional) with orthoses	Knee-ankle-foot orthoses with forearm crutches or walker	As above	Independent
Independent	Independent	Independent	Independent	Potential for independent functional ambulation indoors with orthoses. Some have potential for stairs with railing	Knee-ankle-foot orthoses or ankle-foot orthoses with forearm crutches	As above	Independent
Independent	Independent	Independent	Independent	Independent indoors and outdoors with orthoses	Ankle-foot orthoses with forearm crutches or canes	As above	Independent

General acute-care goals include the following:

1. Prevent the loss of motor power of intact muscle groups, and improve the motor power of weak muscle groups.
2. Prevent the loss of or improvement in range of motion (ROM).
3. Prevent skin breakdown (see the section on skin).
4. Improve respiratory function (see the respiratory section).
5. Mobilize the patient: increase tolerance to the upright position and begin mobilization out of bed.
6. Motivate the patient to assume responsibilty for self-improvement and care.
7. Provide emotional support for the patient and significant others.
8. Provide education to the patient and family regarding SCI.

Early Intervention

The neurologic status of the patient with acute spinal injury can change as the patient recovers from spinal shock. Recovery may vary secondary to the presence or absence of cord edema and can be affected by orthopedic/spinal alignment. Results of neurologic tests such as MMT and sensation can vary depending on the patient's cognitive level of alertness, medical status, pain tolerance, and positioning. It is because of these factors that objective assessments of strength, sensation, and tone should be performed on a daily basis by team members. As previously mentioned, objectivity with MMT often becomes compromised due to the above-mentioned variables and limitations imposed by positioning. As per Daniels and Worthingham, MMT is dependent on positioning in either the antigravity or gravity-eliminated position. It is particularly important to stabilize the extremity to isolate the muscle and prevent substitution. Proper stabilization also allows the tester to more accurately palpate the muscle belly or tendon, which is particularly important if muscle grades are less than 2/5.

Strengthening of the intact musculature begins as soon as possible after a patient's injury—often 48 hours postinjury in order to prevent the effects of bed rest and deconditioning. Specific precautions for active and passive ROM and resistive exercise must be observed in the presence of unstable fractures in order to prevent excessive movement of the spine and to prevent undue stress at the fracture site. These precautions will change depending on the level of injury.

In a study by Hein-Sorensen and Irstrom, it was found that passive shoulder flexion to 45 degrees produced a kyphosis in the lumbar spine.[9] Both passive shoulder flexion to 110 degrees and abduction to 90 degrees produced lordotic movement. Increasing the load on the upper extremities exaggerated the above mentioned spinal movement.

At Thomas Jefferson University Hospital, shoulder flexion is limited to 90 degrees (both actively and passively) regardless of the level of the unstable spinal injury. An exception to this rule is with unstable lumbar injuries, where shoulder flexion should not exceed 45 degrees. With unstable thoracic injuries, hip flexion should not exceed 60 degrees and is limited to 45 degrees for unstable lumbar injuries.

Because of the precautions necessary to protect the unstable spine, isometric exercise of the proximal joints is the recommended strengthening modality. Active ROM can be performed at the distal joints to ensure that the above-mentioned unstable spine precautions are observed. Manual resistance can be applied to the wrist in cervical and high-level thoracic injuries if sufficient strength is present. With low-level thoracic and lumbar injuries minimal bilateral resistance can be applied to the upper extremities, again observing the unstable ROM restrictions. Resistive exercise is restricted for the lower extremities with all unstable injuries; however isometrics can be performed if applicable.

Once the spine is classified as orthopedically stable, full active and passive ROM within the restrictions of the stabilization device can be initiated, and strengthening exercises can become more aggressive by using weights, Theraband, and manual resistance. It should be emphasized that these exercises should begin in the intensive care unit whenever possible (Table 28–4).

Spasticity

Spasticity should not be mistaken for voluntary movement. Spasticity can often mask voluntary motor control and often makes it difficult to assess both motor control and strength. Spasticity can fluctuate with positioning and can increase in the presence of medical complications such as infections, respiratory complications, bowel and bladder dysfunction, and skin breakdown. The consequences of severe spasticity are joint contractures, which can interfere with hygiene and functional activities of daily living (ADL) such as wheelchair seating and management and transfers. Spasticity can also result in skin breakdown from the shearing forces caused by severe muscle spasms. Spasticity often makes the performance of ROM and positioning difficult and leaves the patient at greater risk for skin breakdown (see the section on skin).

Spasticity can also have its advantages. It may increase muscle bulk and decrease edema secondary to the frequent contractions of the muscle. Muscle bulk is particularly important around bony prominences in order to protect the patient from skin breakdown.

An increase in tone may have an occasional functional

TABLE 28–4.

Thomas Jefferson University Hospital Protocol for Muscle Strengthening of Patients With Unstable Spinal Cord Injuries

	Upper Extremities			Lower Extremities		
Lesion Level	PROM*	AROM*	Resisted	PROM	AROM	Resisted
Cervical	Stabilize scapula and shoulder girdle Shoulder F&A* limited to 90 degrees No stretch	To elbow and wrist	Wrist only Isometrics can be done to shoulder	Stabilize pelvis Gentle stretch	Stabilize pelvis Gentle stretch	Isometrics if applicable
Thoracic 1–6	Stabilize scapula and shoulder girdle Shoulder F&A limited to 90 degrees No stretch	To elbow and wrist	Wrist only Isometrics can be done to shoulder	No stretch beyond 90-degree hip flexion	Stabilize pelvis 90-degree hip flexion	Isometrics if applicable
Thoracic 7–12	Stabilize scapula and shoulder girdle Shoulder F&A limited to 90 degrees No stretch	Shoulder, elbow, and wrist Shoulder F&A limited to 90 degrees	No resisted shoulder flexion greater than 90 Bilateral resistance only	Stabilize pelvis 45-degree hip flexion 30-degree SLR*	Stabilize pelvis 45-degree hip flexion	Isometrics if applicable
Lumbar	Shoulder F&A limited to 90 degrees or to pain	Shoulder flexion limit to 45 degrees Shoulder abduction limited to 90 degrees	No shoulder flexion beyond 45 degrees or abduction beyond 90 degrees Minimal bilateral resistance	Stabilize pelvis 45-degree hip flexion 30-degree SLR	No hip motion Ankles OK Knees side-lying	Isometrics if applicable

1. With stable spines, there are no restrictions for the upper or lower extremities other than those imposed by pain or other associated injuries.
2. Patients who are wearing spinal orthoses should have the orthoses on at all times while therapy is being done.
3. We are especially concerned with maintaining *functional* ranges in all extremities.
4. One good isometric contraction held for 6 seconds is sufficient to maintain strength in muscle being strengthened. This contraction should be done 15 times per muscle group being strengthened.

*PROM/AROM = passive/active range of motion; F&A = flexion and abduction; SLR = straight-leg raising.

benefit. For example, an increase in extensor tone may facilitate standing and ambulation, whereas an increase in flexor spasticity may facilitate bed mobility.

Interventions to combat the complications of spasticity begin early with emphasis on the prevention of contractures. Temporary means of controlling and/or inhibiting abnormal tone are passive ROM with the incorporation of slow rhythmic and rotational movements rather than quick stretches, which can recruit the stretch reflex. Weight bearing through proximal joints, such as Bobath positioning, has been clinically proved to be effective in managing abnormal tone. Modalities such as prolonged ice, inhibitive casting, and high-voltage electrical stimulation to induce muscle fatigue of the agonist or to the antagonist muscle to induce reciprocal inhibition are some treatment techniques that can be used in conjunction with passive ROM. Pharmacologic intervention may be indicated as well as selective blocking to motor points or peripheral nerves. The recent use of spinal cord stimulators to modulate muscle tone is still controversial, especially in the complete spinal cord lesion.

Early Mobilization

Orthostatic hypotension is a consequence of prolonged bed rest and a complication associated with acute SCI. Venous return is impaired due to muscle paralysis and decreased vascular tone (see the cardiovascular section). During the acute-care phase, once the spine is considered orthopedically stable, mobilization can be initiated. Mobilization is started by gradually elevating the head of the bed for short periods of time throughout the day while monitoring the vital sign response. Special attention is paid to the blood pressure response with position changes. Abdominal binders and "TED" compression hose (Alba Health Care, Valdese, NC) are used to increase venous return and prevent hypotension. Once the patient is tolerating maximum elevation of the head of the bed for 1 hour, he then can be transferred out of bed to a wheelchair.

In the acute rehabilitation phase the emphasis is on "initiation" of functional activities. However, orthostatic hypotension can continue to have an impact on rehabilitation goals. Therefore, one of the first goals is to increase the patient's tolerance to sitting upright in a wheelchair in order to achieve a 90-degree sitting angle. Tolerance to upright posture can be addressed by beginning out-of-bed activities in a reclining wheelchair, which will allow the patient to gradually achieve a 90-degree sitting angle. The use of abdominal binders, TED hose (compression hose), and elevating wheelchair leg rests will assist with the management of orthostatic hypotension.

Once the patient tolerates an upright position, mobility can be advanced to include such activities as transfer training, wheelchair management, and wheelchair propulsion. In acute rehabilitation, however, goal achievement is often delayed because of restrictions placed on mobility by stabilization devices (i.e., halos, clamshells, etc.), decreased balance, pain, decreased strength and endurance, as well as medical complications inherent with this type of injury. Regardless of these potential limitations, treatment should continue to include strengthening and endurance exercises that were initiated in the acute-care phase. Since the patient may not be able to perform actual functional tasks because of these limitations, the tasks should be broken down into component parts. Those component parts should then be used as treatment modalities until the patient is able to actually perform the functional task.

Transfers

The type and amount of assistance needed for transfers will vary depending on the functional level of the patient. For instance, transfers of high-level quadriplegics (e.g., C5 and above) will involve a dependent lift, whereas C6–7 quadriplegics in the early stages may be able to assist with a side-to-side transfer by using a transfer board. Some C6–7 quadriplegics may become independent with side-to-side transfers later in the rehabilitative process. Certainly paraplegics should progress to independence in side-to-side transfers sooner than a C7 quadriplegic due to an increase in motor power and balance.

Individuals with incomplete injuries may be able to utilize their lower-extremity musculature to assist with a "stand-pivot-sit" transfer. It should not be assumed that patients with incomplete injury will have less difficulty in performing transfers. The presence of spasticity and motor impairment may negate their ability to achieve independence.

Bed mobility skills (such as supine to sitting, sitting to supine, and rolling) will need to be assessed and integrated into the treatment program if necessary.

Progress toward the achievement of functional goals is often complicated by the presence of behavioral, cognitive, and/or perceptual deficits from a variety of causes. It is becoming more apparent that a significant number of spinal cord–injured patients may also have a traumatic brain injury. These two neurologic diagnoses will complicate each other as well as the patient's ability to achieve functional goals.

Balance

Balance reactions are an important component of most functional activities such as transfers, bed mobility, dressing, wheelchair management and propulsion, and certainly ambulation. Paresis or paralysis of the trunk musculature will compromise the patient's ability to sustain and/or regain balance during functional activities.

Balance training is usually begun in a static sitting position with the upper extremities used for support. It is easier for the patient to maintain balance with the upper extremities in either an anterior or posterior weight-bearing position than it is with the arms in a lateral position. Because of the loss of trunk musculature, patients will frequently use their head and neck to pull their trunk in the desired direction in order to avoid a loss of balance.

It is important to practice both static and dynamic balance activities in various positions, such as short (hips and knees flexed) and long sitting (hips flexed and knees extended), standing, and developmental postures as appropriate. This provides the patient several strategies for maintaining balance during functional activities.

Wheelchair Management

The majority of patients beginning acute rehabilitation will rely on a wheelchair as their means of locomotion. A primary goal is to achieve a functional level with wheelchair propulsion and management. Therefore, it is important to advance a patient with acute injury out of reclining wheelchairs as soon as possible to allow for increased function. Reclining wheelchairs are heavy and much harder for patients to propel on their own since the wheel axis is posteriorly placed. For individuals lacking hand function, enhancement with lugs or rubber tubing on the wheelchair rims may facilitate wheelchair propulsion. Adaptive devices such as brake extensions can assist with the management of wheelchair parts.

It is our experience that a lighter-weight chair is a better choice for wheelchair-bound patients. A lighter chair is easier to propel, which helps facilitate endurance training earlier in rehabilitation. This is particularly important for those patients with higher-level cervical lesions and/or significant upper-extremity weakness.

Incompletely injured patients who present with good lower-extremity strength and weak upper extremities (i.e., central cord lesions) often do better in a wheelchair with a lower "seat-to-floor" height so that they can use their feet to propel the chair. For the high-level quadriplegic population, power mobility may need to be considered. Depending on the amount of upper-extremity control, power wheelchairs can be operated by a hand-controlled joystick or via a chin, head, or breath control mechanism.

Ambulation

Most spinal cord–injured patients have a desire to ambulate. There are many factors to take into account when considering ambulation as a realistic functional goal, such as motor power, sensation (primarily proprioception), age, joint deformity, and spasticity.[10] The majority of patients with incomplete injuries will ambulate either as community or household ambulators with the help of the above-mentioned factors. With a complete paraplegic, ambulation may be limited to therapeutic ambulation, which is primarily for exercise and psychological purposes. This is primarily due to the amount of bracing required and the high energy requirements needed for ambulation. Thus, these patients may be more functional from a wheelchair level.

In the acute-care setting, ambulation is a primary goal for the neurologically intact population. "Neurologically intact" patients have typically sustained a traumatic injury resulting in a fracture of the spine with no direct injury to the spinal cord itself. Surgical stabilization and immobilization with a halo, body jacket, or hip spica cast (depending on the level of injury) may be indicated. These patients generally achieve independence with functional activities.

Although the length of admission is short for this population, physical therapy intervention postoperatively is important. Balance reactions can be decreased due to cervical immobilization and the added weight of the halo. Patients undergoing spinal fusion and bone grafting may experience hip (i.e., iliac crest) pain at the graft site. This graft site pain may be the major functional limitation postoperatively. It has been found that a simple hydrocollator pack placed over the graft site followed by gentle stretching is the best intervention. Because of these factors, the use of an assistive device may be indicated at least as a temporary means to increase balance, decrease pain, and achieve a level of independence.

Patients with fractures in the lumbar spine may be immobilized in a body cast with a hip spica. This imposes different limitations. These casts are positioned in trunk and hip extension. Therefore, patients are unable to sit in a standard 90-degree-angle chair. Physical therapy intervention is important to address transfers and bed mobility as well as ambulation. Given good upper- and lower-extremity strength, the neurologically intact population can achieve independence in ambulation despite the restrictions of the body cast and be discharged home without an inpatient rehabilitation stay.

MUSCULOSKELETAL SYSTEM

Dysfunction

Contractures

Immobilization and negligence in performing ROM exercises can cause shortening of the short tissues around a joint and result in joint contractures. Other causes of joint contractures can be immobility secondary to muscle paralysis, the unopposed pull of agonist muscles, spasticity, and bed positioning. Immobilization during the acute phase via traction and specialized beds (e.g., the Rotorest bed) make it especially difficult to achieve full active or passive ROM and effective bed positioning. Contractures can interfere with ADL such as transfers, balance, and dressing, depending on the joints involved. Contractures can also interfere with proper positioning and can lead to skin breakdown.

Range of Motion.—Acutely, daily active and passive ROM exercises are performed primarily for the prevention of contractures. Although ROM may be normal initially, immobilization and neurologic deficits can easily predispose a patient to a loss of joint motion. With unstable spinal fractures active and passive shoulder flexion and abduction will be limited to 90 degrees and hip motion limited to 45 and 60 degrees for lumbar and thoracic injuries, respectively. With an unstable lumbar injury, shoulder flexion is restricted to 45 degrees as well. These limitations are to prevent excessive torque and movement of the spine.

The most commonly found joint limitations in the upper extremity tend to be in shoulder flexion, abduction, and external rotation as well as elbow extension and forearm supination. In the lower extremity decreased hip extension and abduction and ankle dorsiflexion are also likely to develop. Therefore, these movements should be emphasized within the above-mentioned precautions and limitations during ROM exercises. If patients are placed in specialized beds, it is necessary to learn how to work with and around the limitations of the bed itself in order to achieve ROM goals. Once patients are placed in halos, the vests will typically limit full shoulder flexion and abduction from approximately 90 to 140 degrees depending on the fit of the vest. Thoracolumbosacral orthoses (i.e., "clamshells") often limit full shoulder extension and horizontal abduction and adduction as well as full hip flexion and abduction. Thus, a frequent consequence of stabilization is decreased ROM. At this institution, if surgical intervention is delayed secondary to medical instability, patients are sometimes placed in halos and are classified as having "intermediate stability." Mobility restrictions are still observed. However, patients can now be placed in a regular bed, which provides easier access for ROM exercises.

As a result of immobilization the development of soft-tissue tightness at the anterior aspect of the shoulder is common. This results in limited shoulder extension and external rotation. Shoulder flexion and abduction are commonly limited secondary to ROM precautions during the acute phase as well as the limitation placed on motion by the halo vest itself. Halo vests are typically worn for 3 months after stabilization. Therefore, ROM of the upper extremities should emphasize shoulder extension, flexion, abduction, and external rotation; forearm supination; and elbow extension. Biceps brachii tightness is common with spastic quadriplegia/paresis and in C5 quadriplegics due to the unopposed biceps muscle.

Clinicians frequently emphasize shoulder flexion during ROM exercises. However, tightness of the shoulder extensors can have quite a negative impact on functional retraining. Tight shoulder extensors will interfere with wheelchair propulsion. Forward weight shifts also require good shoulder extension and external rotation in order for the patient to loop his arm behind the wheelchair push handle or through a loop around the back of the wheelchair. Balancing in a long sitting position requires adequate shoulder extension as well.

Although it may appear counterproductive, selective shortening of some muscle groups is encouraged in order to enhance function. Shortening of the finger flexors is emphasized with quadriplegics in order to facilitate a grasp response by using wrist extension. This is known as a tenodesis grasp.

In the lower extremities hip flexion and knee extension, straight-leg raising (SLR) to 110 degrees (once orthopedically stable), and ankle dorsiflexion should be emphasized. Hip and knee flexion contractures easily develop secondary to prolonged sitting. Prone positioning is encouraged to prevent hip flexion contractures. Acutely injured patients, once orthopedically stable, should be placed prone as soon as possible. However, high-level quadriplegic patients need monitoring of their respiratory status while prone to ensure that the tracheostomy site is not occluded and that diaphragmatic breathing is not impaired.

Sufficient ankle dorsiflexion is important for proper wheelchair seating and ambulation and should be emphasized from the very start of care. A hamstring length of 110 degrees of SLR in conjunction with selective shortening of the trunk extensor muscles will assist with balance in long-term sitting and enhance the performance of functional activities such as dressing. Self-performed passive ROM exercises are taught to the patient as soon as medical and orthopedic stability have been achieved with emphasis on the above-mentioned motions.

Bed positioning is a key factor in the prevention of contractures. In the upper extremities, foam wedges are used to provide elevation for edema management and positioning into slight shoulder abduction and elbow extension. Dorsal wrist splints are used for high-level quadriplegics above C6 to prevent wrist drop. With quadriplegics, the fingers are positioned in flexion to promote selective shortening for tenodesis.

In the lower extremities, ankle splints, high-top sneakers, or a variety of commercially available foot guards are used to prevent foot drop. Careful skin monitoring is important when any type of splint or sneakers is worn due to the potential for skin breakdown.

In cases of severe spasticity, casting or splinting is indicated. Casting can be used as either static splinting or serial casting, in which case the casts are refabricated every 1 to 2 weeks as ROM increases. Casting/splinting is most typically used for biceps and plantar flexion/inversion spasticity. Careful padding around bony prominences is crucial, and casts are usually bivalved to allow for careful and frequent skin assessment. Wearing time is usually a 2-hour on/off schedule.

Functional electrical stimulation (FES) is another method in which ROM can be facilitated. It can be used for stimulation to the agonist muscle to increase joint motion or to the antagonist muscle to facilitate reciprocal inhibition if spasticity is limiting joint motion.

Shoulder Subluxation

Shoulder subluxations can be seen in individuals with high-level cervical injuries (usually C5 and above) due to paralysis of the deltoid and rotator cuff muscles. The alignment of the scapula is important for mechanical stability and alignment of the glenoid fossa. Paralysis of the scapular muscles will decrease the support of the scapula on the rib cage and change the angulation of the glenoid fossa from its normal position of facing forward, upward, and outward to one where it slopes downward and laterally. This contributes to glenohumeral subluxation. Mechanical seating of the head of the humerus can be decreased due to the paralysis of the supraspinous muscle. Passive support from the superior portion of the capsule can also be decreased due to scapula malalignment. Muscle paralysis and subsequent elongation also contribute to subluxation of the humerus.[2]

Injuries to C6 do not often present with subluxation. The prime rotators of the scapula are the trapezius, innervated by cranial nerve XI, and the innervation of the serratus anterior is formed by C5–7, but primarily C6.[2] This means that the scapula can rotate to maintain mechanical stability of the glenohumeral joint and efficiency of the deltoid muscles, thereby preventing subluxation in most cases.

Positioning is important to decrease the downward and lateral forces on the glenohumeral joint and prevent further elongation of the soft tissues. In bed, pillows or towel rolls can be positioned proximally under the glenohumeral joint and the scapula as well as under the elbow joint in order to increase glenohumeral approximation. This will also help to maintain weight bearing to the shoulder joint, although halos can sometimes make this positioning difficult. When in an upright position, elevating armrests on the wheelchair are helpful in conjunction with lap boards and foam wedges that force the humeral head into the glenohumeral space. Mobilization of the scapula into a more neutral alignment as well as strengthening of the scapular muscles must not be overlooked.

Heterotopic Ossification

The formation of abnormal bone in connective tissue between muscle planes and in tendon, known as heterotopic ossification, is a common complication of SCI. The hips are the most frequently involved joints, although the knees, shoulders, elbows, and spine may also be affected.[26] Heterotopic ossification most often appears 1 to 4 months postinjury but can be detected as early as 19 days. It may also not occur until several years after the initial injury.[26]

The early manifestations of heterotopic ossification are those of inflammation, namely, increased temperature and edema in the involved joint and/or muscle. Fever may also be present. Prior to medical workup one may easily suspect a deep vein thrombosis (DVT) given these clinical signs. Within several days, however, a more localized and firmer mass appears within the tissue itself, and there is frequently a decrease in passive ROM of the involved joint. Ankylosis of the joint can occur in severe cases.

ROM exercise in conjunction with pharmacologic management is the initial method of treatment. However, aggressive ROM is controversial since there is a possibility that ranging will cause bleeding into the joint or muscle. This bleeding is secondary to "fracturing" through the abnormal calcification. It should be noted that physical therapy and drug management may not prevent the ossification once it occurs. Once the bone matures, surgical intervention may then be considered. However, there is a possibility of recurrence postoperatively.

Osteoporosis

Another complication affecting bone that is associated with SCI is osteoporosis. As a result of immobilization and atrophy secondary to paralysis, bone resorption may exceed bone deposition.[20] This bone mass loss progresses rapidly during the first year and remains at a fairly constant state after the first year.[22] Although osteoporosis may not be reversible in this population, it is believed that exercise and weight bearing through the long bones will exert stress and strain on the skeleton and stimulate bone deposition, but it is controversial as to what degree.[22] Patients with SCI often use standing frames as a method of weight bearing and exercise primarily for this purpose. Electrical stimulation to paralyzed muscle is also believed to play a role in the prevention of osteoporosis. It is also important to encourage safety awareness in ADL to prevent falls and other accidents that could easily result in fractures or other associated injuries.

Pain

In managing the acute spinal cord–injured patient, pain is a common and anticipated consequence of the trauma sustained with an SCI. Pain may be a result of trauma to either the soft tissue and bone, the nerve root, or the spinal cord. Most patients with acute SCI experience pain resulting from damage to the bone and soft tissue. This pain is localized to the region of the injured site (since they are usually sensate) and is throbbing and aching in nature. Damage to the nerve roots will cause a more sharp, lancing pain that often radiates to the specific dermatomes. In our experience, transcutaneous electrical nerve stimulation (TENS) seems to be effective in the management of radicular pain. Another type of pain encountered is referred or phantom pain and is described as sharp and burning in nature. It is found more frequently in the lower extremities.[23]

Pain can cause a vicious cycle. Pain can lead to muscle spasm and/or muscle guarding, which will typically cause the patient to assume a position of comfort. This pain will result in immobility, which can lead to tissue shortening and contractures. It is important for the physical therapist to coordinate treatment with the patient's pain medication schedule, if at all possible, in order to obtain the most effective results in treatment.

Relaxation and breathing exercises incorporated with ROM can be used as a method of pain management. Modalities such as heat, ice, ultrasound, and electrical stimulation (including TENS) are used to address muscular spasms and/or to decrease pain. Ice is recommended for acute injuries when tissue inflammation is evident. Heat is indicated for more chronic types of pain.

Pain can also be a result of a poorly fitted halo vest. Pain may occur as a result of pressure over a bony prominence, particularly the scapula. In this case the vest may need to be revised to more evenly distribute pressure.

Shoulder pain is a common occurrence in the SCI population. The effects of immobilization and positioning in the acute quadriplegia population can contribute to soft-tissue tightness and weakness. Muscle imbalance that affects glenohumeral rhythm can result in impingement syndromes and/or tendonitis at the shoulder. Pain can also develop from overuse of the shoulder muscles with functional activities. Treatment should be aimed at strengthening to promote muscle balance as well as flexibility and positioning in order to prevent contractures. It is also imperative that the physical therapist grade the intensity of activities and exercises in order to prevent overuse syndromes.

Measurement

Range of Motion

Evaluation of the musculoskeletal system involves careful ROM assessment. Limitations in passive ROM may indicate abnormalities of the noncontractile tissues (such as heterotopic ossifications) or joint contractures resulting from immobilization or abnormal tone. Limitations in active ROM can indicate abnormalities of the contractile tissues (such as muscle weakness or tendonitis). Palpation and a determination of the presence or absence of pain with passive and/or active ROM can provide objective information regarding musculoskeletal dysfunction.

Other pertinent clinical information can be obtained during ROM evaluation. Skin integrity can easily be assessed in conjunction with ROM. In particular, the assessment of pressure-sensitive areas for redness, breakdown, or necrosis can be easily detected. The finding of soft-tissue inflammation can be indicative of a DVT or heterotopic ossification. Therefore, it is important to communicate with the medical team in order to determine appropriate physical therapy intervention in light of the patient's medical status.

Pain

Pain can be assessed by its location, type (i.e., sharp vs. aching), intensity, and duration. It is recommended that a reliable and useful pain scale be used to document and objectify pain intensity. It has been our clinical experience that a simple 1 to 10 numerical scale that grades pain from minimal (1) to severe (10) is practical and reliable.

Implications

Range of Motion/Positioning

Immobilization as a result of stabilization devices, neurologic impairment, and/or pain can ultimately lead to disuse atrophy, osteoporosis, and contractures. It is the role of the physical therapist to attempt to prevent the sequelae of these complications. Early intervention is imperative. ROM is considered to be the responsibility of nursing, occupational therapy, and physical therapy. Passive and active ROM within unstable SCI precautions is initiated within 24 to 48 hours of admission and is performed one to two times per day. Family members assist with ROM once they have been educated in performing ROM by the occupational or physical therapist. When appropriate, the patient assumes responsibility for daily self-ROM.

Posey foot guards, ankle splints, high-top sneakers, upper-extremity foam wedges, dorsal wrist splints, towel rolls, and pillows are some of the adaptive equipment used to facilitate proper bed positioning. Splinting and casting are also considerations, particularly in the presence of spasticity. However, it is imperative that precautions be taken to avoid peripheral nerve compression when any position device is used, especially in the incomplete SCI population since a peripheral neuropathy could adversely affect recovery.

Pain

Pain often interferes with treatment planning and the achievement of functional goals. Shoulder and neck pain is prevalent in the acute quadriplegic SCI population. It is helpful to determine the etiology of pain in order to implement an appropriate treatment plan. Acutely, most pain is a result of trauma to the bone and soft tissue of the spine. This pain usually subsides as the healing process takes place. Modalities such as ice, which tends to be more effective during the acute phase, or heat can temporarily decrease pain and increase tolerance to an activity. A gradual progression to the upright position as well as gradual progression in activity is often effective in decreasing the patient's pain response to new activities.

Many complaints of pain are secondary to discomfort from stabilization devices such as halo vests and thoracolumbosacral orthoses ("clamshells"). The fit of the device needs to be assessed routinely while noting areas of pressure and pain. Modifications to the device may be indicated to ensure a comfortable fit and skin integrity.

As previously mentioned, shoulder pain is common in the SCI population. However, the etiology of shoulder pain may be difficult to determine due to the many variables contributing to the pain. Muscle imbalance of the shoulder girdle often results in high-level quadriplegia, which therefore impedes smooth glenohumeral rhythm. This factor in combination with the restrictions from the halo vest limitation of full shoulder motion may result in impingement of the supraspinatus tendon and predispose a patient to tendonitis. As patients become more functional, the demands placed on their upper extremities significantly increase, which may predispose patients to tendonitis/overuse syndrome.

RESPIRATORY

Dysfunction

Spinal injuries at the cervical or upper thoracic levels will result in paralysis of the primary muscles of respiration, which are the diaphragm, the intercostal muscles, and the abdominal muscles. Paralysis or weakness of these muscles will compromise respiratory function. Respiratory impairment can be influenced by many factors (e.g., age, past medical history, prior respiratory compromise), including the level of the SCI. The diaphragm is innervated via the phrenic nerve stemming from the C3–5 levels. In a high-level quadriplegic above C5, diaphragmatic paralysis is likely. The intercostal muscles are innervated from T1–12, whereas the abdominals are innervated from T7–11. Therefore, even paraplegics can demonstrate a decrease in respiratory function.

With injuries below the C4 level and above T12, respiratory function will be compromised due to paralysis/

weakness of those muscles that contribute to vital capacity (i.e., forced inhalation and forced exhalation). The tidal volume, on the other hand, will be relatively unchanged as long as the diaphragm is intact. This is because the diaphragm contributes two thirds of the tidal volume in sitting or standing and three quarters of the tidal volume when supine.[7] The intercostals and the neck accessory muscles provide the remainder of the tidal volume.[11]

Since patients with cervical and/or thoracic injuries are at the greatest risk of respiratory compromise, it is important to highlight the inspiratory accessory muscles. These muscles may be left intact postinjury and should be considered as part of the physical therapy care program since they can contribute to an increased vital capacity[7]:

- *Sternocleidomastoids* (accessory nerve and C2).—When the head is held fixed, the muscles act bilaterally to elevate the sternum, which increases the anteroposterior dimension of the chest. These muscles are considered to be the most important accessory muscles of inspiration.
- *Scalenes* (C2–7).—When the head is held fixed, the scalenes raise the first two ribs, which are their insertion.
- *Serratus anterior* (C5–7).—When the scapula is held fixed, the serratus anterior raises its insertion ribs (i.e., ribs 1 through 8).
- *Pectoralis major* (C5–T1).—When the arms are stabilized, the pectoralis major muscles pull the ribs out toward the arms.
- *Trapezius* (accessory nerve and C3–4).—The trapezius is a primary stabilizer of the scapula. When it performs this function, it enhances the ability of the serratus anterior and pectoralis minor to lift the ribs.
- *Erector spinae*.—During deep inhalation, the erector spinae serves to extend the spinal column. This motion allows for greater rib elevation and lung expansion.

Exhalation is normally a passive process that occurs when the intercostals and diaphragm relax. This allows the diaphragm to recoil back to its preinspiratory dome position. The abdominal muscles support the abdominal viscera and keep it in place. This provides counterpressure to the diaphragm and aids in its excursion.

Paralysis of the abdominal muscles results in a paradoxical effect. Normally, the lungs have a smaller volume in the supine position because of the perpendicular effects of gravity on the abdominal contents. Gravity causes the visceral organs to press up against and under the diaphragm, which decreases the lung volume. Individuals with intact abdominal muscles have larger lung volumes in sitting or standing because of the downward pull of the abdominal organs on the diaphragm. It is well known that people with respiratory difficulty are more comfortable sitting than supine.

When there is a loss of abdominal muscle tone, the diaphragm loses its counterpressure. This now allows the diaphragm to descend and compress the abdominal viscera. Because of the lack of counterpressure there is less diaphragmatic excursion (especially during exhalation). A patient with abdominal muscle paralysis finds it easiest to breathe in the supine position. This is because gravity compresses the visceral organs and provides greater diaphragmatic counterpressure. This allows for more effective exhalation and ease of breathing. For this reason, vital capacities in the cervical and high-level thoracic SCI population are greater in the supine than in the upright position. This is the opposite of what is found in the intact population.

Forced exhalation, on the other hand, is an active process essential for an effective cough. Coughing ability is frequently compromised in this population due to paralysis of the abdominals and intercostals.

Paralysis of the respiratory muscles, diaphragmatic fatigue, and decreased rib expansion affect chest wall mobility. Decreased diaphragmatic excursion will result in a decreased vital capacity. Decreased visceral support due to a lack of abdominal tone, decreased cough function that inhibits the ability to clear secretions, and weakness of postural muscles in sitting will contribute to decreased ventilation, which can lead to respiratory complications and failure. The primary cause of death in the acute traumatic spinal cord–injured patient is respiratory compromise secondary to pneumonia, respiratory infection, and atelectasis, which is the most common complication in this population.[6]

Measurement

Because of the significant impact of the SCI on respiratory function, respiratory assessment is an important component of the physical therapy evaluation.

Breathing Pattern

A normal breathing pattern will consist of equal chest expansion/rib elevation and epigastric rise with inspiration.[28] When there is paralysis to the abdominal and intercostal muscles, chest expansion is lost. Therefore there will be a predominance of epigastric rise. If there is weakness of the diaphragm, an increased use of neck accessory muscles is seen. Breathing patterns should be observed in various positions. For instance, in a sitting position diaphragmatic excursion is decreased due to the loss of abdominal tone and the downward pull of gravity as compared with the supine position, where the diaphragm assumes a more normal resting position due to increased abdominal compression. Breathing patterns may change with various activities such as talking due to the increased need for ventilation.

Respiratory Rate

At rest the normal respiratory rate (RR) is 12 to 16 breaths per minute in the adult. However, with an SCI the RR is typically increased at rest and during activity in attempts to compensate for altered oxygenation capabilities.[18] During treatment the RR is assessed at rest to establish baseline values and during activity to monitor the patient's response to the activity. It is also used to compare the patient's RR in the supine vs. the sitting position since the RR tends to be higher when sitting.

Chest Wall Mobility

Paralysis of the external intercostal muscles results in decreased rib elevation and chest wall expansion. Chest wall mobility can be assessed objectively by measuring the difference between maximum inhalation and normal exhalation with a tape measure around the thorax at the level of the xiphoid process and at the axilla.[28] The normal response would be an increased girth of the thorax. In a cervical injury there may be no difference between the inspiration and expiration values. Often a negative difference indicating paradoxical breathing is seen. Paradoxical breathing is defined as epigastric rise and upper thorax depression during inhalation. The opposite pattern occurs with exhalation. This is primarily due to weakness of the abdominal and intercostal musculature.

Cough

Due to the paralysis of the abdominal muscles and internal intercostals (the primary muscles involved in forced expiration), cough function is often affected. A vital capacity of at least 1500 cc is necessary for an effective cough.[11] A cough may be documented as functional if the patient can adequately clear secretions through the mouth or tracheostomy without assistance. With a weak functional cough, the patient will require some type of manual assistance to clear secretions such as a "quad assist cough." An example of this technique is to apply manual pressure to the epigastric area in a downward and upward direction in synchrony with the patient's cough attempt. With a "poor cough" the patient is unable to clear secretions with manual assistance and will require suctioning for effective pulmonary hygiene.

Since respiratory complications are of significant concern in the management of the spinal cord–injured patient, it is important for the therapist to be knowledgeable about the patient's respiratory function and determine what assistance is necessary to maintain good pulmonary hygiene. Pulmonary hygiene should be part of the physical therapy plan of care for any patient with the potential for compromise.

Oxygen Saturation

Normally, the oxygen saturation of arterial blood equals 97%. This represents the percentage of oxygen bound to hemoglobin and corresponds to a 100 mm Hg partial pressure of oxygen. Venous blood normally has a 70% oxygen saturation, which corresponds to a 40 mm Hg partial pressure of oxygen.[8] Pulse oximeters (Ohmeda, Louisville) are used frequently in therapy to monitor the percentage of oxygen bound to hemoglobin in the bloodstream. In the intensive care unit most patients are monitored with pulse oximeters. We have found it helpful to use oximeters for patients who are tolerating more aggressive programs in the rehabilitation unit. The oximeter can be used to identify a patient's tolerance and endurance to activity. As previously discussed, in the presence of impaired ventilation secondary to muscle paralysis, the amount of oxygen available to the working muscles for aerobic metabolism may already be decreased. Therefore with exercise the oxygen saturation may decrease. A decrease in oxygen saturation may also indicate the need for pulmonary hygiene due to decreased ventilation.

Vital Capacity

Vital capacity can be defined as the maximum amount of air that can be forcibly expired after maximal inhalation (approximately 4600 mL).[28] The greater the vital capacity, the greater the ability to move secretions from the alveoli to the larger airways so that secretions can be cleared from the airways.[18] Vital capacities are dependent on height and weight and will vary with the level of the SCI and the degree of muscle paralysis. For instance, a patient with a cervical or high-level thoracic SCI will have a lower vital capacity than will a low-level paraplegic. Vital capacities are one of the many parameters assessed in determining a patient's weaning potential or the need for continued mechanical ventilation. At this institution, a vital capacity of less than 800 mL is considered to be insufficient to maintain ventilation without mechanical support. However, each patient must be evaluated individually since some can survive with lower vital capacities and not need ventilator support.

Vital capacities are assessed weekly in physical therapy and are easily measured by using a hand-held spirometer. Due to the effects of gravity on the position of the diaphragm, it is important to evaluate the vital capacity in the supine and sitting positions. With the quadriplegic and high-level paraplegic populations, vital capacities in the sitting position will be less than in the supine position. It is also important to be as accurate as possible with testing. Air leaks around the mouth, nose, or tracheostomy, status of the tracheostomy cuff (i.e., inflated vs. deflated), as well as the type of inner and outer cannulas will affect test results.

Implications

One of the goals with the traumatic SCI patient is to mobilize the patient as soon as possible in order to prevent the effects of prolonged bed rest, which would further compromise the patient's respiratory function. Early intervention is crucial. Patients with unstable fractures are immobilized in traction and placed in a Rotorest bed (Kinetic Concepts, San Antonio, Tex). These beds rotate from side to side. This continuous motion assists with pulmonary hygiene by mobilizing secretions. This motion is also effective in preventing skin breakdown since the patient's weight is constantly being redistributed, thereby limiting the potential of skin breakdown.

Range of Motion

Prevention of contractures is necessary not only from an orthopedic and functional perspective but from a respiratory perspective as well. It is important to not allow impedance of the patient's inspiratory capacity by chest wall tightness. Upper-extremity exercises that emphasize pectoral stretching and shoulder ROM are important to actively or passively expand the upper part of the thorax. Proprioceptive neuromuscular facilitation (PNF) diagonal patterns incorporating deep breathing with upper-extremity elevation are effective exercise. Exercises incorporating trunk rotation, elongation, and counterrotation will assist in the prevention of chest wall tightness (e.g., lower trunk rotation and side-lying counterrotation). In the acute SCI population some of the trunk rotation exercises may be contraindicated primarily because of stabilization devices such as halos and clamshells. In the absence of a stabilization device, orthopedic clearance must be obtained before proceeding with any trunk rotation activities.

Respiratory Exercises

Respiratory exercises are emphasized in the acute phase as well as in the rehabilitation phase. Inspiratory exercises are initially encouraged via diaphragmatic breathing exercises or by using incentive spirometers such as the Triflow (Sherwood Medical, St. Louis). These exercises emphasize diaphragmatic breathing, chest expansion, and normal timing (i.e., a 1:2 inspiratory-expiratory ratio). Incentive spirometry can be performed through the mouth or through the tracheostomy by using a "trach adapter." Progressions to diaphragmatic breathing exercises can be made by adding manual resistance or by placing weights on the diaphragm. Resistive spirometers are also commercially available. Other activities such as blowing up balloons, blowing bubbles, or using straws with sip and puff games such as "sip and puff shuffleboard" can add some recreation to the exercises. It is necessary to determine the function of the accessory muscles and include them in a strengthening program to enhance respiratory function.

Pulmonary Hygiene

Mobilization of secretions is accomplished by chest percussion in postural drainage positions but can also be achieved simply by changing positions, which is easily accomplished during therapy by changing positions from sitting to supine, rolling, etc. This may necessitate more frequent pulmonary hygiene while in therapy. Patients can be positioned prone for treatment activities but must be closely monitored to ensure that their ventilation is not compromised. Some patients may have poor tolerance for this position secondary to resistance to diaphragmatic excursion due to pressure from the compressed abdominal content while in the prone position.

Wheelchair Seating

When patients begin mobilization out of bed to a wheelchair, abdominal binders are used to support the abdominal contents and assist in diaphragmatic recoil. Patients may initially have more difficulty breathing with the wheelchair in an upright position vs. a reclined position due to the effects of gravity on the diaphragm. Poor sitting trunk posture can affect the patient's inspiratory capacity due to weakness of the paraspinal muscles, kyphotic posturing of the thoracic spine, and protraction of the shoulder girdle. Special attention needs to be paid to wheelchair seating to ensure good upright sitting posture. Strengthening exercises for the neck and/or trunk and shoulder musculature should be initiated as soon as possible to avoid disuse atrophy and weakness.

SKIN

Dysfunction—Pressure Sores

Pressure sores are, unfortunately, a common complication associated with SCI. Pressure sores primarily result from direct pressure. Other contributing factors include time, shearing forces, maceration from urine and feces, increased skin temperature, and altered nutritional status.[25] When pressure exceeds 14 mm Hg on the venous side and 35 mm Hg on the arterial side, obstruction of blood flow occurs and results in tissue injury.[15]

Pressure sores are most common over bony prominences. Susceptible areas for pressure sores are dependent on positioning (Table 28–5).

In addition to the direct tissue pressure sustained in the above positions, the presence of shearing forces will contribute significantly to the size and grade of the pressure sore. Spasticity is the primary cause of shearing forces. Other examples are poor transfer techniques and improper bed mobility.

As previously mentioned, the contributing factors to the development of pressure sores are direct tissue pressure, shearing forces, maceration, skin temperature, and altered nutritional status. The physical therapist should

TABLE 28–5.
Areas Susceptible to Skin Breakdown

Supine	Side-Lying	Semi-Fowler	Sitting
Occiput	Side of head	Sacrum	Scapula
Rim of ear	Shoulder	Lateral malleoli	Sacrum
Scapula	Iliac crest	Heels	Coccyx
Elbow	Trochanter		Ischium
Sacrum	Medial area of knees		Posterior of knees
Heels	Perineum		
	Malleoli		

identify high-risk individuals who are prone to breakdown in order to direct treatment planning.

Impaired or absent sensation is a primary factor contributing to pressure sores. Sensory evaluations of pain discrimination, light touch, and proprioception are routinely performed not only to provide information regarding the level of injury and changes in neurologic status but also to identify individuals who are at risk for skin breakdown. Spasticity also needs to be evaluated and monitored since an increase in spasticity usually increases the shearing forces on the skin. In the acute environment, spasticity does not usually pose a problem until the period of spinal shock subsides. Spasticity may then gradually increase. It has been our clinical experience that patients with incomplete lesions tend to develop spasticity earlier than the population with complete injury.

Patient compliance is a key factor in pressure sore prevention. Once all of the risk factors are identified, the patient needs to be responsible for the management of his skin. If the individual's learning potential is poor or if compliance is low, it should be anticipated that turning and pressure relief are not going to be performed independently by the patient. These activities should then be assigned to a care giver.

Pressure sores can be classified as grades I to IV, which is the scoring system used by the National SCI Data Collection System[15]:

- Grade I.—Limited to the superficial epidermis and dermal layers
- Grade II.—Involving the epidermal and dermal layers and extending into the adipose tissue
- Grade III.—Extending through the superficial structures and adipose tissue down to and including the muscle
- Grade IV.—Destroying all soft tissue down to the bone and communication with bone, joint structures, or both.

Implications

Management of pressure sores involves the entire SCI team—the patient, physical and occupational therapists, nursing, physician, and family. Skin management needs to be a part of the treatment plan from injury onset through acute hospitalization, in the rehabilitation phase, and throughout an individual's lifetime. Prevention of pressure sores is imperative. Pressure sores have an impact on the entire health care delivery system since they result in increased utilization of time, treatment modalities, and cost. Patients may require alternate positioning (such as a prone cart) that may preclude their participation in a full rehabilitative program. This will delay the achievement of the patient's functional goals.

Bed Positioning

It is a goal in acute care to prevent the development of pressure sores so as not to impede the rehabilitation process. Nursing plays a key role during the acute phase of care since it is one of nursing's prime responsibilities to maintain an effective turning schedule while the patient is in bed. Special beds and mattresses such as a water, air, or gel mattress may be indicated for the high-risk patient. However, these are not a substitute for proper turning and positioning.

It is the responsibility of the physical therapist to incorporate bed positioning into the treatment plan (particularly with the acutely injured population) as well as to educate and to communicate with the nursing staff, patient, and family regarding recommendations for effective positioning.

Pressure Relief

Once the patient is orthopedically and medically stable to begin activities out of bed, pressure relief and wheelchair seating are important issues that need to be addressed. Sitting for long periods of time without pressure relief can result in skin breakdown over bony prominences such as the sacrum, ischial tuberosities, and the greater and lesser trochanters. Pressure relief, a method of redistributing weight and decreasing direct pressure, is achieved by performing "weight shifts." During the acute phase when the patient is less mobile, tilt-back wheelchair weight shifts are taught to the patient, family, and nursing staff. This type of weight shift (as well as other methods) is encouraged every 30 minutes and is maintained for 1 to 2 minutes. A tilt-back wheelchair weight shift should not be performed independently by the patient and requires the assistance of another individual. These patients are encouraged to take responsibility for their care by "requesting" their weight shift. As the patient becomes more mobile, alternate methods of pressure relief are taught such as lateral or forward weight shifts. Wheelchair push-ups are most appropriate for the paraplegic population or the incompletely injured quadriparetic population.

Wheelchair Seating

Proper wheelchair seating of a patient with acute SCI is another primary goal of physical therapy. Seating needs to be addressed early since the consequences of improper seating can lead to skin breakdown. These consequences include poor posture and alignment, decreased pressure relief, and decreased functional abilities—all of which could be difficult to correct later in the patient's care.

Seating considerations with the spinal cord–injured patient should include the following[12]:

1. Pressure relief
2. Stability
3. Comfort/pain relief
4. Improvement of functional abilities/endurance
5. Easy maintenance/manageability

As previously mentioned, pressure sores primarily develop as a result of direct pressure over bony prominences. In the sitting position with the pelvis in neutral alignment, the ischial tuberosities bear the majority of the weight and are the most susceptible to breakdown. Therefore, spinal cord–injured patients need to be evaluated for an appropriate wheelchair cushion that will provide adequate pressure relief. There are a variety of cushions on the market today, from simple inexpensive foam cushions to more elaborate and expensive air-filled or air/gel combination cushions. When evaluating a cushion for pressure relief, the physical therapist needs to assess the cushion's ability to accommodate bony prominences. When patients begin acute rehabilitation, they are generally evaluated with either an air-filled cushion such as the "ROHO" (Roho, Inc., Belleville, Ill) or an air/gel (Flolite) cushion such as the "Jay" cushion (Jay Medical, Ltd., Boulder, Colo), both of which allow the bony prominences to enter the cushion without resistance. Foam cushions compress and give resistance back as pressure is applied and have not been clinically effective in providing pressure relief.[12] Cushions also need to be evaluated for their ability to eliminate shearing forces. The Jay and ROHO cushions' structures allow the cushions to move with the patient and prevent the skin from shearing over the surface of the cushion. Patients who are compliant with pressure relief and who are at low risk for breakdown may be able to use a simpler and less expensive cushion. However, it is important to remember that no matter what type of cushion is used, it will not substitute for proper and frequent weight shifts.

Not only must a cushion be evaluated for its ability to provide pressure relief, but it must be evaluated for its ability to provide adequate postural support and stability as well. The SCI population often lacks the appropriate musculature to maintain postural stability and alignment. Even with a less impaired individual, prolonged sitting without appropriate support can contribute to postural deformity. Poor posture is often the result of inadequate pelvic stabilization from a too-flexible cushion. Most wheelchair upholstery tends to "sling" or "hammock" with use. When a soft cushion is used on a stretched seat or if the back upholstery is stretched, the result is poor posture. Poor posture contributes to skin breakdown, postural deformity, decreased respiratory function, and pain. Common postural deformities seen with poor pelvic stabilization are a posterior pelvic tilt (which can increase pressure over the coccyx and the sacrum) and pelvic obliquity (which increases pressure on the weight-bearing ischium and can contribute to scoliotic posturing). Cervical and lower-extremity alignment is also affected as a result of pelvic malalignment.

It is rare for postural deformities to be evident in the acute phase of rehabilitation. However, poor posture can be degenerative. It is imperative to provide early proper positioning because it will facilitate better muscular alignment. Proper alignment is necessary to facilitate maximal function as well as provide stability and comfort, thereby decreasing tone and pain. These issues are addressed by first providing a stable or firm base of support and by ensuring pelvic symmetry/alignment by using a firm, contoured base cushion (such as the Jay products) or by using a solid seat insert with a ROHO cushion. This will eliminate the sling tendencies of the wheelchair seat. Accessories such as build-up foam wedges can be used to accommodate pelvic obliquity. Cushions should be of adequate length, that is, approximately 2 in. from the popliteal fossa to the back of the chair. This will help to load the thighs and distribute pressure more evenly. The thighs can take 80 mm Hg, much more pressure than the coccyx and ischium. The length of the cushion will also facilitate proper lower-extremity positioning. Hip guides and abductor pummels can be used for further positioning to prevent skin breakdown. However, by adding these inserts on the wheelchair, transfers may become more difficult. Contoured solid backs used in conjunction with lateral trunk supports can provide more effective trunk stability/alignment, lumbar support, and cervical alignment.

Wheelchair Frame

It is also necessary to evaluate the wheelchair frame. For instance, a wheelchair that is too narrow can eventually cause skin breakdown over the greater trochanters or lateral aspect of the thighs. Inappropriate height of the foot rests can affect pressure over the ischium and coccyx because if the foot rests are too high, the knees are raised higher than the hips. This contributes to a posterior pelvic tilt that decreases the weight bearing on the distal parts of the thighs and increases the pressure over the sacrum and coccyx.

The height of the wheelchair back also needs to be evaluated. The majority of patients with acute injury require high backs in order to provide maximum support and stability. This is primarily due to the stabilization devices and the patient's fatigue level. If the back height is too low, the patient may slide forward to gain more support from the back of the wheelchair as he fatigues. This contributes to a posterior pelvic tilt and sacral/coccyx weight bearing. Patients with higher-level SCI who are using a lower wheelchair back may present with pressure at the inferior border of the scapula if the back height is not at the appropriate level (i.e., distal to the inferior border of the scapula).

Providing the acutely injured patient with an appropriate seating system that takes into account the wheelchair frame, cushion, and back support can contribute significantly to better skin management and proper positioning. This contributes to a decrease in pain and tone while allowing for increased function. There are many variables and considerations when a cushion is selected for a patient. At the time of discharge a patient's needs may be very different from those at the start of care. One needs to take into consideration not only the pressure relief and postural support afforded by the cushion but also maintenance of the cushion, the weight of the cushion (depending on the activity level of the patient), and finally the cost of the seating system, which often dictates the seating system selection.

CARDIOVASCULAR SYSTEM

Normal Autoregulation

The autonomic nervous system plays a major role in the regulation of the cardiovascular system's pressures and volumes. By altering the diameter of vessel radii in response to metabolic needs, homeostasis is maintained despite stresses placed on the system.

Peripheral vascular control is dominated by the sympathetic autonomic nervous system, with primary outflow coming from the thoracic levels of the spinal cord. The cell bodies lie in the intermediolateral column of the thoracic spine and form a spinal vasomotor center.[19] Via postganglionic fibers, the sympathetic system can cause either vasoconstrictor or vasodilator responses.

Since the control of peripheral vascular resistance is paramount to the maintenance of homeostasis, the sympathetic vasomotor response is subject to many influences. One of the most prominent vasomotor reactions is that of the baroreceptors, which are located in the carotid sinus and the aortic arch. The baroreceptors respond to changes in the magnitude of pressure in the vascular tree. When systemic arterial pressure rises, the baroreceptors respond by causing vasodilation to decrease peripheral resistance and thus cause a decrease in heart rate and contractility. Conversely, when pressure falls, the baroreceptors mediate a vasoconstrictor and tachycardiac response in order to maintain blood pressure via an increase in venous return (i.e., preload) and an increase in cardiac output via an increase in heart rate and contractility. These responses are mediated through the cardioregulatory center of the medulla, which sends efferent impulses to the periphery via the thoracic sympathetic outflow.

Response of the Cardiovascular System to Spinal Cord Injury

The major changes that take place in the cardiovascular system as a result of SCI occur in the peripheral vasculature and not in the heart itself. However, there are some direct cardiac effects of SCI that will be discussed later.

Orthostatic Hypotension

When spinal injuries are above the level of origin of the sympathetic nervous system (i.e., above T5 to T8), there is a loss of resting sympathetic vasoconstrictor tone. Therefore, when events cause a decrease in venous return (e.g., changes in position from supine to sitting/standing) or cause a shunting of blood (e.g., eating or drinking), there is a drop in venous return to the heart (i.e., a decrease in preload).[14] Normally, the baroreceptors would cause a compensatory vasoconstriction peripherally and a central tachycardia. Since there is a disruption of transmission from the brain stem vasomotor center to the peripheral vessels, vasoconstriction does not occur, and the patient experiences a precipitous drop in both the systolic and diastolic blood pressure. These drops in pressure are due to a decrease in cardiac output and peripheral resistance. The normal reflexive tachycardia does occur but is insufficient to maintain peripheral perfusion.

Clinically the patient will present with symptoms of hypoperfusion, that is, dizziness, light-headedness, nausea, etc. The drop in blood pressure may be significant enough to cause loss of consciousness. It is imperative that the clinician familiarize himself with the patient's resting cardiovascular picture and monitor the patient's response to positional changes via blood pressure and heart rate measures throughout an activity.[24]

Noninvasive and/or nonpharmacologic management of orthostatic hypotension involves the use of external pressure advantages to maintain and/or increase venous return so as to increase preload and cardiac output. If the patient experiences sudden symptomatology, the patient should be placed in a recumbent or "tilt-back" position to reduce the gravitational compromise on venous return.

In order to prevent such drops in pressure, the use of thigh-high elastic stockings, elastic bandages, and/or abdominal binders is advocated. It is also preferable to gradually elevate the patient to the upright position by using a tilt table, a reclining wheelchair, and/or the head of the bed. Elevating the leg rests of a wheelchair will also aid in tolerance to the upright position.[14]

Gradually, as the patient becomes tolerant to the upright position and the period of spinal shock resolves, the patient will regain some degree of compensatory responses to positional changes. However, this may take several months to occur.[27]

Deep Vein Thrombosis

It has been well documented that acute spinal cord–injured patients are at high risk for the formation of DVT secondary to an increased coagulability and a decreased venous return secondary to a decrease in vasomotor tone. DVT poses a particular problem for the spinal cord–injured population since DVT detection is at times difficult. The literature cites an incidence of anywhere from 10% to 64% based on clinical criteria. The leading cause of death in this population is pulmonary embolism, with the majority of those emboli originating in the lower extremity. Therefore, many advocate prevention of thrombosis rather than trying to treat it or the pulmonary embolism once it occurs.[13]

Daily clinical assessment for signs of DVT is imperative. Clinicians need to be cognizant of the fact that the quadriplegic patient may not present with the classic signs of DVT or pulmonary embolism secondary to the disruption in sensation. The patient may not complain of calf or thigh tenderness as expected with a sensate patient. Therefore, daily inspection of the lower extremities is called for with circumferential measurements documented. Staas and Formal indicate that a side-to-side difference of 1 cm or more is significant.[24]

Symptoms of pulmonary embolism vary in this population as well. The high-level quadriplegic patient will not complain of the pleuritic pain usually experienced with a pulmonary embolism. Instead, they may present with a sudden onset of shoulder pain that can easily be mistaken for musculoskeletal or radicular pain. Naso and Staas advocate investigating the possibility of pulmonary embolism with any abrupt onset of shoulder pain in this population. The clinician should also be aware of any sudden changes in vital signs, particularly tachycardia and unexplained fever.[14]

Compressive stockings are standardly used in the prophylaxis of DVT. It is also advocated by some that low-dose subcutaneous heparin may be helpful in decreasing the chances of DVT. However, vigilance must be maintained by all clinicians involved with the patient since DVT and pulmonary emboli may occur despite efforts to avoid their development.

If contraindications to heparinization exist, a vena cava filter may be placed to prevent emboli from reaching the lungs. Clinicians should be mindful of the use of the filter since it may remove the necessity for interrupting therapy in the presence of a DVT.

If a filter is not in place and DVT is diagnosed, the patient is routinely placed on bed rest for 7 to 10 days at the discretion of the physician. Once allowed to restart therapy, clinicians should avoid aggressive ROM activities of the lower extremities since the patient is at risk of hemorrhage secondary to anticoagulation.[23]

Autonomic Hyperreflexia

Attention thus far has been directed toward the loss of sympathetic vasoconstrictor tone and the subsequent decrease in peripheral vascular resistance and venous stasis. However, since there is a disruption of the descending regulatory influences of the medullary cardioregulatory center on thoracic sympathetic outflow, reflexive vasoconstriction mediated through the spinal vasomotor center can go unchecked as well.

Autonomic hyperreflexia or dysreflexia is characterized by a sudden onset of hypertension, pounding headache, bradycardia, diaphoresis, piloerection, dilated pupils, nasal stuffiness, and blurred vision. It is most commonly seen in lesions above T6. It usually occurs after spinal shock has subsided (i.e., several months) and usually does not occur after 3 years postinjury. However, patients need to be warned that it may reoccur unexpectedly at any time.[14]

The afferent impulses responsible for autonomic hyperreflexia are usually from visceral organs, especially a distended bowel or bladder. Fecal impactions, rectal stimulation associated with evacuation, decubitus ulcers, or even ingrown toenails can cause dysreflexia. The sensory input to the cord causes segmentally mediated vasoconstriction via the intermediolateral columns that goes unchecked by high inhibitory centers because of the cord lesion. However, the baroreceptor reflexive bradycardia will still occur. It is imperative to find the source of the noxious stimulus and rectify it since the increased vascular pressure can lead to seizures and cerebral hemorrhage. Removing the source of the stimulus will cause an immediate alleviation of the symptoms and return pressure to normal levels.[5]

Clinical signs and symptoms of autonomic hyperreflexia are very overt and should be addressed immediately. As in most cases, no two patients respond exactly the same. It is prudent for the clinician to discuss with the patient his individual clinical signs and symptoms so that the clinician can be on the alert.

Any sudden onset of a pounding headache or diaphoresis should be considered suggestive. If the patient's systolic and/or diastolic blood pressure is 20 mm Hg higher than normal at rest and the patient has a lesion above T8, autonomic hyperreflexia should be considered. Physician assistance should be sought as soon as possible since severe hypertension can readily become a medical emergency.

The easiest thing for a clinician to do is to first elevate the patient's head to 90 degrees. This is intended to cause orthostatic hypotension and start to bring the blood pressure down. Next, the clinician should try to find the cause of the noxious stimulus. In 70% of the cases, the problem is bladder stimulation followed by bowel distension (19%). A common urinary cause is a kink in the catheter tubing or a twisting of the catheter condom. If there appears to be no urine output, the catheter may need to be changed. If the patient does not have a catheter, one can try gentle tapping over the bladder, stroking the inner aspect of the thigh, or pulling a pubic hair to effect bladder emptying.[5]

It is important to monitor the blood pressure throughout the clinical episode. Pharmacologic agents may be necessary if the blood pressure does not respond to the removal of noxious stimuli.

Cardiac Complications

During the first 6 weeks following acute SCI (i.e., during the period of acute spinal shock), the patient may experience reflexive bradycardia that may or may not cause cardiac arrest. This response usually occurs secondary to tracheal stimulation (e.g., during suctioning) and particularly in the presence of hypoxia. This response occurs because tracheal stimulation causes a vagal response that results in sinoatrial suppression. Since there is no sympathetic outflow to contradict this response, bradycardia and possible cardiac arrest ensue. It is therefore prudent to have medical intervention at hand when suctioning a high-level quadriplegic patient. It should be noted that adequate oxygenation prior to suctioning may prevent the bradycardiac response.[24]

The normal sympathetic response to exercise is an increase in the heart rate. However, because of the blunted sympathetic outflow, high-level spinal cord–injured patients will have a lower heart rate response to exercise and lower maximal heart rates. Because of this, patients may experience a wide arteriovenous oxygen difference as well.

Regardless of the cause for muscle inactivitation, be it paralysis or disuse secondary to weakness or immobilization, there is a conversion of slow-twitch to fast-twitch fibers. Since fast-twitch–fiber muscle work has a higher Vo_2 than slow-twitch muscle work, spinal cord–injured patients experience a deconditioning-like syndrome found in immobilized or inactive patients. There is even a decrease in high-density lipoprotein content in this population. In order to improve cardiovascular conditioning, endurance activities should be a consistent part of any spinal cord–injured patient's treatment regimen. Because of the previously described cardiovascular compromises secondary to the SCI, vital sign monitoring is necessary so as to not exceed the ability of the cardiovascular system to meet peripheral oxygen demands.[16, 28]

REFERENCES

1. American Spinal Cord Injury Association: *Standards for Neurologic Classification of Spinal Cord Injury Patients* (revised). American Spinal Cord Association, Chicago, April 1990, pp 3–17.
2. Calliet R: *The Shoulder in Hemiplegia*. Philadelphia, FA Davis, 1980, pp 63–71.
3. Crozier KS, Grazion V, Ditunno JF Jr, et al: Spinal cord injury: Prognosis for ambulation based on sensory examination in patients who are initially motor complete. *Arch Phys Med Rehabil* 1991; 72:119–121.
4. Daniels L, Worthingham C: *Muscle Testing Techniques of Manual Examination*. Philadelphia, WB Saunders, 1980, pp 3–5.
5. Finocchiarro DN, Herzfeld ST: Understanding autonomic dysreflexia. *Am Nurs* 1990; 90:56–59.
6. Fishburn MJ, Marino RJ, Ditunno JF Jr: Atelectasis and pneumonia in acute spinal cord injury. *Arch Phys Med Rehabil* 1990; 71:197–200.
7. Frownfelter DL: *Chest Physical Therapy and Pulmonary Rehabilitation: An Interdisciplinary Approach*. St Louis, Mosby–Year Book, 1978, pp 12–15.
8. Guyton AC: *Textbook of Medical Physiology,* ed 6. Philadelphia, WB Saunders, 1981, pp 507–508.
9. Hein-Sorenson O, Irstrom L: Movements in the lumbar spine during exercise of the upper extremities: A roentgenologic study in paraplegic and tetraplegic patients. *Scand J Rehabil Med* 1979; 11:27.
10. Hussey RW, Stauffer ES: Spinal cord injury: Requirements for ambulation. *Arch Phys Med Rehabil* 1973; 54:544–547.
11. Jacobs SR, Roberts JD: Respiratory system management, in Ruskin AP (ed): *Current Therapy in Physiatry*. Philadelphia, WB Saunders, 1984, p 368.
12. Jay Medical Wheelchair Seating Seminar. Philadelphia, October 1990.
13. Merli GJ, Herbison GJ, Ditunno JD, et al: Deep vein thrombosis: Prophylaxis in acute spinal cord injured patients. *Arch Phys Med Rehabil* 1988; 69:661–664.
14. Naso F, Staas WE: Cardiovascular problems, in Ruskin AP (ed): *Current Therapy in Physiatry*. Philadelphia, WB Saunders, 1984, p 5410.
15. Nawoczenski DA: Pressure sores: Prevention and management, in Buchanon LE, Nazoczenski D (eds): *Spinal Cord Injury: Concepts and Management Approaches*. Baltimore, Williams & Wilkins, 1987, pp 102–105.
16. Pollack SF, Azen K, Spielholz N, et al: Aerobic training effects of electrically induced lower extremity exercise in spinal cord injured people. *Arch Phys Med Rehabil* 1989; 70:214–219.
17. Rieser TV, Mudiyam R, Waters R: Orthopaedic evaluation of spinal cord injury and management of vertebral fractures,

in Adkins HV (ed): *Spinal Cord Injury*. New York, Churchill Livingstone, 1985, p 7.
18. Rinehart ME, Nawoczenski DA: Respiratory care, in Buchanon LE, Nazoczenski D (eds): *Spinal Cord Injury: Concepts and Management Approaches*. Baltimore, Williams & Wilkins, 1987, pp 65–66.
19. Rushmere RF: *Cardiovascular dynamics*, ed 4. Philadelphia, WB Saunders, 1976, p 154.
20. Salter RB: *The Textbook of Disorders and Injuries of the Musculoskeletal System*. Baltimore, Williams & Wilkins, 1970, p 137.
21. Schmitz TJ: Traumatic spinal cord injury, in O'Sullivan SB, Schmitz TJ (eds): *Physical Rehabilitation: Assessment and Treatment*. Philadelphia, FA Davis, 1988, p 550.
22. Schneider FJ: Traumatic spinal cord injury, in Umphred DA (ed): *Neurologic Rehabilitation*. St Louis, Mosby–Year Book, 1985, pp 319–320.
23. Staas WE: Pain, in Ruskin AP (ed): *Current Therapy in Physiatry*. Philadelphia, WB Saunders, 1984, p 423.
24. Staas WE, Formal CS, et al: Rehabilitation of the spinal cord injured patients, in DeLisa JA (ed): *Rehabilitation Medicine: Principles and Practice*. New York, JB Lippincott, 1988, pp 641–642.
25. Staas WE, La Mantia JG: Decubitus ulcers, in Ruskin AP (ed): *Current Therapy in Physiatry*. Philadelphia, WB Saunders, 1984, p 410.
26. Stover SL, Niewmann KMW, Miller JM: Disodium etidromate in the prevention of postoperative recurrence of heterotopic ossification in spinal cord injury patients. *J Bone Joint Surg [Am]* 1976; 58:683–687.
27. Tator CH (ed): Maintaining cardiovascular function and body temperature control, in *Early Management of Acute Spinal Cord Injury*. New York, Raven Press, 1982, p 276.
28. Wetzel J: Respiratory evaluation and treatment, in Adkins HV (ed): *Spinal Cord Injury*. New York, Churchill Livingstone, 1985, pp 78–81.

29

Patient Education and Spinal Cord Trauma

J. Darrell Shea, M.D.

Historically the practice of medicine has been a mystery with few being admitted to the secrets and rites and thereby becoming physicians and surgeons. An awesome responsibility for defending fellow citizens against the onslaughts of disease and aging was accepted by this valiant band. Patients were treated and cured or lost. Treatment alternatives were not considered or proffered. Risks, complications, or results were rarely discussed. Medicine was too complex and potentially dangerous for the uneducated. Proper therapeutic decisions could only be made by a physician relying on training and years of experience. The doctor decided, and the patient consented.

Coincident with recent medical advances, a transformation has occurred in the physician-patient relationship. The modern physician now informs the patient about diagnosis, treatment alternatives, potential risks, and complications. Educating the patient has become acceptable. Experience has demonstrated that expanding patient understanding and participation does not impair but rather improves clinical results.

Today's patient is more informed and educated. There are no secrets in medicine. Popular literature and the press are replete with articles by physicians discussing new and established treatments. Surgical procedures are demonstrated daily on television. Physician talk shows discuss the merits and risks of a variety of medical treatments. Magazines provide lists of questions that every informed patient should ask his physician. Patients are accustomed to making decisions in all aspects of life. Why not make personal medical decisions? The logical progression in medical management is toward increasing patient participation.

Patient involvement in the medical decision presents a dilemma. It is now the physician rather than the patient who is anxious about medical practice. Expanded medical knowledge and success have created an aura of invincibility and a belief that any disorder can be cured. Failure to cure implies that an error was made by the doctor due to a wrong decision. Patients are coming to be regarded as potential adversaries looking for a bad result. The more complicated the medical problem, the more risky the clinical decision. Patients are insisting on being more involved. They want to make decisions.

Although it is accepted that patients should be informed, medical decisions are complex and cannot be made without sufficient information. How is the patient to gain this competence without going to medical school? Expanding medical protocols to include patient education by physicians and allied health professionals is the answer. Education programs thereby allow the patient to acquire increasing understanding and competence to participate in medical management.

PATIENT EDUCATION

The goal of a patient education program is to inform the patient and his family about the nature of the illness and objectives and risks of treatment with a consideration of treatment alternatives. With an increasing knowledge base the patient is encouraged to assume greater responsibility, thus making decisions about his care more effective. Confidence and understanding evolve.

Medical management and patient education progress in an orderly manner. Data are collected through history, clinical examination, and testing. A diagnosis and treatment plan are developed. Patient, family, and significant others are informed. Decisions are made. Treatment is initiated and progress reviewed. As treatment progresses, multiple, informed decisions are made and modified by the physician, patient, and family. A common goal is established. The system is most effective when all parties are involved in the decision-making process. Patient and physician share responsibility in diagnosis, treatment, and compliance.

Taking a medical history is the beginning of the education process. The doctor learns from the patient, and the patient learns by responding to and asking questions. Through the history and physical examination, the trained physician gains specific data about the patient. Although the patient's medical knowledge is less complete, he also learns. As the indications for testing, including radiographs and laboratory work, for example, are explained, the patient learns, and his apprehension decreases. The education process merges imperceptibly with medical treatment. Knowledge alleviates fear and instills confidence. Decisions are not isolated but are relevant. Blind curves are straightened and the remedial road smoothed. Patient education, as in all education, requires organization. A structured curriculum progresses in an orderly manner from basic to complex. At each step a faculty is imparting specific information that must be mastered. Medical education is unique in that the student patient is not matriculating by choice. He brings to the educational situation a knowledge base that is an assortment of previously acquired facts, education, experience, principles, and insights. This knowledge base serves as the foundation upon which new medical knowledge is added. Time constraints and varying clinical environments do not permit an exhaustive assessment and educational presentation. Illness implies a sense of urgency without choice or election. The patient is compelled to learn about his disease. He may be transiently or permanently mentally impaired by disease or drugs. There must be an orderly transition.

EDUCATION FACTORS

Basic components of an education program include (1) time or term of study, (2) classroom, (3) faculty, (4) student, and (5) curriculum. In each phase of medical management, the term or time of study varies from hours to days, weeks, and months. The classroom varies from the accident scene to the emergency room to the hospital and rehabilitation center. The faculty is the treating medical team and is also changing. Only the student as the patient remains a constant. A curriculum, the most crucial and sometimes the least apparent, is developed to permit the patient to progress through each therapeutic phase with increasing understanding and comfort. Testing evaluates comprehension and program efficiency. Continuing education embraces all of the above with the addition of new knowledge and reinforcement or revision of established knowledge. Curriculum suggests a fixed series of studies that are required for progression. This further presumes an educational process in which knowledge is formally acquired through systematic study and teaching. In contrast, learning is universal and refers to the acquisition of knowledge, facts, experiences, or information without relevance or organization.

All patients are learning and acquiring knowledge of the medical process through exposure. Understanding and comprehending the relevance and significance depends on many variables including previous knowledge base, aptitude, environment, and apparent relevance of the facts. An organized education program is essential to avoid confusion. The initial curriculum is simple and expands through subsequent phases as time, faculty, and environment permit. The goal of both medical management and patient education is a patient who has reached maximum medical improvement with an understanding of his disease and the ability to make informed decisions. Misinformation must be avoided and corrected.

MEDICAL MANAGEMENT

The Committee on Trauma of the American College of Surgeons recognizes four primary patient components in a trauma system: (1) access to care, (2) prehospital care, (3) hospital care, and (4) rehabilitation.[1] Surgical management is the focus in each component with emphasis on hospital and prehospital resources. Rehabilitation is a recent addition to the primary concerns of trauma care. Education, prevention, and research are noted to be additional components to be addressed.[1]

Spinal cord injury (SCI) management progresses through four phases: (1) prehospital, (2) hospital, (3) rehabilitation, (4) community reentry. SCI prehospital care includes access and all emergency care prior to hospitalization. Surgery and medical stabilization occur during hospitalization. Functional independence is acquired in rehabilitation while medical treatment continues. Community reentry, the ultimate goal of all injury treatment programs, is characterized by patient independence. An expanding patient education program progresses simultaneously with comprehensive medical management through the four phases. As the patient learns during treatment, his ability to make decisions improves, and reliance on physician medical decisions diminishes (Fig 29–1). Decisions lead to increased responsibility.

Prehospital Phase

The prehospital phase is the patient's personal introduction to medicine (Fig 29–2). With an SCI, an independent, active, decision-making individual is suddenly transformed into a dependent, disabled patient unprepared for an emergency. Independence instantly gives way to dependence. Identity and life are threatened. Strangers appear out of ambulances and make major decisions. Identity is stripped away as catheters and intravenous lines replace clothing and confidence. The emergency medical service paramedics quickly evaluate, immobilize, and transport the patient to an emergency room. The education program has started. Transportation to the emergency room continues the terror and pain as a team bearing needles, catheters, splints, and x-ray devices descends without explanation. A hasty history is extracted and physical examination performed. Judgments are made and the patient transported to the next phase. Everybody seems to know what is happening except the patient for whom this is a first. The patient and his family are forced to trust everybody.

Success of all treatment, present and future, depends on inclusion of the patient. This patient collaboration is accomplished with an organized education plan incorporated

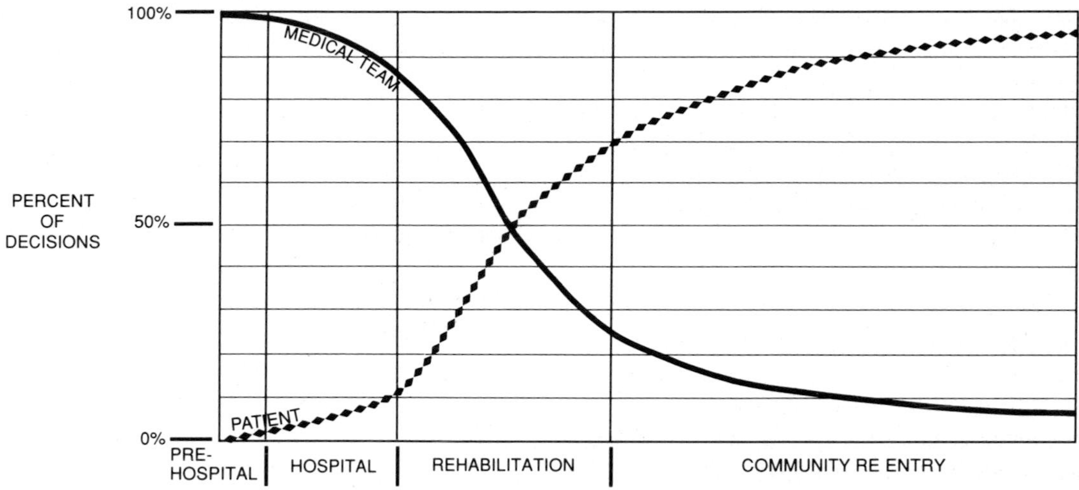

FIG 29–1.
As the patient learns during medical management, his ability to make decisions increases, and reliance on medical team decisions decreases.

into all treatment protocols and understood by all emergency personnel.

Established emergency medical protocols have been demonstrated by the Model System of Spinal Cord Injury Care to have a positive impact on improving patient survival and functional independence. Medical education of providers has caused the incidence of SCI neurologic deficits on admission to decrease from 80% in 1972 to 57.2% in 1988.[2] The next step is to expand prehospital and hospital protocols to include specific patient education. Education is not deferred until the patient is admitted to "rehab."

The increased awareness by patient, family, and hospitals through an education program helps to ensure that patients continue into the rehabilitation phase.

Time: Hours

Prehospital care is only a matter of hours. Admission and discharge are rapid. Education must be simple and appropriate, no slides or diagrams.

Classroom: Accident Scene and Emergency Room

Noise and confusion characterize the scene. Immobilization of the patient in the supine position on a backboard limits the visibility of surroundings, which compounds the turmoil. The patient can see in only one direction, up. The attention span will be short and possibly impaired by associated injuries, alcohol, or medications. Medical priorities require rapid action. This environment is not conducive to a protracted educational program.

Faculty: Emergency Medical Technician, Physicians, Nurses

The number of faculty members is relatively small. The patient/student has a brief encounter with each, but the consequences may have a lifetime effect. Professionalism in all conduct instills confidence. All care providers must be aware that the patient is continuously observing and learning. Sensitivity to the patient's fears will elicit cooperation. Quiet professional confidence and an explanation of each procedure will reduce apprehension and the heart rate. One member of the professional team should be designated to assume responsibility for initiating the education program.

Student: Patient, Family, Friends

Without the patient, there is no need for an emergency team. The present system has tended to emphasize the technical and clinical aspects of injury and treatment at the expense of the patient. Efficiency sometimes overlooks humanity.

Comprehension is blinded by fear and pain. In addi-

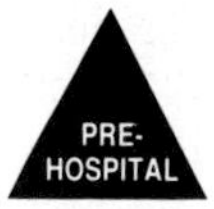

	TIME	CLASSROOM	FACULTY	STUDENT	CURRICULUM
PRE-HOSPITAL	Hours	Accident Scene Emergency Room	EMT MD Nurse	Patient (dependent)	Diagnosis Emergency Treatment Next phase introduced Primary doctor explanation

FIG 29–2.
The prehospital phase includes access and all emergency care prior to hospitalization. This is the patient's introduction to medicine.

tion to concern about the obvious injury, the patient is anxious about work, school, family, and financial responsibilities. He does not live alone in this world and will be relying on others for support. Information will be reinforced, modified, or disputed by family and friends. They are important. They must be recognized, informed, and educated from the beginning. The patient is making very few decisions at this point.

Curriculum

Initial information must be simple. One professional informs the patient of the diagnosis with reinforcement regarding the medical necessity for emergency medical care. Questions are answered with sensitivity. Answers are deferred if in fact no definitive data are available. Unsubstantiated, general statements are avoided. The responsible physician is introduced and directs care reviewing immediate therapeutic plans.

Charting patient education is important for the medical management team. They must know what the patient has been told, thereby providing them a knowledge base on which to build. No assumptions are made. The minimal curriculum content includes the following: (1) the diagnosis has been explained to the patient and family, (2) the emergency treatment rendered has been explained, (3) the next phase of care has been introduced, and (4) the primary physician has spoken to the patient and family about all of the above.

Hospital Phase

The hospital phase includes acute SCI care and hospitalization before transfer to rehabilitation (Fig 29–3). Increased emphasis on improved initial SCI care has resulted in a decreased number of hospital days before transfer to a rehabilitation program. Improved awareness of the total care of SCI by the medical community has helped to reduce the incidence of SCI complications. For example, guidelines and protocols for SCI care have decreased the incidence of pressure sores in the hospital setting from approximately 30% to less than 1%.[2] During the hospital phase, high-intensity medical treatment continues including surgery and intensive care. The patient remains dependent.

Time: Days

Early admission to the SCI system with access to a comprehensive team ensures medical/surgical stabilization and transfer to rehabilitation in a matter of days or weeks. The tempo is slower but ceaseless. More time is available for medical decisions and development of an education program. There is time to initiate a dialogue with the patient and family that outlines the total care plan. Heinemann et al. reported that admission to the model SCI system of care resulted in an average of 27.5 days of acute hospitalization vs. 60.8 days for nonsystem patients.[4]

Classroom: Intensive Care Unit

Continuous medical/nursing surveillance, noise, assessment with monitors, blood tests, catheters, intravenous lines, x-ray equipment, and respirators add to the confusion and anxiety. Sick patients share the intensive care unit and surround the patient with frequent emergencies. Although the patient may be alert and aware of what is going on, the presence of a tracheostomy tube renders him unable to communicate. Sensory and motor deprivation further complicate the patient's response.

Faculty

The medical team has increased to encompass several medical specialties, including a neurosurgeon, orthopedic surgeon, general surgeon, urologist, respiratory medicine specialist, and a physiatrist. The allied health medical team members include nurses, physical therapists, respiratory therapists, and social workers. The patient needs one consistent person from this group with whom to relate: the patient educator. The family and patient have many questions that need answering. All educational encounters should be recorded in the medical record to avoid errors in communication.

Student

The student continues to be a patient with a rather shallow understanding of what is happening. Surgery is a complete mystery. Although the surgeon explained preoperatively and postoperatively what procedures were performed, the patient does not fully understand. He knows that he is in pain and is paralyzed. Rehabilitation is next with the hope of improvement. This is a very emotional and trying time for the patient, family, and friends. All decisions continue to be dependent on professional input. Education is essential.

Curriculum

Initial education in the prehospital phase has covered the basics. With more time available, a more in-depth presentation of the diagnosis, treatment, prognosis, and future medical treatment is explained. Anxiety and pain impair the patient's comprehension, but introduction and confirmation of basic information is necessary. Written material and teaching by a trained professional team member, usually a nurse, helps the patient to begin understanding what is happening. The diagnosis is clarified. It is most important that questions be encouraged and answered. The role of each team member including consultants is described. Nonmedical matters related to the injury such as job, family, spouse, children, and insurance are explored. An introduction to the proposed rehabilitation program is made.

The minimal curriculum content includes the following: (1) the diagnosis has been explained, (2) treatment rendered has been explained, (3) consultants have been introduced and functions explained, (4) the social worker has been introduced to the patient and family, (5) the next

HOSPITAL

TIME	CLASSROOM	FACULTY	STUDENT	CURRICULUM
Days	Intensive Care Unit	MD Specialists Nurses PT, OT Respiratory therapy Patient Educator	Patient Family (dependent)	Diagnosis Treatment explained Consultants introduced Social Worker Next phase introduced

FIG 29–3.
The hospital phase includes acute spinal cord injury care and surgical and medical stabilization. *PT* = physical therapist; *OT* = occupational therapist.

phase of treatment has been explained, and (6) The attending physician has discussed all of the above with the patient and family.

Rehabilitation Phase

Rehabilitation has traditionally been associated with education and the "team approach" to care (Fig 29–4). Rehabilitation is a dynamic, rapidly expanding phase of patient recovery. It is during rehabilitation that the patient grows in understanding of the disability, independence, and confidence with the help of a multidisciplinary team. Patients come to rehabilitation by different paths, with many misconceptions that must be corrected before progress can be made. Some are discharged from a hospital with no rehabilitation or education only to appear months later with severe medical and emotional complications. Others require reinforcement and expansion of previously acquired knowledge. Rehabilitation is the pivotal component of SCI care. Failure of care and education at this stage dooms the patient to a life troubled by multiple complications and hospitalizations.

Time: Weeks/Months

Time is available to develop a progressive education program integrating all disciplines. It is during the rehabilitation phase that the curriculum can be customized to each patient's requirements. The time and expense of rehabilitation depend in part on the quality of care in the preceding two phases. Admission with complications has an adverse effect on hospitalization and costs. For example, pressure sores can impede rehabilitation by 4 to 8 weeks and cost in excess of $90,000.[5] Timely transfer significantly reduces total hospitalization and improves functional outcome.

Classroom

The environment of the rehabilitation unit is conducive to learning. With medical improvement, increased mobility becomes possible. Progression from the bed to the wheelchair allows education in a variety of settings: patient room, therapy gym, classroom, dining room, shopping mall, and home. Daily activities are organized with an agenda. Interaction with other patients promotes growth and confidence. Organized and informal group discussions encourage expression of anxieties and questions. Family access to the patient and program is facilitated.

Faculty

An integrated multidisciplinary team has evolved that unites the skills of many medical specialties with numerous allied health professionals. Medical care is coordinated by a single physician with consultants who have an interest and experience in SCI. One person is given the continuing responsibility for development and coordination of the patient education program. All team members understand that a patient education program exists and know their respective responsibilities. In addition to professional proficiency, the clinical faculty/care team has an overview of the entire education program. Coordination of effort with appropriate reinforcement is essential for success. A health care professional must be discouraged from entering the rehabilitation unit, performing an isolated clinical task, and leaving without explanation to the patient and relevant faculty/team members. Traditionally the physician has visited the patient, rendered care, and left with minimal explanation. The nurse comes behind and explains what just happened and why. It is more effective if the education nurse is aware of the impending visit and procedure and informs the patient before and after the doctor arrives.

Student

By the time the patient has been admitted to rehabilitation he has accumulated considerable experience and knowledge about the disease. If he has progressed in an

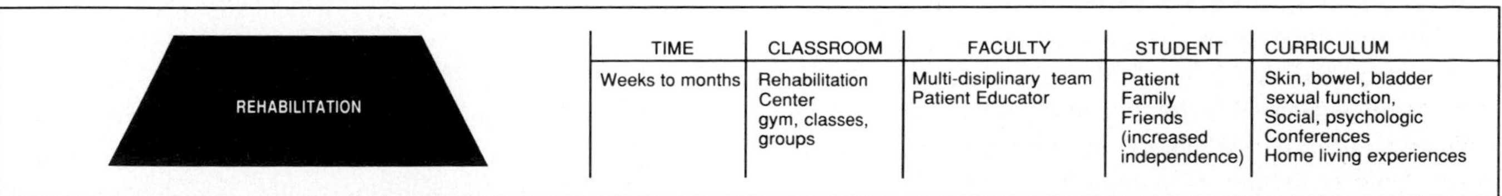

TIME	CLASSROOM	FACULTY	STUDENT	CURRICULUM
Weeks to months	Rehabilitation Center gym, classes, groups	Multi-disiplinary team Patient Educator	Patient Family Friends (increased independence)	Skin, bowel, bladder sexual function, Social, psychologic Conferences Home living experiences

FIG 29–4.
During the rehabilitation phase the patient develops increasing confidence and independence.

orderly manner in a planned education program, the knowledge base is firm. He is maturing from patient to student. If the patient has entered rehabilitation from a different path, the knowledge base will be uncertain and contain much misinformation requiring correction.

Patients have many questions. It is not sufficient to assume that exposure to an education program ensures comprehension or compliance. Not all patients are capable of learning at the same rate. With increasing knowledge and understanding, the patient is making more decisions and observing the consequences in a controlled environment. Education progress is measured and recorded. The family and significant others are essential participants in the patient's education and play an important role in discharge planning. Their education is coordinated with the patient's.

Curriculum

Prior knowledge is evaluated by pretesting. An organized curriculum includes an in-depth discussion of diagnosis, mechanism of injury, surgical procedures, and expected results with time guides. Teaching plans incorporate the following subjects: bowel, bladder, skin, respiratory, cardiovascular, sexual function, neurologic deficits, and function.[3]

Instruction is done in several settings including one on one, group with lecture, slides, and video or unstructured presentations in the patient's room through conversation. Creativity is the byword of success. Teaching tools include books, pamphlets, posters, slides, video and audio tapes, and anatomic models. Participation is important. Lectures without patient response and discussion may be relatively ineffective. Review of all materials on a regular basis fosters reinforcement. Patient interest will vary depending on perception of the relevance of the material. The patient must have an opportunity to use his new knowledge. This is provided through interaction with other patients and staff. Testing of knowledge acquired is essential for assessment of the education program. A grading system documents each patient's understanding, thereby avoiding unrealistic demands being placed for compliance. A patient who achieves a score of 4 out of 10 in skin care is more likely to develop a pressure sore than one who achieves a 9. The latter patient is also more likely to recognize the early stages of skin breakdown and prevent costly surgery and hospitalization. Areas of education that require increased individual emphasis are identified through testing. A tape-recorded admission conference conducted by the primary physician with the patient, family, insurance carrier, and attorney in which the patient's diagnosis, mechanism of injury, treatment, diagnostic studies, and proposed plan of management are presented provides a significant introduction to the rehabilitation education program. Treatment goals are reviewed and agreed upon by the patient and team. Similar progress conferences and a discharge conference reinforce the patient's understanding and participation.

Home living experiences in which the patient is able to leave the rehabilitation center for a day or weekend are excellent means of testing knowledge. Activity and education goals are reviewed before and after each experience to evaluate progress in functional activities of daily living. Results are recorded on the chart. Outings with the rehabilitation team into the community such as to a mall, movies, or airport test and reinforce confidence and community interaction.

By discharge, the patient is more comfortable making medically related decisions and is ready to advance out of the rehabilitation center into the community.

Community Reentry Phase

Upon discharge from rehabilitation, the patient reenters the community (Fig 29–5) and commences the rest of his life. Medicine assumes a secondary role. The ability to cope in this new environment depends on successful completion of the medical and rehabilitation phases. The risk of complications is lessened if he has progressed along the educational path and developed a strong knowledge base. Consistent with the objective of promoting independence, follow-up and counseling characterize the community reentry phase of patient education. Health care, provided initially through the rehabilitation center, progresses to community medical resources. The availability of SCI speciality consultation fosters independence. Nonmedical problems are perceived to be of greater significance. Shelter, work, study, and social development require assistance from many parts of the community. Family and attendant care have an impact on the lives of many beyond the patient. There is a greater involvement of third parties including social agencies, government, insurance carriers, and attorneys. Living at home or at an independent living center is different. Assistance is needed.

Life is forever. Medical care is but a brief interruption in the time line of life.

Time

There are no time constraints after discharge from rehabilitation. The patient establishes the terms of further education. He is ready to get on with life, which will optimally last years. Learning and education are directed toward further independence, which the patient defines. Time is forever.

Classroom

The classroom is the world, the same place from which the patient entered the hospital. Discharge may be to home, a transitional living center, or a nursing home. All the resources of the world are available, but access is difficult. Appropriate attendant care is required. The patient now assumes the role of teacher as he instructs oth-

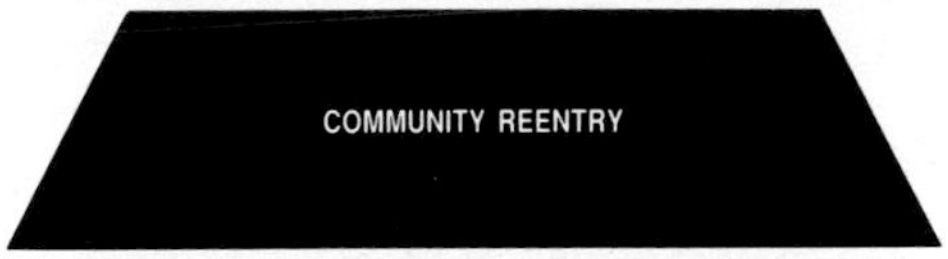

COMMUNITY REENTRY	TIME	CLASSROOM	FACULTY	STUDENT	CURRICULUM
	Lifetime	World Community Outpatient clinic	Family physician Outpatient staff Attendants Employer School	Patient (independent decisions)	Employment Outpatient care Continuing education

FIG 29–5.
With community reentry the patient is responsible for decisions in a less structured environment. Success depends on the quality of the prior education program.

ers and the world about medical, social, economic, and vocational requirements. Community integration with the assistance of the rehabilitation center permits gradual independence and introduction to resources beyond the rehabilitation center. The patient and the world now view each other from different perspectives.

Regular annual visits to the rehabilitation outpatient clinic maintain medical integrity, access to medical progress, and sharing of knowledge.

Faculty

Discharge does not mean an absence of medical care but a change in the character of the team. The family physician progressively assumes greater responsibility for routine medical care and consults the rehabilitation center as needed. Outpatient follow-up at the rehabilitation center with decreasing frequency parallels increasing independence. A rehabilitation team member continues to counsel the patient on community resources by providing financial, social, transportation, housing, insurance, education, and athletic reentry advice. Most patients with SCI require attendant care initially, some forever. The nonmedical faculty, including associates, family, employers, and strangers, is less apparent. Organized agendas do not exist.

Student

The patient is a graduate of an educational/medical program that has prepared him for a new life. Invariably, as with all education programs, the amount of knowledge acquired will vary. Patients discharged from SCI rehabilitation programs have been demonstrated to perform significantly better than nonsystem graduates. Success is also dependent on the student/patient's ability to learn. Realistic goals for independence should be set dependent on ability, performance in the education program, and medical condition. From now on, all decisions are made by the patient. Family involvement and influence progressively diminish as the patient becomes more independent and responsible.

Curriculum

The curriculum of the community is complex and unstructured. Self-rule and independence from medical supervision compete with the necessity for continuing education. Previously acquired knowledge must be reinforced and new information added as the patient's medical/social circumstances change. Discharge from the organized rehabilitation environment does not discharge the patient from the necessity for periodic review. Follow-up outpatient medical care encourages this review and provides access to new information. Although the consequences of SCI are forever, the pressures of meeting the necessities of life tend to displace medical priorities. These must be recognized and provided for through a resource library and reference center at the rehabilitation center. Education is the best prevention program, and remaining within the system is the best insurance for continuous access to medical/social care.

CONCLUSIONS

Patients have anxiety about progression into the unknown. As the pace of therapy decreases and the pace of discussion/education increases, patient comfort and confidence improve. Decisions become easier. Initially data are presented simply with a comfortable first impression. The simple presentation gradually becomes more complex as the patient learns and develops a knowledge base on which to build. Negative emotional implications must be avoided without all the facts. The medical team has an obligation to educate as well as treat the patient at all times.

The patient progresses from total dependence with minimal information to independence, medical stability, and the ability to make sound decisions based on sound medical information gained from a progressive education program that paralleled medical treatment and rehabilitation (Fig 29–6). The content of the patient education program mirrors that of professional medical education. Both share a common vocabulary.

Questions require honest answers based on reliable medical knowledge, data, and experience. The answers and the manner of delivery constitute the initial education process. Initially the family wants simple explanations. As the initial emotional trauma subsides, more substantial, objective information is essential. Reading material must be available. The information imparted is recorded in the chart.

Mandatory, early reporting of SCI in many states introduces patients and families to SCI resources. Minimally involved patients are thus prevented from falling "through

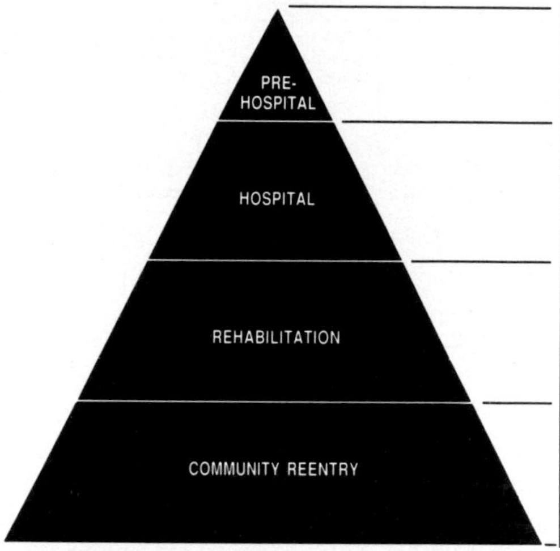

	TIME	CLASSROOM	FACULTY	STUDENT	CURRICULUM
PRE-HOSPITAL	Hours	Accident Scene Emergency Room	EMT MD Nurse	Patient (dependent)	Diagnosis Emergency Treatment Next phase introduced Primary doctor explanation
HOSPITAL	Days	Intensive Care Unit	MD Specialists Nurses PT, OT Respiratory therapy Patient Educator	Patient Family (dependent)	Diagnosis Treatment explained Consultants introduced Social Worker Next phase introduced
REHABILITATION	Weeks to months	Rehabilitation Center gym, classes, groups	Multi-disiplinary team Patient Educator	Patient Family Friends (increased independence)	Skin, bowel, bladder sexual function, Social, psychologic Conferences Home living experiences
COMMUNITY REENTRY	Lifetime	World Community Outpatient clinic	Family physician Outpatient staff Attendants Employer School	Patient (independent decisions)	Employment Outpatient care Continuing education

FIG 29–6.
Patient education and spinal cord trauma management progress through four phases from initial emergency care to community reentry with increasing patient independence.

the cracks" after receiving acute care to reappear later with devastating complications.

REFERENCES

1. American College of Surgeons: *Hospital and Prehospital Resources for Optimal Care of the Injured Patient,* appendices A through J. Chicago, American College of Surgeons, February 1987.
2. Apple DF Jr, Hudson LM: Spinal cord injury: The model. Presented at the National Consensus Conference on Catastrophic Illness and Injury. The spinal cord injury model: Lessons learned and new applications. Atlanta, 1989.
3. Hanak M (ed): *Education Guide for Spinal Cord Injury Nurses.* Jackson Heights, NY, American Association of Spinal Cord Injury Nurses, pp 1170–1178.
4. Heinemann AW, Yarkony GM, Roth EJ, et al: Functional outcome following spinal cord injury: A comparison of specialized spinal cord injury center vs general hospital short term care. *Arch Neurol* 1989; 46:1098–1102.
5. Wharton GW, Milani JC, Dean LS: Pressure sore profile: Cost and management. Presented at the American Spinal Cord Injury Association. Boston, March 1987.

PART VII

SPINAL INFECTIONS

30

Spine Infections

Glenn R. Rechtine, M.D., and Michael Reed, M.D.

At the present time spine infections are considered almost rare; nevertheless, it is very important not to lose sight of the fact that they do occur. The various entities that must be considered, in addition to tuberculosis and fungal infections, are vertebral osteomyelitis, associated epidural and psoas abscesses, discitis, and iatrogenic infections.

PYOGENIC OSTEOMYELITIS

Vertebral Osteomyelitis has increased in incidence over the last several decades and now accounts for between 2% and 4% of all osteomyelitis. This increase may be accounted for by an increase in the number of drug addicts and the large numbers of cases of in-hospital sepsis following procedures.[36] Although the morbidity and mortality of spinal infections are decreasing as a result of appropriate surgical intervention and advances in antibiotic therapy, delay in diagnosis continues to be a major problem. The average delay in initial presentation to diagnosis is 3 months.[11]

Presentation

The clinical picture of the patient presenting with spinal infection can be confusing. Back pain is very common and is localized to the area of infection (Fig 30–1,A and B). The pain is not typical back pain in that the pain of infection is a constant pain not associated with activity. The patient may present with night pain as well. Physical examination reveals point tenderness and decreased range of motion of the involved area. Root tension signs are uncommon. Paralysis has been reported to occur in 4% to 50% of patients, depending on the population studied.[15] In addition to back pain, patients may have loss of hip joint motion, a positive straight-leg raising test, or generalized weakness. The greatest incidence involves the lumbar spine, with the thoracic spine involved somewhat less followed by the cervical spine. Spinal osteomyelitis occurs more frequently in men than in women, and the highest incidence is in the fifth and sixth decade, although it can occur at any age.[23] Risk factors associated with vertebral osteomyelitis are immunocompromised patients, intravenous drug abusers, steroid users, patients undergoing hemodialysis, patients with rheumatoid arthritis, diabetics, patients with tumors, and older patients.[12] Often but not always a recent prior infection can be implicated as a source of pyogenic vertebral osteomyelitis. In children with infectious discitis, a history of ear infections or upper respiratory infections is often elicited. In adults, urinary tract infections are commonly associated with instrumentation, pelvic infection, infected ingrown toenails, bowel disease, furunculosis, or surgery. In approximately 30% of patients no source of infection can be found. Febrile episodes often precede the onset of back symptoms, but may be absent. Leukocytosis may or may not be found.[29, 37]

Blood cultures are positive in 17% to 46% of the patients depending on the series. They are more likely to be positive in the acute phase of the disease when the patient is febrile and indicate a bacteremia. Of all laboratory values, the erythrocyte sedimentation rate (ESR) is the most consistently elevated value in vertebral osteomyelitis.[11] This is not only used in the diagnosis of the condition but also assists in evaluating the effectiveness of treatment. The bacteriology of pyogenic osteomyelitis has been changing, with staphylococcal infections now accounting for only 55% of the cases of adult vertebral osteomyelitis.[18, 19, 36] The remainder of the organisms include a few gram-positive pneumococci, and streptococci, but most are gram-negatives including *Pseudomonas, Klebsiella, Escherichia coli, Salmonella,* and *Corynebacterium.*[16, 29] Tuberculous and fungal infections are occasionally seen. Pyogenic osteomyelitis most commonly involves the vertebral body and adjacent disc space and rarely involves the posterior elements. It is generally agreed upon that the hematogenous route is the most common source of infection when direct inoculation is not a consideration. There is some controversy as to whether spread through Batson's plexus or the arterial route is the most accessible. Whiley and Truetta believe that the arterial route is more easily accessible.[37] The prime focus of the disease is age dependent and explained by the change in the arterial supply to the disc. In children and young adults to about the age of 30 years, the intervertebral disc has a direct arteriole blood supply that allows hematogenous seeding of the infection directly into the disc. Alternatively, the infection can be-

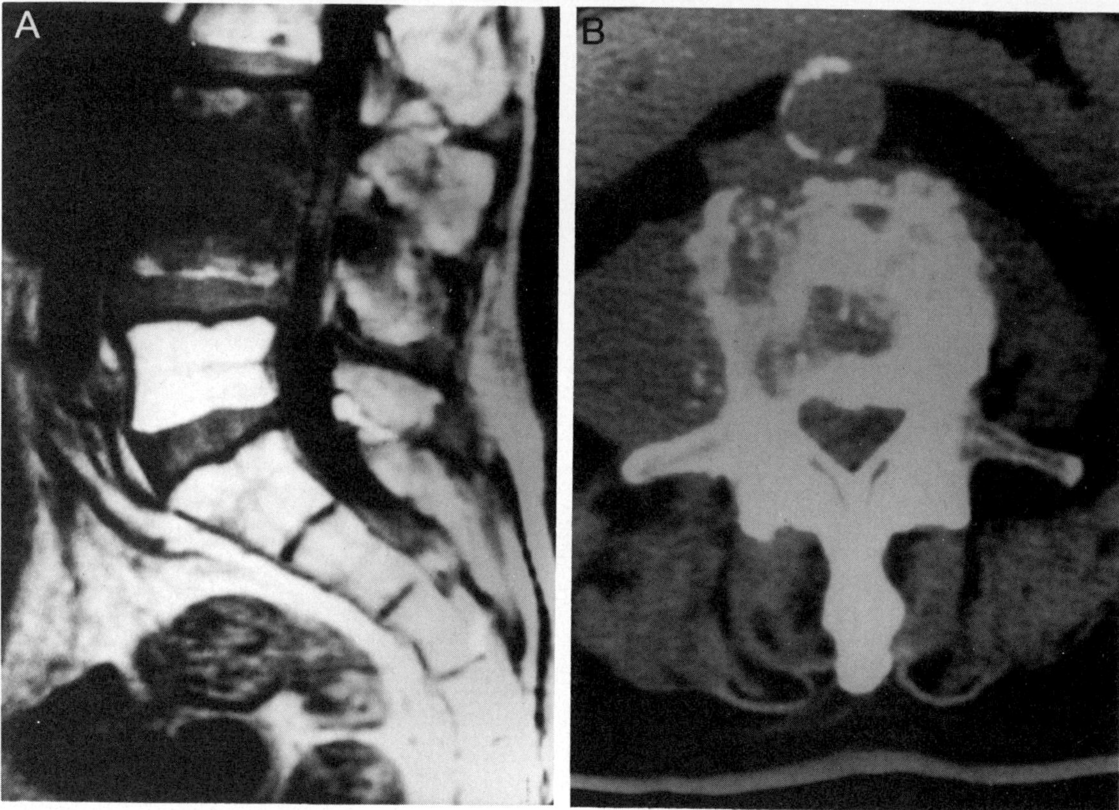

FIG 30–1.
A and **B,** magnetic resonance imaging (MRI) and computed tomography (CT) of the L5 level of the spine in a patient with known prostate malignancy treated empirically with radiation therapy. Subsequent biopsy showed no tumor, and cultures grew *Escherichia coli*.

gin in the metaphysis of the vertebral body, which is highly vascular. Infection can then spread to other levels by erosion through the vertebral end plates or through soft-tissue planes.[9, 37]

Currently there are several excellent studies for the diagnosis of vertebral osteomyelitis and discitis. MRI is very sensitive and accurate in picking up changes early in the vertebral body. Bone scans are also very sensitive, but in some studies they are less accurate anatomically and not as specific as MRI for the diagnosis of vertebral osteomyelitis. In addition, MRI can provide information regarding the thecal sac and neural structures (Fig 30–2) Involvement of the vertebral bodies, discs, and paravertebral regions as separate structures are more readily apparent on MRI. The differentiation of degenerative and neoplastic disease from osteomyelitis is also better appreciated on MRI than on bone scans.[26] Plain radiographs, in the early stages of osteomyelitis, show little radiographic evidence of the disease. At 2 weeks one may see disc space narrowing, and rarefaction of adjacent vertebral bodies may take as long as 6 weeks.

An accurate diagnosis in patients suspected on clinical and radiologic grounds to have spinal infection is often difficult. Even in those cases where there is little doubt regarding the presence of spinal infection, optimal treatment depends on isolating the infecting organism. As already stated, blood cultures are positive in approximately one quarter or fewer of patients with pyogenic infection. In most patients absolute proof of infection and subsequent sensitivities of the organisms to specific antibiotics depends on culturing material obtained directly from the disc space or adjacent bone or soft tissue. Unless the patient is seriously ill, antibiotic therapy should be withheld until results of the cultures and their sensitivities to various antibiotics are known. CT-guided needle aspiration biopsy is a comparatively minor procedure and can be undertaken concurrently with other tests rather than waiting until all investigations are completed, as often is the case with surgery. Needle aspiration biopsy in various series provides a positive diagnostic yield in 50% to 68% of patients. Lower success rates are found in those patients receiving antibiotics prior to needle aspiration.[4] In this procedure material is also obtained for histology, and it is therefore possible to rule out tumor and to confirm the diagnosis of infection in at least some of the patients in whom it proves impossible to isolate the organism. As with all needle biopsy techniques, this cannot be relied upon to exclude pathology. Closed needle biopsy can be performed with fluoroscopic

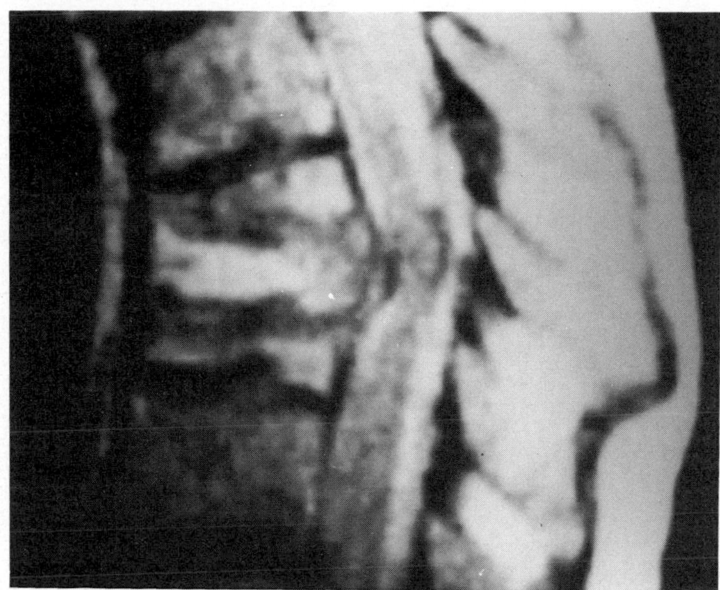

FIG 30–2.
MRI showing increased signal at the disc space with extension into the two adjacent vertebrae and epidural compression.

or CT guidance on all levels of the spine, but it is usually difficult to perform in the cervical area or at the L5 level and is risky in the thoracic spine. Overall complication rates, however, are very low with this procedure, and this should be undertaken early in the course of the patient's workup except where early surgery is indicated.

The goals of treatment for pyogenic osteomyelitis are eradication of infection, osseous fusion, and pain relief.

The primary treatment regimen for spinal infection is rest and antibiotics. Most patients respond very well to nonsurgical treatment after successful needle biopsy or other means of identifying an organism. The use of either a body cast or thoracolumbosacral orthosis (TLSO) for both surgically and nonsurgically treated patients helps to relieve pain, provides stability, and promotes osseous union.[18] There is no clear-cut evidence as to the length of treatment with antibiotics, but most feel that at least 6 weeks of intravenous parenteral antibiotics is recommended. The recurrence of infection with this regimen is only 5% to 10%. If parenteral antibiotics are given for 28 days or less, the recurrence rate for infection rises to approximately 25%. In vivo studies have shown that gentamicin and clindamycin (Cleocin) penetrate the disc space more readily. Oxacillin penetrates at an intermediate level, and cephalothin penetrates extremely poorly.[13] Early surgery is indicated if adequate cultures are not available to obtain material for culture and histology. In addition, abscesses documented by CT or MRI warrant drainage (Fig 30–3). Patients who develop complications secondary to collapse, including spinal deformity and neurologic deficit, require surgical intervention not only for debridement and decompression but also for stabilization. Eismont et al. identified predisposing factors associated with paralysis in spinal infections, including associated diseases such as diabetes mellitus, rheumatoid arthritis, steroid use, increased age, high-level vertebral infection, and *Staphylococcus aureus* infection.[12] Most patients with anterior cord compression require anterior decompression and stabilization. Either anterior and/or posterior stabilization may be required if instability is diagnosed or anticipated.

When radical debridement is indicated, wide exposure should be obtained to expose the active area of involvement. The site of exposure is determined by the specific pathology and the intent of the operation. The rationale for a surgical approach to cervical osteomyelitis includes (1) relief of pressure and pain symptoms by incision and drainage of the paravertebral abscess; (2) relief of compression from epidural extension, abscess formation, or kyphosis; (3) stabilization by debriding destroyed vertebral bodies and performing a fusion; and (4) hastening recovery and reducing the chance for recurrence. Stone et al. reviewed 18 patients with osteomyelitis of the cervical spine who underwent anterior debridement with autogenous iliac graft fusion and intravenous administration of antibiotics. All patients wore a halo for at least 3 months. Patients with two- or three-level vertebrectomies were rigidly immobilized for 4 to 6 months. Successful anterior fusion was accomplished in all patients with follow-up periods ranging from 6 months to 10 years. All patients were ambulatory and free of spinal cord or neurologic deficits.[21, 30, 34]

The supraclavicular approach can be used for lesions

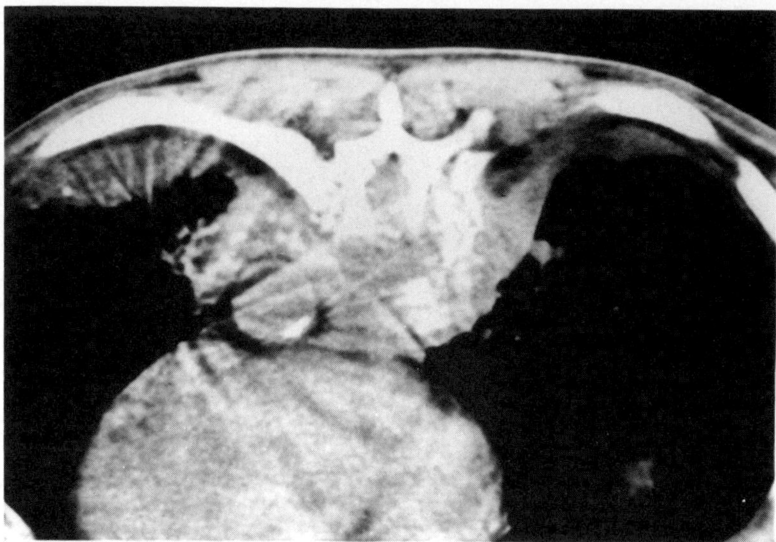

FIG 30–3.
CT of thoracic osteomyelitis with a large soft-tissue extension and bone distraction.

from C6 to T2. The location of the thoracic duct and recurrent laryngeal nerve become important at this level. The approach to the right definitely requires identification and protection of the recurrent laryngeal nerve. Third-rib resection is used for the transthoracic approach to the T1–4 area. Resection of the third rib allows greater spreading of the intercostal area than does second-rib resection. The cephalad extension of the exposure is enhanced with kyphosis deformity of the cervicothoracic junction area. The second rib can be removed if the operative exposure is inadequate.

The standard thoracotomy approach is used for safe exposure of the vertebral levels T4 to L2. Proper rib selection depends on the pathologic process. There are automatic variations at the cervicothoracic and thoracolumbar junction that dictate that the rib be taken. When the condition dictates a direct anterior approach such as a kyphotic deformity from pyogenic destruction, the rib directly horizontal to the vertebral level at the midaxillary line in an anteroposterior costotransverse radiograph should be removed. When direct access to the spinal canal is needed at one disc, resection of the rib that leads directly to that disc is appropriate (i.e., 10th rib to the T9–10 disc). Transthoracic resection of the 9th rib is usually best for maximum exposure of T11–12. A 10th-rib thoracoabdominal approach is preferred for exposure of the T12–L1 area. Both involve detaching the diaphragm at its circumference. A 12th-rib approach is used in cases in which less exposure is needed or when it is imperative that the diaphragm not be taken down. A 12th-rib extrapleural retroperitoneal approach is recommended for exposure of L1–2. A 10th-rib thoracolumbar approach may be used for long exposure of the thoracic and lumbar vertebrae. This allows proximal and distal extension for multilevel operations. Either the transperitoneal or extraperitoneal approach can be used for access to the lower lumbar segments and sacrum. The extraperitoneal approach gives a cleaner exposure to the lower three lumbar vertebrae and upper part of the sacrum.

In patients requiring anterior decompression and primary bone grafting using either an autologous rib strut or iliac crest, 90% to 95% develop solid fusions with a negligible increase in kyphosis at long-term follow-up. Those patients who do not meet the criteria for operative decompression and/or stabilization show a 40% spontaneous fusion rate after 2 years. The chance of spontaneous fusion occurring is better when the destruction is severe and the lesions are located in the upper cervical or thoracic areas.[21]

EPIDURAL ABSCESS

Clinical pyogenic infections of the spinal epidural space are uncommon and represent approximately 10% of spine infections treated surgically. Thirty percent to 40% of epidural abscesses occur secondary to a primary vertebral osteomyelitis and disc space infection. Other routes of infection are hematogenous from foci in the skin or respiratory or urinary tract. In some series the primary source of infection is not found in up to 50% of patients with extradural abscesses. Most spinal epidural abscesses are located posteriorly in the thoracic and lumbar portions of the spine. Epidural abscesses in the cervical spine are rare and may be due to the limitations of the cervical epidural space. Most anteriorly located abscesses are associated with adjacent vertebral osteomyelitis. Clinically the patient presents in four developmental phases of the syndrome described by Heusner: spinal ache, root pain, weakness, and paralysis. Heusner also described two clinical progressions of spinal epidural abscess: acute and chronic. In the acute type, the progression to neurologic deficits was rapid, ranging from a few days to a week, whereas in the chronic type, the progression was delayed, ranging from weeks to months. He stressed prompt recognition of this clinical presentation and noted that the combination of fever, severe spinal pain, and tenderness should help suggest the diagnosis. Other signs and symptoms include loss of the normal spinal curvature, leukocytoses, and elevated ESR values. The late phase is accompanied by paraparesis and bladder and bowel incontinence. The symptomology of an epidural abscess is more extensive than can be accounted for by the mechanical effects of compression alone, although experimental models show that extreme compression is necessary before ischemia results. The organisms cultured are similar to those found with pyogenic vertebral osteomyelitis in adults, with *S. aureus* found in the majority of cases. A frequently delayed diagnosis, more often after the appearance of neurologic signs, appears to be the main cause of the poor prognosis in acute epidural infections.[5, 28] Myelography and puncture of the abscess site have been recommended as important diagnostic studies but may be dangerous in the presence of infection. Recent small series have shown MRI to diagnose and localize the extent and degree of epidural involvement. In these, MRI was conclusive enough to obviate myelography.[3, 27] Treatment of a spinal epidural abscess is considered a relative emergency involving laminectomies at all involved levels. The intraoperative use of spinal sonography may be of benefit in localizing anteriorly located abscesses. Intraoperative sonography also provides immediate information on the adequacy of the decompression. One study reviewed 13 patients treated successfully with parenteral antibiotic therapy alone, but these patients had early diagnosis and no neurologic symptoms at the onset of treatment.[24] The length of treatment with parenteral antibiotic therapy is controversial and ranges from 1 to 8 weeks. The mortality rate for epidural abscesses is 10% to 30% in most series. At long-term follow-up approximately one third of the patients will be neurologically normal, one third will have some degree of paralysis, and one third will have severe paralysis. Recurrence of infection is rare and is usually associated with a vertebral osteomyelitis.[5]

Patients with psoas abscesses will present as patients with discitis or osteomyelitis, but they may have more localized complaints. These symptoms are usually unilateral, but bilateral psoas abscesses have been reported. The patient may complain of hip pain as well as pain and paresthesia in the posterior aspect of the thigh due to pressure on the lumbar or sacral nerve roots. If abscess formation compresses the femoral nerve in the area of the inguinal ligament, radiculopathy may occur over the anterior aspect of the thigh and in the inguinal area. A painful limp often progresses to the point that the patient refuses to bear weight on the involved side. Painful range of motion of the hip is usually present, often with a fixed hip flexion contracture that is usually very painful upon attempts to extend or internally rotate the ipsilateral hip. A palpable mass may be felt in Petit's triangle in the proximal part of the thigh, below the inguinal ligament, intra-abdominally, vaginally, or rectally. In contrast to pyogenic osteomyelitis, the leukocyte count is usually elevated with a shift to the left. The ESR is almost always elevated. Standard radiographs show only indirect evidence of psoas inflammation such as alteration of the psoas margin on supine radiographs of the abdomen, which may be present in normal individuals. MRI is the most sensitive and specific modality for the diagnosis of psoas abscesses. These retrofascial abscesses rarely result from primary muscle infection, trauma, or lymphatic spread. Purpural infections are also a rare cause. Osseous sources are by far the most common, with the spine, ilium, and sacroiliac joint being the most frequent. The treatment of an abscess collection is drainage of the abscess and appropriate antibiotic coverage. Many approaches are described, but a muscle-splitting extraperitoneal approach is optimal.[33] Successful CT-guided percutaneous drainage of psoas abscesses has been described in several small series.[35]

INFECTION OF THE INTERVERTEBRAL DISC

Infection of the intervertebral disc space is a potentially disastrous but not common complication of operative intervention. Direct puncture of the intervertebral disc during the performance of chemonucleolysis of a herniated nucleus pulposus with chymopapain as a result of percutaneous lateral discectomy has been described.[6] The consequences of disc space infection may be devastating to the patient. Patients who return for evaluation of recurrent back pain, especially those who present with paravertebral muscle spasm or fever, should be evaluated by ESR, peripheral white count, and plain roentgenograms of the symptomatic area of the spine. Elevation of the ESR, sclerosis of the adjacent vertebral cortex, or collapse of the interspace is strongly suggestive of discitis. The infecting organism in most cases can be identified and usually is either *Staphylococcus epidermidis* or *S. aureus*. Those infections presenting as discitis can be treated with prolonged antibiotic therapy once a closed biopsy has been performed. Postoperative infections occur in 0.05% to 15% of cases and are increased in reoperative cases and stabilization procedures for patients with myelomeningocele. Several series have shown the efficacy of the use of perioperative antibiotics in decreasing the incidence of spinal infection. Only 30% to 40% of infected postoperative wounds actually look infected and are red, swollen, and/or warm. Definitive diagnosis is with needle aspiration. Broad-spectrum antibiotic treatment is instituted once the culture has been obtained either from needle aspiration of the wound or at surgery. The best results are obtained with aggressive surgical debridement and closure of the wound over drains.[10] Pulsatile irrigation is used intraoperatively. Alternatives include leaving the wound open and using wet-to-dry dressing changes three times a day. This results in increased patient discomfort and poor patient nutrition secondary to fluid loss. With this aggressive regimen 90% to 95% of patients have a satisfactory result with resolution of the infection.

SUMMARY

In summary, an early, accurate diagnosis and appropriate treatment will provide the patient with the best result. Surgery is indicated to (1) drain an abscess, (2) help with the diagnosis, or (3) stabilize an unstable spine. Appropriate long-term antibiotics remain the mainstay of treatment.

REFERENCES

1. Abramovitz J, Batson R, Yablon J: Vertebral osteomyelitis. *Spine* 1986; 11:418–420.
2. Adatepe M, Powel O, Isaacs G: Hematogenous pyogenic vertebral osteomyelitis: Diagnostic value of radionuclide bone imaging. *J Nucl Med* 1986; 27:1860–1885.
3. Angtuaco E, McConnell J, Chadduck W, et al: MR imaging of spinal epidural sepsis. *Am J Nucl Med* 1987; 8:879–883.
4. Armstrong P, Chalmers AH: Needle aspiration/biopsy of the spine in suspected disc space infection. *Br J Radiol* 1975; 53:333–337.
5. Baker A, Ojemann RG, Swartz MN, et al: Spinal epidural abscess. *N Engl J Med* 1975; 193:463–468.
6. Blankstein A, Rubinstein E, Ezra E: Disc space infection and vertebral osteomyelitis as a complication of percutaneous lateral discectomy. *Clin Orthop* 1987; 225:234–237.
7. Bonfiglio M, Lange TA, Kim YM: Pyogenic vertebral osteomyelitis. *Clin Orthop* 1973; 96:234–249.
8. Chan KM, Lang PC, Lee YF: Pyogenic osteomyelitis of the spine—A review of 16 conservative cases. *J Spinal Disorders* 1988; 1:224–331.
9. Coventry MB, Ghromley RK, Kerndran JW: The intervertebral disc, its microscopic anatomy and pathology. Part I. Anatomy, development, and physiology. *J Bone Joint Surg* 1945; 27:105.
10. Dall B, Rowe D, Odette W, et al: Postoperative discitis. *Clin Orthop* 1987; 224:138–146.
11. Digby JM, Kershey TB: Pyogenic non-tuberculosis spinal infection. *J Bone Joint Surg [Br]* 1979; 61:47.
12. Eismont FJ, Bohlman HH, Sony PL, et al: Pyogenic and fungal vertebral osteomyelitis with paralysis. *J Bone Joint Surg [Am]* 1983; 65:19–29.
13. Eismont FJ, Wiesel SW, Brighton CT, et al: Antibiotic penetration into rabbit nucleus pulposus. *Spine* 1987; 12:254–256.
14. Forsythe M, Rothman RH: New concepts in the diagnosis and treatment of infections of the cervical spine. *Orthop Clin North Am* 1978; 9:1039–1051.
15. Garcia A, Grantham SA: Hematogenous pyogenic vertebral osteomyelitis. *J Bone Joint Surg [Am]* 1960; 42:429–436.
16. Goldman AB, Freiberger RH: Localized infections and neuropathic diseases. *Semin Roentgenol* 1979; 14:19–24.
17. Golimbu C, Firooznig H, Rafii M: CT of osteomyelitis of the spine. *AJR* 1984; 142:159–163.
18. Griffiths HED, Jones DM: Pyogenic infection of the spine. *J Bone Joint Surg [Br]* 1971; 53:383–391.
19. Guiri JP: Pyogenic osteomyelitis of the spine. *J Bone Joint Surg* 1946; 28.
20. Horowitz NH, Curtin JA: Prophylactic antibiotics and wound infections following laminectomy for lumbar disk herniation. *J Neurosurg* 1975; 43:727–731.
21. Kemp HBS, Jackson JW, Jeremiaii JD, et al: Anterior fusion of the spine for infective lesions in adults. *J Bone Joint Surg [Br]* 1973; 55:715–734.
22. King DM, Mayo KM: Infective lesions of the vertebral column. *Clin Orthop* 1973; 96:248–253.
23. LaRocca LA: Spinal sepsis, in Rothman PH, Simeone PA (eds): *The Spine,* ed 2, vol 2. Philadelphia, WB Saunders, 1982, p 757.
24. Leys D, Lesoin F, Uavl C: Decreased morbidity from acute bacterial spinal epidural abscesses using computed tomography and nonsurgical treatment in selected patients. *Ann Neurol* 1985; 17:350–355.
25. Lonstein J, Winter R, Moe J, et al: Wound infection with Harrington instrumentation and spine fusion for scoliosis. *Clin Orthop* 1973; 96:222–233.
26. Modic M, Feiglin DH, Piraino D: Vertebral osteomyelitis: Assessment using MRI. *Radiology* 1985; 157:157–166.
27. Patronas N, Mark W, Duda E: Radiographic presentation of spinal abscess in the subdural space. *AJR* 1979; 132:138–139.
28. Post JD, Quencer R, Montalvo B: Spinal infection: Evaluation with MR imaging and intraoperative U.S. *Radiology* 1988; 169:765–771.
29. Resnick D, Niwayama G: *Diagnosis of Bone and Joint Disorders with Emphasis on Articular Abnormalities*. Philadelphia, WB Saunders, 1981, pp 2130–2153.
30. Sanford EE, Chan D, Woodward R: Treatment of hematogenous pyogenic vertebral osteomyelitis with anterior debridement and primary bone grafting. *Spine* 1989; 14:184–219.
31. Sapico FL, Montgomerie JZ: Pyogenic vertebral osteomyelitis: Report of nine cases and review of the literature. *Rev Infect Dis* 1979; 1:754–776.
32. Schofferman L, Schofferman J, Zucherman JM, et al: Occult infections causing persistent low-back pain. *Spine* 1989; 14:417–419.
33. Simons GW, Sty J, Starshak R: Retroperitoneal and retrofascial abscesses. *J Bone Joint Surg [Am]* 1983; 65:1041–1058.

34. Stone J, Cubulski G, Rodriquez J: Anterior cervical debridement and strut-grafting for osteomyelitis of the cervical spine. *J Neurosurg* 1989; 70:879–883.
35. Vatandaslar F, Alemdaroglu A: CT-guided percutaneous drainage of psoas abscess. *Urology* 1987; 29:450–453.
36. Waldvogel FA, Medoff G, Swartz MN: Osteomyelitis: A review of clinical features, therapeutic considerations, and unusual aspects (third part). *N Engl J Med* 1970; 282:316–322.
37. Whiley AM, Truetta J: The vascular anatomy of the spine and its relationship to pyogenic osteomyelitis. *J Bone Joint Surg [Br]* 1959; 41:796.

31

Spinal Tuberculosis

J. Michael Graham, M.D., Ph.D., and Jeffrey A. Kozak, M.D.

Spinal tuberculosis is a relatively uncommon disease in the United States and in other developed countries because of improvements in the distribution of health care and social conditions over the past few decades. However, the apparent incidence of this disease is still significant because of immigration from less developed countries and because of heightened awareness of the medical problems of individuals with chronic immunosuppressive diseases.[6]

Spinal tuberculosis is a secondary infection, usually the result of hematogenous spread from a primary focus of infection in the respiratory or gastrointestinal system. Pathophysiologic studies suggest that the tuberculous bacilli spread to the paradiscal region of the vertebral body via the arterial blood supply. The infection extends under the anterior and posterior longitudinal ligaments and causes disruption of the blood supply to the bone. Several vertebrae are usually affected. The blood supply to the bone is compromised further by endarteritis, which results in bone necrosis and collapse. Destruction of the intervertebral disc follows, and as the disease progresses, tuberculous granulation tissue and an abscess may extend into the paravertebral space. Bone necrosis and collapse of the anterior column may lead to the kyphotic deformity that is the hallmark of advanced spinal tuberculosis, and the neural compression caused by kyphosis and by direct extension of the granulomatous infection into the spinal canal may lead to Pott's paraplegia. Paraplegia may also occur late, after the infection has been eradicated with chemotherapy, as a result of neural compression secondary to the healed kyphos.[3]

DIAGNOSIS

Tuberculous spinal infection occurs most commonly in the thoracic and lumbar vertebrae. Classic clinical features include back pain and a kyphotic deformity, and a neurologic deficit may be present in advanced cases. These findings may be present together or alone, and the symptoms and signs of spinal tuberculous infection may also vary with the degree of involvement, how long the infection has been active, the anatomic location of the principal spinal infection, the amount of deformity present, and the age of the affected host.[5]

Radiographic findings associated with spinal tuberculosis include disc space narrowing, which results from direct extension of infection from the paradiscal bone of the vertebral bodies into the disc space, subchondral bone loss with collapse of the vertebral body due to bone necrosis and lysis, and scalloping of the anterior vertebral body from subligamentous spread of infection. Rarely, tuberculous infection may involve the pedicles, laminae, transverse processes, or spinous processes. Other spinal deformities may be present also, including scoliosis, bayonet deformity, subluxation, spondylolisthesis, and dislocation. Soft-tissue involvement, including paravertebral and psoas abscesses, may be evident on plain radiographs. Computed tomography (CT) and magnetic resonance imaging (MRI) provide invaluable information on the extent of bony and soft-tissue involvement and the degree of encroachment on neural elements.[1]

Laboratory studies confirm the presumptive diagnosis based on clinical history, physical examination, and imaging studies. The serum purified protein derivative (PPD) test is usually positive. Percutaneous biopsy of the affected area may be indicated, and histologic analysis of the material obtained by biopsy may reveal granulomas and bacilli. Treatment should not be delayed until culture results are known if spinal tuberculosis is suspected from the clinical history, physical examination, imaging studies, and histologic data.

TREATMENT

Several reviews have been published recently on the medical and surgical management of spinal tuberculosis, including 3-, 5-, and 10-year reviews of medical and surgical treatment protocols by The Medical Research Council of Britain. In brief, the medical treatment of tuberculosis—triple-drug chemotherapy with rifampicin, isoniazid, and pyrazinamide—has been shown to be very effective in curing bony tuberculosis. However, bone necrosis and lysis can occur despite appropriate chemotherapy and result in late bony deformity, pain, and in some cases, neurologic sequelae. Moreover, kyphosis may continue to progress in children despite apparently solid anterior bony fusion after chemotherapy alone because of continued

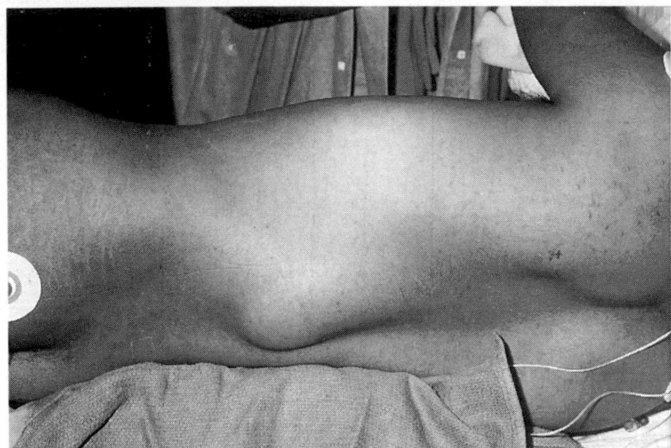

FIG 31–1.
A fluctuant mass was noted on the left side of the thoracic spine.

growth of the posterior elements.[2] These observations, coupled with the superior results of early surgical intervention shown in long-term studies and the suggestion, based on pathologic data, that early surgical intervention may help prevent neurologic damage, have illustrated the advantage of aggressive, early, surgical intervention. Early anterior debridement of the spinal infection facilitates removal of the involved tissue and prevents secondary deformity and complications. The patient's general medical condition improves, the incidence of late disease recurrence is diminished, and often the total hospital stay is reduced. Finally, extensive spread of the tuberculous infection may be prevented by early surgical debridement.[4] The

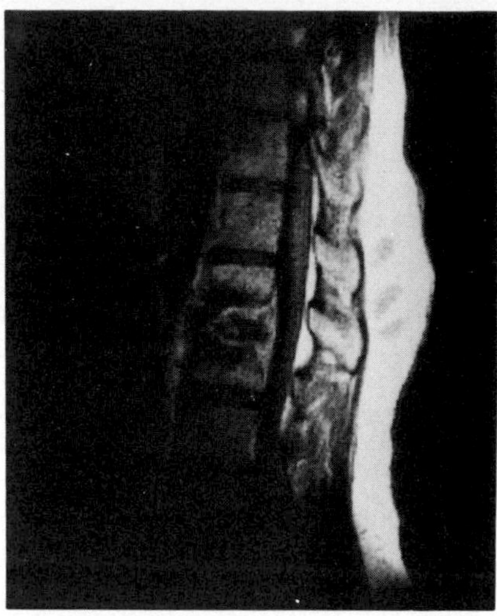

FIG 31–3.
MRI confirmed sequestrum and demonstrated severe destruction of the L1–2 disc.

advantages of early anterior debridement and fusion are clearly shown by the reports of The Medical Research Council, which compared the results of radical debridement and anterior fusion, simple debridement, and chemotherapy alone.[7–11]

CASE REPORT

A healthy 25-year-old college student from India visited the office with a history of pulmonary tuberculosis

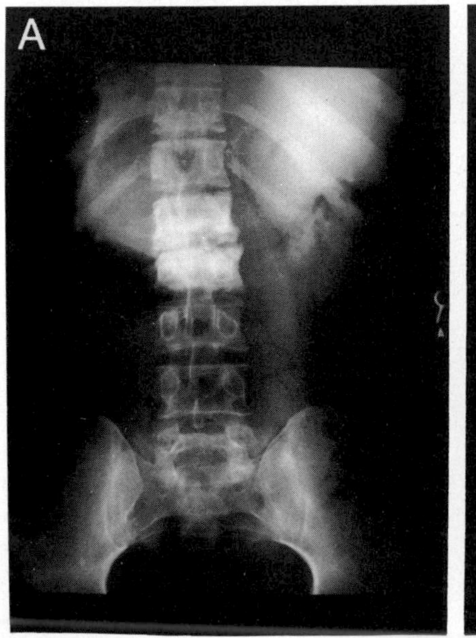

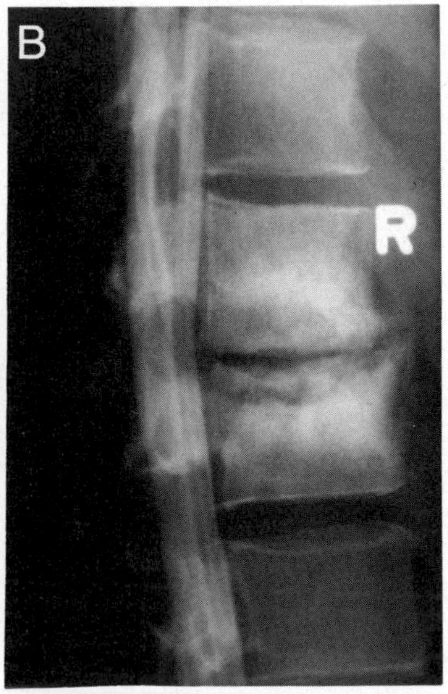

FIG 31–2.
A and **B,** radiographs showed a large density on the left side of the thoracolumbar spine that extended from the L1–2 disc space to the diaphragm.

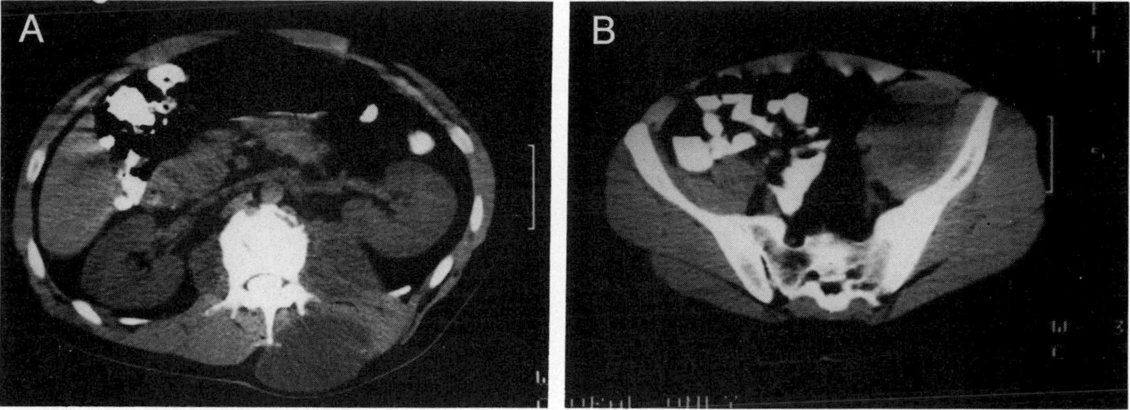

FIG 31–4.
A and **B,** abdominal and pelvic CT scans revealed a psoas abscess from the diaphragm to the pelvis that communicated with a paraspinal abscess.

treated for 6 months with triple-drug chemotherapy. He was completely well, to his knowledge, for several months following completion of the antibiotic regimen. However, he developed a painful mass in the paraspinal musculature on the left side near the thoracolumbar junction over a 3-week period. On physical examination he was noted to have a 10 by 15-cm fluctuant mass at the level of the lower part of the thoracic spine on the left side (Fig 31–1). No motion was noted in the thoracolumbar or lumbar spine on forward and side bending. The neurologic examination and the remainder of the physical examination were within normal limits. There was no history of fever or malaise. Diagnostic studies revealed an intervertebral disc space infection at L1–2 with probable sequestrum formation. Plain radiographs revealed that the psoas margins were increased bilaterally, and a large density was noted on the left side of the thoracolumbar spine that extended from the L1–2 disc to the diaphragm, compatible with the diagnosis of a tuberculous abscess (Fig 31–2,A and B). An MRI scan of the thoracolumbar spine revealed a definite sequestrum and severe destruction at the L1–2 intervertebral disc (Fig 31–3). CT scans of the abdomen and pelvis showed a psoas abscess on the left that extended from the diaphragm to the pelvis and communicated with a left paraspinal abscess (Fig 31–4,A and B).

A subtotal vertebrectomy at L1 and L2 was done with

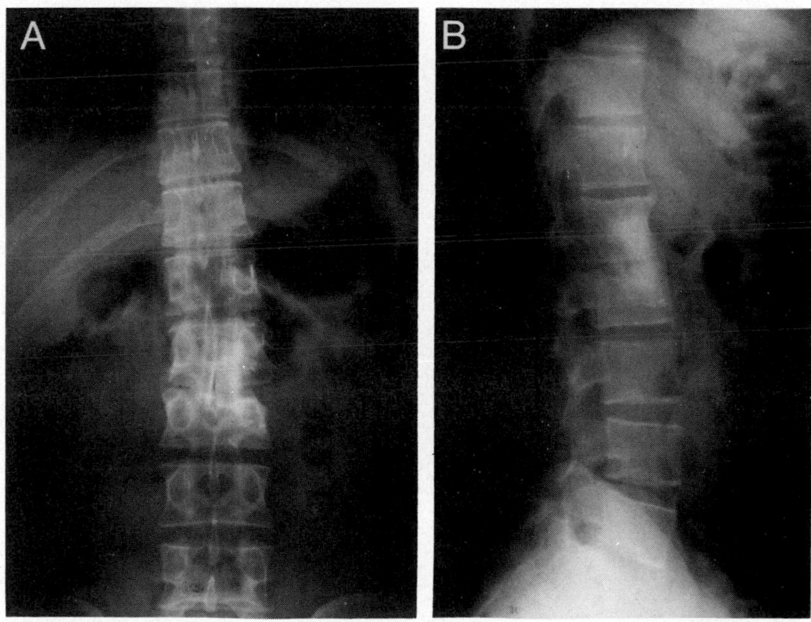

FIG 31–5.
A, anterior-posterior radiograph one year after reconstructive surgery. **B,** lateral radiograph one year after surgery which shows solid arthrodesis and no evidence of recurrent infection.

irrigation and debridement of both abscesses through an 11th-rib thoracoabdominal exposure. Fifteen hundred milliliters of purulent material were evacuated, and reconstruction was accomplished by utilizing strut grafts composed of allograft fibula and autogenous rib material. The left paraspinal abscess was evacuated through the same surgical approach but without a surgical incision since the two abscesses were connected. The patient's postoperative course was uncomplicated, and he subsequently developed a solid fusion and became asymptomatic (Fig 31–5,A and B).

SUMMARY

Although the worldwide incidence of spinal tuberculosis has certainly decreased over the past few decades with improvements in the distribution of medical care and the development of effective chemotherapy regimens, this disease will continue to be common in underdeveloped countries where the diagnosis and treatment of systemic tuberculosis may be delayed. Moreover, as immigration patterns continue to evolve, spinal tuberculosis will be evident in modern, developed countries as well. Appropriate chemotherapy with antituberculous drugs is usually curative, although the morbidity of this disease with regard to spinal deformity, pain, and late neurologic sequelae may be reduced by aggressive early surgical intervention with anterior spinal debridement and fusion.

REFERENCES

1. Bullough PG, Boachie-Adjei O: *Atlas of Spine Disease*. Gower Medical, 1988, p 162.
2. Fountain SS, Hsu LSC, Yau ACM, et al: Progressive kyphosis following solid anterior spinal fusion in children with tuberculosis of the spine. *J Bone Joint Surg [Am]* 1975; 57:1104.
3. Hodgson AR, Skinsnes OK, Leong JCY: The pathogenesis of Pott's paraplegia. *J Bone Joint Surg [Am]* 1967; 49:1147–1156.
4. Hodgson AR, Tack FE: Anterior spine fusion for the treatment of tuberculosis of the spine. *J Bone Joint Surg [Am]* 1960; 42:295.
5. Hodgson AR, Yau A, Kwon JS, et al: A clinical study of 100 consecutive cases of Pott's paraplegia. *Clin Orthop* 1964; 36:128.
6. Hsu LCS, Yau ACMC, Hodgson AR: Tuberculosis of the spine, in Evarts CM (ed): *Surgery of the Musculoskeletal System*. New York, Churchill Livingstone, 1983.
7. Medical Research Council Working Party of Tuberculosis of the Spine (Third Report): A controlled trial of debridement and ambulatory treatment in the management of tuberculosis of the spine in patients on standard chemotherapy. A study in Bulawayo, Rhodesia. *J Trop Med Hyg* 1974; 77:72.
8. Medical Research Council Working Party of Tuberculosis of the Spine (Sixth Report): A five-year assessment of controlled trials of ambulatory treatment, debridement and anterior spinal fusion in the management of tuberculosis of the spine. *J Bone Joint Surg [Br]* 1978; 60:163–177.
9. Medical Research Council Working Party of Tuberculosis of the Spine (Eighth Report): A 10-year assessment of a controlled trial comparing debridement and anterior spinal fusion in the management of tuberculosis of the spine in patients on standard chemotherapy in Hong Kong. *J Bone Joint Surg [Br]* 1982; 64:393–398.
10. Medical Research Council Working Party of Tuberculosis of the Spine (Ninth Report): A 10-year assessment of controlled trials of inpatient and outpatient treatment and of plaster-of-paris jackets for tuberculosis of the spine in children on standard chemotherapy. *J Bone Joint Surg [Br]* 1985; 67:103–110.
11. Medical Research Council Working Party of Tuberculosis of the Spine (Tenth Report): A controlled trial of 6-month and 9-month regimens of chemotherapy in patient undergoing radical surgery for tuberculosis of the spine in Hong Kong. *Tubercle* 1986; 67:243.

PART VIII

SPINAL TUMORS

32

Benign Tumors of the Spine

John J. Regan, M.D.

Benign tumors of the spine are rare. They account for fewer than 10% of all primary bone tumors.[4] In approximately 95% of spinal tumor cases, back pain is the presenting symptom.

Essential in developing a differential diagnosis based on radiographic appearance are the location of the tumor within the vertebra and the pattern and extent of involvement of the disc space and adjacent vertebrae (see Table 32–1). Weinstein and McLain noted that only 24% of primary tumors arising in the vertebral body were malignant whereas 64% of lesions in the posterior elements were malignant.[21] A review of 23 patients by Bohlman et al. found 9 benign and 14 malignant tumors.[2] All patients under 21 years of age had benign tumors. Osteoid osteoma, osteoblastoma, and aneurysmal bone cysts occur most often in the posterior elements. While primary tumors of the spine are typically localized to a single vertebra, osteoblastoma and aneurysmal bone cysts may involve multiple adjacent levels (Fig 32–1).

OSTEOCHONDROMAS

Vertebral involvement occurs in approximately 7% of patients with osteochondromatosis, but neurologic compromise is rarely observed. When symptoms of cord compression do occur,[9] routine imaging studies may not be adequate because the radiolucent cartilage cap producing the compression may not be visualized without magnetic resonance imaging (MRI). In symptomatic osteochondroma, over 60% of the lesions arise in the cervical spine and another 19% in the thoracic spine at or above the T6 level.[4] Because of the very slow progression of the compressive cord lesion, excision of the tumor, en bloc or piecemeal, provides excellent neurologic recovery with little likelihood of recurrence.

Rehabilitation is usually minimal for patients with an osteochondroma. Since symptoms arise from impingement on nearby mobile structures, excision will relieve the problem. A painful bursa may occur over the cartilage cap and result in inflammation. Neurologic compromise is rare and occurs in 0.5% to 1.0% of cases.[12]

Osteochondromas that increase in size or become painful well after puberty should raise suspicion of carcinomatous transformation. Fortunately, malignant transformation is rare in solitary osteochondroma and occurred in fewer than 1% of Dahlin's series[4] (Fig 32–1, A and B).

OSTEOBLASTOMA AND OSTEOID OSTEOMA

Osteoblastoma and osteoid osteoma are benign lesions showing a marked propensity for spinal involvement, especially the posterior elements. Patients present in their second or third decade of life.[4, 13] The frequent complaint is of back pain unrelenting and unrelated to activity, more noticeable at night. Aspirin may provide dramatic relief of pain, but the absence of a response does not rule out the diagnosis.

Computed tomography (CT) usually demonstrates the osteoid osteoma lesion, which is less than 2.0 cm in diameter, but the most sensitive study is the bone scan. Osteoblastomas become considerably larger and may be quite apparent on plain x-ray films. Aside from pain and tenderness, other manifestations include decreased range of motion, gait disturbance, torticollis, headache, neck pain, paraspinal muscle spasm, and extremity pain. Most patients are seen by several physicians before a definitive diagnosis is made. To achieve an earlier diagnosis, Kirwan et al. recommended a CT scan and bone scan in young patients with spinal stiffness, painful scoliosis, and negative radiographic findings.[11] In the Mayo Clinic series, the interval was 35 months in patients diagnosed without the aid of a bone scan and 12 months in patients diagnosed by technetium bone scanning.[4]

Excision is the treatment for either lesion. This provides pain relief and correction of spinal deformity in most cases. Curettage and bone grafting performed when excision is not possible have provided satisfactory long-term results.[7, 13, 16]

Correction of scoliosis is dependent on the age of the patient and the duration of symptoms.[1, 14, 16] Although the critical time frame to make the diagnosis and initiate treatment in order for complete deformity correction to occur has not been exactly identified, it appears to have an upper

A

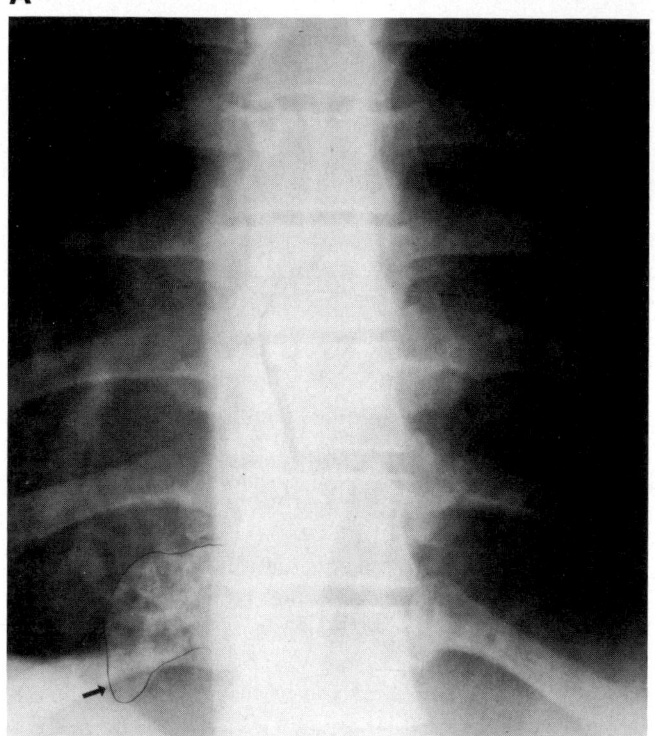

B

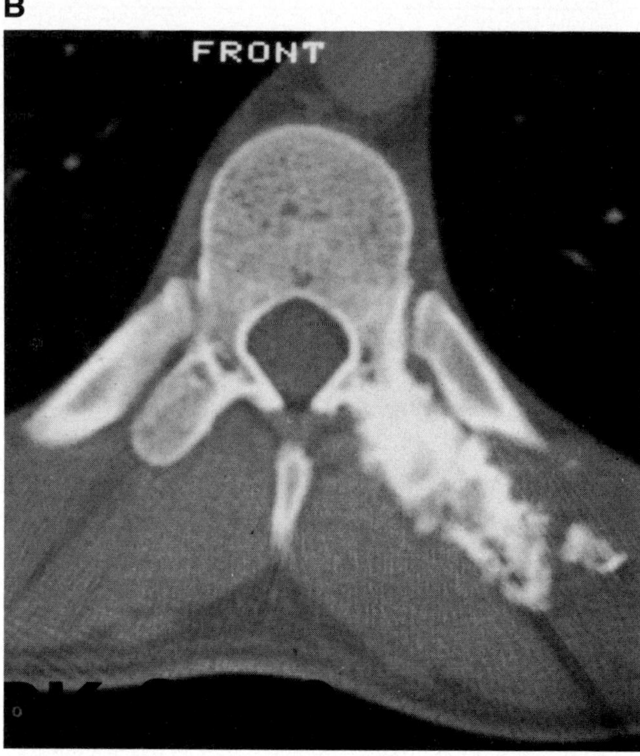

FIG 32–1.
A and **B,** osteochondroma. A 27-year-old man presented with a painless enlarging mass over the right side of the thoracic spine. At the time of surgery, the mass was noted to arise from the transverse process of T9 with the cartilage cap projecting between the ribs against the pleura. Resection was accompanied by an uneventful recovery.

bound of approximately 20 months. If the duration is longer, deformity may not improve, and correction of scoliosis may be difficult. Few patients have actually increased their deformity following treatment requiring either bracing or surgical intervention (Fig 32–2, A–F).

Rehabilitation of osteoid osteoma and osteoblastoma depends primarily upon accurate early diagnosis and definitive surgical treatment. Symptoms attributed to growing pains, a herniated disc, or psychosomatic problems may be treated by manipulation, bed rest, traction, shoe lift, brace, acupuncture, or psychiatric therapy. Once definitive treatment is performed, rehabilitation is centered about the remaining spinal problem, which may be trunk imbalance from prolonged paraspinal spasm. Painful scoliosis results from lesions located in posterior elements at or near the apex of the curve.[11] Following excision, orthotic treatment may be required for the deformity. Most authors do not recommend fusion unless instability is produced.[10, 11]

Patients with osteoblastomas are generally older than those with osteoid osteomas. Of those with osteoid osteoma, 80% are less than 30 years of age, with a peak incidence in the second decade.[13] The nature of spinal deformity is similar to that of osteoid osteoma; however, the deformities may be more structural because of the older age of patients affected. Surgical excision is usually more radical because of the size of the lesion and may lead to spinal instability.

ANEURYSMAL BONE CYSTS

Aneurysmal bone cysts (ABCs) involving the spine are very rare lesions found most commonly in the lumbar spine and involving the posterior elements in 60% of cases.[8] They may involve adjacent vertebrae in up to three or more contiguous levels. Typical radiographs show an expansile osteolytic cavity with strands demonstrating a bubbly appearance. The cortex is eggshell thin and blown out.[19] Curettage provides a high rate of cure when excision is not feasible.[3] Hay et al. reported recurrence in 13% of cases, but all were successfully treated with a second curettage.[8]

Rehabilitation of patients with ABC depends upon their symptoms. As with other benign tumors, loss of range of motion and scoliosis may occur. Neurologic deficit ranging from sensory loss to total paraplegia is more common in ABC than in other benign tumors as a result of its expansile nature. Capanna et al. reported neurologic deficit in 12 of their 22 patients.[3]

Closed needle biopsy is not recommended because

TABLE 32–1.
Radiographic Diagnosis of Primary Spine Tumors According to Age and Location

Diagnosis according to age
0–30 yr
ABC*
Osteoblastoma
Osteoid osteoma
Osteochondroma
Ewing's sarcoma
Giant-cell tumor
Osteosarcoma
Histiocytosis X
30–50 yr
Chondrosarcoma
Chordoma
Hemangioma
Hodgkin's lymphoma
50+ yr
Myeloma
Metastatic carcinoma
Diagnosis according to location
Vertebral body
Chordoma
Giant-cell tumor
Multiple myeloma
Hemangioma
Histiocytosis X
Metastatic carcinoma
Posterior elements
ABC
Osteoblastoma
Osteochondroma
Osteoid osteoma

*ABC = aneurysmal bone cyst.

this may lead to epidural bleeding. Following radical debridement and excision, instability may occur and require fusion. In the cervical spine, a halo vest orthosis may be required. Internal fixation followed by bracing is common in thoracic and lumbar lesions involving facet joints or the vertebral body. Patients should be followed for several years after surgery for recurrence since complete excision of the lesion is difficult in the spine.

HEMANGIOMAS

Vertebral hemangiomas are common lesions that occur in approximately 10% of all patients, but rarely are they symptomatic. Nerve root and cord compression, although rare, have been reported. Abnormal, thickened trabeculae give the classic roentgen picture of vertical striations. If surgical intervention is required, angiography should be performed with embolization of the major arterial supply preoperatively.

Rehabilitation for hemangiomas is rarely required because they are often incidental findings on MRI and x-ray studies. In 1928, Topler studied 2154 autopsies and found 257 vertebral hemangiomas (12%).[20] In virtually all these cases, there was neither clinical nor radiologic evidence to suspect the lesion. Hemangiomas may become symptomatic after pathologic fracture or collapse. Unstable fractures or bony collapse producing neurologic deficit require surgical decompression and fusion. Therapy will be dictated by the level of instability and subsequent orthotic treatment determined at the time of surgery (Fig 32–3).

GIANT-CELL TUMORS

These slow-growing locally aggressive tumors occur in the third and fourth decades and are most commonly found in the vertebral body. Plain x-ray studies may demonstrate focal rarefaction, although some present a geographic lytic appearance with marginal sclerosis. CT is important in evaluation of these tumors because complete excision is key to eradication of the lesion. Early recurrences may also be identified by CT or MRI.

The locally invasive nature of the giant-cell tumor in the spine may explain the particularly poor prognosis. In one small series, two of five patients died as a result of locally invasive disease. Other investigators have reported better results and suggest that lesions of the spine are less aggressive than in the extremities.[17] With aggressive surgical resection, disease-free survival has been reported without the risk of radiation.[17]

Despite their relative rarity in the vertebral column, giant-cell tumors have a predilection for the sacrum. Of the 264 giant-cell tumors in the Mayo Clinic file, 32 involved the vertebral column, and of these, 23 were in the sacrum.[5] The ages ranged from 14 to 66 years. It is considered to be the most frequently encountered tumor of the sacrum after chordoma. In these cases, spinal instability is not a problem, and rehabilitative efforts are usually accomplished with modality treatments (Fig 32–4).

EOSINOPHILIC GRANULOMA

This benign, self-limiting condition is most commonly seen in children before the age of 10 years. In 10% to 15% of cases, vertebrae are involved. Bone destruction may produce a classic vertebra plana following complete collapse of the vertebral body. Severe neurologic symptoms may occur with or without collapse and require irradiation and immobilization.[6]

Radiographs typically demonstrate a flattened vertebra retained between two intact intervertebral discs. A similar appearance can be produced by infection or Ewing's sarcoma. Therefore, the importance of an adequate biopsy cannot be overemphasized. Following confirmation with open biopsy, low-dose radiotherapy (500 to 1000 rads), which has been advocated in the past, may be avoided in

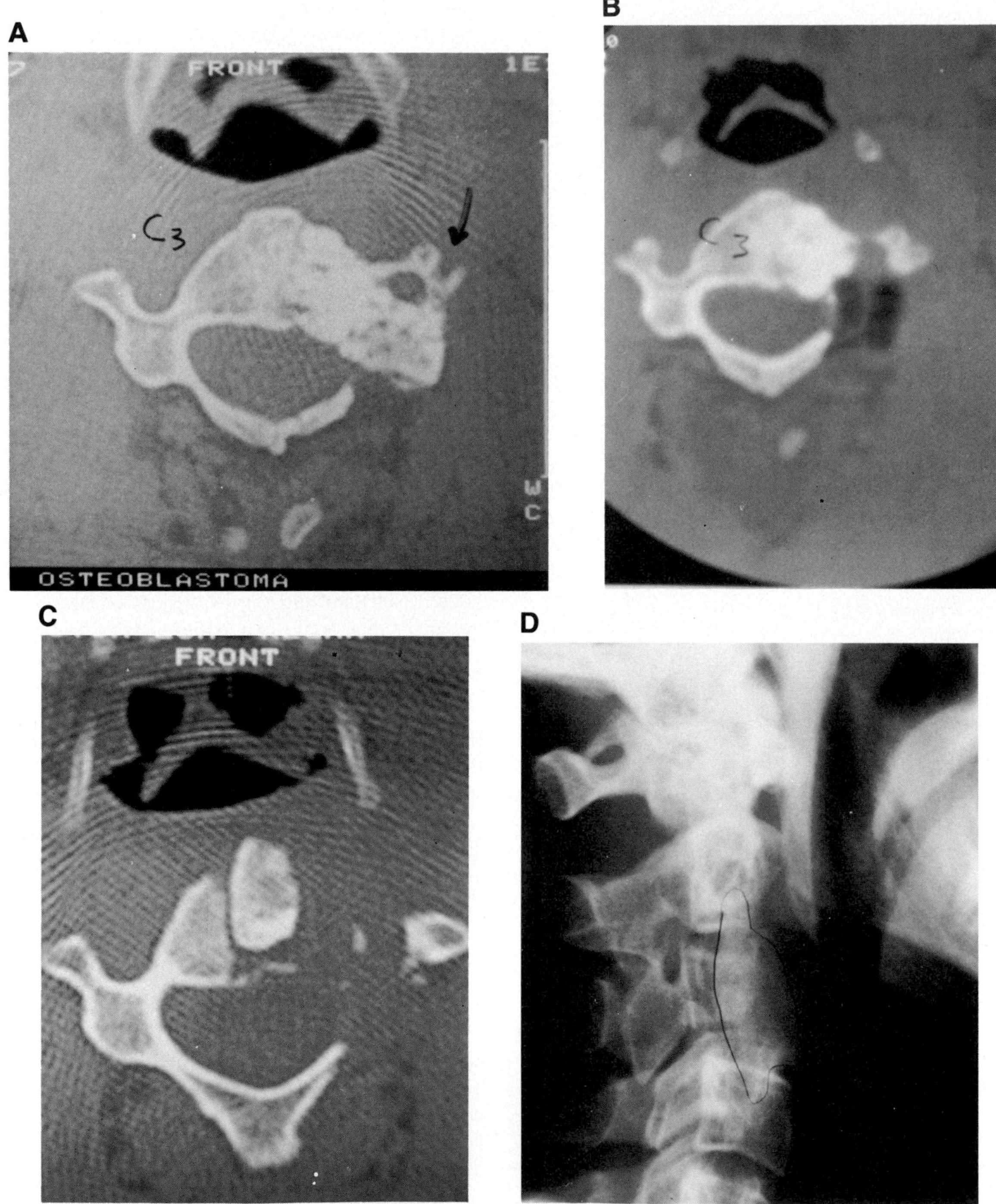

FIG 32–2.
A–F, osteoblastoma. This 26-year-old male computer programmer had seen several physicians with complaints of right shoulder pain for several months. Aspirin and nonsteroidal anti-inflammatory drugs partially relieved this otherwise unremitting pain. Roentgen studies revealed an expansile osteoblastic lesion involving the pedicle, transverse process, and lamina of C3 **(A).** This was treated by a two-stage approach. Initially, the posterior arch was removed unilaterally **(B).** In the second stage, C3 corpectomy was followed by iliac tricortical grafting **(C** and **D).** *Facing page,* the patient was stabilized with a light weight MRI-compatible halo vest for 12 weeks. Following this, a Philadelphia collar was used until consolidation of the graft at 6 months **(E** and **F).**

E

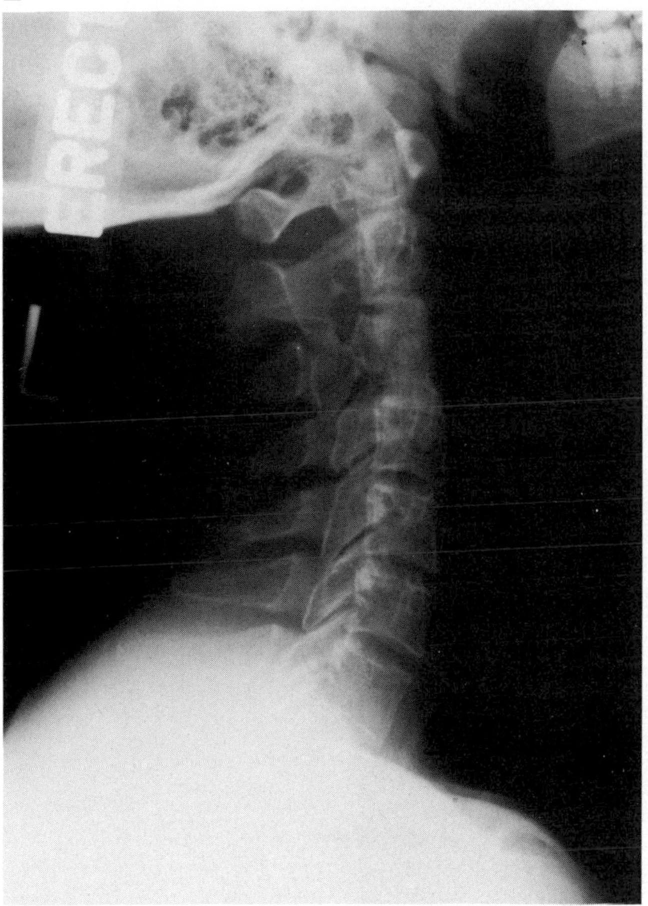

F

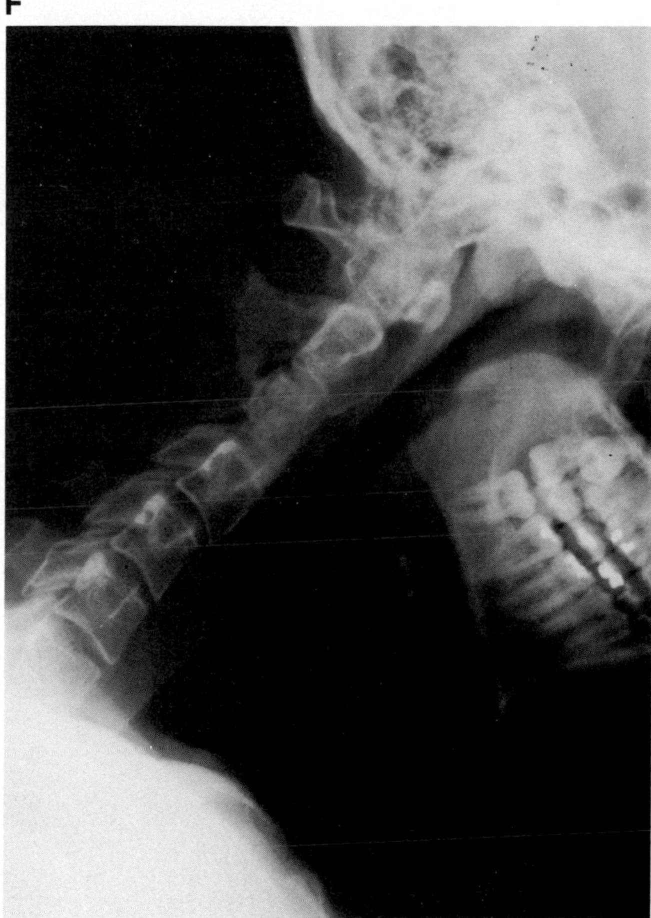

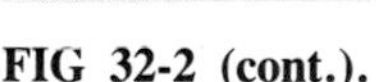

FIG 32-2 (cont.).

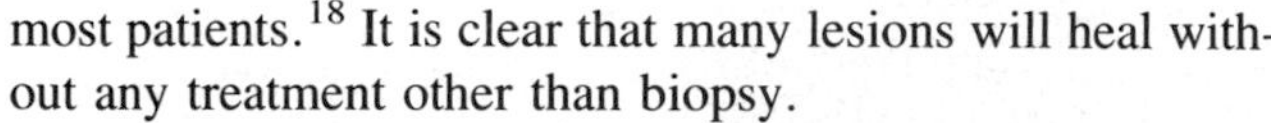

most patients.[18] It is clear that many lesions will heal without any treatment other than biopsy.

Rehabilitation of eosinophilic granuloma depends on the type of histiocytosis X, the presence or absence of neurologic compromise, and the severity of vertebral collapse. In systemic forms of histiocytosis X, medical treatment takes preference over spinal treatment. This consists of various chemotherapeutic agents. With solitary forms of this condition, one must remember that the process is self-limiting and that reconstitution of vertebral height will occur.[15] During the collapse and healing phase, prevention of further collapse and maintenance of alignment can be accomplished with a hyperextension orthosis or cast. If neurologic compression occurs from tumor extension, radiation is usually successful. Bony impingement may require surgical excision, with incumbent rehabilitation efforts depending on the nature of the procedure. Recovery is usually excellent if treatment is instituted without delay.

CHILDREN'S TUMORS

Almost 70% of primary bone tumors in children are benign. Osteoblastomas, osteoid osteomas, ABCs, and osteochondromas account for over 40% of all primary bone lesions observed in children. The added dimension in the care of children's tumors is the management of spinal deformity. Aggressive surgical resection or erosion of bone by tumor may cause more severe deformities than in the adult. Additionally, postlaminectomy kyphosis in the thoracic spine and swan-neck deformity are more common. Irradiation and rib resection may lead to scoliosis. Early paraplegia, especially from high-level cord injury, may lead to severe paralytic scoliosis. The surgeon must anticipate and seek to minimize later deformity.

CONCLUSION

Rehabilitative efforts in benign tumors are dictated by four factors: the location of the tumor, the age predilection, the period between onset and diagnosis, and the extent of surgical excision required. Osteochondromas usually involve posterior elements, which makes complete surgical removal relatively easy with minimal morbidity and thus requires very little rehabilitation. ABCs, on the other hand, may be extensive and involve multiple contiguous vertebrae and frequently result in neurologic deficit.

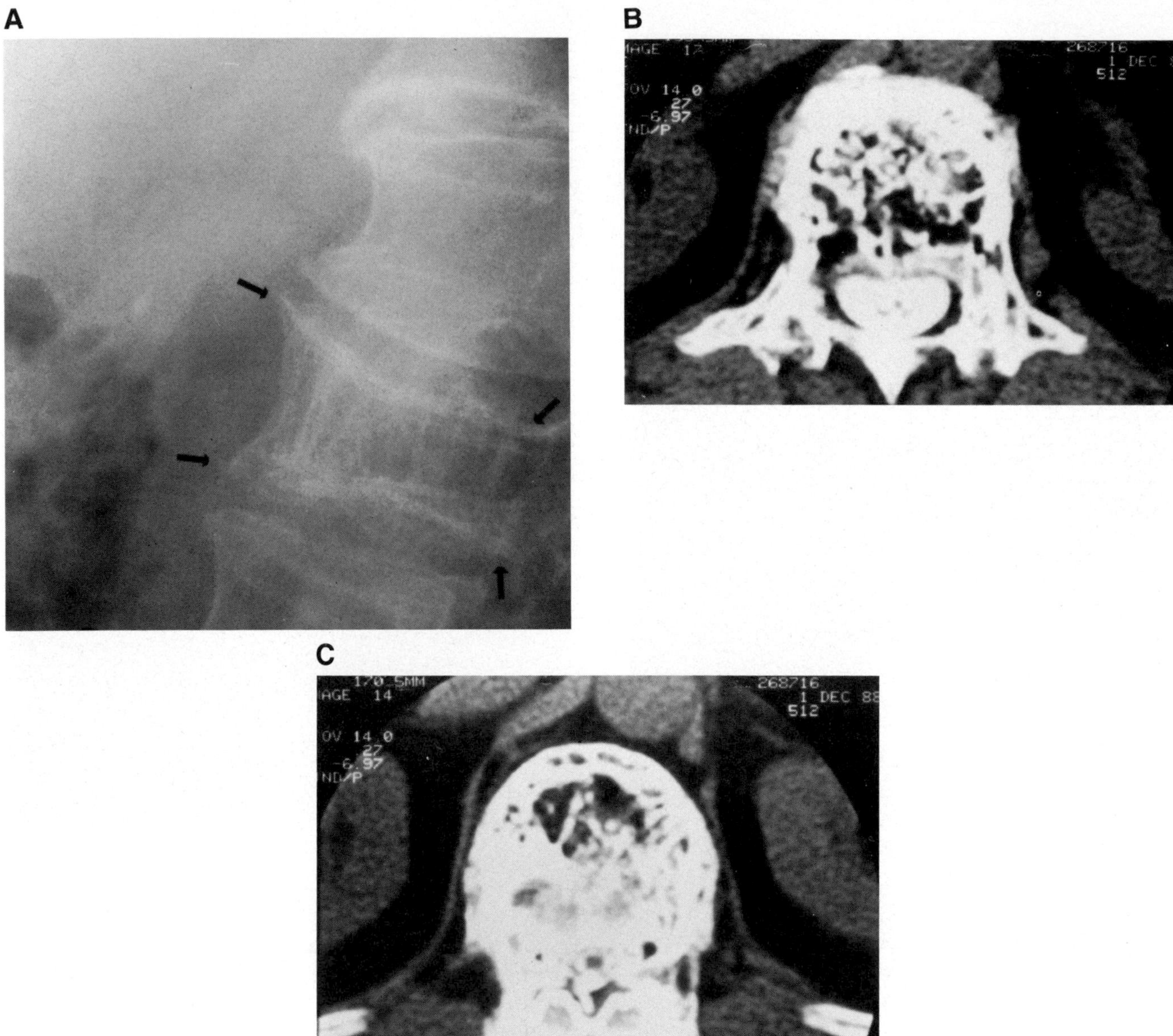

FIG 32–3.
A–C, hemangioma. This 71-year-old man presented with symptoms of spinal claudication. X-ray studies demonstrated a partially collapsed L1 vertebra with characteristic vertical striations **(A).** CT/myelography confirmed canal stenosis secondary to partial vertebral collapse **(B** and **C).** The patient refused surgery and continues to have claudication after one to two blocks. Subsequent studies have remained unchanged. After treatment with a back brace for 4 weeks, he has no further back pain.

The varied presentation may necessitate radical surgery to prevent recurrence with incumbent operative stabilization and postoperative bracing. Therapy may be limited by instability until fusion occurs. Extremity rehabilitation may be required for the neurologically impaired. Osteoid osteoma presents a unique challenge in treating spinal deformity, especially scoliosis. Paraspinous muscle rigidity may be produced as a result of delayed diagnosis, which is common. As in other benign tumors, accurate diagnosis and definitive treatment, usually surgical excision, must precede rehabilitation efforts to ensure a successful outcome. In eosinophilic granuloma, orthotic immobilization in extension may be all that is required until the process abates as spontaneous reconstitution of the vertebral body occurs. Finally, giant-cell tumor represents a unique challenge because recurrence of locally aggressive tumor may result in the patient's demise. Radical excision may be difficult since most giant-cell tumors of the spine occur in the

A

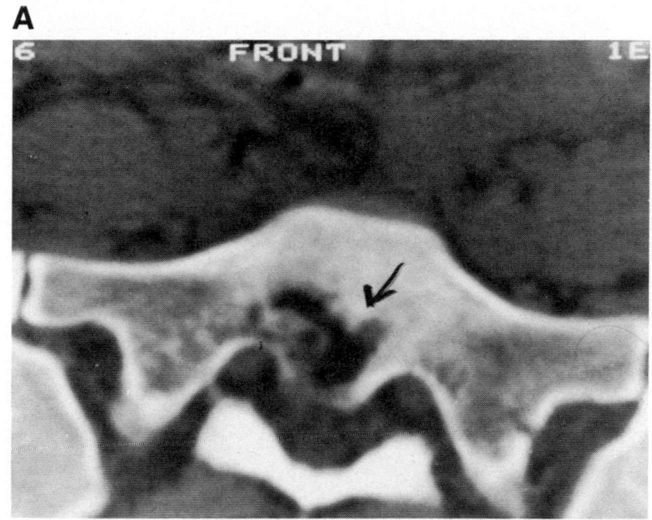

B

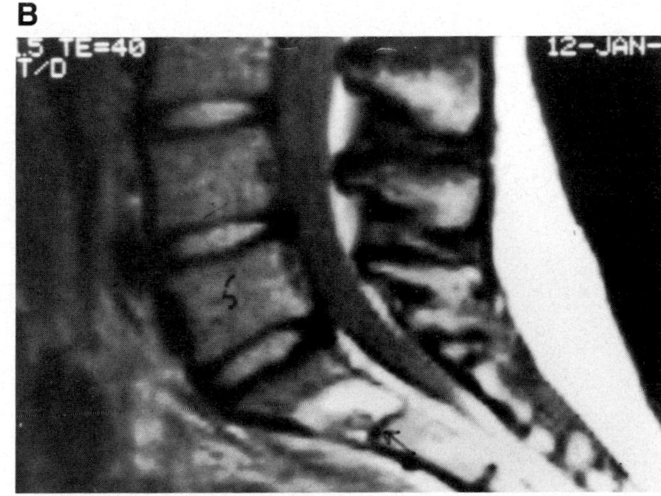

FIG 32–4.
A and **B,** giant-cell tumor of the sacrum. A 29-year-old woman presented with sacral pain radiating into the groin and perineum. The pain was unremitting even at night. After visiting several physicians, the diagnosis was made by MRI **(A),** which demonstrates a low-density lesion surrounded by high-density signal. The computed axial tomography (CAT) scan demonstrates a geographic lesion in the midline with thinning of the cortex posteriorly and toward the left S2 nerve root. The patient was treated by anterior retroperitoneal excision and extension curettage. The S2 nerve root was visualized after curettage of the thinned posterior cortex. The patient complained of dysesthesias in the S2 distribution following surgery, which were treated successfully with nerve blocks. Serial CT scans and MRI yearly have failed to demonstrate recurrence, and the patient is presently asymptomatic.

sacrum. Rehabilitation in this circumstance is directed toward the sacrococcygodynia, which may be associated with radical excision of the sacrum.

REFERENCES

1. Akbarnia BA, Rooholamini SA: Scoliosis caused by benign osteoblasoma of the thoracic or lumbar spine. *J Bone Joint Surg [Am]* 1981; 63:1146–1155.
2. Bohlman HH, Sachs BL, Carter JR, et al: Primary neoplasms of the cervical spine. *J Bone Joint Surg [Am]* 1986; 68:483–494.
3. Capanna R, Albisinni U, Picca P, et al: Aneurysmal bone cyst of the spine. *J Bone Joint Surg [Am]* 1985; 67:527–531.
4. Dahlin DC: *Bone Tumors,* ed 3. Springfield, Ill, Charles C Thomas, 1978.
5. Dahlin DC: Giant cell tumor of vertebrae above the sacrum. *Cancer* 1977; 39:1350–1356.
6. Green NE, Robertson WW Jr, Kilroy AW: Eosinophilic granuloma of the spine associated with neural deficit. Report of three cases. *J Bone Joint Surg [Am]* 1980; 62:1198–1202.
7. Griffin JB: Benign osteoblastoma of the thoracic spine. *J Bone Joint Surg [Am]* 1978; 60:833–835.
8. Hay MC, Paterson D, Taylor TKF: Aneurysmal bone cysts of the spine. *J Bone Joint Surg [Br]* 1978; 60:406–411.
9. Kak VK, Pradhaker S, Khosla VK, et al: Solitary osteochondroma of spine causing spinal cord compression. *Clin Neurol Neurosurg* 1985; 87:135–138.
10. Keim HA, Reina EG: Osteoid osteoma as a cause of scoliosis. *J Bone Joint Surg [Am]* 1975; 57:159–163.
11. Kirwan EO, Hutton PAN, Pozo JL, et al: Osteoid osteoma and benign osteoblastoma of the spine. *J Bone Joint Surg [Br]* 1984; 66:21–26.
12. Malat J, Virapongse C, Levine A: Solitary osteochondroma of the spine. *Spine* 1986; 11:625–628.
13. Marsh BW, Bonfiglio M, Brady CD, et al: Benign osteoblastoma: Range of manifestations. *J Bone Joint Surg [Am]* 1975; 57:1–9.
14. Mehta MH, Murray RO: Scoliosis provoked by painful vertebral lesions. *Skeletal Radiol* 1977; 1:223–230.
15. Nesbit ME, Kieffer S, D'Angio GJ: Reconstruction of vertebral height in histiocytosis X: A long term follow-up. *J Bone Joint Surg [Am]* 1969; 51:1360.
16. Ransford AO, Pozo JL, Hutton PAN, et al: The behavior pattern of scoliosis associated with osteoid osteoma or osteoblastoma of the spine. *J Bone Joint Surg [Br]* 1984; 66:16–20.
17. Savini JR, Gherlinzoni F, Morandi M, et al: Surgical treatment of giant cell tumor of the spine. *J Bone Joint Surg [Am]* 1983; 65:1283–1289.
18. Sherk HH, Nicholason JT, Nixon JE: Vertebral plana and eosinophilic granuloma of the cervical spine in children. *Spine* 1978; 3:116–121.
19. Stillwell WT, Fielding JW: Aneurysmal bone cyst of the cervicodorsal spine. *Clin Orthop* 1984; 187:144–146.
20. Topler D: Zur Kenntnis der Wiebelandiome. *Frank Z Pathol* 1928; 36:537–545.
21. Weinstein JN, McLain RF: Primary tumors of the spine. *Spine* 1987; 12:843–851.

33

Primary Malignant Tumors of the Spine

Alan M. Levine, M.D.

Primary malignant tumors of the spine affecting the adult can be divided into three major groups. These include chordomas, primary round-cell tumors, and sarcomas. Although the range of histologic entities and therefore the range of appropriate treatments is broad, the relative number of patients is quite small as compared with the most common type of spinal tumor: metastatic disease. The presence of a malignant tumor within the spine presents a difficult management problem when the surgeon considers the basic tenets in the management of primary malignancies in general. With the exception of the round-cell tumors, the goals of curative treatment of the patient, both locally and distantly, are best met by a combination of modalities, including radical surgical excision of the primary lesion, followed by appropriate adjuvant and/or neoadjuvant chemotherapy and radiation. The spinal location makes the application of these principles considerably more difficult. Therefore, the treatment of primary non–round-cell malignancies of the spine has, to a large extent, been disappointing because of the significant recurrence rates. The spinal location severely limits the ability to do an en bloc resection with negative margins without compromising either important neural or vascular structures.

CHORDOMAS

Chordomas are primary malignant tumors presumably arising from the embryonic notochord. These tumors are not primarily spinal neoplasms but occur in the axial skeleton. In the majority of series, about 50% of all chordomas are in the sacral-coccygeal region, approximately 30% in the clivus, and approximately 20% in the cervical, thoracic, and lumbar vertebrae.[12, 14, 37, 39, 60] The distribution of lesion within the spine is likewise inconsistent, with the majority either in the high cervical spine or in the midlumbar spine and lesions infrequently occurring in the thoracic spine.[32] These tumors generally present more frequently in males than in females, with a ratio of approximately 2 to 1 in most series. Their peak occurrence is between the fifth and seventh decades of life, although they have been reported to occur in early infancy and childhood.[67] The symptom complex is dependent on the location of the lesion. Lesions occurring in the sacrum have a considerable period during which to enlarge before causing significant symptomatology. They, however, generally present with pain, either in the lower part of the back or over the sacrum with radiation into the buttocks, perineum, and/or legs. Problems with bowel and bladder function occur in only approximately 20% of all patients. Since these can grow quite large before causing significant neural or visceral symptoms, a posterior mass can be noted in some patients. Patients with chordomas involving the vertebral column proper generally have a much shorter duration of symptoms before achieving neural compression. The symptoms are generally of gradual onset and may be mistaken for spinal stenosis, especially in the more elderly osteopenic population. Further growth of the lesion can cause vertebral body fracture and collapse with compression of the dural sac and nerve root symptomatology. Lesions involving the clivus generally present with increased intracranial pressure, including headaches, visual disturbances, and cranial nerve palsies. These tumors generally present at a somewhat earlier age than the sacral chordomas. This is true of the spinal chordomas as well. Spinal chordomas may also be diagnosed on the basis of a mass noted at abdominal exploration for another problem or as asymptomatic masses, especially on a chest or spine radiograph.

The radiologic findings in chordomas are in part dependent on the location of the chordoma. The bony involvement is most frequently lytic, with minor degrees of calcification.[31, 55] The soft-tissue mass associated with the lesion is frequently much larger than the area of bony involvement (Fig 33–1). The lesion generally originates from the vertebral body with infrequent involvement of the posterior elements.[24, 32] Until the recent advent of magnetic resonance imaging (MRI), the most common studies used were myleography, followed then by myelography/computed tomography (CT). The lesion is extremely slow spreading with little reparative function, and therefore radionucleotide scans are frequently negative. MRI clearly allows the tumor to be evaluated in multiple planes with excellent delineation of the soft-tissue components[49] (Fig 33–2). Chordomas infrequently present with metastatic

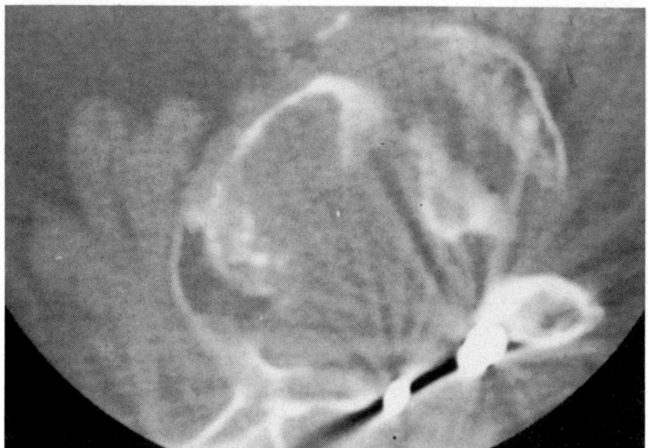

FIG 33–1.
This CT scan demonstrates a recurrent chordoma of an L3 vertebral body in a patient who initially presented with apparent degenerative scoliosis and symptoms of severe spinal stenosis. The patient underwent laminectomy and stabilization with Harrington rods on the assumption that her pathology was spinal stenosis. However, intraoperative biopsy of tissue in the canal demonstrated a chordoma. The patient underwent radiation therapy with relief of symptoms for approximately 18 months. She then had a significant recurrence as noted in this CT scan, with complete destruction of the L3 body and a soft-tissue mass.

disease since these lesions are known more for local recurrence than for a propensity for metastatic disease. Although early series underestimated the occurrence of metastatic disease at approximately 10%,[19] more recent studies have suggested that chordomas may have disseminated metastases. This occurs more frequently in spinal chordomas than in sacrococcygeal chordomas.[61] The metastases can occur in unusual locations such as the heart, brain, or bone.[45]

The treatment of chordomas has evolved over the last two decades. There is general agreement that extralesional excision of the tumor is a desirable goal whether it is in the sacrococcygeal or vertebral region. However, even a marginal resection is not always feasible. Attempts at intralesional control of either the sacrococcygeal or spinal lesions have been met with an unacceptable recurrence rate.[1, 25, 32, 60] Early attempts were made at resection of sacrococcygeal chordomas that significantly antedated any attempts at resection of vertebral chordomas. A differentiation is made between chordomas involving the third sacral segment distally with extension and those involving the proximal portion of the sacrum. The distal chordomas can be excised posteriorly.[27, 35] With en bloc resection and lack of violation of the tumor, the recurrence rate is less than 25%. Violation of the tumor, however, increases the recurrence rate to approximately two thirds. Resection of the distal sacral roots bilaterally results in at least temporary bowel and bladder dysfunction. More proximal involvement of the sacrum and larger tumors (Fig 33–3) requires a more extended approach, generally done through both anterior and posterior incisions.[58] The anterior approach allows anterior dissection of the tumor and appropriate resection of involved rectum. The lesion is resected at least one level proximal to the defined area of involvement. After completion of the anterior osteotomy, the anterior incision is closed, the patient is rolled prone, and the posterior resection is then completed. Although there is sacrifice of bowel and bladder function with high amputation of the sacrum, the loss of such function is clearly inevitable with massive involvement of the tumor. Reconstruction of a high sacral amputation is possible via a number of spondyloiliac fusion techniques.

Chordomas of the vertebral body present an additional level of complexity. Not only do they have soft-tissue masses extending anteriorly that may involve the vascular structures, but they may also extend posteriorly and involve the dural sac. It was originally felt that chordomas involving the vertebral column could not be cured and that surgery should be limited to laminectomy for decompression.[39] Unfortunately, both radiation therapy and chemotherapy have had a limited beneficial effect on this tumor because of its frequently low vascularity. This treatment pattern of simple laminectomy for decompression or limited debulking has been shown to have only a limited period of effectiveness, generally less than 2 years (see Fig 33–1). Complete vertebrectomies now provide a more satisfactory alternative.[28, 50, 56] The role of radiation therapy with this lesion is unclear. It may have an effect as a pallative or adjuvant modality.[13] From Cummings' experience, it is suggested that doses of 6000 to 8000 cGy are most appropriate for this tumor, which limits the ability to treat lesions of the spine as opposed to the sacrum. The overall survival of patients with chordomas has been limited, with few surviving 10 years because of the inability to obtain adequate surgical resections in the past. Inadequate resections with contamination of the resection field will lead to a rather certain recurrence. The initial operative treatment should be sufficient to completely excise the lesion, if only with a marginal resection, and should lead to survival rates in the 50% to 75% range for both spinal and sacrococcygeal chordomas.

ROUND-CELL TUMORS

Round-cell tumors of the spine are likewise infrequently encountered and fall into two major groups. Ewing's sarcoma has been described in the younger age group and, although not reviewed separately, has been encountered in a number of series.[20, 21, 47] The largest series of Ewing's sarcoma involving the spine was reported by Pritchard et al.[44] The patients are generally teenagers, although patients may be in the third decade of life. Ewing's sarcomas are equally divided between the sacrum and the

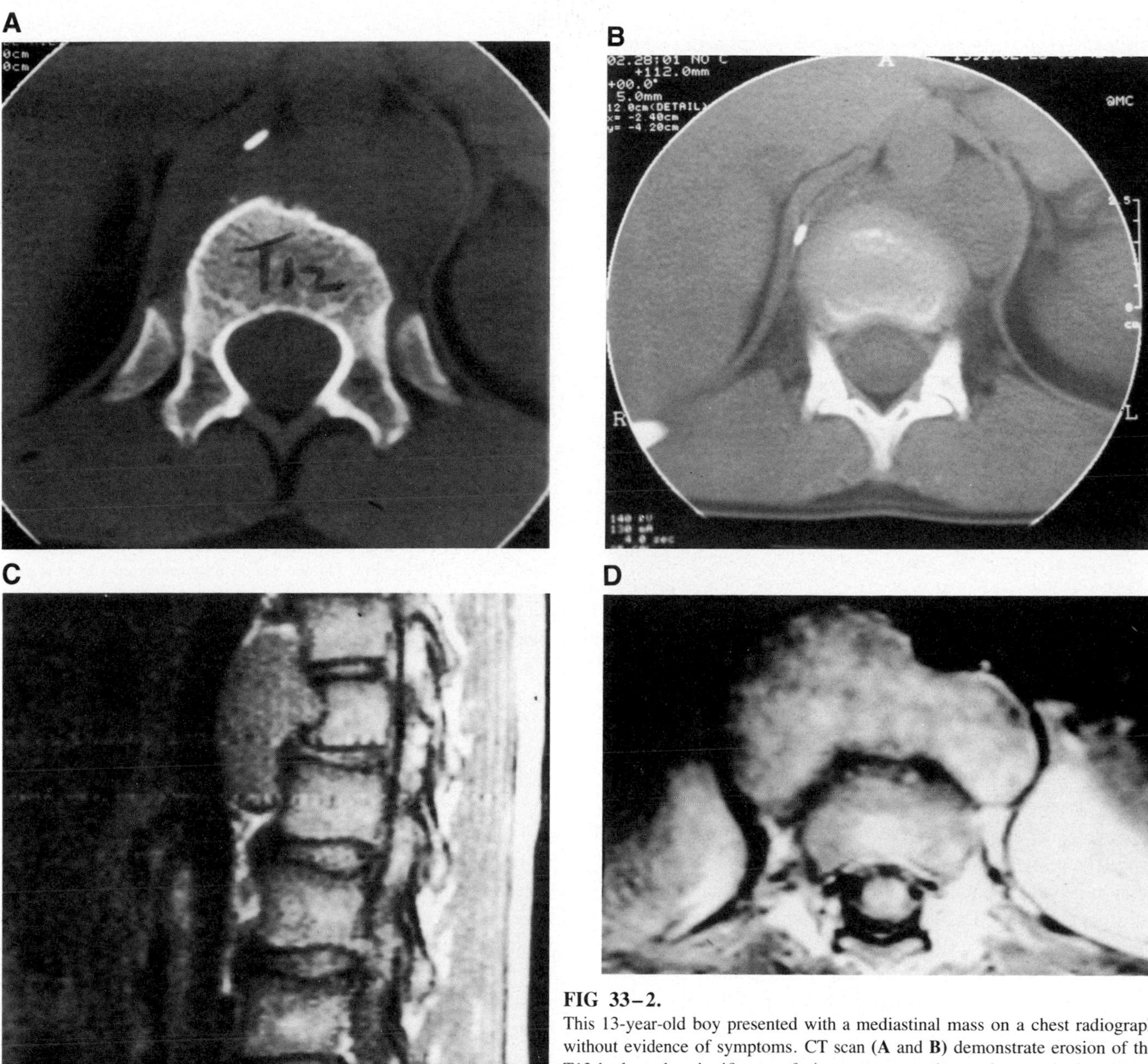

FIG 33–2.
This 13-year-old boy presented with a mediastinal mass on a chest radiograph without evidence of symptoms. CT scan (**A** and **B**) demonstrate erosion of the T12 body and a significant soft-tissue mass anterior to the vertebral body beneath the aorta. Sagittal MRI shows involvement of the T11, T12 and L1 vertebral bodies with a soft-tissue mass anteriorly (**C**). The axial view on MRI shows the full extent of the soft-tissue mass (**D**). The patient underwent an en bloc resection of T11, T12, and L1 through an anterior and posterior approach.

spine. As with other tumors of the spine, the delay in diagnosis may be significant, with a delay from the onset of symptoms to diagnosis of 8 to 10 months. Like other spinal tumors, the most common presenting symptom is pain, which may be accompanied by motor weakness and sensory loss as well as bowel and bladder dysfunction. Radiologic and laboratory findings are similar to other patients with Ewing's sarcomas, which include lysis of the bone and the adjacent soft-tissue mass. The patients will generally also have an elevated alkaline phosphatase level and elevated erythrocyte sedimentation rate (ESR), and some patients present with anemia.

Treatment for Ewing's sarcoma of the spine and sacrum is similar to treatment of any Ewing's sarcoma. The role of surgical treatment is as a part of a combined multimodality approach with radiation and chemotherapy. Similar problems occur with this tumor as with others in the spine in that a resection with free margins is difficult to achieve. The debulking and/or a decompressive laminectomy may be combined with radiation therapy and chemo-

A

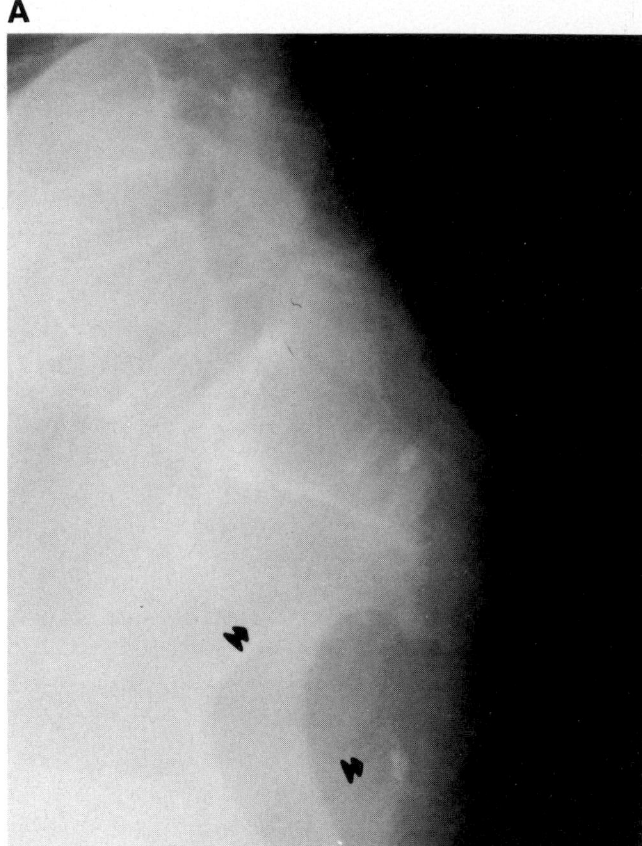

B

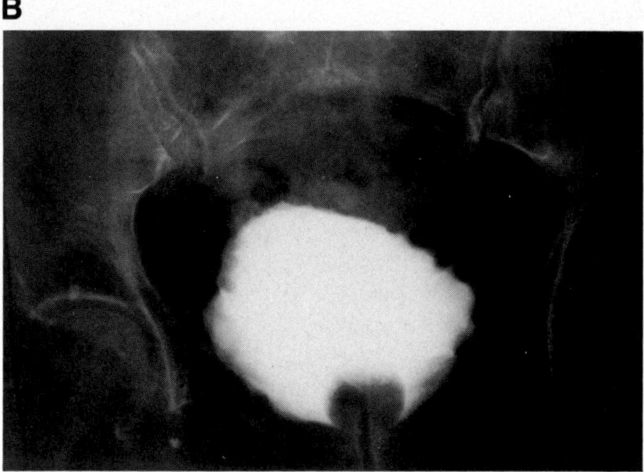

FIG 33–3.
This elderly woman presented with a large, painful mass in her sacrum and bowel and bladder dysfunction. On the lateral roentgenogram **(A)** note the large soft-tissue mass *(arrows)* and complete destruction of the distal end of the sacrum. The anteroposterior (AP) roentgenogram **(B)** during a cystogram shows impression of the dome of the bladder.

therapy, which are both effective with this tumor to achieve a satisfactory result. The combination of resection after cycles of chemotherapy to shrink the tumor may also provide a reasonable adjunct to treatment.[20, 41, 42, 47] The mean survival of patients with Ewing's sarcoma averages less than 5 years.[8] Debulking is not particularly effective. Therefore, currently the treatment of Ewing's sarcoma should be as complete a resection of the spinal lesion as possible in combination with radiation and chemotherapy.

Although involvement of the spine with multiple myeloma is the most common primary tumor, the occurrence of solitary plasmacytoma is not nearly as common. In the older age group, however, a solitary plasmacytoma can present as a lesion of the spine, often with accompanying neurologic deficit.[36] Overall, this presentation of plasma cell tumors represents about 3% of all plasma cell tumors. As with multiple myeloma, the disease is most frequently seen in men (3 to 1)[30] and in those over the age of 50 years.[66] The lesion is most frequently seen in the thoracic spine,[7, 11] with somewhat less frequency in the lumbar spine and seen very infrequently as a solitary lesion in the cervical spine. In the presence of a solitary plasmocytoma, it is not uncommon for these levels to be much lower than in patients with multiple myeloma. Patients most frequently present with back pain, and as a result of the age group, it is frequently mistaken for degenerative arthritis in the absence of radiographic changes. Even with collapse and fracture, the diagnosis may be mistaken for osteopenia and pathologic collapse secondary to osteopenia. Bone marrow specimens should be obtained to exclude the multiple myeloma form of the disease. The radiologic appearance is generally osteopenia and collapse (Fig 33–4). The lesion will frequently begin in a pedicle, with absence of the pedicle on the AP radiograph and significant involvement of the anterior column of the spine with subsequent collapse and the presence of a vertebra plana on a lateral roentgenogram. The lesion is infrequently seen primarily in the sacrum and may not be visible except on CT or MRI (Fig 33–5). Appropriate serum and urinary paraprotein studies should be performed. Evaluation of neural compression should be accomplished by the use of MRI.

Initially, treatment of solitary plasmocytomas is most frequently by radiation therapy.[38, 64] This treatment should be combined with appropriate decompression and stabilization as needed. Therefore, in the patient with an isolated plasmacytoma of the thoracic spine, pain, and minimal collapse, radiation therapy alone may be an adequate initial treatment modality. In the patient with neural compression and/or significant local kyphosis and instability, anterior decompression and stabilization are the preferred initial modality to restore stability (Fig 33–6). Should there be significant posterior element involvement as well,

A

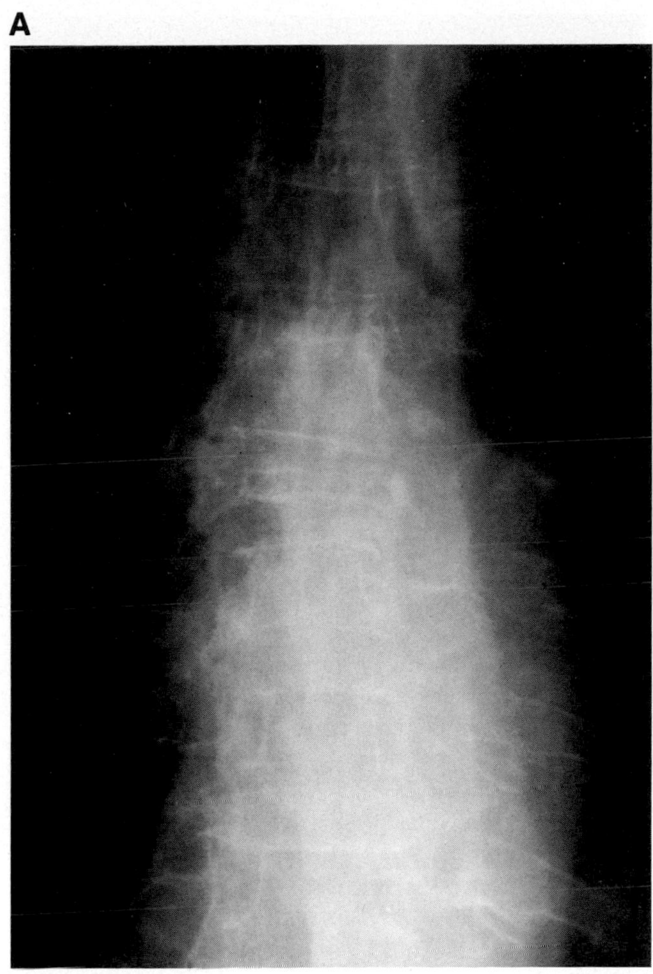

B

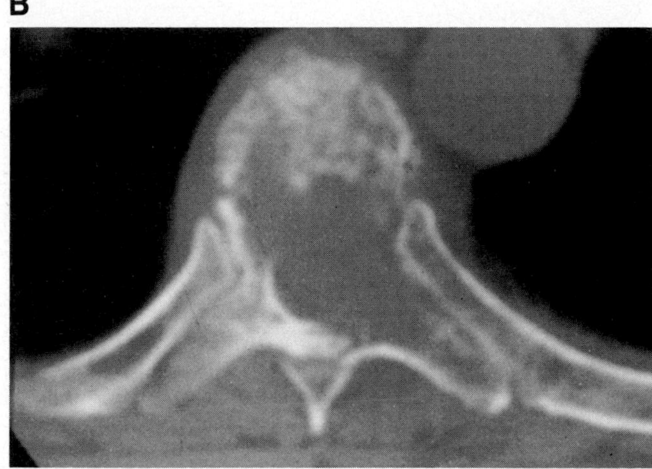

C

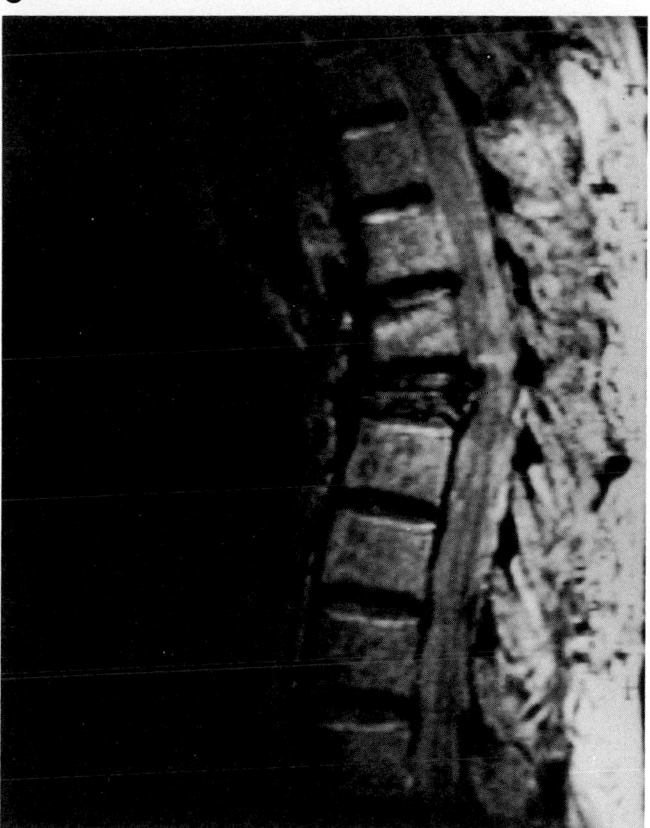

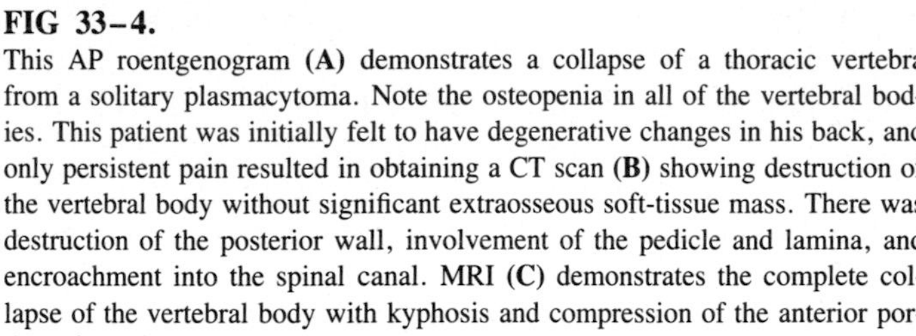

FIG 33–4.
This AP roentgenogram **(A)** demonstrates a collapse of a thoracic vertebra from a solitary plasmacytoma. Note the osteopenia in all of the vertebral bodies. This patient was initially felt to have degenerative changes in his back, and only persistent pain resulted in obtaining a CT scan **(B)** showing destruction of the vertebral body without significant extraosseous soft-tissue mass. There was destruction of the posterior wall, involvement of the pedicle and lamina, and encroachment into the spinal canal. MRI **(C)** demonstrates the complete collapse of the vertebral body with kyphosis and compression of the anterior portion of dural sac.

adjunctive posterior stabilization may frequently be necessary. This initial treatment should be followed by adjuvant radiation therapy to approximately 3500 cGy.[34] The role of adjuvant chemotherapy after the radiation and/or physical therapy intervention remains controversial. Poor prognostic factors for dissemination such as soft-tissue extension, spinal location, pleomorphism, and cellular immaturity may suggest the need for adjuvant chemotherapy. The prognosis for this lesion after treatment is related directly to its development as a precursor of multiple myeloma. Approximately 50% of patients will develop multiple myeloma,[5] but those who retain the solitary form of the disease have a satisfactory long-term survival. As stated previously, spinal location is a poor prognostic factor for the subsequent development of multiple myeloma.

Multiple myeloma (as differentiated from solitary plasmacytoma) occurs in the 50- to 75-year-old age group. The spine is almost universally involved, as are other hematopoietically active areas such as the ribs and pelvis. The treatment of spinal involvement of this type should be

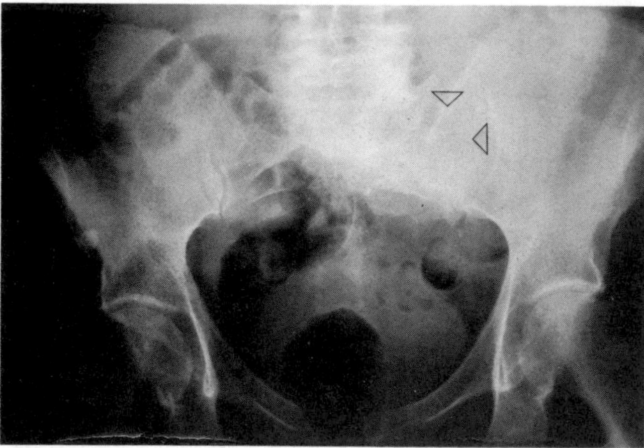

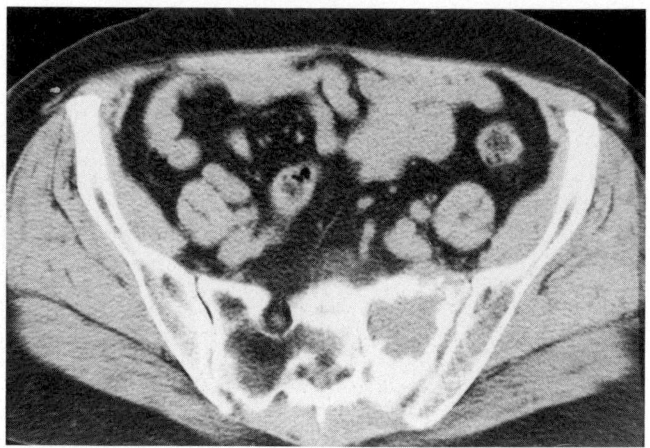

FIG 33–5.
This elderly white female presented with back pain radiating into her right leg. The AP roentgenogram (**A**) demonstrates only some osteopenia and a hint at destruction of the right sacral ala *(arrowheads)*. However, the CT scan (**B**) demonstrates significant destruction of the right sacral ala at S1, S2, and part of S3.

considered along with treatment of other areas of bone involvement. Unfortunately, because of the diffuse nature of the disease involving both the anterior and posterior elements, as well as multiple sequential elements and the universal appearance of osteopenia, many of the surgical modalities that are available for treating metastatic lesions are non-operative in patients with multiple myeloma and significant spinal involvement.

Isolated lymphoma of the spine is infrequent, as with other primary tumors of the spine. Skeletal lesions as a primary presentation of Hodgkin's disease are exceedingly rare, although in non-Hodgkin's lymphoma the bone lesion may either be a solitary focus of disease or may be associated with disseminated disease. Spinal involvement in lymphoma occurs most frequently as a manifestation of relapse, with approximately 3% of patients having spinal cord compression. However, approximately 13% of patients with lymphomas will have bony disease, although only approximately 1% present with skeletal lesions at initial presentation. In primary lymphomas of bone, there is a predilection for the axial skeleton. Approximately 15% of cases occur in the spine.[3, 16, 22, 26, 42, 54] Overall, the survival rate in Hodgkin's lymphoma involving bone is approximately 40% to 50%, but by 10 years it has decreased to approximately 30%. Bone lesions in non-Hodgkin's lymphoma are usually due to histiocytic or poorly differentiated disease rather than a lymphocytic or well-differentiated lymphoma. Patients frequently present with back pain and lumbar involvement in the older age group of 40 to 60 years. Involvement is usually most significant in the anterior column (Fig 33–7), with infrequent involvement in the posterior elements. In the Ann Arbor staging classification, the presence of primary or isolated bony involvement makes the patient automatically stage IV. In view of the marked sensitivity of lymphomas to both radiation and chemotherapy, the treatment is highly dependent on the initial presentation of the patient. If the presentation is an isolated spinal lesion with pain and no significant collapse or instability, needle biopsy followed by appropriate radiation and chemotherapy is the accepted mode of treatment. Additional surgical treatment is generally not necessary. Needle biopsy, however, may be insufficient in patients in whom the diagnosis of Hodgkin's lymphoma as opposed to non-Hodgkin's lymphoma is considered because the biopsy specimen may not be large enough to make a definitive diagnosis. In patients who present with significant du-

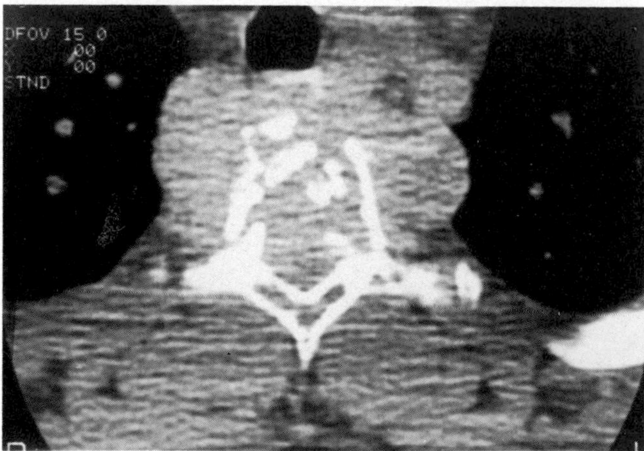

FIG 33–6.
This CT scan demonstrates a large soft-tissue mass associated with an isolated plasmacytoma of the thoracic spine. Note the complete destruction of the vertebral body and posterior wall with significant encroachment on the dural sac. However, the posterior elements are not involved. Anterior decompression and stabilization gave satisfactory relief of neurologic symptoms and stability.

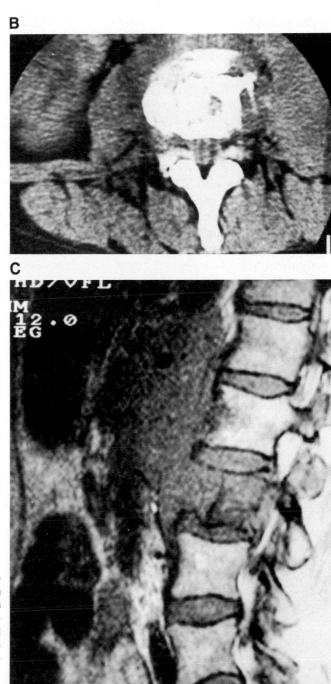

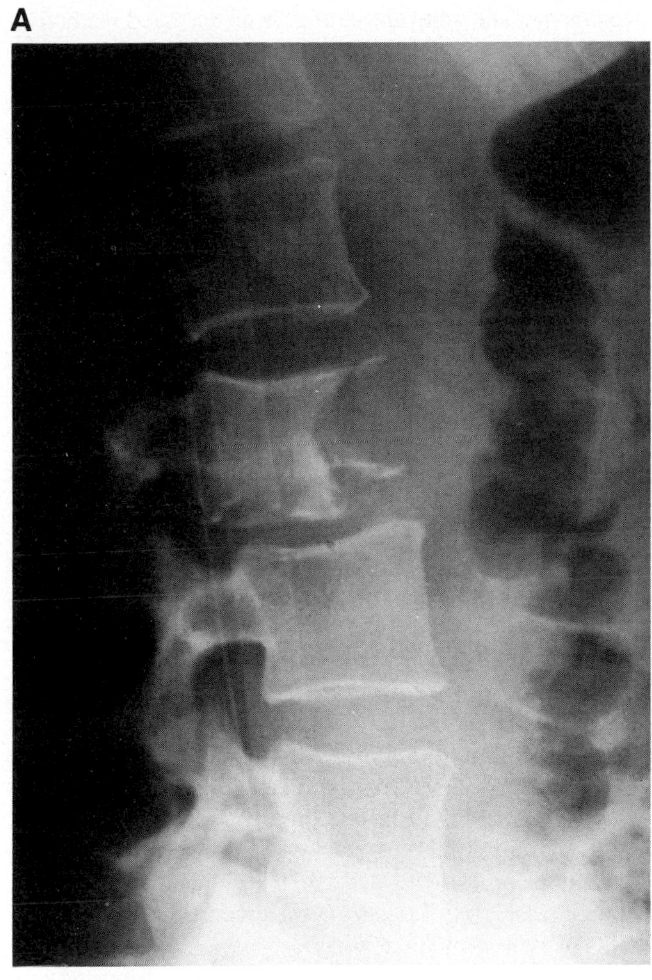

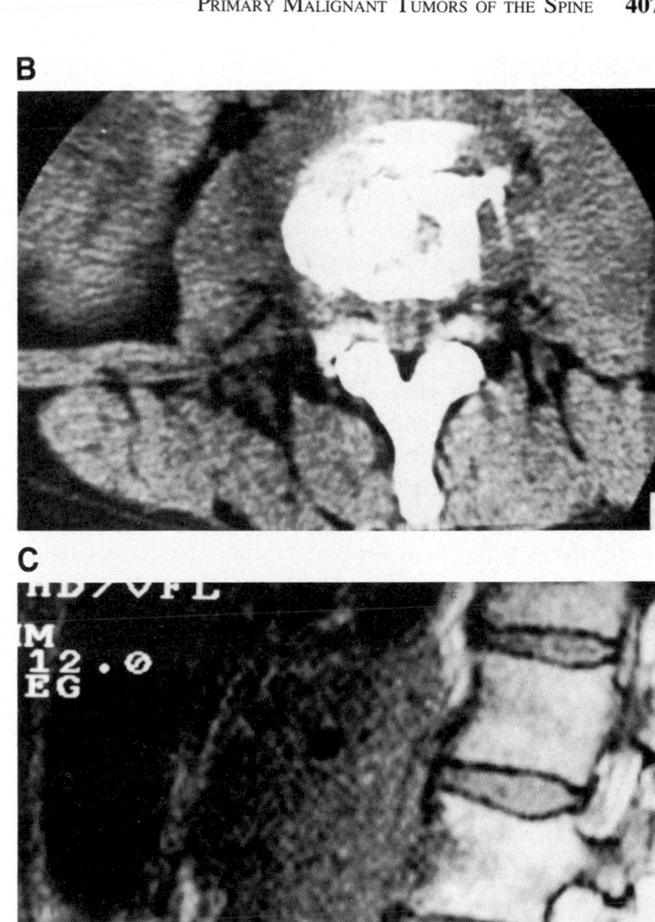

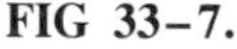

FIG 33–7.
This 54-year-old woman presented with a history of severe back pain and lower-extremity weakness. A lateral roentgenogram **(A)** demonstrates destruction of the L3 vertebra with a loss of height of the L3–4 disc space. The CT scan **(B)** demonstrates destruction of the vertebral body as well as a large surrounding soft-tissue mass. The remainder of her workup failed to reveal additional disease. The sagittal view on MRI **(C)** shows complete involvement of the L3 vertebral body anteriorly, with a large paraspinal mass extending approximately to the L1 level.

ral compression, massive destruction of the vertebral body and pedicles, and/or extension into the posterior elements, surgical intervention may be necessary for either decompression and/or stabilization (see Fig 33–5). Since the predominant involvement is anterior, direct anterior decompression with stabilization will give immediate improved neurologic function and restore stability. This can then be followed by posterior stabilization, if necessary, and radiation and chemotherapy. The role of surgical intervention is predominantly that of decompression and stabilization, as opposed to control of the disease. The current use of combinations, including surgery, radiation, and chemotherapy, may indeed drive the survival rate upward to 60% or 70%.[42]

SARCOMAS

All sarcomas of the spine are exceedingly infrequent as primary lesions. The most commonly seen are osteosarcoma and chondrosarcoma. Osteosarcoma in bone is the most common neoplasm with the exception of myelomas, as previously mentioned. Osteosarcomas of the spine can occur either as primary lesions[6, 53] or as secondary lesions after radiation therapy for other conditions.[17, 52] Overall, the incidence of osteosarcoma of the spine is approximately 1% to 2%.[53, 63] As with other spinal tumors, patients present with pain. This pain may be radiating and therefore deceiving, and the duration of symptoms prior to diagnosis can be extended.[53, 63] Approximately two thirds of the patients reported as either single case reports or in larger series have some degree of neurologic deficit, especially those with cervical involvement. The classic radiographic features seen in osteosarcoma of the long bones, such as Codman's triangle or periosteal elevation, are not as easily identified in the spine. The lesions involve the vertebral bodies primarily but may affect the pedicles and posterior elements as well and are generally osteoblastic in nature except in the presence of telangiectatic osteosarcomas (Fig 33–8). On CT and MRI the soft-tissue involvement of the lesions can be verified.[62] The evaluation of patients with spinal osteosarcoma is the same as for patients with osteosarcoma in any other more common area: bone scans to evaluate other areas of bone involvement and the extent of tumor and CT of the chest to evaluate for the presence or absence of metastatic disease. Prior to resection of the tumor, angiography and embolization may be useful both in determining the vascular supply as well as in decreasing the morbidity of the surgical procedure by excessive blood loss. Although chemotherapy, both in the neoadjuvant and adjuvant setting, is an accepted method of treatment of osteosarcoma, the overwhelming problem in osteosarcoma of the spine has been in achieving adequate margins for resection to eliminate recurrence.[6, 40] The same chemotherapeutic modalities of treatment should be used for osteosarcoma of the spine as for those of the extremities.[2, 4, 33, 46] In spite of the success of neoadjuvant and adjuvant chemotherapy in both the local and distant control of osteosarcoma of the extremities, the anatomy of the spine has limited the success for treatment in that area. Subtotal resection with positive margins has predictably resulted in recurrence of disease complicated by significant neurologic involvement and eventual demise of the patient. The goal is clearly an en bloc resection or complete spondylectomy, which may be technically feasible in the smaller tumor. Overall, there has been limited experience to date with this technique in the setting of neoadjuvant and adjuvant chemotherapy, so results are not yet encouraging. Due to the rarity of this disease, it takes many years to accumulate even a small series of patients on which to report. Over a period of six decades, Barwick et al. indentified 10 patients with the disease.[6] Their mean survival time was 6 months. Similarly, Shives et al. reported a mean survival of 10 months on a group of patients identified over a period of many years.[53] Preliminary results from Memorial Sloan-Kettering suggest that patients treated more recently may show an improved survival rate when it is possible to achieve resections that adhere to modern principles of treatment of sarcomas in combination with chemotherapy.[63]

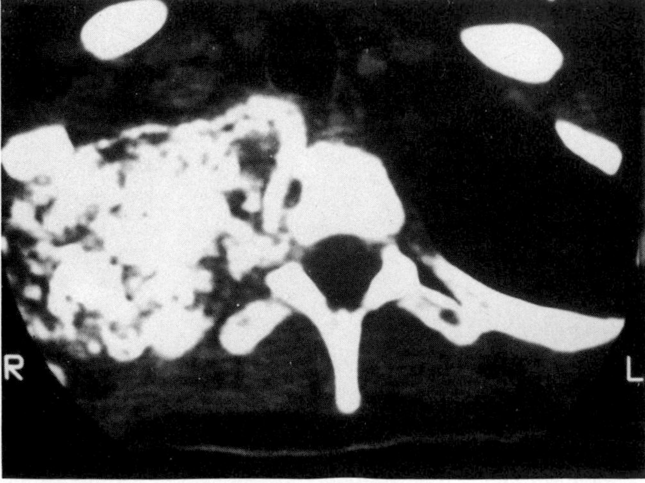

FIG 33–8.
This 18-year-old female presented with right shoulder pain. The diagnosis was delayed approximately 3 months because the source of the shoulder pain was not recognized to be this spinal osteosarcoma.

Overall, chondrosarcomas occur most frequently in the pelvis, femur, and humerus but may infrequently occur in the spine. They show a predilection for males and patients in the fifth and sixth decades of life. The appearance of chondrosarcomas radiographically is related in part to the grade of the lesion. Slowly growing grade I lesions may be extremely lobular, with calcification within the lesion. Grade III lesions are more pleomorphic, often with spotty calcification and significant destruction of the vertebral body. The lesions frequently occur at the costovertebral junction and are well seen on CT[48] (Fig 33–9). Occasionally, a pre-existing lesion from which malignant degeneration occurred may be evident. In large series, approximately 85% of all chondrosarcomas are primary, and 15% result from secondary malignant degeneration.[15] The distribution of chondrosarcomas in the spine is rather uniform, with relatively equal numbers in the cervical, thoracic, lumbar, and sacral areas.[9, 65]

Primary treatment of chondrosarcoma in all locations is surgical excision. The problems with chondrosarcoma in the spine are similar to other malignant tumors. Satisfactory oncologic margins, which generally require wide margins for resection of a high-grade chondrosarcoma and

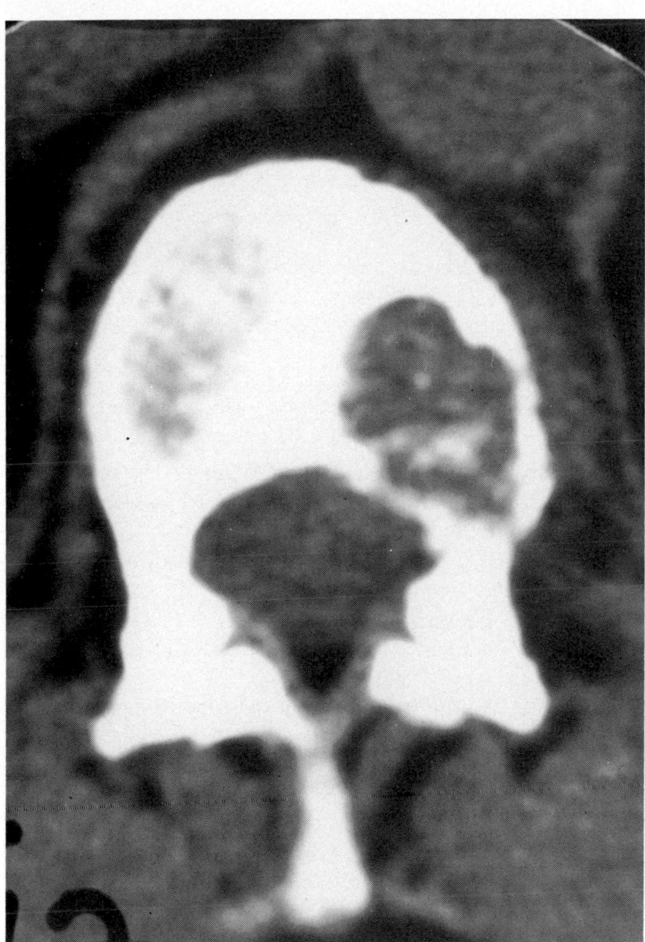

FIG 33–9.
This CT scan demonstrates a chondrosarcoma of T11 with destruction of the body adjacent to the pedicle and extension into the neural canal.

borderline margins for lower-grade lesions, may be difficult to obtain.[18] Because these lesions may surround critical vascular or neural structures, the tendency is to attempt to remove the lesion in an intralesional or piecemeal fashion, which results in a high recurrence rate that is unacceptable in higher-grade lesions. Total spondylectomy as described by Stenner[57] and as practiced by Roy-Camille et al.[51] may yield more satisfactory results. The type of reconstruction is dependent on the extent of involvement of the vertebral element and the necessity for total or subtotal spondylectomy. The use of cryosurgery has been previously reported and was recently reported for use with intralesional procedures in the spine and sacrum.[10] There have been no significant studies demonstrating the use of chemotherapy in this tumor, especially in lower-grade lesions. The use of radiation therapy is controversial, especially since the amount of radiation necessary for adequate treatment cannot be delivered to most regions of the spine. There is some suggestion that it might be of benefit, although high-grade lesions did relatively poorly.[23, 29, 59] Overall, the survival of patients with chondrosarcoma is highly dependent on grade. Those patients with lower-grade lesions have far better survival, both as regards no evidence of disease (NED) and alive with disease (AWD), than those patients with high-grade lesions.

SUMMARY

Although advances have been made in the treatment of malignant tumors of bone with the use of combined multimodality treatment incorporating surgery, radiation, and chemotherapy, these benefits have not translated directly to spinal lesions. As a result of the relative tolerance of the sacrum to large lesions and the delayed diagnosis in patients with spinal lesions, often these lesions are quite large at the time of presentation for treatment. This limits the role of surgery since wide margins or even borderline margins cannot be easily achieved because of the involvement and proximity of vascular and neural structures. In addition, especially in the spine, the role of radiation is severely limited to less than 4000 cGy because of direct radiation toxicity to the spinal cord. Since many of these malignant tumors require radiation doses in the region of 6000 cGy, the optimal doses cannot be delivered. Thus, overall, primary malignant tumors of the spine are infrequent but still remain devastating and difficult lesions to control.

REFERENCES

1. Ariel IM, Verden C: Chordoma: An analysis of 20 cases treated over a 20 year period. *J Surg Oncol* 1975; 7:27–44.
2. Bacci G, Gherlinzoni F, Picci P, et al: Adriamycin-methotrexate high dose vs. Adriamycin-methotrexate moderate dose as adjuvant chemotherapy for osteosarcoma of the extremities: A random study. *Eur J Cancer Clin Oncol* 1986; 22:1337.
3. Bacci G, Jaffe N, Emilini E, et al: Staging, therapy and prognosis of primary non-Hodgkin's lymphoma of bone and comparison of results with localized Ewing's sarcoma: A 10 year experience at the Istituto Ortopedico Rizzoli. *Tumori* 1985; 71:345–354.
4. Bacci G, Picci P, Pignati G: Neoadjuvant chemotherapy for non-metastatic osteosarcoma of the extremities. *Clin Orthop* 1991; 270:87–98.
5. Bacci G, Savini R, Calderoni P, et al: Solitary plasmacytoma of the vertebral column: A report of 15 cases. *Tumori* 1982; 68:271–275.
6. Barwick KW, Huvos AG, Smith J: Primary osteosarcoma of the vertebral column: A clinical pathological correlation of 10 patients. *Cancer* 1980; 46:595–604.
7. Bataille R, Sany J: Solitary myeloma—Clinical and prognostic features: A review of 114 cases. *Cancer* 1981; 48:845–851.
8. Brodway JK, Pritchard DJ: Ewing's tumor of the spine. *Orthop Trans* 1988; 12:746.
9. Camins MB, Duncan AW, Smith J, et al: Chondrosarcoma of the spine. *Spine* 1978; 3:202–209.

10. Camissa F, Glasser D, Lane J, et al: Chondrosarcoma of the spine and sacrum. *Orthop Trans* 1987; 11:578.
11. Chak LY, Cox RS, Bostwick KDG, et al: Solitary plasmacytomas of bone: Treatment, progression and survival. *J Clin Oncol* 1987; 5:1811–1815.
12. Cummings BJ, Esses S, Harwood ARL: The treatment of chordoma. *Cancer Treat Rev* 1982; 9:299–311.
13. Cummings BJ, Hodson DI, Bush RS: Chordoma: The results of megavolt radiation therapy. *Int J Radiat Oncol Biol Phys* 1983; 9:633–642.
14. Dahlin DC, McCarty CS: Chordoma: A study of 59 cases. *Cancer* 1952; 5:1170–1178.
15. Dahlin DC, Unni KK: *Bone Tumors: General Aspects and Data on 8,542 Cases,* ed 4. Springfield, Ill, Charles C Thomas, 1986.
16. Dosoretz D, Raymond K, Murphy G, et al: Primary lymphoma of bone: The relationship of morphologic diversity to clinical behavior. *Cancer* 1982; 50:1009–1019.
17. Dowdle JA, Winter RB, Deaner LP: Post-radiation osteosarcoma of the cervical spine in childhood. *J Bone Joint Surg [Am]* 1977; 59:969–971.
18. Erikson AI, Schiller A, Mankin HJ: The management of chondrosarcoma of bone. *Clin Orthop* 1980; 153:44–66.
19. Erikson B, Gutenberg B, Kindblom LG: Chordoma: A clinical pathologic and prognostic study of Swedish National Services. *Acta Orthop Scand* 1952; 52:49–58.
20. Evans R, Nesbit M, Askin F, et al: Local recurrence rate and site of metastases and time to relapse as a function of treatment regimen, size of primary and surgical history in 62 patients presenting with non-metastatic Ewing's sarcoma of the pelvic bones. *Int J Radiat Oncol Biol Phys* 1985; 11:129–136.
21. Falk KS, Alpert M: A 5 year survival of patients with Ewing's sarcoma. *Surg Gynecol Obstet* 1967; 1224:319–324.
22. Friedman M, Kim TH, Panahon AM: Spinal cord compression in malignant lymphoma: Treatment results. *Cancer* 1976; 37:1485–1491.
23. Harwood AR, Krajbich JI, Fornasier VL: Radiotherapy of chondrosarcoma of bone. *Cancer* 1980; 45:2769–2777.
24. Healy JH, Lane JM: Chordoma: A critical review of diagnosis and treatment. *Orthop Clin North Am* 1989; 10:417.
25. Higginbotham NL, Phillips RF, Farr HW, et al: Chordoma: A 35 year study at Memorial Hospital. *Cancer* 1967; 20:1841–1850.
26. Horan FT: Bone involvement in Hodgkin's disease: A survey of 201 cases. *Br J Surg* 1969; 56:277–281.
27. Kaiser TE, Prichard DJ, Unni KK: Clinical pathologic studies of sacro-coccygeal chordoma. *Cancer* 1984; 54:2574–2578.
28. Kibins NP, Noonan KJ, Weinstein JN: Chordoma of the lumbar spine: Surgical approach and rationale. *Contemp Orthop* 1991; 22:163–172.
29. Kim RY, Salter MM, Brascho DJ: High energy radiation and the management of chondrosarcoma. *South Med J* 1987; 76:729–731.
30. Knowling MA, Harwood AR, Bergsagal DE: Comparison of extramedullary plasmacytomas with solitary and multiple plasma cell tumors of bone. *J Clin Oncol* 1983; 1:255–262.
31. Krol G, Sundaresan N, Deck MDF: Computer tomography of axial chordomas. *J Comput Assist Tomogr* 1983; 7:286–289.
32. Levine AM, Donati D, Bertoni F: Chordomas of the spine. Presented at the Scoliosis Research Society, Kansas City, September 1992.
33. Link MP, Goarin AM, Horowitz M: Adjuvant chemotherapy of high grade osteosarcoma of the extremity: Updated results of a multi-institutional osteosarcoma study. *Clin Orthop* 1991; 270:8–14.
34. Lucantani D, Galzio R, Zenobi M, et al: Spinal cord compression by solitary plasmacytoma. *J Neurosurg Sci* 1983; 27:125–127.
35. McCarty CS, Waugh JM, Mayo CW, et al: The surgical treatment of pre-sacral tumor: A combined problem. *Mayo Clin Proc* 1952; 27:73–84.
36. McClain RF, Weinstein JN: Solitary plasmacytoma of the spine. *Orthop Trans* 1988; 12:528.
37. Meyer JE, Lepkera RA, Lyndfors KK, et al: Chordoma: Their CT appearance in the cervical, thoracic and lumbar spine. *Radiology* 1984; 153:693.
38. Mill WB, Griffith R: The role of radiation therapy in the management of plasma cell tumors. *Cancer* 1980; 45:647–652.
39. Mindell ER: Chordoma. *J Bone Joint Surg [Am]* 1981; 63:501–505.
40. Patel DV, Hammer RA, Levin V, et al: Primary osteosarcoma of the spine. *Skeletal Radiol* 1984; 12:276–279.
41. Perez CA, Tefft M, Nesbit MEJ Jr, et al: Radiation therapy in the multi-modal management of Ewing's sarcoma of the bone: A report of the intergroup Ewing's sarcoma study. *Natl Cancer Inst Monogr* 1981; 56:263–271.
42. Portlock C: Non-Hodgkin's lymphomas: Advances in diagnosis, staging and management. *Cancer* 1992; 65:718–722.
43. Pritchard DJ: Surgical experience of Ewing's sarcoma of bone. *Natl Cancer Inst Monogr* 1981; 56:169–171.
44. Pritchard DJ, Dahlin DC, Dauphine RT: Ewing's sarcoma: A clinical pathological statistical analysis of patients surviving 5 years or longer. *J Bone Joint Surg [Am]* 1975; 57:10.
45. Resnick CS, Young JW, Levine AM, et al: Metastatic chordoma. *Skeletal Radiol* 1989; 18:303–305.
46. Rosen G: Preoperative chemotherapy (neoadjuvant for osteosarcoma): A 10 year experience. *Orthopedics* 1985; 8:659.
47. Rosen G, Caparros B, Nirenberg A, et al: Ewing's sarcoma: A 10 year experience with adjuvant chemotherapy. *Cancer* 1981; 47:2204–2213.
48. Rosenthal D, Shiller AL, Mankin HJ: Chondrosarcoma: Correlation of radiological and histological grade. *Radiology* 1984; 150:21.
49. Rosenthal DI, Scott JA, Mahkin HJ, et al: Sacro-coccygeal chordomas: Magnetic resonance imaging and computed tomography. *Am J Radiol* 1985; 145:143–147.
50. Roy-Camille R, Mazel C: Vertebrectomy through an enlarged posterior approach for tumors and malunion, in Brid-

well K, DeWald R (eds): *Textbook of Spinal Surgery*. Philadelphia, JB Lippincott, 1991, pp 1243–1256.

51. Roy-Camille R, Saillent G, Gagna T, et al: Chondrosarcoma of the spine: Ten cases treated surgically. *Orthop Trans* 1988; 12:201.
52. Shiden R, Oberthaler W: Radiation-induced osteosarcoma of the sacrum following radiation of an undiagnosed bone lesion. *Acta Orthop Trauma Surg* 1987; 102:128–130.
53. Shives TC, Dahlin DC, Sim FH, et al: Osteosarcoma of the spine. *J Bone Joint Surg [Am]* 1986; 68:660–668.
54. Silverberger IJ, Jacobs EM: Treatment of spinal cord compression in Hodgkin's disease. *Cancer* 1971; 27:308–313.
55. Smith J, Ludwig RL, Marcove RC: Clinical radiographic features of chordoma. *Skeletal Radiol* 1987; 16:37–44.
56. Stenner B: Complete removal of vertebra for extirpation of tumors: A 20 year experience. *Clin Orthop* 1989; 245:72–82.
57. Stenner B: Total spondylectomy in chondrosarcoma arising from the 7th thoracic vertebra. *J Bone Joint Surg [Br]* 1971; 53:288.
58. Stenner B, Gutenberg B: High amputation of the sacrum for extirpation of tumors: Principles and techniques. *Spine* 1978; 3:351–366.
59. Suit HD, Goitein M, Munzenrider J, et al: Definitive radiation therapy for chordoma and chondrosarcoma of the base of the skull and cervical spine. *J Neurosurg* 1982; 56:377–385.
60. Sundaresan N, Galicich JH, Chu FC, et al: Spinal chordomas. *Neurosurgery* 1979; 50:312.
61. Sundaresan M, Huvos AG, Krol G, et al: Spinal chordomas: Results of surgical treatment. *Arch Surg* 1989; 122:1478–1482.
62. Sundaresan M, McGuire MH, Herbold D: Magnetic resonance imaging of osteosarcoma. *Skeletal Radiol* 1987; 16:23–29.
63. Sundaresan N, Rosen G, Huvos AG, et al: Combined modality treatment of osteosarcoma of the spine. *Neurosurgery* 1988; 23:714–719.
64. Tony D, Griffin DW, Larrimore G, et al: Solitary plasmacytomas of bone and soft tissues. *Radiology* 1980; 135:195–198.
65. Torma F: Malignant tumors of the spine and spinal extradural space: A study based on 250 histologically verified cases. *Acta Chir Scand Suppl* 1987; 225:176.
66. Wiltshaw E: The natural history of extramedullary plasmacytoma and its relation to solitary myeloma of bone and myelomatosis. *Medicine (Baltimore)* 1976; 55:217–238.
67. Wold LE, Laws ER Jr: Cranial chordomas in children and young adults. *J Neurosurg* 1983; 59:1043–1047.

34

Metastatic Spinal Tumors

Neil A. Schechter, M.D.

Metastatic tumors are the most common of all bone tumors, with the spinal column being the primary site of skeletal involvement.[17, 39] The axial skeleton ranks third among sites of metastatic disease, after the lung and liver, with the lumbar spine constituting the vast majority.[3, 6, 8, 9, 33] As many as 70% of patients with cancer will have evidence of spinal metastases at the time of their death.[39] It has been estimated that 10% to 40% of patients with cancer present initially with spinal involvement.[14, 68, 69] Approximately 5% of cancer patients will develop neurologic deficits attributable to spinal deposits.[8] A similar percentage will exhibit epidural metastases at autopsy.[3]

The majority of metastatic spinal tumors originate in the vertebral body, with the posterior structures involved less often.[39, 77] The principal tumors involving the spine originate in the breast, lung, thyroid, kidney, prostate, and the hematopoietic system.[8, 30, 58, 68]

The actual incidence of vertebral spread in metastatic disease is difficult to detect by plain roentgenographic evaluation. There must be destruction of 30% to 50% of the vertebral body before changes become apparent.[25]

PATHOPHYSIOLOGY

The primary route of tumor spread to the spine or paraspinous tissues is hematogenous. The description of a thin-walled, valveless paravertebral venous plexus by Batson greatly improved the understanding of the dissemination of spinal metastases.[4] Through these vessels, in accordance with the venous drainage of various organ systems, tumor emboli may deposit and proliferate in the vertebrae. Another factor that probably contributes to the predominance of spinal metastases is that vertebral bodies maintain their active red bone marrow throughout life. The adult peripheral skeleton, in contrast, has a relatively avascular yellow marrow. Red marrow, with its vast vascular sinusoidal system, is presumed to be a better milieu for the establishment of tumor growth.[9, 33] The production of degradative enzymes and humoral factors may play a role in the enhancement of metastatic growth in the spinal column.[27, 29] Other theories for the propensity of metastases in the spine include the "seed-and-soil" hypothesis[55] of variable organ susceptibilities to tumor growth, the tenuous medullary vasculature of bone permitting easier penetration by tumor cells and promoting extravasation,[77] and the concept of chemotactic migration of tumor cells to their target site.[44]

CLINICAL PRESENTATION

Patients with metastatic disease of the spine occasionally remain asymptomatic. When clinical symptoms do arise, they are most often a result of one or more of the following: extension of the tumor mass beyond the vertebral cortex with invasion of the local soft tissues, compression or infiltration of the nearby nerve roots, pathologic fracture, development of spinal instability secondary to destruction of anterior and/or posterior elements, or spinal cord compression.[33]

The most frequent presenting symptom of vertebral metastases is pain.[8] In the early stages the pain may be well localized and insidious in its onset. Symptoms may be reproduced by percussion over that particular area. With time, the pain progressively worsens and becomes more diffuse and unrelenting. Incapacitating night pain is often seen and is characteristic of tumor involvement.

With progression of the disease, radicular pain may occur. This is often observed with lumbar or cervical metastases. The location of the tumor may be discerned by the anatomic distribution of the radiculopathy. However, one must also be cautioned that similar symptoms may be seen in patients with disc herniation,[64] which may lead to diagnostic and therapeutic errors. Radicular pain may also portend future development of thoracic cord compression.[34]

Some diagnostic delay may occur when pain is referred to other nonspecific areas. Also, patients with no suspicion of malignancy or incomplete radiologic assessment may cause errors in diagnosis. Early diagnosis of pain secondary to cancer is important since the outcome is improved if the neurologic status remains intact before treatment is undertaken.[57]

Neurologic deficits are rarely the presenting symptoms but are observed frequently in patients with metastatic tumors. Motor deficits will precede sensory loss when anterior cord compression from vertebral body lesions occurs. The incidence of cord compression is reported to be approximately 5%.[3, 14] If unrecognized or if prompt intervention is delayed, progressive and permanent loss of cord function may ensue. Spinal cord compression may be caused by direct pressure from an extruded tumor mass or retropulsed bony fragment, severe angularity deformity after bony collapse, or direct cord or root compression from intradural metastases.[9] Various studies have found that intradural metastases are rarely a source of neurologic symptoms (fewer than 5%).[3, 9, 14] The dura appears to act as an effective deterrent to invading tumor cells.

The rapid progression of muscle weakness is a poor prognostic indicator. The acute onset of paraplegia and a complete deficit before treatment is initiated points toward a poor prognosis for recovery.[10, 32] When the time elapsed from the onset of symptoms and the manifestation of a complete neurologic deficit is less than 24 to 48 hours, the results of treatment are dismal with regard to recovery. On the other hand, those with a more gradual development of neurologic deficits have a more favorable outcome.[33] Approximately 30% of patients will reach a maximal neurologic deficit level in less than 48 hours, while 90% will attain their peak loss in 10 days or less.[63] Rapid deterioration of neurologic function is most commonly seen in thoracic vertebral lesions. This may be a reflection of its tenuous vascular supply as well as the cord-canal ratio. Dysfunction of the bowel and bladder is a late finding. This phenomena usually occurs in patients with major neurologic deficits.[54] In rare situations of conus involvement, isolated loss of sphincter control may occur.[14]

The importance of a thorough history and neurologic assessment cannot be overemphasized because these can help the clinician pinpoint the area of the spinal lesion as well as plan an appropriate diagnostic workup and treatment protocol.

DIAGNOSTIC STUDIES

In order to evaluate a patient with suspected metastatic disease various radiographic studies may be employed. Plain radiographs are usually the initial modality selected. These may aid in delineating the extent and progression of vertebral collapse, local bone reaction to the tumor, pedicle destruction, and abnormal spinal alignment. They are not of value in the earliest phases of destruction and unmask lesions in only 60% of patients with metastases.[63]

Radionuclide bone scanning remains an extremely sensitive test for the detection of spinal tumors.[12, 28, 50] This procedure reveals metastases in more than 95% of cases.[63] In many cases, bone scintigraphy reveals osseous lesions even before patients become symptomatic and may predate plain radiographic changes by 3 to 18 months.[28] Galasko reported that 30% to 50% of tumors detected by scintigraphy are not seen on plain x-ray films.[28] The extent of metastatic spread, i.e., multiple skeletal sites, is also documented well by bone scans. The limitation of this modality lies in its nonspecificity. Fractures secondary to either osteoporosis or trauma, infection, or extensive arthritis may present with findings on bone scans indistinguishable from metastatic disease.[12, 15] False-negative scans may occur in cases of myeloma and thyroid metastases.[40] Radiographs and bone scans are useful as screening and staging tools to provide an overall picture of metastatic involvement.

Myelography is a valuable tool in the diagnosis of epidural metastases and cord compression. The extent of intraspinal disease causing neurologic compromise can be appreciated. Spinal fluid evaluation at the time of puncture may be helpful in suggesting a diagnosis of intraspinal tumor.[37] Unfortunately, myelography is not without its inherent risks. There is a possibility of neurologic deterioration after a lumbar puncture in patients with a complete block.[38] Since the advent of computed tomography (CT) and magnetic resonance imaging (MRI), the indications for myelography have decreased greatly because these noninvasive studies adequately visualize the subarachnoid space and extent of tumor extension.

CT provides greater detail in assessing early bony compromise and soft-tissue extension of the tumor. It is useful in the preoperative planning stages to determine the appropriate surgical approach and the extent of tumor resection. Assessment of spinal canal impingement by tumor can be easily accomplished from CT scans.[24, 56] A disadvantage of this study is the potential failure to visualize a noncontiguous, distant site of involvement.

MRI provides a substantial alternative to standard radiologic assessment, is well tolerated, noninvasive, and readily available. It has proved to be superior for evaluating the soft-tissue extent of a lesion. Its ability to obtain high-quality multiplanar reformations and define areas of extradural compression has been appreciated. MRI may be better than CT and comparable to contrast-enhanced CT in visualizing canal compromise, soft-tissue spread, and bone and vascular infiltration by spinal tumors.[5] A recent study reported a sensitivity of 93%, a specificity of 97%, and an overall accuracy of 95% in the evaluation of metastatic spinal tumors by MRI.[46] In a study of patients with normal plain radiographs, CT, and bone scans, MRI revealed early evidence of metastatic disease in approximately 50% of cases.[1] Gadolinium-enhanced MRI has aided in the differentiation of tumor vs. disc herniation and intramedullary vs. extramedullary disease and aids in following the tumor response to treatment.[72, 73]

Arteriography is employed primarily in evaluating hypervascular tumors such as renal metastases. It can determine vascular anatomy and allow for preoperative embolization to reduce blood loss during surgery.[11, 70]

The final and most definitive of the diagnostic techniques for identifying a tumor is biopsy. The primary role for microscopic analysis is the confirmation of metastatic disease that cannot be traced back to a known primary tumor. It may also assist in planning various treatment protocols. For metastatic disease, biopsies may be performed by either open (incisional) or closed (percutaneously) means.

Percutaneous needle biopsy performed with CT or fluoroscopic guidance is useful in cases of primarily lytic lesions when the differential diagnosis is such that the tumors are easily distinguished by histologic evaluation.[9] One drawback of this technique is that the quantity of specimen may be insufficient to make a definitive diagnosis. Open biopsy is reserved for cases where inadequate material is obtained from closed biopsy and a definitive surgical resection is planned. An adequate amount of tissue should be taken for appropriate histologic and immunologic analysis.

TREATMENT PRINCIPLES

After the diagnosis of vertebral malignancy has been established, a specific treatment protocol must be determined. Patient management must be individualized based on tumor type, extent of disease, the patient's overall medical condition, life expectancy, neurologic impairment, and spinal stability. It must be understood that treatment is palliative and its purpose is to reduce pain, preserve or restore stability, and maintain or improve neurologic function.

Prognostic factors for outcome include the rate and extent of neurologic demise, the nature of the primary tumor, the presence of a complete myelographic block, and the response to steroid treatment.[2, 74] Breast and prostate metastases to bone generally have a good prognosis.[36, 51] Patients with lung tumors have a relatively poor outcome,[61] while the outlook for patients with renal or thyroid tumors is more variable.[20, 31, 52]

Nonoperative Treatment

Most patients with metastases can be treated nonoperatively.[34] In this era of chemotherapy, radiation, and hormonal manipulation, many patients can survive for years with metastatic spinal tumors without further dissemination of the disease. There is some support for prophylactic spinal fixation for lesions occupying more than 50% of the vertebral body.[22] Others have felt that this approach is too aggressive and associated with significant operative risks.[34] The majority of patients do not present with progressive instability or neurologic impairment and can be managed with nonoperative modalities.

Harrington has devised a useful classification scheme for spinal metastases.[33] There are five categories based upon the extent of neurologic deficit or bony involvement:

- Class I—no significant neurologic compromise
- Class II—bone involvement without collapse or instability
- Class III—major neurologic impairment without bony destruction
- Class IV—pain secondary to vertebral collapse and/or instability but intact neurologically
- Class V—bony collapse and instability and major neurologic deficit.

In general, patients in class I or II, with basically intact neurologic function and vertebral structure, obtain some pain relief with nonoperative modalities. Class III patients, who have neurologic impairment without instability, often respond to radiation alone. Patients in classes IV and V usually require surgical intervention.

Chemotherapy and Hormonal Manipulation

In patients with evidence of metastases without vertebral collapse, hormonal manipulation and chemotherapy are advocated to halt the pain progression and the threat of neurologic compromise if the process is left unimpeded.

Hormonal therapy is useful for metastatic breast and prostate carcinoma.[19, 45] It is important at the time of biopsy or surgery of breast metastases to obtain tissue for estrogen receptor (ER) assay. Those patients ER-positive will usually respond to hormonal suppression, while those who are ER-negative are less likely to benefit from hormonal treatment. Spinal lesions of prostatic origin usually respond well to hormonal therapy for at least a short time.

Chemotherapy has been utilized effectively in the treatment of metastatic spinal tumors.[7] There does not appear to be any beneficial consequence of chemotherapy in terms of reestablishing the integrity of bone destroyed by tumor. With breast cancer, the overall survival for patients treated with chemotherapy is greater than for those with untreated disease.[18] Patients with bone marrow spread will often experience significant relief after chemotherapy is introduced. This is most likely why mitigation of symptoms is noted in patients with spinal metastases, even though bony consolidation is absent. Because of the extensive benefits of pain amelioration and increased survival, early chemotherapeutic trials should be instituted for susceptible tumors.[34]

During the course of chemotherapy, one must continue to monitor the patient for pain response. If spinal pain increases, one must consider the possibility of pathologic fracture with vertebral collapse or cord compromise as the cause of such symptoms. It is not appropriate to apply more aggressive chemotherapy protocols in these circumstances. Once the decision to operate is made, bone marrow suppression by the chemotherapeutic drugs may make such intervention impossible.[22] Also, some agents may interfere with bone graft incorporation. Therefore, once operative treatment is considered, chemotherapy may need to be discontinued to provide the best possible results from surgery.

Within the realm of chemotherapy is the use of corticosteroids. In patients with cord compression, steroid therapy is beneficial.[21] Round-cell tumors are also effectively treated with steroids. There does not appear to be any advantage to high-dose steroids over conventional doses.[21] It is important to use steroids appropriately and taper their use as rapidly as possible to maintain efficacy without sustaining deleterious side effects.

Radiotherapy

The use of local irradiation therapy for a spinal tumor with or without operative intervention is controversial. In the past, laminectomy and decompression were performed, but pain relief was poor, and neurologic deterioration ensued.[8, 15, 32] In 1978, Gilbert et al. reported that radiation alone was as effective as laminectomy plus radiation in patients with epidural compression.[30] With either technique, the ability to walk was achieved in fewer than 50% of patients. More pain relief and a lower rate of progressive spinal deformity was achieved with radiotherapy alone.

If metastases are associated with minimal bone destruction but significant pain, radiotherapy is usually effective in providing relief. Patients with disseminated disease can be successfully managed by radiotherapy, in lieu of multilevel decompression. However, when mechanical compression of the cord occurs by bone, ligament, or disc after vertebral collapse, radiotherapy will not be effective in relieving pain. In this situation, operative decompression is indicated.

When radiotherapy is undertaken, its associated complications need to be considered. Radiation myelopathy,[23] osteitis,[34] wound breakdown,[47] and interference with bone graft incorporation are major concerns of the spine surgeon. In order to prevent these potential complications, a dose limitation of 3000 to 5000 cGy is recommended.[34, 76] It is suggested that radiotherapy be delayed for 3 to 4 weeks postoperatively to prevent problems with graft solidification and wound healing. Prior radiation treatment may also increase subsequent surgical morbidity.[48]

The outcome of patients treated with radiation is dependent upon radiosensitivity and neurologic status. Radiosensitive tumors include those of the breast, lymphoreticular system, and prostate. Renal, lung, and thyroid tumors are usually radioresistant. Up to half of patients improve and can ambulate after treatment.[65] While 30% to 40% of nonambulatory patients and 70% of those previously ambulatory will attain the ability to walk following radiotherapy, few frank paraplegics will ambulate again.[75] In terms of pain relief, 80% will have some amelioration, and 50% experience complete relief.[59]

Primary radiotherapy is indicated in the treatment of spinal cord compression.[30, 71] Patients with a history of metastatic cancer presenting with increasing back and neural deficits must be evaluated promptly for cord compression. Those with signs of myelopathy should be administered steroids, obtain proper diagnostic radiographs, and be evaluated by a radiation oncologist. Once the diagnosis is confirmed, radiotherapy should be initiated immediately. In cases of uncertain diagnosis, instability, or previous maximal-dose radiation exposure, surgical decompression should be done before radiotherapy.

Bracing

Treating patients with pathologic thoracic or lumbar fractures secondary to metastases may be similar to treating those with compression fractures secondary to osteoporosis. The initial conservative modalities consisting of bed rest and bracing are initiated. The goal is to immobilize the painful segment(s) while awaiting healing and stabilization of the collapsed vertebrae to occur. The best orthosis is one that is lightweight, easy to wear, and comfortable. A hyperextension, dorsolumbar, or a custom-molded brace is effective for most patients with a thoracolumbar lesion.[71] In the cervical spine, Philadelphia collars, sterno-occipito-mandibular immobilizers (SOMI), cervicothoracic orthoses, and halo orthoses are used depending upon the degree of instability.

Bracing may also be considered when the patient is unable to undergo surgical intervention and external immobilization is warranted. Another role for an orthotic is as a postoperative support following decompression and the implantation of internal fixation. Proper patient selection is important. Older, more frail individuals may have difficulty donning and tolerating a cumbersome brace and thus discard the orthosis early.

Operative Treatment

When the tumor has advanced to the stage of significant vertebral collapse without neurologic deficit or when the collapse causes cord dysfunction secondary to direct mechanical compression (Harrington class IV and V, respectively), no conservative modality will be effective in reducing pain or preventing further deformity. Surgical intervention is indicated for the following[61]: neurologic deterioration or intractable pain during radiotherapy; neurologic compromise caused by bone or soft tissue compressing the cord, a recurrent tumor in a previously radiated area, or a radioresistant lesion; progressive spinal collapse and deformity; and unproven diagnosis.

Surgical Approaches

There is considerable controversy concerning whether an anterior and/or posterior approach and decompression are necessary as well as how to stabilize the spine. In the past, surgical treatment consisted primarily of decompressive laminectomy.[9, 30, 78] Gilbert et al. reported that 49%

of patients treated with laminectomy plus radiation had satisfactory results as compared with 46% of those treated with radiotherapy alone.[30] Other authors have generally reported similar results with radiotherapy alone and 30% satisfactory results with laminectomy.[8, 32, 54] Some still advocate laminectomy, although its role has been curtailed to cases of posterior tumor foci.[68]

The most common reasons for the disappointing results after decompressive laminectomy are the inability to adequately decompress the anterior aspect of the cord and the destabilizing effect of posterior element destruction in cases of vertebral body metastases. Laminectomy is contraindicated in anterior lesions with vertebral collapse or with kyphotic deformity and subluxation.

With the development and proliferation of advanced spinal instrumentation and surgical approaches to the spine, decompression and stability can be achieved through other methods. Since the majority of metastatic compressive lesions originate anteriorly, a direct anterior approach was developed. In 1981, Harrington reported on 14 patients undergoing anterior decompression and cement stabilization.[35] All but 1 patient demonstrated neurologic improvement, and 93% had pain relief. Kostuik, using an anterior approach, noted that all 13 of his patients improved neurologically.[42] Siegel et al. presented 47 patients treated by vertebral body resection and polymethylmethacrylate (PMMA) reconstruction.[62] After surgery, 80% of the survivors were ambulatory, and 93% retained sphincter control.

Anterior decompression involves the performance of a complete vertebrectomy. The main advantage of anterior surgery is the ability to resect the tumor directly and to decompress the cord from the side of its compromise. Stabilization can be accomplished by using corticocancellous bone and bracing until fusion. The advantage of this technique is definitive spinal stability once incorporation has occurred. However, in patients who are physically debilitated and have a limited life expectancy, prolonged immobilization for as long as 3 months may be counterproductive. Also, patients undergoing radiation therapy will have a reduced ability to incorporate the bone graft.[35]

In patients with metastases it is imperative to provide for immediate stabilization to allow early ambulation, thus preventing pulmonary or vascular complications from pro-

A

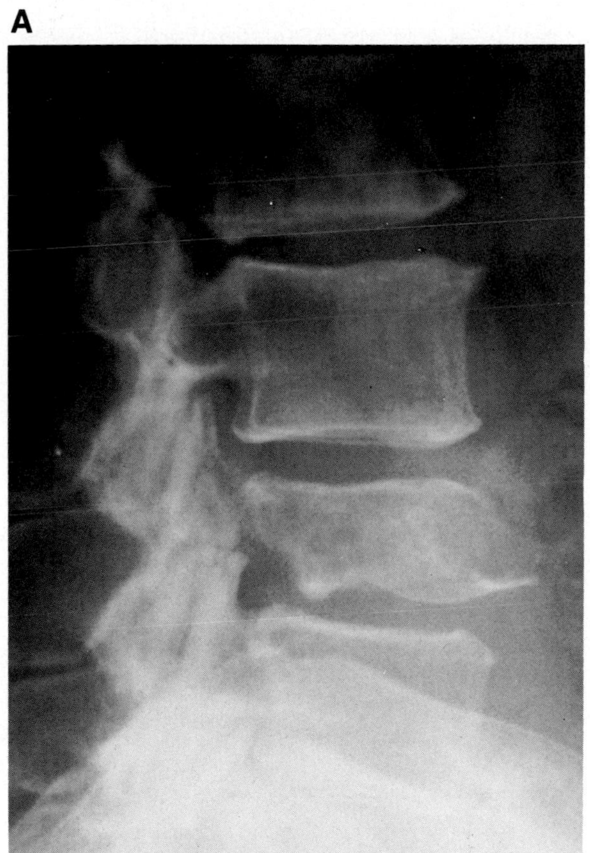

B

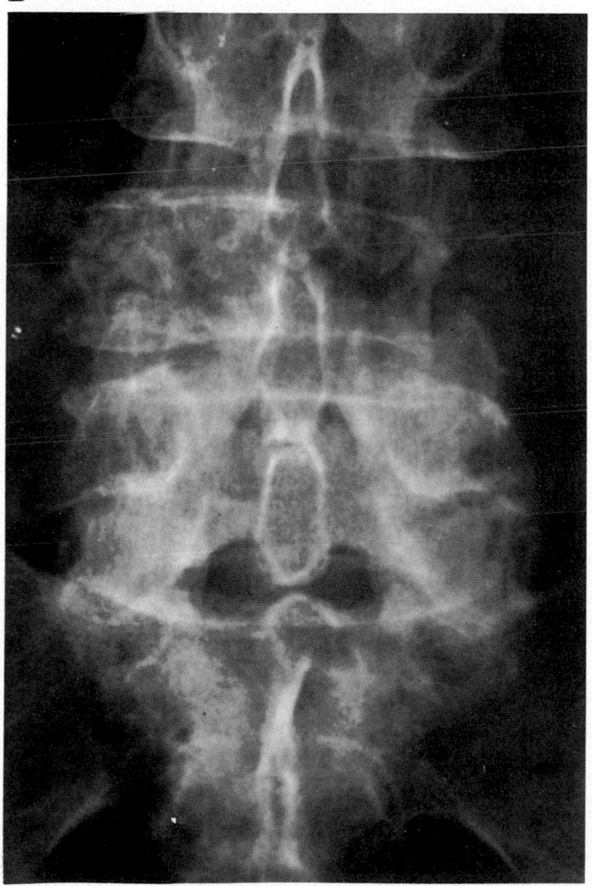

FIG 34–1.
A and **B**, anteroposterior (AP) and lateral radiographs showing collapse of the L4 vertebra secondary to breast carcinoma.

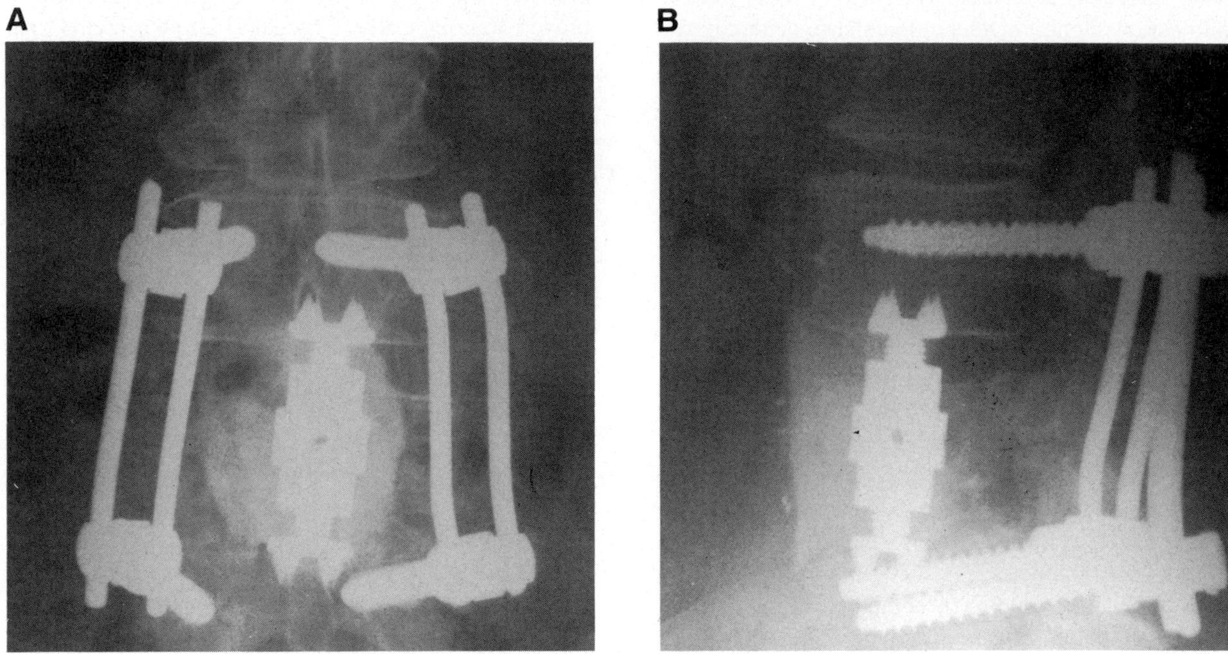

FIG 34–2.
A and **B,** AP and lateral radiographs following L4 anterior corpectomy, placement of a Rezaian device with PMMA reinforcement, and posterior stabilization with pedicle screws in L3 and L5.

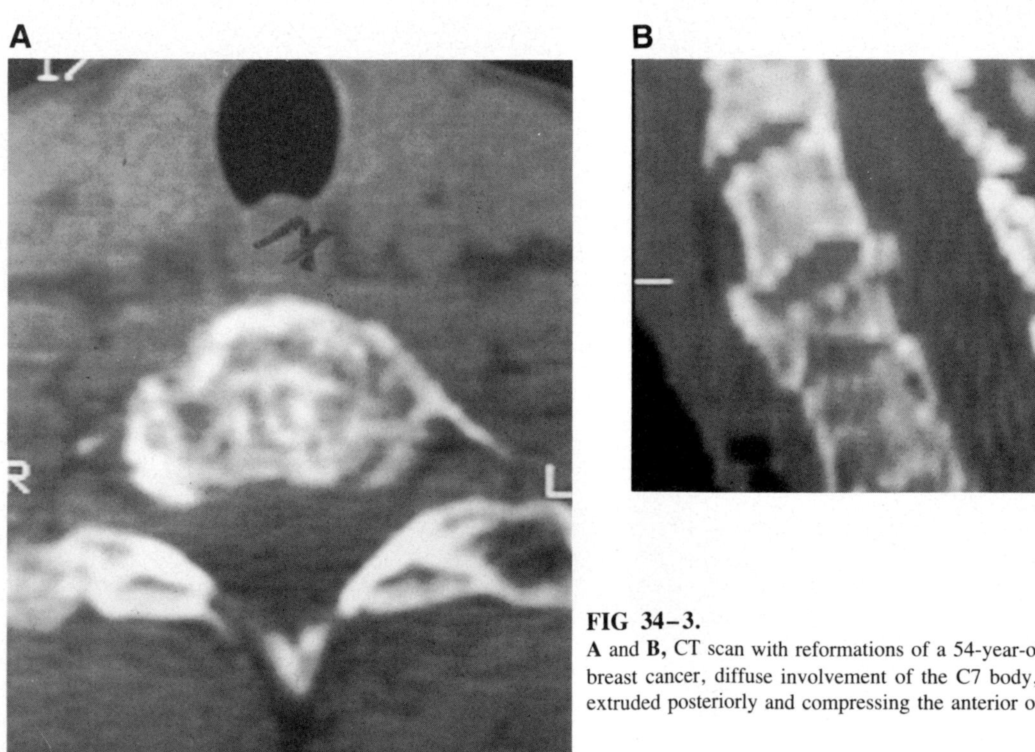

FIG 34–3.
A and **B,** CT scan with reformations of a 54-year-old woman with metastatic breast cancer, diffuse involvement of the C7 body, and a soft-tissue density extruded posteriorly and compressing the anterior of the thecal sac.

A

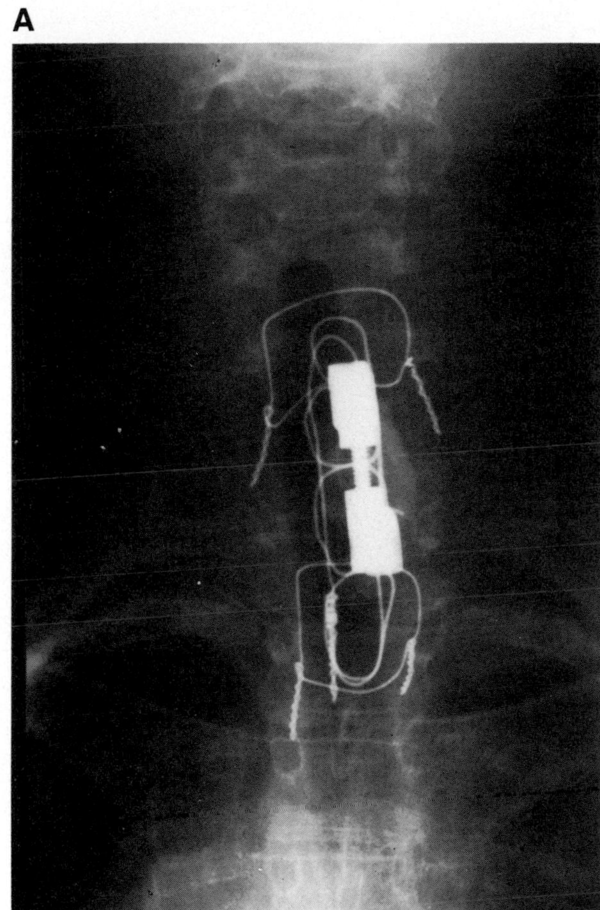

B

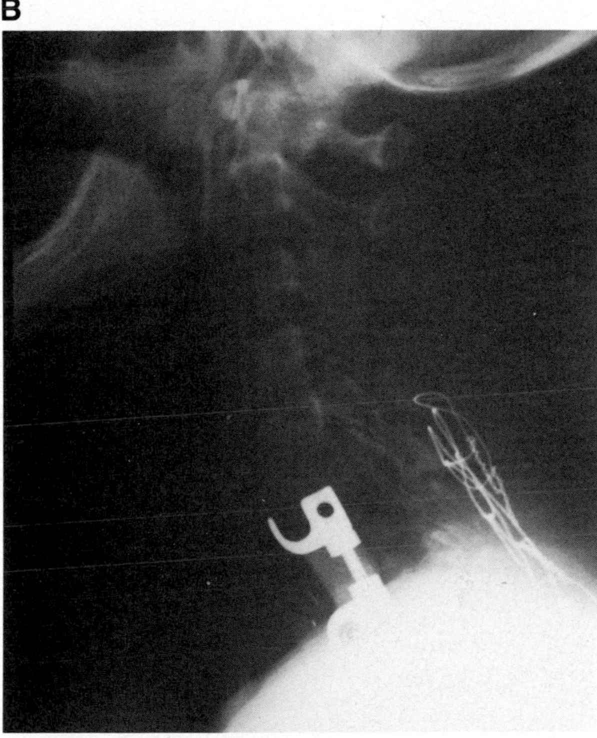

FIG 34–4.
A and **B,** AP and lateral views demonstrating reconstruction using a Harrington compression rod reinforced with methylmethacrylate and posterior wiring from C5 to T2.

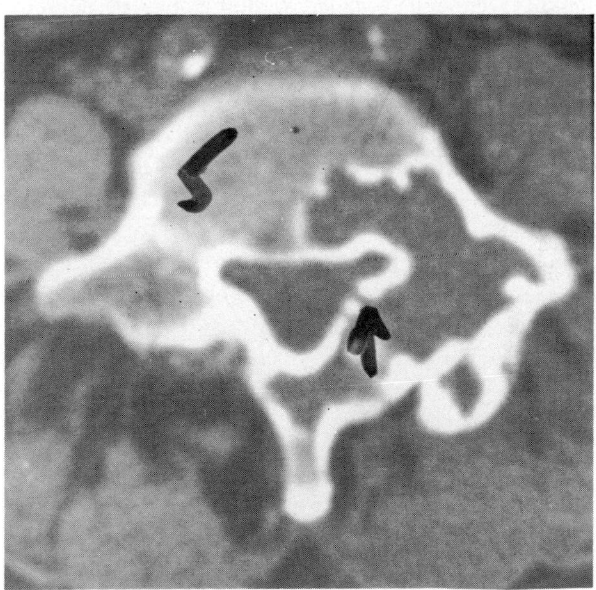

FIG 34–5.
A 57-year-old female with multiple myeloma presenting with intractable left L5 radiculopathy unresponsive to radiotherapy. CT revealed a lytic lesion involving the left L5 vertebral body with extension into the pedicle and posterior elements.

longed inactivity. In light of the decreased life span of tumor patients and the need for adjunctive radiotherapy, PMMA has been used as an effective stabilizer. The presence of acrylic bone cement does not interfere with radiation, and there is no sign of adverse effect on the tissues adjacent to the PMMA.[36] Radiation of PMMA does not cause objective changes in its shear strength, compressibility, or durability.[26, 53] The use of PMMA is advocated by those who want immediate stability that is not dependent on bone grafts or external immobilization. PMMA has superb resistance to compression and is ideal for anterior vertebral stabilization.[13, 35] However, posteriorly placed PMMA is not effective since it cannot resist shear and torque loads.[49]

When used anteriorly as a spacer, there must be a means of securing the cement to the adjacent vertebral bodies in order to prevent displacement. Various implants have been used for incorporation within the cement, including Steinmann pins, semitubular plates, Harrington rods, and Knodt rods.[35, 62, 69] New instrumentation systems such as the Kaneda device,[41] Kostuik-Harrington system,[43] and the Syracuse I-plate[79] have been developed to restore height, prevent collapse, and provide anterior stability.

A

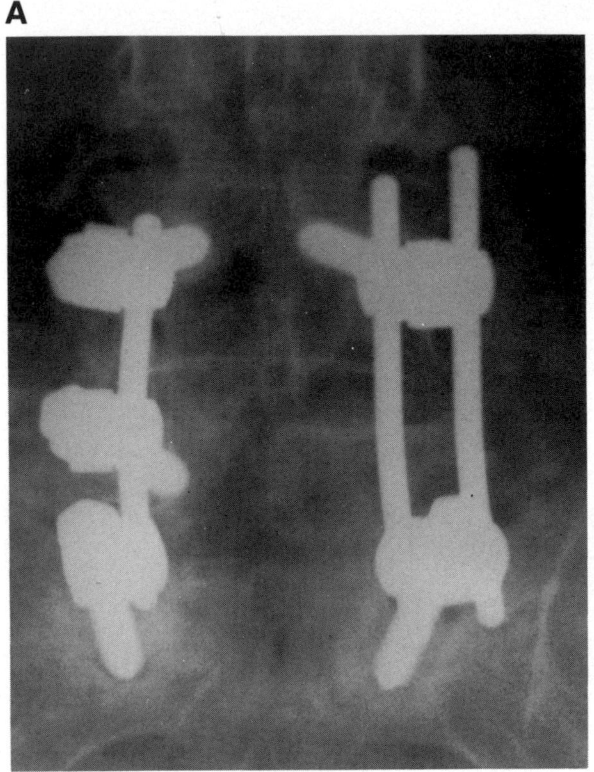

B

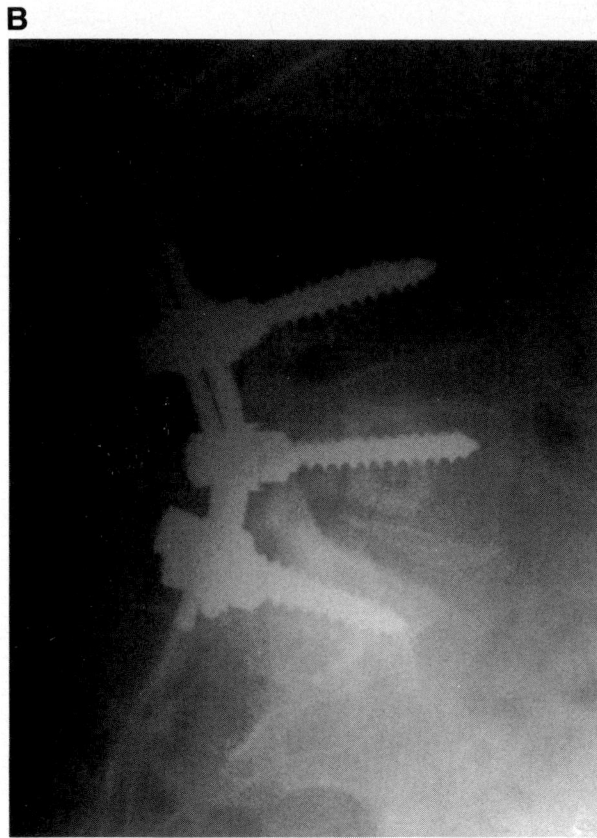

FIG 34–6.
A and **B,** AP and lateral radiographs following posterior decompression and fusion by pedicle screw fixation.

A consideration of the long-term stability of the PMMA-enhanced construct in the absence of bony arthrodesis must be addressed. There is a possibility that these constructs may fail if not reinforced with bone. Therefore, for a patient with a projected survival exceeding 1 to 2 years, the addition of corticocancellous grafting is to be considered.[33]

The final surgical technique combines both anterior and posterior stabilization. This is done in cases of anterior and posterior column disease requiring circumferential decompression, those with anterior destruction and a previous laminectomy, and in some cases of fracture-dislocation due to a pathologic lesion (Figs 34–1 to 34–4).

When posterior stabilization is required to restore alignment and stability, one of several instrumentation systems may be employed. These range from the Harrington rod instrumentation to new devices such as the Cotrel-Dubousset system and pedicle screws[16, 67] (Figs 34–5 and 34–6). As more rigid anterior stabilization is developed, the indications for posterior fixation will decrease.

SUMMARY

Operative decompression is indicated for individuals with metastases and pain secondary to mechanical causes, instability, previously failed radiotherapy, or neurologic deterioration. Most patients can still be managed with bed rest, bracing, local radiation therapy, chemotherapy, or hormonal manipulation. The majority of patients do not present with neural deficits. However, those with minimal neurologic deficit and maintained spinal stability may also respond to radiotherapy and steroids. Another consideration is life expectancy. Those who have less than 3 months to live and those with diffuse spinal involvement do not require operative intervention because the quality of life is not appreciably altered and may even be reduced.

REFERENCES

1. Avraham E, Tadmor R, Dally D, et al: Early MR demonstration of spinal metastasis in patients with normal radiographs and CT and radionucleide bone scans. *J Comput Assist Tomogr* 1987; 4:598–602.
2. Barcena A, Lobatao RD, Rivas JJ, et al: Spinal metastatic disease: Analysis of factors determining functional prognosis and choice of treatment. *Neurosurgery* 1984; 15:820–827.
3. Barron KD, Hisano A, Aradi S, et al: Experiences with metastatic neoplasms involving the spinal cord. *Neurology* 1959; 9:91–106.
4. Batson OV: The function of the vertebral veins and their

role in the spread of metastasis. *Ann Surg* 1940; 112:138–149.
5. Beltram J, Noto AM, Chalceres DW, et al: Tumors of the osseous spine: Staging with MR imaging versus CT. *Radiology* 1987; 162:565–569.
6. Berrettoni BA, Carter JR: Mechanisms of cancer metastasis to bone. *J Bone Joint Surg [Am]* 1986; 68:308–312.
7. Bhardway S, Holland JF: Chemotherapy of metastatic cancer in bone. *Clin Orthop* 1982; 169:28–37.
8. Black P: Spinal metastases: Current status and guidelines for management. *Neurosurgery* 1979; 5:726–746.
9. Boland PJ, Lane JM, Sundaresan N: Metastatic disease of the spine. *Clin Orthop* 1982; 169:95–102.
10. Botterell EH, Fitzgerald GW: Spinal cord compression produced by extradural malignant tumors: Early recognition, treatment, and results. *Can Med Assoc J* 1959; 80:791.
11. Bowers TA, Murray JA: Bone metastases from renal carcinoma: The preoperative use of transcatheter arterial occlusion. *J Bone Joint Surg [Am]* 1982; 64:749–754.
12. Citrin DL, Bessent RG, Greig WR: A comparison of the sensitivity and accuracy of the Tc-99 phosphate bone scan and skeletal radiograph in the diagnosis of bone metastases. *Clin Radiol* 1977; 28:107–117.
13. Clark CC, Keggi KJ, Panjabi MM: Methylmethacrylate stabilization of the cervical spine. *J Bone Joint Surg [Am]* 1986; 68:1145–1157.
14. Constans JP, de Divitiis E, Donzelli R, et al: Spinal metastases with neurological manifestations. *J Neurosurg* 1983; 59:111–118.
15. Corcoran RJ, Thrail JH, Kyle RW, et al: Solitary abnormalities in bone scans of patients with extra-osseous malignancies. *Radiology* 1976; 121:663–667.
16. Cotrel Y, Dubousset J, Guillaumat M: New universal instrumentation in spinal surgery. *Clin Orthop* 1988; 227:10–23.
17. Dahlin DC: *Bone Tumors: General Aspects and Data on 6,221 Cases,* ed 3. Springfield, Ill, Charles C Thomas, 1978.
18. Decker DA, et al: Characterization and analysis of complete regression to chemotherapy in metastatic breast cancer. *Proc Am Assoc Res* 1979; 20:241.
19. Degenshein GA, Bloom N, Ceccarelli F, et al: Estrogen and progesterone receptor site studies as guides to the management of advanced breast cancer. *Cancer* 1977; 3:29.
20. DeKernion JB, Ramming KP, Smith RB: The natural history of metastatic renal cell carcinoma: A computer analysis. *J Urol* 1978; 120:148–152.
21. Delattre JV, Arbit E, Rosenblum MK, et al: High dose versus low dose dexamethasone in experimental epidural spinal cord compression. *Neurosurgery* 1988; 22:1005–1007.
22. DeWald RL, Bridwell KH, Prodromas C, et al: Reconstructive spinal surgery as palliation for metastatic malignancies of the spine. *Spine* 1985; 10:21–26.
23. Dorfman LJ, Donaldson SS, Gupta PR, et al: Electrophysiologic evidence of subclinical injury to the posterior columns of the spinal cord after therapeutic radiation. *Cancer* 1982; 50:2815–2819.
24. Doubilet PM, Seltzer SE, Hessel SJ: Computed tomography in the diagnosis and management of paravertebral masses. *Comput Radiol* 1984; 8:101–106.
25. Edelstyn GA, Gillespie PJ, Grebell ES: The radiologic demonstration of osseous metastases: Experimental observation. *Clin Radiol* 1967; 18:158–164.
26. Eftelchar NS, Thurston CW: Effect of irradiation and acrylic cement with special reference to fixation of pathologic fractures. *J Biomech* 1975; 8:53–56.
27. Fidler IJ, Gersten DM, Hart IR: The biology of cancer invasion and metastasis. *Cancer Res* 1978; 38:651.
28. Galasko CSB: The significance of occult skeletal metastases, detected by skeletal scintigraphy, in patients with otherwise apparent "early" mammary carcinoma. *Br J Surg* 1975; 67:694–696.
29. Galasko CSB, Bennett A: Relationship of bone destruction in skeletal metastases to osteoclast activation and prostaglandins. *Nature* 1976; 263:508–510.
30. Gilbert RW, Kim JH, Posner JB: Epidural spinal cord compression from metastatic tumor; diagnosis and treatment. *Ann Neurol* 1978; 3:949–954.
31. Goldberg LD, Ditchek NT: Thyroid carcinoma with spinal cord compression. *JAMA* 1981; 245:953–954.
32. Hall AJ, MacKay NS: The results of laminectomy for compression of the cord or cauda equina by extradural malignant tumor. *J Bone Joint Surg [Br]* 1973; 55:497–505.
33. Harrington KD: Metastatic disease of the spine. *J Bone Joint Surg [Am]* 1986; 68:1110–1115.
34. Harrington KD: Metastatic disease of the spine, in *Orthopaedic Management of Metastatic Bone Disease*. St Louis, Mosby–Year Book, 1988, pp 308–383.
35. Harrington KD: The use of methylmethacrylate for vertebral body replacement and anterior stabilization of pathological fracture dislocations of the spine due to metastatic malignant disease. *J Bone Joint Surg [Am]* 1981; 63:36–46.
36. Harrington KD, Sim FH, Enis JE, et al: Methylmethacrylate as an adjunct in internal fixation of pathologic fractures: Experience with three hundred seventy-five cases. *J Bone Joint Surg [Am]* 1976; 58:1047–1055.
37. Hirsch LF, Finneson BE: Intradural sacral nerve root metastasis mimicking herniated disc. *J Neurosurg* 1978; 49:764–768.
38. Hollis PH, Malis LI, Zapulla RA: Neurological deterioration after lumbar puncture below complete spinal subarachnoid block. *J Neurosurg* 1986; 64:253–256.
39. Jaffe WL: *Tumors and Tumorous Conditions of the Bones and Joints*. Philadelphia, Lea & Febiger, 1958.
40. Kagan AR, Stekel RJ, Bassett LW: Lytic spine lesion and cold bone scan. *Am J Radiol* 1981; 136:129–131.
41. Kaneda K, Abumi K, Fujuja M: Burst fractures with neurological deficits of the thoraco-lumbar spine: Results of anterior decompression and stabilization with anterior instrumentation. *Spine* 1984; 9:788–795.
42. Kostuik JP: Anterior spinal cord decompression for lesions of the thoracic and lumbar spine, technique, new methods of internal fixation, results. *Spine* 1983; 8:512–530.
43. Kostuik JP, Errico TJ, Gleason TF, et al: Spinal stabilization of vertebral column tumors. *Spine* 1988; 13:250–256.

44. Lam WC, Delikatny JE, Orr FW, et al: The chemothactic response of tumor cells. A model for cancer metastasis. *Am J Pathol* 1981; 104:69–76.
45. Lepor H, Ross A, Walsh P: The influence of hormonal therapy on survival of men with advanced prostatic cancer. *J Urol* 1982; 128:335–340.
46. Li KC, Poon PY: Sensitivity and specificity of MRI in detecting malignant spinal cord compression and in distinguishing malignant from benign compression fractures of vertebrae. *Magn Reson Imaging* 1988; 6:547–556.
47. Luce EA: The irradiated wound. *Surg Clin North Am* 1984; 64:821–829.
48. Macedo N, Sundaresan N, Galicich JH: Decompressive laminectomy for metastatic cancer: What are the current indications? *Proc Am Soc Clin Oncol* 1985; 4:278.
49. McAfee PC, Bohlman HH, Ducker T, et al: Failure of stabilization of the spine with methylmethacrylate. *J Bone Joint Surg [Am]* 1986; 68:1145–1157.
50. McNeil BJ: Value of bone scanning in neoplastic disease. *Semin Nucl Med* 1984; 4:277.
51. Miller F, Whitehill R: Carcinoma of the breast metastatic to the skeleton. *Clin Orthop* 1984; 184:121–127.
52. Muggia RM, Chervu LR: Lung cancer: Diagnosis in metastatic sites. *Semin Oncol* 1974; 1:217–228.
53. Murray JA, Bruels MC, Linberg RD: Irradiation of polymethylmethacrylate. In vitro gamma radiation effect. *J Bone Joint Surg [Am]* 1974; 56:311–312.
54. Nather A, Bose K: The results of decompression of cord or cauda equina from metastatic extradural tumors. *Clin Orthop* 1982; 169:103–108.
55. Paget S: The distribution of secondary growths in cancer of the breast. *Lancet* 1889; 1:571–573.
56. Redmond J, Spring DB, Munderloh SH, et al: Spinal computed tomography in the evaluation of metastatic disease. *Cancer* 1984; 54:253–258.
57. Rodichuk LD, Ruckdeschel JC, Harper GR, et al: Early detection and treatment of spinal epidural metastases: The role of myelography. *Ann Neurol* 1986; 20:696–702.
58. Schaberg J, Gainor BJ: A profile of metastatic carcinoma of the spine. *Spine* 1985; 10:19–20.
59. Seagren SL, Saunders WM: Radiation therapy for spinal cord tumors. *Semin Spine Surg* 1990; 2:197–202.
60. Siegel T, Siegel T: Current considerations in the management of neoplastic spinal cord compression. *Spine* 1989; 14:223–228.
61. Siegel T, Siegel T: Surgical decompression of anterior and posterior malignant epidural tumors compressing the spinal cord: A prospective study. *Neurosurgery* 1985; 17:424–432.
62. Siegel T, Tikva P, Siegel T: Vertebral body resection for epidural compression by malignant tumors. *J Bone Joint Surg [Am]* 1985; 67:373–382.
63. Sim FH: *Diagnosis and Management of Metastatic Bone Disease: A Multidisciplinary Approach*. New York, Raven Press, 1988.
64. Sim FH, Dahlin DC, Stauffer RN, et al: Primary bone tumors simulating lumbar disc syndrome. *Spine* 1977; 2:65–74.
65. Slatkin NE, Posner FB: Management of spinal epidural metastases. *Clin Neurosurg* 1983; 30:698–716.
66. Solini A, Paschero B, Orsini G, et al: The surgical treatment of metastatic tumors of the lumbar spine. *Ital J Orthop Trauma* 1986; 11:427–441.
67. Steffee AD, Biscup RS, Sitkowski DJ: Segmental spine plates with pedicle screw spine fixation: A new internal fixation device for disorders of the lumbar and thoracolumbar spine. *Clin Orthop* 1986; 203:45–53.
68. Sundaresan N, Galicich JH, Bains MS, et al: Vertebral body resection in the treatment of cancer involving the spine. *Cancer* 1984; 53:1393–1396.
69. Sundaresan N, Galicich JH, Lane JM, et al: Treatment of neoplastic epidural cord compression by vertebral body resection and stabilization. *J Neurosurg* 1985; 63:676–684.
70. Sundaresan N, Scher H, Yagoda A, et al: Surgical treatment of spinal metastases in kidney cancer. *J Clin Oncol* 1986; 4:1851–1856.
71. Sypert GW: External spine orthotics. *Neurosurgery* 1987; 20:642–649.
72. Sze G, Abramson A, Krol G: Gadolinium DTPA in the evaluation in intradural extramedullary spinal disease. *Am J Neurol* 1988; 9:153–163.
73. Sze G, Krol G, Zimmerman RD, et al: Malignant extradural tumors: Imaging with Gd-DTPA. *Radiology* 1984; 167:217–223.
74. Tang SG, Byfield JE, Sharp TR: Prognostic factors in the management of metastatic epidural cord compression. *J Neurooncol* 1981; 1:21–28.
75. Tomita T, Galicich JH, Sundaresan N: Radiation therapy for spinal epidural metastases with complete block. *Acta Radiol Oncol* 1983; 22:135–143.
76. Wara WM, Phillips TL, Sheline GE, et al: Radiation tolerance of the spinal cord. *Cancer* 1975; 35:1558–1562.
77. Willis RA: Secondary tumours of bone, in *The Blood Supply of Bone: An Approach to Bone Biology*. Butterworth, London, 1971, pp 67–91.
78. Young RF, Post EM, King GA: Treatment of spinal epidural metastases. Randomized prospective comparison of laminectomy and radiotherapy. *J Neurosurg* 1980; 53:741–748.
79. Yuan HA, Man KA, Found EM, et al: Early clinical experience with the Syracuse I-plate: An anterior spinal fixation device. *Spine* 1988; 13:278–285.

PART IX

DEGENERATIVE DISORDERS OF THE SPINE

35

Degenerative Disc Disease

H.F. Farfan, M.Sc., M.D., C.M., F.R.C.S.(C)

Pathologic changes occur in the spine as it ages. These changes are commonly referred to as degenerative disc disease or degenerative arthrosis. Because degenerative changes increase with aging, the term is used almost as a synonym for getting old.

Heretofore, the pathogenesis of this change was poorly understood, especially the relationship between changes in one part of the body and changes in a distant part. However, with the accumulation of new knowledge, it is now possible to explain and correlate the pathologic reality.

THE AGING SPINE

We are at the beginning of a new understanding of the design of the musculoskeletal system. With this new understanding comes a realization of the true function of its various parts. The spine is made up of passive structures —the bones, joints, and ligaments—none of which can initiate movement. But, these passive parts are manipulated by active muscle contraction to gain an objective with a minimum of energy expenditure. Minimum energy utilization is equivalent to minimum stress. Theoretically, if this is true, then the stress at each of the intervertebral joints must be minimized. Further, to avoid failure of one joint before another, then the ideal is to have the same minimized stress at all joints.

Mathematical deductions based on this theory have shown that this basic principle is correct. We have successfully calculated the electromyograph (EMG) of a person standing upright and during various weight lifts. Numerous other calculations based on the same theory calculate, with fair accuracy, the instantaneous center of motion of the intervertebral joint, or the maximal load supportable in any position of the body.[4] Similar calculations reproduce the EMG of the neck under various loading conditions.[6]

We have also been able to show that this rule extends to the fibers of the disc. Each fiber in the disc is subjected to the same stress. Thus, if we know the angle of the fiber, we can calculate the height of the disc or vice versa.[3]

This theory has not been extended to all parts of the three-joint complex (disc and left and right facets) composing the intervertebral joint. However, we have measured the stress at failure of the pars interarticularis, and this is the same as the stress at failure of the pedicles and the same as the stress at failure of a femur.

Because muscle is the only active member, it follows that muscle is responsible for changing the stress at a joint. Muscle can modify the stress at the joint by direct action at the joint, or it may affect a joint by producing a change in a distant joint. A nod of the head may affect the stress at the lumbosacral joint.

For this system to work, we need to have a sensory system that can read stress and report this to the spinal center, which can in turn cause a muscle response. The presence of such a system for the moment is only a surmise, but there is abundant reason to believe in its reality. The system envisaged is as in Figure 35–1.

There is therefore the possibility that one or another part of this system, if faulty, will cause a change in the mechanism of the spine. For instance, an imbalance between pyramidal and extrapyramidal systems of the central nervous system (CNS) may be the fundamental cause of dyscoordination of the system and of its eventual breakdown.[5]

The array of the stress sensors would naturally be placed in those structures subjected to the most strain, such as the annulus of the disc, the posterior longitudinal ligament, or the periosteum. It is noteworthy that periosteal tissue is loaded with sensors with large myelinated fibers, the function of which is at present unknown but has been assumed to subserve pain. This is also true of the posterior longitudinal ligament, if not in the outer portion of the annulus of the disc. Large myelinated fibers are not normally associated with pain. The transport of stress information should be rapid. This requires a myelinated fiber.

Injury to the sensory organs or to their fibers may also produce changes at the joints. This is seen in diabetes and in congenital absence of pain. In this context, we may understand Paget's disease as a disease of the periosteum instead of a disease of bone.

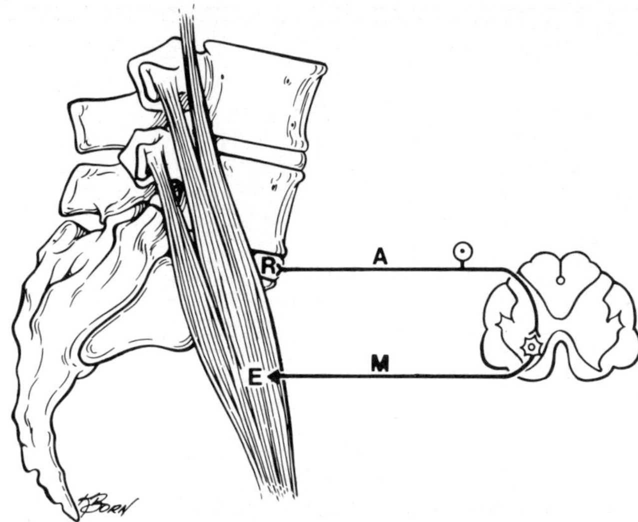

FIG 35–1.
Theoretical model of stress. Damage to any of the components will affect the final behavior. *R* = stress receptor; *A* = afferent fiber; *M* = motor fiber; *E* = efferent fiber.

In an optimized system, we can envisage all the muscles, ligaments, and joints working in a concerted manner to produce a minimum stress at the intervertebral joint that is equal in all joints. Should a member of this system be injured, then the system would have to find a different but still minimal stress. This new minimal stress would be higher than the initial state (Fig 35–2).

Should this member heal and take up its original contribution to the overall strategy, then the system would return to its initial state. Unfortunately, all healing is by scar; therefore, it is not likely that the overall strategy could ever return to the original optimal state. Scar does not have the same physical characteristics as the tissue it replaces.

Theoretically, then, once injured, the injury maintains a permanent deleterious effect on the overall best strategy.

However, in normal life, we calculate that we use less than 60% of our potential, even when functioning at top championship levels. In most common tasks, we seldom strain our joints to more than 10% to 15% of our capacity. We see that the human body has a tremendous reserve of capacity and the individual, after an injury, has room for recovery.

The aim of rehabilitation, therefore, is to preserve what remains after injury. Basically, it is never the muscle that is hurt. It is the passive structures that suffer, particularly the joints. The object must be to maintain joint motion and to make sure that this motion has full muscle control.

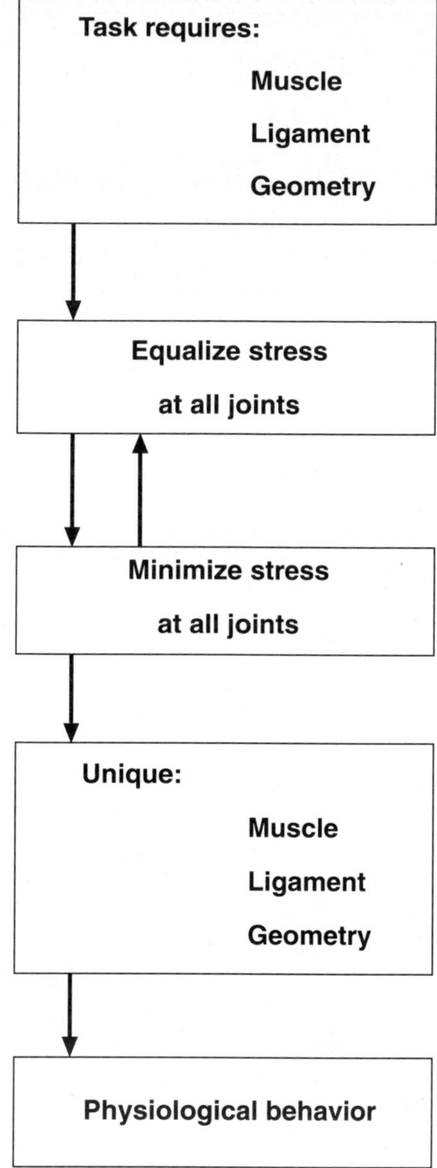

FIG 35–2.
Physiologic behavior and injury. Injury reduces the capacity of one of the components to support stress. Therefore the system has to choose a different strategy to achieve the task, either by choosing a lesser task or by performing the same task at the expense of raising the stress in the uninjured members.

CURVES OF THE AXIAL SKELETON AND POSTURE

The axial skeleton is formed with 34 segments below the head. At first, the axial skeleton is formed as a curved structure from head to tail. The shape or tightness of this curve is influenced by heredity. This may affect what may happen to the spine in adult life.

After birth, the cervical lordosis appears when the infant starts holding his head upright. Lumbar lordosis appears later when the infant starts sitting and standing. The thoracic spine, which is stiffened by the sternum and ribs, and the fixed sacral segments are two fixed curves that have a pronounced effect on the degree of lordosis of the freely moving cervical and lumbar sections.

In the fetus with a tight curve, the degree of lordosis will be increased, and in those with a more open curve, there will be relatively much less lordosis (Fig 35–3).

The combination of curves is crucial to balancing upright on the feet. The median lumbar spine has a lumbosacral joint inclined about 30 degrees to the horizontal. In this shape of the spine, the line of gravity falls in the posterior half of the head of the femur, through the body of L1, and in front of the middle thoracic vertebrae and crosses the thoracic curve at T3 or T4 and generally posterior to the midcervical vertebral bodies (Fig 35–4).

However, natural variations can range from a 10-degree lumbosacral angle to a 90-degree angulation. With the smaller degrees of angulation, the lumbar spine may be totally behind the line of gravity, which passes through the posterior part of the hip. The lumbar as well as the cervical lordosis are much reduced. In the opposite extreme, the line of gravity passes through the posterior aspect of L5 and may be totally behind L3 and cut across the thoracic vertebrae at T5 or T6.

In the median case, the balance is maintained virtually without muscle activity except for an occasional burst from the extensors or the flexers of the spine. In the minimal angle, balance is maintained by continuous activity of the abdominals, while in the increased curve the erectors are found to be continuously active.

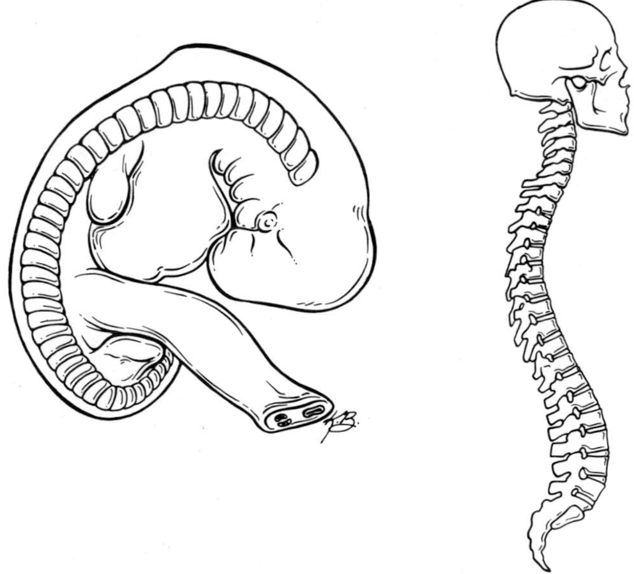

FIG 35–3.
The fetus and the development of adult curves. The thoracic and sacral curves are fixed before birth. When the fetus is "tightly curved," the adult will develop increased lordosis of the cervical and lumbar vertebrae.

It must be stressed that these are variations of normal. We must be able to tell when the posture of the patient has been acquired. In persons with flat backs, the discs themselves as well as the vertebral bodies exhibit small degrees of wedging that may be confined to the lumbosacral joint. On the other hand, those with high curvatures naturally also have a high degree of wedging of the vertebral bodies as well as the discs.

In those spines where the degree of wedging of the vertebral bodies does not correspond to the degree of wedging of the discs, we can suspect a loss of posterior disc thickness. But often we must wait for further evidence. Normally, the center of the facet joint lies on the bisector of the disc. When the inferior facet becomes superior to the end plate of the body above, then it is obvious that there has been a loss of disc height. Accompanying these changes, there may develop evidence of arthrosis of the facet joints.

THE ABDOMINAL MUSCLES AND POSTURE

The female at the age of 20 years and the male at 26 years of age start to lose abdominal tone. There is some reason for this. In the female, it is by training the abdominals out. They have listened to the continuous exhortations of their mothers to "suck the tummy in." This is accomplished by relaxing the abdominals and sticking out the chest. This may do something for the natural charms but has a very deleterious effect on the back (Fig 35–5).

The continuous relaxation of the abdominals effects a change in posture to an increase in the lordosis and to a shift in the line of gravity. This places greater pressure on the posterior part of the intervertebral joint, the posterior part of the disc and the facet joints. The facet joints, which normally bear no weight in the upright position, now acquire the increased pressure of weight bearing. The center of pressure of the disc is normally at the center of the nucleus. It shifts backward and changes appear in the posterior of the annulus that reduce its thickness. This joint loses some of its flexibility.

The process becomes a vicious circle. With the arthritic changes in the facet joint, forced movements become painful and result in muscle guarding by the erectors, which in turn reduces the flexibility even more.

With a pregnancy, very similar changes are common. With the extra stretch of the abdominals and hormonal relaxation of the lower lumbar and pelvic joints, the opportunity for permanent change is ever present. The modern woman is more concerned with regaining her prepregnancy weight than with regaining her original posture. It is commonly said that 20 to 25 years after the birth of the first infant the mother will develop low back pain because

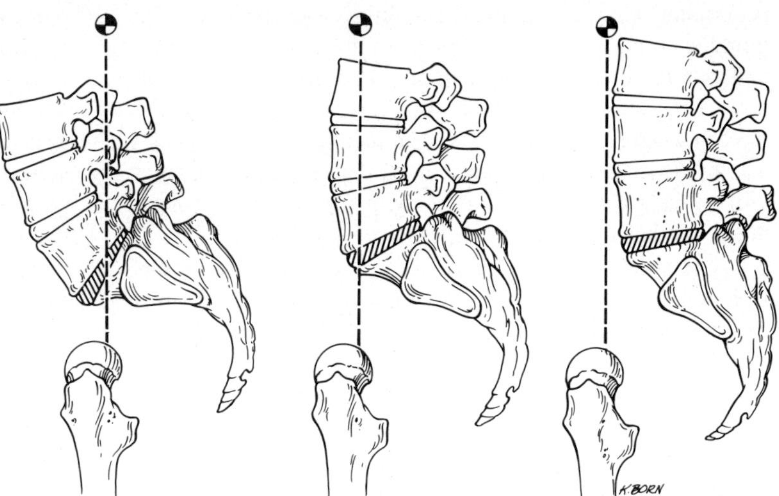

FIG 35–4.
Natural variation in lumbar lordosis: the relationship of the center of gravity, the lumbar spine, and the head of the femur. The median curve for both males and females with lumbosacral joint involvement is 30 to 40 degrees to the horizontal.

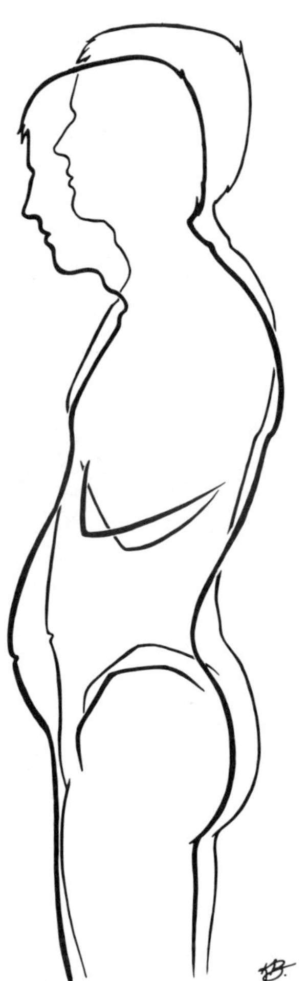

FIG 35–5.
Change in posture with loss of abdominal tone. The increased lordosis is reflected in the new posture of the rib cage, the increased length of the abdominals, and the increased delineation of the pelvis. This change must necessarily affect the posture of the neck.

changes occur in joints that have lost some of their motion.

Diarthrodial joints have an active range of motion that is always somewhat less than the passive range. The same appears to be true of intervertebral joints. The reason for the difference in active and passive motion ranges is for the protection of the joint.

Following injury, it is necessary to regain as full a range of active motion as possible. This requires full muscle control. The tendency to force the range passively can quite frequently result in further injury. When loss of movement occurs in a spinal joint, this is especially true, and the therapist working with "mobilizations" often uses the body weight to force the movement.

The patient would be better served by a coordinated movement of the spine where the muscles actively control the movement of the joint through range.

POSTURAL CHANGES AND THE KINETIC CHAIN

Men and women are different. Changes in posture occur naturally when the hormonal balances in the body change. I realize that this statement is vague, but at this time, specific changes due to specific hormonal influences are not known.

The male reaches his full growth at about 25 years of age and remains without natural posture change until late in life when the change at the neck appears. The lordosis of the neck increases, and he develops a very prominent boss at the top of the thoracic spine, C7 or T1.

The female, on the other hand, attains skeletal maturity at 16 years of age with a very obvious posture change at adolescence accompanying the development of secondary sex characteristics. There is a second postural change with pregnancy, a third with menopause or premenopause, and a final change very similar to that in the male and often referred to as the "dowager" with increased lordosis of the neck.

Similar changes may occur in either males or females taking artificial hormones and in disturbances of the endocrine system. Of particular interest are the postural changes accompanying antipregnancy medication, which do not correct themselves when the medication is stopped.

In women, the sequence of postural change is the increase in lumbar and cervical lordosis and internal rotation of the hips and lower limbs. If one stands with the feet slightly apart and tries to rotate the knees internally, it can be noted that the arches of the feet go down as the foot becomes more pronated. There is a strain felt on the medial sides of the knees. The backside becomes more prominent, and the lumbar lordosis increases. A strain may be felt between the shoulders. The shoulders come forward, and the cervical lordosis is increased.

In the late forties, the female often complains of pain in exactly the same areas. As she goes through premenopause and menopause, these complaints take on more importance.

Thus, we see what has been called the kinetic chain in action, where all parts of the body interact from head to foot. Symptoms in one part of the body may be directly related to another, apparently unrelated asymptomatic part of the chain. For example, a sore heel due to plantar fascitis or a posterior tibial tendonitis may be related to an asymptomatic low back problem because of the gradual weakening of the calf due to an injured nerve root at L5–S1.

We need to recognize the interconnected parts of the chain even though we may not be able to identify the link that caused the symptoms in the first place.

UPPER BACK AND NECK POSTURE CHANGES

We have seen a balanced system in the lumbar spine. There is also a balanced system controlling the posture of head, neck, and shoulders.

The center of gravity of the head falls in front of the cervical spine. The weight of the head must be balanced by a counterweight behind the spine. This counterweight is supported by the levator scapulae and is the weight of the shoulders and arms.

In balance, no muscles work to maintain the posture of the head, and like the lower part of the back, minimal exertion of muscle is necessary to maintain the balance. Slightly greater movement of the head can also be managed. When the head is extended, the shoulders come forward, and when the head is slightly flexed, the tendency is for the shoulders to move back.

However, the system may be unbalanced quite easily: (1) when the head is brought forward, more forward movement is produced than can be compensated by backward motion of the shoulders, and (2) when the shoulders are brought forward, there is no balance position for the neck. It is then necessary to have the shoulder support muscles working. These consist of the levator scapulae and rhomboids, which contract. The lower part of the trapezius must also contract to counteract any tendency of the shoulder blades to rotate (Fig 35–6).

This muscular arrangement, running from C1 to T10, has a double effect. It tends to pull the neck into greater lordosis and the upper part of the dorsal spine into flexion. The smallest intervertebral joint feels the most compression. This joint may become the source of widespread pain

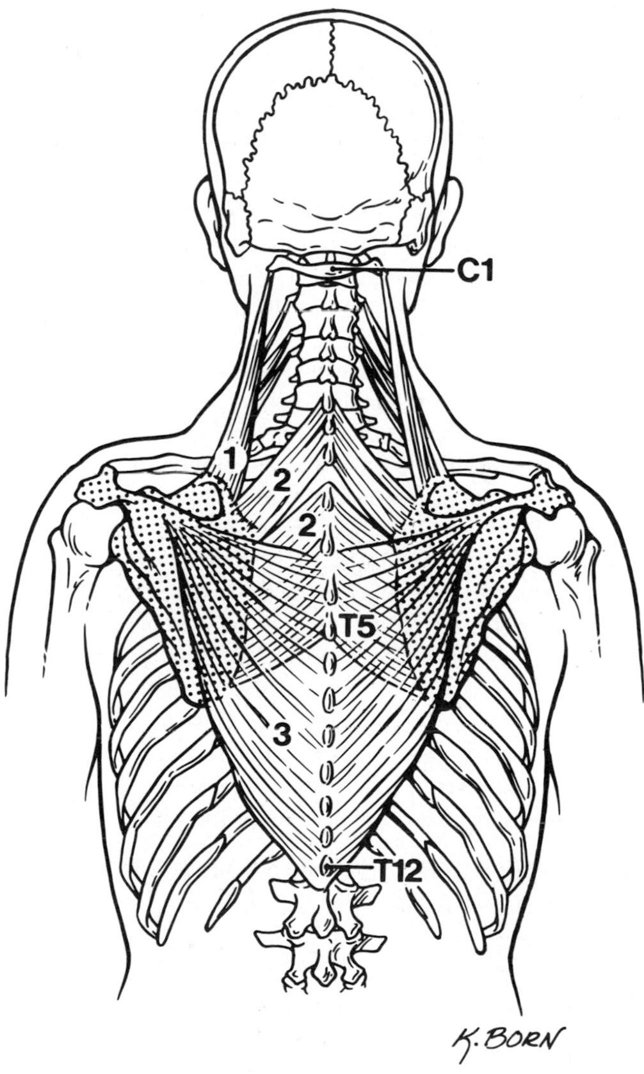

FIG 35–6.
The tired neck syndrome. *1,* levator scapulae; *2,* rhomboids; *3,* lower part of the trapezius. The contraction of the levator scapulae and rhomboids against the contraction of the lower part of the trapezius produces a compression between C1 and T12. The initial vertebral joint to be damaged is the smallest, which is usually at T5.

and is the center of earliest degenerative change in the thoracic spine.

The changes at this joint are osteophytosis of the disc and facet arthrosis. This may extend to involve other joints in the neighborhood.

THE TIRED NECK SYNDROME

This syndrome is not commonly recognized. I call it the tired neck syndrome; others have called it cervicodorsalgia or recurrent strain injury.[2]

Cervical problems, especially those coming from C6–7 and C7–T1, can be shown to radiate pain to a point between the shoulders. Not many realize that a painful source in the upper part of the back can give rise to symptoms in the neck. With the explanation given above, it is easy to see that chronic muscular overwork of the levator scapulae will cause a stiff neck and painful trigger areas along the upper and medial borders of the scapulae. The intense reaction at T5–6 may radiate pain to the epigastrium.

The lordosis of the neck prevents proper closure of the mouth. The person becomes a mouth breather and is subject to nonallergic rhinitis and a dry mouth. The chronic jaw-open posture may cause a temporomandibular dysfunction.

The combination of extension of the neck with a forward and down position of the shoulders may cause the lower and middle cords of the brachial flexors to impinge on the first rib. This, in turn, leads to numbness in the ulna nerve distribution and to a carpal tunnel syndrome.

In 85% of females, there are prominent supraclavicular ribs. This occurs in roughly 10% to 15% of males. This syndrome is therefore much more common in women.

Here again, we see the kinetic chain in action.

The same syndrome may occur following trauma to the neck or following a cervical disc problem. The two conditions are easily distinguished. But the treatment is different. In my opinion, a failure to recognize this problem is the main cause of the prolonged convalescence following whiplash and other injuries of the neck.

THE FACET JOINTS AND SYMMETRY OF THE VERTEBRAE

In the newborn, the facet joints are small and have the same orientation as those of the thoracic spine. With the development of the mamillary processes, the lumbar facet joints acquire their adult orientation. However, there is often considerable variation of one facet joint from its fellow, so Brailsford[1] puts the incidence of asymmetry at 30% of individuals at each level of the lumbar spine.

This easily recognizable asymmetry of the facet joints does not seem to be as important as the asymmetry of the vertebral body that accompanies it.

A vertebra with an asymmetrical facet joint is usually smaller on the side of the more oblique facet, and this facet usually has a smaller surface area than its fellow (Fig 35–7). The line of symmetry that cuts through the spinous process divides the vertebra into unequal halves.

This imbalance of the spine is apparently accommodated by a compensatory muscle mechanism because these individuals seem to function well and do not have a higher incidence of back problems. However, it has been shown that these joints degenerate at an earlier date than normal.

Asymmetry of leg length and asymmetry of the pelvis often accompany asymmetry of the spinal joints and are probably accommodated by a similar mechanism. The asymmetry of the limbs must be greater than 1 to 2 in. to have an effect if occurring naturally. However an acquired short limb of even ½ in. has a demonstrable effect on the back.

An asymmetrical joint may produce a corrective scoliosis that may be one of the mechanisms of compensation.

In true scoliosis, the vertebra seems to have a curved line of asymmetry that divides the vertebra into two equal halves. Scoliotic spines also do not cause more back problems than usual. However, with postural changes due to other causes, e.g., pregnancy, the loss of control of the abdominal muscles can produce severe and often rapid deterioration.

These changes, for the most part, occur at the apex of the curve, which tends to suffer from the greatest leverage and therefore is the first to feel the decompensation.

PATHOLOGIC CHANGES AT THE LUMBAR INTERVERTEBRAL JOINT

The intervertebral joint is a complex of three interconnected joints. Pathologic change in any of the components of the complex is accompanied by pathologic change in the other two.

One of the most common pathologies seen in postmortem specimens is a fissure or a crack in the end plate of the vertebral body. When these are found, the vertebra does not have its normal resistance to compression or torsion and thus has an overall loss of function that extends to all its parts.

This change starts in the attenuated bony trabeculations that support the end plate. These develop microfractures and, as a result, do not contribute to the support of the end plate. The end plate becomes fractured.

The spine is compartmentalized into discs and vertebral bodies. The disc, by virtue of the impervious cartilage surface of the end plate and its annulus, behaves like a hydraulic chamber. It deforms, but with a constant volume. The vertebral body, on the other hand, also fitted with fluid, can be deformed by the extent of blood and intercellular fluid expelled from it. The trabecular bone acts like a

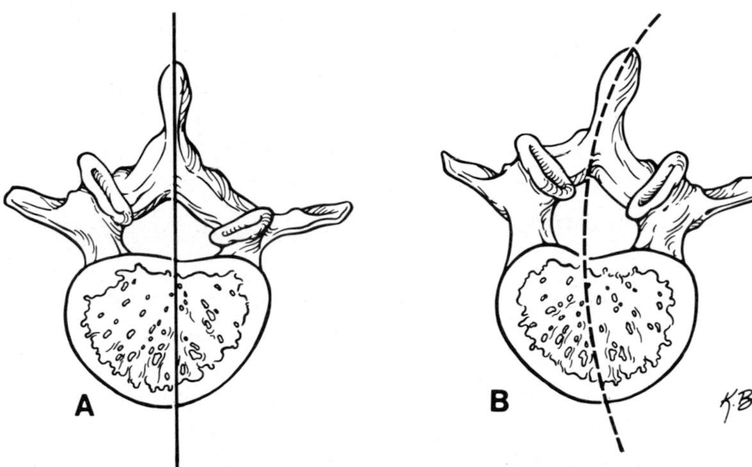

FIG 35–7.
The kinds of asymmetry. In type **A,** the vertebral body is divided into two unequal sections with the more oblique facet on the smaller side. In type **B,** scoliosis, the line of asymmetry appears to divide the vertebral body into two equal areas of much different shape. The facet joints are the same size.

honeycomb and can offer resistance to fluid flow if it is deformed rapidly. In this way, it acts like a shock absorber.

When the integrity of the vertebral end plate is compromised, the fluid compartment must extend to the next enclosing end plates. The new compartment is no longer hydraulic except at high rates of loading.

Thus, a single end-plate fracture may lead to a breakdown of successive end plates. In cadaver material, a skipped intact end plate was never found in a large series of cadaver spines studied by discography.

When first formed, these fractures of the end plate tend to heal and again restore the hydraulic chamber of the disc. But this seal is not as strong as the original and is easily broken by injections under pressure well below that required to cause a leak in a normal disc.

It is understandable that after a while the fractured end plate will not heal in the face of repeated insult. As a matter of fact, the broken end plate often remains an open portal for intercellular disc fluid to directly enter the vascular system via the sinuses of the vertebral body.

The fractured end plate permits another serious effect on the disc. It provides a portal of entry for invasion of the disc by granulation tissue from the vascular vertebral body. This is a well-recognized occurrence when a nonvascularized tissue is exposed to a vascular tissue. The invading vascularized granulation tissue dissolves and replaces the nonvascularized nucleus and inner part of the annulus. Because the vascular supply of the invading tissue is itself tenuous, the replacement may be incomplete, or it may take a long time. The end result is the same. The inner portion of the disc including the cartilaginous end plates are destroyed.

The only part of the disc to survive is the outer portion of the annulus, which is squeezed out of its original location somewhat like a used rubber washer of a faucet.

As the annulus bulges out, it draws with it a ring of osteophytes. This ring of osteophytes, radiographic appearances to the contrary, is never completed between the pedicles of the vertebra.

As the thickness of the disc is lost, the vertebra settles into a new position. The discs in the lumbar and cervical vertebrae settle posteriorly to cause more lordosis. Those in the thoracic area tend to collapse anteriorly and increase the kyphotic curve.

The loss of disc thickness naturally affects the facet joints. They gradually sublimate, lose their cartilaginous surfaces, and become arthrotic. This contributes to the diminishing size of the subarticular recess and the intervertebral canal.

An interesting change occurs in the lamina of the vertebra. The lumbar lamina does not normally support a vertical load. Its function is mainly to support a shear load, and its articular surfaces are arranged transverse to the shearing load. The loss of disc thickness, subluxation of the facet joints, and concomitant loss of facet articular cartilage cause the lower end of the articular process to contact the lamina below. For the first time, the articular processes are carrying up to 25% of the vertical load. The response of the articular process and lamina to this new direction of load is to thicken (Wolff's law). The long-term result is the appearance of stenosis. As similar changes occur in successively higher joints, the spinal stenosis extends upward to affect the other joints.

THE EFFECTS OF TORSIONAL INJURY

As the reader will realize, the changes in the intervertebral joint as aging proceeds are those changes that accompany an overload in compression. This is to be expected because flexion and extension of the spine are the most utilized of all spinal motions. These changes are of course modified and often exaggerated by several other conditions such as obesity, osteoporosis, and vascular supply.

There is a second type of overload—the overload that

occurs with axial rotation. This motion occurs naturally in walking and running and with asymmetrical exertion of the spine such as occurs with one-handed lifts. With this motion, there is almost always an element of compression mixed with the axial rotation. Therefore, the changes are partly due to compression as well as torsion.

The main feature of axial rotation overload is simultaneous damage to the annulus and the facet joints. Neither of these structures are damaged in the initial stages of a compression overload.

It is not surprising, therefore, to find the arthrotic changes in the facet joints to be much more advanced at an earlier age. The annulus develops a radial fissure that allows dye injected into the disc nucleus to escape.

As the rotation injury initially occurs at one joint, usually L4–5, the column above this level is also rotated in relation to the vertebra below. There is an abrupt rotoscoliosis starting at the injured joint. This axial rotation often persists after the injury and causes a compensatory scoliosis at the thoracolumbar junction.

This acquired scoliosis induces a functional disparity in the intrinsic musculature of the spine. This shows itself in a typical torsional pattern of deterioration that increases in degree as we move up the spine. As shown earlier, the progression of change is in the opposite direction with compression injuries.

As can easily be understood, a torsional injury at L4–5 may upset the kinetic chain and affect distant parts of the spine. Theoretically, it can also affect the lower limbs via its effect on rotation and transmission of torque in the lumbar spine and therefore give rise to unequal use of the lower limbs when walking, possibly creating abnormal shearing forces at the hip joints.

PATHOLOGIC CHANGES IN THE CERVICAL INTERVERTEBRAL JOINTS

The cervical intervertebral joints are built in the same plane as the lumbar joints and have a similar lordosis. However, there are some differences. The facet joints support about two thirds of the axial load. The movement at the joint is largely translative rather than rotative. After the age of 9 years, the discs themselves for the most part do not have a nucleus. Fissures in the disc develop at a very early stage in the region of the uncovertebral joints. The fissures spread and extend so that in the adult the disc is a scarred pad between the vertebrae.

With a loss of articular surface cartilage of the facet joints, the joints lose their motion at a relatively early age. Nevertheless, cervical disc problems arise a decade later than lumbar problems. This is probably because of the added stability brought about by the gradual settling of the cervical joints. Motion at the O–C1 and C1–2 joints hide the loss of motion in the other cervical joints.

Loss of cartilage in the facet joints allows a laxity of the ligamentous capsules of these joints. This can lead to an abnormal posterior translation at the joints. Even in the absence of frank disc protrusion, the dorsal root ganglion may be trapped by the posterior translation and cause symptoms.

PATHOLOGIC CHANGE IN THE DORSAL SPINE

Joints in the thoracic spine collapse also. Obvious radiologic effects of this change are seen to occur after changes occur in the lumbar and cervical joints. The process is normally so slow that the osteophytosis is not very marked. However, on occasion, as in the chronic tired neck syndrome, the facet joint may show an intense arthrotic change.

THE EXTREMITIES

We have seen the kinetic chain in action, with change in one part of the spine related to changes in another. We know that conditions in the cervical spine can affect the upper limbs and on rare occasions even the lower limbs. It is common experience that low back conditions may also affect the lower limbs. Do the limbs have a reciprocal effect on the spine?

It is known that a stiff hip has a direct effect on the spine. A flexion deformity at the hip causes a hyperlordosis of the lumbar spine. But does a hyperlordosis of the spine cause a flexion deformity of the hip?

The hip, like all synovial joints, supports only very little shear loads because the joint surfaces are virtually frictionless. When hip motion is lost, at end of its range of motion shearing forces are generated at the cartilage-bone interface, and this can cause damage to the articular cartilage. Theoretically therefore, it is possible that a minimal impairment of the musculature of the hip can produce an arthritis at the hip. This point has been missed in clinical orthopedics. We note the arthritis of the hip and generally ascribe the muscular weakness to stiffness of the hip. This may be putting the cart before the horse.

The effect of knee problems on the back is more difficult to prove. If there is a knee flexion deformity, then a back problem may arise because of the effect of shortening of this limb. However, an arthralgic gait has not been shown to affect the back.

DEGENERATIVE DISC DISEASE

This common diagnosis cannot be maintained in the face of the facts. Numerous pathologic studies have failed to show the presence of degeneration in the true sense of the word. The pathologist needs to see living cells and intercellular ground substance to make this diagnosis. The avascular nature of the disc obviously precludes this possibility.

Everything that happens to the spine happens because of injury. The injuries may be small, certainly subclinical, but each injury heals with a scar that is permanent. The numerous small microtraumas that occur throughout life result in an accumulation of scar tissue.

In a diarthrodial joint, the ligaments and capsule are at the periphery of the joint. However, in the disc, the ligament and capsule are placed between the cartilage surfaces. This is the reason that we see a loss of disc thickness.

"Degenerated" discs, when tested mechanically in forward rotation, exhibit a stiffness that is not seen in normal discs. However, they yield at a lower torque. This is characteristic behavior of scar tissue.

In very old spines, some of the discs test out at values in the range of younger normal values. This would seem to indicate that not all spines show degeneration and, when they do show degeneration, some of the units may still test normal.

All the changes associated with the term "degenerative disc disease" have their basis in injury. This injury may be trivial and produce typical radiographic findings several years later. The kinetic relationship of one part of the spine to another will ensure that when one joint "degenerates," another will certainly follow.

If the injury is less than trivial, the end result may be obtained much more quickly, often with increased symptoms.

The term "degeneration" as a synonym for joint injury is not only unjustified but may also have a discouraging effect on the patient. This problem is intensified when the person is told that he has degenerative arthritis. The first term tells the patient in no uncertain terms that he is falling apart. The second term tells him that he is going to fall apart in his other joints.

How much simpler the truth.

REFERENCES

1. Braisford JF: Deformities of the lumbosacral region of the spine. *Br J Surg* 1929; 16:562.
2. Farfan HF, Baldwin J: The tired neck syndrome, in Karowski EW (ed): *Trends in Ergonomics/Human factors III*. Amsterdam, Elsevier, 1983.
3. Farfan HF, Gracovetsky S: The nature of instability. *Spine* 1984; 9:714.
4. Farfan HF, Gracovetsky S: The optimum spine. *Spine* 1986; 11:543–573.
5. Farfan HH: On the nature of arthritis. *J Rheumatol* 1983; 10(suppl 9):103.
6. Helleur C: *Spine Subjected to Acceleration* (thesis). Concordia University, Montreal, 1983.

36

Arthritides Affecting the Spinal Column

J. Thalgott, M.D., Henry LaRocca, M.D., and Vance O. Gardner, M.D.

Arthritis of the spine is one of the most common diseases that medical practitioners of all types are asked to see and treat. There are a variety of arthritides that affect the spinal column. This chapter will deal with common osteoarthritis, rheumatoid arthritis, and ankylosing spondylitis. Although there are other more esoteric arthritides that affect the spine, these are fairly rare and will not be reviewed in this chapter.

Osteoarthritis of the spine is a disease that affects all members of the population. It should be viewed as a part of the aging process of the human spine and affects all cervical, thoracic, and lumbar levels. The degeneration of the disc and its associated joints produces an entire spectrum of symptomatology. Osteoarthritic changes in the disc and facet joints may be asymptomatic in a large percentage of the population, intermittently symptomatic for mechanical neck and back pain, or completely disabling with intractable pain. Alternatively, this may present with neural encroachment phenomena including myelopathy or radiculopathy. The degree of neural involvement is dictated by the amount and location of the pathology. Cervical spondylosis has a very different natural history and presentation from lumbar spondylosis. This is because of the differential loads carried by the cervical spine as compared with the lumbar region. The cervical and thoracic vertebral encase the spinal cord, where generally the lumbar spine protects the cauda equina.

Cervical spondylosis is a common disease whose natural history is associated with the aging process. Senescent and pathologic changes are essentially indistinguishable in the cervical region. Historically, the Edwin Smith papyrus described a neurologic event after injury to the cervical spine 4000 years ago. Since then, the concepts of cervical spondylosis can be followed through the literature beginning with Key[18] in 1838 who reported on paraplegia from a "spondylytic bar." Stookey[36] in 1940 outlined the clinical spectrum of neurologic changes in severe cervical spondylosis. Later in that decade, Bull[6] described the importance of the neural central joints of Luschka in the generation of radiculopathy from nerve root pressure. Later, O'Connell[29] described three types of lesions from cervical degeneration. First was the classic soft intervertebral disc protrusion. Second was neural encroachment secondary to degeneration of the disc and the zygapophyseal joints. Third was a combination of spondylosis and soft-disc protrusion at a single level. Brain et al.[4] and Mair and Druckman[23] discussed the role of vascular changes in concert with spondylytic compression of neural elements in the cervical spine. Later, it was discussed by Payne and Spillane[31] and Edwards and LaRocca[10] that patients with congenitally small canals may be more prone to neural encroachment from spondylytic changes.

Disc degeneration in the cervical as well as lumbar segments of the spine is a normal aging process. It is quite clear that beginning in the third decade the discs undergo dehydration as a natural aging process. Extensive work has been done by Naylor[28] and Hendry[14] as to the etiology of this dehydration. Other authors[7, 22] have suggested that as a consequence of this dehydration of the discs, the motion segments of the cervical spine become altered, and this leads to either soft-disc herniation or osteophytosis. These events are due to the progressive incompetency of the disc to maintain its normal axial load and motion-dampening function. This sequence of disc dehydration with structural disc incompetence leads to osteophytosis in an attempt by the body to stabilize the segment that is producing the classic cervical spondylytic changes of posterior osteophytes in causing spinal cord compression either in the midline or laterally. Accompanying this are foraminal stenosis and possibly radiculopathy caused by degeneration of the neural central joints of Luschka. These events also produce degenerative changes in the facet itself. The other end of the disc degeneration spectrum is a nuclear herniation giving rise to the "soft disc." A soft-disc herniation may be central, lateral, intraforaminal, dorsal, or ventral. However, disc herniation is not within the scope of this chapter. It suffices to say that soft-disc herniation may be superimposed on a pre-existing spondylosis and add to the neural encroachment disease. Friedenberg and Miller[13] in 1963 discussed the location of cervical spondylosis. They found that below the level of C3–4 there was a higher incidence of degeneration that was more severe than in the upper portion of the cervical spine. It is well known that the C5–6 level is the most frequently involved in cervical spondylosis as well as herniated discs, with the C6–7 level the second most frequent. The cervical levels above C3 are the least frequently involved. In the lower cervical vertebrae, each motion segment carries five distinct joints. These are the intervertebral disc, the zygapophyseal joints posteriorly, and the two joints of Luschka anteriorly. All of these joints are affected by disc degeneration and secondary collapse. In the youthful spine there is a natural tendency toward lordotic positioning secondary to the asymmetry of the disc. As this degenerates, the spine goes from lordosis into kyphosis because of the loss of disc height anteriorly. This movement toward flexion has the effect of producing more posterior displacement of the osteophytes from the superior and inferior end plates and potential lessening of the space within the spinal canal.[19] The C6–7 level is the most frequently associated with posterior osteophyte formation; however, the highest incidence of neural central joint changes causing foraminal stenosis is present at the C5–6 level. There also may be involvement of the zygapophyseal joints as well as subluxation and subsequent neural foraminal encroachment. The most frequent levels involved, because of the degeneration of these three motion segment joints, are C3–4, C4–5, and C5–6.[19] Radiographically, it is noted that the disc spaces begin to narrow and subsequently have anterior or posterior osteophytes. The posterior osteophytes tend to be smaller than the anterior osteophytes; however, it is clear that these osteophytes limit motion in the involved segments. The posterior osteophytes are best seen on the lateral view, and the posterolateral osteophytes are best seen on the oblique x-ray views. The posterolateral osteophytes correlate with the neural central joints and have a tendency to compress the neural foramen and not the central cord. However, the posterior osteophytes may be midline and have a spondylytic bar compressing the spinal cord itself and causing a myelopathy. The posterior zygapophyseal joints are classic synovial joints and may undergo a narrowing of the cartilage, sclerosis of the end plates, and hypertrophy as in any other zygapophyseal joint in the body. It is more common, according to Lestini and Wiesel,[19] that the superior articulating facet undergoes an osteophytic process that if medial in location may cause neural foraminal narrowing as well. If the patient is clinically symptomatic, CT/myelography or MRI may be quite helpful in delineating the specific pathology. However, it is well known that there is no definite correlation between symptoms and radiographic appearance.[15, 40, 41] Other authors[37] have studied groups of asymptomatic and symptomatic patients and found that the only radiographic correlations with symptoms were the neural central joints and narrowing of the intervertebral foramen. However, other authors[13] found no correlation. It is felt that cord compression may be present if the sagittal diameter at any level is less than 10 mm.[26] It is also well known that static films may not be predictive of the amount of cervical cord compromise since there may be a dynamic component to the neural encroachment. Cervical myelopathy can be produced by the intermingling of spondylytic bars, hypertrophic facets, and a pre-existing congenitally small spinal canal. Wilkinson et al.[41] clearly correlated myelopathy with osteophytosis and pre-existing narrow sagittal diameter of the cervical canal. However, they also suggested a vascular etiology as well. The painful zygapophyseal joints of the facets may cause neck pain referred to the trapezius and suprascapular regions. This degenerative process and subsequent facet pain have been clearly delineated by Bogduk and Marslan.[3] An excellent review of cervical spondylytic changes has been performed by Lestini and Wiesel.[19]

LUMBAR DISC DISEASE AND SPINAL STENOSIS AS A MANIFESTATION OF LUMBAR SPONDYLOSIS

Disorders of the lower part of the back are a very common reason for medical treatment. Benn and Wood[2] estimated in 1975 that 1400 days are lost from work each year for every 1000 workers because of low back pain and estimated this to have a staggering financial impact on the world's economy. This loosely correlates with approximately 80% of adults having one or more bouts of serious back pain. In 1969 Horal[16] demonstrated that the majority of patients suffering from low back complaints have nonradiating mechanical low back pain. However, these patients generally respond to conservative management. In contrast to the cervical spine, the lumbar spine is composed of an intervertebral disc and two zygapophyseal joints posteriorly. However, the same type of degenerative process occurs in the lumbar spine, but most likely at a more rapid rate because of the greater loads placed on the lumbar spine in the erect posture. The same dehydration/disc degeneration sequence occurs in the lumbar spine as well as the thoracic and cervical vertebrae. With this deorganization and destabilization of the disc, the subsequent formation of osteophytes posteriorly as well as anteriorly in unstable segments is well described by MacNab,[22] Lestini and Wiesel,[19] and Lipson and Muir.[20] Increasing disc degeneration in the lumbar spine over time and its ability to withstand repetitive trauma and load bearing decreases. The segment becomes increasingly unstable, and the zygapophyseal joints begin to sublux in a craniocaudal fashion. The facet joints begin to overgrow secondary to this increased derangement of the motion segment in an attempt to stabilize the segment. This leads to both medial and lateral overgrowth and widening of the facet. Classic osteoarthritic changes appear in these joints; there is a decrease in the hyaline cartilage and an increase in the periarticular sclerosis with hypertrophy of the lateral margins. The disc itself continues to collapse and cause not only posterior osteophytes but posterior disc bulging and potential neural encroachment. The neural encroachment, as in the cervical spine, may be either secondary to acute disc herniation or a combination of discoligamentous and bony hypertrophy causing either radicular symptoms or spinal stenosis with classic pseudoclaudicatory symptoms.[11] Epstein et al.[11] have clearly described the clinical symptoms of spinal stenosis, and Dyck and Doyle[9] defined a bicycle test for delineating this. There may also be a congenitally small canal in the lumbar spine secondary to short pedicles and thus a predisposition for neural encroachment phenomena secondary to lumbar spondylosis.[39] Arnoldi[1] described acquired stenosis on a degenerative basis as well. There are different locations of stenosis within the spinal canal: central canal, peripheral (lateral recess or subarticular), and foraminal stenosis. Gross degeneration of the disc space with forward subluxation of the facets causes a degenerative spondylolisthesis. This results in high-grade stenosis of the involved segments by narrowing the spinal canal in the presence of degenerative changes. The lateral and foraminal stenosis types of neural encroachment cause predominantly radicular symptoms. This is most common at L4–5 and results in L5 symptomatology secondary to compression by the superior facet of L5 because of bony overgrowth. This may be either bilateral or unilateral. The foraminal stenosis causing L5 radiculopathy may occur at L5–S1. This is caused by a combination of facet hypertrophy and disc degeneration. Narrowing of the neural foramina is caused by decreased disc space height; the facet then settles and causes encroachment of the superior facet on the exiting nerve root against the pedicle. This may occur at multiple levels but is most common at L5–S1 and L4–5. These changes clearly produce neural encroachment with secondary radiculopathy. This pathologic state is best imaged with computed axial tomography (CAT)/myelography combinations. MRI may also be useful in imaging the spinal stenosis as well. There may be symptoms of mechanical back pain that vary with interdiscal pressure from disc degeneration as well. It has been shown by Nachemson[27] that position greatly changes the interdiscal pressure. Patients who suffer from mechanical back pain have discomfort that varies directly with interdiscal pressure. It is worse when they sit or stand and better when they lie down. This pain is often midline back pain radiating to the posterior/superior iliac spines or often into the groin or thighs. This may be generated from the disc itself secondary to symptomatic disc degeneration or internal disc disruption as described by Crock.[8] There also may be back pain that is mediated through the degeneration or injury to the facet joints themselves. This facet pain is generally unilateral and refers to the posterior/superior iliac spine area of the affected side; however, the pain can be bilateral. Facet pain is generally worse with extension and may not vary with interdiscal pressure. The documentation of facet syndrome may be done with evocative facet injections. Management of the specific problems of discogenic pain and facet pain without neural encroachment should be conservative. This should include appropriate physical therapy modalities and anti-inflammatory drugs. This approach is used in the first several weeks of onset. It should progress to a nonmodality functional approach aimed at strengthening abdominal muscles and, in the later stages, the paraspinous and trunk muscles. Also, the use of epidural cortisone blocks and facet joint injections may be helpful adjuvants to the conservative approach. The intermittent use of a lumbar support may be also helpful as well as the continued use of oral anti-inflammatory drugs.

An overwhelming number of patients on a worldwide basis suffer from cervical, thoracic, and lumbar spondylosis. These are diseases that are inseparable from the normal aging process and have a common etiology and natural history. It is quite clear that the congenital size of the spinal canal directly influences whether spinal degeneration will produce symptomatic neural encroachment.[10, 26, 30]

ANKYLOSING SPONDYLITIS

Ankylosing spondylitis is a chronic systemic inflammatory disorder of undetermined etiology (Figs 36–1 to 36–5). This disease predominantly attacks the axial skeletal system, with sacroiliac involvement most common. This inflammatory disorder affects synovial and cartilaginous joints as well as the "entheses," or the sites of ligamentous and muscle attachment to bone. This disease is most commonly seen in predominantly white young men between 15 to 35 years of age and is associated with an

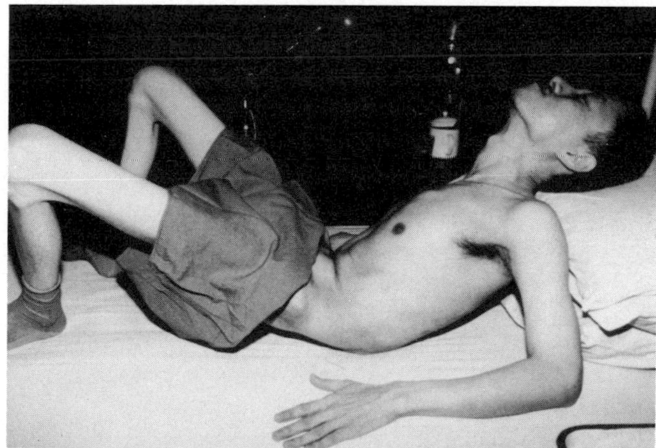

FIG 36–1.
This 32-year-old Oriental man with a long history of ankylosing spondylitis and a fixed midthoracic deformity is neurologically intact but unable to stand erect.

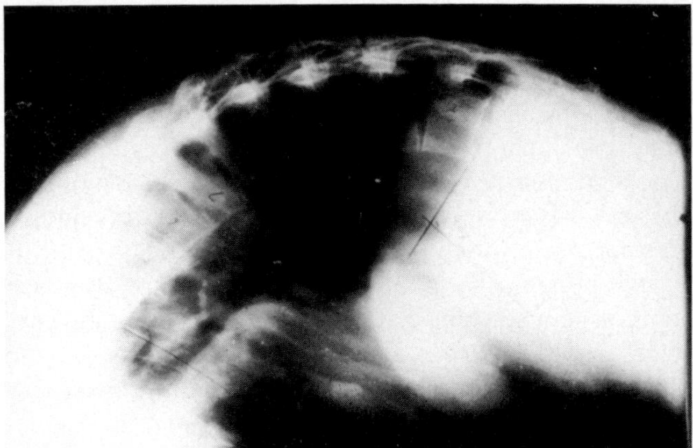

FIG 36-2.
Preoperative lateral radiograph demonstrating a marked kyphos.

HLA-B27 antigen. Clinically, the majority of patients present with insidious low back pain and stiffness. Fifteen percent to 20% of patients present with peripheral joint pain, and sciatic pain occurs in 5% to 15%. Also, involvement of the chest wall with costochondral inflammation and lack of chest expansion is common. This is also associated with pulmonary fibrosis. Iritis, acute and chronic, may affect up to 25% of patients. Also, cardiac manifestations with conductive defects and valvular heart disease may be common in the chronic stages. One of the most common presenting symptoms is sacroiliac joint tenderness. Joint involvement in ankylosing spondylitis appears to originate as subchondral osteitis that invades the overlying cartilage and is accompanied by cartilage metaplasia and ossification. In contrast to rheumatoid arthritis, there is no pannus formation across the joint. One of the classic features of ankylosing spondylitis is that fibrous and bony ankylosis of the involved joints occur and lead to stiffness

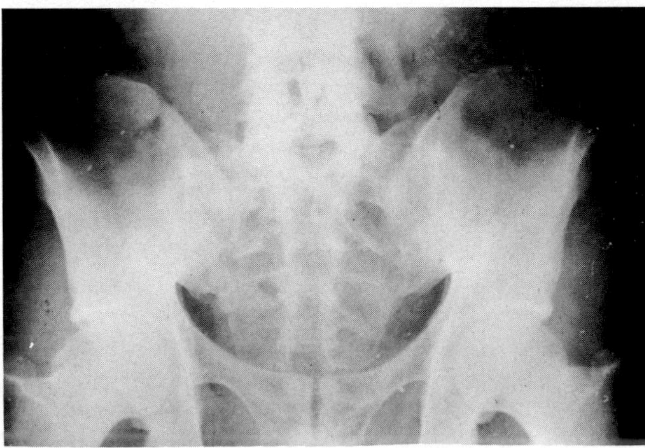

FIG 36-3.
Anteroposterior view of the pelvis showing classic obliteration of the sacroiliac joints from ankylosing spondylitis.

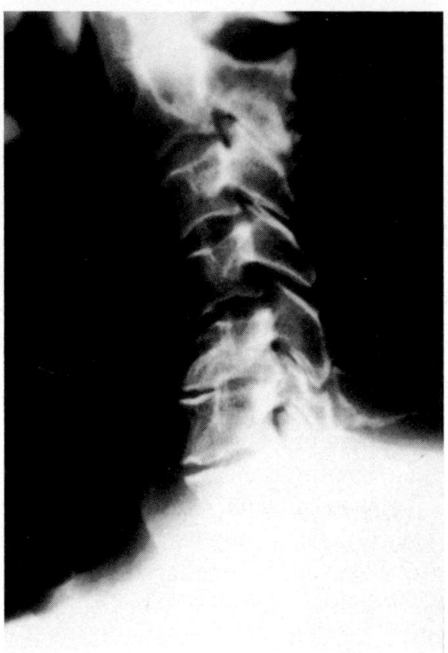

FIG 36-4.
Lateral radiograph showing C5-6 and C6-7 degenerative disc disease with both posterior and anterior osteophytic lipping and degeneration of the facets with foraminal stenosis.

and oftentimes large segments of the spine being solidly fused. Although ankylosing spondylitis is largely a systemic disease, the spine is a frequent site of involvement. Because of the precarious position of the spine in terms of guarding sensitive neural structures, significant complications can be seen from this disease.

Atlantoaxial joint subluxation is quite common with ankylosing spondylitis. Ankylosing spondylitis inflammation may involve the synovial lining of the atlantoaxial joint or the synovial bursa lying between the odontoid process and the transverse ligament. This may lead to erosion of the odontoid process or rupture of the transverse ligament, which will allow forward subluxation of the atlas on the axis. Radiographically, this has shown if the tubercle of C1 to the nearest point on the odontoid is greater than 2.5 mm. Martel[25] in 1961 reported that patients displaying this had disease for more than 10 years and that there were no cases of multiple subluxations such as in the rheumatoid group. Presenting symptoms may be simple neck pain, shoulder pain, or occipital headache. This may have a range of neurologic symptoms from completely normal findings to a myelopathy with sensory loss and weakness in the upper and lower extremities. Also damage to the nucleus of the trigeminal nerve may be present with loss of pain and temperature sensation over the face. Potentially, quadriplegia and death could ensue.[33] Further atlantoaxial subluxation may also cause vertebral artery compression and lead to a variety of central neurologic problems in-

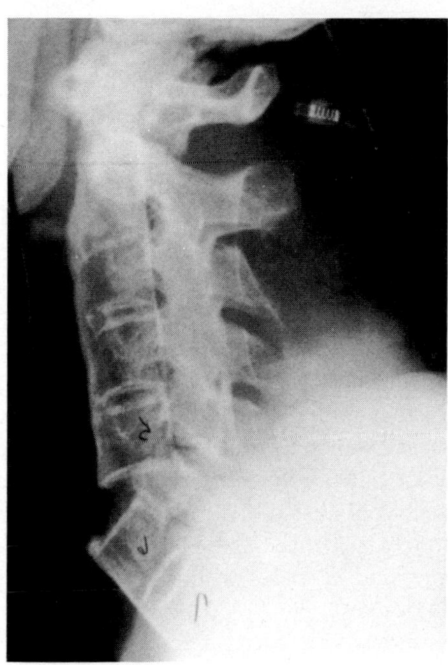

FIG 36–5.
This 47-year-old man with long-standing ankylosing spondylitis was involved in a motor vehicle accident and sustained a hyperextension injury. The patient had a complete transection of his cervical spinal column and was rendered completely quadriplegic at the C5–6 level.

cluding blurred vision and stroke.[21] Generally, a workup of this from a radiographic standpoint includes MRI or CT/myelography. Plain tomograms may also be of benefit in imaging the bony abnormalities. Atlanto-occipital joint subluxation has also been reported.[25] Erosion of the lateral masses of the atlas may be associated with upward subluxation of the axis. In effect this causes the occiput to descend over the cervical spine, which may be demonstrated by lateral tomography showing the top of the odontoid over a line from the hard palate to the inferior margin of the occipital curve.[21] This is a rather uncommon complication of ankylosing spondylitis but may lead to significant medullary compression as in patients with rheumatoid arthritis. Patients with ankylosing spondylitis may also have intervertebral disc lesions secondary to adjacent end-plate erosion. This occurs commonly in the thoracic spine and may be due to excessive stress from the large lever arms of completely ankylosed segments making a stress fracture that does not heal. Hunter and Dubo[17] described this as a spinal "pseudarthrosis" and felt that the apophyseal joints fail to fuse at this level because of increased stress. These lesions may be asymptomatic or symptomatic and cause localized spinal pain. Rarely, spinal cord damage will result from bony instability by proliferation of granulation tissue within the epidural space or from true spinal instability. This condition may also produce an acute angulation or a gibbus formation. The differential diagnosis of these lesions is infection, neoplasm, or Charcot joints of the spine. The major differential is to exclude infections in these patients, who are oftentimes treated with steroids. This could be done by leukocytosis, a high sedimentation rate, and a failure to relieve the spine pain by rest. The treatment of this condition may be surgical stabilization.[12] Spinal fracture is also a significant problem in the osteoporotic ankylosed spine and may be multiple or single level.[17, 38] The majority of patients with ankylosing spondylitis are treated with a rigorous exercise program designed to prevent static deformity and maintain good general conditioning. The use of nonsteroidal anti-inflammatory drugs is also appropriate. Great care must be taken in monitoring all patients with ankylosing spondylitis to anticipate serious spinal complications of this disease.

RHEUMATOID ARTHRITIS

Rheumatoid arthritis is a systemic disease that may be monoarticular or multifocal. Its etiology is unknown, but, there is now good evidence that it is a genetically controlled host immune response to some unknown stimulus. There is also an association with the HLA-Dw4 locus, which is associated with severe seropositive rheumatoid arthritic patients.[35] Currently, more effective therapeutics are aimed at managing the immunologic basis for this disease. The cervical spine is a common target for manifestations of this systemic disease. The thoracic and lumbar vertebrae are generally unhampered by this ailment. This section will concentrate on rheumatoid arthritis of the cervical spine. According to Simmons,[34] the types of involvement of the cervical spine are atlantoaxial subluxation, atlantoaxial subluxation combined with subaxial subluxation, and subaxial subluxation alone. The classic rheumatoid arthritic destruction of joints begins with synovial proliferation and joint effusion and edema. Synovial proliferation causes cartilaginous erosion and destruction. A pannus is formed in the articular cartilage and destroys the architecture of the joint. The periarticular structures such as ligaments and joint capsules are also destroyed and become incompetent at maintaining the position of their respective bony joint structures. This process allows a generalized osteoporosis in the surrounding osseous tissue as well. This makes fixation difficult in the rheumatoid patient because the amount of osteoporosis leads to poor bone quality. Atlantoaxial subluxation in this disease is a hallmark of cervical spine involvement. Initially, erosion of the transverse ligaments allows atlantoaxial subluxation and causes erosion of the periarticular joint capsules, which allows further subluxation and possibly occipitoatlantal involvement as well. With the combination of weakening of the ligamentous stability and local erosive changes within the bone itself, this allows atlantoaxial subluxation with cranial migration of the superior margin of the odontoid into the foramen magnum. These pathologic changes generally present with neck pain and soreness in the suboccipital region. This is exacerbated with flexion and extension, and there is usually some tenderness about the suboccipital regions. As the subluxation advances, the patient may experience some vague paresthesias of the upper and lower extremities and generalized weakness. The atlantoaxial subluxation may be anterior, posterior, or lateral. The anterior is the most common and is found in 11% to 46% of postmortem studies on patients with rheumatoid arthritis. Lateral atlantoaxial subluxation was also observed in the transoral view, where it is found that the lateral masses of C1 have a 2.0-mm or greater shift on those of C2. This was reported to account for 21% of all atlantoaxial subluxation, and 10% of the rheumatoid population was found to have an irreducible head tilt secondary to this problem. Atlantoaxial invagination is also quite common and has been reported in up to 30% of rheumatoid patients. Tomography, CT, and MRI are very useful in imaging this deformity.

Once the diagnosis of atlantoaxial subluxation has been made, the patient should be monitored quite carefully. Most patients can be simply followed conservatively; however, surgical stabilization does play a role. Simmons[34] states that uncontrolled pain is associated with neurologic dysfunction. Pellicci et al.[32] in 1981 graded neurologic involvement: 0 was no neurologic involvement; grade I, hyperreflexia and dysesthesia; grade II, mild weakness and posterior column deficit; and grade III, severe weakness resulting in significant functional disability. The radiographic presence of atlantoaxial subluxation or atlantoaxial invagination does not necessarily mean that surgery is indicated. Only 10% of patients ever require surgery.[32] Even though a solid arthrodesis is obtained, there may be further neurologic progression in some patients.

Most patients can be treated nonsurgically with neck support collars and pain control as well as pharmacologically addressing the rheumatoid disease. However, if surgery is contemplated, then the goal is solid arthrodesis of the involved joints. The surgeon may use wire stabilization or a halo. Most patients with rheumatoid arthritis of this severity are quite debilitated, and halo vest immobilization may not be in the patient's best interest. However, the patients are grossly osteoporotic, and wire fixation may be less than secure. There has been an attempt to use methylmethacrylate to enhance the rigidity of the fixation montage; however, this adds the complications of a higher incidence of wound dehiscence and infection.[5]

Rheumatoid disease may also affect the disc spaces and the posterior zygapophyseal joints of the lower half of the cervical spine. This erosive process destroys periarticular joint capsule stability and the structural integrity of the discs as well as the facet joints. This allows subluxation of the facet joints and increased mobility and decreased structural integrity of the discs. This can lead to subluxation at one or multiple levels of the cervical spine. Generally, these are multiple and give a "stepladder" appearance. Subaxial subluxations can be found in up to 20% of the rheumatoid patient population. Radiographically they do not form osteophytes; however, some patients may have significant neurologic deficits from the secondary spinal stenosis. Generally, this type of instability appears early in the patient's course. These patients' risk factors include cortical steroid use, seropositivity, the presence of rheumatoid nodules, and an aggressive course of the disease. Generally, the patients do not die of their cervical disease but from disease-related processes. However, the subaxial instability can be life-threatening in a small group of patients. There is a higher incidence of cord compression in males with 9.0 mm or greater of atlantoaxial instability.

Most patients with neurologic symptoms and intractable pain may be managed with decompression and fusion. This may be done anteriorly, posteriorly, or combined. The use of internal fixation alleviates the need for a halo; however, fixation in the lower cervical segments is also problematic because of osteoporosis leading to poor fixation. Many of these patients have been taking cortical steroids, which adds to the amount of generalized osteoporosis.

Many other arthritides affect the spinal column. However, the three most common are osteoarthritis, rheumatoid arthritis, and ankylosing spondylitis. The spinal physician must be aware of these entities, how they present clinically, and the principles of management. Surgical intervention for these conditions is rare, and the majority of patients seen by spinal physicians are treated conservatively. However, a basic understanding of the presentation, natural history, and complications of these arthritides as they affect the spinal column is imperative for spinal physicians.

REFERENCES

1. Arnoldi CC: Lumbar spinal stenosis and nerve root entrapment syndrome. *Clin Orthop* 1976; 15:5.
2. Benn RT, Wood PHN: Pain in the back: An attempt to estimate the size of the problem. *Rheumatol Rehabil* 1975; 14:121.
3. Bogduk N, Marslan A: The cervical zygapophysial joints as a source of neck pain. *Spine* 1988; 13:610–617.
4. Brain WR, Northfield D, Wilkinson M: The neurological manifestations of cervical spondylosis. *Brain* 1952; 75:13.
5. Bryan WJ, Inglis AE, Sculco TP, et al: Methylmethacrylate stabilization for enhancement of posterior cervical arthrodesis in rheumatoid arthritis. *J Bone Joint Surg [Am]* 1982; 64:1045–1050.

6. Bull J: Review of cerebral angiography. *Proc R Soc Med* 1949; 42:880.
7. Coventry MB, Ghormley RK, Kernohan JW: The intervertebral disk: Its microscopic anatomy and pathology, Part II. Changes in the intervertebral disk concomitant with age. *J Bone Joint Surg* 1945; 27:460.
8. Crock HV: *Practice of Spinal Surgery*. New York, Springer-Verlag, 1983.
9. Dyck P, Doyle JB: "Bicycle test" of Van Gelderan in diagnosis on intermittent cauda equina compression syndrome. *J Neurosurg* 1977; 46:667.
10. Edwards WC, LaRocca SH: The developmental segmental sagittal diameter in combined cervical and lumbar spondylosis. *Spine* 1985; 10:42.
11. Epstein BS, Epstein JA, Jones MD: Lumbar spinal stenosis. *Radiol Clin North Am* 1977; 15:227.
12. Fang D, Leong JCY, Ho EKW, et al: Spinal pseudarthrosis in ankylosing spondylosis: Clinicopathological correlation and the results of anterior spinal fusion. *J Bone Joint Surg [Br]* 1988; 70:443–447.
13. Friedenberg ZB, Miller WT: Degenerative disk disease of the cervical spine. *J Bone Joint Surg [Am]* 1963; 45:1171.
14. Hendry NG: The hydration of the nucleus pulposus and its relation to the intervertebral disk derangement. *J Bone Joint Surg [Br]* 1958; 40:132.
15. Hitselberger WE, Witten R: Abnormal myelograms in asymptomatic patients. *J Neurosurg* 1968; 28:204.
16. Horal J: The clinical appearance of low back disorders. *Acta Orthop Scand Suppl* 1969; 118:7.
17. Hunter T, Dubo HIC: Spinal fractures complicating ankylosing spondylitics: A longterm follow-up study. *Arthritis Rheum* 1983; 26:751–759.
18. Key CA: On paraplegia depending on the ligaments of the spine. *Guys Hosp Rep* 1838; 3:17.
19. Lestini W, Wiesel S: The pathogenesis of cervical spondylosis. *Clin Orthop* 1989; 239:69–93.
20. Lipson SJ, Muir H: Vertebral osteophyte formation in experimental disk degeneration: Morphologic and proteoglycan changes over time. *Arthritis Rheum* 1980; 23:319.
21. Little H, Swinson DR, Cruickshank B: Upward subluxation of the axis in ankylosing spondylitis: A clinical pathologic report. *Am J Med* 1976; 60:279–285.
22. MacNab I: The traction spur: An indicator of segmental instability. *J Bone Joint Surg [Am]* 1971; 53:663.
23. Mair WG, Druckman R: The pathology of spinal cord lesions and their relations to the clinical features in protrusion of cervical intervertebral disks. *Brain* 1953; 76:70.
24. Martel W: Spinal pseudarthrosis: A complication of ankylosing spondylitis. *Arthritis Rheum* 1978; 21:485–490.
25. Martel W: The occipito-atlanto-axial joints in rheumatoid arthritis and ankylosing spondylitis. *AJR* 1961; 86:223–240.
26. Murone I: The importance of sagittal diameters of the cervical spinal canal in relation to spondylosis and myelopathy. *J Bone Joint Surg [Br]* 1974; 56:30.
27. Nachemson A: The influence of spinal movements in the lumbar intradiskal pressure and on the tensile stresses in the annulus fibrosus. *Acta Orthop Scand* 1963; 33:183.
28. Naylor A: The biophysical and biochemical aspects of intervertebral disk herniation and degeneration. *Ann R Coll Surg Eng* 1962; 31:91.
29. O'Connell JE: Involvement of the spinal cord by intervertebral disk protrusions. *Br Med J* 1953; 2:975.
30. Ogino H, Tada K, Okada K, et al: Canal diameter, anteroposterior compression ratio, and spondylitic myelopathy of the cervical spine. *Spine* 1983; 8:1.
31. Payne EE, Spillane JD: The cervical spine. An anatomicopathological study of 70 specimens (using a special technique) with particular reference to the problem of cervical spondylosis. *Brain* 1957; 80:571.
32. Pellicci PM, Ranawat CS, Tsairis P, et al: A prospective study of the progression of rheumatoid arthritis of the cervical spine. *J Bone Joint Surg* 1981; 63:342–350.
33. Sharp J, Purser DW: Spontaneous atlanto-axial dislocation in ankylosing spondylitis and rheumatoid arthritis. *Ann Rheum Dis* 1961; 20:47–89.
34. Simmons E: Surgery of the spine in rheumatoid arthritis and ankylosing spondylitis. *Surg Musculoskel Sys* 1983; 2:85–151.
35. Stastny P: Rheumatoid arthritis: Relationship with HLA-D. *Am J Med* 1983; 75:9–15.
36. Stookey B: Compression of spinal cord and nerve roots by herniation of nucleus pulposus in cervical region. *Arch Surg* 1940; 40:417.
37. Tapiovarra J, Heinivaara O: Correlation of cervicobrachialgias and roentgenographic findings. *Ann Chir Gynaecol Suppl* 1954; 43:436.
38. Trent G, Armstrong GWD, O'Neill J: Thoracolumbar fractures in ankylosing spondylitis: High risk injuries. *Clin Orthop* 1988; 227:61–66.
39. Verbiest H: Radicular syndrome from developmental narrowing of lumbar vertebral canal. *J Bone Joint Surg [Br]* 1954; 36:230.
40. Wiesel SW, Tsourmas N, Feffer HL, et al: A study of computer-assisted tomography I. The incidence of positive CAT scans in an asymptomatic group of patients. *Spine* 1984; 9:549–551.
41. Wilkinson HA, LaMay ML, Ferris EJ: Clinical-radiographic correlations in cervical spondylosis. *J Neurosurg* 1969; 30:213.

37

Lumbar Spinal Stenosis

Rick B. Delamarter, M.D., and Mark W. Howard, M.D.

Spinal stenosis is characterized by a decrease in the dimensions of the spinal canal and neural foramen. This may result in compression on neural and/or vascular elements. In 1911 Bailey and Casamajor described osteoarthritis of the spine as a cause of compression of lumbosacral nerve roots.[6] In 1931 lumbar neurocompression by thickened ligamenta flava and spondylotic ridges was first described.[66]

The modern-day understanding of spinal stenosis began with Verbiest's 1954 description of the radicular symptoms secondary to cases of developmental narrowing of the lumbar vertebral canal.[69] Since that report multiple studies have helped to advance our understanding of the anatomy, pathology, and pathophysiology of spinal cord and nerve root compression secondary to various causes and types of spinal stenosis.

SPINAL STENOSIS: CLASSIFICATION, DEFINITIONS, AND TERMS

Arnoldi et al. in 1976 gave us the modern-day definition and classification of lumbar spinal stenosis.[3] They defined lumbar spinal stenosis as any type of narrowing of the spinal canal, nerve root canals (or tunnels), or intervertebral foramina. This narrowing may be local, segmental, or generalized and may be caused by bone or soft tissue. This condition may be congenital or acquired or the result of both congenital and acquired factors. A detailed discussion on every cause of spinal stenosis is beyond the scope of this chapter, but Table 37–1 lists the complete classification of lumbar spinal stenosis.[49]

Idiopathic spinal stenosis is generally more common in men and becomes symptomatic between the ages of 35 and 65 years. Presenting symptoms and signs in adults are similar to those of other forms of spinal stenosis. The cervical and lumbar segments of the spine are most often affected, the thoracic spine rarely so. The pedicles may be short and the articular facets and laminae enlarged. The spinal canal may have a trefoil configuration rather than the usual oval configuration (Fig 37–1). The stenosis may be secondary to both bone and soft-tissue hypertrophy. Idiopathic spinal stenosis more commonly affects multiple levels. Archeologic studies of prehistoric North American Indians indicate that developmental idiopathic spinal stenosis may be related to prenatal and infant malnutrition. In addition, genetic factors have been implicated in developmental lumbar stenosis.

Achondroplasia is a type of autosomal dominant, short-limbed dwarfism characterized by vertebral bodies that are short, broad, wedge, or "bowed" shaped. In addition, the pedicles are short and thick with a decreased interpedicular distance commonly causing spinal stenosis. Spinal stenosis is commonly most symptomatic at the lumbar spine and thoracolumbar junction. Achondroplastic dwarfs can demonstrate neurologic deficits as infants but generally present in the fourth or fifth decade when a congenitally narrow canal is further encroached upon by generalized spondylosis or a herniated disk.

Other less frequent congenital or developmental syndromes associated with spinal stenosis include hypophosphatemic vitamin D–resistant rickets, Morquio's mucopolysaccharidosis, cheirolumbar dysostosis, skeletal dysplasias including metatrophic dwarfism, spondyloepiphyseal dysplasia, Kniest's disease, multiple epiphyseal dysplasia, as well as Down's syndrome and congenital spondylolisthesis.

Clinically the most common form of spinal stenosis encountered is the acquired stenosis of a degenerative nature. Other causes of acquired stenosis include postoperative changes and post-traumatic, metabolic/endocrine, and other miscellaneous causes as listed.

Combined spinal stenosis refers to a combination of developmental stenosis, degenerative or acquired stenosis, and/or a herniation of the nucleus pulposus.

Kirkaldy-Willis and coworkers have eloquently summarized the degenerative changes that occur in the intervertebral discs and facet joints of the lumbar spine secondary to the natural evolution of disc degeneration and pathologic changes of spondylosis (Fig 37–2).[35]

Degenerative changes generally begin in the nucleus pulposus. A decrease in its water-binding capacity caused by changes in its proteoglycan structure and composition diminishes the ability of the disc to withstand compression and rotational forces. The disc narrows as a result of loss of nuclear hydration, and this narrowing causes laxity of the annulus fibrosus. With repeated torsional and rotational

TABLE 37–1.
Classification of Spinal Stenosis*

Congenital-developmental stenosis
- Idiopathic
- Achondroplasia/hypochondroplasia
- Hypophosphatemic vitamin D–resistant rickets
- Morquio's mucopolysaccharidosis
- Other congenital disorders
  - Cheirolumbar dysostosis
  - Dysplasias associated with lax atlantoaxial joints (metatropic dwarfism, spondyloepiphyseal dysplasia, Kniest's disease, multiple epiphyseal dysplasia, chondrodysplasia punctata)
  - Down's syndrome
  - Spondylolisthesis
  - Scoliosis

Acquired stenosis
- Degenerative
  - Spondylosis
  - Isolated intervertebral disc resorption
  - Lateral nerve entrapment
  - Spondylolisthesis
  - Scoliosis
  - Calcification or ossification of the posterior longitudinal ligament
  - Calcification or ossification of the ligamentum flavum
  - Intraspinal synovial cyst
  - Spinal dysraphism
- Postoperative
  - Postlaminectomy
  - Postfusion
  - Postchemonucleolysis/postdiscectomy
- Post-traumatic (late changes)
- Metabolic/endocrine
  - Epidural lipomatosis
  - Osteoporosis and vertebral fractures
  - Acromegaly
  - Calcium pyrophosphate dihydrate crystal deposition disease
  - Renal osteodystrophy
  - Hypoparathyroidism
  - Oxalosis
- Miscellaneous
  - Paget's disease of bone
  - Ankylosing spondylitis
  - Diffuse idiopathic skeletal hyperostosis (DISH)
  - Conjoined origin of lumbosacral nerve roots
  - Rheumatoid arthritis
  - Fluorosis
  - Scheurmann's disease
  - Osteopoikilosis

Combined
- Combinations of developmental stenosis, degenerative stenosis, and herniations of the nucleus pulposus
- Tandem spinal stenosis—concurrent stenosis of the lumbar and cervical regions of the spine

*From Moreland, et al: *Semin Arthritis Rheum* 1989; 62:130. Used by permission.

stresses, subsequent annular tears occur. Circumferential annular tears progress to radial tears, and consequently protrusional herniation of the nucleus may result. The subsequent hypermobility of the intervertebral joint may lead to marginal osteophytes at the vertebral margins. These osteophytes along with annular and/or nuclear bulging may contribute to spinal stenosis. As a consequence of disc space narrowing, there may be accompanying subluxation of the facet joints. Relative lengthening of the capsular and ligamentous structures of the motion segment may contribute to "segmental instability" and may be related to "mechanical" or motion-related back pain.

Kirkaldy-Willis believes that there are three phases of degeneration accounting for spondylosis. Initially, there is dysfunction followed by an unstable phase and then restabilization. As the intervertebral disc deteriorates during the dysfunctional phase, there is annular tearing and the disc settles with a progressive loss of nuclear contents and eventually internal disruption of the disc. At this stage there is annular bulging around the periphery of the disc, and the normal stiffness of the disc is completely lost. With further loss of nuclear contents and dehydration, most of the disc height is lost.[10] As a result of this phase of disc deterioration, the vacuum disc phenomenon of Knuttson may be a prominent radiologic feature on a lateral radiograph, particularly with the patient in a hyperextended position. During the restabilization phase, the above changes are accompanied by the formation of osteophytes around the periphery of the disc. This is the "stiffening" phase of the degeneration. In some cases these marginal osteophytes may join to form a bar of bone connecting one vertebral body to the other to produce a stable bony ankylosis. These changes in the disc are accompanied by changes in the posterior facets joints including synovitis, cartilage degeneration, capsular laxity, subluxation, and enlargement of the articular processes. The ligamentum flavum, a passive elastic ligament, shortens with the narrowing of the disc and facet joint subluxation. As a consequence of this shortening, the ligamentum flavum thickens. This thickened ligament can then contribute to neural space narrowing.

All of the above factors may contribute to different types of spinal stenosis. During the unstable phase there may be a dynamic recurrent lateral entrapment secondary to the laxity of the posterior elements and the loss of stiffness of the motion segment. The superior articular process can rock backward and forward in a repetitive fashion as well as sublux in relationship to the inferior articular process to the point of impinging on the undersurface of the upper pedicle. These dynamic changes can narrow the space available for the exiting spinal nerve root both posteriorly and inferiorly, and during the unstable phase the stenosis may be dynamic and positional. During the restabilization phase, a lateral nerve entrapment can become fixed secondary to a progressive loss of disc height, superior articular process subluxation on the inferior articular process, and frank impingement on the next higher pedicle as well as permanent narrowing of the intervertebral fora-

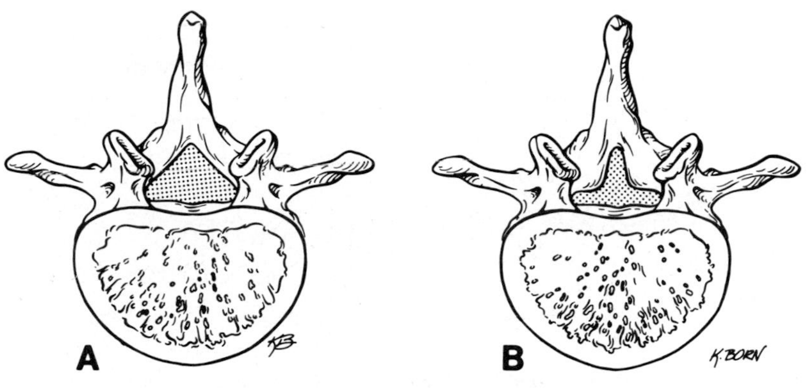

FIG 37–1.
Spinal canal stenosis. **A,** normal axial lumbar spine. **B,** the "flattened" or "trefoil" canal seen in congenital stenosis.

men between the superior articular process and the posterior aspect of the vertebral body. Central spinal stenosis may be caused by enlargement of the facets that encroach upon the central canal in a medial and anterior direction.

ANATOMY

The anatomy of lumbar spinal stenosis has been confused by a proliferation of terms, particularly for lateral lumbar spinal canal stenosis. While central canal stenosis is generally agreed upon, there is commonly misunderstanding in regard to the pathology and anatomy of lateral lumbar spinal canal stenosis. Lee et al. have recently attempted to classify and standardize lateral lumbar stenosis.[39] An example of different terminologies used to describe the stenotic condition include lateral recess stenosis, foraminal canal stenosis, subarticular stenosis, subpedicular stenosis, intervertebral foramen stenosis, and lateral gutter stenosis. The lateral lumbar spinal canal connects the intraspinal space and the extraspinal space. Lee et al. have divided it into an entrance zone (lateral recess), a mid zone (intraforaminal), and an exit zone (extraforaminal) (Fig 37–3). They define the entrance zone as the most cephalad part of the lateral lumbar canal located medial to or underneath the superior articular process. The most common cause for entrance zone stenosis is hypertrophic osteoarthritis of the facet joint, particularly when it in-

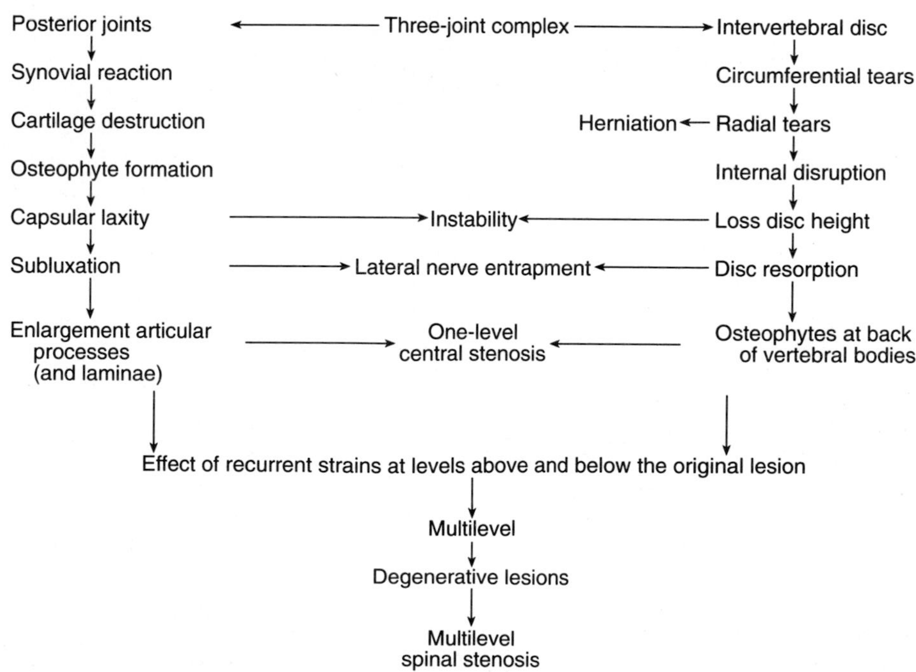

FIG 37–2.
The degenerative changes occurring in the lumbar intervertebral discs and facet joints accompanying disc degeneration and spondylosis. (From Kirkaldy-Willis WH, Wedge IH, Yong-Hing K, et al: *Spine* 1978; 3:320. Used by permission.)

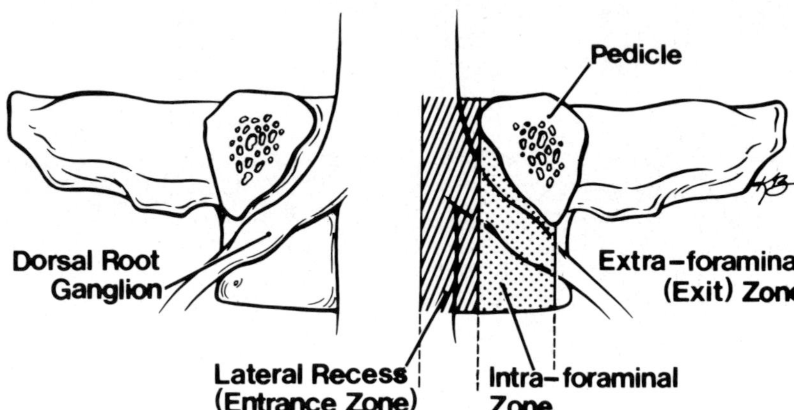

FIG 37–3.
Illustration of the lateral lumbar spinal canal. The three zones of the lateral spinal canal: the lateral recess (entrance) zone, the area just medial to the pedicle; the intraforaminal zone, the area between the medial and lateral pedicle walls; and the extraforaminal (exit) zone, the area lateral to the outer pedicle wall.

volves the superior articular process (Fig 37–4). Causes include developmental variations of the facet joints (shape, size, or orientation), a developmental short pedicle, an osteophytic ridge, or a bulging disc anterior to the nerve root.

The mid zone (intraforaminal) is located under the pars interarticularis part of the lamina and below the pedicle bordered anteriorly by the posterior aspect of the vertebral body and posteriorly by the pars interarticularis. The neural structures contained in the mid zone include the dorsal root ganglion and the ventral motor nerve root (funiculus). These neural structures are bathed in cerebrospinal fluid (CSF). Common causes for mid zone stenosis are osteophyte formation under the pars interarticularis where the ligamentum flavum is attached or fibrocartilaginous or bursal tissue hypertrophy at a spondylolytic defect. Spinal stenosis in the mid zone is most difficult to document on roentgenographic examinations preoperatively.

The exit zone (extraforaminal) is defined as the area surrounding the intervertebral foramen. It is bordered pos-

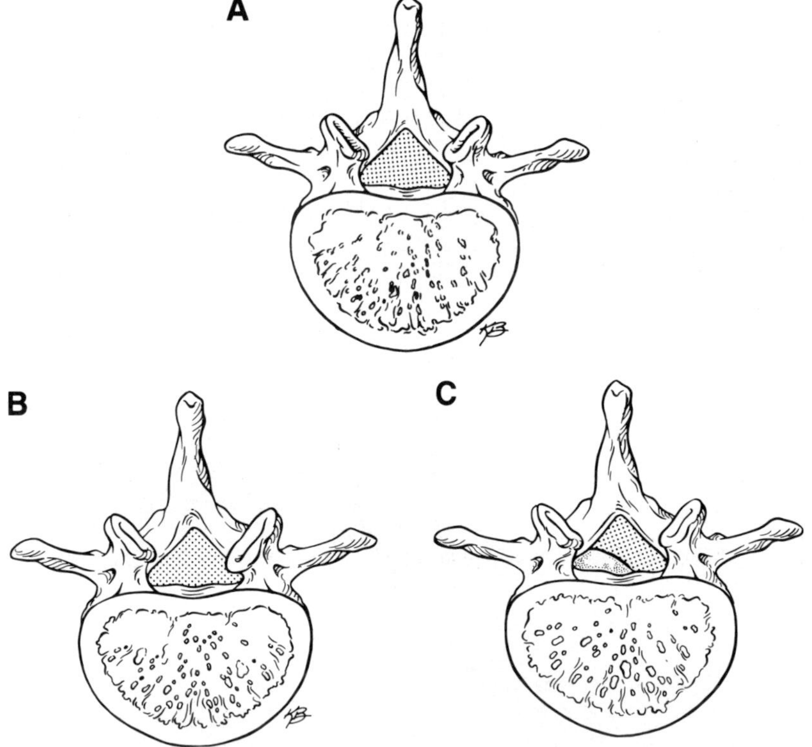

FIG 37–4.
Lateral spinal canal stenosis. **A,** normal axial lumbar spine. **B,** osteophyte hypertrophy of the medial edge of the superior facet causing nerve root impingement most commonly in the lateral recess, less frequently in the mid zone (intraforaminal area). **C,** intraforaminal and/or extraforaminal nerve root compression due to osteophytic formation of the vertebral body or from a lateral disc herniation.

teriorly by the lateral aspect of the facet joint, and the anterior border is the extraforaminal disc. The neural structure contained in the exit zone is the lumbar peripheral nerve, which is covered by perineurium. Exit zone stenosis is caused by hypertrophic osteoarthritic changes of the facet joints with subluxation and osteophytic ridge formation along the superior margin of the disc or by an extraforaminal disc herniation. For example, the L4 lumbar nerve can be entrapped by the subluxed hypertrophic superior articular process of L5 or an osteophytic ridge along the posterior margin of the L4–5 disc.[39]

Having a standardized classification of the anatomy and a clear understanding of the pathophysiology of spinal stenosis allows us to better correlate clinical presentation with planned surgical decompression.

PATHOPHYSIOLOGY

Vague back and leg pains, dysesthesias, and paresthesias distributed over the buttocks and anterior and posterior aspects of the thighs and calves and into the feet are brought on, classically, by ambulation and spinal postures that mechanically compromise the neural canal and foramina. This symptom complex is known as neurogenic claudication.[75]

The etiology of "neurogenic claudication" is not completely understood. Recently, Delamarter et al. have created the first animal model of lumbar spinal stenosis and shed some light on the pathophysiology of lumbar stenosis.[12] In their model, 24 beagle dogs underwent an L6–7 laminectomy, and the cauda equina was constricted 25%, 50%, or 75% to produce chronic compression. The dogs were evaluated with somatosensory evoked potentials (SEPs) and daily neurologic examinations. After 3 months of chronic compression all 24 dogs were studied histologically or had vascular analysis of the cauda equina with a latex injection technique.

The study showed that neurogenic claudication appeared to begin with venous congestion of the nerve root and dorsal root ganglion and that with increasing compression, motor and sensory deficits occurred with blockage of axoplasmic flow. Thus it appears that ischemia of the cauda equina is probably the final pathway precipitating the multiple signs and symptoms of neurogenic claudication.

DIAGNOSIS

The onset of symptoms in patients with spinal stenosis is frequently insidious and spontaneous and can occur in either sex, generally in the fifth to seventh decades. Patients will first complain of vague pains, dysesthesias, and paresthesias in their buttocks and legs with ambulation (neurogenic claudication) but will initially experience excellent relief of the symptoms by sitting or lying supine. As the disease process progresses, the symptoms increase with walking shorter distances. The increased lordotic stance assumed with walking, particularly downhill, commonly exacerbates stenosis symptoms. Recent cadaver and dynamic computed tomography (CT)-myelographic studies have demonstrated significant decreases in the sagittal diameters of the spinal canal in extension.[41, 56] This symptomatic relationship to posture can be verified with the "bicycle test" of Van Gelderan.[14] In this test, claudication symptoms were not produced while patients leaned forward to pedal since there was reduction of the lumbar lordosis and subsequent enlargement of the sagittal dimensions of the central and foraminal spinal canal. Neurogenic claudication from spinal stenosis must be differentiated from vascular claudication because patients with vascular insufficiency also develop leg pain with walking that is generally relieved with rest. In contrast to neurogenic claudication, vascular claudication symptoms are easier to produce with ambulation uphill because of increased metabolic demands. The absence of pulses below the hips combined with rubor and pallor changes with elevation are classic signs of vascular claudication.

Neurogenic claudication pain patterns are generally asymmetrical and are often diffuse and dysesthetic in character. Frequently neurologic examination will reveal no objective findings. Maturation of the syndrome symptoms may even occur at rest. Subtle neurologic changes, for example, sensory reflex or muscular weakness, may be elicited by such maneuvers as the "walk test" or "jackknife test" to dynamically produce an objective neurologic finding only after the patient is stressed. The walk test consists of a neurologic examination before and after walking to the point of symptom appearance. The jackknife test involves having the patient sit in forward flexion with the knees extended and fingers touching the toes for a short time. This position may elicit neurologic signs that would otherwise go undetected. In spinal stenosis a paucity of neurologic findings is the rule. Epstein and Epstein have emphasized, "The history rather than objective findings is the decisive factor in establishing the diagnosis."[17] Table 37–2 outlines the clinical findings that help differentiate neurogenic claudication from vascular claudication.[13]

As previously stated, a herniated nucleus pulposus can contribute to spinal stenosis and is part of the spectrum of the syndrome. Certain clinical features can help differentiate a patient with isolated disc herniation from a patient with spinal stenosis. Patients with disc herniation tend to be less than 50 years of age, while patients with spinal stenosis tend to be older than 50. Back pain can be a more significant element of spinal stenosis. Objective neurologic deficits are more likely to accompany a disc herniation along with positive tension signs.

TABLE 37–2.

Clinical Findings That Help Differentiate Neurogenic Claudication From Vascular Claudication*

Finding	Vascular	Neurogenic
Exercise	Worse	Variable
Stationary bicycle	Worse	Can ride with comfort
Lying flat	Relief	Variable
Standing	Relief	Worse
Sensory	Stocking deficits	Poorly localized
Pulses	Decreased, bruits	Normal
Back motion	No change	Worse with hyperextension
Genitourinary	Impotence	Urinary retention or frequency

*Data from Dodge LD, Bohlman HH, Rhodes RS: *Clin Orthop* 1988; 230:141–148.

RADIOGRAPHIC IMAGING AND DIAGNOSIS

Recent advances in the quality of imaging techniques including CT and magnetic resonance imaging (MRI) have aided greatly in the understanding of spinal stenosis and in the diagnosis of spinal stenosis. Since spinal stenosis may be accompanied by generalized spondylosis, disc resorption and collapse, retrolisthesis, or degenerative spondylolisthesis, plain radiographs are always advisable. Lateral views can demonstrate the sagittal diameter of the lumbar canal, which is normally 15 to 25 mm. If the lateral sagittal canal diameter is less than 12 mm, relative stenosis is generally indicated. Oblique plain radiographs of both the lumbar and cervical vertebrae can demonstrate foraminal stenosis secondary to facet subluxation and osteophytes, disc space narrowing, and laminar thickening with overriding or shingling. Myelography can reveal bone and soft-tissue factors contributing to stenosis, typically an hourglass deformity to partial or complete obstruction of the myelographic dye.

The "gold standard" for diagnosing lumbar spinal stenosis has become myelography followed by high-quality CT scanning. Several recent studies have demonstrated the utility of CT-myelography.[47, 48, 57] CT scanning now allows a precise visualization of all three areas of the lateral lumbar spinal canal including the entrance, mid, and exit zones. CT scanning is also useful in detecting different spinal canal shapes including the trefoil shape of developmental spinal stenosis, facet hypertrophy in isolated disc resorption, neural compression in scoliosis, and retropulsion of fragments in vertebral fractures. CT scanning is invaluable in visualizing levels below a partial or complete myelographic block, and it gives much better definition of the lateral recesses and foramina than plain myelography does because contrast agents often do not diffuse far laterally.[64] There is a risk of overreading CT studies. In a study of 52 asymptomatic patients over the age of 40 years, CT scans demonstrated abnormalities in 50% of these patients, including herniated discs, facet degeneration, and stenosis.[74] One must be mindful that CT scanning has a relatively low specificity but a high sensitivity.

With recent improvements in MRI technology, MRI has become quite popular in diagnosing low back problems because it is noninvasive, has no irradiation, and may replace CT-myelography. It is advantageous in that it allows direct axial and sagittal imaging, being particularly useful in imaging neural foramina. Two recent prospective studies comparing surface coil MRI, CT, and myelography noted that the true-positive rate for MRI was marginally less than that for metrizamide CT-myelography, equal to that for plain CT in the lumbar spine, and superior to that of myelography in both regions.[47–49] Currently it appears that the resolution of CT with or without myelography is better for bony stenosis and MRI is better for soft-tissue and disc pathology.

OTHER DIAGNOSTIC TECHNIQUES

Although most patients with neurogenic claudication may have normal electromyographic (EMG) and nerve conduction studies at rest, EMG and nerve conduction studies have been shown to be 80% to 95% sensitive for myelographically proven spinal stenosis.[27, 30] EMG can provide additional confirmatory evidence of levels of nerve root involvement and is useful in diagnosing other types of nerve pathology (i.e., diabetic polyneuropathy).[13, 16] The finding of a unilateral multiradiculopathy by EMG is indicative of a more diffuse problem than a simple herniated disc. Recent studies have demonstrated SEPs as useful noninvasive techniques for both preoperative diagnosis and intraoperative monitoring to determine the adequacy of lumbar nerve root decompression.[20, 36] Recent studies on dermatomal somatosensory evoked potentials (DSEPs) have demonstrated it to be as accurate as myelography in diagnosing nerve root compression without being invasive[33] as well as a useful technique to be used intraoperatively for assessing the adequacy of neural decompression.[24] These monitoring techniques have resulted in the planned surgical procedure being altered in many patients.*

Initial diagnostic modalities that have not been found to be helpful in the diagnosis of spinal stenosis include the Minnesota Multiphasic Personality Inventory (MMPI)[25] and liquid crystal thermography.[46]

TREATMENT

Conservative

Nonoperative (conservative) treatment should generally be the initial management of patients with spinal stenosis if there are no significant neurologic abnormalities (sphincter disturbances, paralysis, etc.). The initial treat-

*References 15, 21, 30, 34, 37, 45, 62, 68.

ment regimen can include nonsteroidal anti-inflammatory medications, physical therapy, and occasionally a light-weight elastic corset. These measures alone may reverse or delay the early symptoms. Rest, analgesics, muscle relaxants, local heat, and other physical modalities of pain control are often used in the acute stage, after which postural exercises, a lumbosacral corset, and/or transcutaneous nerve stimulation may be used. A back support such as a flexion body jacket to hold the spine in slight flexion and provide abdominal support may provide considerable relief of symptoms in some cases.

One of the most commonly employed techniques of conservative treatment of spinal stenosis remains epidural steroid injections. The administration of steroids for their anti-inflammatory properties can be considered palliative not curative in spinal stenosis. The underlying structural, true nerve entrapment and compression remain; therefore any beneficial effects of epidural steroids is commonly transient. The role of epidural steroids in palliation of the pain of spinal stenosis remains undefined since there are no well-designed prospective, randomized, double-blind studies and most reports evaluating epidural steroid injections do not make clear distinctions between the different causes of low back and leg pain. Following epidural steroid injections, temporary and partial relief of pain should be considered a reasonable outcome.[11, 19, 40, 59, 72]

Surgical Treatment

Unfortunately, in most cases of significant spinal stenosis with neurogenic claudication, conservative treatment is usually unsuccessful. Several studies on the outcome of surgical treatment, however, demonstrate good to excellent results in 75% to 85% of cases.[22, 54, 55, 60, 65, 67, 70] The definition of spinal stenosis denotes an insufficient space in the spinal canal for the neural elements. The aim of any surgery is to completely decompress all neural elements for which there is inadequate room and are therefore symptomatic. The extent of the surgical decompression and the areas to be decompressed depends on the anatomy of the compression as determined on preoperative studies as well as the clinical symptoms. Generally, for central spinal stenosis, a central decompression is done with a total laminectomy brought out laterally to the level of the pedicle (Fig 37–5).[71] Unless a segmental fusion is being performed, care should be taken to preserve as much pars interarticularis and as much of the weight-bearing surface of the facets as possible so as to not create postsurgical instability.

Multiple studies have shown that the primary reason that decompressive spinal surgery fails is inadequate decompression, particularly of the lateral lumbar spinal canal.[8, 9] The lateral lumbar spinal canal deserves special attention, and different decompressive techniques are utilized depending on the pathoanatomy of the compressive lesion. As previously mentioned, the lateral lumbar spinal canal is divided into the entrance zone, the mid zone, and the exit zone. Burton has called these zones the central, foraminal, and extraforaminal zones. The entrance zone (central zone) is that area located just medial to the pedicle, with nerve root compression most often caused by the medial edge of the superior articular process. For an adequate decompression of this area, a medial facetectomy or removal of an osteophytic ridge along the disc provides sufficient room for the nerve root. The mid zone (foraminal zone) is defined as that area under the pars interarticularis part of the lamina and below the pedicle. The neurostructures contained within this zone include the dorsal root ganglion and the ventral motor nerve root. Due to the relatively enlarged size of the dorsal root ganglion, a relatively smaller amount of stenosis can be symptomatic at this level. For an isolated one-level spondylolysis with or without spondylolisthesis, careful cleaning and curettage of the undersurface of the pars defect provides sufficient relief for the neural structures. Most commonly, however, mid zone stenosis is accompanied by either entrance or exit zone stenosis or stenosis at other levels. Wide decompression can be achieved by medial facetectomy (occasionally total facetectomy) and laminectomy. Frequently and more desirably, entrance zone decompression is accomplished by a medial facetectomy, and mid zone decompression requires careful undercutting and curettage of the hypertrophic osteophytic ridge along the margins of the articular surface of the inferior articular process under the pars interarticularis. Technically this undercutting can be achieved by several methods. Some use a high-speed diamond drill, others a sharp chisel. It is also possible to use angled curets and sharp up-biting Kerrson ronguers. We have found that thinning of the distal portion of the rongeur by filing down the tip of commercially available instruments minimizes the chance of inflicting nerve root trauma and allows the instrument to be placed into tighter lateral recesses. Magnification with loupes and the use of a headlamp or an operating microscope is necessary for this type of decompression.

The exit zone (extraforaminal zone) is defined as that area surrounding the intervertebral foramen. Its posterior border is the lateral aspect of the facet joint, and the anterior border is the disc. The neural structure contained here is the lumbar peripheral nerve, which at this point is covered by perineurium and is not surrounded by CSF. Isolated exit zone stenosis is rare and is usually caused by an osteophytic ridge along the disc anterior to the intervertebral foramen. In general, exit stenosis is accompanied by mid zone stenosis and/or entrance stenosis of the next lowest level. Adequate decompression can be achieved by trimming the medial, lateral, and superior margins of the

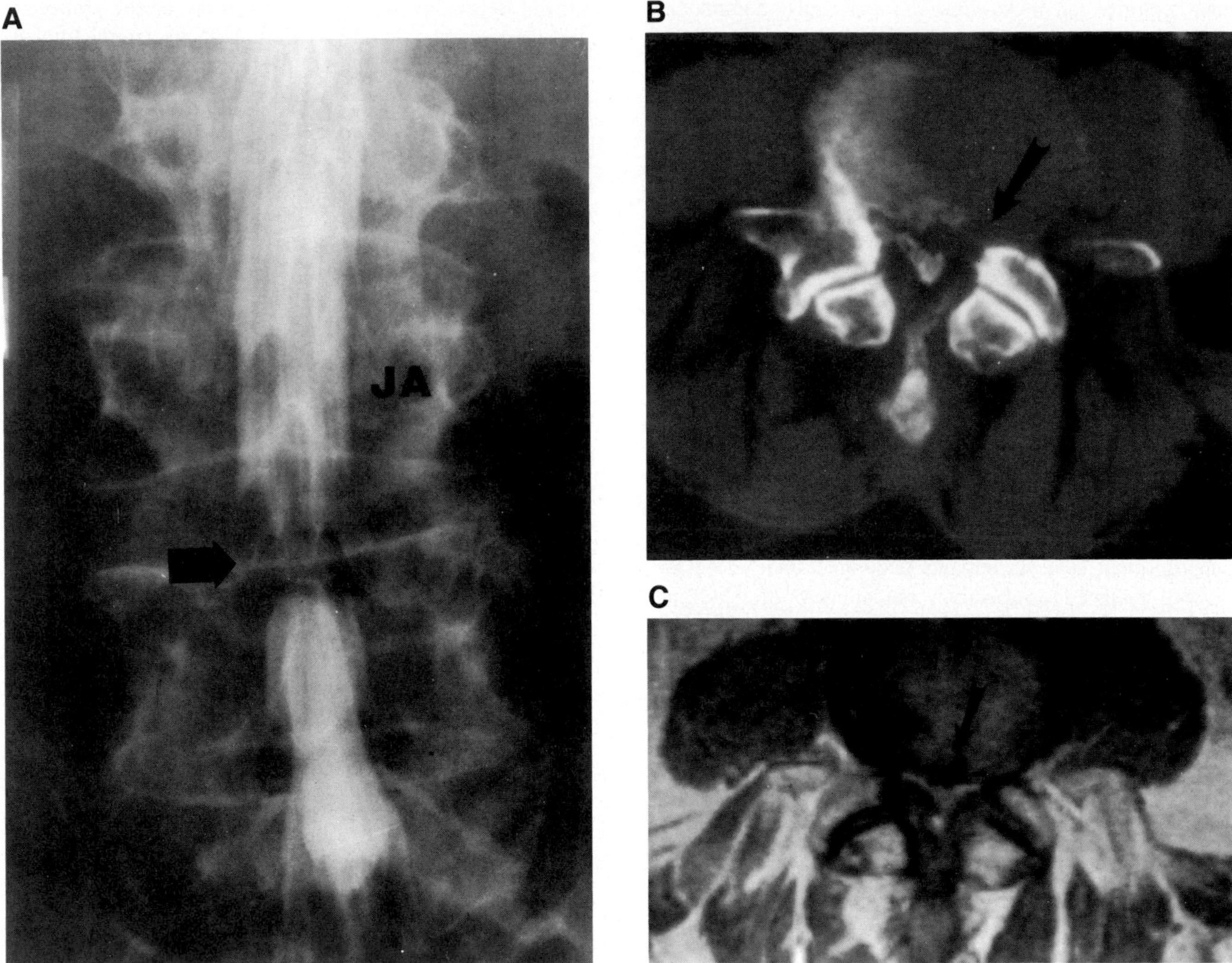

FIG 37–5.
A 69-year-old man presented with bilateral radiating leg pain after walking 10 to 20 m. Sitting in a chair quickly relieved the symptoms. His resting neurologic examination was normal. **A,** an anteroposterior (AP) metrizamide myelogram reveals a nearly total blockage at the L4–5 level *(arrow)*. **B,** computed axial tomography (CAT) following the myelogram through the L4–5 disc space demonstrates moderate lateral recess stenosis, moderate central stenosis, and a central left-sided disc protrusion *(arrow)*. **C,** axial MRI at the same level shows slightly better delineation of the lateral recess stenosis *(arrow)*. Note the "trefoil" canal. A standard laminectomy and discectomy resulted in complete pain relief.

superior articular process and by curettage of the facets under the pars interarticularis or by total facetectomy. If a lateral approach is deemed necessary for adequate exit zone decompression, the lateral half of the superior border of the superior articular process can be removed from a lateral-to-medial approach. The posterior perforating arterial branch of the lumbar artery must be identified and cauterized prior to removal of the lateral osteophytes along the superior articular process. With central or lateral canal stenosis, a herniated disc may need excision to allow complete neurodecompression.

It cannot be overemphasized that clinical symptoms, preoperative diagnostic imaging studies, as well as preoperative electrophysiologic modalities must all be correlated to exactly determine the anatomic area of neural compression so that appropriate surgical planning and decompression will have the highest probability of surgical success.

Recently several authors have reported on more limited hemilaminotomy decompressions for central and lateral canal stenosis, especially for unilateral leg pain, rather than the traditional total laminectomy decompression. Advantages include retention of the supraspinous and intraspinous ligaments and their lumbodorsal attachments for added posterior spinal stability. It has become our practice to perform a wide hemilaminotomy, medial facetectomy, and foraminotomy in the majority of cases of stenosis with unilateral leg pain unless there is significant central stenosis that necessitates a standard total laminectomy.[4, 5, 31, 76] Decompression using a wide hemilaminotomy, medial facetectomy, and foraminotomy in no way implies a keyhole-type approach as has been used for simple discectomy (Fig 37–6). The absolute requirement of all stenosis surgery is to ensure adequate decompression of all neural elements. If this is not possible by any type of laminotomy procedure, then a total laminectomy is indicated.

Indications for Fusion

The most common cause of failure of spinal stenosis surgery is inadequate decompression. A significant number of patients, however, continue to experience disability with back and/or leg pain after adequate spinal decompression. This is often due to unrecognized pre-existing segmental instability or postoperative segmental instability. Segmental instability following lumbar decompression first appeared in the English literature in the late 1970s and early 1980s.[23, 62] Postlaminectomy spondylolisthesis has been reported to range from 0%[61] to 100%[38] but more commonly is reported in the 10% to 12% range.[23, 63, 73] Numerous investigators have recently demonstrated the importance of the posterior elements for axial load bearing and translation shear and rotational resistance.[1, 2, 43, 51, 58]

Posner et al. experimentally excised the posterior elements including the posterior longitudinal ligaments in cadaver specimens loaded to approximate body weight.[58] Annulus failure occurred in all specimens when the forward flexion force reached 75% of body weight. This experiment closely simulated in vivo conditions following radical decompression and disc excision.

The lumbar facet joints are biplanar, with the medial half in the coronal plane and the lateral half in the sagittal plane. The coronal portion acts as a physical stop to forward translation and limits shear forces by transferring forces to the adjacent level. The lateral half of the joint resists axial torsion. Removal of the medial portion of the facet (the standard hemifacetectomy or medial facetectomy) removes some restraint to sagittal translation and thus increases forces in the remaining structures, including the disc. Several investigators have concurred that an abnormal orientation of the plane of the inferior articular process relative to that of the pedicle of the superior vertebra (considered a congenital anomaly) predisposes some people to degenerative spondylolisthesis.[32, 44] If surgical removal of posterior elements (lamina, ligamentum flavum, ligaments, facet joints, and posterior longitudinal ligament) is added to this, disc degeneration may be accelerated. A unilateral or bilateral complete facetectomy removes the resistance to rotatory displacement along with three-dimensional rotatory instability. Hopp and Tsou[26] discussed the concept of the intercrestal line as an anatomic fulcrum and noted that the ilio-lumbar transverse ligaments stabilize the spine generally at the L5 level and transfer forces to the next highest level, generally the L4–5 level.

Nachemson[52] described several clinical clues that may indicate segmental instability, including traction spurs or spondylolisthesis when there has been a previous total laminectomy or in a motion segment adjacent to a previous fusion. A stenosis patient who is middle-aged may exhibit the well-known "instability catch": pain in the lumbosacral area that increases when standing and extending either from a bent or straight position gives sudden exaggerations of the pain, sometimes with leg radiation pain. Several recent studies have attempted to better predict those suffering from clinically significant segmental instability. Johnsson et al., initially in 1986, noted that with acquired degenerative stenosis surgically decompressed, postoperative slipping always meant a poor result, whereas in degenerative spondylolisthesis undergoing surgical decompression, the risk of postoperative slippage was somewhat higher but did not appear to influence the results.[28, 29, 53] In a follow-up study in 1989, they concluded that in spinal stenosis, preoperative instability as revealed by functional myelography seems to be a poor prognostic sign. Radical decompression, without stabilization enhanced the risk of postoperative slipping and a poor outcome.

Postlaminectomy spondylolisthesis appears to worsen the prognosis.[7, 18, 42] Hopp and Tsou[26] offer additional guidelines for determining the indications for spinal fusion in the surgical treatment of lumbar spinal stenosis. They believe that instability is present if spondylolisthesis of 2 mm or greater exists or if a scoliosis and/or wedged disc of more than 10 degrees is present. They recommend fusing all unstable levels. In addition, they note that preoperative evidence of disc damage such as disc space narrowing of 25% or more and/or traction spurs can be indicative of instability preoperatively. They note that the disc level above the iliolumbar transverse ligaments, generally L4–5, is subject to added stresses. If an extensive decompression is to be performed at this level, a fusion should be considered. Finally, complete facetectomy or pars interarticularis excision, unilaterally or bilaterally, renders the decompressed level highly vulnerable, and fusion is strongly recommended. Nasca[53] recommends spinal fusion for patients who have decompression for lumbar stenosis with degenerative spondylolisthesis, isolated disc resorption with degenerative facet joints, or intervertebral disc disease with instability and those with scoliosis with multidirectional instability.

Morris[50] recommends fusion for degenerative spondylolisthesis, which, he notes, is most frequently seen in middle-aged or elderly females and commonly affects the L4–5 level with L5 root findings. Occasionally the L4 root is involved due to traction on it by forward slippage of L4. The pars interarticularis is generally intact in degen-

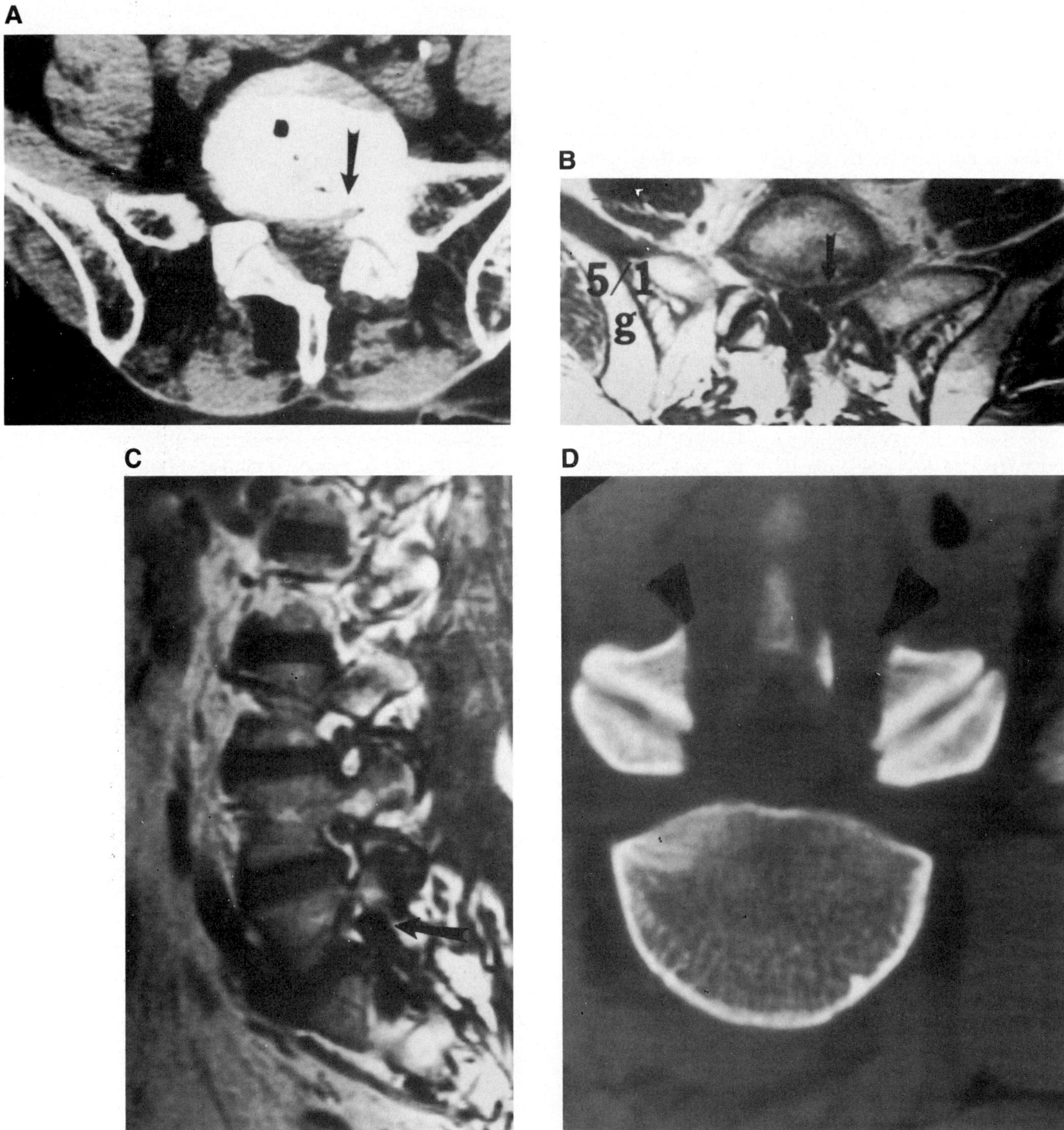

FIG 37–6.
A 67-year-old man presented with progressive bilateral leg pain and weakness over a 2-year period. **A,** this CAT scan reveals lateral recess stenosis *(arrow)* caused by the hypertrophic medial edge of the superior facet compressing the underlying nerve root. **B,** axial MRI also reveals the lateral recess stenosis as well as a small disc herniation *(arrow)*. **C,** sagittal MRI showing the left intraforaminal area. The *arrow* shows the stenotic L5–S1 foramen with compression of the L5 nerve root. This compression is due to cephalad migration and hypertrophy of the S1 superior facet. The patient had a bilateral laminotomy, discectomy, and foraminotomy and remains pain free 3 years following surgery. **D,** this postoperative CT scan shows the bilateral laminotomy, medial facetectomy, and foraminotomy.

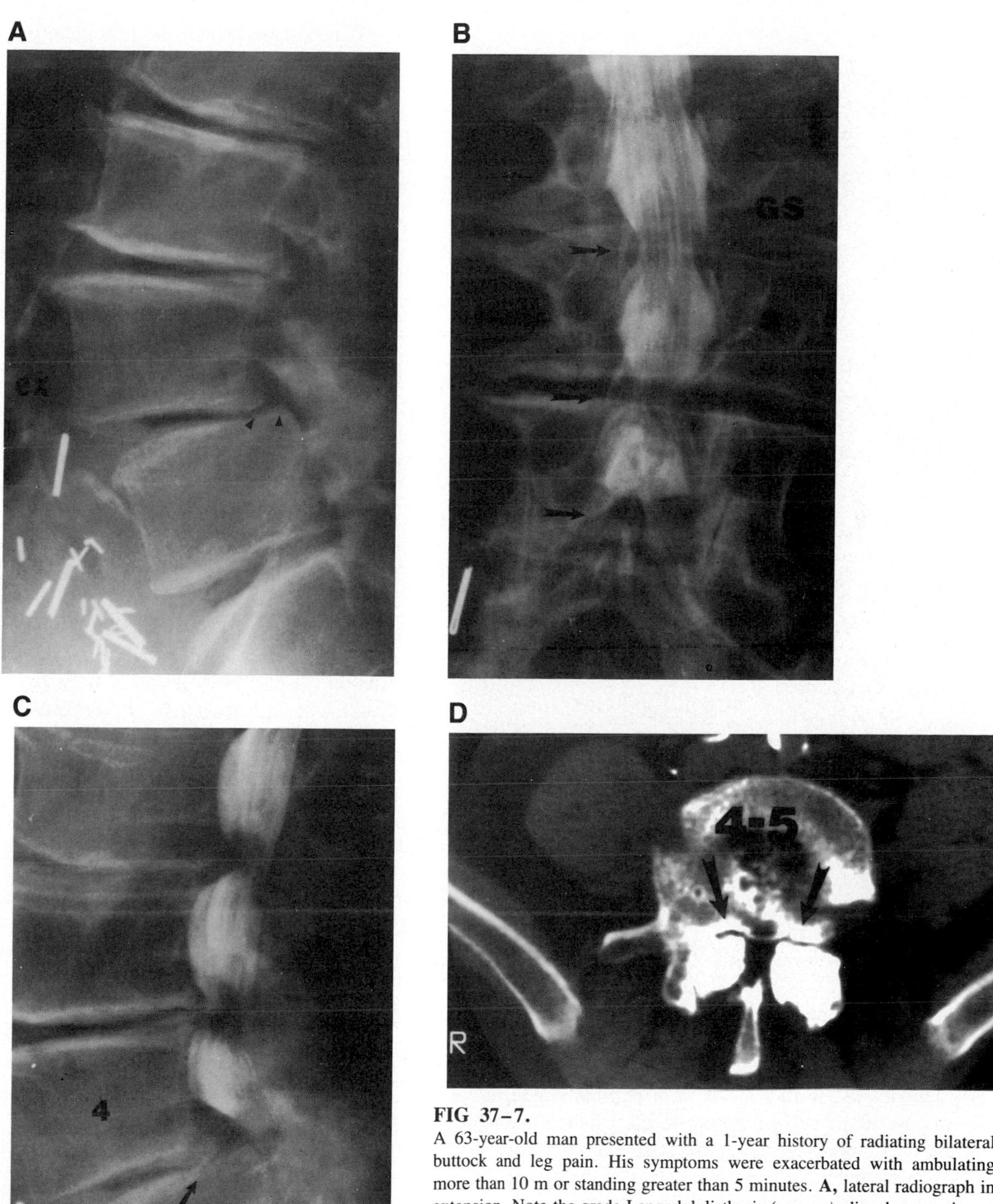

FIG 37–7.
A 63-year-old man presented with a 1-year history of radiating bilateral buttock and leg pain. His symptoms were exacerbated with ambulating more than 10 m or standing greater than 5 minutes. **A,** lateral radiograph in extension. Note the grade I spondylolisthesis *(arrows),* disc degeneration at several levels, as well as anterior and posterior vertebral body osteophytic changes. **B,** AP myelogram showing a complete block at the L4–5 level and "hourglass" narrowing at L2–3 and L3–4. **C,** lateral myelogram showing a complete block at the L4–5 spondylolisthesis level and stenotic narrowing at L3–4 and L2–3. **D,** CAT scan at the L4–5 level revealing severe central and lateral recess stenosis *(arrows),* the result of large hypertrophic facets. **E (facing page),** intraoperative photograph after complete laminectomy, medial facetectomies, and foraminotomies of L2 to L5. A posterior lateral fusion with an iliac crest bone graft was also performed. At the 4-year follow-up, the patient remains symptom free and is working full-time as a contractor.

Continued.

E

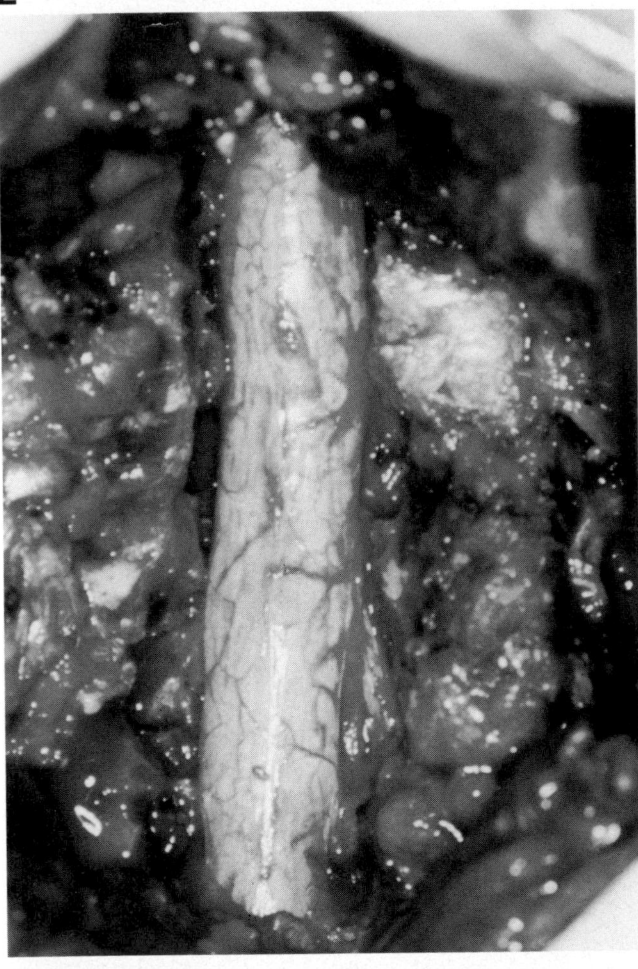

FIG 37–7 (cont.).

erative spondylolisthesis, and CT or MRI demonstrates lateral recess compromise by facet hypertrophy and subluxation.

Morris also recommends fusion for degenerative scoliosis, which he terms multisegmental unstable lumbar spinal stenosis, and notes that this most often occurs in elderly females. This may result from chronic degenerative disc disease or be superimposed on pre-existing scoliosis, and the back pain is generally more severe than lower-extremity symptoms. Radiographs reveal scoliosis with disc space narrowing (or collapse), facet hypertrophy and subluxation, and rotational or translational subluxation of adjacent vertebrae at one or more levels. Spondylolisthesis may also be present. Maximal involvement generally occurs at L3–4, which is usually the apex of the curve. In degenerative scoliosis nerve root symptoms may arise from compression on the concave side of the curve due to facet overriding and foraminal encroachment; they may also occur as a result of traction on the roots that exit from the convex side of the curve.

If fusion is elected, the procedure of choice is a posterolateral intertransverse process fusion utilizing an autologous iliac crest bone graft plus salvaged local laminectomy bone grafting (Fig 37–7). The definitive indication for segmental instrumentation, for example, pedicle screw instrumentation, remains controversial. We reserve pedicle screw instrumentation for fusions of three or more levels, fusion of a degenerated unstable segment above a previously fused level, cases of unstable degenerative spondylolisthesis, and the difficult degenerative scoliotic curves that may require instrumentation to the sacrum and/or ilium.

POSTOPERATIVE CARE

Generally the patient with spinal stenosis is older, and early mobilization is advisable. We attempt to have the patient out of bed the day after surgery and started on progressive ambulation. If only a one- or two-level decompression is performed, generally no spinal support is prescribed. When a one- to two-level fusion has been performed in addition, a lumbosacral corset is worn for a period of 2 to 4 months. If a more extensive fusion procedure is performed such as a multilevel pedicle screw instrumentation, a molded plastic thoracolumbosacral orthotic (TLSO) body jacket is worn from 4 to 6 months. Progressive ambulation is encouraged for general conditioning and aerobic exercise.

REFERENCES

1. Adams MA, Hutton WC: The mechanical function of the lumbar apophyseal joints. *Spine* 1983; 5:327.
2. Adams MA, Hutton WC, Stott J: The resistance to flexion of the lumbar intervertebral joint. *Spine* 1980; 5:245–253.
3. Arnoldi CC, Brodsky AE, Cauchoix J, et al: Lumbar spinal stenosis and nerve root entrapment syndrome. Definition and classification. *Clin Orthop* 1976; 115:4–5.
4. Aryanpur J, Ducker T: Multilevel lumbar laminotomies: An alternative to laminectomy in the treatment of lumbar stenosis. *Neurosurgery* 1990; 26:429–432.
5. Aryanpur J, Ducker T: Multilevel lumbar laminotomies for focal spinal stenosis: Case report. *Neurosurgery* 1988; 23:111–115.
6. Bailey P, Casamajor L: Osteoarthritis of the spine as a cause of compression of the spinal cord and its roots: With report of 5 cases. *J Nerv Ment Dis* 1911; 38:588–609.
7. Bolestra MJ, Bohlman H: Degenerative spondylolisthesis. *Instr Course Lect* 1989; 38:157–165.
8. Burton CV: Successful surgical management of lateral spinal stenosis. *Instr Course Lect* 1985; 34:55–67.
9. Burton CV, Kirkaldy-Willis WH, Yong-Hing K, et al: Causes of failure of surgery on the lumbar spine. *Clin Orthop* 1981; 157:191–199.
10. Crock HV: Isolated lumbar disk resorption as a cause of nerve root canal stenosis. *Clin Orthop* 1976; 115:109–115.
11. Cuckler JM, Bernini PA, Wiesel SW, et al: The use of epi-

dural steroids in the treatment of lumbar radicular pain. *J Bone Joint Surg [Am]* 1985; 67:63–66.

12. Delamarter RB, Bohlman HH, Dodge LD, et al: Experimental lumbar spinal stenosis. *J Bone Joint Surg [Am]* 1990; 72:110–120.
13. Dodge LD, Bohlman HH, Rhodes RS: Concurrent lumbar spinal stenosis and peripheral vascular disease—A report of nine patients. *Clin Orthop* 1988; 230:141–148.
14. Dyck P, Doyle JB: "Bicycle test" of Van Gelderan in diagnosis of intermittent cauda equina compression syndrome. *J Neurosurg* 1977; 46:667.
15. Dvonch V, Scarff T, Bunch WH, et al: Dermatomal somatosensory evoked potentials: Their use in lumbar radiculopathy. *Spine* 1984; 9:291–293.
16. Eisen A, Hoirch M: The electrodiagnostic evaluation of spinal root lesions. *Spine* 1983; 8:98–106.
17. Epstein JA, Epstein NE: Lumbar spondylosis and spinal stenosis, in Wilkins RH, Rengachary SS (eds): *Neurosurgery* New York, McGraw-Hill, 1985, p 2272.
18. Feffer HL, Wiesel SW, Cuckler JM, et al: Degenerative spondylolisthesis: To fuse or not to fuse. *Spine* 1985; 10:287–289.
19. Ferrante FM: Epidural steroids in the management of spinal stenosis. *Semin Spine Surg* 1989; 1:177–181.
20. Gepstein R, Brown MD: Somatosensory-evoked potentials in lumbar nerve root decompression. *Clin Orthop* 1989; 245:69–71.
21. Gonzalez EG, Hajdu M, Bruno R, et al: Lumbar spinal stenosis: Analysis of pre- and postoperative somatosensory evoked potentials. *Arch Phys Med Rehabil* 1985; 66:11–15.
22. Grabis S: The treatment of spinal stenosis. *J Bone Joint Surg [Am]* 1980; 62:308–313.
23. Hazlett JW, Kinnard P: Lumbar apophyseal process excision and spinal instability. *Spine* 1982; 7:171–176.
24. Heron LD, Trippi AC, Gonyeau M: Intraoperative use of dermatomal somatosensory-evoked potentials in lumbar stenosis surgery. *Spine* 1987; 12:379–383.
25. Heron LD, Turner J, Clancy S, et al: The differential utility of the Minnesota Multiphasic Personality Inventory. A prediction of outcome in lumbar laminectomy for disc herniation versus spinal stenosis. *Spine* 1986; 11:847–850.
26. Hopp E, Tsou P: Postdecompression lumbar instability. *Clin Orthop* 1988; 227:143–151.
27. Jacobson RE: Lumbar stenosis, an electromyographic evaluation. *Clin Orthop* 1976; 115:68–71.
28. Johnsson K, Willner S, Johnsson K: Postoperative instability after decompression for lumbar spinal stenosis. *Spine* 1986; 11:107–110.
29. Johnsson KE, Redlund-Johnell I, Uden A, et al: Preoperative and postoperative instability in lumbar spine stenosis. *Spine* 1989; 14:591–593.
30. Johnsson KE, Rosen I, Uden A: Neurophysiologic investigation of patients with spinal stenosis. *Spine* 1987; 12:483–487.
31. Joson RM, McCormick KJ: Preservation of the supraspinous ligament for spinal stenosis: A technical note. *Neurosurgery* 1987; 21:420–422.
32. Junghanns H: Spondylolisthesen ohne Spalt IM Zwischengelenkstuck ("Pseudospondylolisthesen"). *Arch Orthop Unfallchir* 1930; 29:118–127.
33. Katifi HA, Sedgwick EM: Evaluation of the dermatomal somatosensory evoked potential in the disease of lumbosacral root compression. *J Neurol Neurosurg Psychiatry* 1987; 50:1204–1210.
34. Keim HA, Hajdu M, Gonzalez ED, et al: Somatosensory evoked potentials as an aid in the diagnosis and intraoperative management of spinal stenosis. *Spine* 1985; 10:338–344.
35. Kirkaldy-Willis WH, Weoge IH, Yong-Hing K, et al: Pathology and pathogenesis of lumbar spondylosis and stenosis. *Spine* 1978; 3:320.
36. Kondo M, Matsuda H, Kureya S, et al: Electrophysiological studies of intermittent claudication in lumbar stenosis. *Spine* 1989; 14:862–866.
37. Larson SJ: Somatosensory evoked potentials in lumbar stenosis. *Surg Gynecol Obstet* 1983; 157:191–196.
38. Lee CK: Lumbar spinal instability (olisthesis) after extensive posterior spinal decompression. *Spine* 1983; 8:429–433.
39. Lee CK, Rauschning W, Glenn W: Lateral lumbar spinal canal stenosis: Classification, pathologic anatomy and surgical decompression. *Spine* 1988; 13:313–320.
40. Liebergall M, Fast A, Olshwang D, et al: The role of epidural steroid injection in the management of lumbar radiculopathy due to disc disease or spinal stenosis. *Pain Clin* 1986; 1:35–40.
41. Liyang D, Yinkan X, Wienming Z, et al: The effect of flexion-extension motion of the lumbar spine on the capacity of the spinal canal. An experimental study. *Spine* 1989; 14:523–525.
42. Lombardi JS, Wiltse LL, Reynolds J, et al: Treatment of degenerative spondylolisthesis. *Spine* 1985; 10:821–827.
43. Lorenz M, Patwardhand A, Vanderby R: Load bearing characteristics of lumbar facets in normal and surgically altered spinal segments. *Spine* 1983; 8:122.
44. Macnab I: Spondylolisthesis with an insert neural arch: The so-called pseudo-spondylolisthesis. *J Bone Joint Surg [Br]* 1950; 32:325–333.
45. Machida M, Weinstein SL, Yamada T, et al: Spinal cord monitoring, electrophysiological measures of sensory and motor function during spinal surgery. *Spine* 1985; 10:407–413.
46. Mills GH, Davies GK, Getty CJM, et al: The evaluation of liquid crystal thermography in the investigation of nerve root compression due to lumbosacral lateral spinal stenosis. *Spine* 1986; 11:427–432.
47. Modic MT, Masaryk T, Boumphrey F, et al: Lumbar herniated disk disease and canal stenosis: Prospective evaluation by surface coil MR, CT, and myelography. *AJR* 1986; 147:757–765.
48. Modic MT, Masaryk TJ, Mulopulos GP, et al: Cervical radiculopathy; prospective evaluation with surface coil MR imaging, CT metrizamide, and metrizamide myelography. *Radiology* 1986; 161:753–759.
49. Moreland LW, et al: Spinal stenosis: A comprehensive re-

view of the literature. *Semin Arthritis Rheum* 1989; 62:130.
50. Morris JM: Spinal stenosis, in Chapman M (ed): *Operative Orthopaedics*. Philadelphia, JB Lippincott, 1988, pp 2065–2075.
51. Nachemson A: Lumbar intradiscal pressure. *Acta Orthop Scand Suppl* 1960; 43:18.
52. Nachemson A: Lumbar spine instability. A critical update and symposium summary. *Spine* 1985; 10:290–291.
53. Nasca RJ: Rationale for spinal fusion in lumbar spinal stenosis. *Spine* 1989; 14:451–454.
54. Nasca RJ: Surgical management of lumbar spinal stenosis. *Spine* 1987; 12:809–816.
55. Paine KWE: Results of decompression for lumbar spinal stenosis. *Clin Orthop* 1976; 115:96–100.
56. Penning L, Wilmink JT: Posture-dependent bilateral compression of L4 or L5 nerve roots in facet hypertrophy. A CT-myelographic study. *Spine* 1987; 12:488–500.
57. Phytinen J, Lahde S, Tanska EL, et al: Computed tomography after lumbar myelopathy in lower back and extremity pain syndrome. *Diagn Imaging* 1983; 52:19–22.
58. Posner I, White AA, Edwards WT, et al: A biomechanical analysis of the clinical stability of the lumbar and lumbosacral spine. *Spine* 1982; 7:374–389.
59. Rosen CD, Kahanovitz N, Bernstein R, et al: A retrospective analysis of the efficacy of epidural steroid injections. *Clin Orthop* 1988; 228:270–272.
60. San Martino A, D'Andria FM, San Martino C: The surgical treatment of nerve root compression caused by scoliosis of the lumbar spine. *Spine* 1983; 8:261–265.
61. Sarpyener MA: Spina bifida aperta and congenital structure of the spinal canal. *J Bone Joint Surg* 1947; 29:817.
62. Scarff T, et al: Dermatomal somatosensory ekoved potential in the diagnosis of lumbar root entrapment. *Surg Forum* 1981; 32:489–491.
63. Shenkin H, Hash C: Spondylolisthesis after multiple bilateral laminectomies and facetectomies for lumbar spondylosis. *J Neurosurg* 1979; 50:45–47.
64. Simeone FA, Rothman RH: Clinical usefulness of CT scanning in the disease and treatment of lumbar spine disease. *Radiol Clin North Am* 1983; 21:197–200.
65. Simmons EH, Jackson RP: The management of nerve root entrapment syndromes associated with the collapsing scoliosis of idiopathic lumbar and thoracolumbar curves. *Spine* 1979; 4:533–541.
66. Towne EB, Reichert FL: Compression of the lumbosacral roots of the spinal cord by thickened ligamenta flava. *Ann Surg* 1931; 94:327–336.
67. Tile M, McNeil SR, Zarino RK, et al: Spinal stenosis: Results of treatment. *Clin Orthop* 1976; 115:104.
68. Tsitsouplous P, Fotiou F, Papakostopoulos D, et al: Comparative study of clinical and surgical findings and cortical somatosensory evoked potentials in patients with lumbar spinal stenosis and disc protrusion. *Acta Neurochir (Wien)* 1987; 84:54–63.
69. Verbiest H: A radicular syndrome from developmental narrowing of the lumbar vertebral canal. *J Bone Joint Surg [Br]* 1954; 36:230–237.
70. Verbiest H: Results of surgical treatment of idiopathic developmental stenosis of the lumbar vertebral canal, a review of twenty-seven years' experience. *J Bone Joint Surg [Br]* 1977; 59:181–188.
71. Weinstein PR: Diagnosis and management of lumbar spinal stenosis. *Clin Neurosurg* 1983; 30:677–697.
72. White AH, Derby R, Wynne G: Epidural injections for the disease and treatment of low back pain. *Spine* 1980; 5:78–86.
73. White AA, Wiltse LL: Spondylolisthesis after extensive lumbar laminectomy. Presented at the 43rd Annual Meeting of the American Academy of Orthopaedic Surgeons, New Orleans, 1976.
74. Wiesel SW, Tsourmas N, Feffer HI, et al: A study of computer-assisted tomography. The incidence of positive CAT scans in an asymptomatic group of patients. *Spine* 1984; 9:549–551.
75. Wilson CB, Ehni G, Grollmus J: Neurogenic intermittent claudication. *Clin Neurosurg* 1971; 18:62–85.
76. Young S, Veerapen R, O'Laoire S: Relief of lumbar canal stenosis using multilevel subarticular fenestrations as an alternative to wide laminectomy: Preliminary report. *Neurosurgery* 1988; 23:628–633.

38

Rehabilitation of Degenerative Disease of the Spine

Shelly Ritz, P.T., Tom Lorren, P.T., Susan Simpson, P.T., Tammy Mondry, P.T., and Michele Comer, P.T.

Treatment of the spine has as many approaches and protocols as there are medical professionals with opinions. The search for the optimal approach has been hampered by the attitude that "hands-on" conservative care is an art and therefore cannot be measured or quantified. In addition, the large number of treatment variables coupled with a wide array of patient responses has led to a comparative dearth of objective conservative-care research.

Rehabilitation of degenerative disease of the spine requires the same approach as rehabilitation of the spine in sports. The goals and the time frames may be different, but treatment with a sound physiologic basis remains the same.

At the Texas Back Institute, we have developed an interdisciplinary approach to treatment that considers the total patient vs. a sole focus on the predominant disorder. This program is based on the following beliefs:

1. Consistent, progressive activity is a key to restoration of function.
2. While not ignoring pain, increasing activity and maintaining an acceptable level of discomfort are reasonable goals.
3. By targeting the specific tissues most likely involved with the pain and by treating the source of the problem, not the symptoms, a tissue capacity change will occur that will allow increased activity and serve as the groundwork for building more advanced rehabilitation activities.
4. Treatment of the specific dysfunction is a necessity, but no more so than addressing total patient fitness and education.
5. Patient involvement in the goal setting and in the treatment process is the key to avoiding patients returning for treatment for a preventable reason.

This chapter outlines a method that we feel is beneficial and effective in the pursuit of optimal spinal rehabilitation.

EVALUATION

Effective rehabilitation of degenerative spinal disorders is dependent on a comprehensive evaluation of the patient's musculoskeletal and neuromuscular systems. This clarifying examination is used by the physical therapist to assess the nature and extent of the disorder and to determine the most effective method of treatment. The evaluation systematically includes the initial observation, the history and interview, physical examination, the treatment plan, and prognosis.

Initial Observation

The initial observation occurs as the patient walks into the examination room. The therapist observes patient spinal alignment, the presence of guarding or shifts, and the ambulation pattern for the presence of an antalgic gait, neuromotor weakness, or asymmetrical weight bearing. The clinician also notes the patient's facial expression and willingness to move to determine how the patient interprets his problem.

History and Interview

The history and interview allows the patient to communicate to the therapist his own interpretation of the mechanism, duration, frequency, location, nature, intensity, and irritability of the pain and related symptoms. The patient is also questioned about previous episodes and treatments and how past or present problems have affected functional and recreational activities.

In addition to the subjective information being gathered, the therapist assesses the patient's sitting posture. This is done by noting the position of the head and spine and observing whether the patient favors one side or frequently shifts position in the chair.

The interview also sets the stage for the therapist-patient working relationship. The manner in which the questions are delivered helps to determine the level of confidence the patient has in the therapist and affects willingness to cooperate with the treatment plan. The subjective findings gathered during the interview are later correlated with the objective data from the physical examination.

Physical Examination

The objective information collected during the physical examination is quantified whenever possible and used to establish baselines from which progression can be monitored. The physical examination includes structural inspection, selective tissue tension testing, palpation, neurologic screening, and specific mobility testing.

Structural Inspection

In order to perform a structural inspection the patient must be properly disrobed so that the length of the spine and extremities can be viewed. Alignment of bony landmarks are assessed from anterior, posterior, and lateral views starting from the feet and working up to the head.[35] Symmetry of the navicular tubercles, medial malleoli, fibular heads, greater trochanters, ischial tuberosities, posterior and anterior iliac spines, iliac crests, scapular borders, clavicles, and acromions is visually and tactilely assessed to determine possible leg length discrepancies, iliac rotations, or scoliosis. Other notable deviations may include flat or cavus arches of the foot, varus or valgus of the calcaneus, anterior or posterior rotation of the pelvis, excessive or reduced lordotic or kyphotic spinal curves, or forward or sideways positioning of the head on the neck. These structural observations are initial components of the biomechanical examination.

Selective Tissue Tension Testing

This portion of the examination includes active, passive, and resisted movement testing to differentiate between soft-tissue and arthrogenic lesions. This differential evaluation is the contribution of Cyriax.[11] The gross active movements are performed first. Cyriax feels that the active movements alone do not distinguish the type of tissue involved but are helpful in localizing the area to be tested in greater detail.

Active movements are followed by passive movements that indicate the status of the inert or noncontractile tissues, including the joint capsule, ligament, bursa, fascia, dura mater, and nerve roots. The patient is passively moved through the range of motion, thereby eliminating muscular contributions. The therapist assesses the end-feel of the joint. End-feels (the specific sensation transmitted to the examiner's hands at the extreme of each passive movement) may include a rigid, abrupt bone-to-bone feel or a leathery capsular feel. A finding of active and passive motion restricted and/or painful in the same direction indicates an arthrogenic lesion. A finding of active and passive motion restricted and/or painful in the opposite direction indicates a soft-tissue lesion. Cyriax defines soft tissue as muscle, tendon, and bony insertion.[11]

Resisted tests are performed after active and passive tests to determine the state of musculotendinous tissue. The contraction may be weak or strong, painful or painless. A strong and painless response indicates no lesion. A strong and painful response suggests a minor lesion usually involving the tendon. A weak and painless response suggests neurologic involvement or a complete rupture of muscle or tendon, while a weak and painful response indicates a major lesion involving a partial rupture or possibly a fracture or acute inflammation.

Specific selective tissue tests of the spine begin with active flexion, extension, side bending, and rotation. The main purpose of testing active spinal movement is to observe the patient's willingness to move and the quality of the motion. The amount of flexion and extension that occurs in the lumbar spine may also be quantified by utilizing the dual-angle inclinometer technique described by Mayer et al.[52] This measurement differentiates between motion occurring in the pelvis from that occurring in the lumbar spine.

When the patient bends forward, deviations to one side or the other are often observed. Normally during flexion, the superior vertebra glides forward symmetrically on the inferior vertebra. If a facet is limited on one side due to muscle guarding, capsular restriction, or meniscoid locking, it will not glide forward on that side. This results in a sudden shift or "hitching" toward the restricted side followed by a rapid shift back.[65] Conversely, slow, ongoing deviations (as opposed to sudden shifts) with forward bending are associated with disc involvement. With disc prolapse, the patient will tend to laterally shift the trunk as a unit to move the protrusion away from the irritated nerve. Typically the patient will lean away from the involved side if the prolapse is lateral to the nerve root and will list toward the nerve if the protrusion is medial to the root.[22] Forward bending may also be viewed from the lateral aspect to identify flat areas (hypomobilities) and sharp angles (hypermobilities). These flattened areas or sharp angulations of spinal curvature may also be identified during active extension and side bending.

The quality of rotational motion may be assessed by observing the curve created by component side bending. With the spine in a neutral position, lumbar rotation and side bending occur in opposite directions.[43] Normal right rotation is demonstrated by a smooth side-bending curve to the left when the patient actively rotates to the right (Fig 38–1).

Following active movement testing in standing, the patient is seated and passively taken through the available range of motion in all cardinal planes. The therapist assesses resistance to various motions and notes provocation of symptoms throughout the movement and at the end of the range of motion. Overpressure may also be applied at the end of the range to ensure that the full range has been achieved. Quadrant testing (including flexion-side bending-rotation and extension-side bending-rotation combinations) allows for maximal distraction or compression of the facet joints, and any changes in signs or symptoms are noted.[6, 16]

The final stage of selective tissue tension testing is re-

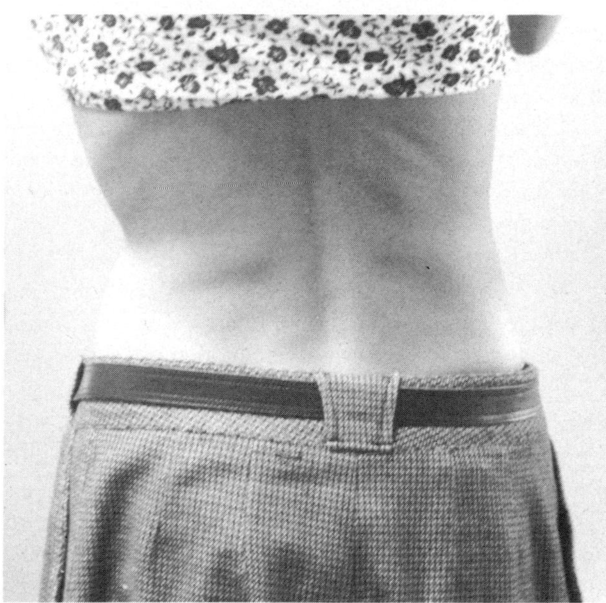

FIG 38–1.
Normal right rotation is demonstrated by a smooth side-bending curve to the left when the patient actively rotates to the right.

sisted movement. Traditionally, resisted tests have been performed isometrically in the mid-range as recommended by Cyriax.[11] He proposes that in the mid-range, the inert tissues around the tested joint are equally relaxed. During muscle contraction, the bones approximate and thereby increase ligamentous and capsular laxity. He negates the possibility of joint compression as a source of pain with muscle contraction since normal cartilage is aneural. This concept is challenged on the premise that degenerated cartilage develops scar tissue as a component of secondary healing.[22] This scar tissue may give rise to pain with joint compression by way of nociceptive mechanoreceptors. Grimsby suggests performing resisted tests not only in the mid-range but also in the inner and outer ranges to open or close the joint spaces to help determine the effect compression has on pain reproduction. Resisted left side bending, for example, may not provoke pain when the patient is in a neutral position or the right side bent position since the facets are relatively distracted. However, resisted left side bending may be painful when the patient is left side bent since this closes the facets on the left and muscle contraction will further increase facet compression on that side and elicit pain. If the contractile tissue were solely at fault, the resisted movements would be somewhat painful when tested at the inner, mid, and outer ranges.

Palpation

Palpation of soft tissues and spinal positional faults follow active, passive, and resisted movement testing. Soft-tissue palpation includes investigating the skin, subcutaneous tissue, muscles, and ligaments for signs of dysfunction. The body's initial reaction to injury involves a local inflammatory response mainly in the connective tissue. This response is characterized by four signs as described by Celsus in the first century A.D.[90] These signs are calor, rubor, tumor, and dolor, which indicate that the involved tissue is warm, red, swollen, and painful. These four signs are helpful in evaluating the presence of dysfunction. The initial reaction to a soft-tissue insult is increased circulation accompanied by increased temperature. Increased blood flow into the capillaries of the traumatized tissue causes redness and eventual penetration of larger molecules into the surrounding soft tissue. The accumulation of extracapillary fluid begins to distort the soft tissue and results in the stimulation of nociceptive mechanoreceptors, which give rise to pain. Finally, the painful area is held still or immobilized, and this leads to dysfunction.

The skin is palpated for temperature and moisture, histamine response, texture, and stretch response. By observing the skin's reaction to specific stimuli, hypomobilities or hypermobilities of the spinal segments may be detected.[22]

Skin Tests.—***Temperature and Moisture.***—This test is performedby placing one's hands with light pressure along the length of the spine and feeling for differences in temperature and moisture from side to side and segment to segment. A cool, clammy area indicates decreased circulation and mobility. A warm, moist area indicates increased circulation and mobility.

Scratch Test.—This test is performed by drawing the thumbnails down the length of the spine to stimulate a histamine response. Histamine released as a result of trauma is proportional to the amount of blood flow in the area. The initial sign should be a blanching due to vasoconstriction followed by a gradual reddening within a few seconds due to capillary dilatation. The nature of the reddening is observed in identifying problem areas. Hypermobile segments have increased redness and stay red longer as opposed to hypomobile segments, which have decrease redness and fade quickly.

Orange Skin Test.—By pinching subcutaneous tissue along the spine, decreased mobility of segments is identified by dimpling from areas of increased subcutaneous tissue.

Skin Rolling.—Folds of skin are rolled along the spine between the thumbs and index fingers. Thick skin that does not roll easily corresponds with hypomobility. Palpation of muscles and ligaments can also signal areas of dysfunction as discussed below.

Muscle Tests.—***Muscular Development.***—Palpation and observation of muscle atrophy or hypertrophy can provide information about mobility and neurologic status. Wasting of paraspinal, gluteal, or pelvic girdle musculature may indicate nerve root entrapment or relative segmental hypomobility. Hypertrophied muscular areas may signal segmental instability. Narrow raised bands of muscle observed at L4 are a possible sign of spondylolithesis of L5 on S1 as muscular activity increases to help stabilize the segment.

Muscle Tone.—Palpation of muscle tone is used to detect reflexogenic guarding. The presence of muscle guarding in the lumbar spine may be assessed with the weight-shift test.[73] With the patient standing, the examiner palpates the lumbar paraspinals with the thumbs. The patient is instructed to shift his weight from one foot to the other. Normally, the paraspinals ipsilateral to the weight-bearing foot will relax, but in the presence of guarding, the paraspinals will not relax with weight shifting.

Muscle Texture.—The spinal, gluteal, and pelvic girdle muscles are palpated for stringy or hardened areas. These fibrotic nodules are indicative of poor circulation secondary to chronic muscular overuse.

Ligament Tests.—***Supraspinous Ligament.***—In order to identify areas of tenderness and localize the involved segments, the area between the spinous processes is palpated with the middle finger.

Interspinuous Ligament.—To differentiate between supraspinous and interspinous ligament tenderness, highly localized pressure is applied with the edge of a coin into the interspinous space.[44]

Spinal Position Fault Tests.—In addition to soft-tissue palpations, the spinous processes of the thoracic and lumbar vertebrae are also palpated to identify any positional faults. Normally the vertebrae line up with equal space between the spinous processes. What appears to be a loss of normal positional relationship may only be asymmetry of bony development; however, it may also indicate that a segment is out of place or subluxed.[26] Positional faults may be rotational, forward bent, or backward bent.

Rotational Fault.—A rotational fault can be palpated by pinching the lateral aspects of adjacent spinous processes with the thumb and index finger. If a vertebra is fixed in a rotated position, its spinous process will move in the opposite direction of the vertebral body and therefore will be out of line with the spinous processes above and below.

Forward-bent Fault.—With forward bending, the superior vertebra glides up and forward on the inferior vertebra. If the vertebra gets fixed in a forward-bent position, there will be a palpable wide gap between the spinous processes at that segment accompanied by a pinching of spinous processes at the segment below.

Backward-bent Fault.—With backward bending, the superior vertebra should glide backward and down on the inferior vertebra. If the vertebra is locked into extension, a narrow space between the spinous processes at that level accompanied by a wide gap between the spinous processes at the segment below may be palpated.

Palpation of the spinous processes may also detect the presence of spondylolisthesis. If L5 slips forward significantly on S1, a "shelf" can be palpated at the level of the L5 spinous process.[21]

Neurologic Screening

The neurologic examination includes sensation, manual muscle, reflex, and nerve root tension testing to assess the status of segmental neural conduction.

Cutaneous Innervation Test.—The sensory test includes light touch with a brush for hypersensitivity and pinprick with a needle for hyposensitivity. Each stimulus is applied to the areas of cutaneous innervation for each spinal segment and the lower extremities compared to determine whether the perceived intensity of stimulus is equal on both sides. The cutaneous innervation areas of the lumbar spine are as follows:

- L1—below the inguinal ligament
- L2—proximal medial aspect of the thigh
- L3—above the patella
- L4—top of the medial arch
- L5—web space between the first and second toes
- S1—lateral edge of the foot
- S2—popliteal fossa

Manual Muscle Test.—Resisted isometric tests are based on myotome stimulation to detect muscle weakness that may result from nerve root compression. The lumbar myotomes are as follows:

- L2—iliopsoas; tested by resisting hip flexion
- L3—quadriceps; tested by resisting knee extension
- L4—tibialis anterior; tested by resisting ankle dorsiflexion and foot inversion
- L5—extensor hallucis longus; tested by resisting big toe extension
- S1—peroneus longus and brevis; tested by resisting foot eversion
- S2—gastrocnemius; tested through walking on the balls of the feet

Reflex Testing.—Deep tendon reflexes at the knee and ankle are observed for symmetry of response from one side to the other to identify segmental neurologic deficits. The lumbar reflex tests are at L3–4, the patellar tendon, and at S1, the Achilles tendon.

Based on the results of the previously described neurologic tests, the nerve root involvement can be categorized as irritation, compression, or combined.[22] With nerve root irritation, the sensation and reflexes may be increased and strength is normal. With nerve root compression, the sensation and reflexes are decreased, and the related muscle groups are weak. Combined involvement may have mixed characteristics.

Nerve Stretch Tests.—The status of the nerve root may be further evaluated through nerve stretch tests. The nerve root may be sensitive to stretch in the presence of pathology, including disc prolapse, adhesions, facet degeneration, or foraminal stenosis.[8, 18, 57]

- **Sciatic nerve stretch tests**
  - *Straight leg raise (SLR)*[88]
    - Position—patient supine.
    - Procedure—passively raise the extended leg.
    - Positive—radicular symptoms produced between 30 and 60 degrees of hip flexion.
    - Comment—posterior thigh pain may indicate hamstring tightness and/or sciatic nerve root tension.
  - *Lasegue's test*[80, 94]
    - Position—patient supine.
    - Procedure—passively raise the extended leg to soft-tissue end-feel, lower slightly, and then passively dorsiflex the ankle.
    - Positive—radicular sign reproduced with ankle dorsiflexion
    - Comment—lowering the leg below end-feel decreases tension on the hamstrings, and dorsiflexion of the ankle increases tension on the sciatic nerve.
  - *Brechterew's test*[21]
    - Position—patient seated.
    - Procedure—passively raise extended leg; ankle dorsiflexion may be added.
    - Positive—radicular signs produced.
    - Comment—the patient may tolerate SLR when sitting because the foramina are relatively open in this position whereas in the supine position the spine is in lordosis, where the foramina are more closed.
  - *Cram's test*[10]
    - Position—patient supine.
    - Procedure—passively flex the hip in slight abduction and internal rotation until a radicular sign is produced. Then flex the knee until pain subsides, and again flex the hip slightly. Finally, apply thumb pressure to the posterior tibial nerve in the popliteal fossa.
    - Positive—radicular sign produced with digital pressure on the nerve.
    - Comments—this is the most reliable of the sciatic nerve stretch tests because the knee flexion component eliminates hamstring tension and direct pressure on the posterior tibial nerve isolates the source of symptoms as true nerve root tension.
- **Femoral nerve stretch tests**
  - *Ely's test*[19]
    - Position—patient prone.
    - Procedure—passively flex the knee and extend the hip.
    - Positive—radicular signs produced.
    - Comment—analogous to SLR; anterior thigh pain may indicate quadricep tightness and/or femoral nerve root tension.

Once the neurologic status has been assessed, specific mobility tests are administered to further isolate the level of involvement.

Specific Mobility Testing

Specific mobility testing of the spine is performed to assess the quantity and quality of motion at each segment. The quality of motion is based on feeling the resistance occurring with passive movement throughout the motion and at the end range. Painful movement in the mid-range that is preceded and followed by painless movement is referred to as a painful arc. According to Cyriax, a painful arc implies that a pain-sensitive tissue is being compressed between hard structures.[13] End-feel at the range limits may also be evaluated. A physiologic end-feel can be classified as soft, due to soft-tissue approximation; as firm, resulting from capsular or ligamentous stretch; or as hard, occurring when bone meets bone. Pathology may be present in the joint if an uncharacteristic or empty end-feel is noted. Quantification of relative segmental mobility is based on the knowledge of anticipated motion provided by Robert[71] and White and Panjabi.[92] Mobility may be graded manually by using the following scale[31, 32]:

Ankylosis	0 = No movement
Hypomobility	1 = Considerable decrease in movement
	2 = Slight decrease in movement
Normal	3 = Normal
	4 = Slight increase in movement
Hypermobility	5 = Considerable increase in movement
	6 = Complete instability

Spinal mobility is determined by digital palpation at the facet joints and interspinous space of each segment while passively maneuvering the spine or extremities. Accurate grading of joint mobility is dependent on the palpation skills of the examiner. As Bourdillon notes, fine-tuned perception of joint motion can be learned with practice, similar to mastering Braille.[5] The reliability of mobility testing can also be improved by performing the movements with the patient in non–weight-bearing positions (supine, prone, and side lying) to reduce the effects of postural tone and muscle guarding. Altered segmental mobility is frequently detected as a stiff or hypomobile segment with a compensatory hypermobile segment nearby.[65]

Evaluation of Related Joints

Physical examination of the lumbar spine should also include a biomechanical screening of the sacroiliac, hip, and pelvis because their function is closely related to the spine.[27, 66, 91]

Correlation of Findings With Other Studies

The subjective data from the history and interview and objective findings from the physical examination may now be correlated with other diagnostic studies. Selective studies in addition to basic roentgenograms may include myelograms, computed tomography (CT), magnetic resonance imaging (MRI), bone scanning, discography, electromyography (EMG), and blood workup. Each test has a specific role in identifying the possible source of symptoms. Other clinical measurements may include computerized isokinetic muscle testing and quantitative evaluation of functional and aerobic capacity.

Treatment Plan

The findings of all relevant evaluative and diagnostic procedures are organized so that short- and long-term treatment goals may be established. The patient is a key member of the rehabilitation team, and his input and involvement in the goal-setting process ensures that all members are working toward the same anticipated outcome. A specific, goal-oriented, treatment plan is outlined. Goals are reviewed at least once a week to ensure that rehabilitation is progressing as anticipated. Any significant deviation is addressed through a reassessment of the patient's program and perhaps in modifying the goals.

Our rehabilitation process involves an interdisciplinary team composed of physicians, psychologists, physical therapists, occupational therapists, exercise physiologists, case managers, and numerous other support personnel. The concept allows the patient to be treated by the individual who has the greatest clinical expertise to deal with the patient's particular immediate need while ensuring a treatment overview that minimizes professional biases.

Rehabilitation of the spine can be divided into three primary phases. These phases will overlap to some extent, but each has a specific function in providing a foundation for advancement to the next level. These phases include protective, active, and resistive.

Phase 1: Protective Phase

Immediately following an injury, the focus is to minimize the extent of the injury, stabilize symptoms, and create an optimal healing environment. It is vital that the patient be involved from the start in sharing the responsibility for achieving a successful treatment outcome. The patient is evaluated thoroughly and involved in the goal setting for short- and long-term needs. The patient is educated in the pathology of the injury, protective activities of daily living (ADL) skills, and his essential role in the rehabilitation process. Advancement to the next phase is contingent upon the following:

1. Ability to performing basic self-care and low-level ADL by using protective modifications and self-treatment concepts for symptom control.
2. Gaining lumbopelvic control (stabilization) during direct spinal movements in unloaded positions.
3. Eliminating abnormal spinal shifts.
4. Ability to ambulate for 15 minutes with a body weight that is mechanically reduced by no more than 20%. This is done to allow exercise and consistent, progressive activity without increasing symptoms.

Phase 2: Active Phase

This phase is critical in the patient's progression through rehabilitation and begins after symptoms have been stabilized and the patient is capable of participating in a supervised high-repetition–low-resistance exercise program. The primary focus is to develop local tissue endurance and provide an optimal tissue stimulus for continued healing while maintaining symptom control. Advancement to the next phase is contingent upon the following:

1. Ability to perform more advanced functional movements such as bending, rotating, squatting, pulling, and pushing without exacerbating symptoms.
2. Maintaining lumbopelvic control (stabilization) during spinal movements in loaded positions.
3. Ability to ambulate for 15 minutes at body weight without increasing symptoms.

Phase 3: Resistive Phase

The final phase of rehabilitation is characterized by cardiovascular conditioning and overall strengthening. It presumes that the patient is able to stabilize symptoms (not necessarily pain free) while functional capacity is restored. Independent preventive maintenance programs of exercise and modified ADL are stressed, and the self-responsibility for long-term success is emphasized. Discharge goals are as follows:

1. The ability to perform complex functional movements such as bending with rotation, pushing, squatting, etc., without exacerbating symptoms (Fig 38–2).
2. Maintaining lumbopelvic control (stabilization) during spinal movements with external loads, such as carrying and lifting.
3. Ambulation for 15 minutes at body weight with an external load without increasing symptoms.

A

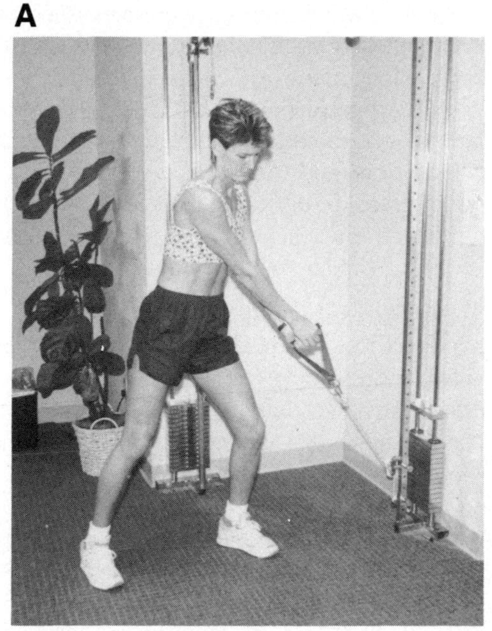

B

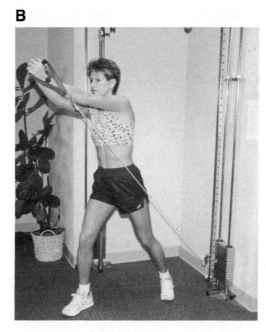

FIG 38–2.
Complex functional movements such as resisted trunk rotation with weight shift (starting from the initial starting position **(A)** and progressing toward the ending position **(B)**) without exacerbating symptoms are a key component in the resistive stage.

4. Trunk strength and endurance appropriate to maintain advanced ADL and recreational activities.

Patients who have progressed through phase 3 and are candidates for progressive work hardening are advanced into such a program to address specific conditioning and work simulation tasks.

The phases listed above are designed to provide the clinician and patient with a road map during rehabilitation. Each phase is defined by measurable, objective data from which patient progress is evaluated. Although none of the data points is a sole determinant of a patient's progression, they are used as indicators to help determine an end point to rehabilitation with the absence of medical contraindications.

During rehabilitation, patients with degenerative spine pathology are treated with a variety of modalities and procedures specific to their particular needs. In an activity-based program, it is recognized that modalities have a place in the restorative process. However, modalities should not constitute a majority of the rehabilitation process. Activity is key, and thus specific activities are designed to enhance the patient's quality of life as well as function.

PROGRAM COMPONENTS

Education

Patient understanding of the pathology present, the impending treatment process, and his role in the rehabilitation process is essential to achieving successful outcomes. Correct body mechanics, protective ADL, self–pain modulation, and a specific exercise program help the patient achieve independence and reinforces his role of responsibility. Education includes the lifetime need of total-body fitness, stress reduction, dietary requirements for adequate nutrition, and the importance of proper body weight. Information cannot be adequately assimilated by most individuals from a lecture setting. For education to be fully effective, it must be interactive, repetitive, and reinforced. Back school is a vital component of any spine rehabilitation program, and its concepts need to be reinforced continually by the treating personnel.

Passive Treatment

The term *passive* in this context is used to describe types of treatment concepts and techniques not requiring the patient to actively participate. These techniques are employed if the patient is unable to achieve the desired effect independently or when an external stimulus is required to elicit a specific physiologic response.

Modalities

The use of modalities and physical agents in the treatment of back pain has often received criticism. This may be due to the philosophy of sports medicine (reactivation through activity) and the view that modalities are passive treatments and therefore incompatible with this philosophy. The criticism may also arise from the unfortunate occurrence of their indiscriminate use as sole hope of returning a patient to a functional level. Given that limiting symptoms last approximately 2 weeks regardless of the treatment rendered,[50, 59] some feel that treatment with modalities is as useful as no treatment at all. Despite some disfavor, modalities play an important role in the treatment of degenerative disease, especially in the treatment of the soft-tissue involvement.

Therapeutic Heat

Heat has been widely used as a pain-relieving agent. Superficial heat modalities such as hot packs and heat lamps are used to assist in the reduction of pain, stiffness, and muscle spasm (through a decrease in gamma efferent activity),[42] to increase the range of motion through increased tissue extensibility, and to improve tissue healing by increasing the flow of blood and nutrients to the injured area.[55] Superficial heat elevates the temperature and provides the greatest effect at 0.5 cm from the surface.[20] Heating to depths of 1 to 2 cm requires longer durations with a limiting degree of efficacy. Due to these limited depths, the thermal agents of choice in many spinal soft-tissue dysfunctions are the deep-heating agents such as ultrasound and diathermy.

Diathermy and ultrasound both heat through the process of conversion whereby electrical current (diathermy) or sound waves (ultrasound) are converted to heat when the energy is passed through tissues. These deep-heating agents can increase tissue temperatures at depths of 3 to 5 cm.[55] Deep-heating agents are of particular use due to their ability to penetrate into deep structures (such as tendons and ligaments) without temperature increases to the overlying skin.[55]

Thermal agents may also cause edema as a result of their vasodilatory effect and should be used at low levels and with caution.

Due to the direct physiologic effects of increased cellular metabolism, vasodilation, pain threshold,[41] and extensibility of collagen (elastic properties), thermal agents are ideally used at the initial phase of the treatment session in preparation for the active and manual procedures to follow.

Cold Therapy

The use of cold in the treatment of soft-tissue injuries has been widely taught and noted in the literature. Its physiologic effects include vasoconstriction (initially), vasodilation (long-term), reduced pain due to decreased sensitivity, reduced inflammation and edema, increased joint range of motion, decreased myospasm (due to a decrease in pain and a decrease in the sensitivity of the muscle spindle fibers to discharge),[55] and a maintained increase in connective tissue length when cold is applied to an already stretched tissue. Little research has been done on the effects specific to spinal musculature and soft tissues.

Cold is applied to the back in the form of ice packs, direct ice massage, or cold gel packs. It is important to monitor its application since surface tissue can be damaged if the intensity or duration of the cold are excessive. Ice is particularly effective in the initial stages of injury due to its effect of vasoconstriction and reduced edema. Its use in later stages should be tempered with the knowledge that hemoglobin holds tighter to oxygen with a drop in tissue temperature. In most stages there is a concern with release of oxygen, and this effect should be considered when determining the appropriate modality.

Electrical Stimulation

Electrical stimulation for therapeutic purposes is divided into two types of current: alternating (faradic) and direct (galvanic). Faradic current is an effective pain modulator due to the stimulation of sensory nerves and for stimulation of motor nerves that are intact to simulate a normal muscle contraction. When muscles are stimulated by electrical discharge, the result is the same as if the muscle was voluntary contracted with a subsequent increase in metabolism and increased waste output and evacuation. Galvanic current, with its positive and negative pole, has physiologic effects that include hardening of the tissues, decreased nerve irritability, and local analgesia, as well as vasoconstriction. The effects at the negative pole include increased nerve root vasodilation. These properties make it very effective for treating soft tissues.[74] As with all electrical stimulation, the effectiveness is based on intensity, duration, and waveform.

Transcutaneous Nerve Stimulation

The use of transcutaneous electrical nerve stimulation (TENS) is based on the gate theory proposed by Melzack and Wall.[54] They theorized that the correct electrical current is capable of interfering with the transmission of pain signals. It is also hypothesized that TENS may act to stimulate the release of endorphins.[33]

TENS is used quite extensively in the treatment of low back dysfunction, especially in those conditions involving soft-tissue pathology. Although TENS provides substantial pain relief in many individuals, its scientific results have been somewhat mixed. Richardson et al. described a group of 15 patients, 6 of whom experienced a 50% reduction in low back pain.[70] However, it was also reported that some patients experienced increased discomfort as well as vertigo and numbness with the initiation of TENS.

Laser

The term *laser* is an acronym for light amplification by simulated emission of radiation. Lasers are classified as either high power or low power. Low-power lasers are also called cold or soft lasers and are primarily associated with wound healing. The use of a cold laser (under 1 mW) will produce only a nonthermal response.[76] Cold laser systems include helium-neon (HeNE) and gallium-arsenide. It is thought that lasers accelerate collagen synthesis, increase vascularization in a healing tissue, and decrease pain sensation.[76] Lasers are relatively new, having been introduced in the 1960s. Through their application in wound healing and pain modulation, the use of lasers may provide a new therapeutic modality.

Biofeedback

Since biofeedback in a mechanism that records, there is no direct physiologic effect derived from its use. However, by utilizing the biofeedback mechanisms, the patient's own neurophysiologic pathways may create many of the physiologic effects as elicited with other modalities. Biofeedback appears to be particularly effective in helping patients understand and manage stress-related muscle tension.

Traction

Traction is an age-old method of providing pain relief through the process of mechanical distraction of the vertebral bodies. It is generally performed with the patient in a comfortable position. The effects of traction also include gliding and distracting of the facet joints, tensing of the segmental ligaments (especially if scarred or bound down), widening of the intervertebral foramina (especially in flexion), alteration of the spinal curves, and stretching of the spinal musculature.[79]

Types of Traction.—Although traction is an apparently simple distraction, there are various types that are appropriate in specific situations. Continuous bed traction, although very rarely used, is effective in that it keeps the patient relatively non–gravity loaded by greatly decreasing mobility. Bed rest has been shown to be effective in the early treatment of an injury, with a recommended dosage of no more than 2 days.[15]

Sustained or static traction is used in cases where there may be an irritable tissue involved. Sustained traction at lower levels may bring temporary relief and is commonly utilized in home traction devices.

Mechanical intermittent traction consists of alternating periods of increased and decreased distraction. It is generally well tolerated by the patient provided that the traction force is never released fully until the end of the treatment. Intermittent traction is an excellent prelude for manual mobilization for areas of hypomobility.

Manual traction has a distinct advantage in that it allows the therapist to assess and accommodate to the patient's responses. Mobilization techniques such as side gliding may be added while traction is taking place to increase the effectiveness of treatment.

Traction may be indicated when forces must be maintained for periods of time or at levels that are beyond the capabilities of the treating therapist. It may also be used when one has been unable to get reduction and maintain it by any other means or to loosen stiff joints. It has also been reported to decrease symptoms of nerve root adhesions.[68]

Traction is contraindicated in structural disease from tumor or infection; in acute strains, sprains, and inflammatory processes; in suspected spinal instability; and in cases where there is increased peripheralization of nerve root impingement signs or symptoms. Traction should also be used with caution in patients with osteoporosis or hiatal hernias. Claustrophobic patients may also need to be treated with a less-confining technique.

Spinal Manipulation

Schools of Thought.—Spinal manipulation is practiced by various medical professionals including osteopathic physicians, chiropractors, medical doctors, and physical therapists. Their philosophies vary, as do their manipulative techniques. The present-day schools of thought on manipulation are based on at least one of three principal characteristics.[62] The first is based on relieving nerve root pressure. The theoretical chiropractic premise is the "law of the nerve," which states that disease results from impaired nerve impulse secondary to impingement via vertebral subluxation. Chiropractors apply direct pressure to the "subluxed" vertebra to cause gapping of the intervetebral foramen and subsequent removal of nerve impingement, thereby restoring normal innervation to the diseased area.[29] Chiropractic techniques are therefore focused on specific movement of vertebrae. Cyriax utilized manipulation for relief of nerve root pressure but proposed that disc displacement (as opposed to vertebral subluxation) is the source of compression.[13] His treatment approach emphasized replacing extruded disc material either by general manipulation (for annular displacement) or by traction to "suck back up" the nucleus pulposus.[75]

The second school of thought is based on relieving pain through manipulation. Maigne developed the concept of utilizing painless and opposite motion in spinal manipulation.[45] His rules of "no pain" and "contrary motion" state that if a passive procedure is painful, it should not be done, and that if a joint is blocked or painful in a certain direction, it may be freed by moving it in the opposite direction. Maitland also emphasizes the pain response to spinal movements and positions.[46] He stresses the use of graduated oscillatory articulations and continual analytical assessment of symptomatic responses before, during, and after treatment.

The third principal characteristic of spinal manipulation is based on normalizing joint mobility. Proponents of this school of thought concur that dysfunctional segmental motion may be relatively hypermobile or hypomobile from the expected norm. Osteopathic physicians have defined these joint derangements as the "osteopathic lesion," which is characterized by hyperesthesia, altered muscular activity, changes in tissue texture and local circulation, and altered visceral and other autonomic functions.[38]

Stoddard stated that "the underlying principle of osteopathy is that structure governs function, that disturbances of structure, in whatever tissue within the body, will lead to disturbances of functioning in that structure and, in turn, of the function of the body as a whole."[81] The main goal of osteopathic manipulation is to restore normal mobility to involved spinal segments in order to relieve abnormal tissue tension, improve circulation, reposition viscera, and facilitate or inhibit the autonomic nervous system. Osteopathic techniques are specific to the level of impaired mobility and are achieved by locking mechanisms including facet opposition and ligamentous tension to protect the segments above and below the one being manipulated.

Norwegian manual therapists also grade joint motion and predominantly use specific stretch articulations at the end of the range of motion to restore normal mobility. They pay particular attention to protecting hypermobilities and to stretching hypomobilities, but at controlled intensities not eliciting the patient's pain.[22] Paris also contends that spinal dysfunction presents as increased, decreased, or aberrant motion.[63] He is primarily concerned with function as it relates to altered segmental mobility and downplays the patient's subjective report of pain since he considers this information to be unreliable.

Definitions.—Spinal manipulation is a "skilled passive movement to a spinal segment either within or beyond its active range of motion."[64] Passive movements are classified as thrust or nonthrust. Thrust manipulation is high-velocity, low-amplitude motion delivered at the end of a range. Nonthrust articulations include distraction (the separation of joint surfaces) and gliding (the translation of joint surfaces). Both distraction and gliding motions may include oscillation throughout and at the end of a range or end-range stretch. The type of joint manipulation used depends on the desired effect.[61]

Mechanical Effects of Joint Manipulation.—Prolonged joint immobilization results in decreased extensibility of the connective tissue, ligaments, muscles, and fascia.[1] The lengthening property of connective tissue is due to water acting as a lubricant between collagen fibrils. Immobilization leads to a loss of water-binding proteoglycans. Decreased fluid volume between connective tissue fibers allows the approximation of collagen fibrils and abnormal cross-link formation.[96] Passive stretch to joint capsules, ligaments, and myofascial tissues is used to restore joint extensibility. Adhesions formed by abnormal cross-links may be ruptured by a high-velocity, short-amplitude thrust.[17] Another possible mechanical effect of manipulation is the release of entrapped tissues such as a meniscoid impacted between articular facets thought to cause the "acute locked back."[3] A more controversial possible mechanical effect is reduction of disc protrusion by spinal manipulation. Matthews and Yates reported reduction of small disc prolapses, confirmed by positive epidurograms, in two patients following spinal rotary manipulation.[48] However, rotation manipulation did not demonstrate a reduction of known disc protrusion determined by myelography in 39 patients studied.[9] Over half the patients (57%) reported relief of sciatic pain within 24 hours of manipulation despite the lack of change in myelographic images. Resolution of pain without reduction of disc material after rotary spinal manipulation apparently requires other mechanisms of pain modulation.

Neurophysiologic Effects of Joint Manipulation.—In addition to the described mechanical effects, joint manipulation is believed to alter neurophysiologic activity and result in inhibition of pain and muscle guarding. How manipulation possibly modulates pain may be explained in a brief review of pain mechanisms and theories.

There are three categories of nerve fibers (A, B, and C) based on fiber diameters, thickness of the myelin sheaths, and conduction velocities. In general, the greater the diameter of the fiber, the thicker the myelin sheath and the faster the conduction velocity. A fibers are large, myelinated, and fast conducting. Of the four subgroups of A fibers, one, A-alpha, is responsible for vibration sense and proprioception. Another, A-delta, is associated with temperature and sharp, localized, "fast" pain.

B fibers are smaller, myelinated, and slow conducting. They regulate preganglionic sympathetics. C fibers are the smallest, nonmyelinated, and slowest in conduction. They mediate temperature and burning, less localized "slow" pain.

Nociceptive, small-diameter fibers (C and A-delta) enter the spinal cord and synapse with interneurons of the substantia gelatinosa in the dorsal horn before ascending to the brain. Proprioceptive, large-diameter fibers carry sensory impulses from muscles, tendons, ligaments, and joints to the posterior spinal cord before ascending to the brain.

A restatement of the gate control theory proposed that the brain receives information about pain depending on injury signals from small-diameter fibers, input from other peripheral afferents, and impulses descending from the brain.[89] The interneurons in the substantia gelatinosa regulate the position of the "gate" of pain transmission to the brain as determined by the balance between large- and small-fiber input and possibly by descending inhibitory pathways from the brain. Stimulation of mechanoreceptors inhibit presynaptic cells of the substantia gelatinosa thereby closing the gate to pain perception.

Four types of joint receptors have been described.[97] Type I, II, and III receptors are mechanoreceptors that provide positional and kinesthetic information, and type IV receptors are nociceptors responsible for signaling pain. Type I are tonic receptors located in the superficial layers of joint capsules, predominantly in the neck, shoulder, and hip. They are slow adapting and provide information concerning postural muscle tone and kinesthetic sense. Type II are dynamic receptors located in the deeper layers of joint capsules, predominantly in the lower part of the back, foot, hand, and jaw. They are fast adapting and regulate initiation, acceleration, and deceleration of joint movement. Type III are inhibitive receptors located in the superficial and deep layers of joint capsules of the lumbar spine. They are very slow adapting and have reflex-inhibitory effects on muscle tone to protect joints from injurious overstretch. Type IV are nociceptive receptors located in fibrous joint capsules, superficial and deep ligaments, fat pads, periosteum, anterior dura mater, and blood vessels. They are absent in articular cartilage, intra-articular fibrocartilage, synovium, and muscles. Nociceptors are non-adapting and signal pain when noxious mechanical or chemical stimulation reaches a specific threshold.

Joint mechanoreceptor stimulation generated by spinal manipulation is thought to increase proprioceptive, large-fiber input, thus decreasing nociceptive, small-fiber transmission. Type I postural receptors respond to stretch articulations at the end of a range. Type II dynamic receptors are activated by oscillations at beginning and midrange of tension. Type III inhibitory receptors fire during a strong stretch or thrust manipulation that has a reflex-inhibitory effect and produces muscle relaxation about the joint.

Psychological Effects of Joint Manipulation.—Pain has been defined as an "unpleasant emotional disorder evoked by sufficient activity of the nociceptive receptor system."[98] Therefore, pain is not just a reaction to a nociceptive stimulus but a perception composed of sensory, behavioral, and affective components. Spinal manipulation is also considered to diminish the perception of pain due to a psychological effect. Paris supports the idea that the "laying on of intelligent hands" acts as a placebo in pain relief, especially when an audible pop or snap occurs with the manipulation.[62] McKenzie warns that overuse of manipulation by the clinician creates patient dependency and suggests that patients be taught self-mobilization techniques whenever possible.[53]

Soft-Tissue Mobilization

The role of soft tissue as a primary or secondary source of pain in spinal disorders is often overlooked. A wide variety of soft-tissue mobilization techniques including massage, muscle energy procedures, trigger point therapy, and myofascial release are useful in treating spinal pain and dysfunction related to the myofascial system.

Massage.—Traditional massage was originated by the Chinese and introduced to Western medicine by the French.[83] French terminology is used to describe massage strokes including effleurage and petrissage (kneading of soft tissue). The effects of massage include improved circulation and metabolic balance within the muscle and inhibition of pain and reflexogenic guarding.

Under normal conditions, intermittent muscle contraction during activity creates a pumping action that facilitates venous blood flow toward the heart. When a trauma is sustained, the injured area is often immobilized due to pain leading to decreased circulation and lymphatic drainage. Deep stroking along the superficial veins in the direction of venous flow decreases venous pressure and increases lymphatic flow.[40]

Muscular contraction during normal activity mechanically assists elimination of toxic products into the lymphatic and venous flow. The metabolic balance of muscles can be disturbed due to overactivity or underactivity. Too much muscular activity creates insufficient relaxation time for nutritive substances to flow in and by-products to flow out. Too little muscular activity reduces the "milking" effect and results in an accumulation of irritant acids within the muscle. Although not as effective as normal muscular activity, massage can mechanically assist the flow of waste products into the venous and lymphatic systems when active exercise is still too painful.

Sustained muscle contraction due to reflexogenic guarding or neuromuscular tension can cause ischemia and subsequent pain. Frequently the primary local arthrogenic pain is minimal and overridden by the secondary soft-tissue pain. Massage may relieve this pain via three proposed mechanisms.[28] Pain may be modulated by increased circulation provided by the mechanical effect of massage on the venous and lymphatic flow. Pain may also be inhibited through increased circulation by reflex vasodilation resulting from facilitation of cutaneous afferents mediating touch and pressure. Finally, deep massage may alter pain through stimulation of mechanoreceptors in the tendons and fascia during stretching and compressing strokes and result in the inhibition of sustained muscle contraction.

Deep friction is another form of massage commonly used on ligaments and tendons. These tissues are quite susceptible to breakdown manifested by overuse, mainly because they have a low metabolic rate and relatively poor vascularity. Tendons and ligaments also tend to develop adhesions secondary to protective immobilization. Tissue degeneration must be addressed by decreasing stress and/or increasing nutrition to the tissue. Cyriax and Coldham advocate the use of direct manipulation at the site of the lesion in a direction perpendicular to the normal orientation of the fibers.[12] This technique, known as deep transverse friction massage, is believed to increase interfibrous mobility and vascularity of connective tissue.

Muscle Energy Procedures.—Muscle energy procedures are contract-relax techniques utilized to promote muscle inhibition and subsequent improved mobility.[56] Relaxation is achieved through manual resistance to isotonic contraction of the antagonistic pattern followed by passive motion of the agonistic pattern to the point of antagonistic limitation. This procedure is repeated several times to achieve progressive relaxation and greater range of the antagonistic pattern.[37] This relaxation, or inhibition, of the antagonist during facilitation of the agonist is dependent on reciprocal innervation.[30]

Trigger Point Therapy.—Simons and Travell consider trigger points to be a major component of myofascial pain syndromes.[78] They define myofascial trigger points as "self-sustaining hyperirritable foci located in skeletal muscle or its associated fascia." Trigger points may be active or latent. Active trigger points give rise to referred pain with sustained digital pressure, whereas latent trigger points are only locally tender to palpation. Specific characteristics help identify the presence of myofascial trigger points:

1. Active trigger points cause referred pain in distinctive patterns described as pain reference zones. These reference zones do not correspond with segmental patterns or peripheral nerve distributions. Each muscle has a predictable referred pain pattern that assists in identifying the trigger point from which pain originates.
2. The muscle containing a trigger point often has a palpable band of taut fibers or nodules that is painful with tension due to stretch or contraction of the muscle.
3. A snapping palpation over a taut band may elicit a brief contraction of fibers within the band.[86] This reaction is called a local twitch response, which is a unique characteristic of a trigger point.[14]
4. Deep pressure exerted on a trigger point may also evoke a jump sign in which the patient moves suddenly and verbalizes discomfort in response to hyperalgesia.[39]

Active trigger points that have been identified by the methods described may be treated manually in two ways. Stretch and spray is a technique performed by passively stretching the muscle containing the active trigger point to its normal maximum length. The stretch is immediately followed by a stream of vapocoolant spray onto the skin overlying the muscle to inhibit pain and guarding secondary to tension on the muscle.[84] A second manual treatment for trigger points is known as ischemic compression.[78] Direct finger pressure is applied to the active trigger point with a progressive increase in downward force as the hypersensitivity of the trigger point fades. Both techniques are directed primarily at the trigger point where pain originates rather than the reference zone where pain is felt.[85]

Myofascial Release.—Myofascial release is a method of soft-tissue mobilization focusing on the fascial component of musculoskeletal pain and dysfunction. Barnes defines fascia as a "three dimensional web of connective tissue surrounding and infusing every structure of our body all the way down to the cellular level."[2] Fascia is composed of collagenous fibers that coil around elastic fibers. Collagen fibers have a plastic quality in that they are not very extensible but pliable. The elastic fibers are more easily stretched. Fascia also contains a ground substance that provides lubrication allowing free gliding between muscles. The connective tissue fibers that compose fascia are interwoven rather than parallel like tendinous fibers, and this gives fascia the ability to resist tension in all directions.

Normally fascia is slightly mobile but, according to Barnes, tends to shorten and tighten secondary to inflammation or poor posture over time.[2] Fascial restrictions may generate enormous pressure on pain-sensitive structures. Fascia is richly innervated but poorly vascularized, which results in pain and slow healing capacity.[7] Prolonged shrinkage of fascial tissues may result in poor postural alignment and affect the quality of movement.[87]

Myofascial release techniques involve stretching along the line of fibers of the restricted muscle until resistance to further stretch is felt. The stretch is held in the lengthened position until the soft tissue is felt to relax or "release" (Fig 38–3).[47] The slack is taken up after the initial release, and a new stretch position is held. This procedure is repeated several times until the tissues are fully elongated. Myofascial release techniques may be utilized to elongate collagenous fibers and improve the viscosity of ground substance for the purpose of reducing pain, increasing mobility, and correcting posture.

External Assists

As indicated from clinical findings, it may be necessary to provide external support via a cervical collar or lumbosacral support. This should always be done with a plan to wean the patient out of the support. The wearing of an external support may allow the patient to be successful with the indicated exercise prescription without overloading tissue tolerance.

Active Treatment

The term *active* in this context is used to define treatment in which the patient may assist or independently perform activities. These treatments include unloading activities, self-mobilization, stabilization, strengthening, and conditioning exercises.

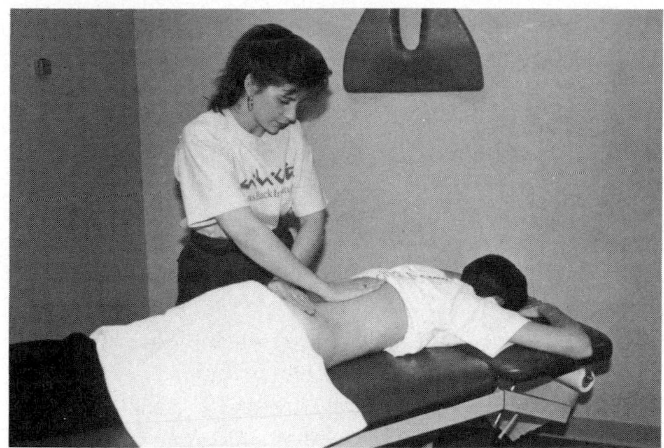

FIG 38–3.
Myofascial release techniques involve stretching the restricted muscle until resistance is felt. The stretch is held in a lengthened position until the soft tissue is felt to relax or "release."

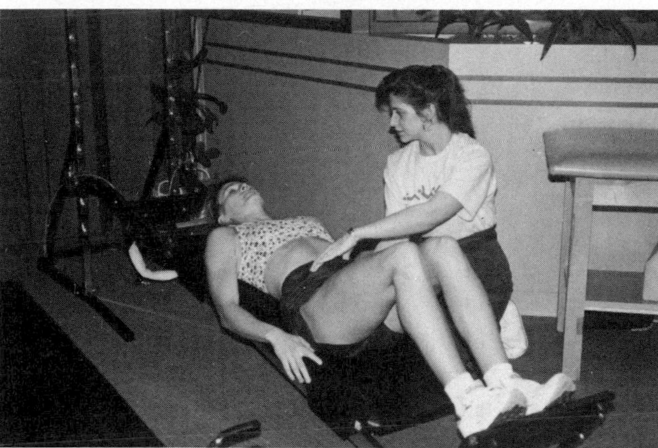

FIG 38–4.
Unloading performed by using an inclined board that is adjusted to a specific percentage of the patient's body weight.

Unloading

The basic principle of unloading the spine is found in the centuries-old practice of assigning the patient to bed rest following an injury. Although full unloading of the spine in acute conditions may be beneficial for a short period of time,[93] it is generally recognized that long-term full unloading is deleterious to cartilage. Full unloading for most of the spine would be supine with the knees slightly flexed. This full unloading allows the spine to be subjected only to those forces that are inherent within the soft-tissue structures surrounding and in the spine.

Unloading, as used in this chapter, describes a method of exercise in which the body or part of the body's weight is controlled to a point that is less than the normal gravitational weight. Unloading should not be confused with traction, in which a body part's gravitational weight is exceeded by the distraction force. This concept of unloading is an integral part of the Norwegian spinal treatment techniques called medical exercise training. This type of unloading may occur by exercising on an inclined board (Fig 38–4) or by assisting with the upper extremities while performing squats or step-ups.

During unloading, the body's weight is offset to alter energy system use and allow aerobic activity to occur. It improves the body's ability to control and stabilize in a weight-bearing position with reduced body weight and decreases the nociceptive input while allowing the affected tissues to adapt at a tolerable level.

The use of upright unloading with the body weight offset mechanically by utilizing pulleys and harnesses is a concept developed and refined by Kelsey and allows for a very precise dosage of exercise to be delivered to healing tissue (Fig 38–5).[34] This concept was developed in conversations with Norwegian physical therapists and with introduction through the work of Holten.[25] The description below of unloading is based on the work of these individuals with changes specific to our clinic.

Most health professionals generally progress patients through exercise programs with a selected dosage to allow healing and adaptation of the tissues to increased stress. Holm and Nachemson found that nutrition to the intervertebral disc was enhanced by mechanical stimuli.[24]

If a patient demonstrates pain and weakness in gait or functional movements, he would not be expected to perform many normal activities in a standing or upright position. To do so would result in increased discomfort for the

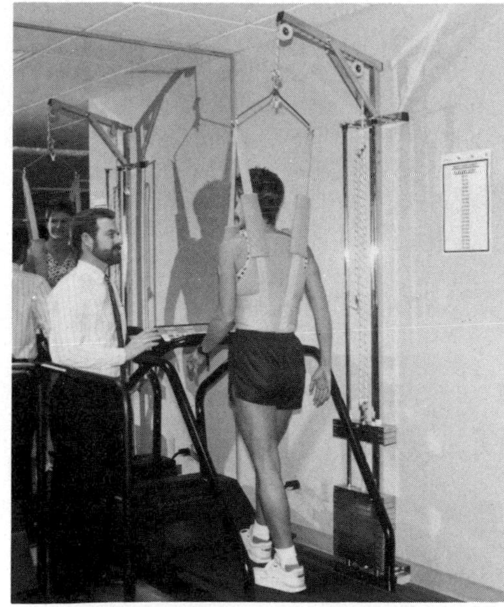

FIG 38–5.
Unloading a patient with low back pain by utilizing an 80-kg latissimus pull and unloading harness to allow the patient to walk with decreased load on the injured tissue.

spine and involved extremities. Also, those patients who are severely deconditioned may be prevented from exercising at required levels in functional positions since this level of activity would require too much energy expenditure. It is possible to perform the required activities in isolated movements; however, it is preferable for the patient to exercise and train in a weight-bearing position for maximal functional restoration. To do this in the initial phase of treatment, many patients must be unloaded. The amount of body weight that is in excess of what the patient can tolerate is removed to allow the patient to train at acceptable levels in a weight-bearing position.

Hydrotherapy for Unloading.—One of the more common methods of unloading the spine is through hydrotherapy. Pool immersion decreases the body's weight due to the buoyant forces of the water.[77] Our hydrotherapy program utilizes traditional pool therapy with timed, and measured exercise protocols and incorporates stabilization principles.[49]

Indications for Unloading Therapy.—Unloading is indicated for most spinal dysfunction patients with disc derangement, degenerative disc disease, hypomobilities, strains and sprains, or radicular syndromes. Since the effect is one of decreasing the load as opposed to applying traction, it provides an extremely safe and useful procedure.

Contraindications for Unloading Therapy.—Contraindications to unloading include structural disease secondary to tumor or infection, recent fractures, osteoporosis, pregnancy, hiatial hernia, increased peripheralization of symptoms, or indications that the patient's symptoms are increasing. Many of the contraindications are not a direct result of unloading but are contraindications to the use of the harness and its attachment to the thorax. Cardiovascular conditions and respiratory problems should be screened and monitored as with any aerobic or exertional exercise program.

Dosage for Unloading Therapy.—The amount of unloading required to produce the desired result may be roughly calculated for each patient. Since the head, neck, upper extremities, and trunk account for approximately 65% of the body weight, one would not want to exceed this level if traction is to be avoided. The average 150-lb individual unloaded by 15% to 20% may have relatively asymptomatic ambulation for 20 to 30 minutes. The unloading session generally will run for 30 minutes but may be terminated for any of the following signs:

1. Substitution patterns.—The patient is observed for the use of other body parts as an attempt to compensate for fatigue. This may include upper-extremity as well as excessive trunk movements.

2. Pain that increases.—This is pain greater than the pain present at rest. Patients are told that if the pain stays the same, the unloading has been successful.

3. Loss of range of motion during activity. If this occurs due to fatigue of the primary muscle groups, the dosage should be adjusted.[34]

Procedure for Unloading Therapy.—After a patient has been evaluated for possible unloading and possible contraindications have been eliminated, the patient is taken to the unloading station for a determination of the amount of force necessary to provide proper unloading. The station for unloading consists of a treadmill, an 80-kg pulley system for a latissimus pull, and an unloading harness. Initially, the unloading pulley is set at maximum poundage to provide a stable and relatively unmovable suspension. A latissimus pull bar is attached to the end of the cable, and the patient is instructed on how to ambulate on the treadmill. This latissimus pull bar is placed at shoulder height in front of the patient, and he is instructed to gently pull down on the bar while ambulating to a point that eliminates or substantially diminishes discomfort. Between the latissimus pull cable and the latissimus pull handle, a force gauge similar to the Chatillian (Chatillian; Greensboro, NC) is installed to register the amount of force required to produce the desired effect. This force is noted by the staff and recorded to be used during the treatment process.

Unloading to the point where the patient can ambulate 20 to 30 minutes without increased pain is considered an adequate response. Once the initial unloading amount has been determined, the patient is instructed to lie down on an appropriate level surface, and an unloading harness is applied. The harness, produced by Chattanooga (JA Preston Corp., Clifton, NJ) as a gravity–lumbar reduction unit, is selected by the patient's size and is attached by moving caudally to cranially. It is essential that the initial lower straps be tightened to prevent the unit from riding up and impinging in the patient's axilla. Once the harness is in place, it is attached to the pulley via a spreader bar of the type that is used for static traction units. This bar should be rather substantial since it will be required to bear significant poundage. The patient is attached to the unloading harness, and the desired weight, as determined through the testing method, is selected. The patient is instructed in the use of the treadmill, and the ambulation process is initiated. The treadmill is initially set at 2 miles per hour or at a speed that will provide a comfortable walking pace. The patient is instructed not to grab the siderails tightly but is allowed to rest his fingers lightly on the siderails for stability. Since ambulating in a harness with weights attached is initially an unusual sensation, the therapist is with the patient during the initial treatment as the patient reaches a level of comfort allowing independent operation.

The patient initially ambulates for 20 to 30 minutes at a rate that allows the development of aerobic capacity. In Holm and Nachemson's study, the duration of exercise that produced the greatest response was 2 hours, but no significant difference was found between daily exercise of 2 hours and daily exercise of 30 minutes' duration.[24] Exercise is terminated when the patient demonstrates substitution patterns, shows an increase in pain, begins to lose range of motion, or has reached the duration assigned.

Progressions in Unloading Therapy.—For the purpose of training discal cartilage, the goal is to achieve a steady state of exercise that may be tolerated for a sustained (20 to 45 minutes) period of time. The cartilage being treated generally does not need the rest stops; however, the patients are often so deconditioned that even in the presence of a decreased body weight they may require additional recovery times.

Most patients are progressed approximately 3% to 5% each week in load, with some patients progressing after every visit. Since the goal of the program is to build endurance through high-repetition, low-load work, a 5-day/week program is recommended.

Problems in Unloading Therapy.—Besides the contraindications to general aerobic exercise for some individuals and the contraindications given previously, there are problems that are uniquely inherent to mechanical unloading. One such problem is motor learning. The ability to ambulate on a motorized treadmill is a motor skill that must often be learned. This is compounded by the unloading requirement of being attached to a pulley via an upper-body harness. Some individuals have experienced difficulty in walking smoothly under these circumstances and require the use of handrails attached to the treadmills. The patients are allowed to lay their hands flat on the handrail for balance but are requested not to grip the rail to avoid facilitating an unwanted muscle contraction. The second problem that may be encountered is harmonic resonance. Since the human gait pattern demonstrates a systematic rise and fall of the trunk with ambulation, it is no surprise that the weight stack of the unloading pulley mirrors this action in an opposition movement. This normally causes no problems unless the weights are a low percentage of the body weight and the treadmill speed is high (3 to 4 mph). The result is an "out-of-phase" phenomenon, with the weight being accelerated up and free-falling within the confines of the pulley system. This usually ends with the weight reaching the end of the rope and a rather abrupt deceleration that is often unpleasant to the patient. This may usually be avoided through adjustment of the treadmill speed or the weight of the pulley. Soma (Soma, Austin, Tex) has develop a device called the ZUNI that eliminates this undesired effect while leaving the unloading concept intact.

Overprogression in Unloading Therapy.—As with any exercise program, there are patients who are overprogressed with resultant signs and symptoms. Complaints that are accompanied by swelling, loss of range of motion, or loss of strength should be evaluated and the program revised to accommodate the problem. Pain complaints of ache and stiffness in the morning, especially early morning, and some pain at night are indicative of overprogression and overloading and should be heeded. Overload of low-metabolic tissues may result in pain following activity and should not be discounted because of their latency.

Benefits of Unloading Therapy.—Unloading offers great potential benefits in that it allows patients to engage in activity at a reduced percentage of body weight and not develop chronic problems, poor postural patterns and deviations due to nociceptive input, and adverse tissue changes. Although a relatively new concept as previously described, it offers great potential to medically increase patient compliance and progression through a program of return to activity and work.

Self-Mobilization Exercises

The purpose of self-mobilization exercises is to increase joint mobility at specific levels where hypomobile segments have been identified. Specificity of motion (localizing) may be accomplished through ligamentous or facet positional locking techniques to limit motion in adjacent segments. For example, if L5–S1 is hypermobile and T12–L1 is hypomobile into extension, a simple ligamentous locking technique may be utilized. The patient is seated in a chair with the T12–L1 level at the top of the backrest and the knees and hip flexed and supported beyond 120 degrees. The patient is then asked to extend the spine over the backrest while ensuring that the lumbar spine remains in contact with the chair back. Thoracolumbar extension occurs from above (craniocaudal) without creating unwanted extension at the lumbosacral junction (Fig 38–6).

Hypomobile joints should be trained with endurance exercises (30 repetitions, 60% of their 1 resistance maximum [RM]) initially to provide an increased capillarization and to promote increased mobility and control through low-intensity repetitive movements. This is followed by training for strength/endurance (15 to 30 repetitions, 60% to 75% of their 1 RM) in the outer range of motion, which allows increased strength to maintain the gained range of motion. Finally, patients should be trained with 8 to 12 repititions at 80% or more of their 1 RM for pure strength.[25]

Conservative treatment of degenerative spinal disorders in the form of active exercise is felt to be very effective given that the involved structures have been identified through a comprehensive diagnostic and biomechanical evaluation. Once certain tissues are targeted as the source

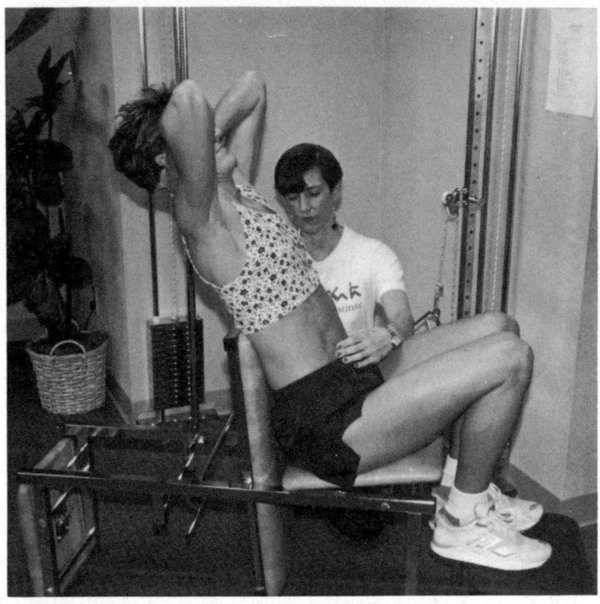

FIG 38–6.
In a self-mobilization exercise, the patient extends his back over the backrest while the lumbar spine remains in contact with the chair back. This allows thoracolumbar extension to occur from above without creating unwanted extension in the lumbosacral junction.

of symptoms, a specific exercise program with a physiologic basis may be designed to provide not only pain modulation but, more importantly, optimal stimulus for the regeneration of tissue.

Vertebrae.—The vertebral bodies perform the weight-bearing function of the vertebrae. Bone loss due to prolonged non–weight bearing and immobilization reduces the load-bearing capacity of the vertebrae. Bone absorbs biomechanical energy through its trabecular formations and, according to Wolff's law, will change its internal architecture depending on the forces placed upon it.[95] Since load bearing is the primary function of the vertebrae, continual stimulus is necessary to maintain its architecture. The optimal stimulus for regeneration of bone is biomechanical energy in the line of stress (longitudinal axis of the bone). This biomechanical energy is transmitted to the bone through intermittent compression and distraction by way of antigravity muscular contraction and through the forces of gravity and body weight in upright postures. Exercises involving repeated high-force movements in weight-bearing positions produce greater bone densities.[82]

Degenerative disease is often compounded by abnormal bone growth (spurring). Exercise applied indiscriminately may actually compound the problem through irritation of already-compromised soft tissue. Care must be taken to tailor the exercise to the constraints of the pathology while still proceeding toward the treatment goals.

Ligaments.—Ligaments are composed of collagen, proteoglycans and fibroblasts. Fibroblasts are responsible for synthesizing collagen and proteoglycans. Proteoglycans, stated simply, are a combination of protein and sugar molecules that make up the ground substance of connective tissue. Proteoglycans bind collagen fibers and provide increased tensile strength, and they have a significant water-binding capacity facilitating the diffusion of nutrients.

Ligaments contain predominantly type I collagen fibers that are arranged in a highly ordered pattern and resist tension according to their location. The anterior longitudinal ligament (ALL) resists vertical separation of the anterior ends of the vertebral bodies during extension, while the posterior longitudinal ligament (PLL) resists separation of the posterior ends of the vertebral bodies during flexion. The ligamentum flavum prevents the anterior capsule of the zygapophyseal joint from being trapped within the joint cavity during movement. The interspinous (ISL) and supraspinous (SSL) ligaments resist separation of the spinous processes (flexion). The iliolumbar ligament prevents the fifth lumbar vertebrae from displacing forward on the sacrum and thereby stabilizes lumbar lordosis.[4]

Joint immobilization results in reduced synthesis of proteoglycans and plasticity of ligaments over time. Ligamentous laxity tends to be prominent in the lumbar spine secondary to chronic improper postural loading or traumatic ligamentous strain. If ligaments are torn or overstretched, they may remain lax, in which case neutral postures and muscular stabilization is required.

Ligaments with reduced elasticity respond well to modified tension in the line of stress.[22] This modified tension may be applied to the ligaments through selected exercises designed to target the specific ligament. Tension to the PLL, SSL, and ISL, for example, is applied by flexion of the lumbar spine at the end range (knees to the chest; Fig 38–7).

Zygapophyseal Joints.—The inferior and superior articular facets are covered by articular cartilage that serves to distribute loads and reduced wear over the bony surfaces. The articular facets are compressed bilaterally in extension and unilaterally in rotation or side bending of the lumbar spine. Articular cartilage is prone to degeneration from continuous compression. Cartilage is dependent on synovial fluid for nutrition, and the chondrosynovial membrane is only permeable to synovial fluid low in viscosity. Repeated motion, especially gliding, decreases the viscosity of synovial fluid. The optimal stimulus for regeneration of articular cartilage is intermittent compression/decompression and gliding, which can be achieved through specific active movements of the lumbar spine while avoiding static loading.[22]

Intervertebral Disc.—The intervertebral discs contain two basic components: the nucleus pulposus, which is

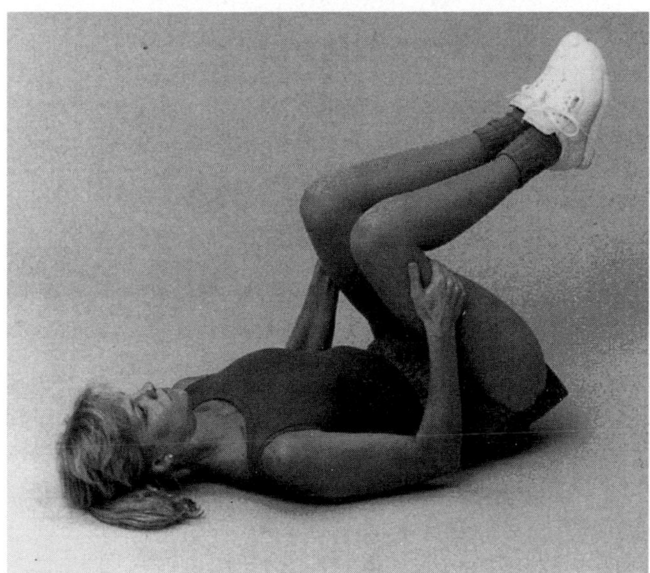

FIG 38–7.
Tension to the posterior longitudinal, supraspinous, and interspinous ligaments is applied by flexion of the lumbar spine at the end range (knees to chest).

centrally located and is surrounded by the second component, the annulus fibrosus. The annulus, like ligaments, contains mainly type I collagen fibers that are highly organized and resist tension. These collagen fibers make up sheetlike lamellae arranged in concentric rings surrounding the nucleus. The collagen fibers within each lamella are parallel to one another and oriented at 65 to 70 degrees from the vertical.[23] The angle remains the same from one lamella to the next, but the direction alternates.

The nucleus pulposus has a greater concentration of water and proteoglycans than the annulus and contains mainly irregularly arranged type II collagen fibers that respond to pressure. The semifluid nature of the nucleus allows deformation under pressure transmitting forces outward toward the annulus.

The main role of the intervertebral discs is to accommodate motion between vertebral bodies and to transfer loads from one vertebra to the next. The discs confer stability to the intervertebral joints during movement. Distraction, sliding, and twisting movements are restrained by the annulus to varying degrees depending on the orientation of individual collagen fibers with respect to the direction of movement. The nucleus and annulus together permit deformation to accommodate rocking or bending motions.[4] When the discs are compressed with weight bearing, the nucleus expands outward to exert pressure on the annulus. The annulus develops tension to oppose the radial pressure of the nucleus. In this sense, the discs act as "shock absorbers" due to their turgid and tensile properties.

The exercise of choice for stimulating disc repair is lumbar rotation (Fig 38–8,A B). The reason for this is twofold. First, modified tension in the line of stress stimulates protein synthesis of type I collagen of the annulus. Second, intermittent compression and distraction promote regeneration of type II collagen and proteoglycans. Lumbar rotation creates tension of every other lamella of the annulus in one direction. The tension on the collagen fibers creates a screw-home mechanism that applies compression to the nucleus. As the direction of the rotation is reversed, the tension is released, and the nucleus is momentarily decompressed. Full rotation in the opposite direction then applies tensile forces to the remaining lamallae, and the nucleus once again sustains compression. Since excessive rotational torque to the disc may be detrimental to its structural integrity, care must be taken to ensure that the forces used are within the tissues' tolerance to loading.

Muscles.—Muscles may be generally classified as either tonic (slow twitch) or phasic (fast twitch). Tonic muscles such as the multifidi act as stabilizers, and phasic muscles such as the erector spinae (iliocostalis lumborum and lumbar longissimus) act as movers of the lumbar spine.

Muscles will atrophy as a result of disuse, immobilization, and starvation. Tonic fibers are particularly prone to atrophy because they are totally dependent on oxygen from the capillary systems, whereas phasic fibers utilize their stores of sugar and fat for energy.

The optimal stimulus for the regeneration of tonic fibers is high-repetition, low-resistance exercise to improve capillarization to the muscle. The optimal stimulus for regeneration of phasic fibers is low-repetition, high-resistance exercise with increasing speed. Since tonic muscles atrophy first, muscular endurance exercises should be performed initially, followed by strengthening exercises.[22]

Based on the Holton medicine training theory, muscular endurance is enhanced by performing approximately 30 repetitions at 60% of one resistance maximal (1 RM).[25] One RM is defined as the amount of resistance required to allow only one repetition of a given movement. Holton purposed that 20 to 25 repetitions at 70% of 1 RM stimulates a combination of strength and endurance. Pure strength is achieved by 8 to 12 or fewer repetitions at 80% to 100% of 1 RM.

Self-Stabilization Exercises

Stabilization exercises for the spine provide the trunk with a means to limit the repetitive microtrauma occurring in pathologic motion segments. These exercises, specifically designed to provide a "muscle corset," limit the undesirable motions and allow healing to occur. They also allow individuals with previous problems to lead active

A

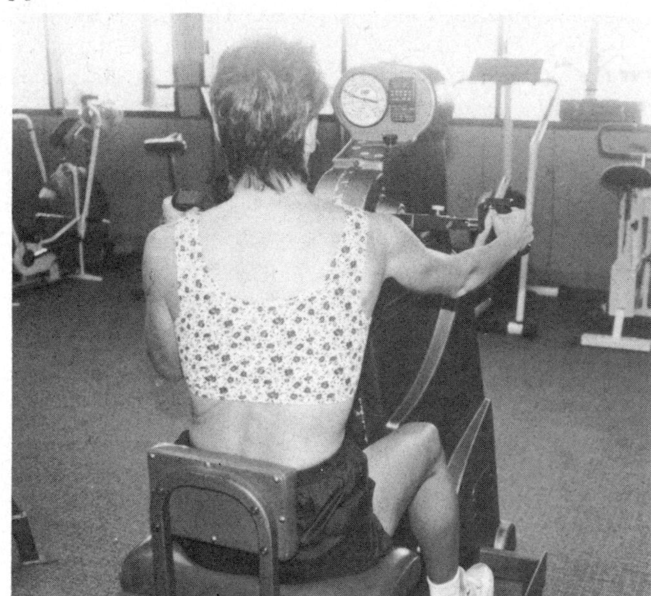

B

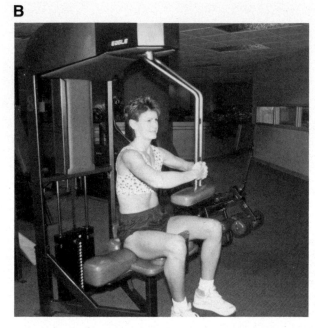

FIG 38–8.
Disc repair is stimulated by lumbar rotation through activities such as upper-body ergometry **(A)** and resistive equipment for craniocaudal rotation **(B)**.

lives without continued stress to the involved area that may lead to flare-ups or rapid degenerative changes. Whether the application of these exercises in a healthy population will prevent or significantly alter the degenerative process has yet to be shown. Stabilization exercises provide the trunk with a method of control. Saal described the anatomic basis for this method of control.[72] He stated that "the abdominal mechanism, which couples the midline ligament as well as the dorsolumbar fascia, combined with a slight reduction in lumbar lordosis, can eliminate shear stress to the lumbar intervertebral segments." Saal felt that the coupled action of this musculature together with the latissimus dorsi allows a "muscle fusion" for spinal protection. Spinal extensors, particularly the multifidus, are essential for balancing the stress to the intervertebral segments.

Neuromuscular Control.—Although patients may have adequate flexibility and strength, they may fail to control the spine if they have not learned to contract the appropriate muscles in the desired sequence. An important goal of stabilization exercise is to promote muscle sensitivity to stretch (particularly of the deep rotators such as the multifidi). This sensitivity to stretch occurs via stimulation of the muscle spindle that is responsible for the muscle's sense of position and provides a stimulus to avoid excessive movement. High tension–producing contractions such as eccentrics should eventually be utilized to facilitate further neurmuscular feedback via stimulation of the Golgi tendon organs. With eccentrics, the greatest tension occurs in 80% of the inner range of motion. Consequently, an example of an indicated exercise to reduce hypermobility in right rotation would be to work the right multifidus eccentrically. The left multifidus performs right rotation, and the right multifidus needs to control the movement. The indicated exercise would be controlled right rotation via inner-range eccentrics to facilitate tension.

Stabilization, particularly during complex functional movements, relies heavily on a learned response by the patient to control the movement. This kinesthetic awareness is necessary to control the fine subtle movements of the spine. The learned sequence is the consequence of multiple sessions of repetition training with attention to correct technique. The "unconscious" carryover to daily activity is the result of making the movement pattern a habit. Particular emphasis is generally placed on aspects of the individual's activity that have the highest potential to produce injuries. These are often lifting, pushing, pulling, as well as transitional activities such as getting in and out of bed or a vehicle.

Neutral Pelvis Exercises.—In working with the patient to establish trunk control, the first component to be addressed is the position of the pelvis. The pelvis is the base of support for the spine and as such must be stable for controlled activity to occur. An anteriorly tilted pelvic and lordotic lumbar curve is generally contraindicated for those with degenerative spinal disorders of the spine because this position increases the shearing forces on the lumbar intervertebral discs and increases compression on the zygapophyseal joints. Patients are instructed to posteriorly tilt the pelvic girdle to neutral to create relative lumbar "flat

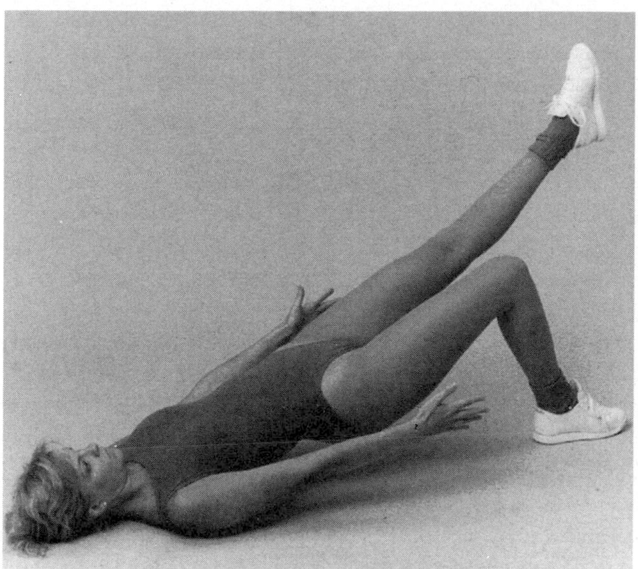

FIG 38–9.
Progression to more advanced activities of stabilization requires the patient to maintain a neutral pelvis during combined spinal and extremity movements.

backs" by way of cocontraction of the abdominal and gluteal musculature. The neutral pelvis is practiced first in supported and then nonsupported static positions. Once the patient has learned basic lumbopelvic control in a regulated environment, the therapist can begin to add additional challenges to the patient's dynamic exercise program. Progression to more advanced activities requires the patient to maintain a neutral pelvis during combination spinal and extremity movements (Fig 38–9).

Contrary to some beliefs, spinal stabilization is not about maintaining a static position. This may be desirable for a particular posture, but the concept is really about maintaining a controlled range of motion that varies with the position and with the activity being preformed.

Control Progressions.—Morgan has described several methods or stages for limiting and controlling spinal movement.[58] He refers to them as passive prepositioning, active prepositioning, dynamic control, and transitional control.

Passive prepositioning involves placing the patient in a position that requires very little muscular effort and will avoid movement into a possibly painful range of motion. An example (Fig 38–10) would be to combine the flexed position of the pelvis with support from the floor to minimize the patient's ability to achieve a painful lumbar extension while working the arms overhead.

Active prepositioning involves utilizing muscular control to the previously described example to preposition the pelvis rather than relying on a hip-flexed posture to limit the extension. Morgan also recommends facilitation of the desired muscle group through associated movements, e.g., neck flexion to facilitate abdominal muscle contraction to assist the patient in active prepositioning.

Dynamic control is described as "continually altering the muscle tension to accommodate the changing stresses and loads."[58] This allows the use of a more midrange position rather than a preposition placement. This is somewhat more difficult since it requires continuous fine motor system adjustments while the activity is being performed. Figure 38–11 demonstrates the trunk and pelvic muscles continually responding to maintain the appropriate pain-free range of pelvic motion.

Transitional control is defined as "the change in the primary muscle stabilizers from agonist to antagonist."[58] Morgan cites the example of reaching from overhead to below the waist. In this case the transitional shift would be from flexion stabilizers to extension stabilizers to provide the low back with protection.

Exercise Progressions.—After the appropriate initial dosage of exercise has been determined, the intensity of the exercise should be consistently progressed to facilitate increasing tissue tolerance and stability. There are, however, different ways to progress exercise. One is to alter the position in which the exercise is performed, i.e., to go from a horizontal position to a weight-bearing position.

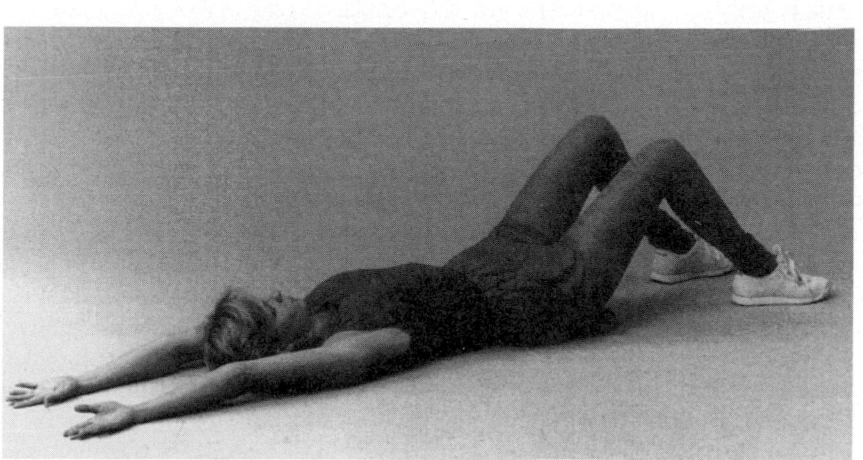

FIG 38–10.
Passive prepositioning combines the flexed position of the pelvis with support from the floor to minimize painful lumbar extension while working the arms overhead.

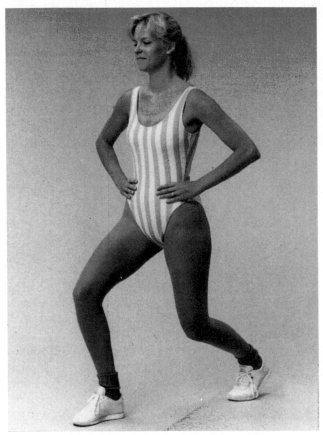

FIG 38–11.
Stabilization during dynamic movements requires the pelvic and trunk muscles to continually respond to maintain the appropriate pain-free range of pelvic motion.

All patients should eventually be progressed to weight-bearing exercise since humans function in this posture. Additionally, eventual exercise should encompass activities that replicate the patient's individual needs relative to work, exercise, sports, or hobby requirements.

Second, if the exercise is assisted, the amount of assistance can be reduced. The eventual goal for the patient should be to perform the exercise unassisted. Additionally, resisted movements should be considered on the basis of the patient's individual work and activity requirements.

Third, the type of muscle contraction utilized in the exercise can be modified, i.e., less tension is produced with a high-repetition concentric than with an eccentric contraction. Specifically, the following progression involves increasing tension production: high-repetition concentric contractions progressing to concentrics with a hold progressing to low-speed eccentrics progressing to fast eccentrics, with the speed utilized with the concentrics dependent on the coordination needs.[25] Other considerations in exercise progression include repetition number, speed of movement, length and number of resting intervals, and training frequency. Frequency of progression should be as tolerated, with each treatment progressing if the prior dosage was appropriate.

General Conditioning

General conditioning is total-body development, the improvement of physical capability through the use of an exercise program. Fitness has long been recognized as an important factor in decreasing the incidence of low back pain. In theory, exercise raises endorphin levels to increase pain thresholds. High levels of physical activity increase endurance and strength, augment the amount of calcium deposited in the skeleton, improve the flow of nutrients into the discs, and contribute to a sense of well-being.[60]

The philosophy of an exercise approach is to maintain balance between muscle groups in terms of flexibility and strength, coupled with coordinated, controlled motion and an energy-efficient posture. Exercise also promotes psychological benefits by improving self-confidence and decreasing stress levels by reducing the resting heart rate.[67] Patients who participate in supervised exercise programs have been found to have increased aerobic fitness, increased strength, decreased body fat, decreased subjective pain levels, and increased compliance, all of which are related to increased psychological benefits.[69] Deconditioning is a progressive process, and if uninterrupted, becomes a vicious cycle in which lower physical capacity predisposes to pain recurrence with progressively lower levels of physical activity.[51] When an exercise program is initiated to terminate this cycle, it is very important that a physical therapist monitor the progression of the physical activity. Often a lack of coordination in combination with impulsiveness predisposes to recurrent injury if the patient is not carefully monitored and kept within the limits of a graduated program.[51] It is crucial that there be detailed communication between the patient and the therapist about the different types of pain that may be experienced. The patient should understand that he may experience fatigue and/or muscle soreness secondary to the exercise program and that these perceptions are unrelated to the initial pain complaint. The patient should be encouraged to work through the fatigue or soreness but should cease exercising if the initial symptoms increase. The therapist must rely on objective functional capacity assessment for mobility, strength, and endurance as well as subjective pain complaints for progression in the treatment program.

Initially, a conditioning program focuses on mobility. This is followed by progressive resistive exercise training for strengthening to include both resistive and repetitive low-load exercises. Endurance is then improved through aerobic training, followed by protocols to improve whole-body coordination and agility.[51] Exercise parameters needing to be specifically addressed are intensity, duration, frequency, and mode. Intensity is a measure of "stress," usually relative to the patient's maximum abilities. Duration is how long the patient is to continue the specific activity, usually measured in time or number of repetitions. Frequency refers to how often the patient is to perform the activity, as in the number of sessions per day or week. The mode is the specific activity or exercise. A warm-up period should always be included to increase muscle temperature and blood flow and decrease the risk of musculotendinous injury. Following each exercise session, a cool-down period of low-intensity exercise should be incorporated to prevent blood pooling in the lower extremities and to reduce muscle soreness.

Flexibility is determined by the ability of muscles and surrounding soft tissues to lengthen and allow normal ranges of motion of the joints involved. Mobility is dependent upon the degree of flexibility present. Mobility of soft tissues and joints is necessary for the performance of normal functional movements. Mobility exercises include passive or active stretching and joint mobilization.[36] The patient should be instructed to perform all stretches in a gradual, slow, pain-free manner and avoid ballistic movements of short duration. All stretches should be initiated and completed in a gradual fashion.

Strength is the maximum force exerted by a muscle at a given point in the range of motion. The capacity of a muscle to produce tension can be improved in two ways: by using high resistance with low repetitions or by using low resistance with high repetitions. In order to achieve adaptive increases in strength, the muscle must be exercised to the point of fatigue, and the load used must exceed the metabolic capacity of the muscle being used.[36] Injury prevention is enhanced when muscle strengthening occurs at all positions within the full range of available motion. Endurance is the ability to perform a repetitive movement continuously over a prolonged period of time. An active exercise performed repeatedly against a moderate load to the point of fatigue will increase the endurance of a muscle. In order to increase general endurance, exercise should be directed at large muscle groups, as in aerobic exercise.[36] Aerobic exercise is the physical activity that results from energy generated by metabolic processes using oxygen. Different types of aerobic activity include running, jogging, cycling, walking, and swimming. Aerobic exercise should be performed for 15 to 60 minutes, three to five times per week, at an intensity of 70% to 85% of the maximum heart rate.

It is important not only to regain muscle flexibility, endurance, and strength but also to ensure that the patient has proper coordination and motor control of muscle activity. General principles of coordination exercises involve constant repetition of specific motor activities while utilizing sensory cues to enhance motor performance. The speed of motor activities should be increased over time.[36] It is important that each specific activity be mastered before progressing to the next level of complexity.

When planning a program to improve balance, exercises are progressed in a proximal-to-distal sequence with emphasis on developing stability first, followed by mobility. Components of coordinated activity include volition, perception, and the development of motor programs. Volition is the ability to initiate activity, to continue it, and to stop it on command. Perception is the ability to monitor the activity by using the proprioceptive, visual, and tactile systems. Motor programs are preprogrammed patterns of activity developed by repetition. An example would be walking. Some methods to improve balance and coordination include Frenkel's exercises and Swiss ball activities.[36] Balance can be assessed by either observation or simple timed tests.

Physical activity as a whole is responsible for restoring, improving, or maintaining normal function. It must be made clear to the patient that it is critical to continue to improve physical capacity by utilizing a home maintenance program of exercise.

Home Programs

Stabilization concepts and exercises are an important part of the rehabilitation program. All patients are given a specific home exercise program to enhance the rehabilitation regimen for their particular dysfunction. This program, called "Back at Home" consists of written specific exercises in a format that allows easy patient visualization and understanding (Fig 38–12). As the patient progresses and masters the desired techniques, the program is advanced with new exercises being issued to continually challenge increased mobility and ability. The exercises are designed to not only build on the patient's initial rehabilitation program but also serve as the basis for an ongoing maintenance program of preventive exercises.

CONCLUSION

Patients with degenerative spinal disorders are commonly encoutered in an orthopedic spine practice. Treatment of these patients is a process of not only addressing the physical condition but also treating the emotional aspects of pain. A holistic interdisciplinary approach with the patient included as a team member deals with the core of what has driven him to seek assistance. Even more importantly, continuous education will create an informed patient who will, it is hoped, understand the degenerative process and the steps of self-care that will enable him to

Back At Home

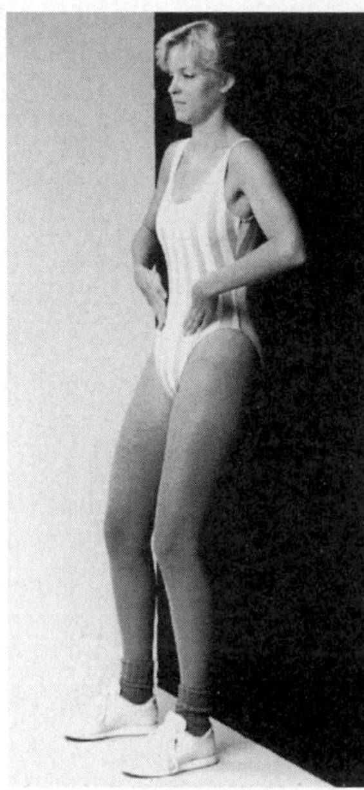

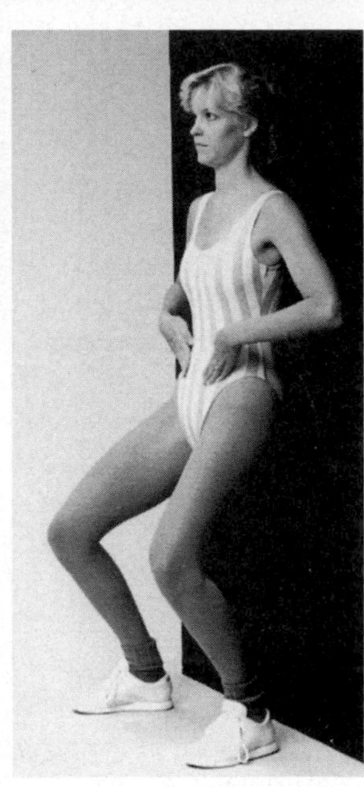

Wall Slide with Pelvic Stability

Starting Position: *Stand with back and head against the wall. Place feet 6-8" away from the wall. Hold pelvis in neutral.*

Instructions: *Keeping pelvis stable, bend your knees to lower yourself into a sitting position. Hold that position. Again, keeping pelvis stable, return to full standing position.*

Purpose: *Pelvic stability. Leg strengthening.*

REPETITIONS	SETS	HOLD (seconds)	TIMES (per day)
3 5 10 15 20 Other ___	1 2 3 4 5 Other ___	3 5 10 30 60 Other ___	1 2 3 4 6 Other ___
□ □ □ □ □ □	□ □ □ □ □ □	□ □ □ □ □ □	□ □ □ □ □ □

NOTES:

Texas Back Institute

FIG 38–12.
The "back at home" exercise program consists of written specific exercises in an easy-to-understand format.

have personal control over an improved quality of life. To the extent that we can achieve this, our treatment goals are considered to have been met.

REFERENCES

1. Akeson WH, Amiel D, Woo SL: Immobility effects of synovial joints: The pathomechanics of joint contracture. *Biorheology* 1980; 17:95.
2. Barnes JF: Myofascial release: Questions, concepts and the future, in *Progress Report No. 4*. Alexandria, Va, American Physical Therapy Association, 1988.
3. Bogduk N, Jull G: The theoretical pathology of acute locked back: A basis for manipulative therapy. *Manual Med* 1985; 1:78–82.
4. Bogduk N, Twomey LT: *Clinical Anatomy of the Lumbar Spine*. New York, Churchill Livingstone, 1989, pp 11–24.
5. Bourdillon JF: *Spinal Manipulation,* ed 3. London, William Heinemann, 1970.
6. Brown L: An introduction for the treatment and examina-

tion of the spine by combined movements. *Physiotherapy* 1984; 74:347–353.

7. Calliet R: *Soft Tissue Pain and Disability*. Philadelphia, FA Davis, 1977, pp 3–8.
8. Charnley J: Orthopaedic signs in the diagnosis of disc protrusion with specific reference to straight leg raising test. *Lancet* 1951; 1:186–192.
9. Chrisman OD, Mittnacht A, Snook SA: A study of the results following rotary manipulation in the lumbar intervertebral disc syndrome. *J Bone Joint Surg [Am]* 1964; 46:517.
10. Cram RH: A sign of sciatic root pressure. *J Bone Joint Surg [Br]* 1953; 35:192.
11. Cyriax J: *Textbook of Orthopaedic Medicine,* ed 8, vol 1, *Diagnosis of Soft Tissue Lesions*. London, Bailliere Tindall, 1982, pp 64–103.
12. Cyriax J, Coldham M: *Textbook of Orthopaedic Medicine,* vol 2, *Treatment by Massage, Manipulation and Injection,* ed 11. London, Bailliere Tindall, 1984, pp 8–12.
13. Cyriax JH: *Illustrated Manual of Orthopaedic Medicine*. London, Butterworths, 1983, p 30.
14. Dexter JR, Simons DG: Local twitch response in human muscle evoked by palpation and needle penetration of a trigger point. *Arch Phys Med Rehabil* 1981; 62:521.
15. Deyo RA, Diehl AK, Rosenthal M: How many days of bed rest for acute low back pain? A randomized clinical trial. *N Engl J Med* 1986; 315:1064–1070.
16. Edwards BC: Clinical assessment: The use of combined movements in assessment and treatment, in Twomey LT, Taylor JR (eds): *Physiotherapy of the Low Back*. New York, Churchill Livingstone, 1987, pp 81–109.
17. Enneking W, Horowitz M: The intra-articular effects of immobilization on the human knee. *J Bone Joint Surg [Am]* 1980; 42:973.
18. Epstein JA, Epstein BS, Lavine LS, et al: Lumbar nerve root compression at the intervertebral foramina caused by arthritis of the posterior facets. *J Neurosurg* 1973; 39:362–369.
19. Estridge MN, Rouke SA, Johnson NG: The femoral stretching test. *J Neurosurg* 1982; 57:813–817.
20. Greenberg RS: The effects of hot packs and exercise on local blood flow. *Phys Ther* 1972; 52:273.
21. Grimsby O: *Course Notes, 1990 Manual Therapy Residency Program*. Dallas.
22. Grimsby O: *Fundamental of Manual Therapy—A Course Workbook,* ed 3. Norway, Sorlandets Fusikalske Institutt, 1981.
23. Hickey DS, Hukins SWL: X-ray diffraction studies of the arrangement of collagen fibers in human fetal intervertebral disc. *J Anat* 1980; 131:81–90.
24. Holm S, Nachemson A: Variations in the nutrition of the canine intervertebral disc induced by motion. *Spine* 1983; 8:866–874.
25. Holten O: *Course Notes From Medical Training Therapy*. Loma Linda, Calif, 1987.
26. Homewood AE: *The Neurodynamics of the Vertebral Subluxation,* ed 2. Ontario, Chiropractic Publishers, 1973.
27. Hoppenfield S: Physical examination of the hip and pelvis, in Hoppenfield S (ed): *Physical Examination of the Spine and Extremities*. New York, Appleton-Century-Croft, 1976, pp 143–169.
28. Jacobs M: Massage for the relief of pain: Anatomical and physiological consideration. *Phys Ther Rev* 1960; 40:96–97.
29. Janse J, Houser RH, Wells BF: *Chiropractic Principles and Technique*. Chicago, National College of Chiropractic, 1947.
30. Kabat H: Proprioceptive facilitation in therapeutic exercise, in Licht S (ed): *Therapeutic Exercise,* ed 2. New Haven, Conn, E. Licht, 1961, p 21.
31. Kaltenborn FM: *Manual Therapy for the Extremity Joints*. Oslo, Olaf Norlis Bokhandel, 1976.
32. Kaltenborn FM: *Test Segment: Moblis Columbia Vertebris*. Oslo, Freddy Kaltenborn, 1975.
33. Kellett J: Acute soft tissue injuries—a review of the literature. *Med Sci Sports Exerc* 1986; 18:489–500.
34. Kelsey D: *Medical Exercise Training With Unloading. Course Notes* 1991. Austin, 1991.
35. Kendall FP, McCreary EK: Muscle function in relation to posture, in Kendall FP, McCreary EK (eds): *Muscle Testing and Function,* ed 3. Baltimore, Williams & Wilkins, 1983, pp 270–316.
36. Kisner C, Colby LA: *Therapeutic Exercise: Foundations and Techniques*. Philadelphia, FA Davis, 1988.
37. Knott M, Voss DE: *Proprioceptive Neuromuscular Facilitation: Patterns and Techniques,* ed 2. Philadelphia, Harper & Row, 1968, p 98.
38. Korr IM: The neural basis of the osteopathic lesion, in *The Collected Papers of Irvin M. Korr*. Newark, NJ, American Academy of Osteopathy, 1989, pp 120–127.
39. Kraft GH, Johnson EW, Laban MM: The fibrositis syndrome. *Arch Phys Med Rehabil* 1968; 49:155–162.
40. Ladd MP, Kottke FJ, Blanchard RS: Studies of the effect of massage on the flow of lymph from the foreleg of the dog. *Arch Phys Med* 1952; 33:604–612.
41. Leahmann JF: Therapeutic heat and cold. *Clin Orthop* 1974; 99:205–207.
42. Licht S: *Therapeutic Heat and Cold,* ed 2. Baltimore, Everly Press, 1965.
43. Lovett RW: The mechanics of lateral curvature of the spine. MSJ 1900; 97:622–627.
44. Maigne R: *Orthopaedic Medicine*. Springfield Ill, Charles C Thomas, 1976.
45. Maigne R: The concept of painless and opposite motion in spinal manipulation. *Am J Phys Med* 1965; 44:55–69.
46. Maitland GD: *Vertebral Manipulation,* ed 5. London. Butterworths, 1986, pp 1–13.
47. Manheim CJ, Lavett DK: The myofascial release manual. Thorofare NJ, Slack, 1989, pp 1–4.
48. Matthews JA, Yates DAH: Reduction of lumbar disc prolapse by manipulation. *Br Med J* 1969; 20:696.
49. Maxwell C, Speigel A: The rehabilitation of athletes following spinal injuries. *Spine State Art Rev* 1990; 4:485–488.
50. Mayer TG: Rehabilitation of the patient with spinal pain. *Orthop Clin North Am* 1983; 14:623–637.
51. Mayer TG, Gatchel R: *Functional Restoration for Spinal*

Disorders: The Sports Medicine Approach. Philadelphia, Lea & Febiger, 1988.

52. Mayer TG, Tencer AF, Kristoferson S, et al: Use of noninvasive techniques for quantification of spinal range of motion in normal subjects and chronic low-back dysfunction patients. *Spine* 1984; 9:588–595.
53. McKenzie RA: A perspective on manipulative therapy. *Physiotherapy* 1989; 75:440–444.
54. Melzack R, Wall PD: Pain mechanism: A new theory. *Science* 1965; 150:971–979.
55. Michlovitz S: Biophysical principles of heating and superficial heat agents, in Michlovitz SL (ed): *Thermal Agents in Rehabilitation*. Philadelphia, FA Davis, 1986, p 99.
56. Mitchell FL, Moran PS, Pruzzo NA: *An Evaluation and Treatment Manual of Osteopathic Muscle Energy Procedures*. Valley Park, Mo, Mitchell, Moran, & Pruzzo, 1979.
57. Mooney V, Robertson J: The facet syndrome. *Clin Orthop* 1976; 115:149–156.
58. Morgan D: *Training the Patient With Low Back Dysfunction: Course Notes*. Folsom, Calif, 1990.
59. Nachemson A: A critical look at conservative treatment of low back pain, in Jayson MIV (ed): *The Lumbar Spine and Back Pain*. Turnbridge Wells, England, Pitman, 1980, pp 453–466.
60. Nachemson AL: Advances in low back pain. *Clin Orthop* 1985; 200:266–278.
61. Nyberg R: Role of physical therapists in spinal manipulation, in Basmajian J (ed): *Manipulation, Traction, and Massage*, ed 3. Baltimore, Williams & Wilkins, 1985, pp 22–46.
62. Paris SV: *Course Notes: The Spine, Etiology and Treatment of Dysfunction Including Joint Manipulation*. 1979, pp 28–34, 259.
63. Paris SV: Mobilization of the spine. *Phys Ther* 1979; 59:988–995.
64. Paris SV: Spinal manipulative therapy. *Clin Orthop* 1983; 179:55–61.
65. Paris SV: *The Spinal Lesion*. New Zealand, Degasus Press, 1965.
66. Porterfield JA: The sacroiliac joint, in Gould JA, Davies GJ (eds): *Therapy*. St Louis, Mosby–Year Book, 1985, pp 550–580.
67. Raithel KS: Chronic pain and exercise therapy. *Physician Sports Med* 1989; 17:203–209.
68. Rath WW: *Cervical Traction: A Clinical Perspective*. Minneapolis, Lossing Orthopaedic, 1984.
69. Reilly K, et al: Differences between a supervised and independent strength and conditioning program with chronic low back syndromes. *J Occup Med* 1989; 31:547–550.
70. Richardson RR, Arbit J, Siqueira EB, et al: Transcutaneous electrical neurostimulation in functional pain. *Spine* 1981; 6:185–188.
71. Robert WH: Testing intervertebral joint movement. *J Am Osteopath Assoc* 1962; 61:635–639.
72. Saal JA: Lumbar injuries in gymnastics, in Hochschuler SH (ed): *The Spine in Sports*. Philadelphia, Hanley & Belfus, 1990, pp 192–206.
73. Saunders DH: *Evaluation, Treatment and Prevention of Musculoskeletal Disorders*. Minneapolis, Viking Press, 1985.
74. Sawyer M, Zbieranek C: The treatment of soft tissue after spinal injury. *Clin Sports Med* 1986; 5:387–405.
75. Schiotz E, Cyriax J: *Manipulation Past and Present*. London, Heinemann, 1975.
76. Seitz LM, Kleinkort JA: Low power laser: Its applications in physical therapy, in *Thermal Agents in Rehabilitation*. Philadelphia, FA Davis, 1986, pp 217–240.
77. Sheldahl L: Special ergometric techniques and weight reduction. *Med Sci Sports Exerc* 1985; 18:25–30.
78. Simons DG, Travell JG: Myofascial origins of low back pain: Principles of diagnosis and treatment. *Postgrad Med* 1983; 73:66–73.
79. Sprague R: *Course Notes: PT Instruction Assessment and Treatment of Spinal Dysfunction*. 1990, p 46.
80. Sprangfort EV: Lasègue's in patients with lumbar disc herniation. *Acta Orthop Scand* 1971; 42:459–460.
81. Stoddard A: *Manual of Osteopathic Practice*. London, Hutchinson, 1969.
82. Stone MH: Implications of connective tissue and bone alterations resulting from resistance exercise training. *Med Sci Sports Exerc* 1988; 20(suppl):162–168.
83. Tappan FM: *Healing Massage Techniques: A Study of Eastern and Western Methods*. Reston, Va, Reston Publishing, 1978, pp 3–27.
84. Travell JG: Ethylchloride spray for painful muscle spasm. *Arch Phys Med Rehabil* 1952; 33:291–298.
85. Travell JG: Myofascial trigger points: Clinical view, in Bonica JJ, Albe-Fessard D (eds): *Advances in Pain Research and Therapy*, vol 1. New York, Raven Press, 1976, pp 419–426.
86. Travell JG, Simons DG: *Myofascial Pain and Dysfunction: The Trigger Point Manual*. Baltimore, Williams & Wilkins, 1983.
87. Upledger JE, Vredevoogd JD: *Craniosacral Therapy*. Seattle, Eastland Press, 1984.
88. Urban LM: The straight-leg raising test: A review. *J Orthop Sports Phys Ther* 1981; 2:117–133.
89. Wall PD: The gate control theory of pain mechanisms—A re-examination and restatement. *Brain* 1978; 101:1–18.
90. Walter JB: *An Introduction to the Principles of Disease*, ed 2. Philadelphia, WB Saunders, 1982, p 63.
91. Wells PE: The examination of the pelvic joints, in Greive GP (ed): *Modern Manual Therapy of the Vertebral Column*. New York, Churchill Livingstone, 1986, pp 590–964.
92. White AA III, Panjabi MM: The basic kinematics of the human spine. A review of the past and current knowledge. *Spine* 1978; 3:16.
93. Wiesel SW, Cuckler JM, Deluca F, et al: Acute low back pain: An objective analysis of conservative therapy. *Spine* 1980; 5:324–330.
94. Wilins RH: Lasègue's sign. *Arch Neurol* 1969; 21:219–220.
95. Woo SLY, Kuei SC, Amiel D, et al: The effect of prolonged physical training on the properties of long bone: A

study of Wolff's law. *J Bone Joint Surg [Am]* 1981; 63:780–787.

96. Woo SL, Matthews JV, Akeson WH, et al: Connective tissue response to immobility. *Arthritis Rheum* 1975; 18:257–264.
97. Wyke BD: Neurological aspects of low back pain, in Jayson MIV (ed): *The Lumbar Spine and Back Pain*. London, Sector Publishing, 1976, pp 265–314.
98. Wyke BD: The neurology of joints. *Ann R Coll Surg Engl* 1967; 41:25–50.

PART X

ADULT DEFORMITY

39

Adult Scoliosis

Jean-Jacques Abitbol, M.D., F.R.C.S.C., John P. Kostuik, M.D., F.R.C.S.C., and Steven R. Garfin, M.D.

Adult scoliosis has been defined as the presentation of deformity past skeletal maturity. The curve may have its onset prior to maturity or arise later in adult life de novo secondary to metabolic bone disease or other causes such as degenerative changes.

The past two decades have witnessed an increasing interest in the problems of the deformed adult spine. The increasing number of mature scoliotics presenting to physicians is related to a number of factors. One is the improved ability of the physician to deal with these often complicated deformities and frequently compromised individuals. Additionally, the fact that salvage procedures are becoming increasingly common and successful in correcting failures of previous surgery in the treatment of a spinal deformity has prompted yet others to seek help. Although there are comparatively few long-term follow-up investigations of idiopathic scoliosis following maturity, several reports have provided much needed information and contributed to our current understanding of adult deformity.

PREVALENCE

Studies investigating the prevalence of scoliosis report varying statistics depending on the method used for diagnosis, the minimum deformity required to report a significant scoliosis or a positive screening test, and in adults, the definitions of maturity used by the author. Most existing data on prevalence are based on adolescent populations with only scant statistics available for mature patients. Strayer studied routine postpartum roentgenograms of 928 women and obtained standing anteroposterior (AP) views of the spines in those appearing to have scoliosis.[45] Of this group, 5% had curves measuring 10 to 19 degrees, and 2% had curves of 20 degrees or more. Of the patients with curves, 77% were thought to have an idiopathic pattern. Shands and Eisberg reviewed 50,000 chest minifilms taken during a survey for tuberculosis.[36] They noted a deformity measuring 5 degrees or more in 1.4% over 14 years of age. Of the patients found to have a deformity in the first 15,000 cases reviewed, 65% were suspected of having a postural etiology.

The report by Kostuik and Bentivoglio is the only study providing insight concerning the prevalence of adult scoliosis in North America.[19] The authors studied the intravenous pyelograms of 5000 patients over the age of 20 years. Based on these radiographs, 3.9% of the patients were found to have thoracolumbar or lumbar curves measuring more than 10 degrees. The authors felt that the prevalence may have been higher if chest roentgenograms were available for the same group. Vanderpool et al. appreciated a higher frequency of scoliosis in adults over 50 years of age.[46] The authors could not account for the increased incidence based on pre-existing idiopathic curves. They believed that curves can arise "de novo" in adults and that their etiology may be related to metabolic bone disease.

NATURAL HISTORY

An understanding of the natural history of scoliosis in adults is essential for the development of an optimal treatment program. Although the present widespread application concerning the principles of early detection and treatment of adolescent idiopathic scoliosis makes natural history studies of this type difficult, several reports with long-term follow-up have provided insight into the outcome of untreated mature patients.

The original belief has been refuted that when skeletal maturity is reached, scoliotic curves stabilize. The phenomenon of curve progression after skeletal maturity has been clearly established.[8, 9] Later, in a 40-year follow-up study looking at curve progression in idiopathic scoliotics, Weinstein and Ponseti noted an average curve increase of 13.4 degrees past skeletal maturity.[47] Although curves measuring less than 30 degrees at maturity tended not to progress regardless of curve pattern, thoracic curves measuring between 50 and 75 degrees at the completion of growth demonstrated the most marked progression. Deterioration of thoracolumbar and lumbar curves appeared to be affected by the magnitude of the curve, vertebral rotation, and translatory shifts. In addition, the authors noted that combined curves tended to balance with age, with slightly greater progression in the lumbar component than in the initially larger thoracic component. These findings were similar to those reported by Ascani et al. in a study with an average follow-up of 33 years.[1] These authors also noted that the greatest deterioration occurred in thoracic curves followed by lumbar and thoracolumbar deformities. Combined curves appeared to be the most benign. In an investigation of scoliosis surgery in adults, Kostuik and coauthors reported that 55% of patients required surgery because of continued progression of the curve after maturity.[22]

Although there is general agreement concerning the pattern of progression in adult life, differences of opinion exist regarding the incidence of back pain, psychosocial aspects, cardiorespiratory complications, and mortality rate.* Complaints of back symptoms are common among patients with adult deformity and have been documented in up to 90% of patients with idiopathic curves. Long-term follow-up studies suggest that the incidence of back pain in scoliotics is no greater than that in the general population.[1, 8, 13, 19, 30, 32]

Separately, the studies by Collis and Ponseti and Edgar and Mehta were unable to find a correlation between the degree or type of curvature and the severity of back symptoms.[8, 11] In contrast, the series by Kostuik and Bentivoglio and by Fowles et al. found a definite relationship between the magnitude of the curve and the presence and severity of back pain.[13, 19] The paper by Kostuik et al. reported that in curves greater than 45 degrees, the incidence of pain increased significantly. Although the papers by Nachemson and by Collis and Ponseti found severe low back pain to be unusual, other authors have described incapacitating back symptoms severe enough to warrant surgery.[8, 30] These series, however, lacked control patients and long-term follow-up.

The connection between scoliosis and "respiratory embarrassment" was suggested by Hippocrates. A number of long-term follow-up studies have confirmed this association. Nilsonne and Lundgren, reporting on 102 patients with idiopathic scoliosis observed for up to 50 years, noted a mortality rate that was twice that of the general population.[34] Respiratory failure or right heart failure (cor pulmonale) accounted for 60% percent of the deaths. Similar results were reported by Nachemson in his long-term follow-up of 117 patients with untreated scoliosis.[32] Of 117 patients, 20 were dead, 16 having died of cardiopulmonary disease probably related to the deformity of the spine. The diagnoses in this study included idiopathic deformity and congenital, poliomyelitic, and miscellaneous curves.[1] The increased mortality rate in the untreated scoliotic population was first corroborated in a recent long-term follow-up study by Ascani et al.[1] The authors documented a death rate of 17% in a group of patients with idiopathic scoliosis that was nearly twice as high as the mortality rate of the general population. All patients had severe thoracic scoliosis and died as a result of cardiopulmonary complications. In contrast, the authors of the Iowa study found the death rate to be similar for scoliotics and the normal population.[47, 48] The inclusion of only idiopathic curves in a younger population in their study may explain the lower death rate as opposed to other studies on scoliosis.

Psychological and social factors in scoliotics have been considered by a number of investigators. Nilsonne and Lundgren found that almost half of their patients were unable to work, particularly those with severe deformity, in addition to a low marriage rate for the females.[34] Nachemson's review found that 30% of the patients were on disability pensions.[30] Of those engaged in full-time work, none were employed in heavy manual labor. Ascani and coworkers identified real psychological disturbances in 19% of their cases, particularly in patients with severe thoracic curves and in females.[1] Most curves measured greater than 40 degrees. They also commented on the low marriage rate in females, particularly those with thoracic curves. Similar psychosocial disturbances were documented by other investigators.[13, 22] In contrast, Collis and Ponseti noted few psychiatric reactions to back deformity.[8] Ninety percent of their patients married, and most led active, productive lives despite spinal curves of more than 50 degrees in 71%. Nineteen percent of the group admitted psychological reactions to their deformities, but none were severe enough to require psychiatric treatment.

The possible association between pregnancy and curve progression is of interest. A study by Nachemson in brace-treated patients suggests that multiple pregnancies before the age of 23 years may be associated with an increased likelihood of curve progression.[33] Ascani et al. found curve progression to be significantly greater in women with one or more pregnancies vs. females with no pregnancies.[1] In contrast, Blount and Mellenkamp found that in those patients in whom the curve had been stable prior to pregnancy, no progression was noted during gestation.[5] However, in patients in whom the curve had been progressing when they became pregnant, there was some acceleration of the deformity.

More recently, Betz et al., in studying the effects of pregnancy on scoliosis, concluded that pregnancy did not increase the likelihood of progression in skeletally mature patients with mild to moderate curves.[3] In addition, the incidence of cesarean section and health problems in children of women with scoliosis was no greater than that for a nonscoliotic population.

Patients with idiopathic scoliosis whose curves measure more than 30 to 40 degrees at skeletal maturity are at risk for curve progression as adults. Thoracic curves more than 50 degree are most likely to deteriorate. Although the incidence of back pain is similar to that in a nonscoliotic group, the degree of discomfort and implications for man-

*References 1, 4, 7, 8, 13, 16, 18, 22, 31.

agement may be different. Pregnancy does not predictably appear to influence curve progression. Pulmonary volumes are abnormal in patients with severe thoracic curves and may lead to further cardiopulmonary morbidity. In addition to these issues, psychosocial aspects in the adult scoliotic population must not be ignored.

PATIENT PRESENTATION

Mature patients with deformity present with a variety of complaints. These include pain, curve progression, structural disabilities, cardiorespiratory problems, neurologic complications, and cosmesis. In addition, patients may present with problems arising from previous failed surgery in adolescence or adult life.

Pain is classically the most common presenting symptom. Those with lumbar or thoracolumbar curves complain much more frequently of discomfort in comparison to patients with primarily thoracic or combined curves. Patterns of pain are not dissimilar to those encountered in degenerative disease of the lumbar spine. Typically, pain begins over the convexity of the deformity. As degeneration of the discs and facet joints progress, the pain may migrate to the concavity and occasionally lead to a radicular pattern on that side. The exact cause of discomfort, however, is unclear. Muscle spasm, disc degeneration, facet arthrosis, or more likely, a combination of these has been implicated. The radicular pattern is probably related to structurally narrowed neuroforamina as a result of lateral vertebral subluxations, facet hypertrophy, and bulging degenerative discs along the concavity.

Although pain is the most common presenting complaint, curve progression is the most widely accepted indication for surgery. Patients may note this by describing a greater hump on their back, increasing asymmetry in their flank folds, a shorter height, or alterations in their clothes size or length. In addition, curve deterioration may be associated with pain. In general, deformities under 30 degrees rarely progress. In our experience, the curve with the worse prognosis in adult life is in a young adult or adolescent who presents with an unbalanced lumbar or thoracolumbar curve where a fifth lumbar vertebra not parallel with the sacrum leads to a lumbosacral "takeoff" (Fig 39–1). Other curves with a poor prognosis for progression include those with an apex below L2 to L3, curves with a significant rotation, imbalanced deformities, or those with a secondary compensatory curve that is sharp and angular at the L4–5 or L5–S1 area. If surgically treated early, fusions can often be limited to one or two levels rather than dealing with entire, more complex curves later.

Occasionally, curves originally dismissed in adult life progress. Additionally, they may become painful in association with degenerative changes. Separately, studies have shown that deformities can arise "de novo" in the adult. In 1969, Vanderpool and coauthors documented a sixfold increase in the incidence of scoliosis in adults over 50 years old having osteoporosis or osteomalacia as compared with a controlled population.[46] Robin et al. confirmed the de novo development of lumbar scoliosis in a patient group aged 50 years or more.[35] In contrast to the findings of Vanderpool et al., these authors found no correlation between osteoporosis, radiographic signs of degeneration, back pain, and scoliosis. Although the precise cause is unknown, there are patients who develop adult-onset scoliosis with progression not associated with metabolic bone disease but with severe degenerative disc disease of the spine. The role of asymmetrical degeneration of lumbar discs as a cause of late-onset deformity has been suggested by some. Occasionally, a more serious underlying pathologic process such as tumor or infection may cause the onset and/or progression of the curve. These etiologies must be sought. Access to previous roentgenograms to help document progression is invaluable. In addition, as surgical options and interventions to treat scoliosis increase, failed surgery has developed as an increasing cause of curve deterioration. In these circumstances, the physician should carefully examine the patient for pseudarthrosis and/or progression of the curve beyond a short fusion. As a result of the possible disfiguring aspects of scoliosis, cosmesis is an additional presenting complaint. Presently, the psychological disturbances as a result of significant deformity are more frequently expressed by the patient, possibly due to an increasing awareness of treatment possibilities. In view of the possible complications, surgery performed for appearance alone remains controversial.

Structural disabilities are more common in patients with neuromuscular scoliosis. These patients may present with difficulty sitting at a desk or in a wheelchair as a result of pre-existing scoliosis and/or progression. In addition, pain and deteriorating cardiorespiratory function are sometimes found in combination with curve progression.

Neurologic demise arising from curve progression is more commonly seen in patients with congenital curves. These curves may subsequently progress as a result of degenerative disease or trauma. Patients with idiopathic scoliosis occasionally present with radicular signs/symptoms as a result of superimposed degenerative disease. This is more commonly associated with lumbar deformities in combination with neuroforaminal encroachment occurring primarily on the concavity of the curve.

Although the association of severe thoracic deformity with cardiopulmonary decompensation is well recognized, patients presenting with signs and symptoms of cardiopulmonary insufficiency are unusual. Abnormalities have been documented in both lung mechanics and volumes, especially decreased vital capacity, alveolar hypoventilation,

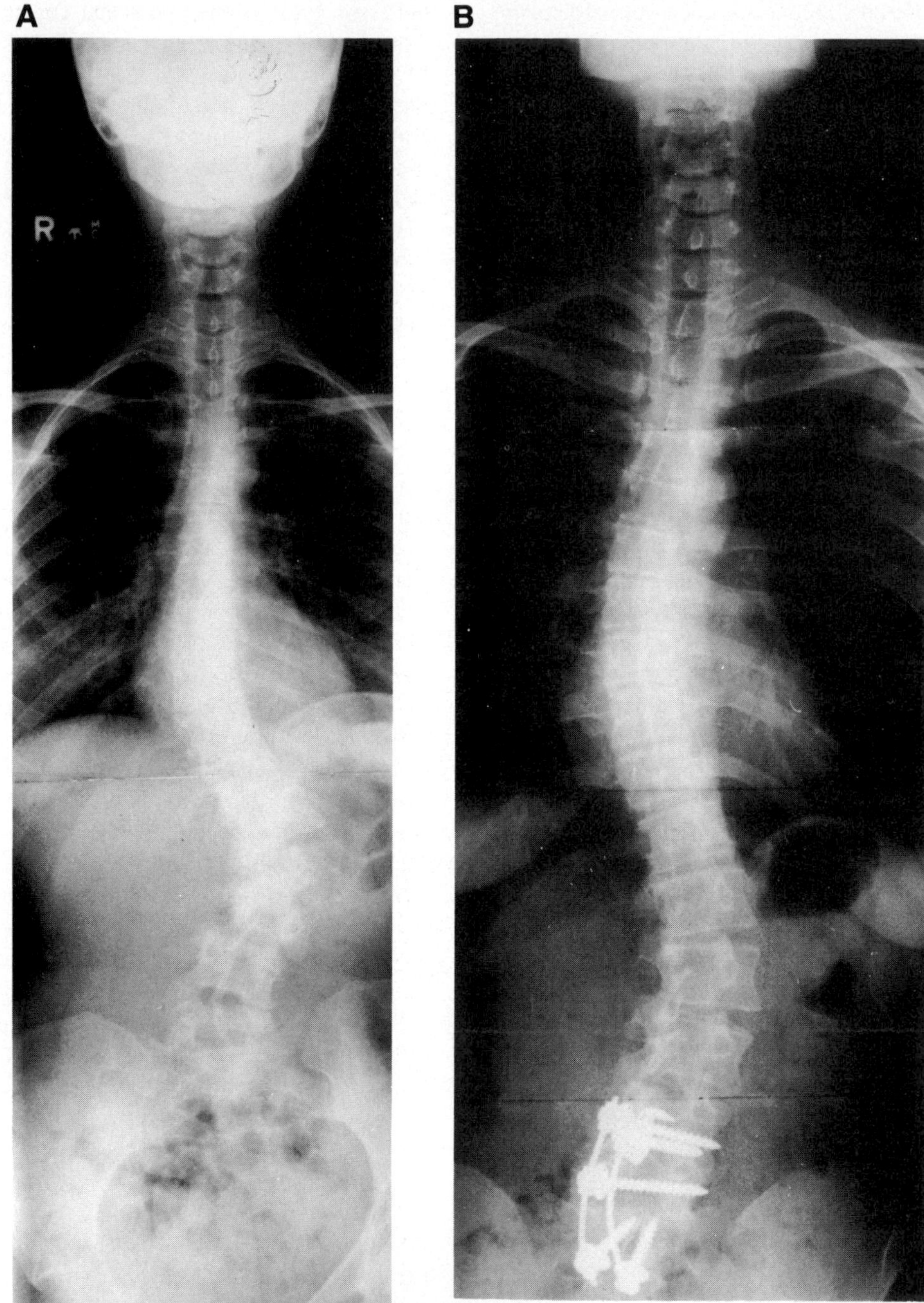

FIG 39–1.
A, posteroanterior (PA) radiograph of a 26-year-old woman with a progressive, painful scoliosis. The L4 and L5 vertebrae are not parallel with the sacrum, which leads to a "lumbosacral" takeoff. **B,** the deformity was corrected by using Zielke instrumentation from L4 to S1 to diminish the lumbosacral takeoff and effect a significant reduction of the primary lumbar curve above. Note the double Zielke rods to control rotational forces.

abnormal ventilation perfusion distribution, in addition to increased heart and respiratory rates.* These findings apply mostly to thoracic curves measuring more than 60 degrees, particularly if combined with thoracic lordosis. Lung mechanics demonstrate purely restrictive ventilatory impairment. Significant suppression of respiratory function is most significant in patients who have paralytic and congenital curves. Whether surgical correction of the scoliosis improves lung function remains debatable. A review of 200 consecutive adults with idiopathic scoliosis revealed no cases of significant pulmonary dysfunction, even with severe curves.[22] Arterial blood gas values were often nor-

*References 2, 6, 12, 14, 15, 26, 29, 30, 37, 49, 50, 52.

mal. In the authors' experience, presentation with severe cardiopulmonary problems often underlines the presence of a congenital scoliosis.

As more corrective surgery is being performed, the adult presenting with symptoms related to a failed procedure is more common. Presenting complaints are similar to those mentioned above, including pain, progression of deformity, or dyspnea, but more commonly, a combination of these is present. This group of patients presents a difficult diagnostic and treatment problem. Careful assessment as to the origin of their symptoms is required. Other etiologies for pain such as tumor or infection should be considered. Presently, approximately one third of our patients present after a failed procedure. In addition, we have observed that pseudarthroses that were asymptomatic for many years can become painful in later life. Furthermore, pain developing below a previously fused curve with or without progression of the deformity, particularly with instrumentation into the lumbar segments, has been described. In a long-term anatomic and functional review of patients with adolescent idiopathic scoliosis treated by Harrington rod instrumentation and fusion, Cochran et al. have reported an increased incidence of degenerative changes and pain with more distal fusion.[7] These findings were corroborated in a study by Edgar and Mehta who similarly found an increased incidence of degenerative changes associated with pain at levels below a posterior fusion that extended to L3 or L4.[11]

Spinal instrumentation for scoliosis may lead to a potentially disabling symptom complex, the "flat back" syndrome, if the lordosis is flattened sufficiently.[20, 24, 25] This disorder is characterized by straightening of the lumbar spine and forward tilting of the trunk with compensatory flexion at the knees to balance the body. Back pain is often an accompaniment of this problem. Patients often complain of increased forward stooping and upper back pain as the day progresses. Numerous etiologies leading to this condition have been implicated. The most common contributing factor to loss of lumbar lordosis is distraction instrumentation extending to the lower lumbar vertebrae or sacrum. Other causes include thoracolumbar kyphosis, thoracic hyperkyphosis, and hip flexor contractures. In patients with previous surgery, pseudarthrosis is often encountered and should be sought. The authors have also noted this syndrome to occur as a result of the degenerative changes and loss of disc height below a fusion mass and ending in the lower lumbar segments.

PATIENT EVALUATION

A detailed history and physical examination followed by proper roentgenographic studies are necessary in all patients presenting with spinal deformity. If pain is a predominant complaint, it is important to rule out other possible causes of back discomfort. Particularly in older age groups, pain and progression can be related to tumor or infection. The medical evaluation should initially be directed to rule out all of these abnormalities before embarking on the treatment of scoliosis.

A detailed history should be obtained with specific questions related to presenting symptoms. In addition, a relevant family history of deformity may give some indication of prognosis. For example, an older and close relative to the patient who has a progressive and severe deformity may give some insight to the patient's future. The date of onset of the curve should be considered but is usually not in itself important.

A pain questionnaire and diagram are helpful in localizing and understanding a patient's symptoms. Questions pertaining to the character, location, severity, and aggravating or relieving factors of the pain as well as its effects on the quality of life are essential. Radicular symptoms are suggestive of nerve root irritation. True sciatica typically radiates below the knee, while referred pain from the lumbar region remains above the knee. With associated spinal stenosis, a history of bowel and bladder dysfunction may be elicited. A history of curve progression should be obtained from both the patient and available family members. Deterioration of the deformity may be suggested by an increasing rib hump, a loss of height, asymmetry in the waistline, or a necessity for change in clothing. Ideally, progression is best documented through serial radiographs, but past radiographic studies are often unavailable. Cardiopulmonary symptoms are rarely seen as a presenting problem. The presence of dyspnea, tiredness, or disorders of cardiac function must, however, be documented. Furthermore, progressive compromise of the respiratory and/or cardiac systems should be noted since further deterioration may lead to increasing morbidity and/or mortality.

Physical Examination

The physical examination should be carried out with the patient completely undressed beneath an examining gown. This diminishes the risk of missing important findings suggestive of intraspinal pathology such as café au lait spots, nevi, or a hairy patch. Careful documentation of the patient's height, body balance, rib hump, and asymmetry of the trunk measured with the use of a plumb line are essential. A complete clinical assessment should include an evaluation of rigidity of the curves and a determination of the three-dimensional nature of the deformity.

Documentation of a precise neurologic examination is imperative and should be compared with previous testing whenever possible. The physical examination is incomplete without a general examination including a full cardiopulmonary assessment. If surgery is being contemplated, psychiatric evaluation is useful to assess any underlying psychiatric dysfunction that may be related to long-term deformity.

RADIOLOGIC EVALUATION

Radiographs are an integral component of a complete patient evaluation. If possible, previous studies should be retrieved for comparison purposes, even if taken for other reasons (e.g., chest radiographs or scout films for an intravenous pyelogram). Patients are increasingly aware of the potential risks of radiation exposure. Organs particularly susceptible to tumor induction are the bone marrow, thyroid gland, and the breast. Recommendations to limit radiation hazards must be followed. Most important is to limit the number of radiographs to only those necessary for diagnosis and/or treatment. Roentgenographic techniques that produce the lowest radiation exposure to the patient are based on proper beam collimation, gonadal shielding, beam filtration, and kilovoltage potential technique. Furthermore, because of improved information on radiation dosage and concerns regarding exposure to the breast, posteroanterior radiographs are presently recommended.

Initial standing, PA, and lateral radiographs should be obtained on 3-ft cassettes. They are part of a routine primary examination. Sitting views are obtained for patients who are unable to remain erect. With severe curves, it may not be possible to appreciate the true magnitude of the deformity on PA roentgenograms because of the significant rotation usually associated with large deformities. Stagnara et al. have suggested eliminating the rotatory component by taking an oblique view with the cassette positioned parallel to the medial aspect of the prominence of the rib hump.[40–44] This results in a "derotated," more reliable AP view of the spine.

When surgery is being considered, views assessing flexibility of the curves are helpful in planning instrumentation and fusion levels. These usually consist of recumbent lateral bending films with the patient giving maximum bending efforts to each side. In patients with absent trunk muscle power (neuromuscular scoliosis), a supine AP radiograph with traction applied is recommended to assess curve flexibility. Hyperextension views for kyphosis and flexion views for lordosis may be helpful for investigating flexibility in these deformities. However, these should be carefully assessed in order to not mistake correction above and below the deformity for an intrinsically flexible curve. Other special views may occasionally be necessary and include oblique and "coned-down" lateral views of the lumbosacral spine in order to further evaluate degenerative pathology and/or other disorders such as spondylolisthesis. A bone scan may be helpful in situations where pain follows an inexplicable pattern. Occasionally, an occult lesion not seen on routine radiographs will be demonstrated on this study. In patients being considered for surgical treatment, other investigations may prove beneficial in determining fusion levels and the necessity for decompression. In addition, it may influence a surgeon's decision concerning the surgical approach.

Myelography has traditionally been used when intraspinal pathology is suspected, particularly in the presence of high-degree curves where it is difficult to rule out a congenital etiology. It is especially helpful in adult patients presenting with radicular symptomatology when root compression is suspected.

Computed tomographic (CT) scans have been helpful in delineating bony pathology. Occasionally, the CT scan may define a focal destructive process not seen on plain roentgenograms. It is valuable in further delineating spinal stenosis, particularly when combined with myelography.

Magnetic resonance imaging (MRI), although only recently introduced, has already demonstrated its ability to show detailed intraspinal anatomy and pathology. Interpretation of the results when imaging severe curves may be difficult and possibly require other investigations. As experience with MRI evolves, its future in diagnosing abnormal anatomy in patients with scoliosis appears limitless and may replace myelography and CT scans.

The role of discography in diagnosing symptoms from degenerative discs continues to be controversial. The usefulness of discography in the preoperative assessment of painful disc levels has previously been shown in a prospective study using discograms to help differentiate sources of pain.[22] Currently, the authors use this test to assess lower levels of the lumbar spine, particularly L3–4, L4–5, and the lumbosacral junction. Discograms are rarely performed at the apex of the curve. Discography is primarily used as a provocative test in an attempt to reproduce the patient's pain pattern, thus helping to determine the lower end point of the fusion.

Similar objections concerning the use of facet joint injections in localizing the source of pain have been raised. Theoretically, this study should differentiate facet joint pain from discogenic pain if they occur independently. It is recognized that levels other than the L5–S1 articulation have multiple innervations, and if the L4–5 level is to be assessed, then the L3–4 level must be infiltrated as well. The authors have found this test to be particularly useful at the L5–S1 level and routinely infiltrate the L4–5 joints as well. If relief of pain is experienced with local anesthetic injection of the joint, steroid injection into the joints may occasionally prove therapeutic as well as diagnostic. If facet blocks relieve pain and discography reproduces the discomfort at the lumbosacral junction, then it is the author's feeling that the fusion should be extended to the sacrum. Conversely, should discograms not reproduce the patient's typical pain pattern and facet blocks at the lumbosacral junction not relieve the discomfort, then it is assumed that the pain arises predominantly from within the curve itself. Therefore, if the lumbosacral junction is not part of the structural curve, the deformity above is corrected and the lumbosacral junction not fused.

Pulmonary function tests in conjunction with arterial blood gas determinations are routinely recommended in those patients with cardiorespiratory symptoms and/or a thoracic deformity. They are particularly important when patients are being considered for surgery. The data collected provide additional information concerning the possible risks of surgery and help predict the need for postoperative mechanical ventilation.

TREATMENT

Although frequently discussed, adult scoliosis requiring surgical management is relatively uncommon and accounts for only 20% to 25% in most scoliosis series. In addition, certain patients may have conditions precluding operative intervention such as serious cardiac and/or respiratory disease or psychological dysfunction.

The nonoperative management of adult idiopathic scoliosis with back pain is not unlike that suggested for back pain with degenerative disc disease. Initially, nonsteroidal anti-inflammatory drugs (NSAIDs), nonnarcotic analgesics, physical therapy, and possibly orthotic devices are recommended. Enteric coated aspirin is often as valuable as more expensive NSAIDs and can be used long-term. If the initial NSAID therapy is unsuccessful, patients may respond to another type of anti-inflammatory medication. A few should be tried prior to abandoning this modality. Nonnarcotic analgesic medications may be used in conjunction with anti-inflammatories. Muscle relaxants and narcotics should not be used routinely to avoid the possibility of drug dependence because pain is often the chronic problem.

Physiotherapy, particularly exercise, is not usually successful in controlling pain. However, certain therapeutic modalities for pain relief such as applications of heat, ultrasound, transcutaneous electrical nerve stimulation (TENS) units, etc., may be helpful in a few patients, particularly the high surgical risk, osteoporotic, elderly patient. With the pain controlled, specific exercises promoting motion of the spine may not be as useful as emphasizing postural exercises, maintenance of muscle tone, general instruction in back care, and aerobic activities, particularly in females. Since osteoporosis is thought to play a role in progression of deformity in the postmenopausal female, 20 minutes of general low-impact aerobic exercise four times a week in the premenopausal years diminishes this risk. In addition, calcium replacement and hormonal therapy, under the supervision of a physician should be started in the early postmenopausal years.

The activity program should be tailored to the patient in an effort to avoid a sedentary life-style. If obesity is a problem, the patient should be encouraged to lose weight. Consultation with a dietician may be necessary and useful. Smoking should be discontinued as soon as possible. Its contribution to respiratory dysfunction and possibly osteoporosis is known.

Although orthoses have not been found to prevent curve progression in patients with adult scoliosis, its immobilizing effects may prove beneficial in pain relief. These need to be rigid and formed to the patient's deformity. They should be worn while the patient is ambulatory. Concomitant strengthening exercises should be recommended with brace wear. In the author's experience, many adults do not tolerate rigid orthoses.

A medical workup should be initiated in those patients with atypical pain patterns or severe discomfort unresponsive to nonoperative management in order to rule out other sources of pain (tumor, infections). Regardless of the outcome with nonoperative management, continued follow-up for the adult with spinal deformity is recommended.

SURGICAL INDICATIONS: LUMBAR AND THORACOLUMBAR VERTEBRAE

Indications for surgery in the adult include pain, progression of deformity, neurologic disability, cosmesis, progression associated with pain below previous fusions for spinal deformity, and finally iatrogenic flat back (kyphosis).

The younger adult presenting prior to 35 years of age without discomfort but with documented increasing deformity and a lumbar or thoracolumbar curve measuring 40 to 50 degrees is best treated surgically. Curves of this magnitude will often progress and possibly lead to a painful lower part of the back. This is particularly true of female patients, primarily because degenerative changes and age may convert the condition from a primary scoliosis, with retention of lumbar lordosis, to a rigid kyphoscoliosis. If disabling enough, both anterior and posterior surgery may be indicated in order to correct this deformity.

Lumbar and thoracolumbar curves can often be adequately treated with a one-stage anterior release and Zielke instrumentation (Fig 39–2). The status of the discs below the fusion levels remains a concern following anterior and/or posterior instrumentation and fusion. Other authors have discussed the increased incidence of degenerative changes below the fusion, often associated with pain, following posterior instrumentation extended to L3 or below.[7, 11] If possible, these patients should be encouraged to continue to maintain a satisfactory level of physical fitness. In addition, good back hygiene and low back exercises should be routinely performed. Exercises are tailored to the individual's age and tolerance level.

An unbalanced curve extending to L3 or L4 with a

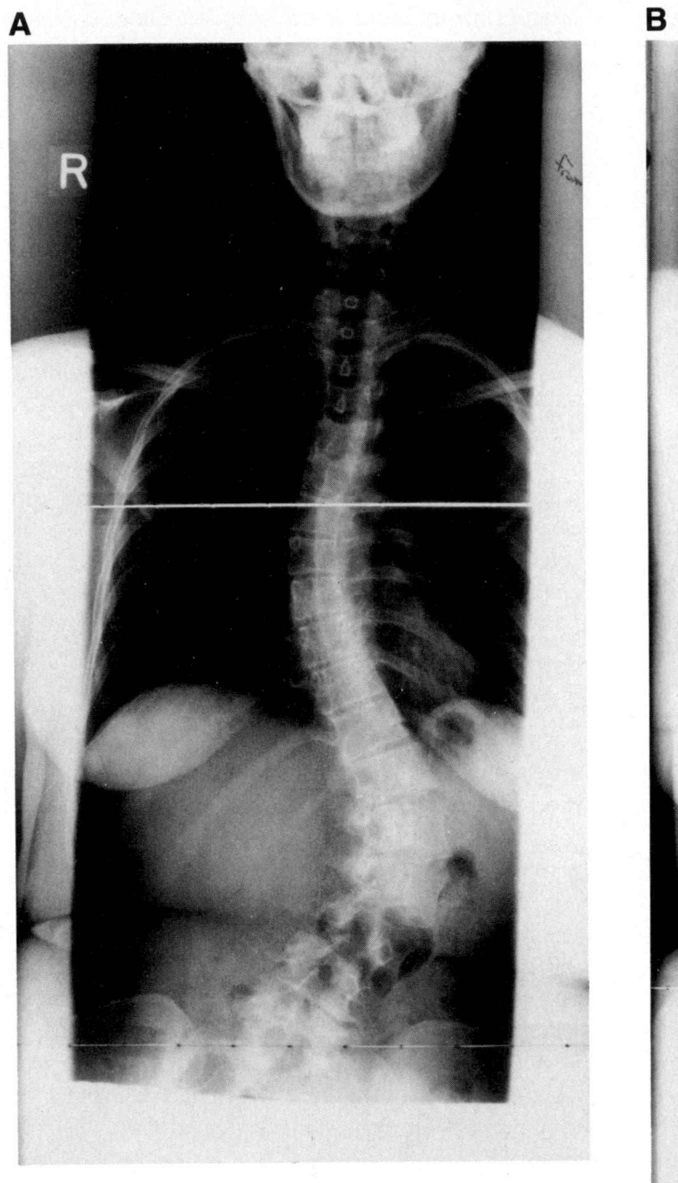

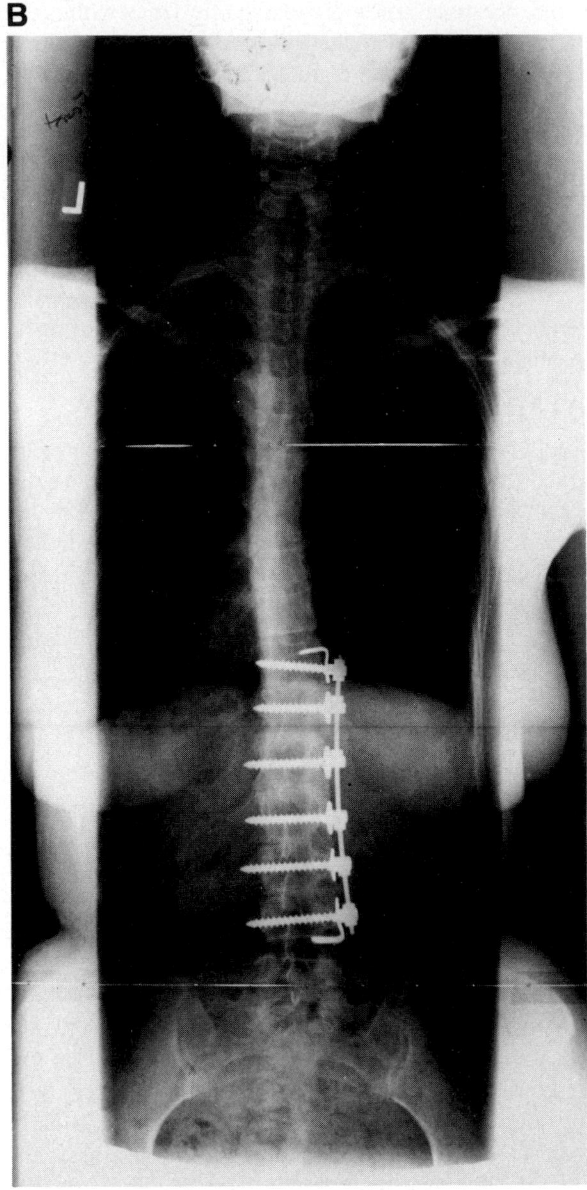

FIG 39–2.
A, PA radiograph of a 77-year-old woman with a severe, incapacitating, painful curve measuring 75 degrees. **B,** the postoperative curve measures 15 degrees. Methylmethacrylate was used to hold the screws. The patient was pain free 1 year postoperatively.

compensatory curve below in a younger patient whose major deformity measures 40 degrees or more may often be balanced by reducing the lower curve (see Fig 39–1). This should be attempted only in patients whose lower curve is felt to be symptomatic. Separately, if corrected, they should be warned of the risk of progression of the upper curve at a later date, with possible proximal extension of their fusion needed. To date, this technique has been found to be effective in a small number of patients.[16] Although the follow-up is of short duration, mean correction of the major curve was more than 50%. Painful patterns may be delineated preoperatively with the use of discography and/or facet blocks.

In our experience with more than 1000 adults with deformity treated surgically, neurologic deficit as an indication for surgical intervention was unusual. However, with an aging population, increasing numbers of patients present with associated spinal stenosis. Laminectomy with associated correction of the curve was rarely indicated in 1979 in the review by Kostuik, with only 5 of 220 patients requiring associated laminectomy.[16]

Patients complaining of significant pain should undergo investigation preoperatively in order to rule out other, more serious causes of pain such as tumor. In addition, those adults with significant lumbar or thoracolumbar curves of more than 45 degrees should undergo preoperative myelography or MRI, particularly in the presence of pain, to rule out the possibility of spinal stenosis. This is primarily a problem in patients over the age of 60 years.

Surgical Techniques

With the advent of segmental fixation devices, Harrington instrumentation is rarely used in the treatment of adult scoliosis. Distraction instrumentation into the lower lumbar segments often leads to a loss of lumbar lordosis and possibly a flat back syndrome. Today, lumbar and thoracolumbar curves can be corrected by a variety of techniques discussed below.

Lumbar and thoracolumbar curves can often be corrected by using the instrumentation and technique described by Zielke and Pellin.[51] However, a major contraindication is the presence of significant kyphosis. In this situation, the kyphosis is exaggerated with the use of Zielke rods and screws.

Kyphoscoliosis, which is often encountered in patients over 50 years of age with deformity, requires the restoration of lumbar lordosis in order to improve balance and relieve pain. In the presence of a rigid kyphos, a two-stage procedure is often required. An anterior release is performed with multiple-level discectomies and fusion followed by segmental instrumentation from the posterior aspect. However, if the kyphoscoliosis is mobile as shown on preoperative bending films, correction may be achieved through a single-stage posterior procedure using Cotrel-Dubousset (C-D) instrumentation, which will derotate and restore the normal lumbar contours.

The introduction of Luque instrumentation in 1976 has popularized the use of segmental fixation posteriorly. Others have combined Harrington instrumentation with segmental wiring in order to correct lumbar or thoracolumbar curves.[28] However, the authors believe that this is often not sufficient to restore normal sagittal contours. Fixation to the pelvis with Luque rods by using the Galveston technique is widely used today. However, more recent studies indicate that perhaps patients develop pain related to the sacroiliac joint, even in the presence of a solid fusion of the lumbar spine. Because of the significant risk to the spinal cord and the inability of the Luque rods to derotate the spine, this instrumentation should be avoided when correcting deformity in a neurologically intact patient.[27]

Zielke Instrumentation

Zielke instrumentation is primarily indicated for mobile thoracolumbar or lumbar curves that are not kyphotic and do not require fusion to the sacrum. In mature patients, the entire curve is usually incorporated with the instrumentation. However, in younger adults, fewer levels may need to be fused as determined on preoperative bending films. From a technical standpoint, osteoporosis may be a major problem when inserting the vertebral body screws. Methylmethacrylate has successfully been used by the authors after drilling the screw holes (Fig 39–2). If possible, the screws should be angled and directed toward the contralateral junction of the pedicle with the vertebral body. This requires careful cleaning of the disc space, including the end plates, posteriorly to the longitudinal ligament in order to directly visualize and safely determine the trajectory for insertion of the screws. For maximal strength, the opposite cortex should be penetrated and a depth gauge used to ensure penetration. In addition, 2 mm can be added to the length of the chosen screw in order to ensure that the far cortex is engaged. The screw tips can be directly palpated, and if there is any doubt about their position, an intraoperative radiograph is recommended.

Cooling the methylmethacrylate or using low-viscosity cement will allow increased working time for injection of the material into the screw holes. Frequently, the authors use a cure inside the hole to enlarge the space, followed by injection of the cement under pressure to enhance fixation of the screws. Pullout has been a significant problem at the most proximal screw site (Fig 39–3). Although some recommend extending the instrumentation across a nonfused space to prevent this problem, the authors do not believe that this is necessary. In postmenopausal women, bone cement at the upper level may prove useful in avoiding this problem.

Although little difficulty is usually encountered in achieving instrumentation and fusion proximal to L5, extension of a Zielke device to the sacrum is difficult and challenging[21] (see Fig 39–1). The iliolumbar veins at the L5 level must be ligated to allow mobilization of the common iliac system. This is often necessary even when fusing and/or instrumenting to the L5 vertebral body level. When fusing to the sacrum, a posterior fusion is recommended in addition to achieve optimal fusion rates. Extension above T9 or T10 has not been of significant value in our experience because the disc spaces are so narrow with minimal correction possible. The use of a derotator should be routine in reducing the kyphosis at the thoracolumbar junction. Autogenous bone grafting is primarily used, with the grafts carefully placed anteriorly in order to minimize the risks of exaggerating the kyphosis.

Hypotensive anesthesia and cell savers are useful in minimizing blood loss. In addition, patients are routinely allowed to donate their own blood or arrange for donor-specific products prior to surgery. Hypotensive anesthesia

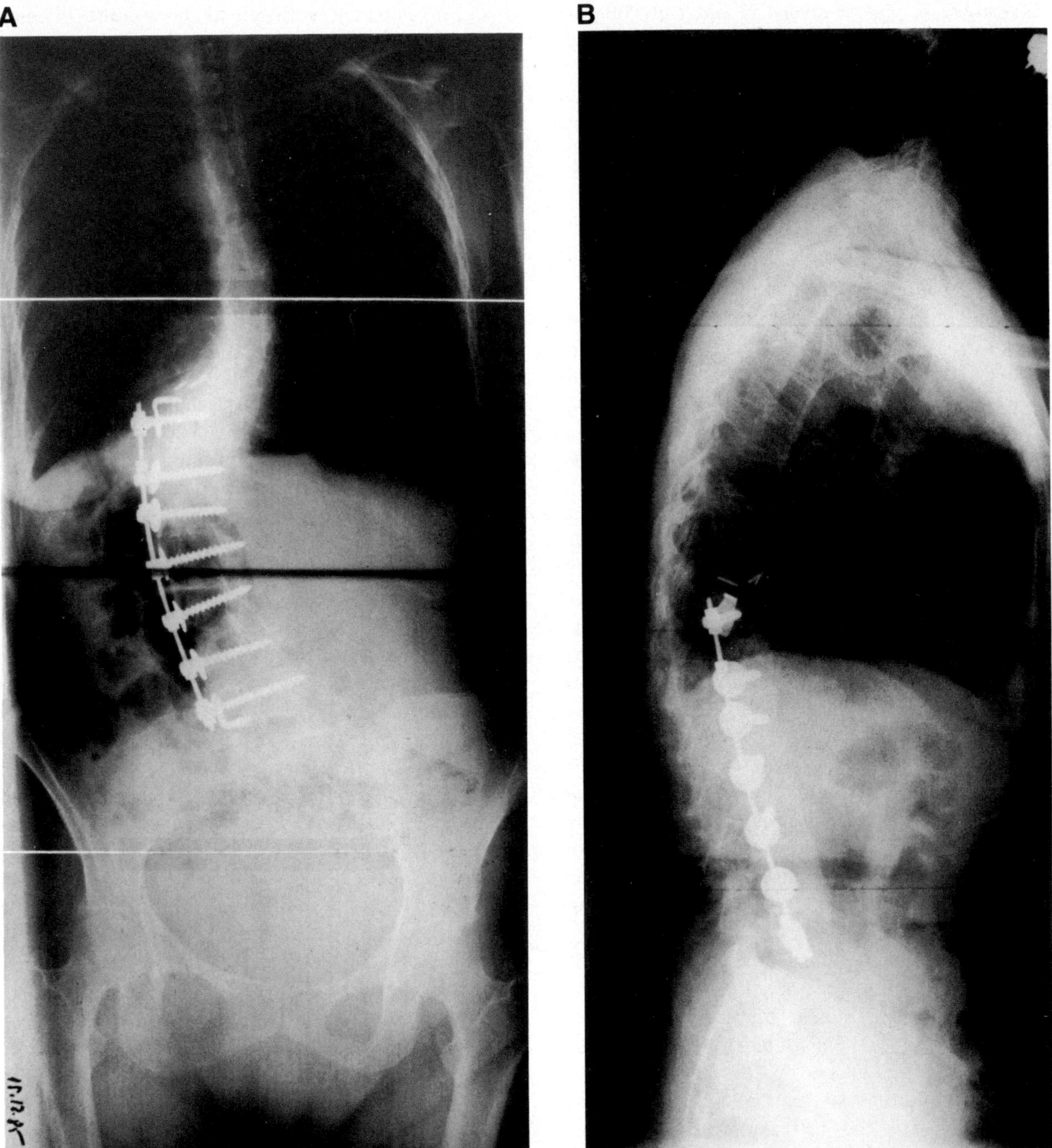

FIG 39–3.
A and B, postoperative AP and lateral radiographs of a 52-year-old woman presenting with a painful, progressive scoliosis initially measuring 68 degrees. Postoperatively, the curve measures 34 degrees. Note the proximal hook pullout. The patient was managed in a molded body jacket with a good long-term result.

is best avoided in elderly patients or those with a significant cardiovascular history.

Correction using Zielke instrumentation is superior to that previously possible with the Dwyer device.[10] A long-term review of 57 patients showed an average correction of 70% with Zielke instrumentation vs. 45% improvement with the Dwyer instrumentation.[18] The use of the derotational device improved correction of the curve in both the sagittal and coronal planes. Intraoperative complications included 5 fractured vertebral bodies. Fixation in these cases was secured with methylmethacrylate. Postoperative complications included 3 lateral femoral cutaneous nerve entrapments, 1 of which required surgical decompression. Two post-thoracotomy syndromes were encountered, and these resolved with time. Ten cases of atelectasis and pleural effusions were encountered but gradually resolved. In 1 case, the instrumentation failed, and subsequent posterior surgery was required. Proximal staple pullout occurred at two levels. Nuts backing off the screw head were noted in 10 patients without any curve deterioration or rod displacement. Rod disengagement from intermediate screw heads was reported in 6 patients without loss of correction seen on the postoperative radiographs. Six patients had proximal staple disengagement. At the 2-year follow-up, the average loss of correction was less than 1 degree. In double idiopathic curves, the average correction was 62%. At 24 months the mean loss was 3.4 degrees (4%). The noninstrumented proximal thoracic curve improved 38% after correction of the distal lumbar curve without deterioration at follow-up. In all cases, improvement of 50% over that anticipated from preoperative bending AP radiographs was noted.

An analysis of Zielke rods with pedicle fixation used posteriorly for degenerative scoliosis has shown a high incidence of rod breakage. The introduction of C-D instrumentation posteriorly makes this unnecessary. Zielke instrumentation has also been used by one of the authors (J.K.) in six patients with significant unbalance as a result of an acute lumbosacral takeoff (see Fig 39–1). This resulted in a more than 50% correction of the proximal major curve. This was done only in patients in whom the distal fractional curve was proved to be painful and in whom balance had not been shown to be restored on bending x-ray films of the major curve. The authors recommend that this technique be reserved only for fractional curves in the lower lumbar and lumbosacral segments of the spine in which the source of pain has been proved by discography and for facet blocks in a patient with trunk imbalance.

Treatment of Kyphoscoliosis

As mentioned previously, rigid kyphoscoliosis usually requires both anterior and posterior surgery. Multiple anterior discectomies and associated bone graft placement at the interbody spaces is followed by posterior surgery either on the same day, if possible, or 1 to 2 weeks later. C-D instrumentation has proved to be invaluable in restoring lordosis and maintaining rigid fixation (Figs 39–4 and 39–5). Sublaminar wiring, described by Luque, is rarely used anymore and would preclude any decompression that would be possible with the C-D device. One author's (J.K.) experience to date has been encouraging, particularly in elderly patients.

Fusions to the Sacrum

A 1983 review of Harrington rod fusions to the sacrum by Kostuik and Hall revealed a loss of lumbar lordosis in about 50% of patients with clinically significant deformity requiring corrective surgery.[21] The concept that distraction instrumentation to the lumbar spine leads to kyphosis was not recognized until the late 1970s. This was noticed even with contoured Harrington rods in addition to the use of square-ended Moe rods and sacroalar hooks. Consequently, the use of Luque L-rods across the sacroiliac joint, with further refinement by using the Galveston technique, was believed to result in an improved maintenance of lordosis and an enhanced rate of fusion for posterior instrumentation to the sacrum. Initially, the incidence of pseudarthrosis of the sacrum when Harrington rods were used with either a sacral bar or alar hooks was reportedly as high as 40%.[21] A more recent review of Luque instrumentation to the sacrum revealed that the incidence of pseudarthrosis had decreased to 15%. However, the incidence of flat back and fusion to the sacrum was reduced to only 25%.[28] This occurred despite contouring of the L-rods into lordosis and was believed to be due to simple loss of mobility. It occurred in only those patients who were kyphoscoliotic. The resulting kyphosis was generally not as severe as that encountered when Harrington instrumentation was used. The introduction of derotation using the C-D device has made this problem less frequent.

In order to enhance fusion rates to the sacrum, the authors generally recommend a two-stage procedure when correcting adult deformity (Fig 39–6). In the presence of scoliosis with lordosis and a mobile curve, a procedure involving multiple anterior discectomies followed by Zielke instrumentation is usually successful. Although the use of Zielke instrumentation anterior to the sacrum is technically demanding, it has not resulted in any problems related to the common iliac vessels in Kostuik's experience. The technique involves carefully placing the screw heads into the vertebral bodies to avoid any major vessels. The rods are safely passed beneath the common iliac vessels and kept close to the vertebral body. Occasionally, two rods at the distal two or three levels are used in order to help control rotation at the lumbosacral junction. A second-stage procedure using posterior C-D instrumentation is then performed.

In the presence of kyphoscoliosis requiring fusion to the sacrum, the first stage consists of multiple anterior discectomies with minced bone graft used at the interbody spaces, preferably from an autogenous source. This is also followed by posterior C-D instrumentation to derotate the spine and reduce lordosis. On the contrary, if the curve is mobile with good preservation of lordosis, then anterior Zielke instrumentation to the sacrum is followed by posterior C-D instrumentation.

Bicortical grafts from the iliac crests of younger adult patients or a tricortical piece in the more osteoporotic elderly patients are used to maintain disc height at L4–5 and at L5–S1 in addition to enhancing restoration and/or maintenance of lordosis. Internal fixation is used to enhance

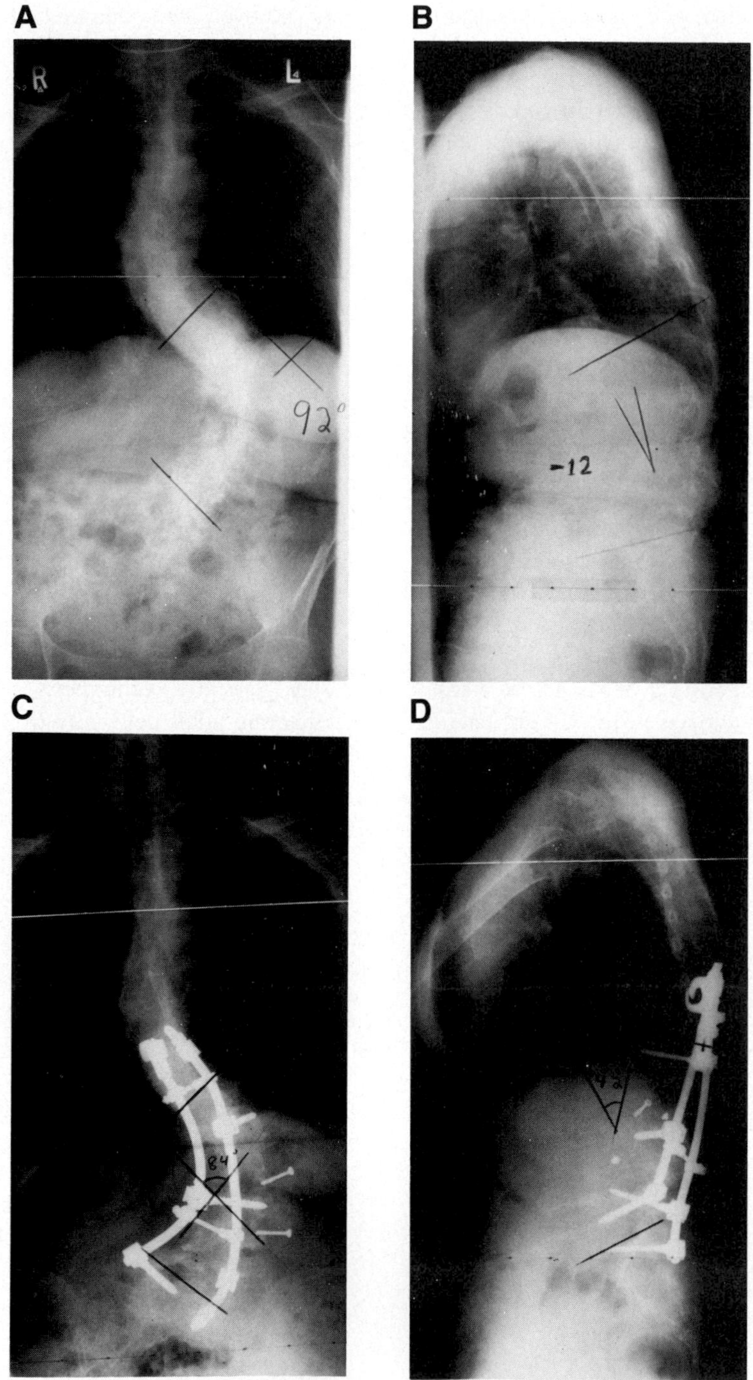

FIG 39–4.

A, a 63-year-old woman with a progressive kyphoscoliosis curve measuring 92 degrees. Stage 1, multiple anterior discectomies with bone graft; stage 2, Cotrel-Dubousset instrumentation and fusion. **B,** preoperative lateral view. Note the kyphotic lumbar spine measuring −12 degrees. **C,** postoperative AP view. There is only a small amount of correction in the coronal plane. **D,** postoperative lateral view. Note the marked restoration of lordosis to 42 degrees (a gain of 54 degrees).

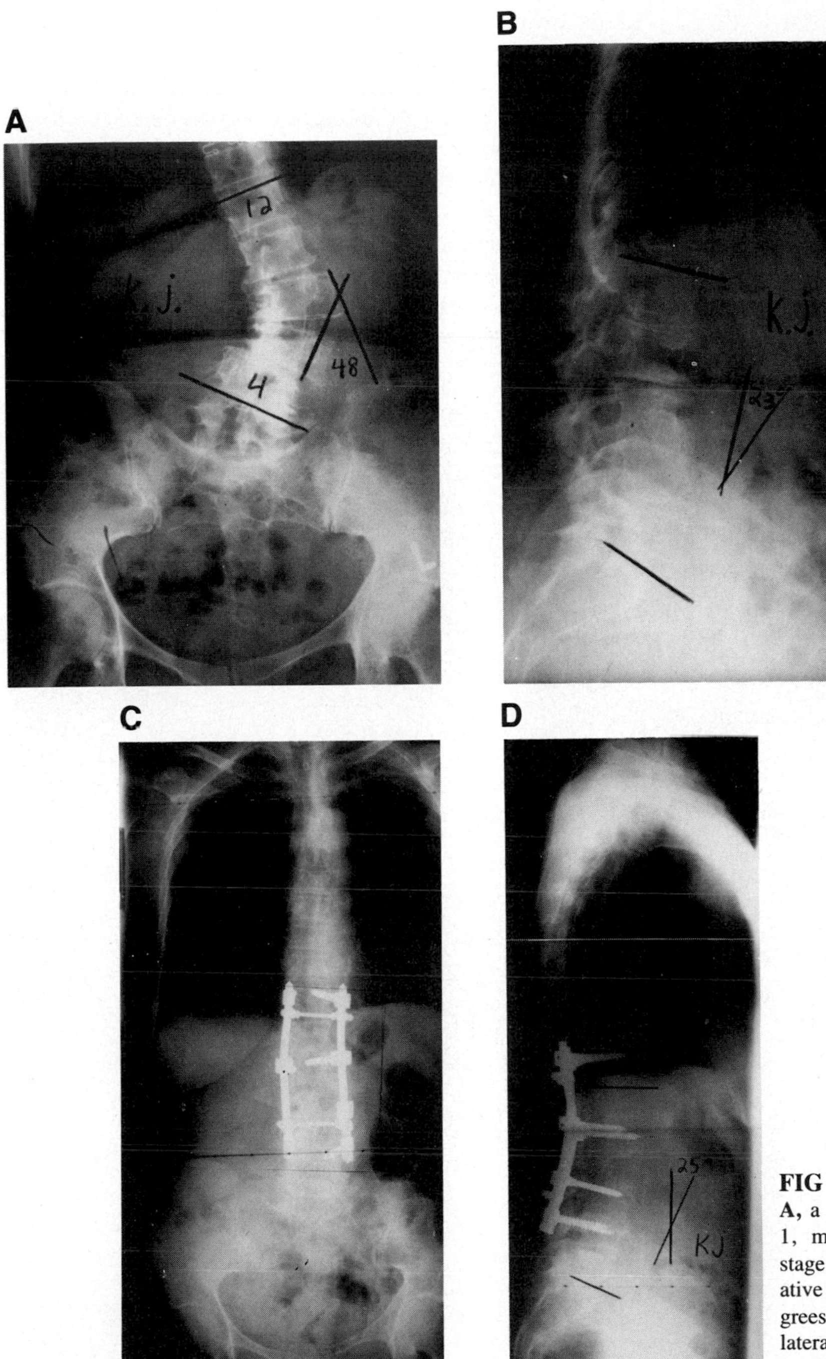

FIG 39–5.
A, a 58-year-old woman with a progressive, painful curve. Stage 1, multiple anterior discectomies with morselized bone graft; stage 2, Cotrel-Dubousset instrumentation and fusion. **B,** preoperative lateral view. Note the significant loss of lordosis (−23 degrees from L1 to S1). **C,** postoperative AP view. **D,** postoperative lateral view. Note the significant return of lumbar lordosis due to derotation following anterior release.

stability and prevent graft extrusion. In addition, combined anterior and posterior approaches minimize the risk of pseudarthrosis and enable more difficult revisions to be performed.

Extensions and Fusions in the Lumbar Spine

Reports reviewing patients who have previously been fused to L2, L3, or L4 noted an increased risk of developing degenerative changes below the previous fusion level.[7, 11] These patients may require extension of the fusion if nonoperative means fail to control their pain and their problem becomes a progressive one (Fig 39–7). In addition, spinal stenosis may be associated with the painful levels. Diagnostic investigations of patients possibly requiring extension of fusion into the lumbosacral spine may include a combination of the following investigations: myelography, CT, MRI, facet blocks, and discography. If it is determined after these tests and a complete physical examination that fusion does not require extension to the sacrum, then posterior or anterior instrumentation alone may suffice. However, if extension of the fusion to the sacrum is required, then a combined approach is recommended by the authors. Extension of fusion to the sacrum is usually carried out in a single stage. One of the authors (J.K.) has had much success with posterior pedicle fixation and anterior Zielke instrumentation. In order to improve lordosis, the posterior lamina between L3 to S1 may be removed and compression applied in order to increase extension of the lower lumbar segments. Anteriorly, interbody grafts are placed after the disc space is opened as widely as possible. Subsequently, two Zielke rods are used to control rotation at the lumbosacral junction.

A recent review of 24 cases of fusion extension to the sacrum demonstrated 6 cases of fusion with Harrington rods.[21] Only 5 failed owing to the development of pseudarthrosis in the flat back. Nine were fused anteriorly in situ with interbody grafts and instrumentation used to maintain lordosis; these were supplemented either at the same stage or second stage with posterior instrumentation and fusion. With this technique, 3 pseudarthroses with as-

A

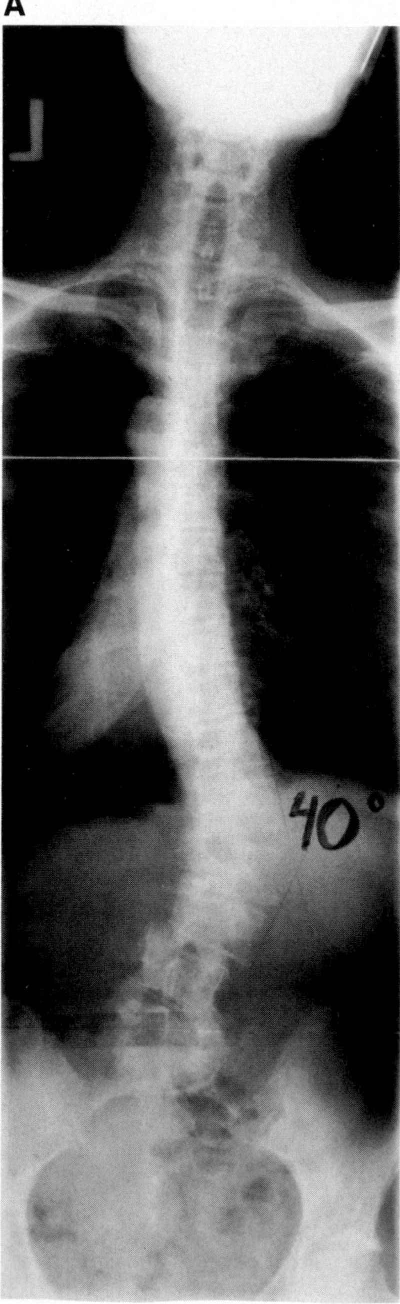

B

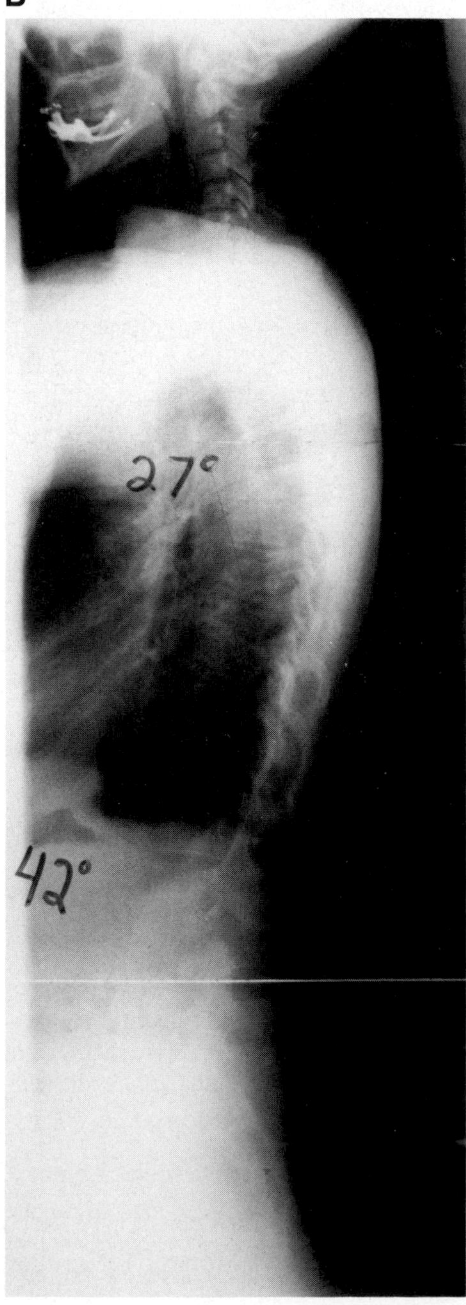

FIG 39–6.
A, a 53-year-old woman with a progressive, painful scoliosis measuring 40 degrees. **B,** the curve was flexible. Preoperative discography revealed painful degenerative L4–5 and L5–S1 discs. **C** and **D (facing page),** in order to achieve solid fusion, a two-stage surgery was performed. The first stage consisted of anterior L4–5 and L5–S1 discectomies, interbody iliac crest grafts, internal fixation with a Yuan I beam plate at L4 to S1, and two AO (Arbeitsgemeinschaft für Osteosynthesefragen) 6.5-mm screws at L5 to S1. The second stage, Cotrel-Dubousset instrumentation and fusion, derotated the spine and increased lordosis. Pain was significantly relieved at follow-up.

C

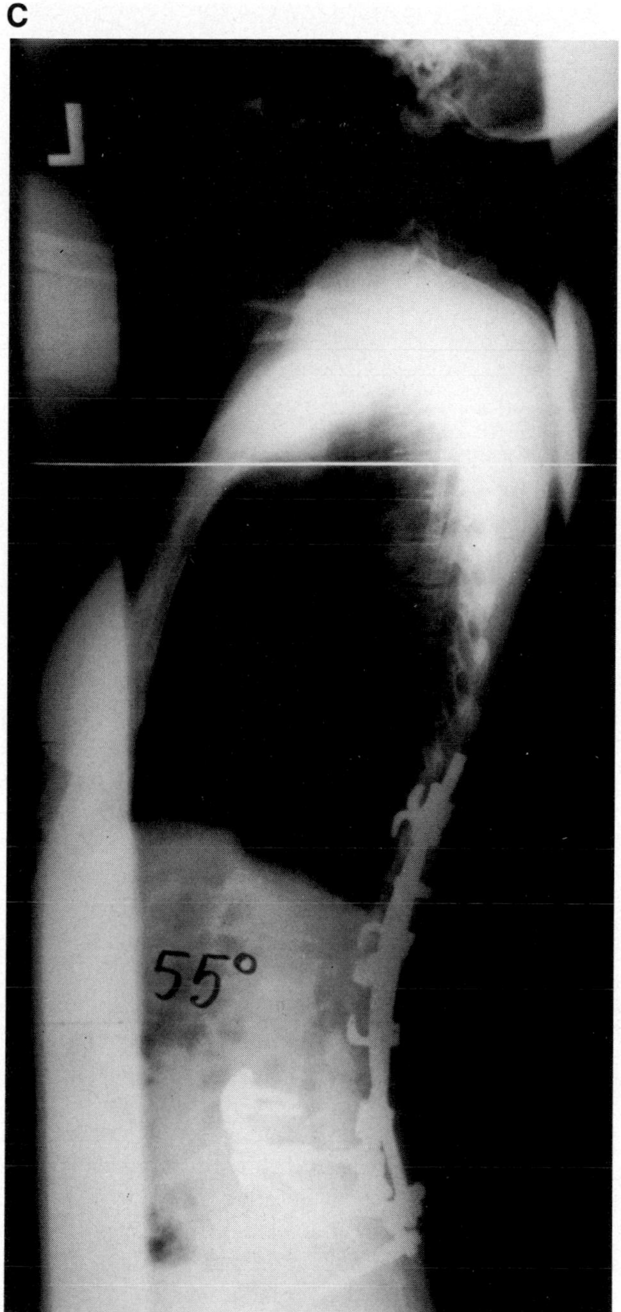

D

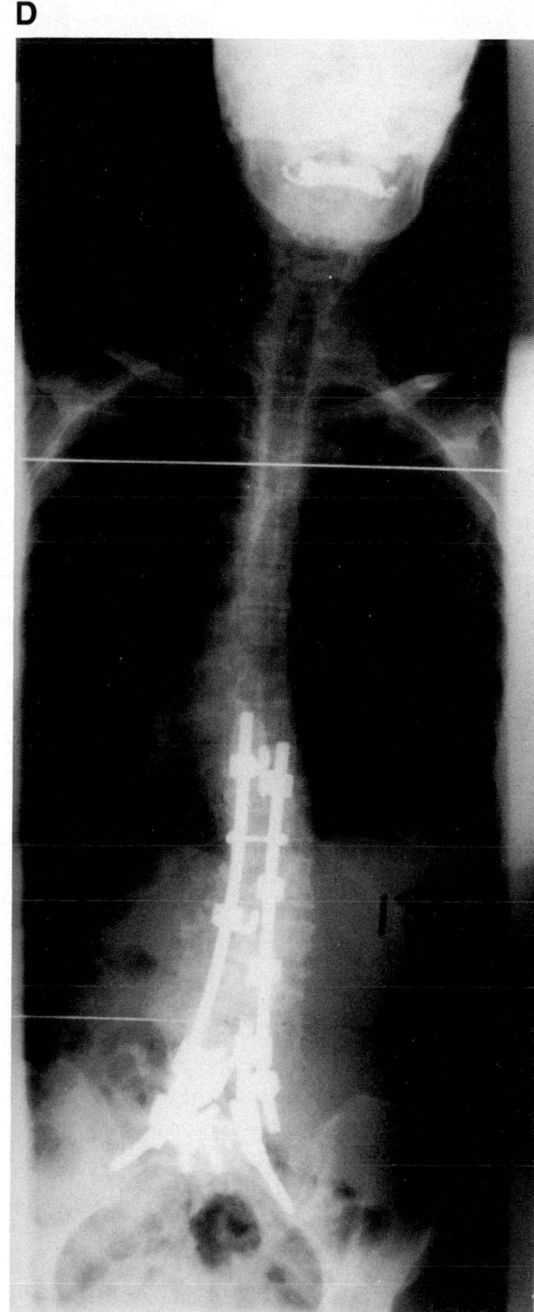

FIG 39–6 (cont.).

sociated flat back occurred. Separately, 10 fusions were performed at a single stage with associated removal of bone posteriorly through the pars interarticularis; except for 1 instance of pseudarthrosis, all patients had satisfactory results manifested by an increased ability to open the interbody space anteriorly in addition to the instrumentation.

Treatment of Severe Rigid Scoliotic Deformities

In 1980, Kostuik reported on 85 patients with severe, rigid deformities measuring 90 degrees or greater.[18] Fifteen of these patients were primarily kyphotic, 42 had idiopathic curves, and 28 were reportedly congenital. The majority of curves were thoracic or thoracolumbar. There were 28 congenital fusions as a result of failure of segmentation and 4 resulting from spontaneous fusions. Thirty-three untreated patients were shown to be rigid on bending x-ray films and at the time of surgery were found to have no evidence for spontaneous fusion. Twenty patients with previous fusions presented with progressive deformity and pain. All patients underwent posterior releases including, if necessary, osteotomies of previous fusion masses or

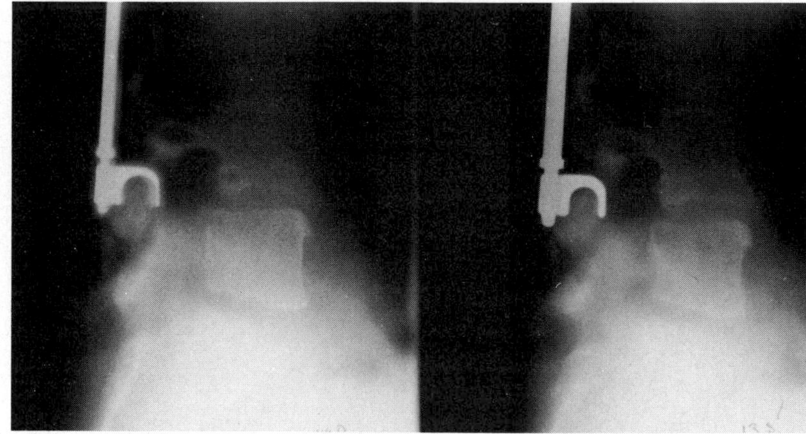

FIG 39–7.
Lateral tomograms at the L4–5 disc space in a 33-year-old woman who had undergone Harrington instrumentation 12 years earlier. Note the severe degeneration of the disc space with forward subluxation of L4 on L5.

congenitally fused spines. If done, posture osteotomies were carried out at multiple levels averaging four in number. In addition, rib releases were carried out over three to four levels on the concavity with transverse process osteotomies and rib resections on the convexity. All patients had anterior osteotomies performed as well. Ages ranged from 20 to 55 years, and curve magnitudes measured anywhere from 75 to 180 degrees.

At the time of primary release, as described previously, patients were additionally placed in traction in one of two forms: In 32 patients halo femoral traction was used, and in the latter part of the study halo pelvic traction was applied.[17] The latter form of traction continues to be used in very severe curves. Following these releases, the final procedure performed 2 weeks later consisted of posterior instrumentation. In the initial part of the study, Harrington rods were used but were later replaced by Luque sublaminar wiring techniques. In the latter part of the study and today, C-D instrumentation is almost exclusively used. Today, when indicated, most types of traction are carried out by halo-dependent methods in a circolectric bed at 30 degrees dependency or in association with a wheelchair.

When these techniques were used, the extent of correction averaged 40% with halo pelvic traction and 32% with halo femoral traction techniques. Harrington instrumentation added a further 8% to the correction. As regards idiopathic curves, correction averaged 48% vs. 33% mean correction in the congenital group.

Cosmesis

Correction of deformity for primarily cosmetic reasons is more common than previously thought. In a review of 1000 patients with scoliosis, 10% were operated on for cosmesis. Deformities were primarily in the thoracic region and ranged from 45% to 75%. Ninety percent of patients in this group were female with an age range of 20 to 42 years.

With the newer techniques available today, surgical correction should be seriously considered in patients unhappy with disfiguring curves. In their review, Kostuik et al. found that not all patients were single; many were happily married.[22] However, despite their marital status, they continued to be concerned about cosmesis. Surgery should only be carried out after carefully assessing the patient's desire for surgery and if necessary using a psychologist. After a careful explanation of the procedure, its postoperative course, and possible complications, surgery can be successfully carried out in the majority of patients provided that the surgeon is experienced in this field and has full support of institutional facilities and care.

The past few years has seen a resurgence of rib resections in the hump region. This is especially gratifying in severe rigid curves of the thoracic spine, particularly when hypokyphosis is noted in the sagittal plane. In more mobile curves, the use of C-D instrumentation to derotate the spine also helps to decrease the rib hump. If the hump is thought to be severe, an associated rib excision can be performed at the same time as the posterior instrumentation.

One author's (J.K.) review of 20 patients undergoing rib excision primarily consisting of five to six excised ribs on the convexity revealed minimal morbidity. Curves in these patients were very rigid and measured 90 degrees or greater. There were no changes noted when comparing preoperative and postoperative ventilation studies. Of great importance, the excision resulted in a markedly improved cosmetic result when compared with a control group. Patients with lumbar or thoracolumbar curves less commonly complain of cosmetically displeasing figures. Usually other factors will determine surgical suitability, particularly in the young adult who is unbalanced or in the elderly individual with kyphoscoliosis and complaints of pain.

Treatment of Structural Disabilities

Patients with a paralytic scoliosis may complain of a seating imbalance that is often due to a marked pelvic obliquity, an associated kyphosis in a collapsing spine, or hyperlordosis. The latter is encountered more commonly in patients who have had lumbar peritoneal shunts placed in childhood. Patients with paralytic scoliosis are still best treated by a combined anterior and posterior approach, thus eliminating the need for external postoperative immobilization and allowing for early mobilization in a wheelchair.

Deteriorating respiratory function in those individuals with a collapsing spine as a result of paralysis can be significantly improved following correction of their curves. This usually results in improved diaphragmatic breathing. A preoperative trial of halo–dependent traction may show an improvement in respiratory function and demonstrate, with little morbidity, the advantages of surgical correction of the deformity and improving respiratory function by "lifting" the diaphragm out of the abdomen.

In one of the authors' (J.K.) experience, the use of C-D instrumentation alone posteriorly has not yet proved to be sufficient in the treatment of paralytic curves that extend into the distal part of the lumbar spine. Presently, we recommend both an anterior and posterior procedure. Although in children Luque instrumentation to the pelvis with the Galveston modification has proved to be of value in achieving a solid fusion, this has not been our experience with adults, where superior results have been noted with a two-stage anterior and posterior procedure.

Treatment of Spinal Deformities in Patients Older Than 50 Years

Managing spinal deformities in adults over 50 years of age is often a challenging problem. The curves are often rigid and usually imbalanced. In addition, loss of the normal sagittal contours is often encountered. The bone is frequently osteopenic, and associated neurologic problems related to spinal stenosis are not uncommon. The major indication for presentation in this group is pain. Prior to the newer fixation techniques, correction was often carried out by using Harrington instrumentation, which potentially placed neurologic structures at risk in this group of patients.

With improved devices such as the anterior Zielke instrumentation and the posterior C-D device, curve reduction is more safely achieved. As mentioned previously with thoracolumbar or lumbar deformity and preservation of lordosis, anterior Zielke instrumentation can be effectively used. With a more rigid curve and minimal lumbar lordosis or kyphosis, a two-stage procedure is preferable. Posteriorly, derotation is most effectively carried out by using C-D instrumentation to correct the curve in both the coronal and sagittal planes.

In a recent review by Kostuik of 80 patients over 50 years of age who underwent surgery for scoliosis, results were good to excellent in 69% of patients. Fair and poor results were noted in 31%. Twenty-seven patients complained of minimal to no pain (34%).

Surgical decompression of spinal stenosis in the presence of significant deformity should be associated with a stabilization procedure, particularly if more than one level is decompressed.[38, 39] A major decompression in the presence of scoliosis but no stabilization procedure will often lead to significant collapsing as well as progressive and painful scoliosis. Further surgery in these patients is often difficult as a result of the inadequacies of bone stock and scarring, which often require both an anterior and posterior procedure for salvage.

Treatment of Iatrogenic Lumbar Kyphosis

Instrumentation for scoliosis into the lower lumbar segments may result in a significant loss of lumbar lordosis. If sufficiently flattened, a potentially disabling symptom complex, "flat back" syndrome, may result. Patients with this disorder often walk with their knees and hips flexed in order to balance the pathologic forward tilt of the trunk. Despite a potentially solid fusion, back pain is often an accompaniment. Kostuik et al. reported their early experience with 33 patients in which a combined anterior and posterior osteotomy was used for restoration of lordosis.[23, 24] The combined approach offered improved correction and fusion rates when confined to a single approach. The causes of lumbar kyphosis include distraction instrumentation extending to the lower lumbar vertebral or sacrum and kyphosis at the thoracolumbar junction; in addition, degenerative changes above and/or below the previous fusion mass were commonly seen at fusions ending between L3 and L5 (Fig 39–8). If loss of lumbar lordosis is associated with a pseudarthrosis, a repair of the pseudarthrosis alone does not usually suffice in relieving the patient's symptoms.

The surgical technique involves a simultaneous anterior and posterior approach with the patient positioned in the lateral decubitus position (Fig 39–9). An anterior and posterior osteotomy is carried out at the same level in order to restore lordosis. Typically, the osteotomy is carried out at the L3 level but may be performed at the level of the pseudarthrosis. The nerve roots at the level of the posterior osteotomy must be clearly identified and freed prior to extending the spine. Dwyer screws and cables are used in a lateral fusion mass posteriorly after closing the osteotomy sites. Four screws proximal and distal to the osteotomy site are usually placed. A midline contoured AO plate is used to help control rotation posteriorly. Anteriorly, the osteotomy is opened simultaneously with posterior closure of the osteotomy by Kostuik-Harrington instrumentation. A tricortical or bicortical iliac crest graft is then used anteriorly to fill the gap.

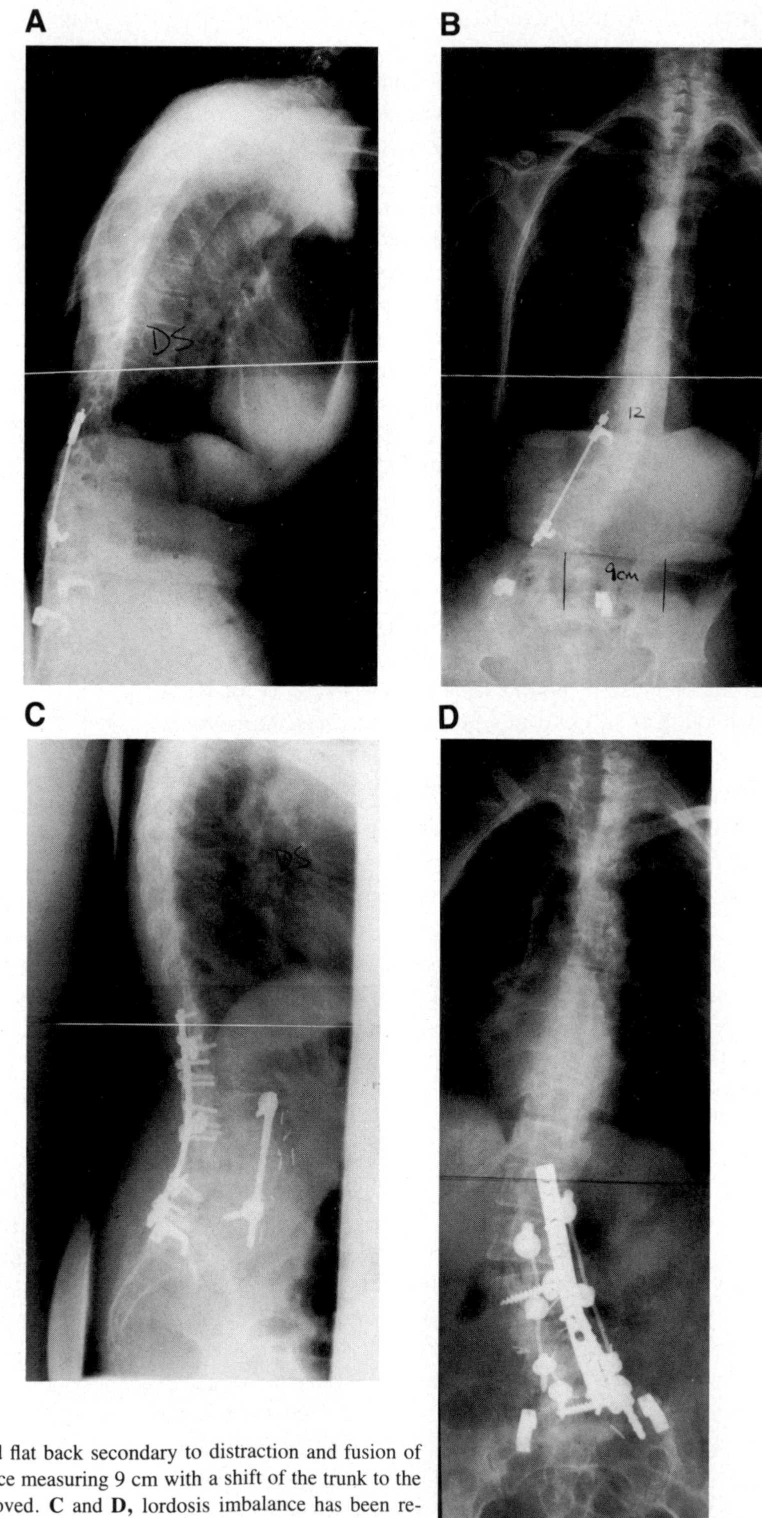

FIG 39–8.
A, a 45-year-old woman with a loss of lordosis and a marked flat back secondary to distraction and fusion of the lumbar spine. **B,** AP radiograph demonstrating an imbalance measuring 9 cm with a shift of the trunk to the right. A Harrington distraction rod had previously been removed. **C** and **D,** lordosis imbalance has been restored following a single-stage anterior and posterior osteotomy.

A

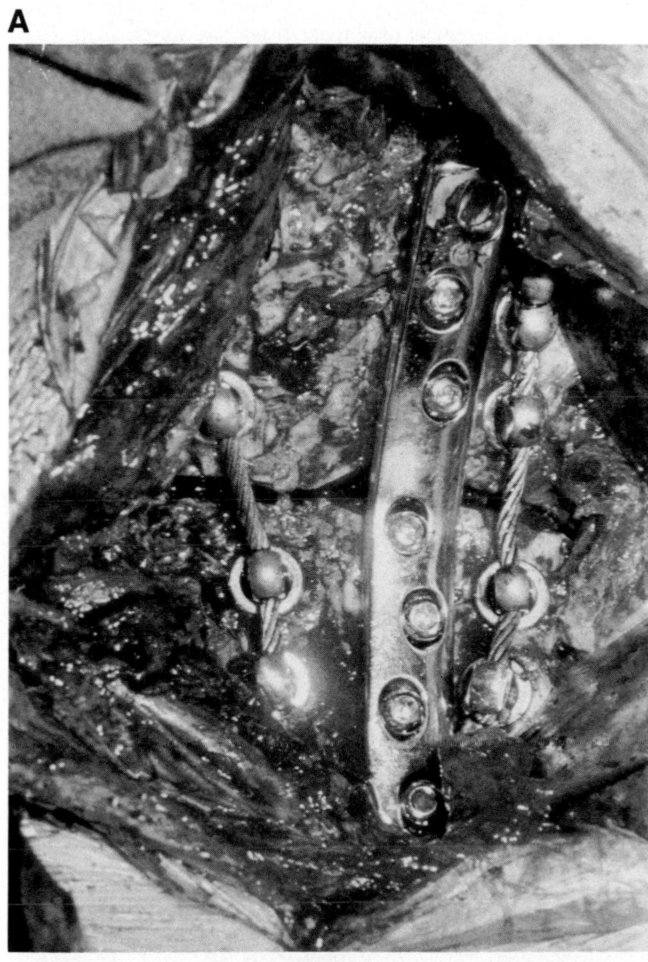

B

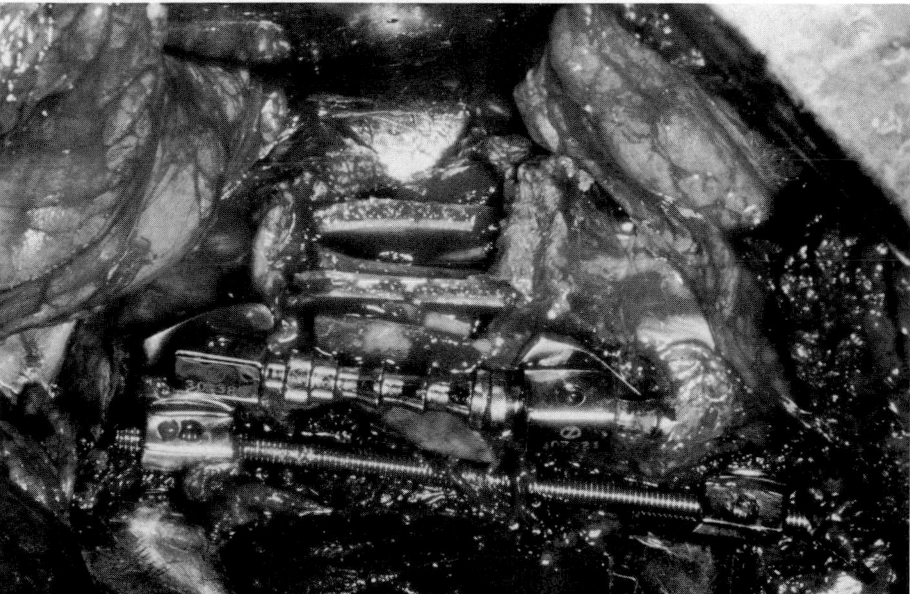

FIG 39–9.
A, this posterior osteotomy has been closed by the application of Dwyer screws in the lateral fusion mass, and an AO plate has been added in the midline to help control rotation. **B,** simultaneous with posterior closure, the anterior osteotomy site is opened with Kostuik-Harrington instrumentation. Iliac crest grafts are added, and a second Kostuik-Harrington compression rod is added to enhance stability.

MORBIDITY AND MORTALITY

The treatment of spinal deformities in adults is not without risk. Neurologic complications in adolescents are reported to occur in 1%; in adults, the incidence of neurologic complications is reported to be between 2% and 3%. In a review by Kostuik of his first 1000 patients, the incidence of paraparesis was 0.7%. The incidence of motor weakness as a result of nerve root injury was 3%. The author further commented that the majority of these were covered. Other potentially life-threatening complications include pulmonary emboli. If not contraindicated, routine prophylaxis is recommended. The deep-infection rate was reportedly 1% with no major sequelae. Prophylactic antibiotics are routinely recommended. A mortality rate of 0.8% was noted in this group of patients, 2 resulting from pulmonary emboli, 3 from adult respiratory distress syndrome, 1 from a disseminated intravascular coagulopathy, and 2 from vascular problems.

REFERENCES

1. Ascani E, Bartolozzi P, Logroscino CA, et al: Natural history of untreated scoliosis after skeletal maturity. Presented at a Symposium on Epidemiology, Natural History and Non-Operative Treatment of Idiopathic Scoliosis at the Annual Meeting of the Scoliosis Research Society, Orlando, Fla, 1984.
2. Bergofsky EH, Turino GM, Fishman AP: Cardiorespiratory failure in kyphoscoliosis. *Medicine (Baltimore)* 1959; 38:263–317.
3. Betz R, Bunnel W, Lambrecht-Mulier E, et al: Scoliosis and pregnancy. *J Bone Joint Surg [Am]* 1987; 69:90.
4. Bjure J, Nachemson A: Non-treated scoliosis. *Clin Orthop* 1973; 93:44–52.
5. Blount WP, Mellencamp DD: The effect of pregnancy on idiopathic scoliosis. *J Bone Joint Surg [Am]* 1980; 62:1083–1087.
6. Chapman EH, Dill BD, Graybiel A: The decrease in functional capacity of the lungs and heart resulting from deformities of the chest pulmocardiac failure. *Medicine (Baltimore)* 1939; 18:167–202.
7. Cochran T, Irstram L, Nachemson A: Longterm anatomic and functional changes in patients with adolescent idiopathic scoliosis treated by Harrington rod fusion. *Spine* 1983; 8:576–584.
8. Collis DK, Ponseti IV: Long-term follow-up of patients with idiopathic scoliosis not treated surgically. *J Bone Joint Surg [Am]* 1969; 51:425–445.
9. Duriez J: Evolution de la scoliose idiopathique chez l'adulte. *Acta Orthop Belg* 1967; 33:547–550.
10. Dwyer AF: Experience of anterior correction of scoliosis. *Clin Orthop* 1973; 93:191.
11. Edgar MA, Mehta MH: A long-term review of adults with fused and unfused idiopathic scoliosis. *Orthop Trans* 1982; 6:462–463.
12. Flagstad A, Kollman S: Vital capacity and muscle study in 100 cases of scoliosis. *J Bone Joint Surg* 1928; 10:724.
13. Fowles JV, Drummond DS, L'Ecuzer S, et al: The prognosis and management of untreated scoliosis in the adult. Presented at the Annual Meeting of the Scoliosis Research Society, Louisville, Ky, 1973.
14. Godfrey S: Respiratory and cardiovascular consequences of scoliosis. *Respiration* 1970; 27:67.
15. Gucker T III: Changes in vital capacity in scoliosis. *J Bone Joint Surg [Am]* 1962; 44:469.
16. Kostuik JP: Decision making in adult scoliosis. *Spine* 1979; 4:521–525.
17. Kostuik JP: Halo–pelvic traction in the surgical management of adult scoliosis. *J Bone Joint Surg [Br]* 1973; 55:232.
18. Kostuik JP: Recent advances in the treatment of painful adult scoliosis. *Clin Orthop* 1980; 147:238–252.
19. Kostuik JP, Bentivoglio J: The incidence of low back pain in adult scoliosis. *Spine* 1981; 6:268–273.
20. Kostuik JP, Gleason TF, Errico TJ, et al: The surgical correction of flat back syndrome (iatrogenic lumbar kyphosis). *Orthop Trans* 1985; 9:131.
21. Kostuik JP, Hall BB: Spinal fusions to the sacrum in adults with scoliosis. *Spine* 1983; 8:489–500.
22. Kostuik JP, Israel J, Hall JE: Scoliosis surgery in adults. *Clin Orthop* 1973; 93:225–234.
23. Kostuik JP, Matsusaki H: Anterior stabilization, instrumentation and decompression for post-traumatic kyphosis. *Spine* 1989; 14:379–386.
24. Kostuik JP, Maurais GR, Richardson WJ, et al: Combined single stage anterior and posterior osteotomy for correction of iatrogenic lumbar kyphosis. *Spine* 1988; 13:257–266.
25. Lagrone MO, Bradford DS, Moe JH, et al: Treatment of symptomatic flatback after spinal fusion. *J Bone Joint Surg [Am]* 1988; 70:569–580.
26. Lamarre A, Hall J, Weng T, et al: Pulmonary functions in scoliosis one year after surgical correction. *J Bone Joint Surg [Am]* 1971; 53:195.
27. Lowe T: The morbidity and mortality report. Presented at the 21st Annual Meeting of the Scoliosis Research Society, Bermuda, 1986.
28. Luque ER: *Segmental Spinal Instrumentation*. Thorofare, NJ, Slack, 1984.
29. Mankin H, Graham J, Schack J: Cardiopulmonary function in mild and moderate idiopathic scoliosis. *J Bone Joint Surg [Am]* 1964; 46:53.
30. Nachemson A: Adult scoliosis and back pain. *Spine* 1979; 4:512–517.
31. Nachemson A: A long-term follow-up study of non-treated scoliosis. *Acta Orthop Scand* 1968; 39:466–476.
32. Nachemson A: A long-term follow-up study of non-treated scoliosis. *J Bone Joint Surg [Am]* 1969; 50:203.
33. Nachemson A, Cochran RP, Irstram L, et al: Pregnancy after scoliosis treatment. *Orthop Trans* 1982; 6:5.
34. Nilsonne U, Lundgren KD: Long-term prognosis in idiopathic scoliosis. *Acta Orthop Scand* 1968; 39:455–565.
35. Robin G, Span Y, Steinberg R, et al: Scoliosis in the elderly: A follow-up study. *Spine* 1982; 7:355.
36. Shands AR, Eisberg HB: The incidence of scoliosis in the state of Delaware: A study of 50,000 minifilms made dur-

ing a survey for tuberculosis. *J Bone Joint Surg [Am]* 1955; 37:1243.

37. Shannon D, Riseborough E, Kazemi H: Ventilation perfusion relationships following correction of kyphoscoliosis. *JAMA* 1971; 217:579.
38. Simmons EH, Jackson RP: The management of nerve root entrapment syndromes associated with the collapsing scoliosis of idiopathic lumbar and thoracolumbar curves. *Spine* 1979; 4:533–541.
39. Simmons EH, Jackson RP, Stripinus D: Incidence and severity of back pain in adult idiopathic scoliosis. *Spine* 1983; 8:749–756.
40. Stagnara P: *Scoliosis in Adults: Surgical Treatment of Severe Forms*. Paris, Excerpta Medica Foundation International Congress Series No. 192, 1969.
41. Stagnara P: Traitment chirugical des scoliosis cyphosantes ches l'adulte. *Acta Orthop Belg* 1981; 47:721–739.
42. Stagnara P, Fleury D, Pauchet R, et al: Scolioses majeures de l'adultes superieures a 100–183 cas traites chirurgicalement. *Rev Chir Orthop* 1975; 61:101–122.
43. Stagnara P, Gonon GP, Faucher P: Surgical treatment of idiopathic rigid lumbar scoliosis in the adult, in *Management of Spinal Deformities (Orthopaedics 2)*. London, Butterworths, 1984, pp 303–321.
44. Stagnara P, Jouvinroux P, Pelous J, et al: Cyphoscolioses essentielles de l'adulte: Formes severes de plus de 100°. Redressement partial et arthrodese. XI Sicot Congress, Mexico City, 1969, pp 206–233.
45. Strayer LM III: The incidence of scoliosis in the postpartum female on Cape Cod. *J Bone Joint Surg [Am]* 1973; 55:436.
46. Vanderpool DW, James JIP, Wynne-Davies R: Scoliosis in the elderly. *J Bone Joint Surg [Am]* 1969; 51:446–455.
47. Weinstein SL, Ponseti IV: Curve progression in idiopathic scoliosis. *J Bone Joint Surg [Am]* 1983; 65:447–455.
48. Weinstein SL, Zavala DC, Ponseti IV: Idiopathic scoliosis—long term followup and prognosis in untreated patients. *J Bone Joint Surg [Am]* 1981; 63:702–711.
49. Westgate H: Pulmonary function in thoracic scoliosis, before and after corrective surgery. *Minn Med* 1970; 53:839.
50. Winter R, Lovell W, Moe J: Excessive thoracic lordosis and loss of pulmonary function in patients with idiopathic scoliosis. *J Bone Joint Surg [Am]* 1975; 57:972.
51. Zielke K, Pellin B: Ergebnisse operativer Skoliosen- und Kyphoskoliosen-behandlung beim Adoleszenten über 18 Jahre und beim Erwachsenen. *Z Orthop* 1975; 113:157–174.
52. Zorab PA: Assessment of cardio-respiratory function, in Zorab PA (ed): *Proceedings of a Symposium on Scoliosis*. London, The National Fund for Research Into Poliomyelitis and Other Crippling Diseases, Vincent House, 1964, p 54.

PART XI

REFLEX SYMPATHETIC DYSTROPHY

40

Reflex Sympathetic Dystrophy

Aaron K. Calodney, M.D., and Prithvi Raj, M.D.

Reflex sympathetic dystrophy (RSD) is the term applied to a variety of seemingly unrelated disorders having strikingly similar clinical features and manifesting the same fundamental disturbed physiology. The term *reflex* indicates a response to a primary, exciting mechanism that is traumatic, medical, infectious, or vascular; the term *sympathetic* indicates the neurologic pathway subserving the development and maintenance of these syndromes; and the term *dystrophy* indicates that if untreated, these syndromes can lead to irreversible and disabling trophic changes.

As seen in Table 40–1, there have been many terms used to describe the syndrome that we now refer to as RSD. Causalgia, which means "burning pain," is a term describing an RSD following partial or, more rarely, complete injury to a peripheral nerve.[62] It is characterized by constant, spontaneous burning pain and is usually associated with sensory disturbances along with vasomotor and sudomotor disturbances that if persistent, result in trophic changes. RSD need not be initiated by damage to a peripheral nerve. Other etiologies listed in Table 40–2 are characterized by similar although perhaps less severe symptomatology. Regardless of the etiology, RSD can be defined[40] as a syndrome of diffuse limb pain often burning in nature and usually consequent to injury or a noxious stimulus with variable sensory, motor, autonomic, and trophic changes. The syndrome may spread independently of the source or site of the precipitating event and often presents in a pattern inconsistent with dermatomal or peripheral nerve distributions. Clinical findings usually include the following:

- *Autonomic dysregulation* (e.g., alterations in blood flow, hyperhidrosis, edema)
- *Sensory abnormalities* (e.g., hypoesthesia or hyperesthesia, allodynia to cold and mechanical stimulation)
- *Motor dysfunction* (e.g., weakness, tremor, joint stiffness)
- *Reactive psychological* disturbances (e.g., anxiety, hopelessness, depression)
- *Trophic changes* (e.g., muscle atrophy, osteopenia, arthropathy, glossy skin, brittle nails, and altered hair growth)

Regardless of the etiology or severity of presentation, the underlying pathophysiologic mechanism is extremely similar if not identical in all of these disorders. The common etiologic denominator appears to be local tissue damage, which apparently initiates a reflex response that in some way involves the sympathetic nervous system. Furthermore, the pain and vasomotor disturbances, with minor exceptions, are improved, cured, or otherwise modified by interruption of the involved sympathetic pathways.

Rarely is the diagnosis of severe RSD difficult to make, both because the initiating mechanism is usually related to obvious trauma to major nerve trunks or tissues in close proximity and because the resultant syndrome and particularly the burning pain are so characteristic. However, a less severe RSD, without obvious injury or etiology, is frequently misdiagnosed and hence often mismanaged or neglected. In many of these cases, the clinical presentation is so bizarre in its distribution and apparently so unrelated to any precipitating factor that not infrequently the physician doubts an organic basis and attributes the signs and symptoms to psychogenic factors. It is to be emphasized that severe degrees of pain and/or vasomotor changes may occur following a seemingly insignificant injury, even in the absence of infection or other post-traumatic sequelae. As a result, this group of patients is in danger of being misunderstood, discredited, and certainly mismanaged or neglected for long enough that the disease progresses from a reversible to an irreversible state.

In this chapter an understanding of RSD and its management is developed through a review of the autonomic nervous system, historical perspectives, consideration of the theories of pathogenesis, detailing of the clinical presentation and course of the disease, and finally a discussion of current management.

For the surgeon who manages skeletal trauma, understanding RSD will promote the most important factor in successful treatment, i.e., a short interval between the onset of symptoms and the administration of therapy.[77]

TABLE 40–1.
Terms Used to Describe Reflex Sympathetic Dystrophy

Acute atrophy of bone
Algodystrophy
Algodystrophy mineures
Algodystrophy reflexes
Causalgia
Chronic traumatic edema
Mimo-causalgia
Minor causalgia
Neurodystrophy
Pain-dysfunction syndrome
Post-traumatic syndrome
Post-traumatic dystrophy
Post-traumatic osteoporosis
Post-traumatic pain syndrome
Reflex sympathetic dystrophy
Shoulder-hand syndrome
Sudek's atrophy
Sympathalgia
Traumatic vasospasm

REVIEW OF THE AUTONOMIC NERVOUS SYSTEM

Since RSD represents aberrant sympathetic activity, detailed knowledge of the autonomic nervous system is essential. In 1954, the great anatomist and surgeon Dr. Joseph Pick wrote the following description.[74]

> We find in those animals which are threatened with moments of extreme emergency, not only by heat or cold, but also when facing an enemy, that the homeostatic mechanisms of the sympathetic nervous system are thrown into sudden and complete activity. This profuse sympathetic discharge, dilated pupils, rapid heartbeat, deepened respiration, color change in the skin, sweating, and dry mouth, is characteristic of a frightened animal. All resources of the body are mobilized for combat or for flight.
>
> As soon as the emergency is over, the energies which were dissipated during moments of stress must be restored and further reserves gradually built up for the next emergency. Herein lies the significance of the parasympathetic, the other grand division of the autonomic nervous system. There must be also proper homeostatic balance between the parasympathetic, the accumulator of reserves, and that of the sympathetic, the spender of energies. If the body spends too much, it goes bankrupt. If it is too thrifty, incapable or afraid to spend, it will be overwhelmed by some enemy, be it another organism, extremes of temperature, or an excess of material retained in the body, whether salt or sugar. Adequate spending, therefore, helps to free the body from the restrictions of environment and upholds the constancy of the "milieu interieur" of the body.[74]

Phylogenetically, the parasympathetic system appeared first and has been designated "paleoautonomic."

TABLE 40–2.
Etiology of Reflex Sympathetic Dystrophy*

Trauma
- Accidental injury
  - Sprain, dislocation, fracture, usually of the hands, feet, or wrists
  - Minor cuts or pricks, lacerations, contusions
  - Crush injury of fingers, hands, or wrists; traumatic amputation of fingers
  - Burns
- Surgical
  - Procedures in the extremities
  - Excision of small tumors, ganglia of the wrist
  - Forceful manipulation, tight casts
  - Surgical scars
  - Damage to small peripheral nerves with a needle (e.g., during its insertion for infusion, transfusion injection therapy, or analgesic block)
  - Injections or irritants

Diseases
- Visceral disease
  - Myocardial infarction
- Neurologic disease
  - Cerebral: vascular accidents (posthemiplegic dystrophy), tumors, post-traumatic
  - Spinal cord: poliomyelitis, combined degeneration, tumors, syringomyelia, and others
  - Spinal nerves or their roots: herpes zoster, radiculitis
  - Brachial plexus
  - Infiltrating carcinoma from the breast, apex of the lung (upper extremity), or pelvis (lower extremity)
  - Glomus tumor
- Infections
  - Extremity skin and other soft tissues
  - Periarticular
- Vascular disease
  - Generalized: periarteritis nodosa, diffuse arteritis, arteriosclerosis
  - Peripheral: thrombophlebitis, frostbite
- Musculoskeletal disorders
  - Postural defects
  - Myofascial syndromes

Idiopathic

*Adapted from Bonica JJ: *The Management of Pain,* Philadelphia, Lea & Febiger, 1953.

The sympathetic system, or "neoautonomic," developed next when animals became terrestrial because they then required inhibition of intestinal activity, especially of the sphincter mechanisms of rectal and urinary passages.[73]

Anatomic Aspects of the Autonomic Nervous System

The autonomic nervous system consists of a central and peripheral component.

Central Component

Although the brain stem and spinal cord largely constitute the central component, the hypothalamus is regarded as the principal area of integration of the entire autonomic system. In its regulation of body temperature, water balance, carbohydrate and fat metabolism, blood

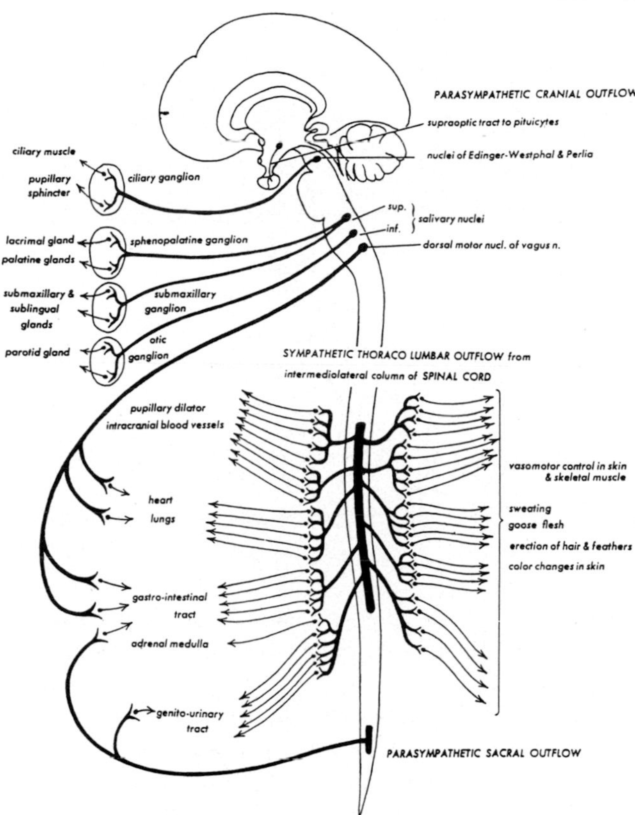

FIG 40–1.
The origin and distribution of the two great divisions of the autonomic nervous system. (From Pick J: *The Autonomic Nervous System; Morphological, Comparative, Clinical, and Surgical Aspects*. Philadelphia, JB Lippincott, 1970. Used by permission.)

pressure, emotions, sleep, and sexual reflexes, it also has connections with the cerebral cortex and the limbic system.

The parasympathetic, or craniosacral, outflow is from four areas: (1) hypothalamus: supraoptic nucleus; (2) midbrain: Edinger-Westphal nucleus (cranial nerve III); (3) brain stem: superior salivary nucleus (VII), inferior salivary nucleus (IX), and the dorsal vagal nucleus (X); and (4) the sacral spinal cord. The sympathetic outflow is from the intermediolateral column of the thoracic and upper lumbar vertebral (T1–2 or L3 and more rarely C8, C7, or L4)[16, 73] (Fig 40–1).

The autonomic nervous system differs from the Somatic nervous system in that it innervates all bodily structures, except skeletal muscle, and reflex arcs synapse in ganglia outside the central nervous system (CNS) without apparent conscious control.

Peripheral Component

This portion of the autonomic nervous system consists of afferent sensory fibers and efferent motor fibers. Sensory neurons are considered as autonomic whenever they mediate afferent impulses from viscera and blood vessels. They synapse in dorsal root ganglia before flowing into the CNS. The efferent motor fibers, which course to glands, the heart, other visceral organs, and smooth muscles, consist of two neurons. The sympathetic preganglionic neuron fibers are short with numerous collaterals that synapse with many long postganglionic neuronal fibers in the paravertebral sympathetic chain. The parasympathetic system is the reverse: long preganglionic fibers with few collaterals that synapse with few short postganglionic fibers, usually at the innervated organ. This anatomic arrangement enables sympathetic discharge to spread widely throughout the body, whereas parasympathetic impulses remain confined to more limited areas. More specifically, the sympathetic outflow (Fig 40–2)[73] begins with a myelinated preganglionic nerve that travels with the spinal nerve out of the cord and then through the white ramus communicans to a ganglion either paravertebral, prevertebral, or terminal. An unmyelinated postganglionic fiber exits through the gray ramus communicans back to the spinal nerve and then with it to the organ, or it exits alone directly from a prevertebral ganglion to the organ.

Regionally, the peripheral sympathetic component essential for management of RSD consists of (1) the stellate ganglion and (2) the lumbar sympathetic chain. The stellate ganglion is composed of the 1st thoracic and inferior cervical ganglions in the fascial space just anterior to the prevertebral muscle at the level of the seventh cervical vertebra. The lumbar sympathetic plexus is formed by the anterior (ventral) divisions of the 1st, 2nd, 3rd, and 4th lumbar nerves with a branch from the 12th thoracic and the 5th lumbar nerves. It is located anterior to the transverse processes of the respective lumbar vertebrae.

Pharmacologic Aspects of the Autonomic Nervous System

At the adrenergic nerve terminal, norepinephrine is synthesized from tyrosine and hydroxylated to dopa; dopa is then decarboxylated to dopamine, which is hydroxylated to norepinephrine. In the adrenal medulla norepinephrine in the presence of phenylethanolamine-*N*-methyl transferase becomes epinephrine, which constitutes 80% of the catecholamine content in this gland. Norepinephrine is stored in vesicles along with a small amount of epinephrine, which may accumulate from the circulation. With electrical stimulation in the presence of calcium, catecholamines are released. Norepinephrine is recaptured by active transport into the terminal, which simultaneously terminates its effect. Its action is also terminated via dilution by diffusion out of the synaptic junction and by metabolic transformation. Monoamine oxidase (MAO) associated with the mitochondria works principally within the terminal, and catechol-*o*-methyl transferase (COMT) works in the cytoplasm to produce metanephrine or norme-

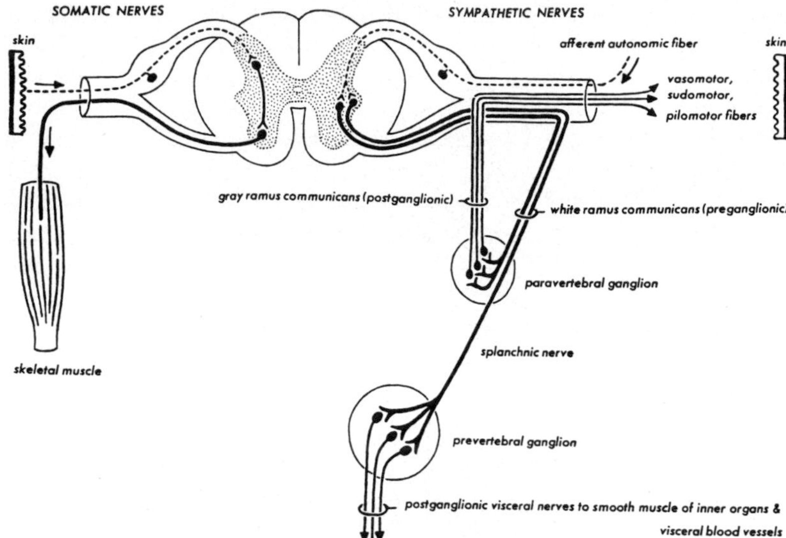

FIG 40-2.
Diagram illustrating the sympathetic outflow tract. (From Pick J: *The Autonomic Nervous System; Morphological, Comparative, Clinical, and Surgical Aspects*. Philadelphia, JB Lippincott, 1970, p 28. Used by permission.)

tanephrine. The metabolic product of both enzymes is 3-methoxy-4-hydroxymandelic acid, called vanillylmandelic acid (VMA), which is excreted in the urine.

Cocaine and imipramine (a tricyclic antidepressant) inhibit norepinephrine uptake and potentiate its effects. MAO inhibitors cause an increase of norepinephrine in the tissue but do not directly potentiate its effect. Reserpine depletes norepinephrine from the nerve terminal. Guanethidine and bretylium, which prevent the release of norepinephrine, however, transiently stimulate the release of norepinephrine by displacing it from storage sites.

Physiology of the Autonomic Nervous System

Functionally, *parasympathetic nerves* promote the secretion of the posterior lobe of the pituitary, shade the eye by causing the pupillary sphincter to contract, accommodate the ocular lens to near objects through the ciliary muscle, and protect the cornea from drying by lacrimal secretion. The parasympathetic component furthers the activity of the digestive system by inducing secretion of the salivary glands of the mouth, the pancreas, and the liver and by increasing the peristaltic movements of the intestine. Cardiac and pulmonary functions are inhibited by parasympathetic vagal fibers because they decrease the rate and force of the heart and produce contraction of the small bronchioli in the lungs. The significance of the parasympathetic component of the autonomic nervous system is essentially anabolic because it is directed toward the preservation, accumulation, and storage of energies in the body.

Sympathetic nerves widen the pupil through contraction of the pupillary dilator and inhibit peristalsis of the alimentary tract except for the contractions of the intestinal sphincters; however, they also accelerate the rate and force of the heart beat, elevate the blood pressure by vasoconstriction of wide areas of the body, and promote the secretory activity of the adrenal medulla and the exchange of gases in the pulmonary circulation by dilating the bronchioli of the lung.

The general effect of the sympathetic discharge, then, is catabolic because it causes expenditure of bodily energies and inhibits the intake and assimilation of nutrient matter. The body is thus endowed with several controllers of homeostasis, of which the autonomic nervous system is one.[73]

Historical Review of Reflex Sympathetic Dystrophy

Among the earliest descriptions of severe burning pain following peripheral nerve injury is that of the surgeon Ambroise Paré in the 17th century.[72] King Charles IX, ill with smallpox fever, was subjected to the current treatment of the day: bleeding induced by a lancet wound to the arm. Following this therapy, the king suffered from persistent pain, muscle contracture, and the inability to flex or extend his arm. Paré was called upon to treat the king, whose symptoms finally disappeared.

Severe burning pain in an extremity following nerve injuries was described in 1864 in soldiers by Mitchell and associates.[63] Mitchell subsequently introduced the term *causalgia* (from the Greek, meaning "burning pain") to describe the syndrome.[62] In the 1920s it was demonstrated that the pain of causalgia was often relieved by sympathetic blockade and that sympathectomy could effect permanent relief.[51, 52] It later became apparent that similar types of pain occurred after trauma or surgery in nonmilitary patients, many of whom had no obvious nerve injury.

The literature on causalgic pain is confusing not only because the pathophysiology is poorly understood but also because the terminology is far from uniform. The International Association for the Study of Pain (IASP)[39] proposed a taxonomy that defines RSD as "continuous pain in a portion of an extremity after trauma which may include fracture but does not involve a major nerve, associated with sympathetic hyperactivity. [11] The IASP regards causalgia as a similar but separate entity defined as "burning pain, allodynia, and hyperpathia, usually in the hand or foot, after partial injury of a nerve or one of its major branches." We adopt the terminology drawn up at the 1988 international symposium on RSD held in Mainz, Germany[40] which uses the term "reflex sympathetic dystrophy" to describe all of the syndromes listed in Table 40–1. Under this taxonomy, causalgia is included in RSD.

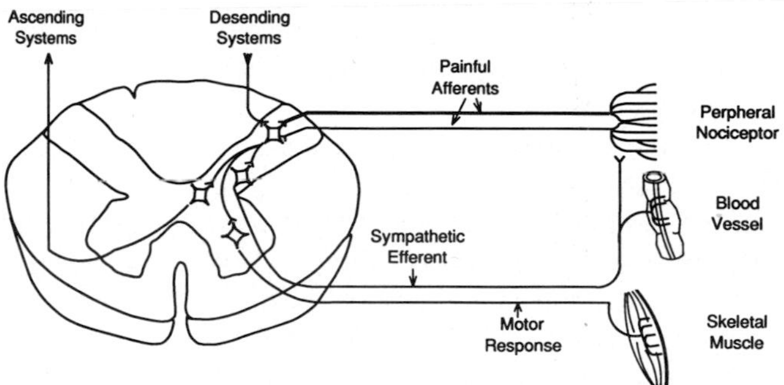

FIG 40–3.
A reflex arc is set into motion following a painful stimulus. Both an efferent sympathetic reflex and an efferent motor reflex may be initiated. This is a normal response to injury. Note the sensitization of the peripheral nociceptor by efferent sympathetic activity.

Mechanism of Reflex Sympathetic Dystrophy

The pathogenesis of RSD has been the subject of much attention. Many theories have been proposed to explain this disease, although none has proved conclusive, and it is likely that the explanation may involve mechanisms from several of the current theories. Mitchell[63] in 1864 suggested that the syndrome he would later name causalgia was the result of an ascending neuritis affecting a damaged peripheral nerve. The frequently observed failure of peripheral nerve block or surgery to abolish the pain indicated that more than a simple irritating peripheral lesion is involved. Section of the peripheral nerve at successively higher levels and even cutting the sensory pathway at a multitude of sites from the peripheral receptors to the somatosensory cortex has been attempted in the treatment of RSD; the initial results were encouraging, but there was a frustrating tendency for the pain to return.[16, 60, 89, 99]

Any proposed explanation for the pathophysiology of RSD must be able to explain the character of the pain, the relief of pain by sympathetic block in the early stages of the disease, and the observation that sympathectomy often fails to relieve pain in the later stages.[19, 50]

RSD may be thought of as a prolongation of the normal sympathetic response to injury.[13] A sympathetic reflex arc is the normal response to any traumatic injury. Painful afferent impulses from the periphery travel along A-delta and C fibers via the peripheral nerves to enter the spinal cord through the dorsal roots and synapse in the dorsal horn with interneurons carrying the impulses to either (1) ascending tracts, where they are then projected further to the thalamus and finally the somatosensory cortex; (2) to the anterior horn, where a motor reflex may be initiated via efferent motor fibers causing muscle contraction; or (3) to the intermediolateral cell column, where the painful message is relayed to the sympathetic nerve cell bodies. A sympathetic reflex (Fig 40–3) is activated by efferent sympathetic impulses sent out of the spinal cord via the ventral roots to a white ramus communicans and then into the sympathetic chain to synapse in a sympathetic ganglion. The postganglionic sympathetic fiber leaves the ganglia by way of the gray ramus where it travels with the peripheral nerve to the extremity to produce vasoconstriction. This is a normal reflex that usually gives way to vasodilatation as part of the orderly progression toward healing.[13, 48, 109] If this sympathetic reflex arc does not shut down but continues to function and accelerate, a sympathetic hyperdynamic state ensues. This results in increased vasoconstriction and tissue ischemia causing more pain and thus increasing the barrage of afferent pain impulses traveling to the spinal cord and reactivating the sympathetic reflex. This sympathetic efferent stimulation enhances the sensitivity of the nociceptor by causing vasoconstriction and ischemia, changes in vascular permeability, and smooth muscle contraction around the nociceptor; it also enhances nociceptor sensitivity by the direct action of locally released substances including norepinephrine, histamine, substance P, prostaglandins, and bradykinin. Thus sympathetic efferent activation of primary afferent nociceptors appears to be important in the development of RSD.

Why the hyperdynamic sympathetic state continues after the initial tissue injury has healed and why the critical pathophysiologic process seems to progress from the periphery to the CNS in the later stages of the disease[13, 60, 104] are not known, although many theories have been proposed to explain these phenomena.

These theories may be conveniently divided as to the site of origin of the pain impulses into peripheral tissue, peripheral nerve, and CNS abnormalities.[13, 98, 100]

Peripheral Tissues

Vasoconstriction and Vasodilatation.—Changes at the peripheral tissue level have been implicated by several authors as the cause of this persistent painful state. Both vasodilated and vasoconstricted states have been suggested.[26, 48, 52, 89] Leriche felt that vasoconstriction at the site of injury led to tissue ischemia and pain. Abnormal vasomotor reflexes were stated to be the cause of the vasospasm.[51] Lewis postulated that causalgia was a state of painful vasodilatation due to the liberation of pain-producing vasodilator substances in response to antidromic impulses arising from the area of nerve injury.[52]

Peripheral Nerve

Artificial Synapse.—Doupe and colleagues ascribed the peculiar qualities of causalgic pain to stimulation of afferent sensory fibers by crossover of impulses carried by efferent sympathetic fibers[29] (Fig 40–4). This theory states that an artificial synapse or ephapse is created at the damaged segment of the nerve by a breakdown in the normal insulation between adjacent fibers. Efferent sympathetic impulses, which are tonically active, can cross over to sensory fibers in the area of injury, travel centrally, and be interpreted as pain. Experimental support for this theory, unfortunately, is thin, although Granit and colleagues demonstrated that motor impulses can be "short-circuited" to sensory fibers in damaged nerve segments in cats.[33]

Fiber Dissociation.—An imbalance between fiber types that results from damage to a peripheral nerve is the basis for the "fiber dissociation" theory of Noordenbos[67] and the "gate control" theory of Melzack and Wall.[61]

Noordenbos proposed that within a nerve the large fibers are subject to proportionally more damage from a variety of injuries than are the smaller fiber types.[67] This produces an imbalance between the smaller pain-producing fibers and the now-decreased, larger inhibitory fibers. The result is a facilitation of small-fiber activity and finally an abnormal central response, which is felt to be the basis of causalgia.

Gate Theory.—Melzack and Wall introduced the "gate theory" of pain in 1965,[61] which is a refinement of the fiber dissociation theory[98, 109] (Fig 40–5). This theory proposed a balance of input by large A-beta and small A-delta and C fibers to the CNS. This balance could be upset by any number of pathologic processes including soft-tissue or peripheral nerve injury as in the reflex sympathetic dystrophies. According to this theory, large-fiber input inhibits (closes the gate) while small-fiber input facilitates (opens the gate) the spinal cord transmission of afferent impulses. Causalgia is felt to be due to selective damage to these large myelinated fibers that allows the balance to favor small-fiber activity and increases central transmission of the painful afferent impulses. Large-fiber stimulation may form the basis for the use of transcutaneous electrical nerve stimulation (TENS). TENS preferentially stimulates large fibers to "close" the gate and afford pain relief.[60, 66]

Neuroma Formation and Sprout Growth.—The observation that properties of nerves change markedly following injury has led to a model of RSD based upon neuroma formation.[13, 27, 61, 105]

Sensory fibers have their cell bodies in the dorsal root ganglia, just outside the spinal cord. When a nerve fiber is transected, the distal portion degenerates, for it is now separated from its cell body. As the distal part of the fiber degenerates, the debris is absorbed by neighboring cells. The proximal portion of the fiber sprouts in an attempt to reinnervate target organs. The sprouts advance at approximately 1 in. per month. The functional result is dependent upon the number of sprouts reaching specific target organs and the number of sprouts that instead become mired in fibrous tissue and form a neuroma.[58]

Wall and Gutnick have investigated the properties of these regenerating sprouts.[105] Several unusual properties were observed that may play a role in the pathogenesis of RSD. First, these sprouts are extremely sensitive to mechanical stimulation. This is the basis for Tinel's sign, where tapping gently over a neuroma or sprouts will produce a shooting pain. Second, some of these fibers originating in the neuroma are capable of generating impulses in the absence of any obvious stimulation. The midportion of an axon is normally only capable of impulse propagation; however, following injury it becomes capable of impulse generation. Third, these fibers were found to be easily excited by small amounts of epinephrine and norepinephrine. Norepinephrine is the neurotransmitter re-

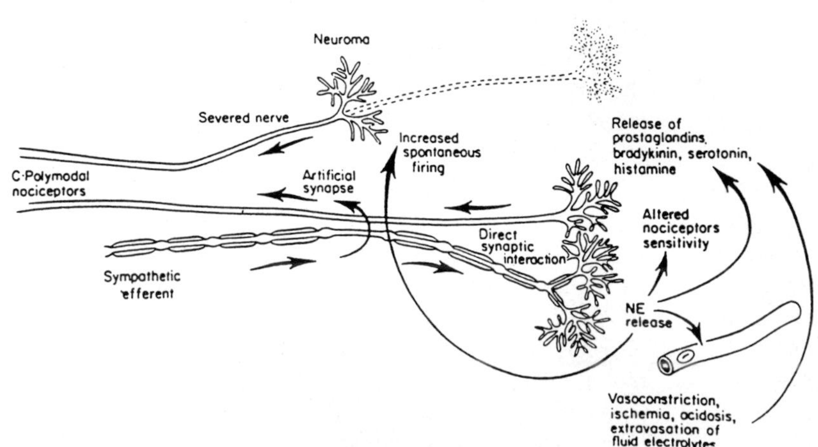

FIG 40–4.
Some proposed mechanisms of interaction between sympathetic efferent and nociceptive afferent fibers in causalgia. (From Raj PP: *Practical Management of Pain.* St Louis, Mosby–Year Book, 1986, p 211. Used by permission.)

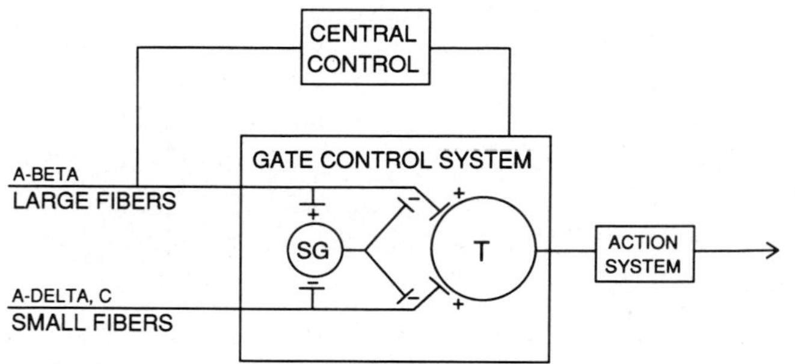

FIG 40–5.
The gate control theory. Large-fiber input inhibits while small-fiber input facilitates the transmission in the spinal cord of all afferent information. (From Melzack R, Wall PD: Pain mechanisms: A new theory. *Science* 1965; 150:971–979. Used by permission.)

leased by the sympathetic nerve fibers. The sympathetic fibers are in close proximity to the afferent pain-conducting fibers, and sympathetic stimulation may liberate substances that can excite the regenerating sprouts. Finally, the proximity of these sprouts and the lack of an intact endoneural sheath provide an opportunity for cross talk or ephaptic transmission between fibers as described earlier.

Central Mechanisms

Vicious Circle Hypothesis.—Livingston proposed a central mechanism for causalgia and related states.[54] He stated that distorted information processing in the spinal cord caused by abnormal firing patterns in the internuncial pool of neurons[25] sets up a vicious circle of reflexes responsible for causalgia. Livingston suggested that a partial nerve injury creates an irritative focus[54] (Fig 40–6). This

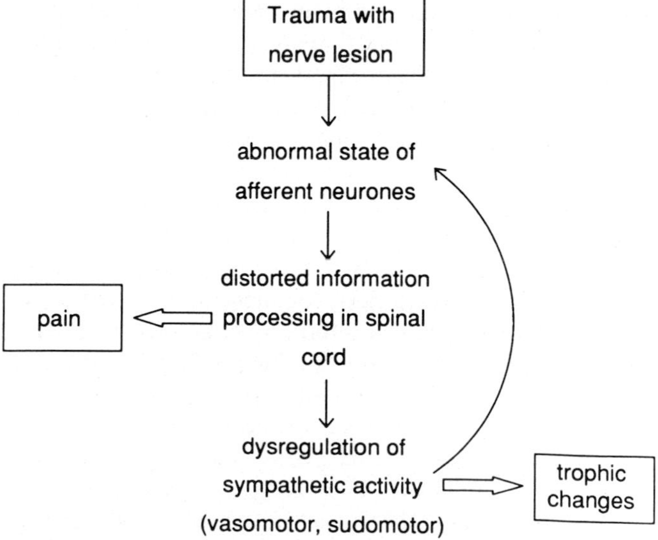

FIG 40–6.
Schematic expression of Livingston's hypothesis about the mechanism of generation of the syndrome of reflex sympathetic dystrophy. (From Blumberg H, Janig W: *J Auton Nerv Syst* 1983; 7:399–411. Used by permission.)

painful focus then serves to present the spinal cord with a constant bombardment of noxious impulses that overwhelm and upset the normal functioning of the internuncial pool. Abnormal firing patterns are initiated and spawn self-exciting neuronal loops in the dorsal horn of the spinal cord. Reverberating activity sends nerve impulses to higher centers, which are recognized as pain, and continued pool activity spreads to neurons in the anterior and lateral horns to give rise to reflex skeletal muscle spasm and sympathetic activation. This reinforces the painful peripheral focus that supports and augments the abnormal central activity. In time, this process becomes a self-sustaining, "vicious circle."

Turbulence Hypothesis.—Sunderland[98] supported Livingston's theory of a self-sustaining circle. Sunderland proposed that causalgia is the "functional expression of the retrograde neuronal reaction which follows nerve injury." When a peripheral nerve is injured, the distal portion degenerates. The proximal portion may also undergo retrograde changes that can affect the structure and function of parent cell bodies. The greater the violence causing the injury, the greater the retrograde reaction; thus an avulsion injury causes a more intense reaction than does surgical section of a nerve. Sunderland argues that the retrograde reaction can in fact cross a synapse and effect changes in neurons with which the initial damaged neuron communicates.[98] This transynaptic reaction may distort synaptic transmission and account for the derangement in internuncial pool activity. Thus, causalgia may be the result of peripheral nerve damage and lead to retrograde neuronal reaction with injury or death of the parent sensory ganglion cells and further transynaptic damage to the dorsal horn cells with which they are connected. This may generate abnormal spinal cord activity that becomes self-sustaining.

Spinal Cord Hyperexcitability.—The assumption that sympathetic efferent activation of primary afferent nociceptors forms the basis for RSD was questioned by Loh and Nathan[55] and later by Roberts.[84] Attempts to demonstrate sympathetic activation of primary afferent nociceptors have been largely unsuccessful according to Roberts.[85] He proposed that low-threshold mechanoreceptors and not nociceptors were responsible for the pain and allodynia in RSD. This is supported by the observation that a selective large (mechanoreceptor) fiber block can abolish the spontaneous pain and mechanical allodynia (touch-evoked pain) in patients with RSD.[15] Some spinal sensory neurons receive converging sensory input from both low- and high-threshold primary afferents. These are called wide–dynamic range (WDR) or convergent neurons. These neurons show increased responses to afferent activity following brief periods of noxious stimuli. They essentially become hyperexcitable, fire excessively in response

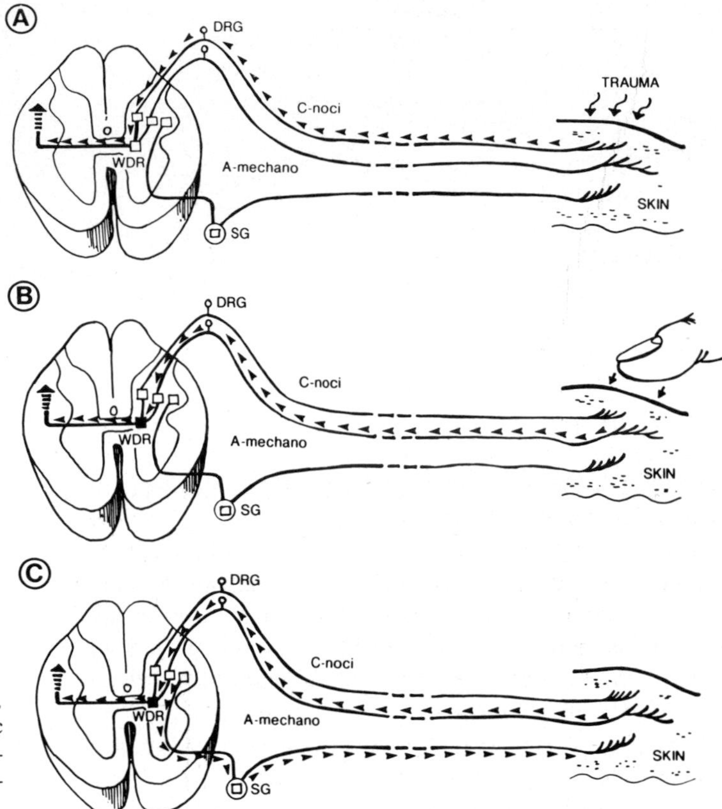

FIG 40–7.
Schematic of the relationship of the skin, dorsal root ganglion *(DRG)*, and sympathetic ganglion *(SG)*. Trauma sensitizes the wide–dynamic range *(WDR)* neurons. Activation of large A-beta fibers leads to excessive firing of hyperexcitable WDR neurons, which results in sympathetically mediated pain.

to subsequent stimulation, and thus produce pain.[86, 87] Roberts proposed the following hypothesis (Fig 40–7):

1. Trauma leads to the sensitization of spinal WDR neurons.

2. Subsequent sympathetic activation of low-threshold mechanoreceptor (large A-beta) fibers results in excessive firing of these sensitized or hyperexcitable WDR neurons and therefore spontaneous pain or "sympathetically mediated pain."

3. Mechanical (touch) activation of low-threshold mechanoreceptors results in excessive firing of these hyperexcitable neurons and therefore pain (allodynia or touch-evoked pain).

This theory explains the effectiveness of sympathetic blocks in RSD but cannot explain why TENS which stimulates large fibers, is often helpful in these patients.

CLINICAL PRESENTATION

Etiology

Traumatic

RSD can be produced after any of the etiologic agents tabulated in Table 40–2. Trauma secondary to accidental (or intentional) injury is probably the most common cause. Peculiar to sympathetic dystrophy is the lack of correlation between the severity of the initial injury and the subsequent incidence and severity of the resultant syndrome. In fact, severe trauma causing fractures of long bones and transection of nerves and blood vessels is less likely to be followed by RSD than are minor injuries to regions rich in nerve endings such as the skin and pulp of the fingertips, the skin of the hands, and the periarticular structures of the interphalangeal, wrist, and ankle joints. For example, RSD is a more common sequela of a Colles' fracture than previously recognized.[7, 8] In the majority of cases the precipitating injury may be so minor and to the patient so insignificant that one may forget the incident until or unless questioned by the physician. On the other hand, while accidental injuries are the most common cause of RSD, surgical procedures represent a form of tissue trauma, so they may also produce this syndrome, and both the patient and the physician may fail to consider surgery as an etiologic mechanism. RSD of the knee has been reported as a consistent complication of arthroscopy and total-knee arthroplasty.[6, 9, 41] Similarly, other therapeutic procedures may produce sufficient trauma to result in RSD. For example, this syndrome has developed after the application of casts, the accidental insertion of infusion needles into nerves, accidental extravasation of thiopental during induction of anesthesia, and injection of alcohol into or around a nerve in an attempt at chemical neurolysis.

Medical

The classic concept of RSD following some form of external violence has been so firmly established in the past that a history of trauma was expected or assumed when manifestations of RSD were present in an extremity. However, in recent years it has become obvious that while injury is the most common cause, many visceral, neurologic, vascular, and musculoskeletal disorders may also produce RSD, presumably by producing an injury to nerves that initiates a physiopathologic mechanism similar to if not identical with that produced by external trauma. Perhaps the most notable disease process that produces RSD is myocardial infarction, although other thoracic disorders such as pneumonitis, carcinoma, and embolism may be followed several months later by a full-blown RSD of the upper extremity. Similarly, RSD may develop in patients with lesions of the CNS. Of these, vascular accidents involving the brain, more particularly the thalamic region with consequent hemiplegia, are the most common, but the same syndrome may be produced by tumors and diseases involving the brain, brain stem, or spinal cord. Infectious processes may be the inciting agent that results in RSD almost without respect to the system involved in the infection, and certain peripheral vascular diseases such as thrombophlebitis often produce pain, edema, and vasomotor phenomena typical of RSD. In short, RSD can follow virtually any pathologic process that can befall the body, regardless of the magnitude of the process.

Signs and Symptoms

RSD is manifested by pain, hyperesthesia, vasomotor and sudomotor disturbances, increased muscular tone, and later weakness, atrophy, and trophic changes involving the skin, its appendages, muscles, bones, and joints.

Pain is certainly the most prominent and characteristic feature, and while it usually has a burning quality, not infrequently the patient describes it as an aching pain. It may vary in severity from mild discomfort to excruciating and intolerable pain such as what occurs with classic causalgia. The pain is usually constant but with recurrent paroxysmal aggravations. Initially the pain is localized to the site of injury, but typically with time it spreads to involve the entire extremity, and in certain cases, with the progression of time the pain even spreads beyond the affected extremity to the contralateral limb and sometimes even to the ipsilateral extremity or the entire side of the body. Hyperesthesia is almost invariably a part of the syndrome, and the patient characteristically protects the involved extremity in one way or another. Not infrequently, a patient will appear for treatment with the involved extremity wrapped in a protective cloth and one arm cradled in the other. If the examining physician attempts to touch the affected extremity, the patient characteristically withdraws and refuses to allow anything to make contact with it.

Disturbance of vasomotor function is the common denominator of all of the various types of sympathetic dystrophy and may be manifested by either signs of vasoconstriction, which produces cyanosis and coldness of the skin, or vasodilation, which results in a warm and erythematous extremity. In addition, not infrequently edema and sudomotor disturbances, usually hyperhidrosis, are also evident. As the disease progresses, trophic changes develop insidiously and include thin glossy skin, atrophy of muscle, decalcification of bones, and usually the loss of hair.[92]

The severity of the signs and symptoms vary from patient to patient and in the same patient in different stages of the disease. However, common to all cases of sympathetic dystrophy is the fact that the pain and physical signs do not conform to known patterns of nerve distribution, either segmental (dermatomes, myotomes, and sclerotomes) or peripheral. Moreover, they have a tendency to spread proximally so as to involve the contralateral and ipsilateral extremity. Once an RSD has become established, the entire syndrome will continue even after the etiologic mechanism has healed or disappeared. An important characteristic common to all of the sympathetic dystrophies is the fact that the symptoms can be abolished by sympathetic block at an appropriate level, and if carried out prior to the development of irreversibility, repetitive interruption of the sympathetic pathways involved can result in resolution of the entire syndrome.

COURSE OF THE DISEASE

The onset of RSD varies considerably: when provoked by external trauma, the onset is usually rapid, with the onset of symptoms immediately to several weeks after the injury. When the condition follows systemic disease, the onset may be slower and more insidious and may remain unrecognized until it becomes an irreversible process.

Stages

Sympathetic dystrophy has three stages, and the presenting signs and symptoms will vary somewhat depending upon the stage at the time the patient is first seen (Table 40–3).

Acute (Hyperemic) Stage

This stage commences at the time of injury or may be delayed for several weeks. It is characterized by constant pain, usually of a burning quality, of moderate severity, and localized to the area of injury. The pain is aggravated by movement and is associated with hyperpathia (delayed overreaction to a stimulus, particularly repetitive) and allodynia (pain elicited by a normally nonnoxious stimulus, particularly if repetitive or prolonged). Hyperesthesia (increased sensitivity) and hypoesthesia (decreased sensitivity) may also be present. The results are localized edema, muscle spasm, and tenderness. At this stage the skin is

TABLE 40–3.
Reflex Sympathetic Dystrophy: Clinical Staging Criteria

Feature	Stage 1, Acute	Stage 2, Dystrophic	Stage 3, Atrophic
1. Pain*	Burning+++	Burning+++	Burning+++
2. Sensory disturbance*	++	+++	+
3. Function deficit*	++	+++	++++
4. Blood flow*	Increased	Same or decreased	Decreased
1. Temperature†	Increased	Decreased	Decreased or no change
2. Appearance†	Erythematous	Mottled	Cyanotic
3. Sudomotor†	Minimal	++	+++
4. Edema†	++	+++	+
5. Trophic changes†	0	++	++++

*Must have three of four.
†Must have three of five.

usually warm, red, and dry because of vasodilatation, although signs of vasoconstriction sometimes predominate late in this stage. Toward the end of this stage the skin becomes smooth and taut, with a decrease or loss of normal wrinkles and creases. Radiographs taken in this stage usually show slight if any osteoporosis. In mild cases the first stage lasts only a few weeks, while in severe cases this stage may last as long as 6 months. During this stage, the syndrome can often be completely reversed by sympathetic blockade.

Dystrophic (Ischemic) Stage

If the acute stage is untreated, it can be expected to progress to the second (dystrophic) stage. This stage is characterized by spreading of the edema, increasing stiffness of the joints, and muscular wasting. Pain remains the major symptom and is usually spontaneous and burning in nature. It may radiate proximally or distally from the site of injury and may involve the whole extremity. Hyperpathia and allodynia are usually more pronounced than in the first stage. The skin is moist, cyanotic, and cold; the hair is coarse, and the nails show ridges and are brittle. Signs of atrophy become more prominent, and radiographs usually reveal patchy osteoporosis. During this stage, sympathetic blocks may still be effective in reversing the process, although the response to blockade may be less pronounced and short-lived. A larger series of blocks or prolonged sympathetic blockade may be necessary to provide permanent relief.

Atrophic Stage

The third stage is characterized by marked trophic changes that eventually progress to irreversibility. Pain is a less prominent feature. The skin becomes smooth, glossy, and tight; its temperature is lowered, and it appears pale or cyanotic in color. While the hair has become long as this stage is entered, by the end of the third stage, the hair has usually fallen out. The subcutaneous tissues are atrophic, as are the muscles, particularly the interossei. There is extreme weakness and limitation of motion at virtually all of the involved joints, which finally become ankylosed. Contractions of the flexor tendons often occur at this stage; osteoporosis is more advanced, and the pain is aggravated by weight bearing, movement, and frequently by exposure to cold. At this point many of the trophic changes produced by the syndrome become irreversible, and while interruption of sympathetic pathways by blocks may still provide temporary relief, repetitive sympathetic blocks alone are no longer effective in terminating the process permanently. An aggressive approach including physical therapy, psychological counseling, and sympathetic and somatic nerve blockade is needed to reverse the process as much as possible. No longer is the pathophysiology confined to an aberrant sympathetic reflex arc. Other nerve fiber types are now involved, including A-beta (mechanoreceptors), A-delta, and C (nociceptor) fibers. At this point the process may not respond to neural blockade, either chemical or surgical, performed at any point in the neuraxis because the self-sustaining mechanism may have moved to higher CNS centers out of reach of scalpel or syringe.

Diagnosis

A diagnosis of RSD may be obvious if (1) there is a history of recent or remote trauma, infection, or disease; (2) there is persistent, spontaneous pain that may be burning, aching, or throbbing in character; (3) there are vasomotor and/or sudomotor disturbances; and (4) there are obvious trophic changes. However, while the "typical" case of RSD can be diagnosed without difficulty, many cases do not present with classic signs and symptoms, but with vague and confusing symptomatology that not infrequently simulates other diseases. A number of diagnostic RSD scales have been proposed.[5] Current criteria under investigation by Wilson are shown in Table 40–4.[107] We use a scoring system devised by Raj et al.,[82] which allows for both the diagnosis and also the staging of the patient's disease (Table 40–3).

TABLE 40–4.
Putative Diagnostic Criteria for Reflex Sympathetic Dystrophy*

Clinical symptoms and signs
  Burning pain
  Hyperpathia/allodynia
  Temperature/color changes
  Edema
  Hair/nail growth changes
Laboratory results
  Thermography/thermometry
  Bone x-ray
  Three-phase bone scan
  Quantitative sweat test
  Response to sympathetic blockade
Interpretation
  >6, probable RSD
  3–5, possible RSD
  <3, unlikely RSD

*From Wilson P: Sympathetically maintained pain, in *Sympathetic Pain*, Boston, Kluwer, 1989. Used by permission.

Differential Diagnosis

Several postoperative or post-traumatic conditions have symptoms in common with causalgia and RSD. Peripheral nerve injuries may produce burning dysesthetic pain without a sympathetic nervous system component. Hyperpathia is frequently encountered within the distribution of transected or entrapped nerves. Pain is limited to the distribution of the involved nerve, and a positive Tinel sign is often elicited over the site of nerve injury.

Inflammatory lesions such as tenosynovitis or bursitis may produce post-traumatic pain that may be burning in quality and may persist for months. Myofascial pain often develops after injury or surgery. It is nondermatomal in distribution, may be burning in nature, and is characterized by sensitive trigger points in affected muscles.[59] Although the truncal musculature is most often affected, such problems may also involve the extremities.

Raynaud's disease produces vasospasm of the extremities along with cold skin, pallor, and often cyanosis. The condition is bilateral and involves the hands and sometime all four extremities. The vasospasm may be relieved by sympathetic blocks, but most patients are not helped by such treatment. Patients who experience transient vasodilation with sympathetic blocks may benefit from sympathectomy or systemic α-adrenergic blocking agents.

Raynaud's phenomenon, a similar vasospastic disorder, is associated with an underlying pathologic process, frequently one of the connective tissue diseases such as scleroderma, and is often unilateral. As with Raynaud's disease, sympathetic blocks are helpful in a minority of patients.

Establishing an absolute diagnosis for a chronic pain problem is usually difficult since multiple pain mechanisms often exist. It is often possible, however, to assess the importance of sympathetic mechanisms by comparing the degree and duration of pain relief achieved by sympathetic blocks with that produced by somatic blocks and placebo injections.

The response to a placebo injection (e.g., intramuscular saline) is often helpful diagnostically. A true placebo response, which is elicited in about one third of patients with chronic pain, is usually brief (10 to 30 minutes). Pain relief persisting for days or weeks probably signifies a psychogenic pain mechanism. A very transitory response to the placebo and a prolonged analgesic effect from a sympathetic block (hours or days) provides some assurance that sympathetics are involved in the pathogenesis of the pain. If no analgesia occurs after sympathetic blockade and pain is relieved by blocking the appropriate somatic nerves, then a somatic pain mechanism such as neuralgia, myofascial syndrome, or radiculopathy is likely. Failure of both sympathetic and somatic blockade to produce analgesia points to a central type of pain mechanism, which may be psychogenic or may result from neuronal activity within the CNS that is independent of peripheral input.

For lower-extremity pain, a differential spinal block may be used to distinguish among sympathetic, somatic, and central pain mechanisms. After the needle is placed in the subarachnoid space and the patient is positioned laterally, 10 mL of normal saline is injected. Relief of pain is interpreted as a placebo response. If no analgesia occurs, 10 mL of 0.25% procaine is injected, which should block preganglionic sympathetic fibers while sparing somatic fibers. If signs of sympathetic blockade develop and pain relief ensues, a sympathetic pain mechanism is likely. If no analgesia occurs, 10 mL of 0.5% procaine is injected, and the pain is reassessed after the onset of somatic blockage. Analgesia is interpreted as evidence of a somatic mechanism. A lack of pain relief points to a central or psychogenic mechanism.

Winnie has suggested a simpler differential block procedure done in retrograde fashion.[108] The placebo saline injection is first carried out. Subsequently, 2 mL of 5% procaine is injected to produce motor, sensory, and sympathetic blockade. If the block produces analgesia and the pain recurs as the somatic block wears off while the sympathetic blockade persists, a somatic mechanism is likely. If it recurs only after the sympathetic blockade regresses, a sympathetic mechanism is assumed to be responsible for the pain.

This retrograde differential study can also be done as an epidural block, with less chance of post–lumbar puncture headache.[80] Table 40–5 shows data from a retrograde differential epidural block in a 22-year-old man who developed RSD following a traumatic medial malleolar fracture.

TABLE 40–5.
Retrograde Differential Epidural Block*†

				Objective Findings					
				Motor Power			Temperature (°F)		
Time (min)	BP (mm Hg)	Pulse (Beats/min)	Subjective Feelings	Leg	Knee Bend	Toes	Sensation on Pinprick	R Leg	L Leg
Control	134/84	60	Burning pain in left foot					91	86
0	148/80	64	Burning pain in left foot	X	X	X	X	90	86
10	120/80	88	75% pain relief	25%	X	X	T10	95	90
20	114/82	76	Total pain relief				T8	95	92
60	140/96	64	Total pain relief	X	X	X	T12	95	92
70	140/96	64	Total pain relief	X	X	X	X	94	92
80	138/94	64	Total pain relief	X	X	X	X	92	90

*From Raj PP: *Practical Management of Pain*. St Louis, Mosby–Year Book, 1986. Used by permission.
†The results of a differential block (20 mL of 3% 2-chloroprocaine) in a 22-year-old man with pain in the left foot. At first evaluation at the pain control center the patient gave the history of a motor vehicle accident 6 months previously. He sustained a medial malleolar fracture at the ankle that was surgically corrected and put in a cast. The fracture healed normally, but the patient complained of burning pain in his left foot, especially after weight bearing. A diagnosis of reflex sympathetic dystrophy of the left leg was made, and a retrograde differential epidural block was done to confirm the diagnosis. The findings seen above show that total relief of pain was obtained by blocking the C fibers only. A-delta and A-alpha nerve fibers did not transmit the nociceptive impulses. A series of six lumbar sympathetic blocks were done at 2-week intervals with adjuvant physical therapy. The patient recovered completely.

Investigations

Several clinical measurements and laboratory investigations are helpful in the diagnosis and treatment of patients with RSD. These studies are helpful in confirming the diagnosis, determining the stage and severity of the disease, and obtaining objective baseline information that can then be used to monitor the patient's response to therapy.

Temperature Measurement

Temperature changes in the affected extremity are a simple but important observation to record during examination of the patient with suspected RSD. Skin temperature is dependent upon cutaneous blood flow, and this in turn is under the control of the sympathetic nervous system. Early in the course of RSD (hyperemic stage), the affected extremity may be warmer, while later in the course skin blood flow and temperature may be reduced. While the examiner's perception of a temperature difference between the two extremities by touch offers a gross qualitative temperature measurement, surface thermistors and hand-held infrared thermometers allow for quantification and baseline recordings.[21]

Thermography

Thermography is a noninvasive procedure that images the temperature distribution of the body surface. In contrast to radiography, computed tomography (CT), or myelography, which show only anatomic changes, thermography demonstrates functional changes in circulation consequent to damage to nerves, ligaments, muscles, or joints.[75, 76, 101, 107]

Fine-Detail Radiography

The earliest radiographic evidence of sympathetic hyperdysfunction includes patchy demineralization of the epiphyses and short bones of the hands and feet. Subperiosteal resorption, striation, and tunneling of the cortex may occur. However, these unilateral changes are not diagnostic of RSD and may occur in any condition producing disuse of one limb. This patchy osteopenia is generally not appreciated until the disease advances to the second stage.[5, 31, 37]

Triple-Phase Scintigraphy/Bone Scan and Bone Density

Three-phase radionuclide bone scanning is helpful in both confirming the diagnosis of RSD and excluding other conditions that could be a cause of symptoms.[107] The sensitivity and specificity of this technique have varied, largely due to a lack of common diagnostic criteria.[20, 34, 47] The scan pattern most commonly associated with RSD is that of increased flow to the involved extremity and delayed static images that show diffusely increased activity throughout the involved extremity, usually in a periarticular distribution.[20]

Based on more recent refinement of bone scan criteria, grading of RSD was performed by evaluating both early (flow and blood pool) images and delayed (static) images according to the system in Table 40–6.[107]

Interpretation of Bone Scans.—In a study of 24 patients with RSD by Raj and Lowry et al., bone scans were obtained as part of the initial workup.[107] Most of the scans clearly defined as consistent with RSD had the features of stage 1 RSD (i.e., increased activity on both early and delayed images, with static images showing diffusely increased uptake in a somewhat periarticular distribution). A differential diagnosis is not usually a problem since few conditions mimic this scan appearance and clinical information provides specificity. However, somewhat similar

TABLE 40–6.

Triple-Phase Bone Scan Findings in Reflex Sympathetic Dystrophy at Various Stages of the Disease*

Stage	Flow†	Early (Blood Pool Phase)†	Delayed Static Phase†
1	↓	↑	↑
2	N	N	↑
3	↓	↓	N

*From Raj P, Cannella J, Kelly J, et al: Management protocol of reflex sympathetic dystrophy, in Stanton-Hicks M, Janig WP (eds): *Reflex Sympathetic Dystrophy* Boston, Kluwer, 1989. Used by permission.
†Uptake of radioisotope: ↑ = increased; N = normal; ↓ = decreased.

scan appearances may occur in several conditions, including disuse, cellulitis, degenerative joint disease, recent trauma, and osteomyelitis. The clinical presentation, time course of the disease, and scan appearance should help differentiate these conditions.

False-negative bone scan results may be fairly common. Many "normal" scans correspond to stage 2 RSD as determined on clinical grounds. The most likely explanation is that as the condition progresses, the initial state of hyperemia becomes, in later stages, that of decreased flow. Because this change occurs gradually, the disease passes through an intermediate stage of "normal" perfusion, at which time the bone scan appearance may be entirely normal as well. In these cases, the diagnosis remains an entirely clinical one, and the bone scan is helpful only to rule out other causes of the patient's pain (i.e., occult fracture, infection, etc.). Magnetic resonance imaging (MRI), although not helpful in establishing the diagnosis of RSD, may improve the diagnostic sensitivity of scintigraphy.[46]

Bone Density Measurement.—Nuclear bone density measurements provide a quantitative measure of bone density as a baseline.

Electromyography

There is no evidence that peripheral neuromuscular function is abnormal in sympathetic pain states. Abnormalities seen on electromyography (EMG) may reflect the initial injury, although evidence for EMG changes as RSD develops is lacking.[5, 27]

Tests of Sudomotor Function

Sympathetic cholinergics control sweating, and an estimate of sweat production can be made by a variety of methods. Surface moisture can be demonstrated by the application of triketohydrindene hydrate (Ninhydrin), cobalt blue, or starch-iodide to the skin. A quantitative method has recently been devised: the quantitative sudomotor axon reflex test (Q-SART). A Perspex capsule is placed on the skin, and the increase in humidity of air blown through the capsule is measured. Sweat output can then be stimulated by iontophoresis of acetylcholine into the skin, and stimulated sweat output can be measured. The stimulated output is greater and prolonged when sympathetic hyperfunction is present.[56]

Differential Studies

Mixed peripheral nerves contain a variety of fiber types classified as A, B, and C fibers based on the work of Gasser and Erlanger who demonstrated that the compound action potential of a mixed peripheral nerve changes with varying distance of the stimulating electrode.[30] The A fibers have been further separated into alpha, beta, gamma, and delta subtypes. A-delta fibers carry sharp pain, while C fibers carry dull burning pain, and preganglionic autonomic fibers are called B fibers. Susceptibility to local anesthetic agents follows a fairly well-ordered progression of B (preganglionic autonomic) fibers followed by C fibers and then A-delta fibers. This differential is the basis for this investigation, which helps to pinpoint the fiber type carrying the painful impulse, and thus aids in the diagnosis and treatment.

Intravenous Phentolamine

Raja and colleagues have described the use of intravenous phentolamine (total dose, 25 to 35 mg) as a diagnostic test for sympathetically maintained pain (SMP).[83] By comparing the effects on pain of local anesthetic sympathetic ganglion blocks (LASB) of the stellate or lumbar sympathetic chain with intravenous phentolamine, an α-adrenergic blocking agent, a close correlation ($r = 0.84$) was found between the use of LASB and phentolamine. Thus, α-adrenergic blockade with intravenous phentolamine seems to be a sensitive alternative to LASB to identify patients with RSD.

Psychological Evaluation

The psychological assessment is conducted in order to obtain an understanding of the psychosocial stressors that may adversely affect treatment or to obtain information about the psychological distress patients may be experiencing as a result of the pain and subsequent loss of functioning. The evaluation should consist of a structured clinical interview and personality measures such as the Minnesota Multiphasic Personality Inventory (MMPI) and the hopelessness index.

Previous pilot research indicate that as the RSD progresses, the patients' MMPI profiles tend to resemble those of patients experiencing chronic pain, as revealed by the increasing elevations on the hypochondriasis, depression, and hysteria scales. Stage 1 patients also report more pessimism than do patients in the second and third stages of the disorder, which suggests that the patients have more difficulty adjusting to the disorder in the early stages. Younger patients with RSD tend to report more pessimism and symptoms of depression than do older patients.[107]

CURRENT TREATMENT

Since the pathophysiology of RSD is predominantly hyperactivity of the regional sympathetic nervous system, it is rational for management of pain in such patients to focus treatment on interrupting the activity of the sympathetic nervous system. This interruption can be produced by different modalities. These modalities are classified as pharmacologic, nerve blocks, surgical and chemical sympathectomy, physical therapy, and psychology. In addition, a serious effort has to be made toward maintaining function and alleviating the stresses produced by the syndrome on the CNS.

Reports of treatment efficacy in RSD are plagued by the lack of uniform quantification of treatment outcome, as defined by a change in pain or improvement in function. This nonuniformity of outcome measurement as well as inconsistent diagnostic criteria makes it difficult to draw hard inferences from many published therapeutic trials in patients with RSD.[23]

Pharmacologic Treatment

Many drugs have been used in the treatment of RSD. Drugs from all of the classes seen in Table 40–7 have been utilized. The reason why such a wide variety of unrelated agents have been used in treating RSD is that patients suffering from this syndrome can go through periods of severe pain, limited function, and depression and eventually develop the characteristics of the "chronic pain syndrome," defined as involving chronic intractable pain with major behavioral changes, multiple nonproductive treatments, and the absence of a clear relationship of complaints to organic findings.[17, 95]

For example, a patient with RSD may have severe pain requiring analgesics, often opiates, which are particularly difficult to wean in these patients. As the disease progresses, anxiety mounts concerning the chronicity of the illness, loss of work, and social and familial dysfunction, and anxiolytics are required. Sleep is lost to pain and worry, which prompts the use of a sedative-hypnotic. Exhaustion develops both physically and emotionally. The situation magnifies, and hope for improvement dampens with increasing depression. Tricyclic antidepressants may be then prescribed. Sympathetic hyperdysfunction causes vasoconstriction, pain, and swelling as detailed above, and this necessitates sympathetic blockade with local anesthetics, sympathetic blocking drugs, or vasodilatation with vasodilating drugs. A myofascial pain component is common in RSD; thus a nonsteroidal anti-inflammatory agent and a muscle relaxant are often utilized. At times, anticonvulsants are used to quiet a painful peripheral or central focus of lancinating or shooting pain. Rarely, neurolytic agents are used to destroy the sympathetic pathways.

TABLE 40–7.
Drugs Used in the Treatment of Reflex Sympathetic Dystrophy

Antidepressants
Sedative-hypnotics
Anxiolytics
Anticonvulsants
Muscle relaxants
Narcotic analgesics
Nonnarcotic analgesics
Nonsteroidal anti-inflammatory agents
Corticosteroids
Local anesthetics
Sympathetic blocking agents
Vasodilators
Neurolytics

Antidepressants

Three effects of tricyclic antidepressants make this class valuable in the treatment of RSD: sedation, analgesia, and mood elevation. Amitriptyline is used most commonly in a dose of 25 to 100 mg orally at bedtime. The analgesic action of the tricyclics may be related to inhibition of serotonin reuptake at nerve terminals of neurons, which acts to suppress pain transmission, with resultant prolongation of serotonin activity at the receptor.[38] If that indeed is the mechanism, then amitriptyline, which has the most potent effect on the amine pump, should be the most effective of the tricyclics. Others, however, are used for their varying anticholinergic, weight gain, and sexual dysfunction properties.[2, 69, 71]

Narcotic Analgesics

Systemic narcotics are often abused by those with chronic pain and eventually do little to treat sympathetic pain because tolerance develops and alternate pathways may be used by nociceptive impulses. In an acute inpatient setting, however, when given epidurally in combination with local anesthetics, narcotics are extremely effective analgesics.[4, 90]

In addition, this route allows maximum narcotic effect in the dorsal horn with very low plasma concentrations and thus minimizes toxicity. Both morphine and fentanyl have been used by continuous infusion in doses of 0.5 mg/hr and 0.03 to 0.05 mg/hr, respectively. For chronic oral therapy, narcotics are used sparingly and only if other nonnarcotic agents have been tried without success. However, in an inpatient setting a carefully ordered narcotic regimen may be necessary in order to promote effective physical therapy in patients otherwise restricted by pain. In this setting morphine and methadone have both been used with success.

Oral Nifedipine

Following reports of the use of oral nifedipine in the treatment of Raynaud's phenomenon[88] and RSD,[68, 79] we have begun using orally administered nifedipine to relieve the symptoms of RSD. Nifedipine, a calcium entry blocker, relaxes smooth muscle, increases peripheral blood flow, and antagonizes the effect of norepinephrine on arterial and venous smooth muscle. Thus, it induces peripheral vasodilation. Experience with this technique suggests that nifedipine in an oral dose of 30 to 90 mg daily may be an effective therapeutic option for the treatment of patients with RSD. In a series of 13 patients with RSD treated with nifedipine,[69] 7 had complete relief of symptoms, 2 had partial relief, and 1 patient failed to obtain any degree of relief. Nifedipine therapy was withdrawn from 3 other patients because of the side effect of headache. Symptoms of lesser intensity may recur when the drug is withdrawn and are usually relieved upon reinstitution of the drug. Although a number of side effects of nifedipine have been reported, the only frequent and troubling side effect observed is that of headache.

The newer therapeutic techniques for management of patients with RSD provide options that are less invasive and generally better tolerated by patients. It is difficult to predict which technique will be most efficacious in any given patient. One would suppose that patients who are not responsive to one of these forms of therapy would similarly be unresponsive to the other forms of therapy. However, it is not uncommon for a patient to be unresponsive to one technique and yet derive benefits, either transient or permanent, from one of the other alternatives discussed.

Systemic Corticosteroids

Kozin et al.[47] advocate a several-day course of high-dose systemic corticosteroids. They reported an 82% success rate in patients with "definite" RSD. Their criteria, however, were not very rigid, and three of the most important ones, burning pain, hyperpathia, and response to sympathetic blockade, were not among them. Many of the patients who responded to steroids had very chronic pain (the mean duration of pain for the group was 25 weeks), and a trial of steroids might be a reasonable form of treatment for patients with long-standing pain who have failed to respond to blocks.

Adrenergic Blocking Agents

The systemic use of adrenergic blocking agents has met with only limited success. Several patients treated by McLeskey, all of whom had pain for more than 6 months, experienced moderate improvement in pain, swelling, and vasoconstriction with oral prazosin. The most gratifying response was in a patient with recurrent foot pain after sympathectomy. Intravenous phentolamine appears to be useful in predicting favorable responses to prazosin because only those patients who experienced pain relief and increased skin temperature in the affected limb responded to the oral medication. Orthostatic dizziness was seen occasionally with prazosin and precluded its continued use in a few patients. Propranolol has been reported to be effective in the management of RSD.[94, 103]

Nerve Blocks

Although the causal mechanisms of RSD are not limited purely to sympathetic hyperactivity, sympathetic blockade along with physical therapy is the mainstay of current therapeutic management. Most patients respond in an impressive manner to sympathetic blockade, and permanent resolution is possible if therapy is instituted before irreversible changes have occurred.

A series of sympathetic blocks should be performed and continued until minimal discomfort persists. If repeat injections in this manner are not possible, e.g., the patient's reluctance for multiple needle sticks or the inability of the patient to travel because of injury or distance, then admission to the hospital for continuous infusion of local anesthetic at the appropriate site is an alternative. For the upper extremity the site of block is either at the stellate ganglion level or on the brachial plexus (Fig 40–8,A and B). Continuous stellate ganglion blockade has been reported with the use of an indwelling catheter. In a series of 29 patients with upper-extremity RSD, improvement was seen in all but 2 patients with regard to pain. Long-term follow-up demonstrated a relapse rate of 25%, but marked improvement persisted in the rest of the patients.[53] There are numerous approaches available for blockade of the brachial plexus (Figs 40–9 to 40–12). For repetitive blocks, the axillary approach is the most convenient. The infraclavicular approach as described by Raj et al.[81] is excellent for continuous infusion techniques. The thoracic sympathetic chain is not a convenient site for repeated injections, is technically difficult, and requires the use of radiographic guidance. For lower-extremity disease, the lumbar sympathetic chain or epidural space is the preferred site for sympathetic blockade (Fig 40–13). Either of these sites can be used with repetitive injection and continuous infusion techniques. Wang et al. treated 71 patients with lower-extremity RSD.[106] Of the 27 patients treated by conservative means, 41% showed improvement at 3 years. Of the 43 patients treated with sympathetic blockade, 65% experienced progress at the 3-year evaluation.

Neurolytic sympathetic blockade for RSD of the upper extremity is not commonly performed because of the close proximity of the cervical nerve roots to the cervical sympathetic chain. However, lumbar sympathetics are very amenable to neurolytic blockade and may be chosen as an alternative to surgical sympathectomy for persistent lower-extremity involvement.

Treatment methods gaining popularity include the intravenous regional block (Bier block) technique employing reserpine, guanethidine, and bretylium, as well as the use of nifedipine, a calcium channel blocker as a vasodilator.[14, 24, 42, 77, 96, 102]

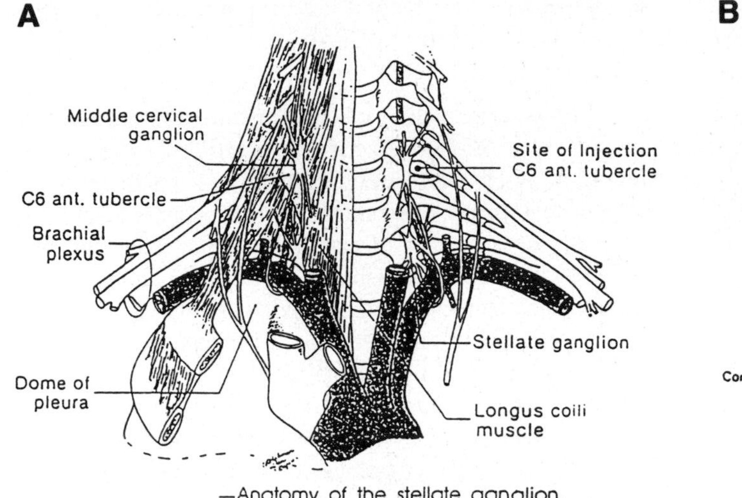

FIG 40–8.
Surface landmarks and needle position for a stellate ganglion block. Note that the head is well extended. The anesthetist's fingers retract the carotid sheath laterally with the needle at the C6 level in the paratracheal space. (From Raj PP: *The Practical Management of Pain*. St Louis, Mosby–Year Book, 1986, p 662. Used by permission.)

Intravenous Regional Block (Bier Block)

Intravenous or intra-arterial infusion of ganglionic blocking agents into the affected extremity have recently gained prominence.[11, 14, 42] There are two reasons why the intravenous administration of ganglionic blockers is superior to intra-arterial injection for the treatment of RSD. First, the likelihood of systemic side effects from an injection of these vasodilating agents is significantly greater if administered intra-arterially than if administered in an intravenous regional block (Bier block) technique. Second, it has been proposed that when these drugs are administered by an intravenous regional anesthetic technique, they are permitted to have more protracted contact with the affected extremity to allow them to fix to the tissue and, optimally, produce more significant and prolonged improvement in symptomatology. Experience with intravenous

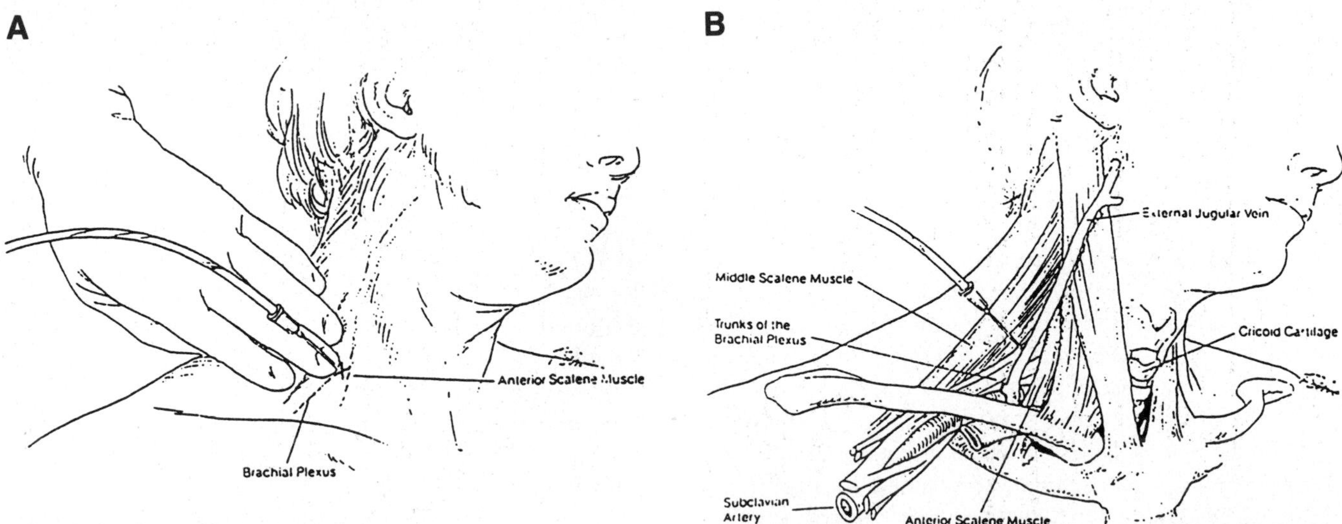

FIG 40–9.
A and **B,** superficial landmarks, site of entry, and position of the needle for the interscalene approach to a brachial plexus block. Note that in **B** the needle usually contracts the upper part of the trunk. (From Raj PP, Pai U: Techniques of nerve blocking, in Raj PP (ed): *Handbook of Regional Anesthesia,* New York, Churchill Livingstone, 1985. Used by permission.)

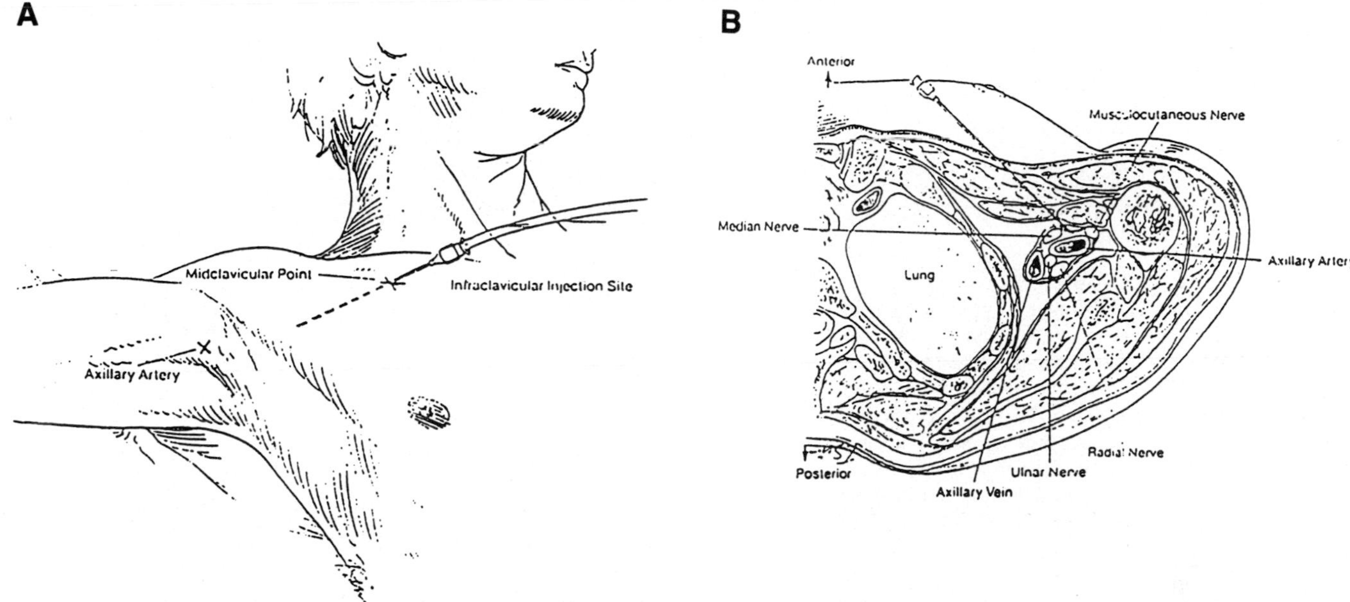

FIG 40–10.
A, technique of a brachial plexus block by the intraclavicular approach. A 22-gauge, 3½-in. needle is directed from 1 in. below the midpoint of the clavicle toward the brachial artery in the upper part of the arm. The needle is at a 45-degree angle to the skin. **B,** horizontal section of the axillary space showing the relationship of the axilla and the direction of the needle laterally from the point of entry. (From Raj PP, Pai U: Techniques of nerve blocking, in Raj PP (ed): *Handbook of Regional Anesthesia*. New York, Churchill Livingstone, 1985. Used by permission.)

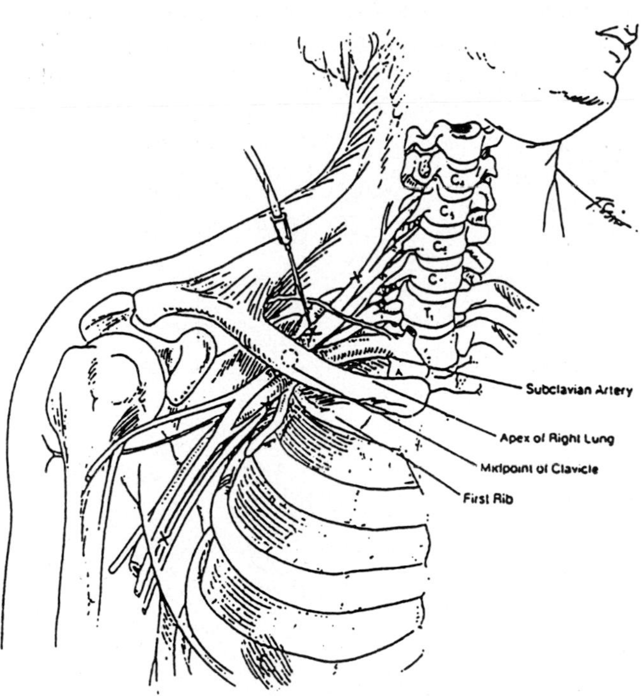

FIG 40–11.
Direction of the needle (backward, inward, and downward) for the supraclavicular approach to a brachial plexus block. The point of entry is 1 cm superior to the upper border of the clavicle at its midpoint. (From Raj PP, Pai U: Techniques of nerve blocking, in Raj PP (ed): *Handbook of Regional Anesthesia*. New York, Churchill Livingstone, Inc., 1985)

regional reserpine techniques is controversial. Abrams[1] and Brown[14] have found the results of this technique to be sporadic and side effects including postural hypotension, facial flushing, and burning on injection to be relatively common.

In an attempt to improve results and lessen side effects during the treatment of patients with RSD, guanethidine has been substituted for reserpine in the intravenous regional block (Brier block) format. Results with intravenous regional guanethidine techniques from Europe and selected North American centers appear to be more consistent and more reliable than those with intravenous regional reserpine.[36, 47, 96] Twenty milligrams of guanethidine is diluted in 40 mL of 0.25% lidocaine for upper-extremity blocks or 50 mL of 0.25% lidocaine for lower-extremity blocks. The solution is injected into an exsanguinated extremity with drug contact permitted for 30 to 45 minutes by tourniquet inflation. McLeskey et al. found partial or complete success in the treatment of painful symptoms in 25 of 35 patients treated in this manner. Repeat blocks were required in 4 of these patients. The average duration of improvement of symptomatology was 17 days, with complete, permanent relief of symptoms in 3 patients. Side effects following intravenous regional guanethidine blockade are less often seen than with intravenous regional reserpine blocks. However, patients frequently complaining of a burning pain in the extremity during injection of the drug that lasts for approximately 4 to 5 minutes.

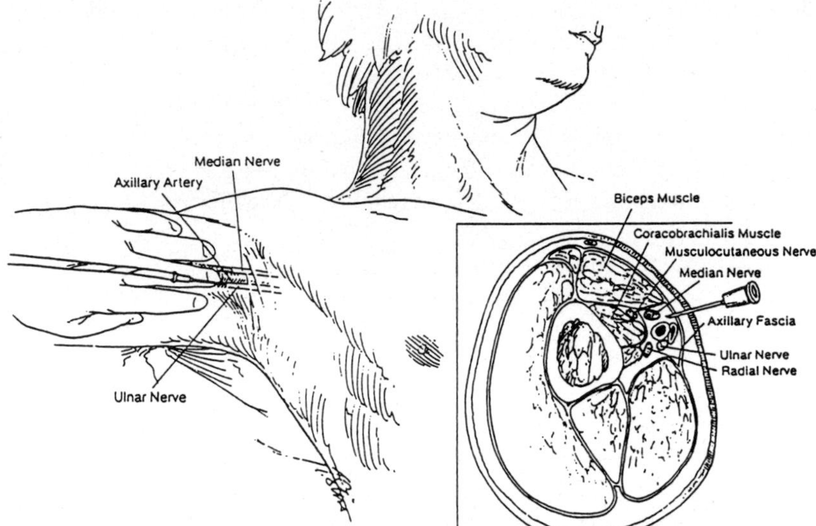

FIG 40–12.
Axillary approach to a brachial plexus block. The middle finger of the anesthetist's nondominant hand is on the axillary artery. A 25-gauge, 1-in. needle is directed toward the axilla. The inset shows the needle in the neurovascular bundle close to the brachial artery. The musculocutaneous nerve lies in the coracobrachialis muscle, outside the brachial plexus sheath at this site. (From Raj PP, Pai U: Techniques of nerve blocking, in Raj PP (ed): *Handbook of Regional Anesthesia*. New York, Churchill Livingstone, 1985. Used by permission.)

Orthostatic hypotension was not seen, although precautions to lessen the likelihood of this problem should be employed. This drug continues to remain for investigational use only in the United States and is not clinically available.

Intravenous regional bretylium has been used in this manner because of its ability to accumulate in adrenergic nerves and block norepinephrine release. In a report of four patients with RSD, Ford et al. noted good to excellent pain relief in all of the patients for up to 7 months after treatment.[32] In addition, bretylium produced objective signs of prolonged sympatholytic activity and improved function in all four cases. Side effects were minimal; thus bretylium appears to be an attractive alternative to guanethidine or reserpine as an adrenergic blocking agent.

Surgical Sympathectomy

Surgical sympathectomy has been advocated for patients who do not experience permanent relief from blocks or other conservative measures. Kleinert et al. reported on

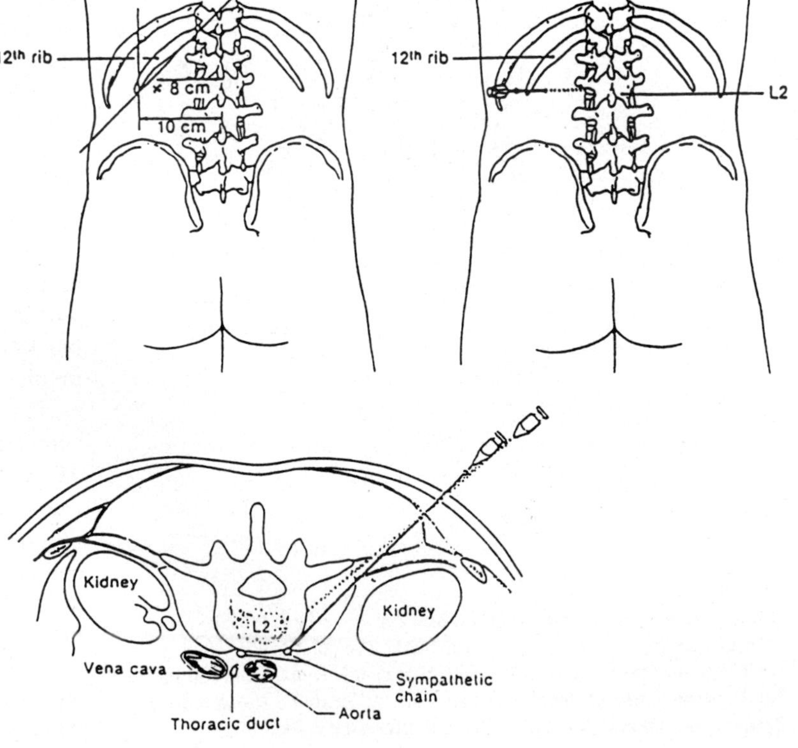

FIG 40–13.
Reid's technique of lumbar sympathetic blockade. **A,** with the patient prone, a line is drawn along the lower border of the 12th rib. A second line is dropped 10 cm lateral and parallel to the middle of the spine. The lines will intersect at the L2 vertebra. The point of entry of the needle is 8 cm from the L2 vertebra at this level. **B,** needle in position. **C,** initially the needle is advanced anteriorly at a 45-degree angle. It will touch the vertebral body. The needle is withdrawn to the skin and reinserted more acutely 1 in. deeper than the initial insertion to lie at the anterior lateral surface of the vertebral body. (From Raj PP: *The Practical Management of Pain*. St Louis, Mosby–Year Book, 1986. Used by permission.)

a series of 183 patients with upper-extremity sympathetic dystrophy who were initially treated with sympathetic blocks.[45] No demonstrable improvement was seen in 39 patients. Permanent improvement was achieved in 121 patients. In the remaining 23 patients, who experienced only transient relief from blocks, surgical sympathectomy was performed and produced permanent relief in all but four patients.

A study of 34 sympathectomies for causalgic pain by Mockus et al. resulted in satisfactory relief of pain in 97% of patients immediately postoperatively.[64] Postsympathectomy neuralgia was seen in 40% of patients and lasted just over 1 month on the average, and a 10% wound complication rate was seen. Extended follow-up showed satisfactory pain relief in 94% of the patients, with 84% reporting the same degree of relief that they experienced immediately postoperatively.

Immediate or delayed failure of sympathectomy to relieve pain in RSD may be due to reinnervation from the contralateral lumbar sympathetic chain.[44, 65]

Anatomic studies of the lumbar sympathetic chain have displayed cross communications of fibers.[57]

Prior to electing sympathectomy, several criteria should be met:

1. The patient should experience pain relief from sympathetic blocks on several occasions.
2. Pain relief should last at least as long as the vascular effects of the block.
3. Placebo injection should produce no pain relief, or the relief should be less pronounced and of shorter duration than that achieved with local anesthetic sympathetic blocks.
4. Possible secondary gain motives and significant psychopathology should be ruled out as possible causes of pain complaints.

Chemical Sympathectomy

Neurolytic lumbar sympathetic blockade may be chosen as an alternative to surgical sympathectomy for lower-extremity sympathetic dystrophy. Boas et al.[12] cite 100% success in five patients treated with phenol sympathetic blocks. Because of the proximity of the roots of the brachial plexus to the cervical sympathetic chain, neurolytic sympathetic blockade for upper-extremity pain is too hazardous.

Sympathectomy is not without potential problems. Patients are occasionally bothered by dermatologic problems associated with skin dryness. A painful condition, sometimes termed sympathalgia, may begin in the second or third postoperative week. Patients experience muscle fatigue, heaviness, deep pain, and tenderness in the limb, which may continue for weeks. When sympathectomy includes ablation of the stellate ganglion, the resultant ptosis, conjunctival injection, and nasal congestion may be distressing but can usually be controlled by the use of 10% phenylephrine eye drops.

Spinal Cord Stimulation

Electrical stimulation of the dorsal column in an attempt to inhibit pain was initially reported by Shealy et al. in 1967.[91] Placement of electrodes into the epidural space either percutaneously or via laminotomy has been used to treat a variety of chronic pain states in a large number of patients.[28] This technique has been used to treat RSD in patients who fail otherwise conventional conservative therapies. Dorsal column stimulation (DCS) can be time intensive because the affected area must be covered by paresthesias during stimulation and optimal stimulus parameters determined for each patient. Available data to date suggest a valid role of DCS in the treatment of RSD. Selection criteria for this procedure, however, are not well established. Patients in the later stages of the disease who have been through appropriate treatment programs including sympathetic blockade, physical therapy, and psychological assessment and treatment without response are candidates for the procedure.

Physical Therapy

Physical therapy is the cornerstone of treatment along with sympathetic interruption and may be effective alone for the treatment of mild cases of RSD.[70] For long-standing cases, extensive physical rehabilitation may be necessary. Active and active-assisted range-of-motion exercises, muscle strengthening and conditioning, massage, and heat (whirlpool, paraffin, radiant heat) are particularly useful. Low-dose ultrasound (0.5 W/cm^2 for 5 minutes) has been used by Portwood et al.[78] in three patients with RSD of the lower extremity. Two of the three patients had been refractory to pharmacologic therapy, and all three preferred a more conservative approach than surgical sympathectomy. All three patients were symptom free, and no complications were observed at the end of the study period. It is hypothesized that ultrasound may affect the peripheral sympathetic nerve fibers in addition to increasing blood flow to the limb.

Exercises are best performed during analgesic periods following sympathetic blocks. Frequently the pain is so severe as to interfere with the patient's ability to do meaningful physical therapy. These patients may require hospital admission and aggressive analgesia via the epidural, intravenous, or oral routes in order to engage them in an effective physical therapy program.

Transcutaneous Electrical Nerve Stimulation

TENS has been effective as the sole treatment[43, 97] and as adjunctive therapy for sympathetic dystrophy. Increased skin temperature has been documented during

TENS therapy.[3] Pain control may be achieved with the regular use of TENS in some patients with long-standing sympathetic dystrophy who have not responded to sympathetic blocks.

Continuous Passive Motion

The use of continuous passive motion (CPM) has been helpful in the treatment of RSD.[18, 22] CPM can be used to enhance the patient's ongoing program of physical therapy. The device is used to maximize range of motion and keep the affected extremity moving. The patient can use the device while resting or during sleep, and in severe RSD, this can accelerate progress made while the patient is under an epidural or other nerve block. These patients may require some degree of motor block initially in order to provide analgesia. This makes active exercise difficult. CPM can be used to provide passive motion of the injured part. For patients with disease involving the hand, small ambulatory devices are available that can be used at home.

Psychology

Psychological intervention in patients with RSD should be threefold:

1. To help them deal with the psychic distress (e.g., depression, anxiety) that resulted from the prolonged pain experience
2. To address psychosocial factors that may adversely affect the patient's response to treatment
3. To teach effective coping strategies

The various interventions consist of psychotherapy, family therapy, stress management training, biofeedback, and relaxation training. Psychotherapy and family therapy are aimed at helping patients deal with the adverse effects of pain on their functioning as well as the factors that could have a negative impact on their response to treatment. Stress management training, which may include biofeedback and relaxation training, helps the patient learn effective methods of dealing with the pain or factors that could cause the pain symptomatology to exacerbate (i.e., stress).[10, 35, 49, 93, 107]

OVERALL MANAGEMENT OF THE PATIENT WITH MODERATE TO SEVERE REFLEX SYMPATHETIC DYSTROPHY

Even though a small number of patients with RSD can get better spontaneously or with minimal medical procedures, the majority of them suffer for 6 to 12 months before they are close to normal and productive. Patients in the second and third stages of the syndrome require a multidisciplinary approach to manage pain, depression, functional disability, and possible drug abuse.[107] At our institution, we have found a 3-week intensive inpatient, multidisciplinary treatment very effective to bring the patient to the stage of 50% functional and emotional recovery. Following this, an outpatient program of physical therapy and continued psychological support continues to help them progress toward full recovery.

Case Report

A 14-year-old female competitive gymnast was referred to The University Center for Pain Medicine (UCPM) in Houston with severe right leg pain of 2 months' duration. During a training session she had landed with full weight on her right leg and sustained a mild strain injury of the right knee. Over the next several days, the knee became swollen and painful, and the pain and swelling progressed distally. The pain was described as a throbbing, burning pain, and weight bearing was not tolerated.

Prior to coming to the UCPM, the patient had a workup consisting of plain films showing patchy demineralization, a bone scan to rule out osteomyelitis, a venogram to rule out deep vein thrombosis (DVT), and multiple physician consultations culminating in a diagnosis of RSD. A series of lumbar sympathetic blocks was performed but provided only temporary relief.

At her initial UCPM evaluation, she was noted to be anxious, in considerable distress, and unable to weight bear or even touch the foot to the floor. The lower part of the leg appeared mottled and was edematous from the knee distally including the foot. She was extremely sensitive to even a light touch and would jump and cry out with pain even before the examiner's hands contacted her skin on the affected limb. The lower part of the leg was warm to the touch, and loss of hair was noted on the medial aspect. She was unable to move the foot and had only slight movement of the toes on the affected side. A diagnosis of RSD stage I-II was made, and the patient was admitted to the hospital for aggressive management.

After admission, a lumbar epidural catheter was inserted and an infusion of bupivacaine and morphine sulfate started after a test dose and bolus. Even with dense epidural blockade, the patient would not tolerate passive range of motion of the affected extremity. A subarachnoid catheter was placed, and with dense spinal anesthesia along with heavy intravenous sedation we were able to initiate physical therapy. One week later, with a marked decrease in swelling and a similar decrease in her level of anxiety, the subarachnoid catheter was replaced with an epidural catheter, and physical therapy continued with slow but steady progress. During the last hospital week, the catheter was removed, and the patient continued on her accelerated physical therapy program.

Physical therapy was initially possible only with the aid of either epidural or subarachnoid analgesia along with intravenous sedation because of the intense afferent nociceptive barrage and the high level of anxiety displayed. Passive, assisted active, and finally active exercises were performed, initially without weight bearing and then with increasing amounts of weight bearing.

At discharge, the patient had a normal appearance of both lower extremities, without swelling or discoloration. Active range of motion of 90 degrees at the ankle was obtained. Light touch of the extremity by the patient or examiner was tolerable, and ambulation with crutches was possible. Discharge instructions for rigorous physical therapy toward weight bearing were followed by the patient with the help of her family; however, it was 12 to 18 months before she was able to return to her prior activities.

This case illustrates that a young and healthy patient who has developed RSD can rapidly become dysfunctional and display marked psychogenic changes requiring aggressive therapy for pain management, exercise, and coping strategies. After 3 weeks of hospitalization and in spite of such aggressive treatment, this patient was only partially recovered at discharge. It is doubtful that she would have recovered further if she had not continued with her home exercise program for the following 18 months. This observation is significant for the fact that quite often physicians treating such patients, as well as the patients themselves, expect dramatic and complete recovery within a very short time and with minimal medical intervention. Unfortunately, this does not usually occur. More often one finds that patients with RSD who progress rapidly from stage 1 to stage 2 or 3 require 6 to 12 months of medically monitored multidisciplinary treatment to reach full functional recovery.

SUMMARY

This chapter has tried to present the current thoughts on RSD and its management so as to reflect the thinking of basic scientists and clinicians deeply interested in this syndrome today. Although we have come a long way in our understanding of this syndrome, no definitive treatment is as yet available that can provide total recovery of all patients suffering from RSD. It does emphasize, however, the need for continuous comprehensive management initiated as early as possible in the course of the disease in order to obtain optimal recovery for our patients.

REFERENCES

1. Abrams SE: Intravenous reserpine. *Anesth Analg* 1980; 59:889–890.
2. Abrams SE: Pain of sympathetic origin, in Raj PP (ed): *The Practical Management of Pain*. St Louis, Mosby–Year Book, 1986.
3. Abrams SE, Aisddao CB, Reynolds AC: Increased skin temperature during transcutaneous electrical stimulation. *Anesth Analg* 1980; 59:22–25.
4. Ackerman B, Arwestrom E, Post C: Local anesthetics potentiate spinal morphine antinociception. *Anesth Analg* 1988; 67:943–948.
5. Amadio P, MacKinnon S: Reflex sympathetic dystrophy syndrome. *Plast Reconstr Surg* 1991; 87:371–375.
6. Arthroscopic Association of North America, Committee on Complications: Complications of arthroscopy and arthroscopic surgery: Results of a national survey. *Arthroscopy* 1985; 1:214–220.
7. Atkins R: Algodystrophy after Colles fracture. *J Hand Surg [Br]* 1989; 14:161–164.
8. Atkins R: Features of algodystrophy after Colles fracture. *J Bone Joint Surg [Br]* 1990; 72:105–110.
9. Barber F, et al: Complications of ankle arthroscopy. *Foot Ankle* 1990; 10:263–266.
10. Barowsky E, Zwieg J, Moskowitz J: Thermal biofeedback in the treatment of symptoms associated with reflex sympathetic dystrophy. *J Clin Neurol* 1987; 2:229–232.
11. Benzon HT, Chomka CM, Brenner EA: Treatment of reflex sympathetic dystrophy with regional intravenous reserpine. *Anesth Analg* 1980; 59:500–502.
12. Boas RA, Hatangdi VS, Richards EG: Lumbar sympathectomy—a percutaneous technique, in Bonica JJ, Albe-Fessard D (eds): *Advances in Pain Research and Therapy*. New York, Raven Press, 1976, pp 485–490.
13. Bonica JJ: Causalgia and other reflex sympathetic dystrophies, in Bonica JJ, et al (eds): *Advances in Pain Research and Therapy,* vol 3. New York, Raven Press, 1979, pp 141–166.
14. Brown BR: Intra-arterial reserpine. *Anesth Analg* 1980; 59:889.
15. Campbell JN, Raja SN, et al: Myelinated afferents signal the hyperalgesia associated with nerve injury. *Pain* 1988; 32:89–94.
16. Cannon WB: Some aspects of the physiology of animals surviving complete exclusion of sympathetic impulses. *Am J Physiol* 1929; 89:84.
17. Chapman SL: Chronic pain and the injured worker, in Lynch NT, Vasudevan SV (eds): *Persistent Pain: Psychosocial Assessment and Intervention*. Boston, Kluwer, 1988.
18. Chow J, Schenck RR: Early continuous passive movement in hand surgery. *Curr Surg* 1989; 46:97–100.
19. Cicala RS: Causalgic pain responding to epidural but not to sympathetic nerve blockade. *Anesth Analg* 1990; 70:218–219.
20. Constantinesco A, Brunot B, Demangeat JL, et al: Three phase bone scanning as an aid to early diagnosis in reflex sympathetic dystrophy of the hand: A study of 89 cases. *Ann Chir Main* 1986; 5:93–104.
21. Cooke E, Glick E: Reflex sympathetic dystrophy algoneurodystrophy temperature studies in the upper limb. *Br J Rheumatol* 1989; 28:399–403.
22. Cooper DE, DeLee JC, Ramamurthy S: Reflex sympathetic dystrophy of the knee: Treatment using continuous epidural anesthesia. *J Bone Joint Surg [Am]* 1989; 71:365–369.
23. Davidoff G, Morey K, Stamps J: Pain measurement in reflex sympathetic dystrophy syndrome. *Pain* 1988; 32:27–34.
24. Davies JAH, Beswick T, Dickson G: Ketanserin and guanethidine in the treatment of causalgia. *Anesth Analg* 1987; 66:575–576.
25. de No RL: Analysis of the activity of the chains of internuncial neurons. *J Neurophysiol* 1938; 1:208–242.

26. de Takats G: Causalgic states in peace and war. *JAMA* 1945; 128:699–704.
27. Devor M: Nerve pathophysiology and mechanisms of pain in causalgia. *J Auton Nerv Syst* 1983; 7:371–384.
28. Devulder J, et al: Spinal cord stimulation in chronic pain therapy. *Clin J Pain* 1990; 6:51–56.
29. Doupe J, Cullen CR, Chance GQ: Post-traumatic pain and the causalgic syndromes. *J Neurol Neurosurg Psychiatry* 1944; 7:33–48.
30. Erlanger J, Gasser HS: Nobel prize award: High differentiation of the functions of various nerve fibres. 1944.
31. Fahr LM, Sauser DD: Imaging of peripheral nerve lesions. *Orthop Clin North Am* 1988; 19:27–41.
32. Ford S, Forrest W, Eltherington L: The treatment of reflex sympathetic dystrophy with intravenous regional guanethidine. *Anesthesiology* 1988; 68:137–140.
33. Ganit R, Leksell L, Skoglund CR: Fibre interaction in injured or compressed region of nerve. *Brain* 1944; 67:125–140.
34. Greyson ND, Tepperman PS: Three phase bone studies in hemiplegia with reflex sympathetic dystrophy and the effect of disuse. *J Nucl Med* 1984; 25:423–429.
35. Grunert B: Thermal self regulation for pain control in reflex sympathetic dystrophy syndrome. *J Hand Surg [Am]* 1990; 15:615–618.
36. Hannington-Kiff JG: Intravenous regional sympathetic block with guanethidine. *Lancet* 1974; 1:1019–1020.
37. Herman LG, Reineke HG, Caldwell JA: Post-traumatic painful osteoporosis: A clinical and roentgenological entity. *AJR* 1942; 47:353–361.
38. Hollister L: Tricyclic antidepressants. *N Engl J Med* 1978; 299:1106–1109.
39. International Association for the Study of Pain, Subcommittee on Taxonomy: Reflex sympathetic dystrophy (1-5). *Pain* 1986; 3(suppl):29–30.
40. International Symposium on Reflex Sympathetic Dystrophy. Mainz, Germany. 1988.
41. Katz M, Hungerford D, et al: Reflex sympathetic dystrophy as a cause of poor results after total knee arthroplasty. *J Arthroplasty* 1986; 1:117–124.
42. Kepes ER, Raj PP, Vemulapalli R, et al: Regional intravenous guanethidine for sympathetic blockade. Report of 10 cases. *Reg Anesth* 1982; 7:52–54.
43. Kesler RW, Saulsbery F, Miller LT, et al: Reflex sympathetic dystrophy in children: Treatment with transcutaneous electric nerve stimulation. *Pediatrics* 1988; 82:728–732.
44. Kleiman A: Evidence of the existence of crossed sensory sympathetic fibers. *Am J Surg* 1954; 87:839–841.
45. Kleinert HE, Cole NM, Wayne L, et al: Post-traumatic sympathetic dystrophy. *Orthop Clin North Am* 1973; 4:917–927.
46. Koche: Failure of MR imaging to detect reflex sympathetic dystrophy of the extremities. *AJR* 1991; 156:113–115.
47. Kozin R, Ryan LM, Carerra GF, et al: The reflex sympathetic dystrophy syndrome (RSDS), III. Scintigraphic studies, further evidence for the therapeutic efficacy of systemic corticosteroids, and proposed diagnostic criteria. *Am J Med* 1981; 70:23–30.
48. Lankford LL: Reflex sympathetic dystrophy, in Huner JM, et al (eds): *Rehabilitation of the Hand*. St Louis, Mosby–Year Book, 1984, pp 509–532.
49. Lebovitz A: Reflex sympathetic dystrophy and posttraumatic stress disorder: Multidisciplinary evaluation and treatment. *Clin J Pain* 1990; 6:153–157.
50. Lee V: Neuropathic pain may not respond to sympathetic blockade (letter). *Anesth Analg* 1990; 70:313–314.
51. Leriche R: In Young A (ed): *The Surgery of Pain*. London, Bailliere, Tindall, & Cox, 1939.
52. Lewis D, Gatewood W: Treatment of causalgia: Results of intraneural injections of 60% alcohol. *JAMA* 1920; 74:4.
53. Linson M, Leffort R, Todd D: The treatment of upper extremity reflex sympathetic dystrophy with prolonged continuous stellate ganglion blockade. *J Hand Surg* 1983; 8:153–159.
54. Livingston WK: *Pain Mechanisms: A Physiological Interpretation of Causalgia and Its Related States*. New York, MacMillan, 1943.
55. Loh L, Nathan PW: Painful peripheral states and sympathetic blocks. *J Neurol Neurosurg Psychiatry* 1978; 41:664–672.
56. Low PA, Caskey PE, Tuck RR, et al: Quantitative pseudomotor axon reflex test in normal and neuropathic subjects. *Ann Neurol* 1983; 14:573–580.
57. Lowenberg R, Morton D: The anatomic and surgical significance of the lumbar sympathetic nervous system. *Ann Surg* 1951; 144:525–532.
58. Mackinnon S, Dellon AL: Surgery of the peripheral nerve, in *Surgery of the Hand*. New York, Thieme Medical, 1988.
59. McCain G, Scudds R: The concept of primary fibromyalgia. *Pain* 1988; 33:273–287.
60. Melzack R: Clinical aspects of pain, in *The Puzzle of Pain*. New York, Basic Books, 1973, pp 60–65.
61. Melzack R, Wall PD: Pain mechanisms: A new theory. *Science* 1965; 150:971–978.
62. Mitchell SW: On the diseases of nerves resulting from injuries, in Flint A (ed): *Contributions Relating to the Causation and Prevention of Disease, and to Camp Disease*. New York, United States Sanitary Commission Memoirs, 1967, pp 412–468.
63. Mitchell SW, Morehouse GR, Keen WW: *Gunshot Wounds and Other Injuries of Nerves*. Philadelphia, JB Lippincott, 1864, p 164.
64. Mockus MM, Rutherford R, Rosales C, et al: Sympathectomy for causalgia. *Arch Surg* 1987; 122:668–672.
65. Munn J, Baker W: Recurrent RSD: Successful treatment by contralateral sympathectomy. *Surgery* 1987; 1:102–105.
66. Nathan PW: The gate control theory and pain: A critical review. *Brain* 1976; 99:123–158.
67. Noordenbos W: *1955 Pain: Problems Pertaining to the Transmission of Nervous Impulses Which Give Rise to Pain: Preliminary Statements*. Amsterdam, Elsevier, 1959.

68. Ohta S: A case report of reflex sympathetic dystrophy treated with nifedipine. *Jpn J Anesth* 1989; 38:679–683.
69. Oxman T, Denson D: Antidepressants and adjunctive psychotropic drugs, in Raj PP (ed): *The Practical Management of Pain*. St Louis, Mosby–Year Book, 1986.
70. Pak TJ, Martin GM, Magness JL, et al: Reflex sympathetic dystrophy: Review of 140 cases. *Minn Med* 1970; 53:507–512.
71. Panerai AE, Monza G, Movilia P, et al: Psychotrophic drugs, in Raj PP (ed): *The Practical Management of Pain*. St Louis, Mosby–Year Book, 1986.
72. Paré A: Of the cure of wounds of the nervous parts, in Johnson T (translator): *Collected Works of Ambroise Paré*. Pound Ridge, Milford House, 1634, pp 400–402.
73. Pick J: *The Autonomic Nervous System: Morphological, Comparative, Clinical and Surgical Aspects*. Philadelphia, JB Lippincott, 1970, p 362.
74. Pick J: The evolution of homeostasis. The phylogenetic development of the regulation of bodily and mental activities by the autonomic nervous system. Presented at the American Philosophical Society, 1954, p 298.
75. Pochaczevsky R: Thermography in skeletal and soft tissue trauma, in Taveras J, Ferrucci J (eds): *Radiology*. Philadelphia, JB Lippincott, 1987.
76. Pochaczevsky R, et al: Liquid crystal thermography of the spine and extremities. *J Neurosurg* 1982; 56:386–395.
77. Poplawski ZJ: Post-traumatic dystrophy of the extremities: A clinical review and trial of treatment. *J Bone Joint Surg [Am]* 1983; 65:642–655.
78. Portwood M, Liberman JS, Taylor RG: Ultrasound treatment of reflex sympathetic dystrophy. *Arch Phys Med Rehabil* 1987; 68:116–118.
79. Prough DS, McLeskey CH, Weeks DB, et al: Efficacy of oral nifedipine in the treatment of reflex sympathetic dystrophy (abstract). *Anesthesiology* 1983; 61:3.
80. Raj PP: *Case Histories (2): Nesacaine for Retrograde Differential Blocking: Nesacaine, in Case Studies in Obstetrical and Surgical Regional Anesthesia*. New York, Pennwalt Corp, 1979, pp 8–12.
81. Raj PP, et al: Infraclavicular brachial plexus block. A new approach. *Anesth Analg* 1973; 52:897–904.
82. Raj P, Cannella J, Kelly J, et al: Multi-disciplinary management of reflex sympathetic dystrophy, in Stanton-Hicks M, et al (eds): *Reflex Sympathetic Dystrophy*. Boston, Kluwer, 1989.
83. Raja SN, Treede RD, Davis KD, et al: Systemic alpha-adrenergic blockade with phentolamine: A diagnostic test for sympathetically maintained pain. *Anesthesiology* 1991; 74:691–698.
84. Roberts W: A hypothesis on the physiological basis for causalgia and related pains. *Pain* 1986; 24:297–311.
85. Roberts WJ: Spinal hyperexcitability in sympathetically maintained pain, in Stanton-Hicks M, et al (eds): *Reflex Sympathetic Dystrophy*. Boston, Kluwer, 1989.
86. Roberts WJ, et al: I. Spinal recordings indicate that wide dynamic range neurons mediate sympathetically maintained pain. *Pain* 1988; 34:289–304.
87. Roberts WJ, et al: II. Identification of afferents contributing to sympathetically evoked activity in wide dynamic range neurons. *Pain* 1988; 34:305–314.
88. Rodeheffer RJ, Rommer JA, Wigley F, et al: Controlled double-blind trial of nidefedipine in the treatment of Raynaud's phenomenon. *N Engl J Med* 1983; 308:880–883.
89. Santo J, Arias L, Barolat G, et al: Bilateral cingulumotomy in the treatment of reflex sympathetic dystrophy. *Pain* 1990; 41:55–59.
90. Schulze S, Roikjaer O, Hasselstrom L, et al: Epidural bupivacaine and morphine plus systemic response and convalescence after cholecystectomy. *Surgery* 1988; 103:321–327.
91. Shealy CN, et al: Electrical inhibition of pain by stimulation of the dorsal column. *Anesth Analg* 1967; 46:489–491.
92. Shelton R, Lewis CJ: Reflex sympathetic dystrophy: A review. *Am Acad Dermatol* 1990; 22:513–520.
93. Sherry D, Weisman R: Psychologic aspects of childhood reflex neurovascular dystrophy. *Pediatrics* 1988; 88:572–578.
94. Sison G: Propranolol for causalgia and Sudek's atrophy. *JAMA* 1974; 227:327.
95. Social Security Administration: *Report of the Commission on Evaluation of Pain*. Washington, DC, Dept of Health and Human Services, 1986.
96. Sonneveld GJ, Vander Muelen JC, Smith AR: Quantitative oxygen measurements before and after intravascular guanethidine blocks. *J Hand Surg* 1983; 8:435–442.
97. Stilz RJ, Carren H, Sanders DB: Reflex sympathetic dystrophy in a 6-year old. Successful treatment by transcutaneous nerve stimulation. *Anesth Analg* 1977; 56:438–443.
98. Sunderland S: Pain mechanisms in causalgia. *J Neurol Neurosurg Psychiatry* 1976; 39:471–480.
99. Sweet W: Deafferentation pain. *Man Appl Neurophysiol* 1988; 51:117–127.
100. Tahmoush AJ: Causalgia: Redefinition as a clinical pain syndrome. *Pain* 1981; 10:187–197.
101. Thomas PS, Zauder HL: Thermography, in Raj PP (ed): *The Practical Management of Pain*. St Louis, Mosby–Year Book, 1986.
102. Thomsen MB, Bengtsson M, Llassvi C, et al: Changes in human foramen blood flow after intravenous regional sympathetic blockade with guanethidine. *Acta Chir Scand* 1982; 48:657–661.
103. Visitunthorn U, Prete P: Reflex sympathetic dystrophy of the lower extremity. A complication of herpes zoster with dramatic response to propranolol. *West J Med* 1981; 135:62–66.
104. Wall PD: The prevention of postoperative pain. *Pain* 1988; 33:289–290.
105. Wall PD, Gutnick M: Ongoing activity in peripheral nerves. The physiology and pharmacology of impulses originating from a neuroma by stimulation of the sympathetic supply in the rat (letter). *Neuroscience* 1981; 24:43–47.

106. Wang J, Johnson K, Ilstrup D: Sympathetic blocks for reflex sympathetic dystrophy. *Pain* 1985; 23:13–17.
107. Wilson P: Sympathetically maintained pain, in Stanton-Hicks M (ed): *Sympathetic Pain*. Boston, Kluwer, 1989.
108. Winnie AP: Differential diagnosis of pain mechanisms: Refresher courses. *Anesthesiology* 1978; 6:171–186.
109. Zimmerman M: Peripheral and central nervous mechanisms of nociception, pain, and pain therapy. Facts and hypotheses, in Bonica JJ, et al (eds): *Advances in Pain Research and Therapy,* vol 3. New York, Raven Press, 1979, pp 3:3–32.

PART XII

SPONDYLOLYSIS AND SPONDYLOLISTHESIS

41

Spondylolysis and Spondylolisthesis

Leon L. Wiltse, M.D., and Stephen L.G. Rothman, M.D.

Spondylolisthesis is the slipping forward of all or part of one vertebra on the one below. The classification presented here has been derived from several previous published classifications. It is both an anatomic and an etiologic classification.[37, 38] The order of the last three types (postsurgical, traumatic, and pathologic) has been changed from previously published classifications by the author and is listed here in order of clinical importance.

CLASSIFICATION OF SPONDYLOLISTHESIS

I. Congenital

Spondylolisthesis due to congenital anomalies of the lumbosacral junction can be divided into three subtypes, as follows.

Subtype A

This subtype has dysplastic axially oriented articular processes at the level of olisthesis. Spina bifida (Fig 41–1,A–C) is also frequently associated.

Subtype B

This subtype has a sagittal orientation of the articular processes that causes instability at the affected level (Fig 41–2).

Subtype C

There are other congenital anomalies of the lumbar spine that permit spondylolisthesis to occur. Congenital kyphosis is the principal one[71] (Fig 41–3).

II. Isthmic

Spondylolysis is the basic lesion in this type. The lesion is in the pars interarticularis. Three subtypes can be recognized (Fig 41–4,A).

Subtype A

Lytic: stress fracture of the pars[64] (Fig 41–4,B).

Subtype B

Elongated but intact pars secondary to healed stress fractures (Fig 41–5,A–D).

Subtype C

Acute fracture of the pars due to major trauma.

III. Degenerative

Due to long-standing intersegmental instability (Fig 41–6,A and B).

IV. Postsurgical

A partial or complete loss of posterior bony and/or discogenic support secondary to surgery or to stress fractures of the inferior articular processes may permit olisthesis[6] (Fig 41–7).

V. Traumatic

Due to acute fractures of the supporting structures other than the pars (Fig 41–8,A–E).

VI. Pathologic

Due to generalized or localized bone disease.

DISCUSSION OF TYPES OF SPONDYLOLISTHESIS

Before discussing the types of spondylolisthesis, I would like to define the various descriptive words used. The terms "hereditary," "genetic," "developmental," "degenerative," and "acquired" are rather nonspecific. I found wide differences of opinion among various authorities as to the meaning of these terms. The following definitions were formulated by using *Stedman's Medical Dictionary* (22nd edition),[58] Webster's third edition,[62] the *Oxford Dictionary,*[39] and consultation with the professor of genetics at the Long Beach State University.

In this chapter, I will consider the meanings to be as follows.

1. Hereditary.—Transmitted from parent to offspring by the genes; synonymous with "genetic."
2. Congenital.—Existing at birth; may be either hereditary (genetic) or due to some influence arising during gestation, that is, from conception to birth.
3. Developmental.—Arising during the extrauterine development of the person from birth to skeletal maturity.
4. Degenerative.—Generally arising after skeletal maturity due to changes secondary to injury, wear and tear, aging, or various combinations of each.
5. Acquired.—This term probably has no place in a classification such as this since strictly speaking, every trait, good or bad, is acquired some time between conception and death.

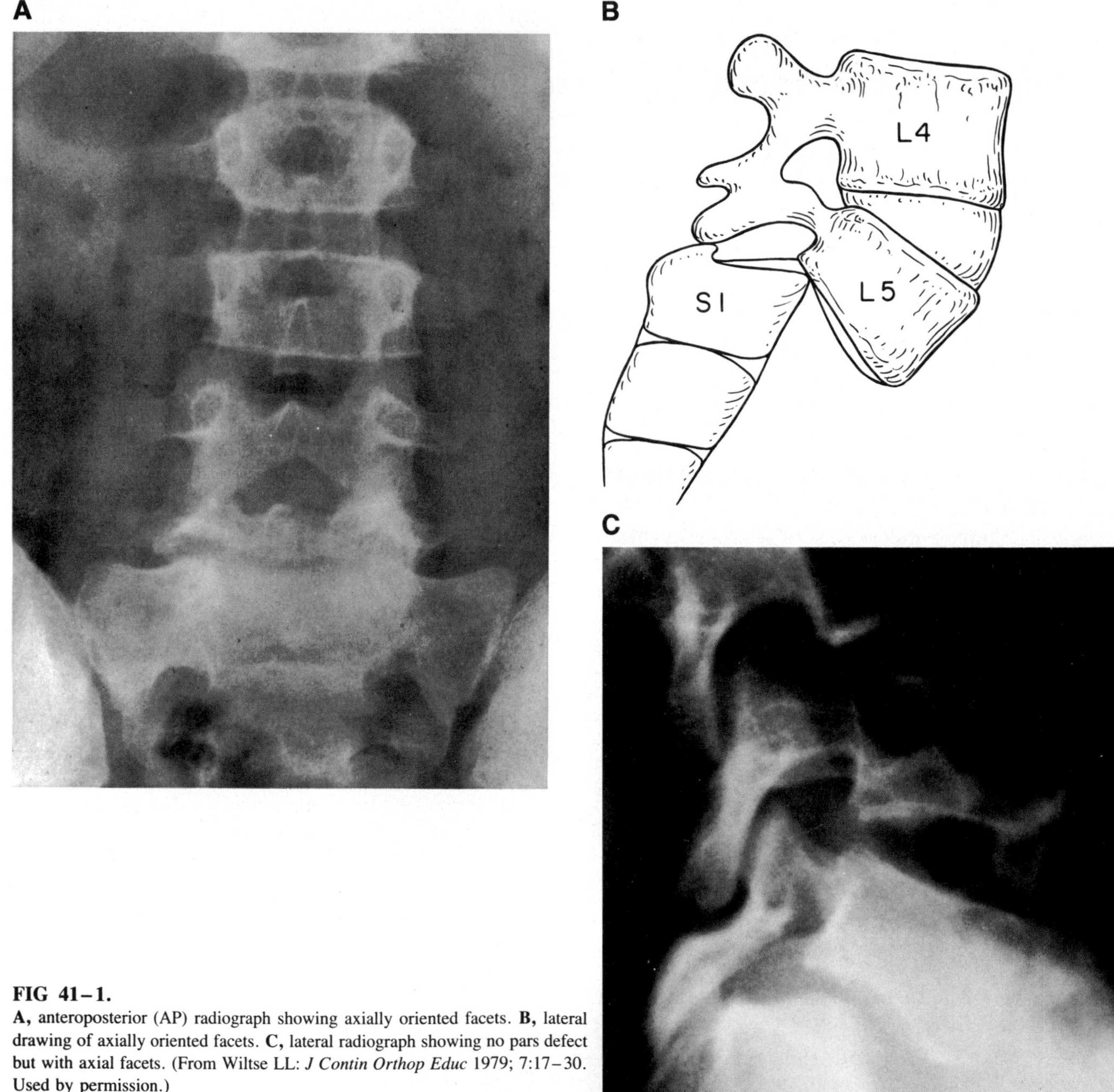

FIG 41–1.
A, anteroposterior (AP) radiograph showing axially oriented facets. **B,** lateral drawing of axially oriented facets. **C,** lateral radiograph showing no pars defect but with axial facets. (From Wiltse LL: *J Contin Orthop Educ* 1979; 7:17–30. Used by permission.)

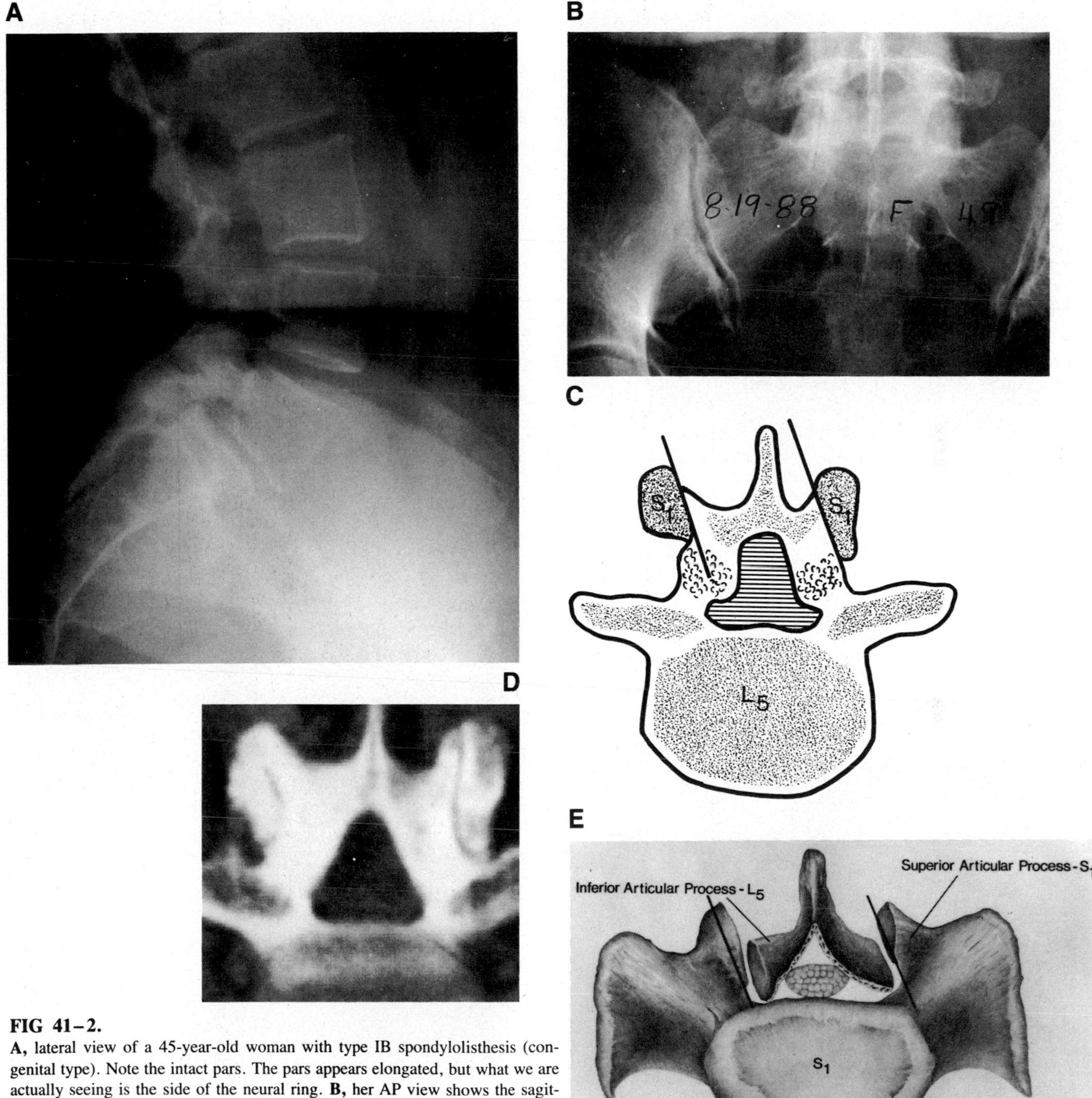

FIG 41–2.
A, lateral view of a 45-year-old woman with type IB spondylolisthesis (congenital type). Note the intact pars. The pars appears elongated, but what we are actually seeing is the side of the neural ring. **B,** her AP view shows the sagittally oriented facets. **C,** drawing of her axial computed tomographic (CT) section through the lower fourth of the body of L5. **D,** axial CT section through the lower fourth of the body of L5. Note the sagittal orientation of the facets. Also note how the facets on the right are rotated so that the more posterior tip of the facet is more medial than the anterior tip. This peculiar rotation effectively removes the stability normally supplied by the facets. **E,** drawing of the cephalic end of the sacrum in the same 45-year-old white woman with type IB spondylolisthesis. This shows the sagittal orientation of the facets. Note that the left facet is rotated in the opposite direction from the one on the right. This peculiar rotation effectively removes the stability normally supplied by the facets. (From Wiltse L, Rothman S: Spondylolisthesis: Classification, diagnosis, and natural history, in Weinstein J, Weisel S (eds): *The Lumbar Spine* Philadelphia, WB Saunders, 1990, p 478. Used by permission.)

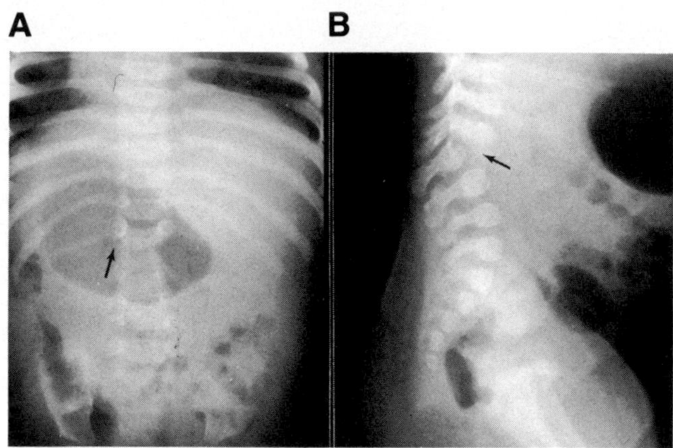

FIG 41–3.
Anteroposterior (**A**) and lateral (**B**) radiographs showing congenital kyphosis at the level of L2–3 in a 3-year-old girl.

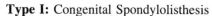

Type I: Congenital Spondylolisthesis

This is due to congenital anomalies of the lumbosacral junction.

Subtype A

In this subtype, the dysplastic articular processes have an axial orientation, usually more on one side than the other.[64] The combination of dysplastic articular process, axial (horizontal) orientation of the facets, and frequently wide spina bifida of L5 and S1 makes the area unable to support the superincumbent weight, and spondylolisthesis results. The pars interarticularis may remain unchanged. If it remains completely unchanged and the neural ring is intact, no spina bifida being present, slip cannot exceed more than about 35%, or there will be too much pressure on the cauda equina. Severe tightness of the hamstrings is likely to result (Fig 41–9,A and B).

Spina bifida is very frequently associated with this type. Often there is wide spina bifida of L5, S1, or both. This wide defect in the posterior arch permits a severe slip forward to occur without compression of the cauda. Thus a very high degree of olisthesis may occur, and the patient may still function satisfactorily.

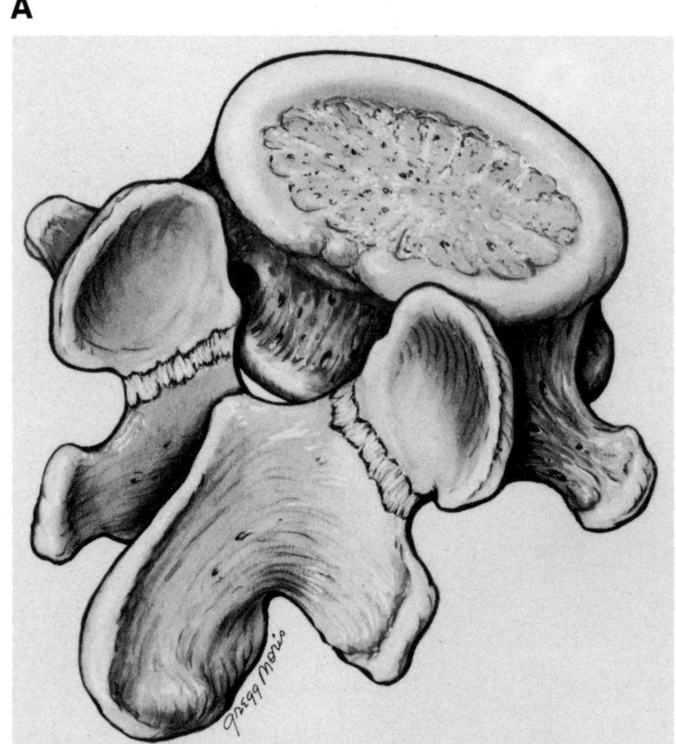

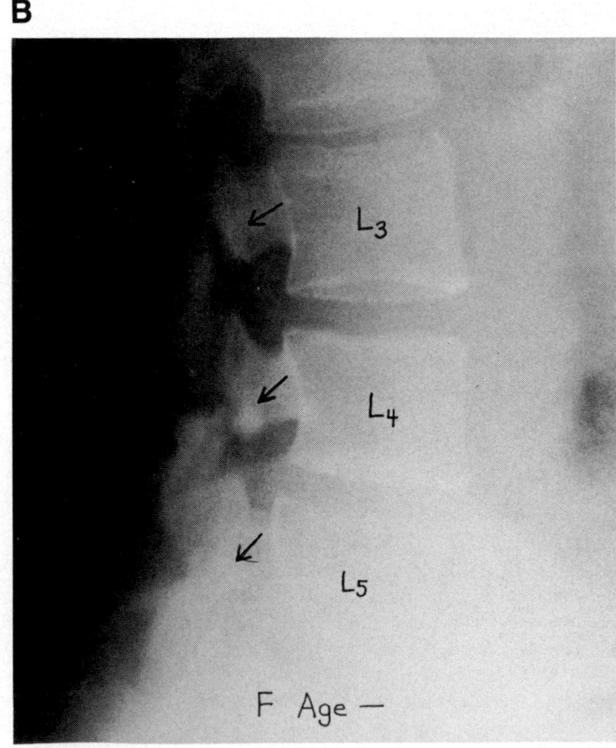

FIG 41–4.
A, drawing showing the defect in isthmic spondylolysis, classification IIA. (From Ruge D, Wiltse L: Spondylolisthesis and its treatment: Conservative treatment, fusion with and without reduction, in *Spinal Disorders—Diagnosis and Treatment*. Philadelphia, Lea & Febiger, 1977. Used by permission.) **B,** stress fractures of the pars in a 19-year-old female equestrian competing for the Olympic games. The L3 lesion is older than the L4 lesion. L5 is intact. (From Wiltse L, Rothman S: Lumbar and lumbosacral spondylolisthesis, in Weinstein J, Weisel S (eds): *The Lumbar Spine*. Philadelphia, WB Saunders, 1990, pp 471–498. Used by permission.)

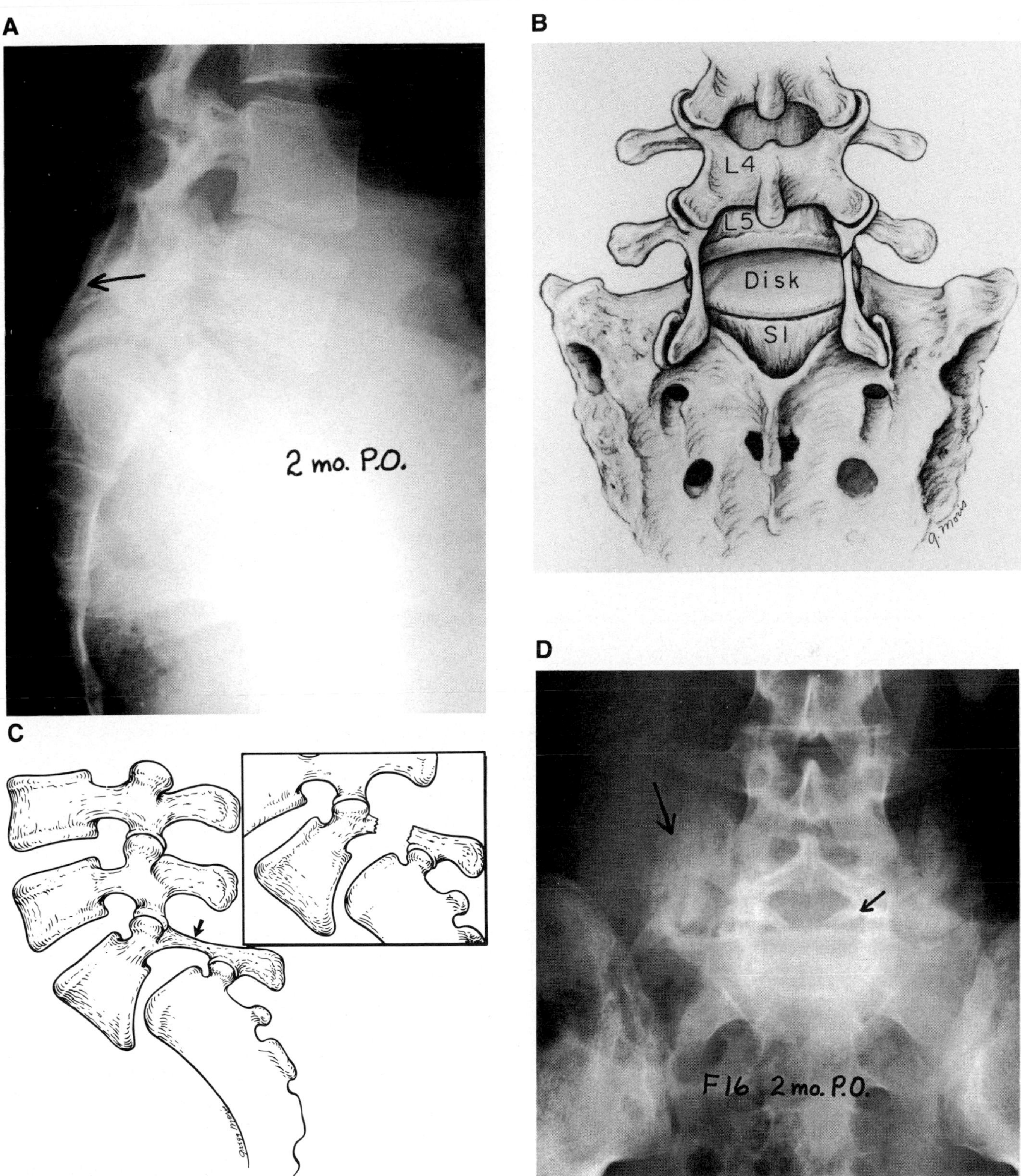

FIG 41–5.

Elongated but intact pars. **A,** preoperative lateral radiograph of a patient with elongated but intact pars due to repeated stress fractures with healing in an elongated position. **B,** drawing made at surgery of the elongated but intact pars. The right pars has cracked through, and the left has elongated but remained intact. It might have healed even if the fusion had not been done. **C,** lateral drawing of type IIB. The pars may stretch for years and then crack and come apart. **D,** postfusion AP radiograph of the patient in the drawing. (From Ruge D, Wiltse L: Spondylolisthesis and its treatment: Conservative treatment, fusion with and without reduction, in *Spinal Disorders—Diagnosis and Treatment*. Philadelphia, Lea & Febiger, 1977. Used by permission.)

A

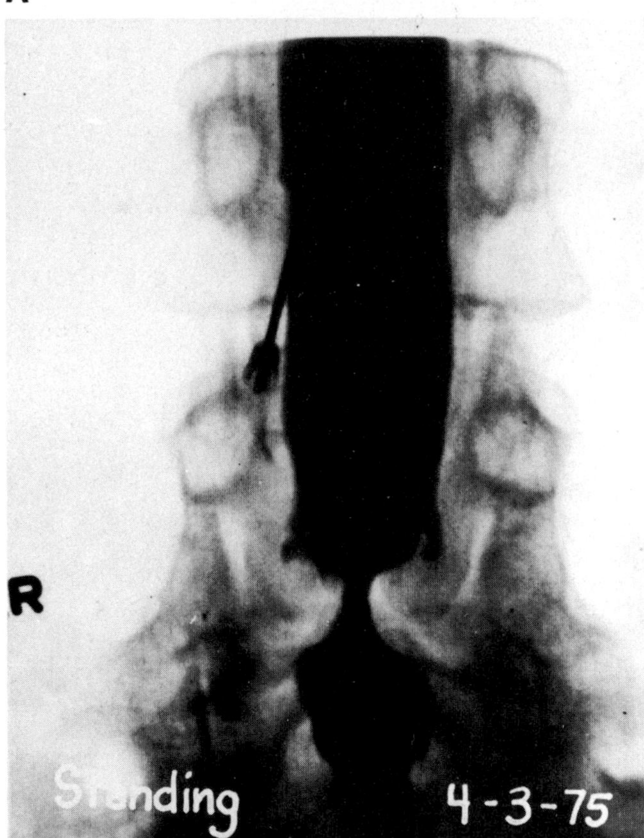

B

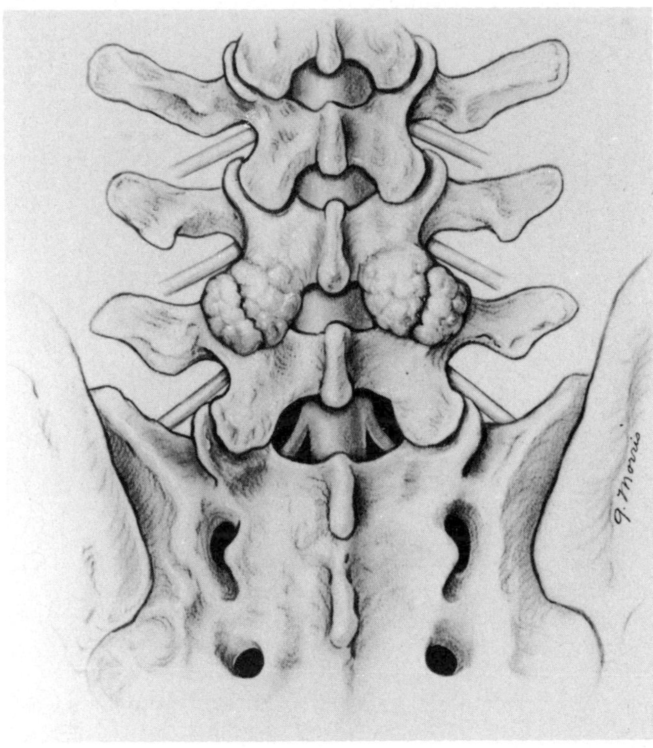

FIG 41–6.
A, typical AP myelogram of degenerative spondylolisthesis. The hourglass deformity is due to forward slippage of L4 on L5, plus the enlarged articular processes and bunching up of the ligaments, particularly the ligamentum flavum. **B,** drawing showing the deformed articular processes at the L4–5 level. (From Wiltse LL: *J Contin Orthop Educ* 1979; 7:17–30. Used by permission.)

Subtype B

In this subtype, there is sagittal malorientation of the articular processes. As in type A, the posterior elements are often poorly developed. It is probably because of the unstable orientation of the facets and the fact that not only are the articular processes at the olisthetic level sagittally oriented but also a form of tropism is present so that the facets on one side are rotated such that the posterior tip on one side is more medial than the anterior tip. This unstable situation allows the slip to occur. This type seldom progresses to an extremely high degree of olisthesis because the neural ring is usually intact.[25]

Subtype C

Other congenital abnormalities of the lumbar spine that cause spondylolisthesis are grouped in subtype C and are included only for completeness:

1. Congenital kyphosis is due to a congenital failure of vertebral body formation.
2. Anterior or posterior angulation of the sacrum, as described by Armstrong and Chen, is a rare cause of spondylolisthesis.[1]

Type II: Isthmic Spondylolisthesis

This type always has a fracture in the pars interarticularis.[70] Changes (e.g., alteration in the shape of the body of L5) may occur, but these are secondary changes and not fundamental to its etiology. There may, however, be some changes in the articular processes that are congenital.

Subtype A: Lytic

Lytic spondylolisthesis is due to separation or dissolution of the pars from a stress fracture. It is seldom seen below 5 years of age. In this type with a fracture in the pars, if the anterior elements slip forward, the spinous process, inferior facets, and caudal part of the pars usually remain in a fairly normal position, in which case there is plenty of room for the neural elements between the arch and the posterior rim of the sacrum. However, in some cases[7] the soft tissue between the ends of the fractured

A

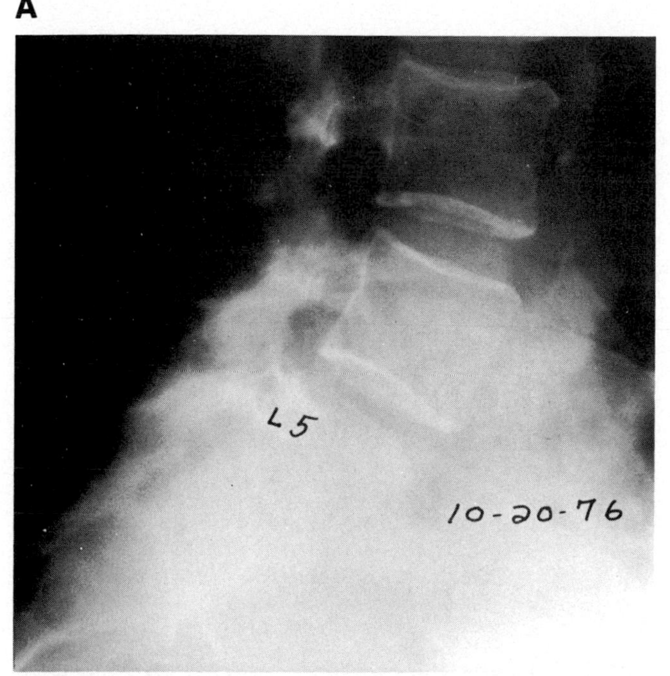

B

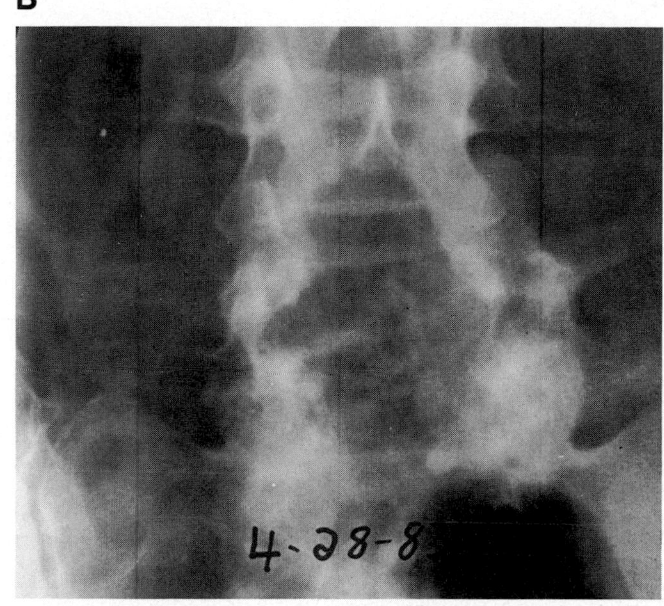

C

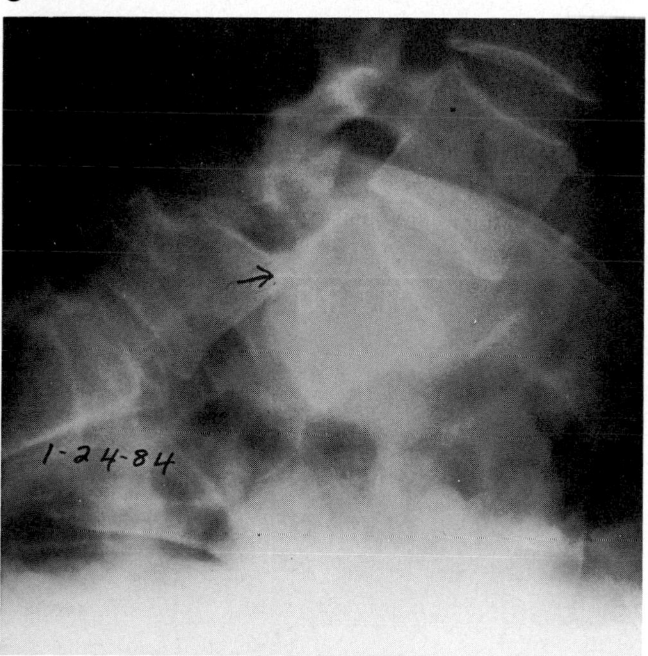

FIG 41–7.
A, preoperative lateral radiograph. **B,** after the patient had endured several years of back pain, a large midline decompression was done as above. Note that lateral masses have been removed. **C,** during the next 6 months, severe spondylolisthesis developed. We consider this a case of postoperative spondylolisthesis. (From Wiltse LL, Rothman, SLG: Spondylolisthesis—classification, diagnosis and natural history. In Evarts M (ed): *Surgery of the Musculoskeletal System,* vol 2. New York, Churchill Livingstone, 1990, p 2104. Used by permission.)

pars is very tough and strong, plus being strongly attached to the bone. In this case, as slip progresses, the posterior elements are pulled forward along with the anterior elements, and thus the patient's symptoms will resemble those of congenital spondylolisthesis.

Subtype B

There is elongation of the pars without separation. Because of cracking and healing as the vertebral body slides forward, the pars elongates but remains in continuity. This is the same disease as subtype A.

A Theory Supporting a Common Mechanism of Etiology for Both the Congenital and Isthmic Types of Spondylolisthesis

It is likely that except in the case of the young athlete, there is a common congenital component in the etiology of all variations of both the congenital and isthmic types of

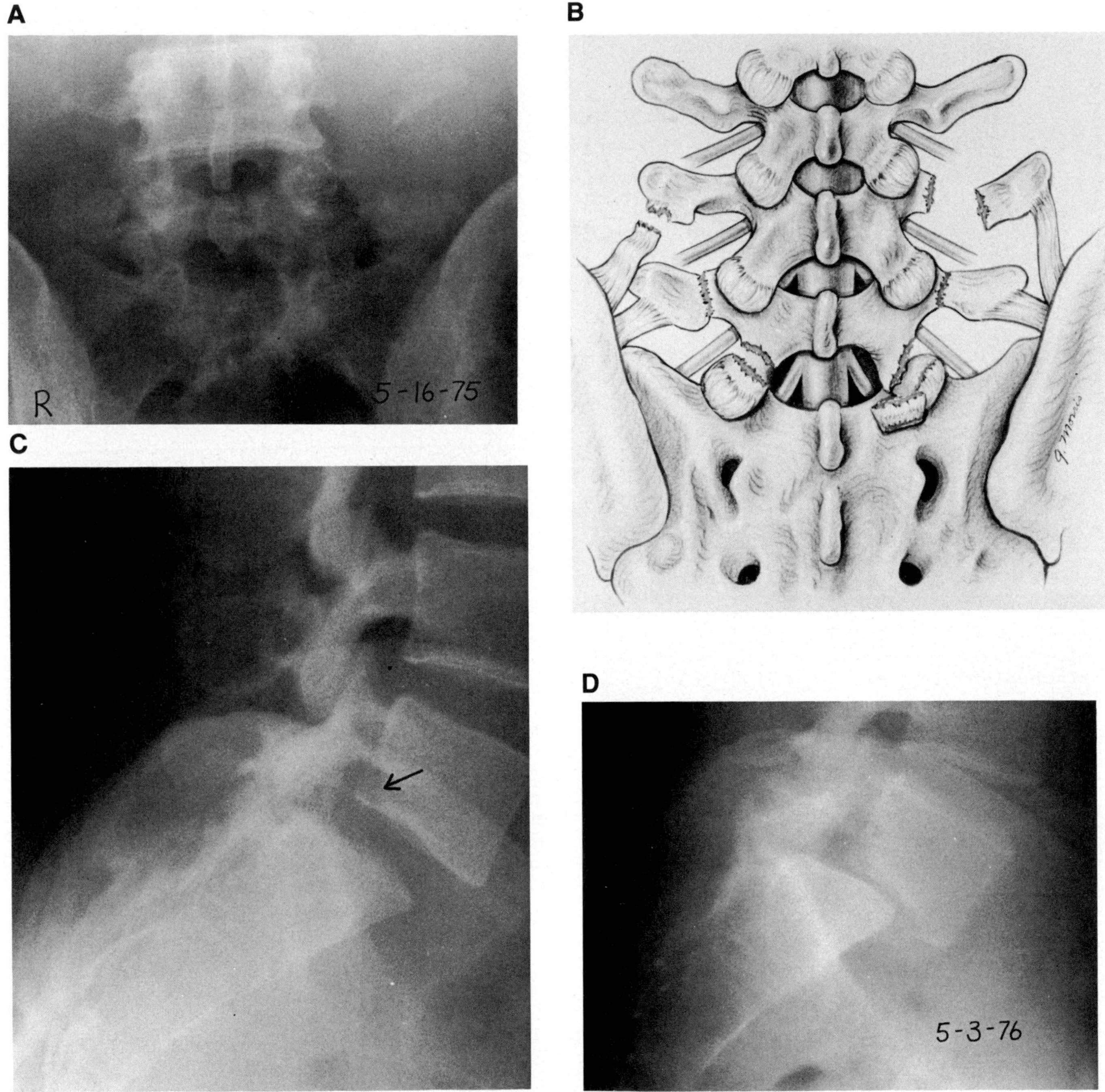

FIG 41–8.
Traumatic spondylolisthesis. **A,** AP radiograph of a 25-year-old man who was involved in a severe automobile accident. Note the multiple fractures but no pars fracture. **B,** drawing showing the injuries. **C,** lateral view taken 14 days postinjury. **D,** lateral view taken 1 year postinjury and after solid fusion. Note that the slip had progressed. This case demonstrates the low progression of olisthesis after severe injury, typical of traumatic spondylolisthesis. (From Wiltse LL: *J Contin Orthop Educ* 1979; 7:17–30. Used by permission.)

spondylolisthesis. I have come to believe this because consanguinity studies of patients with a clear-cut congenital type have a high frequency among close relatives of persons who have the isthmic type. The reverse is true among the close relatives (parents, siblings, children) of patients with the isthmic type. Here we find an incidence of congenital spondylolisthesis that is far above what would be expected by pure chance. For this reason, the following hypothesis regarding etiology is presented.

CT scans demonstrate hypoplasia of the superior artic-

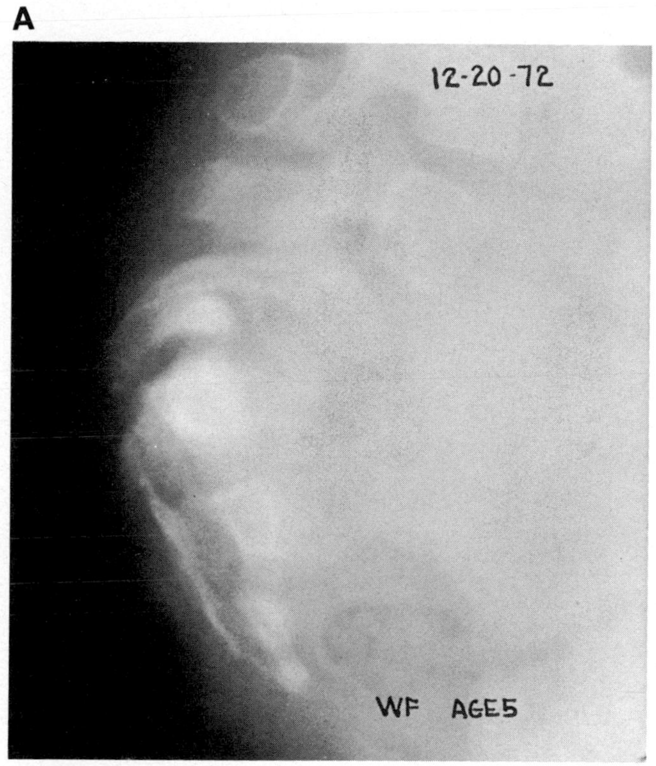

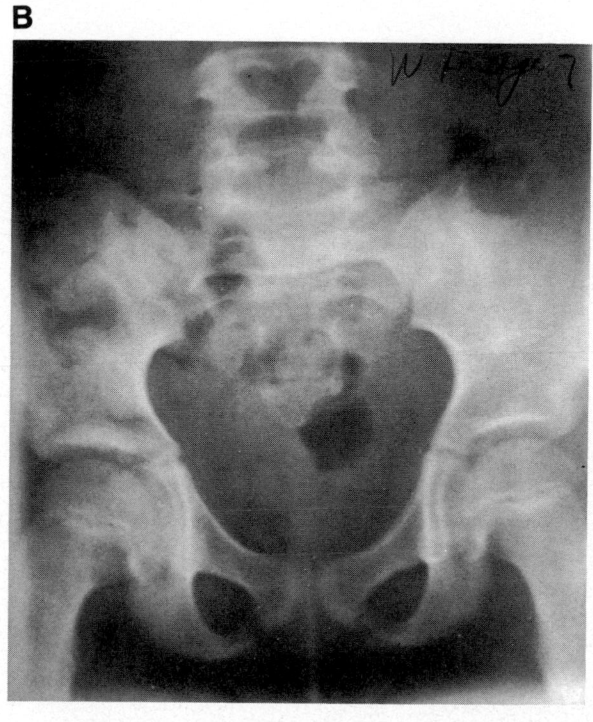

FIG 41–9.
A, very high-grade slip in a 5-year-old child with a wide posterior defect in L5 and S1. **B,** an AP radiograph of a 7-year-old girl with wide posterior defects (spina bifida occulta) in L5 and S1. (From Wiltse LL: *J Contin Orthop Educ* 1979; 7:17–30. Used by permission.)

ular process of S1 in most patients with either type of spondylolisthesis. With this in mind, we suggest that the congenital propensity for fracture at the pars in the isthmic type and also for the slip in the dysplastic type is hypoplasia of the posterior arches of L5, S1, or both. This situation is usually combined with an unstable orientation of the facets.

In the presence of hypoplasia of the facets, because the area of interfacet contact is small, the L5 pars is predisposed to stress fractures because the fulcrum, which should be through the middle of the pars, is displaced caudally. The increased length of the lever arm puts greater stress on the pars, thus predisposing it to fractures.

The facets may be sagittally or axially oriented, but never coronally oriented. If they were coronally oriented, olisthesis would be impeded by the direct bony contact between the facets. With sagittally or axially oriented facets, especially when tropism is present and the facet on one side is more medial at its posterior tip than at its anterior (windblown), only the ligamentous structures check forward gliding. Add to this a wide spina bifida, and luxation is likely to occur.

The question might be asked, is the stress fracture of the pars that develops in the young athlete also etiologically related to congenital spondylolisthesis. It appears not to be. In a very recent study[68] of six young athletes with fresh pars fractures, except for a possible increased incidence of spina bifida all had normal bony anatomy. This leads us to surmise that this one type comes on in teenagers who have unquestionable stress fractures in normal vertebrae. It is likely that the extreme stress placed on the pars causes the fracture and that no underlying dysplasia is necessary. To my knowledge there have been no studies to determine whether or not the relatives of these teenage athletes who develop stress fractures of the pars have a higher incidence of pars defects than is present in the general population. It seems likely that it is simply that the pars, being the most vulnerable point, is the area that breaks. The pars in the young athlete who has spina bifida may be slightly more prone to develop a stress fracture than the pars in athletes with totally normal bony architecture. This explains the increased incidence of spina bifida in the young athlete with fresh pars fractures. Spina bifida is clearly hereditary (Fig 41–10,A and B).

Type III: Degenerative Spondylolisthesis

The lesion is due to long-standing intersegmental instability. There is remodeling of the articular processes at the level of involvement. It is the belief of Farfan[13] that there are multiple small compression fractures of the infe-

A

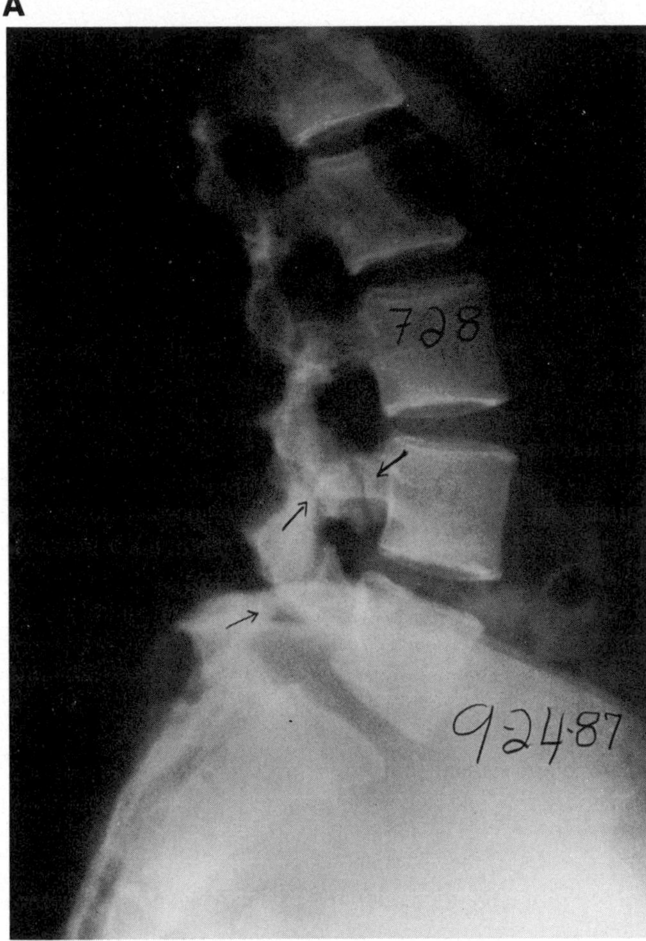

B

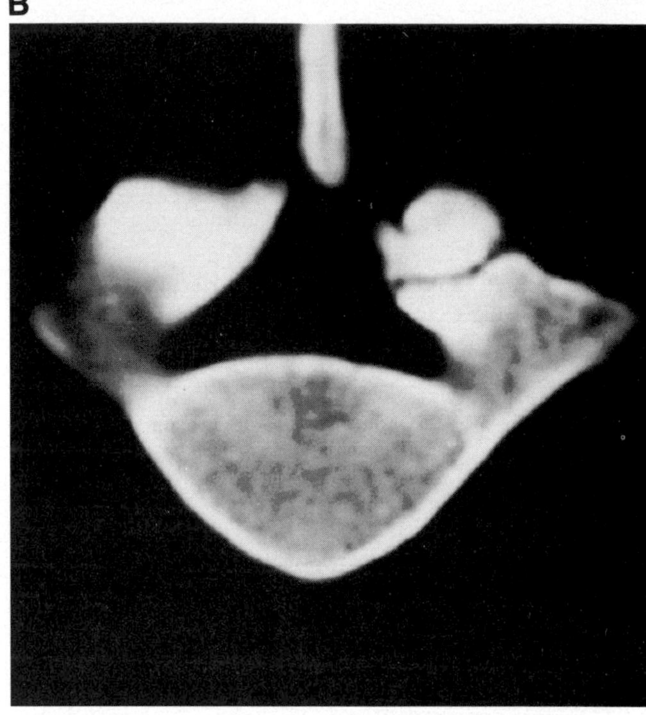

FIG 41–10.
A, 28-year-old woman with bilateral L5 pars defects and a defect in the right pars and left pedicle. **B,** 14-year-old male little league pitcher. On the right, the pars remains unhealed. On the left the pars is healed with evidence of bone thickening and sclerosis.

rior articular processes of the vertebra that slips forward. As the slip progresses, the articular processes change direction and become more horizontal.[46, 47] Rotary instability is a part of degenerative spondylolisthesis, as is tropism. Tropism of the facets is very common and may account for the fact that one side virtually always slips more than the other, and rotation of the vertebra at the level of olisthesis is also an integral characteristic. The subluxation is more severe on the side of the more sagittally oriented facet.

Degenerative spondylolisthesis occurs six times as frequently in females as in males, six to nine times more frequently at the L4 interspace than at adjoining levels, and four times more frequently when the L5 is sacralized than when it is not. When the lesion is at L4, the L5 vertebra is more stable and in less lordosis than average. A horizontal line drawn between the cephalic borders of the iliac crests (intercristal line) on the average passes through a more caudal level in the spines of patients who develop degenerative spondylolisthesis than in others. The slip seldom exceeds 33% slip unless there has been surgical intervention. It might be asked whether the condition is hereditary. I know of no studies that address this question, but we know that severe degenerative disc disease is, so it is very likely that there is a familial predisposition to the condition.

Type IV: Postsurgical Spondylolisthesis

This is a fairly frequent type of spondylolisthesis.[30] The incidence varies in different reported series but was about 3% to 5% in the series reported by White and Wiltse.[63] The slip occurs because too much of the supporting structure has been removed in an effort to decompress adequately. This group should not include patients developing further olisthesis after decompression of degenerative spondylolisthesis or olisthesis following the removal of the loose element in isthmic spondylolisthesis, but the etiologies are very similar. This group includes patients seen after extensive decompression for spinal stenosis, after laminectomy for disc removal, or after any other spine surgery, which in an effort to decompress adequately the spine is destabilized.[57] Several authors have used the term "iatrogenic spondylolisthesis" to describe this type. It is my belief that this word is far too harsh because it implies fault on the part of the surgeon, which is not necessarily so. Often, a minor degree of instability was present before surgery but could not be detected by ordinary x-ray examination. If a rather wide laminectomy is performed, as is often necessary to adequately decompress, postoperative olisthesis is a common sequela. Also, in the presence of osteoporosis and poor ligamentous support, unanticipated olisthesis may occur. To call this "iatrogenic" is to invite an undeserved malpractice suit.

In a study of CT scans made by one of us (S.L.G.R.)[48] for patients who had undergone laminectomy, more than 10% were noted to have stress fractures in the area where the pars becomes the inferior articular process at the level of decompression. Mild postsurgical spondylolisthesis is common in these patients. This is somewhat different from instances in which too much bone has been removed. It is suggested that in these cases surgical weakening occurs because too much bone is removed at the base of the articular process and fracture occurs during normal activity.

Type V: Traumatic Spondylolisthesis

The traumatic type is secondary to a severe acute injury that fractures parts of the supporting bone other than the pars and allows forward slip of the upper vertebra on the one below as a secondary phenomenon.[9] Fracture of the pedicle may also be present in this type.[67]

This type of spondylolisthesis is always due to severe trauma. Essential to this type is that slip occurs gradually, over a period of weeks or longer. Otherwise, it would be an acute fracture-dislocation. The pathology may be virtually the same, but we do not normally call an acute fracture-dislocation "spondylolisthesis."

Type VI: Pathologic Spondylolisthesis

Because of local or generalized bone disease, the bony mechanism (consisting of the pedicle, the pars, the superior and inferior articular processes) fails to hold the forward thrust of the superincumbent body weight, and forward slip of the vertebra on the one below occurs. It is a fairly rare type.[44]

Subtype A: Generalized

In this type, there are widespread generalized bony changes, as in the following examples.

1. Abers-Shoenberg disease (osteoporosis).
2. Arthrogryposis. In a type of arthrogryposis called Kuskokwim disease, several pedicles (but L5 in particular) may be elongated and produce spondylolisthesis of L5 on S1.
3. Syphilitic disease.[28]

Subtype B: Localized

This subtype is due to localized bone infection, tumor, or some other localized destructive process.

NATURAL HISTORY OF SPONDYLOLISTHESIS AND SPONDYLOLYSIS

The natural history of the three most important types of spondylolisthesis (congenital, isthmic, and degenerative) is summarized as follows.

Type I: Congenital

Subtype A

In subtype A the facets are axially oriented, wide spina bifida of L5, S1, or both is often present, and the following features may be seen:

1. Olisthesis often appears earlier than in others.[37]
2. Slip may be very severe if there is associated wide spina bifida.
3. These patients may have severe hamstring spasm but fare better neurologically if there is wide spina bifida present, in which case the cauda equina is not compressed very much. These patients probably need fusion earlier than others.

Subtype B

A sagittal facet orientation with tropism and a fairly intact posterior ring (Fig 41–11) are seen with the following:

1. High-grade slip is less common.
2. Leg pain, back spasm, hamstring spasm, and altered gait bring the patient to the doctor. Newman[37] has reported that he believes this altered posture to be due to an attempt by the patient to find a comfortable position of his trunk.
3. In an L5–S1 slip, it is the part of the cauda equina caudal to the L5 nerve that is compressed.
4. If fusion in situ without decompression is done on these patients, they will be slow in getting over their tight hamstrings and altered gait, but usually do eventually. Decompression can be done after the fusion is solid.

Type II: Isthmic

These have either a separated fracture in the pars (subtype A), or the pars has elongated as the vertebral body slips forward with the posterior elements left in a normal position (subtype B). The following tendencies are seen:

1. There are few cases before 5 years of age.
2. Most develop during the first year of school.

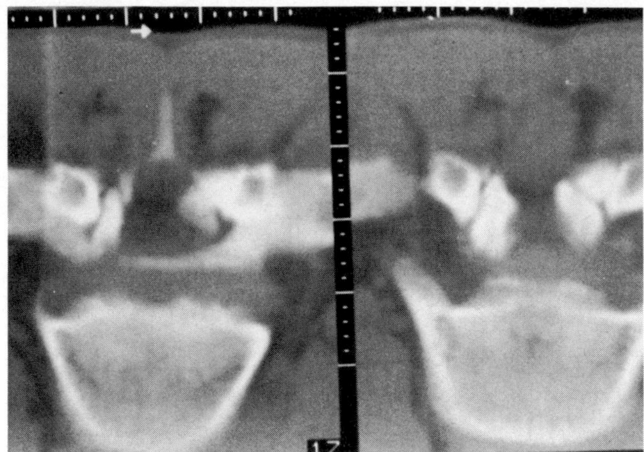

FIG 41-11.
This 14-year-old boy with sagittally oriented facets permitting moderate olisthesis was still able to participate in sports.

3. By 7 years of age, 4% of the cases will have appeared.

4. Another 1.4% will appear before adulthood. Most of this 1.4% will appear between the ages of 11 to 15 years, and these occur in very athletic youngsters.[2]

5. In persons engaged in very strenuous athletics, new cases appear even into early adulthood.

6. Olisthesis develops any time after the pars fractures occur, but the majority of high grades of slip develop from 10 to 14 years of age (in girls, a year or so earlier than in boys). For some reason, these only rarely develop high-grade slip.

7. High-grade slip is four times as likely in girls as in boys, yet pars defects are only half as frequent in girls as in boys.[26]

8. Back and leg pain commonly bring the patient to the doctor. Changes in the body contour alone seldom bring the child to the doctor.

9. A significant increase in olisthesis after adulthood does occur, but it is uncommon enough that it can be ignored as an important problem.

10. Olisthesis up to 10%[34] appears not to increase the likelihood of back problems even with heavy work. With slip between 10% and 25%, there may be some question, and beyond 25% it quite clearly does increase the likelihood of a patient having low back symptoms over what would be expected in a population without pars defects.[50]

11. There is considerable controversy as to what conditions portend further slip, but youth of the patient, wedging of the olisthestic vertebra, being female, rounding of the top of the sacrum, and a diminished AP diameter of the S1 body appear to.[49]

12. An increase in sagittal rotation causes more change in body contour than does an increase in olisthesis.

13. Olisthesis, even high grade, or sagittal rotations cause no problem with pregnancy.[51]

Type III: Degenerative Spondylolisthesis

The following are noted in degenerative spondylolisthesis:

1. It is seldom seen before 40 years of age, but the incidence increases with age and is very common in the very elderly.[45]

2. Women are more commonly affected than men.[46, 47]

3. Pain is of two types: the claudicant, characterized by pain in the calves brought on by walking,[45] and the much more common sciatic type, where there is pain down one leg that resembles the pain from a herniated disc.

4. Slip seldom progresses to more than 33% if no surgery is done.

5. Severe paralysis is rare, but foot drop, unilateral or rarely bilateral, does occur.

6. Sciatic tension signs are often absent even in the sciatic type.

7. Most patients can be treated nonoperatively. It has been reported that only one in ten who come to the doctor showing slip needs surgery.

TREATMENT OF SPONDYLOLISTHESIS IN CHILDREN

In children the principal types of spondylolisthesis are congenital (dysplastic) and isthmic. Treatment can usually be conservative, but if symptoms persist, surgery should be undertaken. Persistent symptoms in a child will require surgery more often than the same symptoms in an adult because symptoms that appear early in life mean years of trouble at an age when a child wishes to engage in the more strenuous activities usual for children and young adults. The older a person is when symptoms begin, the more likely that person is to be satisfied to follow a nonoperative regimen and live with some discomfort without resorting to surgery.

Before surgery is elected, several months should elapse after the onset of symptoms to see whether they will disappear spontaneously. The symptoms may have an unrelated cause (e.g., degenerative disc disease), and the spondylolisthesis may be only an incidental finding.

When a growing child with pars defects is first seen, a standing spot lateral radiograph of the lumbosacral joint should be taken for future reference. This type of radiograph is repeated at 4- to 6-month intervals to detect further slip. Once all growth has been attained, no additional slip is likely to occur, and no further radiographs are necessary.[53]

Risk Factors for Further Slip and for Increased Sagittal Rotation

The risk factors for further slip and sagittal rotation of L5 on S1 are listed below. When these are present, the surgeon should watch the child very carefully and perform a fusion if in doubt.[31]

1. Age.—The younger the child, the greater the risk of further olisthesis. Once growth stops, further slip is unlikely, but the patient should be watched for another few years.[4, 5]
2. Sex.—Girls have at least four times the likelihood of developing severe slip as do boys.[4, 5]
3. Presence of spina bifida.—This slightly increases the likelihood of further slip.[44]
4. Wedging of L5.—A markedly trapezoid-shaped L5 body is a bad prognostic sign. The degree of wedging is calculated as follows:

$$\frac{\text{Posterior height of body of L5}}{\text{Anterior height of body of L5}} \times 100 = \%\text{ of wedging}$$

5. Rounding of the anterior portion of S1.—Marked rounding of the anterior portion of S1 or a changed superior sacral contour is a bad prognostic sign. The further posterior the start of rounding, the worse the prognosis.
6. Diminished AP dimension of the S1 vertebral body: Patients with high-grade slip nearly all have significant narrowing of the AP dimension of the body of S1.

Relevant Measurements

Sacral inclination usually decreases as the L5 vertebra slips forward, in which case the sacrum becomes more vertical because the pelvis becomes more flexed. Figure 41–12 shows the method we use to measure the percentage of olisthesis. We prefer to use the widest point of S1. Sacral wedging is shown in Figure 41–12,A–C.

Sagittal rotation has been called the roll or slip angle. As L5 slides forward, it usually rolls (Fig 41–13,A–D).

The superior sacral contour is evaluated by the method shown in Figure 41–14,A and B for calculating the percentage of the top of S1 that is rounded. The farther back the rounding starts, the greater the likelihood of further slippage.

Indications for Surgery

The indications for spinal fusion in the child are as follows.

1. Symptoms severe enough to interfere with usual activities over 8 months or more
2. Very severe tightness of the hamstrings
3. Progressive olisthesis or increasing sagittal rotation
4. Even mild symptoms in a very young child (aged 10 or certainly below 7 years of age) with over a first-degree slip, particularly if the slip is progressing[21]

Authors' Preferred Technique

We have used a paraspinal incision since the late 1950s. I believe that we can attribute a good share of our success with fusion in these patients to this approach.[65, 69]

Position and Surgical Approach

The patient is placed in a kneeling position on any type of frame that allows the abdomen to swing free. In addition to the kneeling frame, in certain cases we have been using the frame designed by Homer Pheasant, along with a crank-up chest support designed by us. The patient is prepared and draped in the routine orthopedic manner. A midline skin incision is made[65] (Fig 41–15); previously, we had recommended two lateral skin incisions,[65] but since 1970 we have used a midline skin incision because we find it to be cosmetically more desirable than the two lateral skin incisions or even a transverse incision.[69] Since a skin incision has often been made for a previous operation, it is not desirable to make two more. The skin incision is carried down to thc level of the deep fascia, and the skin is retracted about two finger breadths laterally on either side.[65] This is done so that the fascial incisions can be made in their proper place, which is 2 cm lateral to the midline as shown. Previously we had recommended angulating these fascial incisions medially at their caudal ends, but this angulation is unnecessary.

The posterior layer of the thoracolumbar fascia is in two layers, a rather flimsy posterior one and a very heavy one covering the muscle.[69] Once the heavy layer has been cut through, two ordinary Gelpi retractors are placed so as to separate the fascia a few centimeters. There is a natural cleavage plane between the multifidus and the longissimus muscles (Fig 41–16,A–H). The finger can be plunged between these muscles at any point at or above the L4 level. We previously recommended going down onto the sacrum and then sliding the finger down the cranial border of the sacral ala; however, at this level fibers of the multifidus swing laterally, and the approach is much bloodier. At the L4–5 level, when the finger is passed down between the two muscles, the top of the finger comes right to the facet joint between L4 and L5. Gelpi retractors that have been bent to 90 degrees 5 cm from their tips are now placed between the two muscle groups. As mentioned above, beginning at the L4–5 level, when the finger is passed down between the two muscles, the top of the finger comes right to the facet joint between the two vertebrae. As also mentioned above, beginning at the L4–5 facet level, the muscle fibers can be seen to traverse laterally from the multifidus and go about 45 degrees and attach to the heavy

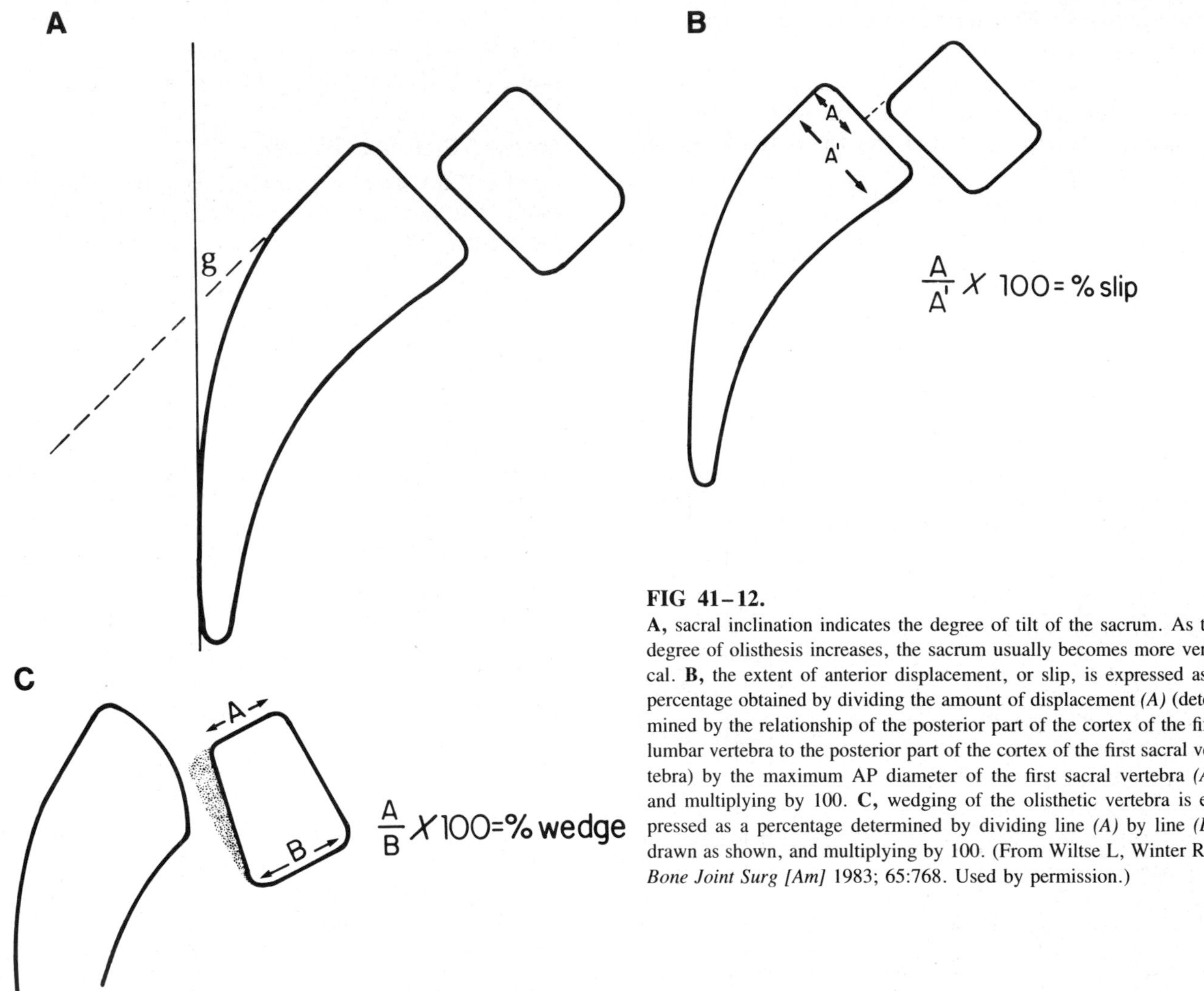

FIG 41–12.
A, sacral inclination indicates the degree of tilt of the sacrum. As the degree of olisthesis increases, the sacrum usually becomes more vertical. **B,** the extent of anterior displacement, or slip, is expressed as a percentage obtained by dividing the amount of displacement *(A)* (determined by the relationship of the posterior part of the cortex of the fifth lumbar vertebra to the posterior part of the cortex of the first sacral vertebra) by the maximum AP diameter of the first sacral vertebra *(A')* and multiplying by 100. **C,** wedging of the olisthetic vertebra is expressed as a percentage determined by dividing line *(A)* by line *(B)*, drawn as shown, and multiplying by 100. (From Wiltse L, Winter R: *J Bone Joint Surg [Am]* 1983; 65:768. Used by permission.)

fascia, which is the distal extension of the combined longissimus and iliocostalis muscles. These oblique muscle fibers can be easily separated from this heavy, almost tendinous fascia either with a scalpel, by cutting cautery, or even with a Cobb elevator.[69]

We find that if care is taken, very little blood need be lost, and it is a far better method of separating the muscles than to start from the sacrum and proceed upward. For best exposure, the bent Gelpi need to be repositioned frequently. Extra soft tissue in the bottom of the wound is removed with a very large pituitary rongeur or a Leksell rongeur. The laminae of the vertebrae to be fused are exposed well up onto the sloping bases of the adjacent spinous processes. The lumbar transverse processes should also be denuded of soft tissue out to their tips and well around their superior and inferior borders.

We never place bone in front of the transverse processes. The spinal nerves are just in front of the transverse processes and may be injured if the exposure is continued around anteriorly. Injury to these nerves is also possible if bone is packed hard between the transverse processes. In our experience, there seems to be little danger of damaging these spinal nerves if the dissection is kept posterior to the transverse processes. The lumbar arteries and veins pass just above the bases of the transverse processes and also at the angle of the medial point of the sacral ala. These often bleed freely and can be difficult to stop with cautery, but the bleeding areas can be plugged with a wad of Surgicil. The vessels coming out of the superior sacral foramen may also bleed profusely, and this bleeding can also be stopped with Surgicil. The Surgicil should be removed before closing: however, no harm is done if a small wad of it is inadvertently left in place. If cautery is to be used here, it should be the bipolar type because unipolar cautery may damage the adjacent spinal nerve.

Only the lateral surface of the superior articular process of the most cephalad vertebra to be included in the fusion should be denuded.[65] Care should be taken not to re-

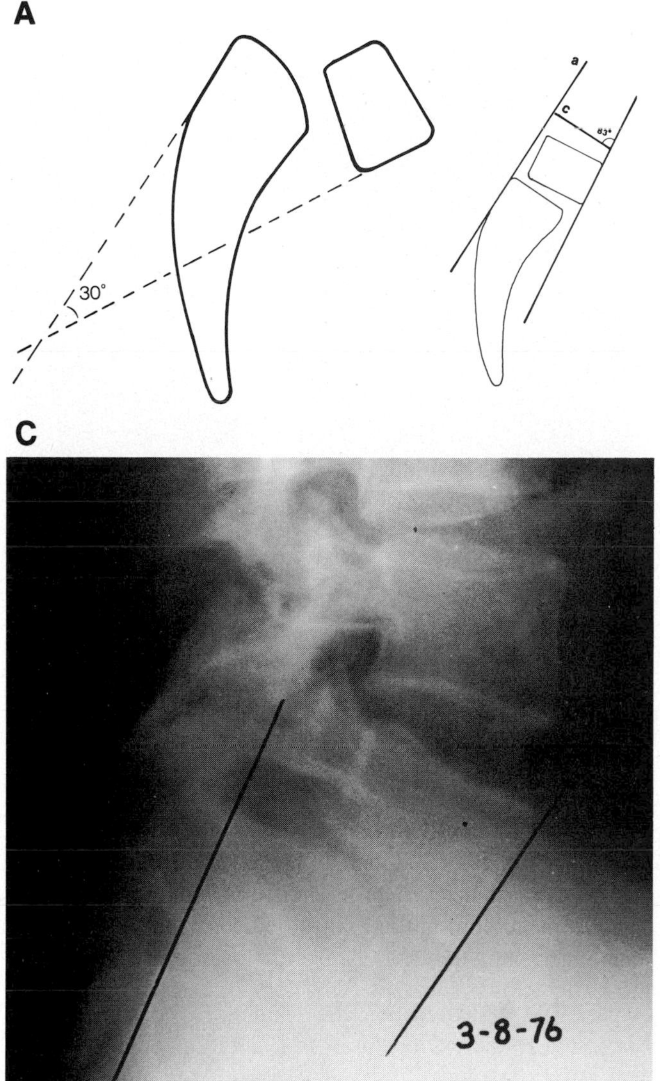

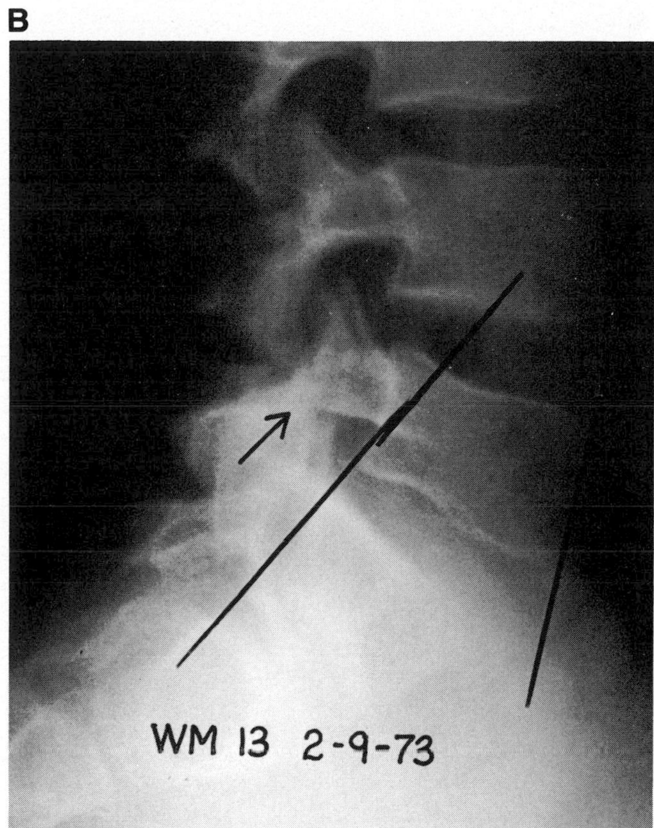

FIG 41–13.
A, *sagittal rotation* is the term used to express the angular relationship between the fifth lumbar and first sacral vertebrae. It is determined by extending a line along the anterior border of the body of the fifth lumbar vertebra until it intersects a line drawn along the posterior border of the body of the first sacral vertebrae. The drawing on the right shows an alternative method of measuring sagittal rotation that should be used when the degree of olisthesis is small and lines *a* and *b* do not intersect. A third line, *c*, is added perpendicular to line *a*. Lines *c* and *b* intersect to form the angle of sagittal rotation. **B,** 13-year-old boy fractured his pars in 1973 due to excessive lifting while working on a hay baler. **C,** note that the slip and sagittal rotation increased, and he underwent a fusion procedure. The fusion became solid and he did well. (**A** from Wiltse L, Winter R: *J Bone Joint Surg [Am]* 1983; 65:768. Used by permission.)

move the capsule or damage the adjacent joint at this level. Neither should the surgeon expose any part of the lamina of the vertebra immediately above the area to be fused. By observing these precautions any tendency for the fusion to extend upward will be avoided. Incidentally, we also believe that damage to these facets may account for some of the cases of postfusion spondylolisthesis and other problems seen at the upper ends of the fusions as years go by. Often there is no more than a few square centimeters of area available for fusion, but every bit of this area should be used. Not only the lateral surfaces of the superior articular process but also the dorsal and lateral areas of the pars interarticularis should be denuded. The laminae, as far medially as the sides of the spinous processes, should also be meticulously denuded. The spinous processes themselves are not exposed, so their ligamentous attachments and some of their blood supply are preserved. Crock[11] is of the opinion that preservation of these midline structures is of very great importance.

The intervertebral joints within the fusion area are carefully exposed.

If the surgeon wishes, the posterior two thirds of the joint cartilage can be removed and packed with cancellous bone. In the case of spondylolisthesis involving a loose element, the joint cartilage between the loose element and the facet below should not be removed because this would further destabilize an already unstable area. In spondylolisthesis we always fuse the loose element to S1 since otherwise it may rock about with muscle contractions and cause pain. This loose element often lies against the posterior

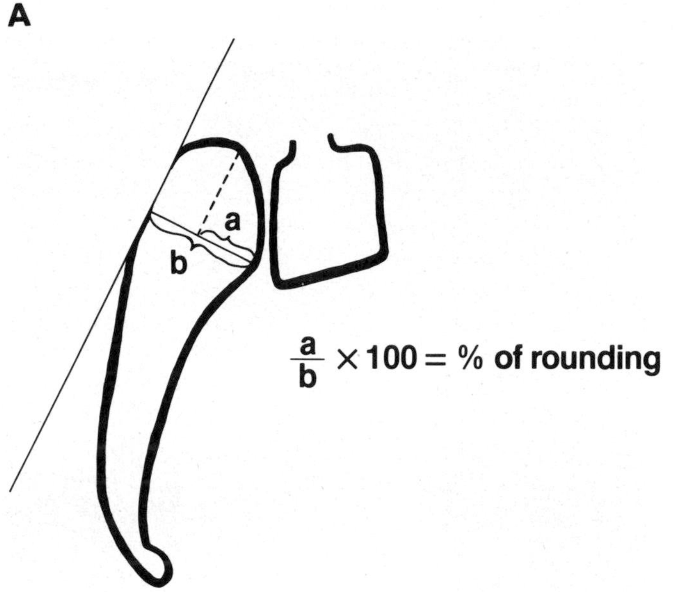

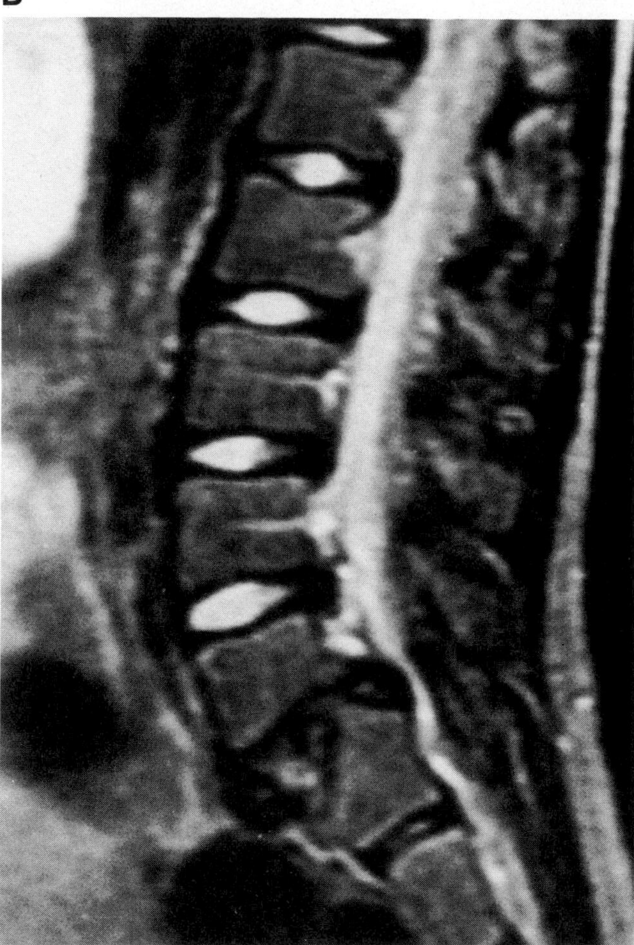

FIG 41–14.
A, rounding of the top of the centrum of the first sacral vertebra is expressed as the relationship between lines *a* and *b,* drawn as shown. The result, when multiplied by 100, gives the percentage of rounding of the first sacral vertebra. **B,** sagittal magnetic resonance imaging (MRI) of 9-year-old girl. Note the shape of the top of the sacrum. (**A** from Wiltse L, Winter R: *J Bone Joint Surg [Am]* 1983; 65:768. Used by permission.)

rim of the sacrum. Thus it should be prepared with a rongeur; a hammer and gouge should never be used because this has been known to damage the underlying nerves. Even when using a Leksell, care should be taken not to push down hard when getting a bit of bone because even this may be too much for the nerves. We are even cautious with a high-speed burr in this area because the vibration may be too severe. Maurice and Mosley[33] and Bradford[5] have reported some cases of severe cauda equina lesions following in situ fusion for severe spondylolisthesis. I have no completely satisfactory explanation for this but theorize that the damage to the cauda has resulted from swelling of the neural tissues in a stenotic canal where there is very little room for swelling. I believe that the chances of this complication can be minimized by the following.

1. Extreme care should be taken in working on the posterior element of the slipped vertebra.
2. If the patient has been having a lot of sciatica before surgery, he should be kept horizontal for 6 weeks postsurgery.
3. The patient should be watched carefully postsurgery, and if he develops a lot of sciatica or burning in the feet during the first 21 days, he should be maintained on complete bed rest for 3 weeks or longer until all pain is gone.
4. Decompression should be performed if there is more than minimal neurologic change. This decompression must include removing the posterior portion of the S1 body and tracing the L5 nerves out beyond the compressed area. It may be necessary to use pedicle screws for stability. An anterior interbody fusion of the Freebody type might also be necessary later.

Bone from the iliac crest is tamped into place. We put in soft cancellous bone first. A large Cobb elevator is placed at the cranial end of the area to be fused. The edge of the elevator can be hooked over the cranial border of the superior articular process. Often another instrument such as a transverse process retractor is hooked over the tip of the transverse process. This makes it easy to tamp bone into place with no danger of the bone creeping cephalad or even out laterally further than desired.

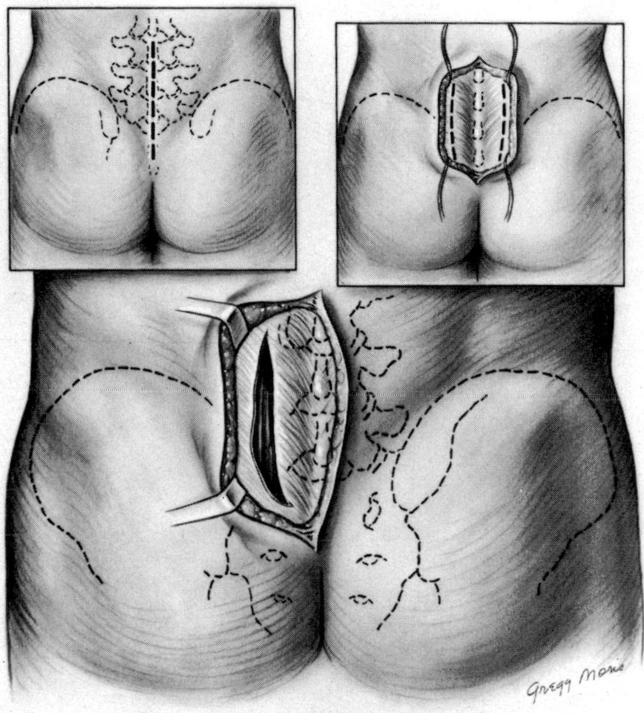

FIG 41-15.
Composite drawing of the paraspinal approach. A midline skin incision is made, but once it is through the skin, the skin flap is pulled two finger breadths to one side, and the fascial incision is made 2 cm lateral to the midline. (From Wiltse LL: *Clin Orthop* 1973; 91:48-57. Used by permission.)

When should the fusion be limited to L5-S1, and when should L4 be included? Based on the degree of slip and roll, ignoring for the moment such factors as a ruptured disc at that level, we use the rule of thumb that if the angle of the superior border of L5 with the horizontal (the new sacrohorizontal angle) is smaller than 55 degrees, we fuse only L5 to S1. If this angle is greater than 55 degrees, we include L4 in the fusion.[68]

Wound Closure

Before closure, any small tags of muscle are snipped off. The muscle itself is closed extremely loosely with small sutures. Both layers of the fascia are closed securely. The thoracolumbar fascia is essential to the stability of the lumbar spine. At least some nonabsorbable sutures should probably be used.[3] In cases in which a laminectomy has been done and bone graft laid over the transverse processes, we often put a suture through the muscle and attach it to the remnants of capsule to eliminate the danger of bone creeping medially.[65]

It is important to suture the skin edges to the underlying deep fascia, or blood and serum will collect under the portion of the skin that has been undermined, and the area will balloon out. If this occurs, it may need to be aspirated.

Postoperative Management

After paraspinal fusion, patients are encouraged to get out of bed when able, usually in a few days, and allowed to walk as much as they like. Patients should sit in straight-backed chairs and avoid twisting and should be trained to squat rather than bend their backs. No corsets or braces are used in children. In adults, we may use a brace or a cast with a thigh extension on one side.

It is our practice in children with high-grade slip to always take a standing spot lateral radiograph of the lumbosacral joint just before surgery to use as a baseline and precaution. Then, after the patient has been out of bed for 3 or 4 days, another standing spot lateral film is taken of L5-S1 and repeated 1 week later. If there is any sign of slip, the child should be put to bed until the fusion becomes partially solid, usually in about 2 or 3 months. In 20 years of experience with this technique, our patients have never needed bed rest because of increased slip.

If the loose posterior element has been removed in a patient with spondylolisthesis, further slip may occur. If the annulus has been incised for removal of a ruptured disc at the same level and the loose element has been removed, progression of slip is a virtual certainty if the patient is allowed up before the fusion is solidified. A few children who have had extremely tight hamstrings and sciatic scoliosis have been kept horizontal for 2 weeks to 2 months to allow the spasms and tightness to go away. This bed rest was given not for fear of further slip but simply to let the severe pain subside.

Summary of Treatment of Types I and II in the Child

In a child, regardless of the type of spondylolisthesis, the degree of slip, and the presence of sciatica, neurologic change, or tight hamstrings, we usually perform fusion in situ with no decompression. If sciatica is very severe, the patient is kept horizontal for a few (3 to 6) weeks until pain subsides.

In the case of the congenital type in which the arch is intact and in a normal position, the cauda equina may be being choked off rather severely. In these cases the tightness in the hamstrings will be slow to disappear. Once a wide fusion is solid, decompression is easy and safe, and thus late decompression can be done. The patient will still benefit because if decompression is done before fusion, a successful fusion will be difficult to achieve unless pedicle screws and rods or plates are used and an anterior interbody fusion added. Unless internal fixation is added, the patient must be kept horizontal in a cast, or the slip is likely to progress. We have never used pedicle screws in a child. Rapid postsurgical progression of a slip seems to be very painful. We have had to do (postsurgical) decompression in only one child, and her tight hamstrings became normal in 3 weeks. Several others have been slow to ob-

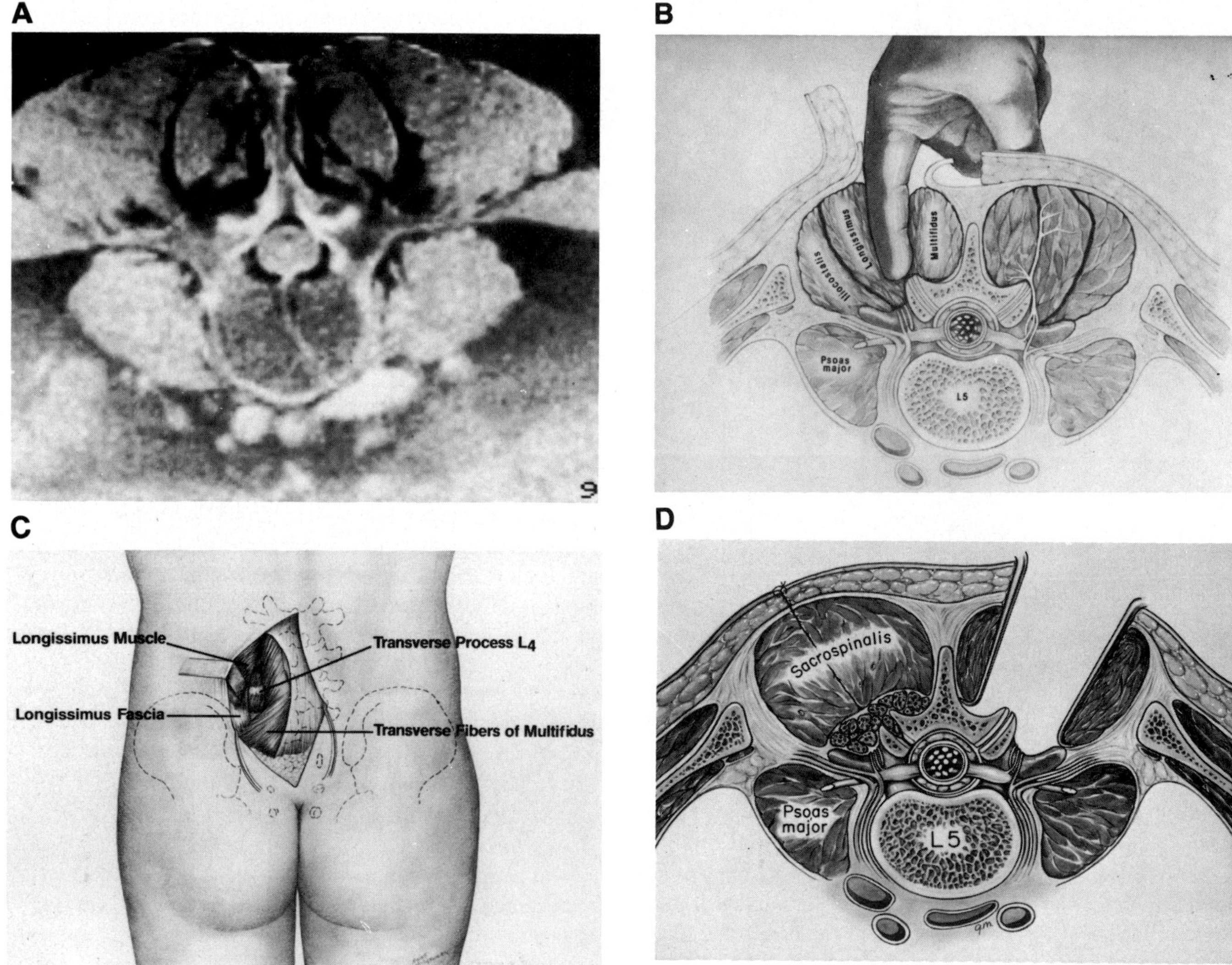

FIG 41–16.

A, note the cleavage plane between the multifidus and longissimus muscles. This plane moves a bit closer to the midline as we progress cranialward from L4. **B,** note the cleavage plane between the multifidus and longissimus muscles. This plane moves a bit closer to the midline as we progress craniad from L4. The surgeon's finger has been plunged between the multifidus and longissimus to the joint between L4 and L5. **C,** note that from the level of the L4–5 joint and caudalward the fibers of the multifidus turn laterally and attach to the tendinous extension of the two lateral muscles, the longissimus and the iliocostalis. With a cautery knife, the muscle fibers can be separated from the aponeuroses rather bloodlessly. **D,** two Gelpi retractors bent to 90 degrees 5 cm from their tips seem to be the best instruments for retraction. The standard large spinal retractors are virtually useless in this approach. **E,** extent of bone graft used by us. Note that the graft covers the lateral surface of the superior articular process of the first sacral vertebra and that the joint between the fifth lumbar and first sacral vertebrae is fused. The joint between L4 and L5 is not injured, but the graft extends onto the lateral aspect of the superior articular process of the fifth lumbar vertebra. An identical area is fused on the opposite side also. Note that on the reader's right, a flap of bone is turned upward from the ala of the sacrum so that it bridges the gap between the ala and the transverse process of L5. **F,** the sacrohorizontal angle is the angle between a line drawn across the cranial border of the body of the first sacral vertebra and the horizontal. It has also been termed "sacral" angle, "lumbosacral" angle, "sacral lumbosacral" angle, and "Ferguson's" angle. When L5 is fused to the sacrum in a one-level fusion, the "new" sacrohorizontal angle is that made by the top of L5 with the horizontal. We have arbitrarily chosen a 55-degree sacrohorizontal angle as the point at which the L4 vertebra will be included when a fusion is done for high-grade spondylolisthesis. **G,** the skin flaps are sutured to the underlying fascia. This prevents a postoperative hematoma from forming and causing ballooning out of the wound area. **H,** a one-level fusion in a patient with 20% slip. Note that bone has not crept cephalad, as it often does if care is not taken. (From Wiltse LL, Spencer CW: *Spine* 1988; 13:696–706. Used by permission.)

E

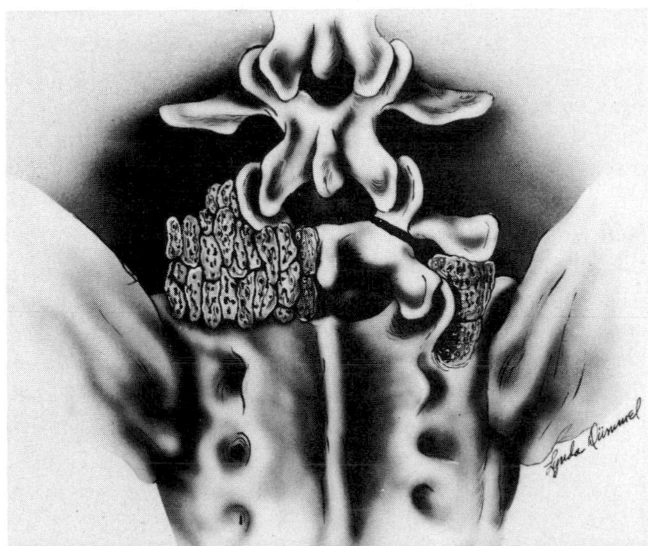

F

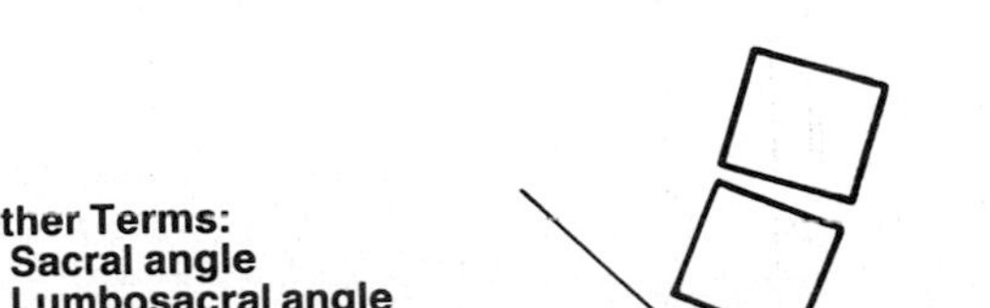

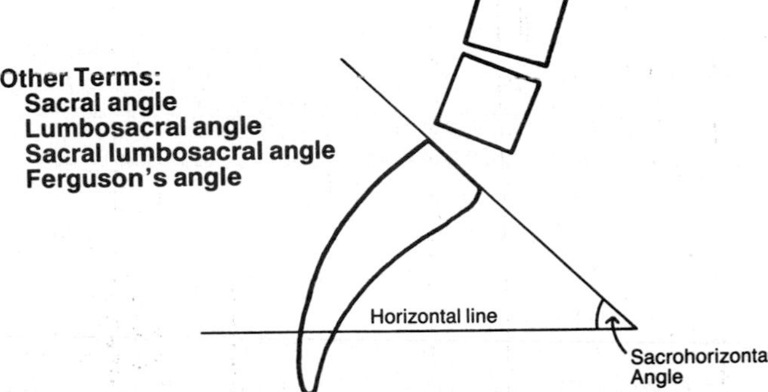

G

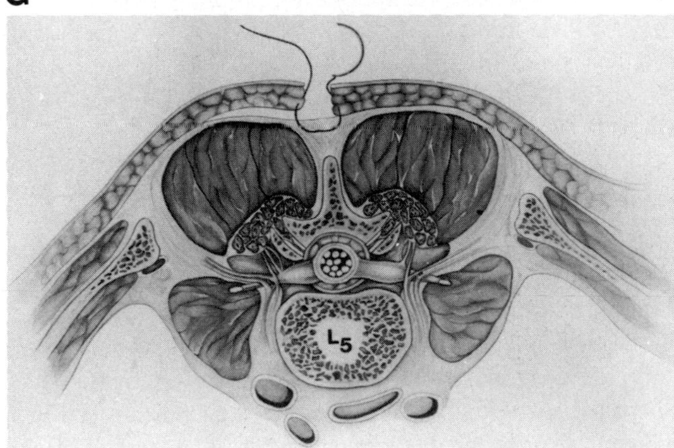

H

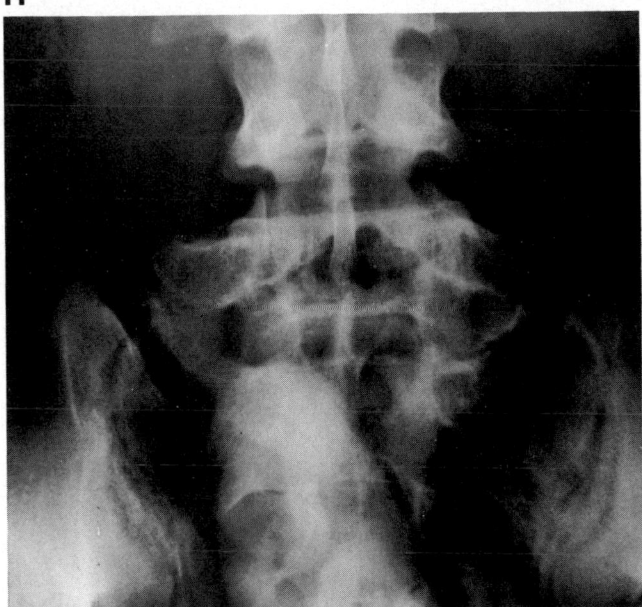

FIG 41–16 cont'd.

tain relief from their tight hamstrings but did eventually without decompression. If one is concerned about the fusion not becoming solid, a one-legged pantaloon case may be used to good advantage. We have not actually used this on primary cases. In addition, the electronic transcutaneous bone stimulator may be of value.

The Midline Approach for Arthrodesis in Spondylolisthesis

We have not used the midline approach to fuse isthmic or congenital spondylolisthesis since the mid 1960s. However, we usually perform a midline decompression and then an arthrodesis for the degenerative type of spondylolisthesis, and in this type we use a midline approach.

TREATMENT OF ISTHMIC SPONDYLOLISTHESIS IN ADULTS

The "conservative" treatment for adult isthmic spondylolisthesis is much the same as that for backache from any other cause, particularly chronic strain or disc disease. The same exercises are prescribed, although we have found them to be less effective in spondylolisthesis than in disc disease. The same type of corset is used with about the same chance of success. The low back school is of value.

Surgical Treatment

The principal reason for surgical treatment in the adult is relief of pain, not (as is the occasional misconception) to prevent progression of slip.[41–43] Slip rarely increases in the adult when there has been no surgical intervention.

When it does progress, the increase is small and is not in itself an indication for surgery.

A one-level fusion is usually all that is needed. Whether to extend the fusion to L4 depends on the status of the L4–5 disc, which should be ascertained. MRI is of great value in determining the status of the L4–5 disc, and discography with the pain reproduction test has been of real value.

The surgical treatment of types I and II can be summarized as follows for patients with up to 25% slip.

1. No leg pain.—Fuse in situ without decompression.
2. Mild to moderate leg pain.—Fuse in situ without decompression.
3. Severe leg pain.—If the surgeon chooses to fuse in situ with no decompression, the patient should be kept horizontal for 3 to 6 weeks until the leg pain subsides and then be allowed up walking with a one-thigh pantaloon brace or cast. Alternatively, the surgeon may do a limited decompression by tracing the L5 nerve out to where it ceases to be compressed and then fusing both sides and allowing the patient out of bed in a one-thigh pantaloon cast. The surgeon may also choose to do a total decompression on the painful side by sacrificing the articular processes and tracing the nerve far out laterally, in which case pedicle screws should be used at the one level only.

Spinal Stenosis in Types I and II

If the surgeon intends to do a decompression, it is important for him to know preoperatively just where the nerve pressure is in order to avoid unnecessarily destabilizing that segment.

Congenital

Type A.—In this type, as slip progresses, the lateral canals for the L5 nerve do not close down severely, but because the lamina is in place, the space between the laminae and the posterosuperior rim of the sacrum instead decreases, and the entire remaining cauda equina at that level becomes compressed (Fig 41–17). These patients often walk with a very poor gait and may occasionally even develop bowel and bladder trouble. If surgery is elected in cases with a lot of leg pain and gait changes, the entire lamina should be removed to decompress the cauda. If pain and sciatica are limited to one side only, only that side need be decompressed. If fused in situ without decompression, eventually almost all hamstring tightness disappears, but this can take years, and the patients often continue to have trouble bending over to touch the floor for an indefinite time.

If surgery is done in a child with severe stenosis, the lamina of L5 is removed, and a lateral fusion is performed, the child is placed in a knee-to-nipple cast for 8 weeks. Otherwise, further slip is likely to occur. In an adult, pedicle screws should be used—then the patient can remain ambulatory. Fusion of only L5 to S1 should be performed if the top border of L5 is less than 55 degrees with the horizontal in the standing position. If the top of the border of L5 is greater than 55 degrees, L4 should be included.

If there is wide spina bifida of L5, one need not decompress.

Type B.—The area of stenosis is between the posterior arch of L5 and the posterior rim of the body of S1. Also in these cases, since the inferior articular process of L5 slips forward, it compresses the S1 spinal nerve, and any decompression must take this into account. Since these patients are usually females in their thirties to fifties, decompression and pedicle screws would be in order if they come to surgery. These patients seldom have spina bifida.

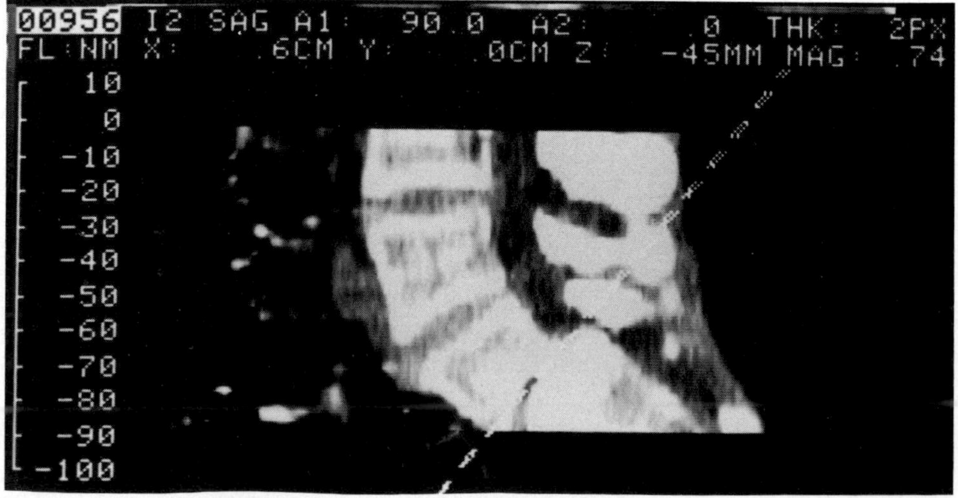

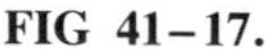
FIG 41–17.
Sagittal CT of a patient with congenital type II spondylolisthesis. The pars are intact; thus, the lamina of L5 is pulled forward until it presses on the posterosuperior border of S1. Severe neurologic change can occur but seldom does.

Isthmic (Type II)

Type IIA.—If the loose posterior element stays somewhere near its normal position, no stenosis occurs between the arch and thc posterior rim of the body of S1. Since there is a defect in the pars of L5, when the body and lateral masses of L5 slip forward, especially if they rotate, the proximal stump of the pars and lateral masses of L5 settle down onto the L5 spinal nerve and cause pain and hamstring spasm.

Burski and McCall[7] have recognized two types of situation as regards the posterior elements: (1) the loose element stays in a more or less normal position, and the defect opens or the pars stretches as it comes apart, and (2) because of tough scar tissue between the broken tips of the pars, the posterior element is dragged forward, in which case the areas of nerve pressure are similar to those in congenital spondylolisthesis in that there is stenosis between the loose element and the posterosuperior body of the sacrum.

Type IIB.—In these cases, the pars is elongated but intact, and the posterior element remains in a normal position. The area of stenosis is similar to those with a fractured pars (isthmic type IIA).

Stress Fracture of the Pars in the Young Athlete

Over the past two decades, the number of young people engaging in highly competitive individual and team sports has skyrocketed.[19] As a result, the incidence of stress fractures of the pars in the young athlete has increased markedly. When a young athlete in his early teens who has been engaged in very vigorous athletics is seen in the doctor's office with back pain, a stress fracture of the pars should be suspected. While ages 11 to 15 are the years of greatest risk, new stress fractures appear even in the senior years of college.[19] Table 41–1 summarizes the nonoperative treatment of these patients (Fig 41–18).

Fusion of the Pars Fracture Only

What is the place of fusion of the pars interarticularis only? We have used the following rules:

1. It must be used in isthmic-type spondylolisthesis.
2. It should be used in patients in whom it is important to save the motion segment.[19]
3. The patient should be a young person, no more than 30 years old. Results are better below 20 years of age.
4. There should be no significant spina bifida in the segment to be operated.
5. The disc at the defective level and at neighboring areas should be normal or ncarly normal by MRI.
6. The disc above should be nearly painless on injection.

TABLE 41–1.
Nonoperative Treatment of Stress Fracture of the Pars in Young Athletes

X-Ray	Bone Scan	Treatment	Repeat X-Ray	Repeat Bone Scan	Likelihood of Pars Healing	Length of Immobilization	Time Off Athletics
Negative	Unilateral pars uptake	Off athletics; wear corset	3 mo	6 mo	Nearly 100%	Until bone scan "cools" down significantly	Until bone scan "cools" down significantly; probably 6 mo
Possible unilateral pars fracture	Bilateral pars uptake	Off athletics; wear corset	3 mo	6 mo	Nearly 100%	Until bone scan "cools" down significantly	Until bone scan "cools" down significantly; probably 6–9 mo
Possible bilateral pars fracture	Bilateral pars uptake	Off athletics; wear corset	3 mo	6 mo	Fair	Until pars are healed by plane x-ray and scan cooling or else it is clear healing will not take place	Until pars are healed by plane x-ray and scan cooling or else it is clear healing will not take place
Definite bilateral pars fracture appearing fresh	Still very "hot"	off athletics; wear corset	3 mo	6 mo	Poor	Until pars are healed by plane x-ray and scan cooling or else it is clear healing will not take place	Until pars are healed by plain x-ray and scan cooling or else it is clear healing will not take place
Fracture appears old	Negative or only mildly positive	Treat symptomatically, posterior fusion or pars repair	—	—	Poor; Nearly nonexistent	May choose not to use a corset	Only until symptoms allow return

A

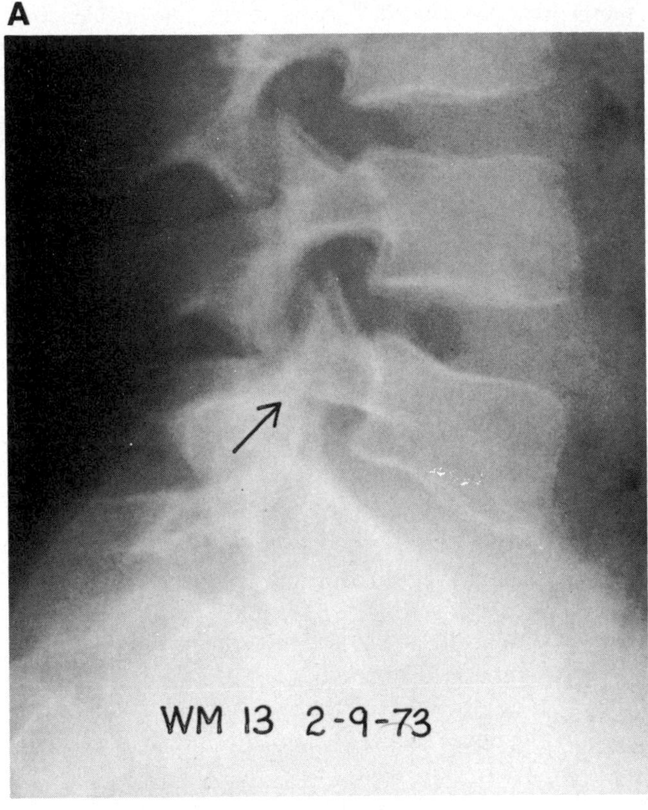

B

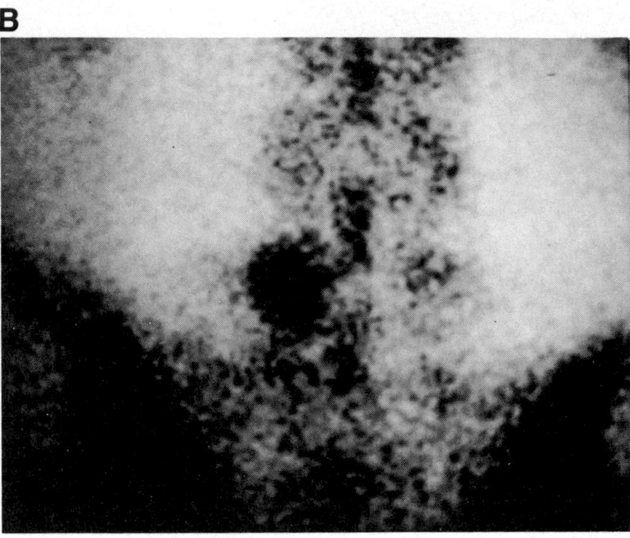

FIG 41–18.
A, 13-year-old boy with fresh pars fractures. **B,** bone scan "hot" on one side but not on the other. The "hot" side indicates bone regeneration. The "cold" side can indicate that no stress reaction has started yet or that the lesion is so old on that side that is has cooled off. This was taken at least a year and a half after injury.

7. The patient should experience definite temporary relief upon injection of the pars defect with local anesthetic.
8. There should be no more than 10% slip on standing lateral radiographs.
9. From a symptomatic standpoint, fusion should be performed if the young person with defects cannot live comfortably when not engaged in athletics.
10. A high-grade athlete who cannot practice his sport because of pain and has had an adequate trial with conservative therapy should undergo spinal fusion.
11. There should be no chance of the pars healing.

There are at least three principal methods of fusing the pars. The earliest was described by Buck,[6] who passed a screw down the pars interarticularis to draw the fragments together and then grafted. Scott[52] of Edinburgh advocated a method of passing wires around the base of the transverse processes and tying them around the spinous processes. Morscher et al.[36] (Fig 41–19) of Switzerland has developed another method using a tiny Harrington-type hook around the loose element and a screw into the superior articular process of L5. All require the addition of a fusion at that level. All these methods work, and all require a fairly demanding surgical technique. The obvious problem is to determine when it is appropriate to perform this rather major operation for a condition from which the patient will probably recover and go on to live a nearly pain-free life.

I have never used the Buck system, so I can make no valuable comment on this technique, but I do note that it has not been used to any great extent by others. I have used the Morscher technique and find that it works well; however, as of this writing, the instruments have not been readily available in the United States.

We have used the Scott technique on several occasions and like the technique quite well. The clinical results have been surprisingly good. I know of no failure of healing in our small series.

In the past year we have been using the Scott technique with a small modification by Hambly and Wiltse.[18] The details of this operation are as follows.

The patient is in the kneeling position, and a paraspinal approach is used (Fig 41–20,A–C). Gelpi retractors of various sizes are used to expose both sides. An 18-gauge wire is passed around the transverse process from below upward. I use a curved Cloward ligamentum flavum dissector to get around the transverse process. It is sometimes difficult to get around the transverse process, in which case it is permissible to remove the ligament from the end of the transverse process, as suggested by Hambly and Wiltse[18] and loop the wire around. The wires are

A

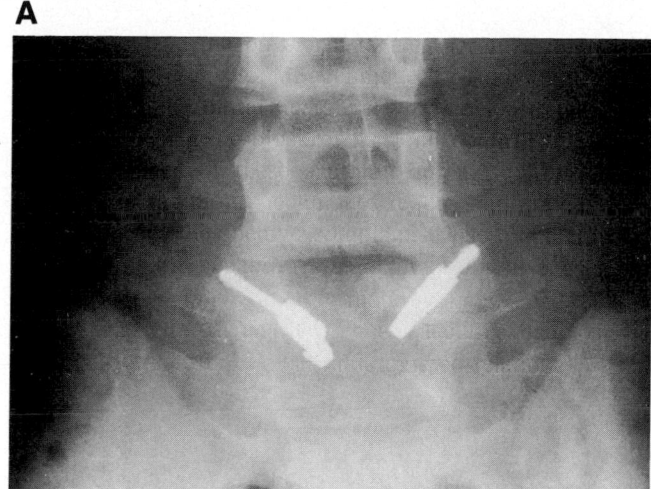

B

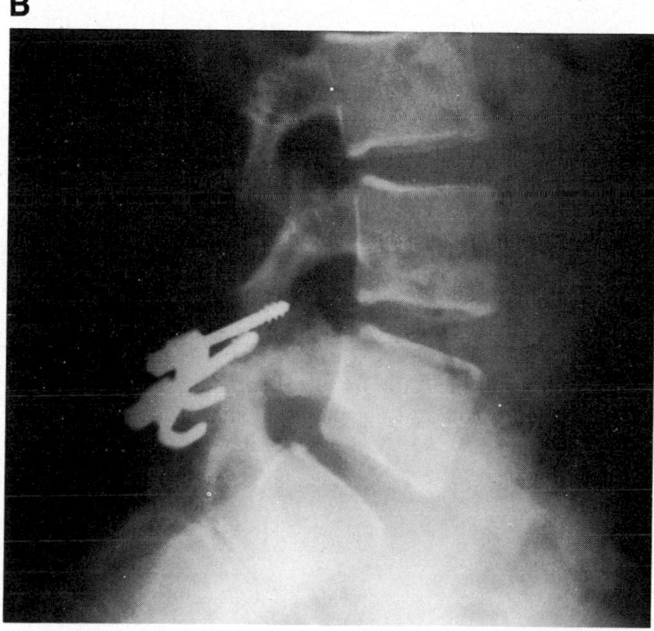

FIG 41–19.
A, AP radiograph of the Morscher system for pars fixation. **B,** lateral view.

tightened and the patient allowed up immediately. The fusion rate has been very good in our experience, and the patient has been able to return to athletics in most cases.[19]

Reduction in Spondylolisthesis

We have not performed reduction on a significant number of patients with spondylolisthesis, but there are many reports of this procedure in the literature, the first of which was by Jenkins[27] in 1936. Since then, others have reported on different reduction methods, in particular, Bradford,[4, 5] Steffee,[60] Dick,[12] and Pederson[40] and their colleagues.

At the present state of the art, it is my opinion that reduction is never necessary in a spine that has never undergone surgery if the slip is less than 60%. Many patients with even more than 60% slip show relatively little change in bodily contour and do well with fusion in situ. The reduction procedure should be attempted only by a surgeon who has made a very careful study of all available methods and has a good deal of experience in spine surgery. An orthopedist who only occasionally reduces spondylolisthesis is likely to run into severe trouble.

For cases with spondyloptosis, vertebrectomy of L5 may be indicated. Steffee[59] states that if the caudal border of L4 is level with or below the top of S1, he will do a vertebrectomy according to the technique of Gaines and Nichols[16] rather than trying to stretch the patient enough to place the L5 body on the top of S1.

Treatment of Traumatic Spondylolisthesis

Cases of traumatic spondylolisthesis in which the slip has been fairly rapid can often be reduced very easily.[67] Often nothing more than the kneeling position on the operating table will cause the vertebrae to slip into a position of near reduction; in these cases internal fixation is desirable to hold the reduction. Because the deformity is recent, there is often a good deal of sciatic pain present in traumatic cases, and reduction is very desirable. Pedicle screws work well to hold the reduction. Long-established traumatic olisthesis should be treated as any other case of spondylolisthesis.

Removal of the Loose Element Only

In 1950 Gill[17] at the annual meeting of the Western Orthopaedic Association in Portland, Oregon, described an operation in which the loose element is removed along with any fibrocartilaginous mass or bony fragments that might be impinging on the L5 spinal nerve (Fig 41–21). Over the years since his original description, the only significant change in the technique is that the nerve is channeled more widely after the stump of pars is removed and even the lower half of the base of the transverse process of L5. Normally, we would always fuse after a Gill operation and virtually always use internal fixation. In an adult, a Gill operation might be done if the patient has very severe bilateral leg pain with neurologic change. In such a case, one could do a Gill operation and fix just the one level with pedicle screws. We would go in anteriorly immediately or a week or so later and put in an anterior graft. Bank bone works well in such cases.[54] We would never do a complete Gill operation for unilateral leg pain; instead, we would decompress only the L5 nerve on one side and follow with a fusion. If the nerve must be traced all the way out to the muscle, we would use pedicle screws at the one level.

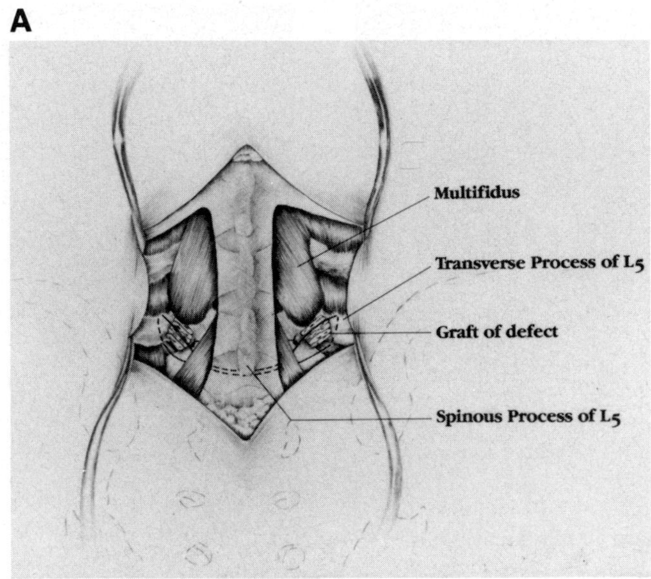

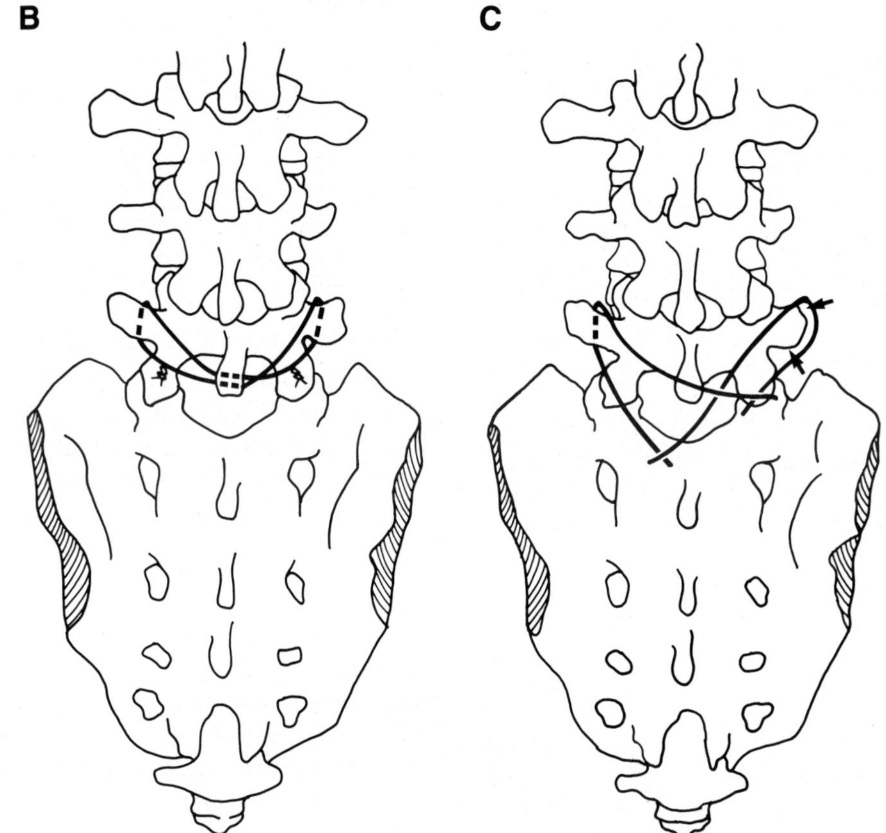

FIG 41–20.
A, Mark Hambly of Sacramento, Calif, has modified the Scott system. He uses a paraspinal approach and uses two wires that he passes around each transverse process but puts the knots one on either side. **B,** this can be tightened and at the same time draws the pars together more evenly. **C,** he believes that it is permissible to detach the ligament from the tip of the transverse process to make placing the wire around the tip of the transverse process easier. (From Hambly MF, Wiltse LL: A modification of Scott wiring. 1991. Submitted for publication. Used by permission.)

A

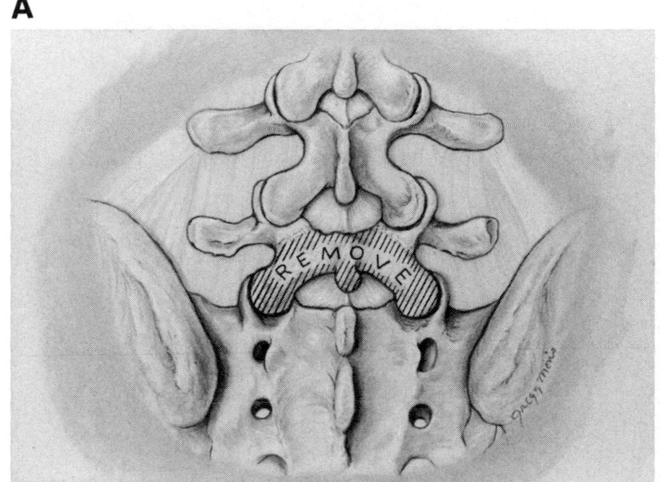

B

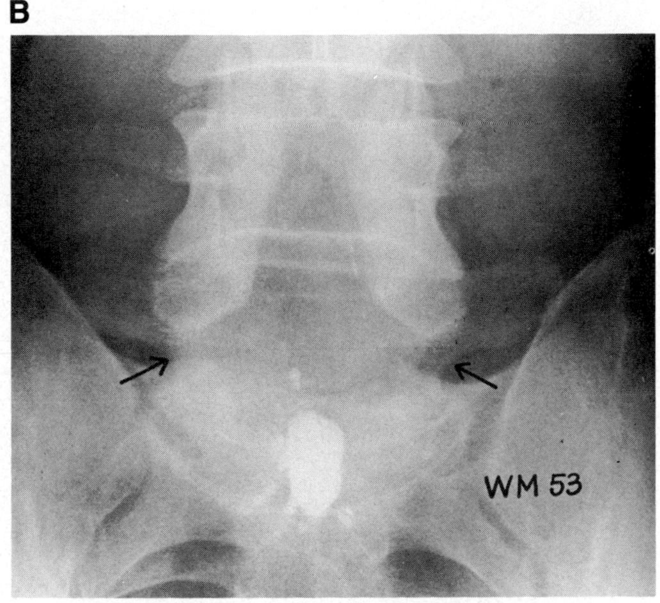

C

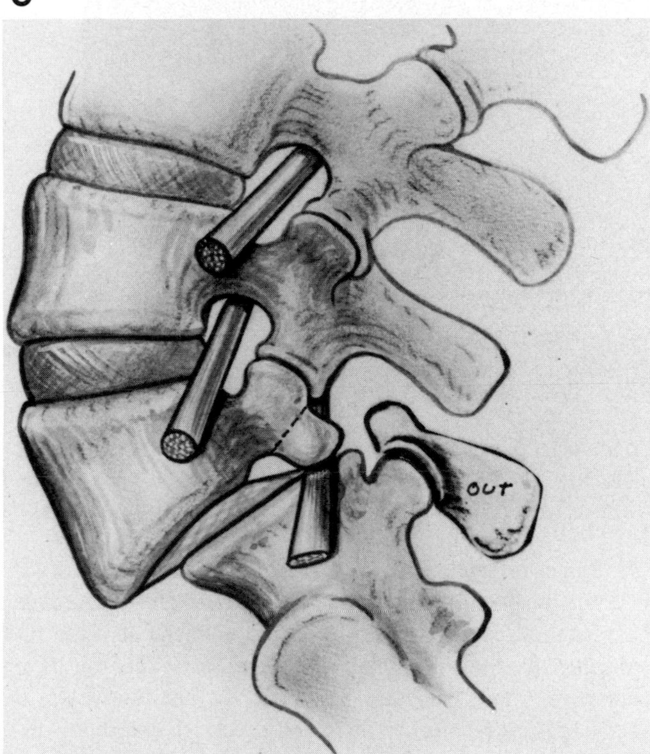

FIG 41–21.
A, loose element in isthmic spondylolisthesis. **B,** typical AP radiograph after a Gill operation. If a Gill operation is done, the proximal stump of the pars and often the distal third of the pedicle must be removed to adequately decompress the nerve. This will destabilize the lumbosacral joint, and either internal fixation should be added, or an interbody fusion is added, in which case the patient must be kept horizontal for 8 weeks (otherwise further slip will occur in a large percentage of cases). **C,** if one elects to do a Gill operation, he should do a very complete decompression and then a fusion, generally by using pedicle screws. Many would add an interbody fusion also. (From Wiltse LL: *J Contin Orthop Educ* 1979; 7:30. Used by permission.)

Unless rods have been inserted, which would hold the graft bone out laterally so that it does not creep over on the nerve, we would not recommend laying bone over a wide gap with exposed nerve.[66]

Use of Pedicle Screws

We have been using pedicle screws in the adult with spondylolisthesis in whom there has been a failure of previous surgery. We have not made a point of reducing the slip except in cases of alar transverse process impingement, in which situation we may avoid a decompression by lifting L5 off the sacrum. Pedicle screws have been especially useful in these cases.[29]

With pedicle screws the L5 can be jacked cranially and posteriorly, thus lifting the lateral masses off the nerve. Only the one level need be fused. This is the type that will need an added interbody fusion to take the stress off the screws. If the surgeon prefers, he can decompress the nerve by channeling far out laterally and then fix in situ with rods and pedicle screws with an added in situ fusion (Fig 41–22). These do not require an interbody graft since no reduction was done. In these cases, the approach can be either from the midline or paraspinally, as shown in Figure 41–22.

A

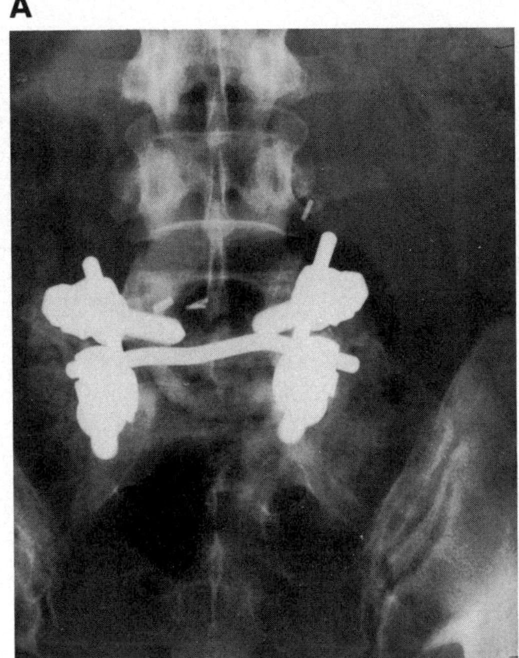

B

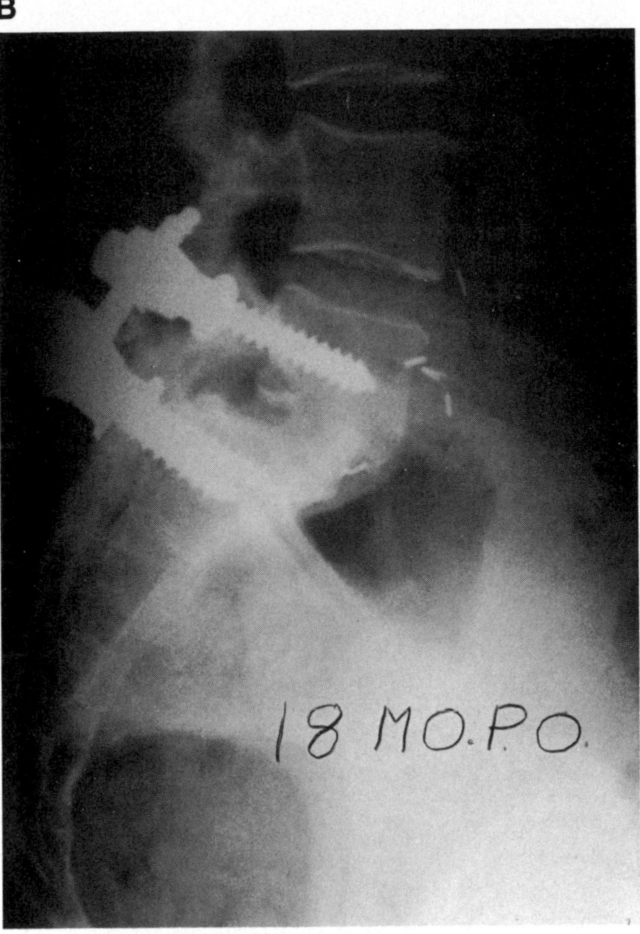

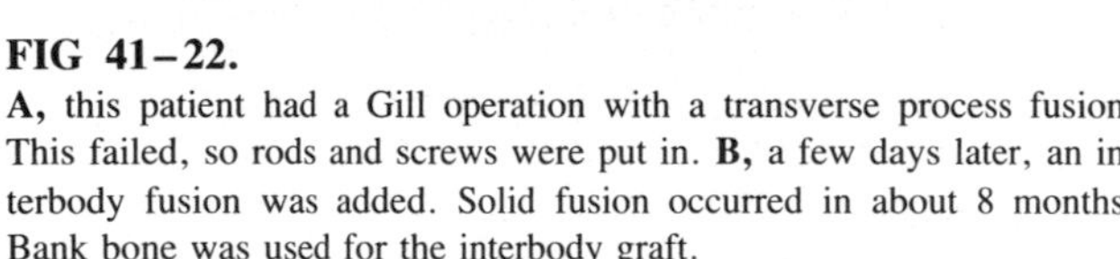

FIG 41–22.
A, this patient had a Gill operation with a transverse process fusion. This failed, so rods and screws were put in. **B,** a few days later, an interbody fusion was added. Solid fusion occurred in about 8 months. Bank bone was used for the interbody graft.

The Alar Transverse Process Impingement Syndrome in Isthmic Spondylolisthesis With the Far-Out Syndrome

Impingement of the L5 spinal nerve is common in spondylolisthesis where there is more than 20% slip.[66] The leg symptoms may be either unilateral or bilateral. As the body of L5 slips forward, owing to a combination of the olisthesis, disc bulging laterally, and disc space narrowing, it settles down onto the nerve. The annulus is drawn taut posteriorly but bulges posterolaterally. The combination of the bulging lateral disc, the stump of the pars, the lateral mass, and even the transverse process pushes the nerve against the S1 body and ala. Because the nerve is tethered out laterally, there may also be some traction on it, which may explain the severe dermatomal pain. Also the corpora–transverse process ligament may compress the nerve.

Surgery can relieve the impingement in two ways: (1) the nerve can be decompressed by channeling out beyond the cycle ligament, and (2) the slip can be at least partially reduced in combination with lifting of the L5 vertebra cranially along with fixation by pedicle screws.[66] If this is done, it is likely that an interbody fusion should be done also (Fig 41–23).

Interbody Fusion

Since the late 1940s we have often used interbody fusion for the treatment of spondylolisthesis. Our preference has generally been for only a posterior intertransverse fusion through the paraspinal approach. However, we have been using more interbody fusions in the last few years. It is my belief that the incidence of failure of interbody fusion of the lumbar spine in most surgeons' hands is high when used alone without a posterior fusion. However, some techniques yield an adequate success rate, including Freebody's. We have never used this technique except in the presence of high-grade olisthesis following one or two failures of posterior surgery and where gross instability is noted on flexion or extension.

Freebody Technique

In Freebody's technique[15] (Fig 41–24), a midline incision is made in the lower part of the abdomen. A longitudinal incision is made in the posterior peritoneum overlying the vertebrae to be fused. Great care is used to avoid

A

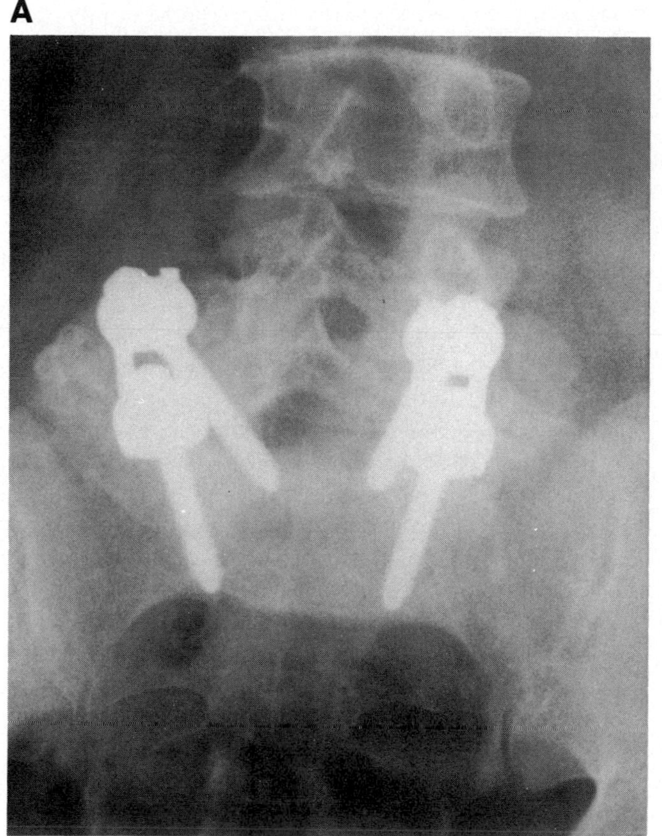

B

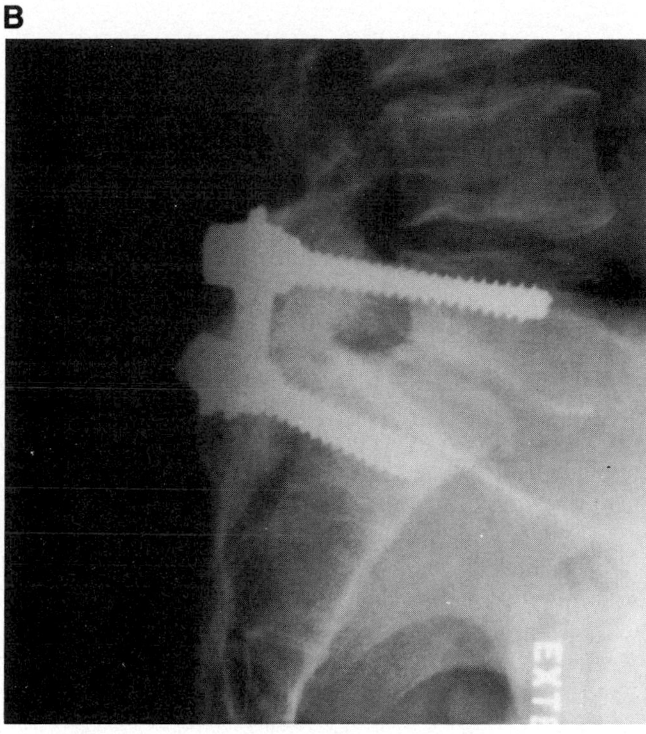

FIG 41–23.
A and **B,** this patient had a far-out syndrome on both sides due to far-out compression of the L5 nerve. Decompression and fusion using rods and pedicle screws were performed. Today we would probably do an interbody fusion first, jack the vertebrae apart, and then fuse posteriorly with rods and screws.

damaging the presacral nerve. Electrocoagulation should not be used here.

A "trapdoor" is removed from the front of the body of L5. A point on the front of the body of S1 is selected. Three guide pins are inserted, each about a distance of 2 cm but in different directions. Radiography or fluoroscopy is used to check the direction. One can usually be selected as being properly directed. This pin is driven in farther and the others removed with a curet. The hole is cnlarged. It passes through S1 to the top of S2. A full-thickness bone graft measuring 2.5 × 6 cm is then removed from the top of the iliac crest at its thickest point. It is driven into the prepared slot across L5 into S1. The use of fibular grafts driven across from L5 to S1 instead of the piece of ilium in the Freebody technique has not worked well. These grafts are very slow in becoming incorporated when healing is expected from side to side.

Freebody recommended that the patient be kept horizontal for 6 weeks, but the advent of pedicle screws has made it possible to allow our patients out of bed immediately.

Other Grafts

Horseshoe-Shaped Iliac Crest Grafts

Grafts such as those shown in Figure 41–25 work fairly well.[35] When they are used, it is important to jack the vertebrae apart strongly and fill the space very full with bone. If possible, five grafts should be used. The surgeon should remove enough of the surface of the end plate to reach raw, bleeding bone but remain within the hard cortical portion if possible.

The system cannot be used if the slip is more than 40% because there is not enough contact remaining between the vertebrae.

Dowel Grafts

Dowel grafts have been used extensively by Harmon.[20] Crock[10] has developed a technique using two dowel grafts, and he reports a good success rate. Recently, Selby[55] has refined the technique. Dowel grafts have the very distinct advantage of making the operation easier to perform than with other grafts. They often cannot be used in cases of spondylolisthesis because (1) the symphysis pu-

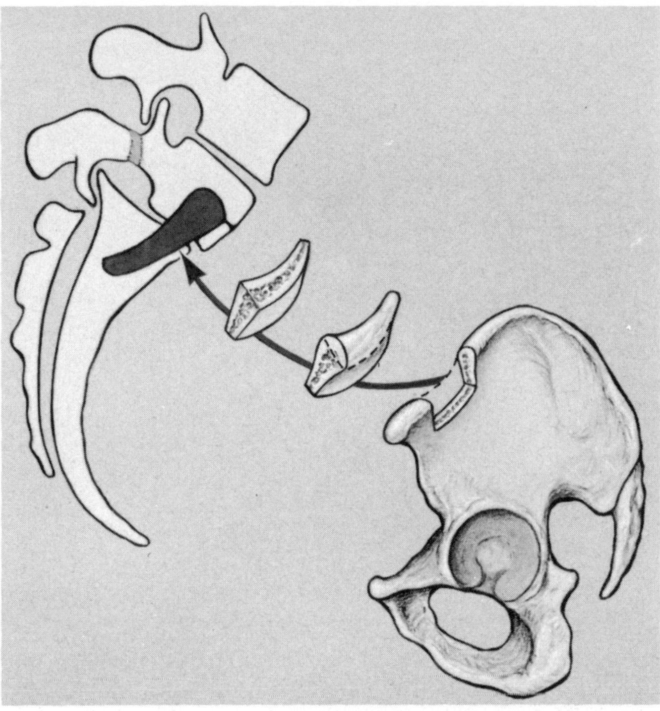

FIG 41–24.
Freebody graft. (From Ruge D, Wiltse LL: Spondylolisthesis and its treatment: Conservative treatment, fusion with and without reduction, in *Spinal Disorders—Diagnosis and Treatment*. Philadelphia, Lea & Febiger, 1977. Used by permission.)

bis is in the way of the drill, and (2) there is not enough remaining contact between the bodies.

The graft site in the ilium can be filled with Proplast, as recommended by Hochschuler et al.[24]

Fibular Grafts

Fibular grafts can be used to good advantage. The vertebral end plates are only partially excised, good hard bone being preserved, and the vertebrae are spread evenly. The segments of fibula are sawed with a reciprocating saw and impacted securely in place, standing on end. These fibular grafts must be held in place in a straight up-and-down position between the vertebral bodies. If they tip over, fusion may not occur (Fig 41–26). Great care must be used in taking out the fibula. We use Henry's approach. It is very easy to injure the superficial branch of the peroneal nerve because it passes distally along the front of the proximal 3 cm of the shaft of the fibula. Even vigorous retraction can injure this nerve. Small periosteal strippers should be used and retraction carefully done. Fibula should not be removed distal to the top of the lower third, and the interosseous membrane below this should not be preserved. We usually preserve at least 4 cm of the upper end of the fibula.

Often a sensory nerve crosses where the incision is to be made. A scalpel with a no. 15 blade should be used to incise the skin and all sensory nerves saved. Again, this system of grafting only works well in cases of low-grade slip.

Anterior Extraperitoneal Approach to the Lumbar Spine

We find the approach described by Harmon[20] and later modified by Fraser[14] and recently by Selby[55] to be the best. The skin incision is made overlying the left rectus muscle just below the umbilicus when exposing the L4–5 level and approximately halfway between the umbilicus and the symphysis pubis when exposing the L5–S1 level. Once through the skin, exposure is carried down to the rectus sheath, which is then incised transversely. The fascial incision is extended 4 cm caudad on the medial end and 4 cm cephalad on the lateral end. The rectus muscle is then freed hemostatically (with electrocautery) from the

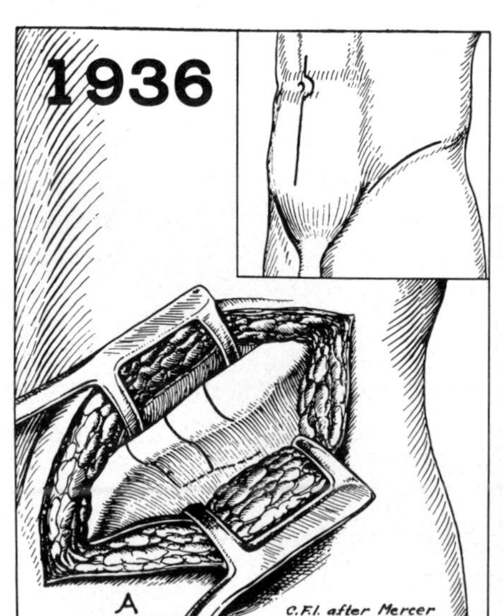

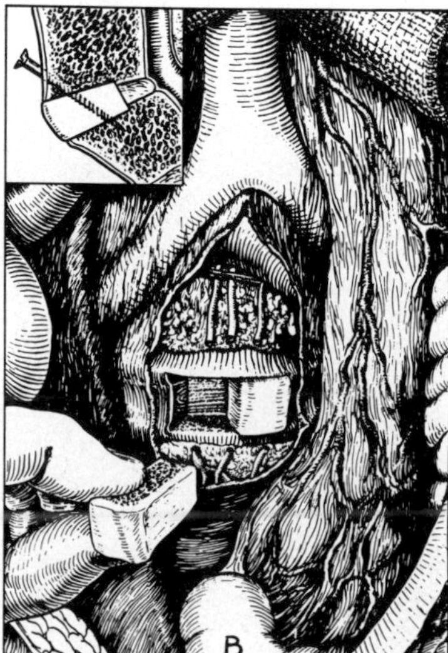

FIG 41–25.
Grafts are cut from the crest of the ilium. The vertebral bodies are spread with a lamina spreader. At the same time the kidney rest of the operating table is elevated. If possible, four grafts are inserted. (From Mercer W: *Educ Med J* 1936; 43:545. Used by permission.)

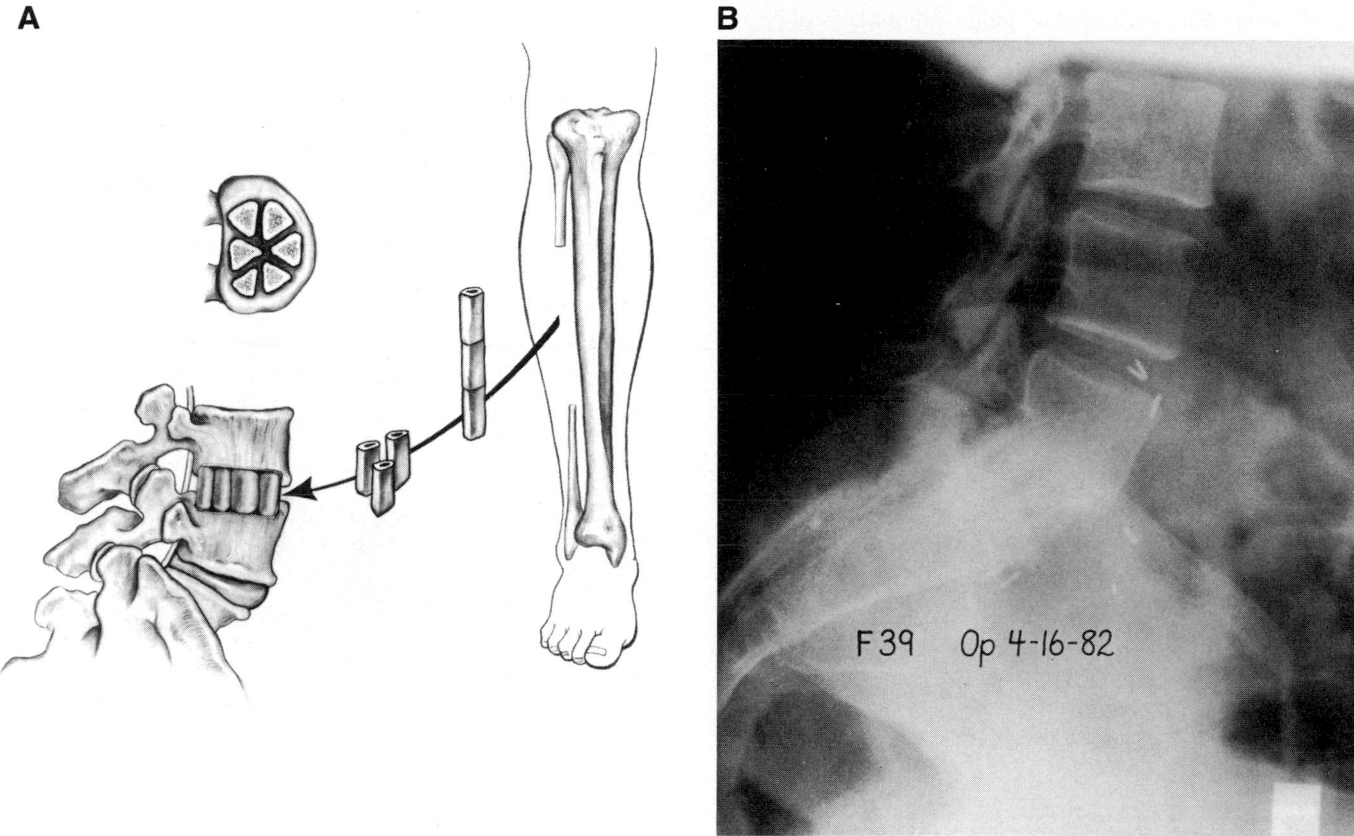

FIG 41–26.
A, struts of fibula are placed standing on end in the disc space. The vertebral bodies are separated severely. **B,** lateral radiograph of a typical L5-to-S1 interbody fusion using fibular struts. (**A** from Wiltse LL: *Instr Course Lect* 1979, vol 7. Used by permission.)

anterior rectus sheath, which is then incised on a vertical plane down to the peritoneal sac. Blunt finger dissection is used to mobilize the left hemiperitoneal sac from its attachments. It is important to not dissect behind the psoas muscles and to not disturb the genitofemoral or ilioinguinal nerves. As the iliac vessels are exposed, they are left in situ, but the left ureter is mobilized with the peritoneal sac. Long Hibbs' retractors as modified by Selby are valuable. If desired, spike retractors or simple Steinmann pins covered with a rubber tube can be driven into the vertebral bodies and also serve well as retractors.

With the kidney rest extended and the interspaces thus opened, manual palpation identifies the appropriate interspaces, counting up from the sacral promontory. Even so, radiographic verification should always be obtained.

In very large patients a midline transperitoneal approach will often be necessary, and in patients with high-grade slip, a midline approach should be used. Since pedicle screws are being used extensively, use of the dowel graft is likely to add the "third leg to the stool." Where reduction of deformity has been done, pedicle screws used posteriorly especially need support anteriorly.

Lumbar Interbody Fusion by the Posterior Route

Cloward[8] was one of the first to describe a method of posterior lumbar interbody fusion (PLIF) through a posterior midline approach. In his operation the laminae are approached as in a classic laminectomy. In isthmic spondylolisthesis, all posterior elements of L5 are removed, including the proximal stump of the pars. The superior articular process of L5 is saved so that the joint between L4 and L5 remains intact. The cauda equina is retracted to one side. The cortical surfaces of the adjacent vertebral bodies are removed as far as raw, bleeding bone by using special chisels. Full-thickness iliac grafts, autologous or homologous, are then driven into place, two in each side, to fill the disc space completely.

Several different PLIF techniques have been described in the literature. However, all PLIF operations have the problem of scar formation in the epidural area, all have an increased complication rate, and all require a high level of surgical skill. There is a great revival of interest in PLIF in recent years because of the fact that it works well in conjunction with pedicle screws. There is recent evidence that the approach for the PLIF does not, in fact, produce painful scarring and spinal nerve pain. Thomas et al.[61] reviewed 14 patients who had had an approach for a PLIF made on the side having no leg pain or sciatica. All had a simultaneous posterior fixation with pedicle screws and rods. On the 18-month follow-up, 12 had not developed any pain on that side. Two had developed mild pain but seem to be recovering. If this observation is confirmed by others, I predict that it will change the indications for PLIF in association with posterior internal fixation. I am hopeful that it will find its rightful place. I would not recommend use of a PLIF in the presence of pars defects unless posterior pedicle screw fixation is used in conjunction with it.

Treatment of Degenerative Spondylolisthesis

Symptomatic therapy is adequate in the vast majority of patients with degenerative spondylolisthesis, but when the pain is unrelenting and constant, surgery is most gratifying. Advanced age is not a contraindication. The myelogram is characteristically dramatically abnormal. The L4 spinal nerve, which passes out laterally at the level of slip (when the olisthesis is at L4), is seldom involved; it is the L5 spinal nerve that is compressed.[22]

It has been our custom to perform decompression and fusion in these cases. With decompression, the lateral two thirds of the zygapophyseal joint is preserved at the level of the olisthesis.[45] Even so, further olisthesis at this level usually occurs. Occasionally, in removing the lamina the inferior articular process of the vertebra is broken off. To avoid this, a high-speed, side-cutting, air-driven burr can be used to cut part way through at the proposed level of osteotomy (Fig 41–27,A).

The surgeon may prefer to use a smaller decompression as shown in Figure 41–27,B. However, the advantage of the smaller decompression, as long as all articular processes are saved, might be questioned.

In a study of 48 patients with degenerative spondylolisthesis operated on by us,[32] the following findings were noted.

1. The pain was predominately of the sciatic type in 70% and the claudicant type in 30% of patients.
2. The electromyogram (EMG) was abnormal in 41%. In every case of L4–5 olisthesis, it was the L5 spinal nerve that showed EMG changes and not the L4 nerve, as might be expected.
3. The degree of olisthesis ranged from 2 to 14 mm, with a mode of 4 mm.

A

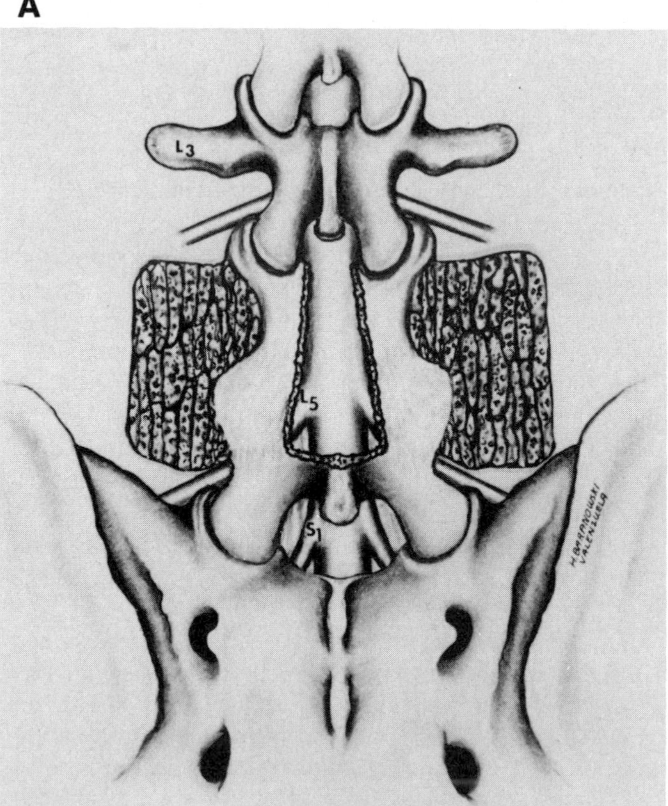

B

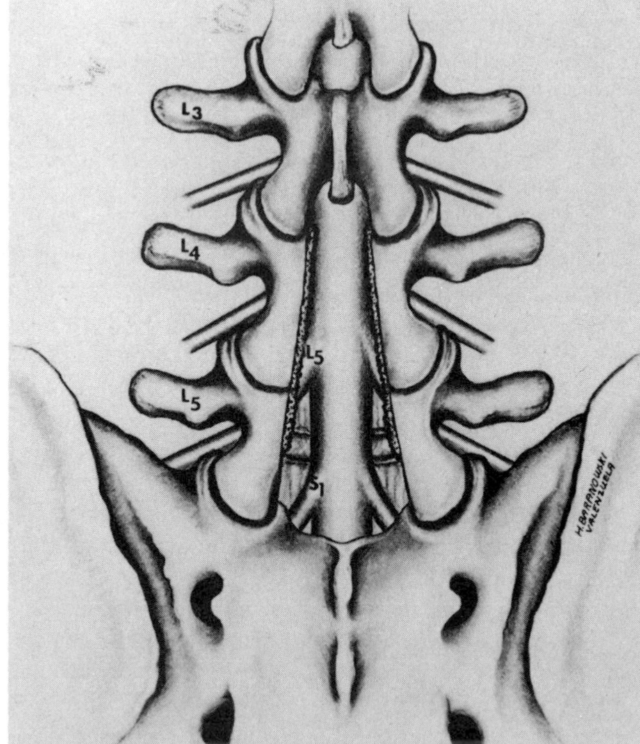

FIG 41–27.
A, a typical decompression done for degenerative spondylolisthesis. **B,** typical area of fusion. A smaller area of decompression may be done if there is no stenosis at L5. (From Lombardi J, Wiltse LL, Reynolds J, et al: *Spine* 1985; 10:821. Used by permission.)

4. There was no correlation between the following and the amount of pain relief: age, degree of preoperative slip, degree of preoperative hourglass constriction, and degree of further slip after surgery.[32]

5. There was no correlation between the degree of hourglass constriction and elevation of the cerebrospinal fluid protein content.[32] However, elevated cerebrospinal fluid protein levels portended a poorer result.

6. Slip progressed for at least 2 years and perhaps longer after surgery in some patients.

7. The level of the intercristal line (a line drawn between the tops of the iliac crests) was characteristically low and fell at the level of or below the L4 disc in 76% of the patients.

There was a great difference in the degree of pain relief as to whether a total posterior element removal was done or a midline decompression with preservation of the articular processes. If the entire posterior element (i.e., spinous process, laminae, and articular processes of L4) was removed, a good or excellent long-range result was obtained in only 33% of patients. If a midline decompression was done and the pars and articular processes saved, the result was good or excellent 80% of the time.

To summarize, degenerative spondylolisthesis is seldom seen in patients under 40 years of age and is symptomatic principally in women. The results of surgical decompression are good. We prefer a midline decompression to save the pars and articular processes. Fusion is usually done, and we limit it to one level, the olisthetic level. It is the L5 spinal nerve that is compressed in an L4–5 olisthesis. The nerve is compressed between the facets of L4 and L5 and the upper margin of the body of L5.

Lombardi et al.[32] studied patients with degenerative spondylolisthesis from our office and concluded that patients who had a one-level floating fusion did about 10% better than matched patients who underwent decompression but not fusion. However, Herron and Trippi,[22, 23] in a similar study, found that those left without fusion did about as well as similar patients who underwent fusion. We plan to continue to perform fusion in most patients but may be less inclined to do so in the very elderly.

Internal Fixation in Degenerative Spondylolisthesis

Shulman et al.[56] studied 27 cases of primary one-level degenerative spondylolisthesis. These were compared with identical cases in the Lombardi study where an identical operation was done but no internal fixation used. Pedicle screws and rods were used at one level only, the L4–5 level. By using internal fixation, the fusion rate was 100% as compared with 90% in the patients without fixation. The subjective clinical results were not quite as good in the group with fixation, and there were more complications in the group with fixation as compared with the group without fixation (Fig 41–28).

Point of Stenosis in Degenerative Spondylolisthesis

In considering the point of stenosis in degenerative spondylolisthesis, I will use as an example an L4–5 slip because it is the most common.

With an L4–5 slip, it is the L5 spinal nerve that is compressed. The pressure points are as follows. Where the L5 nerve comes over the posterior rim of the body of L5, it is the inferior articular process of L4 that compresses the nerve. As the nerve progresses distally, it becomes trapped between the superior articular process of L5 and the middle of the body of L5. One might question the proposition that a nerve could be trapped between two parts of the same vertebra, but in this case, we believe that the inferior articular process of L4 erodes the superior articular process of L5, and bone builds up in front of the superior articular process of L5 and traps the nerve (Fig 41–29). The nerve may swell a little and is tethered so that it cannot move. Then with flexion and extension, traction is put on the nerve, and pain results. It is well known that in degenerative spondylolisthesis at L4–5, when the patient bends forward, the body of L4 slips forward on L5. If there is a tethered nerve, pain could result.

To decompress adequately, the surgeon must unroof this area of compression but still save as much of the articulation between the facets as possible. Also, the pars should be saved.

When the pars breaks, as it does quite often after decompression, it usually slips forward at least a few millimeters. In this case the proximal stumps of the fractured pars may compress the L4 nerve between themselves and the posterosuperior border of the body of L5.

In cases of very high-grade slip, beyond 30% (which happens rarely in degenerative spondylolisthesis), the L4 as well as the L5 nerve may be compressed at the olisthetic level. The same mechanisms are present when the olisthesis is at levels other than L4–5.

SUMMARY

In the classification that we have presented, we recognize that there is great overlap in the fundamental etiology of types I and II. For example, we find in our consanguinity studies that both have a strong hereditary component. Both are characterized by dysplasia of the facets and an increased incidence of spina bifida.

There are, however, important anatomic differences that affect prognosis and treatment. For this reason, we have chosen to continue to separate the congenital (dysplastic) from the isthmic and have presented a classification that is largely anatomic. We believe that this division

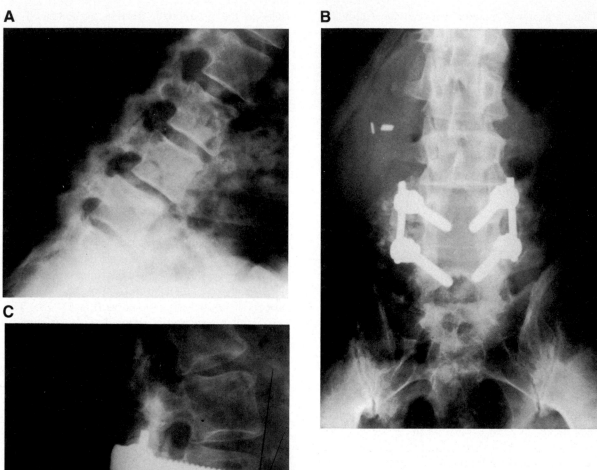

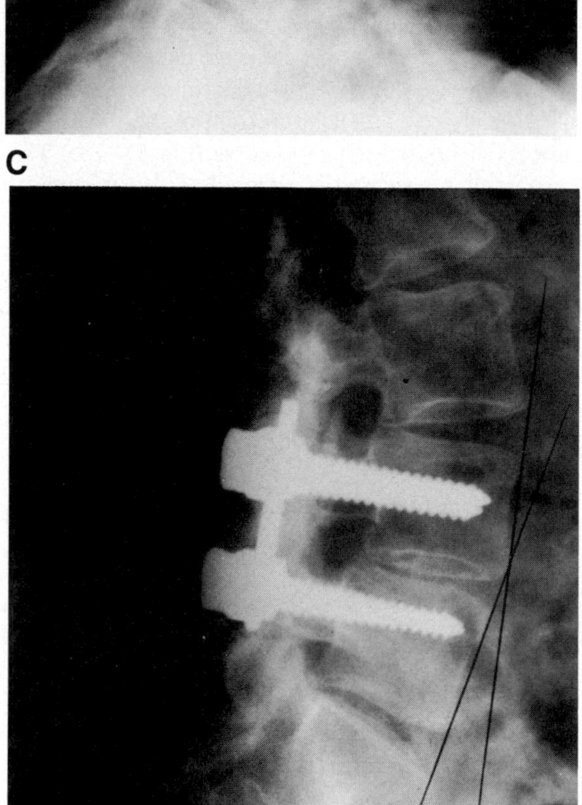

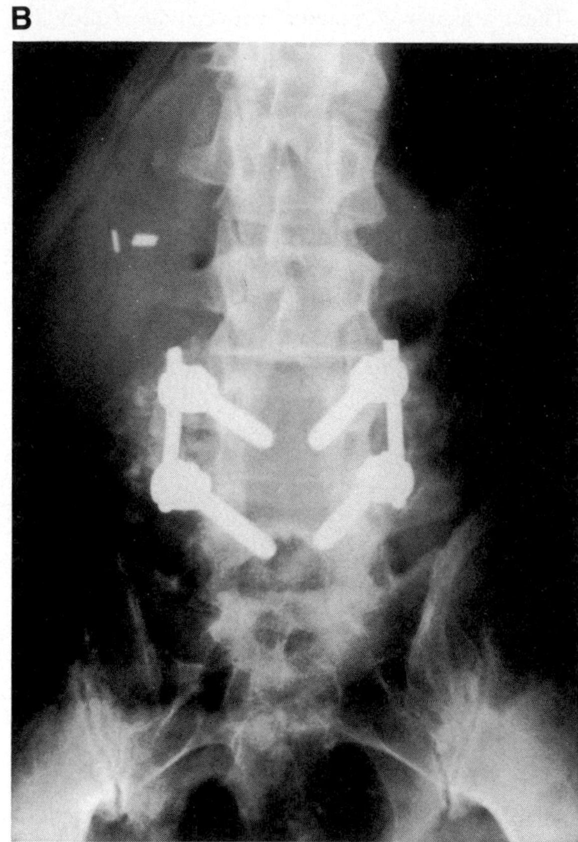

FIG 41–28.
A, preoperative flexion view of a case of degenerative spondylolisthesis. **B,** internal fixation with rods and screws. **C,** lateral view showing rods and pedicle screws in place.

will help the physician in the surgical treatment of the patient. We have also chosen to use the word "congenital" instead of "dysplastic" since both types of spondylolisthesis involve dysplastic articular processes and the dysplasia is considered congenital.

The section on surgical treatment presents the methods we have used for many years, which we believe give generally good results. The reduction of spondylolisthesis is discussed only briefly. I would refer you to the writings of Bradford, O'Brien, Gainer, Steffee, and others for more on this subject.

The use of pedicle screws and other methods of fixation are very likely over the next few years to alter some of the recommendations made in this part.

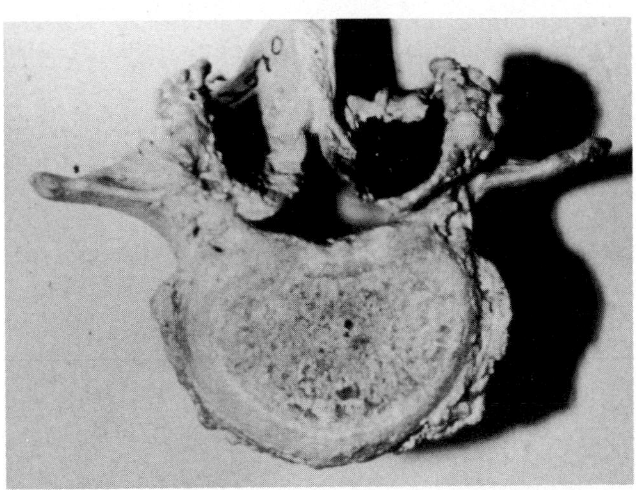

FIG 41–29.
Photograph of L5 from a case of degenerative spondylolisthesis with severe slip (30%). Note how the anterior portion of the superior articular process of L5 has eroded posteriorly and built up anteriorly so that the passageway for the L5 nerve is small. (Courtesy of Norman Rosenberg slide collection, 1975.)

Surgical procedures for spondylolisthesis that are generally contraindicated are as follows:

1. Gill operation in a child (there is such a phenomenon as "spondylolytic crisis," in which case a wide decompression would be advisable).
2. Gill operation at any age without fusion.
3. Gill operation and fusion in an adult and immediate anterior interbody fusion. Unless the patient is kept horizontal in a cast for at least 10 weeks, severe slip may occur. The reason is that the Gill operation, if properly carried out, removes all posterior support. If an anterior interbody fusion is performed, a large share of the anterior support is removed also. It may be that dowel grafts can prove adequate in such cases since these do not compromise the stability very much. Also, pedicle screws can be used to give immediate stability.

REFERENCES

1. Armstrong GWD, Chen BY: Sacral configuration in dysplastic spondylolisthesis (abstract). *J Bone Joint Surg [Br]* 1985; 67:335.
2. Baker DR, McHolick W: Spondylolisthesis and spondylolysis in children. *J Bone Joint Surg [Am]* 1956; 38:933.
3. Bogduk N, Twomey L: *Clinical Anatomy of the Lumbar Spine*. New York, Churchill Livingstone, 1987, pp 84–89.
4. Bradford D, Boachie-Adjii O: Treatment of severe spondylolisthesis by posterior reduction and stabilization. *J Bone Joint Surg [Am]* 1990; 72:1060–1073.
5. Bradford DD: Treatment of severe spondylolisthesis: A combined approach for reduction and stabilization. *Spine* 1979; 4:423–429.
6. Buck JE: Direct repair of the defect in spondylolysis. *J Bone Joint Surg [Br]* 1970; 52:432–437.
7. Burski G, McCall I, O'Brien J: Myelography in severe lumbosacral spondylolisthesis. *Br J Radiol* 1984; 57:1067–1072.
8. Cloward RB: The treatment of ruptured lumbar intervertebral discs by vertebral body fusion: Techniques and afterfare. *J Neurosurg* 1952; 10:154.
9. Cop R: Acute traumatic spondylolisthesis. *Clin Orthop* 1988; 230:162–165.
10. Crock HV: Anterior lumbar interbody fusion. *Clin Orthop* 1982; 165:157.
11. Crock HV: Personal communication, 1989.
12. Dick W, Schnebel B: Severe spondylolisthesis reduction and internal fixation. *Clin Orthop* 1988; 232:70–79.
13. Farfan HF: *Mechanical Disorders of the Low Back*. Philadelphia, Lea & Febiger, 1973.
14. Fraser: Personal communication, 1984.
15. Freebody D: Treatment of spondylolisthesis by anterior fusion via the transperitoneal route. *J Bone Joint Surg [Br]* 1964; 47:788.
16. Gaines RW, Nichols WK: Treatment of spondyloptosis by two stage L5 vertebrectomy and reduction of L4 and S1. *Spine* 1985; 10:680–686.
17. Gill GG, Manning JG, White HL: Surgical treatment of spondylolisthesis without spinal fusion. *J Bone Joint Surg [Am]* 1955; 33:493.
18. Hambly MF, Wiltse LL: A modification of Scott wiring technique. Submitted for publication.
19. Hambly MF, Wiltse LL, Peek RD: Spondylolisthesis in athletes, in Watkins R (ed): *The Spine in Sports*. St Louis, Mosby-Year Book, in press.
20. Harmon PH: Anterior extra peritoneal lumbar disc excision and vertebral body fusion. *Clin Orthop* 1960; 18:169.
21. Harris I, Weinstein S: Long-term follow-up of spondylolisthesis. *J Bone Joint Surg [Am]* 1987; 69:960–969.
22. Herron L, Trippi A: Degenerative spondylolisthesis. *Spine* 1989; 14:53–54.
23. Herron L, Trippi A: L4–L5 degenerative spondylolisthesis: The results of treatment by decompressive laminectomy without fusion. *Spine* 1989; 14:534.
24. Hochschuler SH, Guyer RD, Stith WJ, et al: Proplast reconstruction of iliac crest defects. *Spine* 1988; 13:378–379.
25. Hutton WC, Cyron BM: Spondylolysis: The role of the posterior elements in resisting the intervertebral compressive force. *Acta Orhop Scand Suppl* 1954; vol 16.
26. Jackson DW, Wiltse LL, Cirincione RJ: Spondylolisthesis in the female gymnast. *Clin Orthop* 1976; 117:68–73.
27. Jenkins JA: Spondylolisthesis. *Br J Surg* 1936; 24:80.
28. Karaharjii E, Hunnuksela M: Possible syphilitic spondylitis. *Acta Orthop Scand* 1973; 44:289.
29. Karlstrom G, Olerud S: Segmental fixation. *Orthopedics* 1988; 11:689–692.
30. Lee CK: Lumbar instability (olisthesis) after extensive posterior spinal decompression. *Spine* 1983; 8:429–433.
31. Lindholm T, Tagni P, Yukowski M, et al: Lumbar isthmic spondylolisthesis in children and adolescents. *Spine* 1990; 15:1352–1355.

32. Lombardi J, Wiltse LL, Reynolds J, et al: Treatment of degenerative spondylolisthesis. *Spine* 1985; 10:821–827.
33. Maurice HD, Morley TR: Proceedings BOA. Cauda equina lesions following fusion in situ for severe spondylolisthesis. *J Bone Joint Surg [Br]* 1989; 71:335.
34. McCarroll JR, Miller JM, Ritter MA: Lumbar spondylolysis and spondylolisthesis in college football players. *Am J Sports Med* 1986; 14:404–406.
35. Mercer W: Spondylolisthesis. *Educ Med J* 1936; 43:545–572.
36. Morscher E, Gerber B, Fasel J: Surgical treatment of spondylolysis by bone grafting and direct stabilization of the spondylolysis by means of a hook screw. *Arch Orthop Trauma Surg* 1984; 103:175.
37. Newman PH: A clinical syndrome associated with severe lumbosacral subluxation. *J Bone Joint Surg [Br]* 1965; 47:472.
38. Newman PH: The etiology of spondylolisthesis. *J Bone Joint Surg [Br]* 1963; 45:39.
39. *Oxford Dictionary*. Oxford University Press, 1977.
40. Pedersen AK, Hagen R: Spondylolysis and spondylolisthesis: Treatment by internal fixation of the pars and bone grafting of the defect. *J Bone Joint Surg [Am]* 1988; 70:15–24.
41. Peek RD, Wiltse LL, Reynolds JB: In situ arthrodesis without decompression in grade III or IV spondylolisthesis in adults who have severe sciatica. *J Bone Joint Surg [Am]* 1989; 71:62–68.
42. Pizzutillo PD, Humes CD: Nonoperative treatment of painful adolescent spondylolysis or spondylolisthesis. *J Pediatr Orthop* 1989; 9:538–540.
43. Postacclini F: The evaluation of spondylolysis to spondylolisthesis during adulthood. *Ital J Orthop Traumatol* 1989; 15:210.
44. Rask MR: Spondylolisthesis resulting from osteogenesis imperfecta. *Clin Orthop* 1979; 139:164.
45. Reynolds JR, Wiltse LL: Degenerative spondylolisthesis. Presented at a meeting of the International Society for the Study of the Lumbar Spine, San Francisco, June 1978.
46. Rosenberg NJ: Degenerative spondylolisthesis, predisposing factors. *J Bone Joint Surg [Am]* 1975; 57:467.
47. Rosenberg NJ: Degenerative spondylolisthesis, surgical treatment. *Clin Orthop* 1976; 117:112.
48. Rothman SLG, Glenn WV: CT multiplanar reconstruction in 253 cases of lumbar spondylolysis. *Am J Neuroradiol* 1984; 5:81–90.
49. Saraste H: Long term clinical results: A radiological follow up of spondylolysis and spondylolisthesis. *J Pediatr Orthop* 1987; 7:631–638.
50. Sarasta H: Prognostic radiologic aspects of spondylolisthesis. *Acta Radiol* 1984; 25:427.
51. Sarasta H: Spondylolysis of pregnancy: A risk factor analysis. *Acta Obstet Gynecol Scand* 1986; 65:727.
52. Scott J: Fixation of spondylolisthesis with circumferential wire around the transverse processes and spinous processes. Presented at the Combined Meeting of the English Speaking World, Great Britain, 1970.
53. Seitsalo S, Osterman K, Hyvarinen H, et al: Severe spondylolisthesis in children and adolescents—a long term follow up of fusion in situ. *J Bone Joint Surg [Am]* 1987; 72:369–377.
54. Selby D: Personal communication, 1988.
55. Selby D, Henderson R, Blumenthal S, et al: Anterior lumbar fusion, in White AH, Rothman SLG, Ray CD (eds): *Lumbar Spine Surgery*. St Louis, Mosby–Year Book, 1987.
56. Shulman GK, Wiltse LL, Banta CJ II, et al: Surgical treatment of degenerative spondylolisthesis with and without pedicle screw fixation. Presented to the North American Spine Society, Keystone, Colo, 1991.
57. Sienkiewicz PJ, Flatley TJ: Post operative spondylolisthesis. *Clin Orthop* 1987; 221:172–180.
58. *Stedman's Medical Dictionary,* ed 22. Baltimore, Williams & Wilkins, 1972.
59. Steffee A: Personal communication, 1989.
60. Steffee A, Sitkowski DJ: Reduction and stabilization of grade V spondylolisthesis. *Clin Orthop* 1988; 227:82–89.
61. Thomas JC, Wiltse LL, Haye W: Does posterior lumbar interbody fusion cause iatrogenic leg pain? Presented at the Fifth Annual Meeting of the North American Spine Society, Keystone, Colo, July 1990.
62. *Webster's Dictionary,* ed 3. Springfield, Mass, Merriam-Webster, 1971.
63. White AH, Wiltse LL: Spondylolisthesis after extensive lumbar laminectomy (proceedings). *J Bone Joint Surg [Am]* 1975; 57:727.
64. Wiltse LL: Etiology of spondylolisthesis. *J Bone Joint Surg [Am]* 1962; 44:539.
65. Wiltse LL, Bateman JG, Hutchinson RH: The paraspinal sacrospinalis-splitting approach to the lumbar spine. *J Bone Joint Surg [Am]* 1968; 50:919.
66. Wiltse LL, Guyer RD, Spencer CW, et al: Alar transverse process impingement of the L5 spinal nerve: The far out syndrome. *Spine* 1984; 9:31–41.
67. Wiltse LL, Newman PH, Macnab I: Classification of spondylolysis and spondylolisthesis. *Clin Orthop* 1976; 117:23–29.
68. Wiltse LL, Rothman SLG: Lumbar and lumbosacral spondylolisthesis, in Weinstein J, Weisel S (eds): *The Lumbar Spine*. Philadelphia, WB Saunders, 1990, pp 471–498.
69. Wiltse LL, Spencer CW: New uses and refinements of the paraspinal approach. *Spine* 1988; 696–706.
70. Wiltse LL, Winter RB: Terminology and measurement in spondylolisthesis. *J Bone Joint Surg [Am]* 1983; 65:768–772.
71. Winter RB: Congenital kyphosis. *J Bone Joint Surg [Am]* 1973; 55:223.

PART XIII

OSTEOPOROSIS: TREATMENT AND REHABILITATION

42

Osteoporosis

Joseph M. Lane, M.D., Richard S. Bockman, M.D., and Stuart A. Weinerman, M.D.

Osteoporosis defines a group of entities that have a common feature of decreased skeletal bone mass.[3, 25] The resultant structural and mechanical incompetence brings about fatigue and fragility of the bone in the range of stresses generated by normal activities and low-energy falls. When this low-set inherent threshold is exceeded, osteoporotic fractures occur. Osteoporosis per se and a series of other entities that have concurrent osteopenia (less bone mass) result in pathologic fractures of the axial spine. This chapter will discuss the general concepts of bone metabolism, the pathophysiology of osteopenia, and common entities other than osteoporosis that can lead to bone fragility, and finally, the remaining segments of this chapter will be devoted to a fuller discussion of osteoporosis and the various modes of accepted and experimental therapy.

Osteoporosis is a major public health problem since more than 20 million individuals in the United States have osteoporosis.[25, 32] As the population ages, the absolute number and the percentage within the population will increase. Recently, reports of 1.2 million fractures annually have been attributed to osteoporosis, including over 500,000 vertebral crush fractures.[21, 25] Osteoporosis is greatly feared among the elderly because of the inherent spinal deformity, pain, disability, and finally the significant mortality rate from hip fractures (12% to 20% higher than cohorts without hip fractures).[5, 10, 18, 23, 25, 30] The financial cost of osteoporosis is estimated at over 6 billion dollars in 1983 and will only increase as the population ages.[25, 29]

Primary osteoporosis is an age-related disorder characterized by decreased bone mass and increased fracture risk (Fig 42–1,A and B) in the absence of other recognizable causes of bone loss.[3, 25, 32] Inherent in the definition is the dependence upon an understanding of bone mass homeostasis, particularly those metabolic events that play critical roles in the establishment, maintenance, and removal of the skeleton.

BONE METABOLISM

Bone Matrix

Bone matrixes consist primarily of an inorganic phase, hydroxyapatite (calcium, phosphate, hydroxy ion), and an organic phase, type I collagen. Ninety-eight percent of the body calcium and 85% of the body phosphorus is deposited in inorganic matrix.[3, 25, 35] Type 1 collagen is the predominant organic component (90%),[13, 25] but numerous other noncollagenous proteins such as osteocalcin, osteonectin, and bone growth factors are critical components.[25, 26, 46] Only recently have the roles for these noncollagenous proteins been described, and they have been identified as critical control proteins for bone formation, maintenance, and resorption. Bone is a composite structure in which the strength of the bone is related to the architectural design, quality, and the absolute mass of bone. Collagen predominantly provides tensile strength, and hydroxyapaptite, the compressive strength.

Bone Cells

Bone is a living matrix that is constantly in flux and under direct cellular control (Fig 42–2). Bone formation is charged to the osteoblast.[25, 40] This cell arises from a marrow stromal cell origin. The osteoblast produces the organic matrix that is subsequently mineralized.[25, 34] Alkaline phosphatase and bone Gla protein are hallmarks of osteoblast formation. Bone resorption is under the predominant control of osteoclasts. They arise from macrophage line, isolate a segment of the bone surface (Howship's lacunae), lower the pH to solubilize the mineral phase, and produce acid proteases that enzymatically degrade the organic components. Osteoblasts that become subsequently encased within the bone matrix are known as osteocytes. They have direct connections to the other surface through microcanaliculi and play a critical role in calcium flux. Frost described the bone metabolic unit as a process that consists of a sequence in which resorption precedes formation and is coupled.[9, 10, 25] Recent investigations identify a direct biological communication in function between the osteoblast and osteoclast. An example of this phenomenon is the direct binding of parathyroid hormone on osteoblasts, their subsequent release of some unidentified paracrine factor, and the secondary activation of the osteoclast. The osteoclast itself has no direct binding site for parathyroid but responds to its control through this indirect coupled pathway.[2, 25, 31, 39, 45]

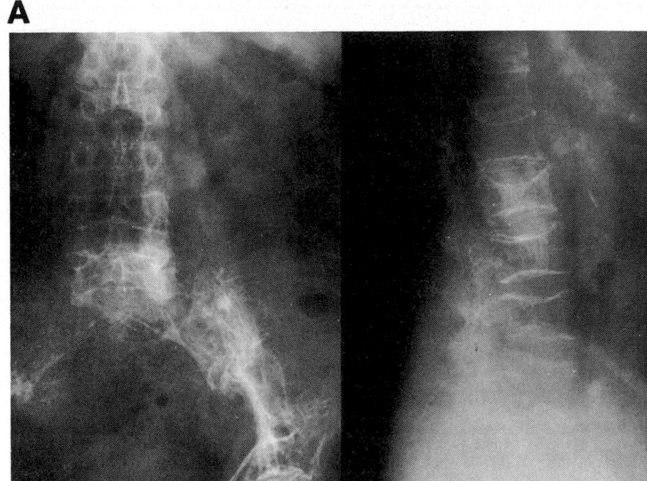

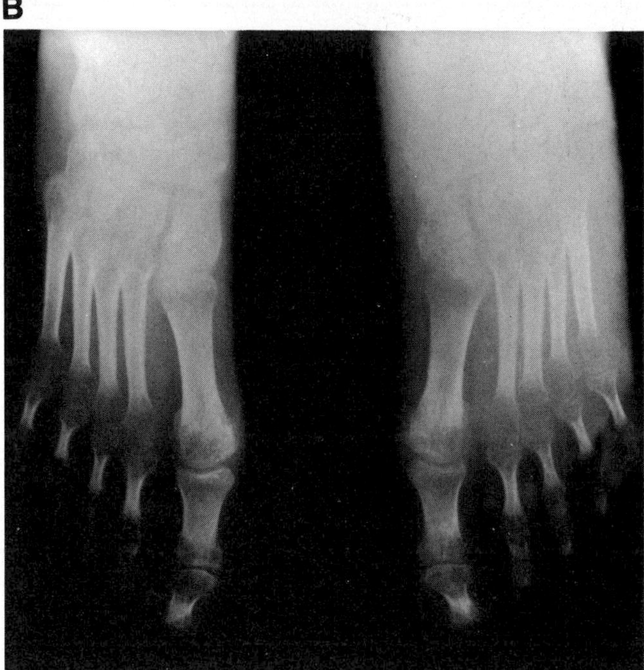

FIG 42–1.
A, anteroposterior and lateral radiographs of the lumbar spine of a 71-year-old osteoporotic female with a typical "codfish" deformity. **B,** AP view of the feet of a patient with disuse osteoporosis secondary to dermatitis. Note the decreased bone density at the metaphyses of the metatarsal.

Calcitropic Hormones

Numerous hormones have direct effects on bone metabolism. A predominant hormone is parathyroid hormone (PTH).[25, 48] It responds to a low ionic calcium level by retaining calcium and excreting phosphate in the kidney. It stimulates the conversion of 25-hydroxyvitamin D to the active vitamin D metabolite 1,25-dihydroxyvitamin D in the medullary portion of the kidney. Indirectly via the 1,25-dihydroxyvitamin D, parathyroid increases gut absorption of calcium. Indirectly via the osteoblast (coupling factor leading to increased osteoclast activation), PTH leads to bone resorption. Hence, PTH directly or indirectly will lead to increased absorption of calcium across the gut, increased resorption of calcium from the bone, and increased retention of calcium within the kidney.

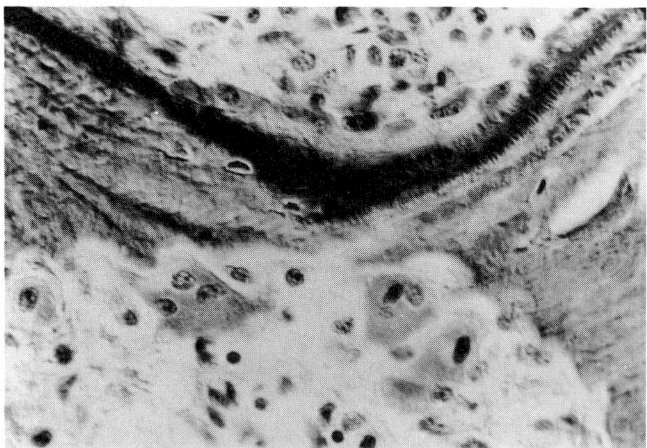

FIG 42–2.
Photomicrograph showing osteoblasts (bone-forming cells) at one surface *(top)* and osteoclasts (bone-resorbing cells) at the other surface *(bottom)* (Goldner stain, × 25).

Calcitonin[1, 25] is a calcitropic peptide produced within the parafollicular cells of the thyroid gland. It responds to high ionic calcium levels by decreasing the number and activity of the bone-resorbing osteoclasts directly. Thus, it lowers the ionic calcium concentration. Calcitonin has secondary functions by being a neuropeptide and has analgesic effects. This component will be discussed during therapy for painful osteoporosis. Its primary pharmacologic activity is therefore to decrease bone resorption. It secondarily increases bone formation temporarily, possibly by a still-to-be-described coupling mechanism.

Vitamin D is a sterol hormone that plays a critical role in calcium metabolism.[6, 7, 25] The active metabolic form 1,25-dihydroxyvitamin D is produced by a response to hypocalcemia stimulation by PTH stimulation of the medullary portion of the kidney. Vitamin D is synthesized from 7-dehydrocholesterol in the skin by ultraviolet light. 25-Hydroxyvitamin D is formed from the vitamin D in the liver by the P-450 hydrolase system and has a 3-day half-life. 25-Hydroxyvitamin D is converted to 1,25-dihydroxyvitamin D in the kidney following PTH stimulation and has an 8-hour half-life. 1,25-Dihydroxyvitamin D is the active metabolic form of vitamin D.[3, 6, 7, 24, 25] It functions as a maturation hormone to increase calcium absorption across the gut via the maturation of the villus lining cells of the intestine and their production of calcium-binding protein. It augments PTH recruitment of osteoclasts for bone resorption by acting as a maturation hormone for the macrophage stem cell. It does not directly stimulate bone formation.

CALCIUM METABOLISM

Not only does calcium function in numerous areas in achieving peak bone mass and maintenance of the skeleton, as we will discuss further in the treatment of osteoporosis, but it also plays a critical role in the teeth, cell function, maintenance of blood pressure, muscle contraction, nerve impulse transmission, and intracellular functioning. Calcium is injested in the upper part of the gut, with approximately 25% of the dietary dose absorbed.[10, 25] The calcium requirement changes throughout life depending on the bone mass requirements and the efficiency of the intestine[10, 14–17, 25] (Table 42–1): children, 400 to 700 mg of elemental calcium or two to three dairy equivalents; adolesence to the age of 25 years, 1300 mg or five dairy equivalents; premenopausal adults, 500 mg or two dairy equivalents; pregnancy, 1500 mg or six dairy equivalents; lactation, 2000 mg or eight dairy equivalents; postmenopausal women, 1500 mg or six dairy equivalents; and major fracture, 1500 mg or six dairy equivalents. Facilitators of calcium absorption include an appropriate gastric pH, adequate 1,25-dihydroxyvitamin D, and an appropriate calcium phosphate ratio of 1:1 to 1:2. Inhibitors of calcium absorption include achlorhydria, decreased vitamin D, increased phosphates, increased fat, phytates, oxylates (spinach), sprue, blind loop syndrome, and renal disorders. Inadequate intake of calcium is widespread in the United States, particularly among the adolescent females and the elderly.[4, 11, 25]

Phosphate is ingested in the lower portion of the gut.[11, 25] It is easily assimilated in the gut, with the majority of the dietary portion being absorbed and excess ultimately being excreted from the kidney. The requirement of phosphate is 1000 to 1500 mg/day, and in most modern American diets phosphates are never a limiting factor. Specific inhibitors include aluminum and beryllium; excretion is increased by PTH.

Table 42–2 includes a series of common abnormal mineral metabolic states.

TABLE 42–1.
Calcium Requirements

Population	Requirement
Young children	400–700 mg/day (2–3 dairy equivalents/day)
Growing adolescents to age 25 yr	1300 mg/day (5 dairy equivalents/day)
Premenopausal women	800 mg/day
Pregnant women	1500 mg/day
Lactating women	2000 mg/day

TABLE 42–2.
Common Abnormal Mineral States

Calcium—hypercalcemia (common)
- Primary hyperparathyroidism
- Hyperthyroidism
- Sarcoidosis
- Cancer—primary or metastatic (myeloma, hypernephroma, breast cancer)
- Mild alkaline syndrome

Calcium—hypocalcemia (common)
- Vitamin D deficiency (rickets/osteomalacia)
- Hypoparathyroidism
- Pseudohypoparathyroidism
- Malnutrition (low albumin)
- Secondary hyperparathyroidism

Calcium—normal calcemia (common)
- Osteoporosis
- Vitamin D–resistant rickets
- Paget's disease (unless immobilized)
- Osteogenesis imperfecta
- Osteopetrosis (increased acid phosphatase)
- Fibrous dysplasia

Phosphorus—hyperphosphatemia (common)
- Renal insufficiency
- Hypoparathyroidism

Phosphorus—hypophosphatemia (common)
- Hyperparathyroidism
- Vitamin D deficiency/resistant rickets
- Malabsorption

Alkaline phosphatase—increased
- Paget's disease
- Osteomalacia/rickets
- Hyperparathyroidism
- Osteoblastic sarcoma/carcinoma

Alkaline phosphatase—decreased
- Hypophosphatasia (phosphoethanolamine increased)

NONINVASIVE BONE MASS DETERMINATIONS

Bone mass can be determined by a number of noninvasive methodologies.[3, 25] Critical components of any system include accuracy, precision, and sensitivity to change in bone mass. Classic radiographic analyses of the spine demonstrate fractures and osteopenic changes when 30% of the skeleton has been removed.[19, 25] A large degree of artifact is noted due to technical considerations. The hypertrophy of the vertical trabeculae may further highlight changes within the bone mass. Specific changes associated with fractures have been well described elsewhere. Minimal changes in asymptomatic fractures are not fully defined, and controversy exists. Riggs has postulated a fracture as that in which either the anterior central or posterior vertical measurement has changed by 15%.[25, 36] This will include a very large percentage of asymptomatic individuals. Conversely, Genant's classification requires a 25% change in dimension or a 40% change in total cross-sectional area.[44, 47] These correlated much more with symptomatic changes and are preferred by this author.

Single-beam densitometry measures bone mass classically at the distal third of the forearm.[22, 25] Measurements made at the extreme distal end of the radius are more sensitive to the trabecular bone changes; however, it is difficult to measure reproducibly in that location. Consequently, the precision decreases as one goes to the extreme distal location. Other major limitations of the wrist are its anatomic and functional differences from the axial spine. Clearly, patients with profound osteopenia have decreased bone masses in both locations; however, the wrist is very strongly affected by occupation and function, and therefore, particularly in men, the correlation between the two locations can be poor. Due to the high concentration of cortical bone at the distal third it is also not very sensitive to changes in active bone metabolism.

Dual-beam absorptiometry of the spine and femur with an x-ray source has now achieved 1% to 2% and 3% to 4% precision rates respectively, and have extremely low radiation (half that of a quantitative computed tomographic [QCT] scan).[22, 27] Fifty percent of the vertebral body still remains cortical, and osteocytes and spurs will artificially increase the bone mass. New investigation utilizing lateral densitometry appears to be more sensitive due to its ability to decrease the amount of cortical bone under study. Scoliosis and rotational changes further complicate the ability of densitometry. It will never read low values but may artificially elevate some values due to to the osteocytes and artifacts. QCT sets a window width within the body of the spinal vertebra and measures the spinal trabecular bone mass. It is clearly the most sensitive to change; however, precisions have been reported from 3% to 15%. There is a 20-fold increase in radiation as compared with dual-beam absorptiometry. Artifacts caused by the vertebral veins within the body field and the change in bone marrow need to be recognized. As the marrow fat increases with aging, it artificially decreases the apparent amount of bone mass.

With the newer changes in the densitometry, it is the author's impression that the dual-beam absorptiometry techniques will become the predominant method for determining bone mass. It appears to have its primary goal in testing the efficacy of treatment and a secondary goal in segregating patients. The "fracture threshold" that has been created both for QCT and dual-beam absorptiometry are set at levels at which fractures begin to become common but not dominant. In addition, in all studies some patients with profoundly low bone mass can remain fracture free throughout their life. This brings to mind the observation that the strength of a bone is not only related to its mass but to the distribution of its mass (structure) as well. At the Hospital for Special Surgery[3, 25] (Table 42–3), the prevalence of spinal fractures increased as bone mass decreased; however, even in the lowest bone mass grouping, three out of eight patients failed to have spinal fractures. Consequently, the "fracture threshold" should only be utilized as a risk guide but not a certainty.

TABLE 42–3.
Prevalence of Spinal Fractures

Bone Density* (g/cm^2)	Fracture (%)
0.8–0.9	26
0.7–0.8	33
0.6–0.7	51
0.5–0.6	63

*Measured by dual-photon absorptiometry.

LABORATORY ANALYSES

Numerous laboratory studies are currently available for evaluating bone metabolism. A detailed description will not be the subject of this chapter, but the reader is referred to more traditional textbooks on endocrinology and internal medicine.[38] The critical functions[3, 25] to measure, however, remain calcium, phosphorus, alkaline phosphatase, serum protein electrophoresis, thyroid function, parathyroid function, 25(OH) vitamin D, cortisol, glucose, complete blood count, sedimentation rate, 24-hour urinary calcium, creatinine, and hydroxyproline. An algorithm has been created that utilizes these various laboratory maneuvers to define the osteopenic patient. Newer assays such as bone Gla protein and collagen cross-linking products may provide powerful diagnostic tools in the future but are currently still under investigation. The algorithm that is proposed is based on a segregation of patients presenting with pathologic fractures of the spine into endocrinopathy, bone marrow abnormality, osteomalacia, or osteoporosis. In those individuals whose condition is not a clear case of high-energy trauma, a differential diagnosis must be made between local pathology and generalized osteopenia. The vertebral body must be screened carefully for a structural defect secondary to local pathology, and the general skeleton must undergo bone density determination to ascertain osteopenia. Patients with normal bone density and/or structural defects require careful localized analyses of the vertebral body in question by bone scan, computed tomography (CT), and magnetic resonance imaging (MRI) among other choices. Patients with a structurally intact vertebral body (no localized defect) and evidence of osteopenia needs segregation into the appropriate category of osteopenia as mentioned above.

Bone marrow abnormalities account for 2% of osteopenic patients. They can be identified on either a complete blood count, differential, elevation of the sedimentation rate, or serum protein electrophoresis. Half of the bone marrow abnormalities masquerading as osteopenia are multiple myeloma. Fifteen percent of the patients with multiple myeloma will have normal serum protein electrophoresis results; they can only be identified by bone marrow biopsy or urinary changes. All these patients should manifest a low hemoglobin value or an elevated sedimentation rate. In the presence of these latter findings, even with normal protein electrophoresis, a bone marrow analysis is warranted to identify some underlying bone marrow abnormality.

If no bone marrow abnormality is present, the patient should next be screened for endocrinopathy. Unstable diabetes and iatrogenic Cushing's disease are clearly associated with osteoporosis. Adrenal tumors, although they produce Cushing's disease, are extraordinarily rare, and a check of 24-hour urinary blood cortisol levels has such a low yield that they should not be considered as the first line of investigation. Conversely, hyperparathyroidism is common[25, 48] and can occur even in the presence of normal calcium concentrations; therefore, an intact PTH determination, the most sensitive test today for parathyroid dysfunction, should be ordered. Patients with hyperthyroidism commonly present in the guise of an individual with extremely great body weight loss coupled with osteopenia. Iatrogenic hyperthyroidism is common in women who are slightly obese and have been placed on thyroid medication for borderline indications of hypothyroidism. Patients frequently utilize the thyroid medications to control weight gain. Their triiodothyronine (T3) and thyroxine (T4) levels are often in the upper limits of normal, depending on the preparation of thyroid supplementation. The key to their diagnosis is a markedly suppressed thyroid-stimulating hormone by immunoradiometic assay (TSH-IRMA).

With endocrinopathy eliminated as well as bone marrow abnormality, the two leading causes of osteopenia that remain are osteomalacia and osteoporosis. In the New York City environment 8% of patients presenting with osteopenia have varying degrees of osteomalacia. Half of those patients clearly have abnormal blood studies, most notably decreased urinary calcium, decreased 25-hydroxyvitamin D, low to normal serum calcium, low phosphorus, elevated alkaline phosphatase, and elevated PTH (secondary hyperparathyroidism) levels. The remaining mild osteomalacic patients will fit within the broad ranges of "normal" laboratory values and can only be diagnosed by a transilial bone biopsy. Patients with osteoporosis per se and normal-appearing osteomalacic patients can be differentiated by a transilial bone biopsy that evaluates not only bone quantitity but the dynamics of bone formation, bone resorption, and the quality of bone.[25, 33] By utilizing a double tetracycline-labeling program (Table 42–4) a bone biopsy can generate information as to bone formation, bone resorption, and mineralization parameters. Osteoporosis itself can clearly be divided into high-turnover and quiescent osteoporosis. High-turnover osteopenia accounts for a third of osteoporotic patients with high resorptive rates and high formation rates. Quiescent osteoporosis in which bone formation and resorption are both markedly dampened accounts for the remaining two thirds of patients with osteoporosis. Treatment programs differ for these two forms of osteoporosis as they do for the entities of osteomalacia, endocrinopathies, and bone marrow abnormalities.

TABLE 42–4.

Double Tetracycline Labeling Program for Dynamic Measurements

1. Take oxytetracycline, 250 mg (1 capsule), 4 times a day for 3 days.

_________ _________ _________

2. *Do not take* either of the medications for 12 days.

_________ _________ _________
_________ _________ _________
_________ _________ _________
_________ _________ _________

3. Take demeclocycline (Declomycin), 300 mg (1 tablet), 3 times a day (morning, afternoon, evening).

_________ _________ _________

4. Bone biopsy will be performed on_________, 7 days after the Declomycin is finished.

RICKETS AND OSTEOMALACIA

Rickets and osteomalacia represent respectively a failure to mineralize epiphyseal cartilage with an increased hypertrophic zone and a decreased mineralizion rate of trabeculae with increased unmineralized osteoid[8] (Fig 42–3,A–D). Clinical rickets and osteomalacia represent apathetic, irritable, shortened individuals with a positive Gower test, laxities, frontal bossing, ricketic rosary, Harrison grooves, and enlarged epiphyses. Clinical signs of osteomalacia are localized bone pain and muscle weakness. The radiographic findings of rickets include a widened epiphyseal plate with a paintbrush phenomenon and cupping with an indistinct zone of provisional calcification (Fig 42–3,C and D). Stress fractures (Looser's lines), long-bone bowing, genu valgum, and genu varum are other abnormalities. Osteomalacia is best seen with Looser's lines and other radiographic findings such as the rugby jersey spine. In the hands of the radiologists at The Hospital for Special Surgery, other than the presence of Looser's lines, osteomalacia is indistinguishable from osteoporosis radiographically. Laboratory findings include normal or decreased calcium, phosphorus is decreased except where it is increased with renal osteodystrophy, alkaline phosphatase is increased, and 25-hydroxyvitamin D is decreased in vitamin D deficiency syndromes. (Table 42–5 illustrates specific disorders of vitamin D). The treatments vary for the etiologies of osteomalacia. Vitamin D deficiency is treated with 50,000 units of vitamin D plus calcium, vitamin D–resistant osteomalacia requires phosphate plus 1,25-dihyroxyvitamin D (low dose). Renal

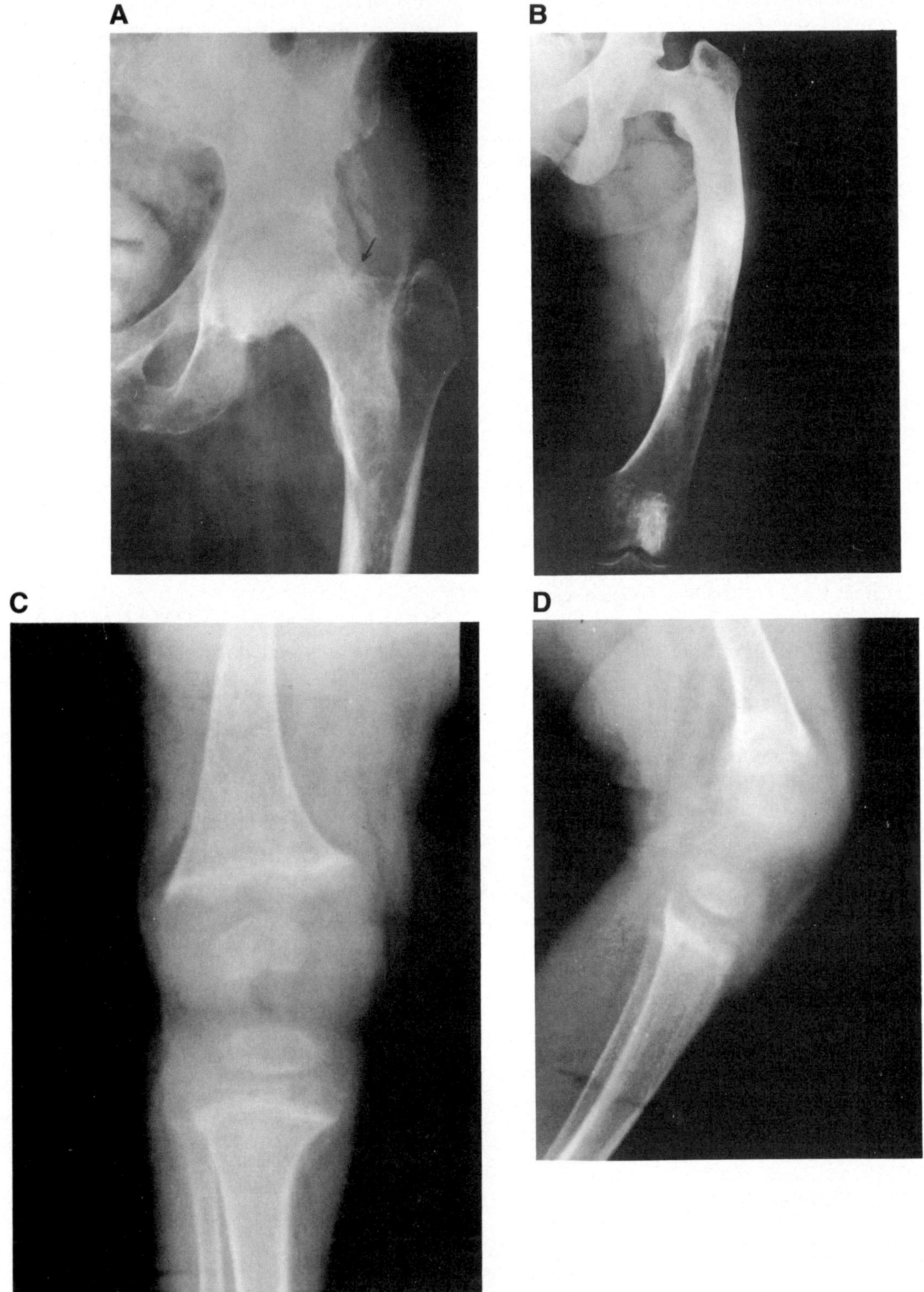

FIG 42–3.
A, patient with osteomalacia and a Looser line in neck of the femur. **B,** Looser line and deformity of the femur in a patient with osteomalacia secondary to "milkman's" syndrome. **C** and **D,** AP and lateral views of rickets demonstrating osteopenia and epiphyseal cupping.

TABLE 42–5.
Disorders of Vitamin D

Disorder	Ca	PO_4	PTH*	Alk Ph*	25 (OH)	1,25(OH)	Ur Ca*
Vitamin D deficiency	Nl, Dec*	Dec	Inc*	Inc	Dec	Any	Dec
Vitamin D resistant	Nl	Dec	Nl	Inc	Nl	Nl, Dec	Nl
Renal osteodystrophy	Dec	Inc	Inc	Inc	Nl	Dec	Dec
Hypophosphatemic	Nl	Dec	Nl	Inc	Nl	Nl	Nl

*PTH = parathyroid hormone; Alk Ph = alkaline phosphatase; Ur Ca = urinary calcium; Nl = normal; Dec = decreased; Inc = increased.

osteodystrophy is treated with increased calcium, low phosphate, phosphate binders, and the use of sodium bicarbonate to control the calcium phosphorus ratio. Selective parathyroidectomy may be indicated. Orthopedic treatments include bracing and osteotomies for frank rickets. Spinal disorders are addressed by bracing and correction of the underlying etiologic factor.

HYPERPARATHYROIDISM

Primary hyperparathyroidism is most commonly associated with, in decreasing order, parathyroid adenoma, parathyroid hyperplasia, and parathyroid cancer. Secondary hyperparathyroidism occurs in osteomalacia, rickets, and renal osteodystrophy. Clinical findings are those of bone pain: brown tumors, pathologic fractures, renal stones, and ulcers. Hypercalcemia today is the most common single entity that brings attention to this diagnosis. The radiographic findings include those of a brown tumor, salt-and-pepper skull, osteopenia, occasionally osteosclerosis, soft-tissue calcification, scalloping of the phalangeals, loss of the phalangeal tuft, clavicular erosions laterally, and decreased bone density (Fig 42–4,A–C). Laboratory findings (Table 42–6) in primary hyperparathyroidism include elevated serum calcium, low serum phosphate, and elevated PTH levels; in secondary hyperparathyroidism, findings are decreased calcium, decreased phosphate, and increased PTH levels; in secondary hyperparathyroidism specifically related to renal osteodystrophy, decreased calcium, increased phosphate, and increased PTH levels can be seen; and in hypercalcemia of malignancy, increased calcium, decreased phosphorus, and decreased PTH levels are noted.

TABLE 42–6.
Laboratory: Hyperparathyroidism

Type	Calcium	Phosphate	PTH*
Primary	Increased	Decreased	Increased
Secondary	Decreased	Decreased Increased (renal)	Increased
Hypercalcemia of malignancy	Increased	Decreased	Decreased

*PTH = parathyroid hormone.

OSTEOPOROSIS

Osteoporosis is defined as a loss of bone mass and resultant bone fragility. Contributing factors for bone loss include (1) decreased peak bone mass achieved by the age of 25 years; (2) the associated physiologic bone loss at 0.5% per year for both men and women after the age of 30 years; (3) the accelerated bone loss in the postmenopausal phase (10 years) of approximately 2% per year, (8% per year trabecular and 0.5% per year cortical); and (4) resumption of gradual slow bone loss during later life (0.5% per year).[25, 28, 32, 42]

Blacks have greater bone mass than Caucasians do, but the loss rates are equally corrected for sexes. Risk factors that contribute to osteoporosis include early menopause; episodes of amenorrhea and oligomenorrhea; alcohol, which is toxic to the osteoblasts; smoking, which increases estrogen degradation; chronic low calcium intake; malnutrition; the use of steroids; calcium-losing diuretics; and genetic factors such as fair complexion, northwest European ancestry, thin small bones, hypermobility, scoliosis, and a strong family history. At the osteoporosis center of the Hospital for Special Surgery, one third of osteoporotic patients have extremely strong family history and genetic correlations.

Riggs and Melton[25, 37] have defined a subclassification of involutional osteoporosis based on fracture and the pattern of bone loss. "Postmenopausal osteoporosis" (type I) is characterized by the rapid bone loss seen in recent postmenopausal females. There is a rapid phase of loss predominantly in trabecular bone as well as an association with vertebral and wrist fractures, and type I responds to antiresorptive treatment (estrogen). "Senile osteoporosis" (type II) affects women 2:1 over males and is related to aging and chronic calcium deficiency, increased PTH activity, and decreased bone formation.

The radiologic findings of osteoporosis include osteopenia (more than 30% of the mineral is absent), loss of the vertebral horizontal trabeculae, wedge fractures of the thoracic spine, crushed or end-plate fractures of the lumbar spine, stress fractures of the pelvis, and appendicular fractures, most notably of the humerus, wrist, hips, supracondylar femur, and tibial plateau.

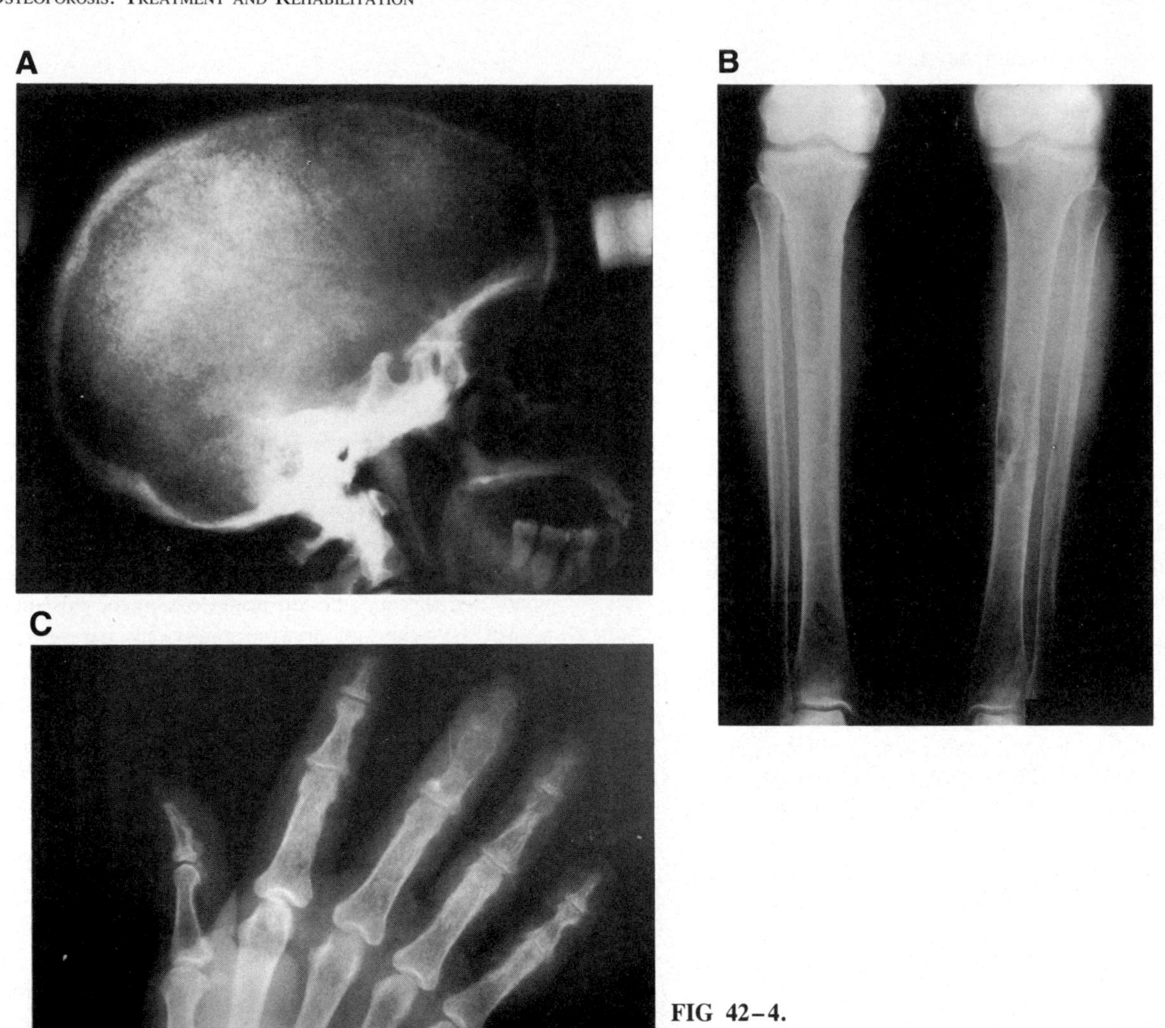

FIG 42–4.
A, this patient with parathyroid adenoma has developed a "salt-and-pepper" skull. **B,** hyperparathyroidism in a patient who has developed small "brown tumors" in the right/left tibias. **C,** hand film of hyperparathyroidism with brown tumor in the metacarpal, subperiosteal resorption, and thinning of the terminal tuffs.

Bone scans will be positive in fractures that are less than 2 years in duration. Bone density will be decreased on dual-beam absorptiometry and QCT. Laboratory studies are within normal limits for calcium, phosphorus, and alkaline phosphatase except that levels of the latter will be elevated within 1 week of a significant new fracture.

The differential diagnosis of osteoporosis includes osteomalacia in which there is a decreased to normal calcium content, decreased phosphorus, and increased alkaline phosphatase level in half the patients with osteomalacia. Five percent to 10% of osteopenic patients have mild to moderate osteomalacia in the northern urban environments. Hyperparathyroidism will have an increased PTH level and elevated calcium and alkaline phosphatase concentrations. Hyperthyroidism will have decreased TSH-IRMA values and increased T_3 and T_4 concentrations. In primary hyperthyroidism there is significant weight loss. Iatrogenic hyperthyroidism usually occurs in obese individuals who utilize thyroid supplements to control their weight. Hyperglucosteroidism will lead to osteopenia, and over 99% of cases are iatrogenic. This occurs when prednisone doses are greater than 7.5 mg/day. Diabetes (juvenile) is associated with increased hypercalciuria and a negative nitrogen balance, which lead to osteopenia. Premature estrogen deficiency, whether primary or secondary amenorrhea or premature menopause, is associated with osteopenia. Disturbances in collagen metabolism such as osteogenesis imperfecta and scurvy cause osteoporosis. Hematologic disorders will lead to osteopenia, most notably thalassemia or any disorder within this family that leads to bone marrow expansion at the expense of trabecular bone mass. Neoplastic disorders can account for osteopenia. Two percent of osteopenic patients will have bone marrow abnormalities, half of which will be multiple myeloma. The abnormal laboratory findings will include decreased hemoglobin, an increased sedimentation rate, and abnormal serum and/or urinary protein electrolytes. Male testosterone deficiencies will be present in more than 50% of osteopenic males.

The elements of treatment of osteoporosis are based on adequate nutrition and appropriate exercise stimulation, prevention of rapid bone resorption when indicated, and selective use of stimulatory agents for augmentation. Clear evidence has been demonstrated that calcium plays a critical role in achieving peak bone mass at the age of 25 years. It has been demonstrated at The Hospital for Special Surgery that physiologic levels of calcium can maintain bone mass in the premenopausal individual and in those over 65 years of age. Bone mass in the spine will continue to decrease at approximately 2% per year in patients who recently became postmenopausal. However, additional information has now suggested that these patients fall into three groups: one group will lose no bone mass in the face of calcium supplementation; the second group will lose only 2% per year; and the third group, approximately one third of the individuals, will be rapid losers even in the face of calcium supplementation. This latter group requires additional treatment to prevent their loss of bone mass. Exercise has also been indicated as a very strong stimulus to the maintenance of bone structure. The osteoblasts respond to stimuli by maintaining those trabeculae that are stressed. Work by Rubin and Lanyon[41] demonstrated that a small period of minimal exercise can be translated into a 24- to 48-hour protection mode for those trabeculae. Working with these concepts, Smith et al.[43] have shown that simple exercises such as square dancing can markedly decrease the rate of bone loss in postmenopausal individuals and in some selective studies have actually led to a small augmentation of bone mass. The consequence of these studies has suggested that a combination of calcium and exercise would be universally beneficial to all individuals not only as a preventive program but as a treatment modality as well. Superimposed on this foundation are additional therapies that are available and will be discussed by category (Table 42–7).

The premenopausal individual aged 13 to 25 years who is achieving peak bone mass should be maintained on a program of elemental calcium of approximately 1200 mg/day, 400 units of vitamin D, and a reasonable impact exercise program. If these individuals develop amenorrhea or oligomenorrhea, cyclical estrogen and progesterone programs should be added in an effort to reestablish normal and biological ovarian function. Not only do young individuals who are amenorrheic fail to gain bone during their period of amenorrhea, but they can actually go into a negative balance. They can never make up for the period of amenorrhea. Thus, it is critical to keep these periods as limited as possible, and an aggressive corrective program is warranted. Exercise per se has been suggested as causing amenorrhea; however, it has now been shown that individuals who can maintain a normal menstrual cycle in the face of excessive exercise are in no jeopardy. Conversely, individuals who develop amenorrhea cannot be protected by exercise.

Premenopausal women 25 years of age or older can be maintained on a low calcium intake of 800 to 1000 mg/day and 400 units of vitamin D. They too need a reasonable exercise program. Bone loss can be terminated with this program and will only accelerate as they approach their perimenopausal period. Postmenopausal women up to the age of 65 years require an elemental calcium program of 1500 mg/day and vitamin D, 400 to 800 units/day. If they have a strong family history of osteoporosis, present with a bone mass more than 1.5 SD below their peers, or demonstrate on serial bone density determinations a loss of bone of 4% or more per year, they would be strong candidates for an antiresorptive program. In order of recommendation by the federal government, the treatments of choice include an estrogen/progesterone program or calcitonin. Estrogen by itself is associated with a ninefold increase in uterine cancer and a slightly increased risk of breast cancer.[20] The addition of progesterone seems to eliminate the increased incidence of uterine cancer and may blunt some of the changes regarding the breast. Nevertheless, women who have a strong family history of breast cancer, thrombophlebitis, or cerebral vascular disease are contraindicated from estrogen therapy. Mammograms should be taken at least on a yearly basis if not at closer periods, and these patients should be under the direct observation of an experienced internist or gynecologist. Calcitonin is an antiresorptive agent but at this time requires injections in a subcutaneous fashion. It is associated with flushing, and

TABLE 42–7.
Medical Therapies for Osteoporosis

Drugs and Dosage	Side Effects
Accepted therapies	
Calcium, 1–1.5 g/day	Mild GI upset, bloating
Vitamin D, 400–800 IU/day	Well tolerated
Estrogen:	Resumption of menses
Conjugated equine estrogens, 0.625–1.25 mg/day (days 1–25)	Possible increased risk of breast cancer Alteration of hepatic protein production (oral Rx)
or	
Transdermal patch, 0.05 mg BIW (days 1–25)	Skin irritation (patch)
plus	
Medroxyprogesterone acetate: 5–10 mg/day (days 14–25)	
Off all Rx (days 25–30)	
Salmon calcitonin: 50–100 units SC daily; can decrease to TIW	Flushing, nausea, vomiting, local irritations
Experimental therapies	
Sodium fluoride, 1 mg/kg/day	GI upset, leg pains, increased hip fractures?
Calcitriol, 0.25 μg/day	Hypercalcemia Hypercalciuria
Bisphosphonates	
EHDP,* 5–20 mg/kg/day	Osteomalacia
ADP,* 150–300 mg/day	Pyrexia, neutropenia
Thiazide diuretics, (25–50 mg/day of HCTZ*)	Electrolyte changes, volume depletion, hypercalcemia
Anabolic steroids	Virilization Liver abnormalities

*EHDP = ethane-1-hydroxy-1,1-diphosphate; ADP = adenosine diphosphate; HCTZ = hydrochlorothiazide.

95% of individuals experience nausea when the injections are too deep. Forty percent of people develop antibodies, but this does not preclude the benefit from calcitonin. Pretesting with small doses would be warranted. Although the original studies by Gruber et al.[12] suggested 100 units on a daily basis, other investigators have shown that 50 units three times a week appears to be quite beneficial. Calcitonin should only be reserved for rapid losers of bone who cannot tolerate estrogen or for osteoporotic fractures associated with a major component of back pain. The analgesic benefits of calcitonin may be beneficial in this setting.

Postmenopausal women aged 65 years or older with no fractures and a bone density by dual-beam absorptiometry greater than 0.75 g/cm^2 could be maintained easily with just elemental calcium, 1500 mg/day; Vitamin D, 400 to 800 units/day; and a reasonable impact exercise program (walking 1 mile/day).

Postmenopausal individuals with spinal fractures, especially if more than one and new, or a bone density by dual-beam absorptiometry less than 0.75 g/cm^2 in the age group 50 to 65 years old require a more in-depth evaluation and a selective treatment program. If a transilial bone biopsy demonstrates significant active trabecular resorption by osteoclasts but less than 5% osteoid volume, the diagnosis will be considered high-turnover or active osteoporosis. The treatment of choice would include elemental calcium, 1500 mg/day; vitamin D, 400 to 800 units/day; and an antiresorptive program. If the patient is less than 65 years old, cyclical estrogen/progesterone would be the treatment of choice. If they are over 65 years old or have bone pain, calcitonin would be recommended at 50 units three times a week. Recent information regarding the unapproved agent etidronate[44, 47] would suggest that this bisphosphonate is also quite effective in this setting. Etidronate requires a dose of 400 mg to be given for the first 14 days of each quarter on an absolutely empty stomach, preferably 4 hours after eating and before the next meal. Personal communications would suggest that etidronate may not be as effective as the estrogen/progesterone combination or calcitonin; however, it essentially has no side effects other than some slightly rare cases of minimal diarrhea. Newer bisphosphonates promise to be more effective and may well have equal potency of the estrogen/progesterone program.

If biopsy samples of the individual demonstrate more than a 5% osteoid volume, the individual should be investigated for osteomalacia and the therapy individualized for that diagnosis.

If the biopsy specimen demonstrates suppressed resorption and less than 5% osteoid volume, the individual would be classified as a quiescent or low-turnover osteoporotic. Treatment of this patient would consist of elemental calcium, 1500 mg/day; vitamin D, 400 to 800 units/day; and a bone augmentation program. At this time, no technique has been demonstrated to be unequivocally without complications and approved by the federal government. Antiresorptive maneuvers will have minimal effect on this population and will augment their bone mass only 1% to 2% per year. At The Hospital for Special Surgery, patients have been treated with sodium fluoride, 45 mg/kg/day, since the 1960s. They are cyclically treated for 3 months and then have an antiresorptive rest period for 3 months. By utilizing this alternate series one would sequentially stimulate the bone and then allow a period of normalization. Normalization is accomplished by treatment with an antiresorptive agent, and this could include cyclical estrogen/progesterone or calcitonin, 50 units three times a week, or etidronate during the 3-month rest period (400 mg the first 14 days of that quarter). It should be noted that this technique is clearly experimental. Large doses of fluoride alone in high-turnover osteoporosis are contraindicated. Work by Riggs and his coworkers[36] has suggested that patients receiving high doses of sodium fluoride, 75 mg/day, although they markedly increased their bone mass, demonstrated no statistically significant decrease in spinal fractures over calcium treatment alone. Riggs' definition of spinal fractures was extremely broad in that a change of as little as 15% in any parameter was considered a fracture. From personal experience at The Hospital for Special Surgery, patients with high-turnover osteoporosis have large histomorphometric parameters of bone formation and resorption. The addition of sodium fluoride further aggravates these dynamic values and impairs bone quality. Sodium fluoride should not be utilized for high-turnover forms of osteoporosis but should be reserved for the quiescent types where osteoblastic stimulation is indicated. Normalization periods are still needed to ensure an improved bone product. Utilizing this technique in quiescent osteoporotic patients has largely resulted in freedom from spinal fractures and markedly improved symptomatology.

Finally, there is a unique role for calcitonin as an analgesic agent. A multicenter study is currently under way that utilizes this hormone for patients with fresh spinal fractures. Calcitonin is a neuropeptide with an analgesic function as well as an antiresorptive activity. It appears to be extremely effective in providing pain relief in an individual with an acute fracture and has been used by our fracture service for the first 6 weeks after a fresh fracture even in patients who may have low-turnover osteoporosis. Its benefits also include the ability to prevent loss of bone in immobilized patients until they can be rehabilitated into the ambulatory phase again.

Osteoporosis has traditionally been slow to capture the interest of the orthopedic community. Attention is given to the individual fracture episodes and then wanes as the acute injury heals, with the result that diagnosis and treatment are often slighted. This chapter has highlighted the advances in understanding osteoporosis and associated disorders, including its origin, pathomechanics, treatment, and prevention. The treating physician and his patients can rest assured that there now exists the capacity to successfully intervene actively in the disease process.

REFERENCES

1. Austin LA, Heath H III: Calcitonin: Physiology and pathophysiology. *N Engl J Med* 1981; 304:269–278.
2. Baron R: Anatomy and ultrastructure of bone, in *Primer on the Metabolic Bone Diseases and Disorders of Mineral Metabolism,* ed 1. Kelseyville, Calif, American Society of Bone and Mineral Research, 1990, pp 3–7.
3. Barth RW, Lane JM: Osteoporosis. *Orthop Clin North Am* 1988; 19:845–848.
4. Birge SJ Jr, Keutman HT, Cuatrecasas P, et al: Osteoporosis, intestinal lactase deficiency and low dietary calcium intake. *N Engl J Med* 1967; 276:445–448.
5. Cummings SR, Kelsey JL, Nevitt MC, et al: Epidemiology of osteoporosis and osteoporotic fractures. *Epidemiol Rev* 1985; 7:178–208.
6. De Luca HF: Metabolism and action of vitamin D, in Peck WA (ed): *Bone and Mineral Research,* annual 1. Amsterdam, Excerpta Medica, 1982, pp 7–73.
7. De Luca HF, Schnoes HK: Metabolism and mechanism of action of vitamin D. *Annu Rev Biochem* 1976; 45:631.
8. Doppelt SH: Vitamin D, rickets and osteomalacia. *Orthop Clin North Am* 1984; 15:671.
9. Frost HM: *Bone Remodeling Dynamics.* Springfield, Ill, Charles C Thomas, 1963.
10. Gallagher JC, Melton LJ III, Riggs BL, et al: Epidemiology of fractures of the proximal femur in Rochester, Minnesota. *Clin Orthop* 1980; 150:163–171.
11. Gallagher JC, Riggs BL: Current Concepts in nutrition and bone disease. *N Engl J Med* 1978; 298:183–195.
12. Gruber H, Ivey JL, Baylink DJ, et al: Long-term calcitonin therapy in postmenopausal osteoporosis. *Metabolism* 1984; 33:295–298.
13. Guterman IA, Boman TE, Wang GJ, et al: Bone induction in intra-muscular implants by demineralized bone matrix: Sequential changes of collagen synthesis. *Collagen Rel Res* 1988; 8:419–431.
14. Heaney RP: Calcium, bone health, and osteoporosis, in Peck WA (ed): *Bone and Mineral Research,* ed 4. Amsterdam, Elsevier, 1987.
15. Heaney RP: Calcium intake and bone health, in Coissac P (ed): *Postmenopausal Osteoporosis: Prevention and Treatment.* Davos, Switzerland, Sandoz, 1985.
16. Heaney RP, Recker RR, Saville PD: Calcium balance and calcium requirements in middle-aged women. *Am J Clin Nutr* 1977; 30:1603–1611.

17. Heaney RP, Recker RR, Saville PD: Menopausal changes in calcium balance performance. *J Lab Clin Med* 1978; 92:953–963.
18. Jensen JS, Tondevold E: Mortality after hip fractures. *Acta Orthop Scand* 1979; 50:161–167.
19. Johnston CC Jr, Epstein S: Clinical, biochemical, epidemiologic, and economic features of osteoporosis. *Orthop Clin North Am* 1981; 12:559–569.
20. Kaufman DW, Miller DR, Rosenberg L, et al: Noncontraceptive estrogen use and the risk of breast cancer. *JAMA* 1984; 252:63–67.
21. Kelsey JF: Osteoporosis: Prevalence and incidence. Presented at the NIH Concensus Development Conference, April 2–4, 1984, pp 25–28.
22. Kimmel PL: Radiologic methods to evaluate bone mineral content. *Ann Intern Med* 1984; 100:908–911.
23. Lewinnek GE, Kelsey J, Lane AA, et al: The significance of osteoporosis and a comparative analysis of the epidemiology of hip fractures. *Clin Orthop* 1980; 152:35–43.
24. Lane JM, Bockman RS, Buss DD: *Bone Metabolism and Metabolic Bone Disease. Orthopaedic Knowledge Update 3. Home Study Syllabus*. Park Ridge, Ill, American Academy of Orthopaedic Surgeons, 1990, pp 29–46.
25. Lane JM, Cornell CN, Healey JH: Orthopaedic consequences of osteoporosis, in Riggs BL, Melton LJ III (eds): *Osteoporosis: Etiology, Diagnosis and Management*. New York, Raven Press, 1988, pp 433–455.
26. Lane JM, Sandhu HS: Current approaches to experimental bone grafting. *Orthop Clin North Am* 1987; 18:213–225.
27. Mazess RB: Bone densitometry of the axial skeleton. *Orthop Clin North Am* 1990; 21:51–63.
28. Mazess RB: On aging bone loss. *Clin Orthop* 1982; 165:239–252.
29. Melton LJ III, Riggs BL: Epidemiology of age-related fractures, in Avioli L (ed): *The Osteoporotic Syndrome*. New York, Grune & Stratton, 1987, pp 1–30.
30. Minaire P, Meunier P, Eduoard C, et al: Quantitative histological data on disuse osteoporosis: Comparison with biological data. *Calcif Tissue Res* 1974; 17:57–73.
31. Mundy GR: Bone Resorbing Cells, in *Primer on the Metabolic Bone Diseases and Disorders of Mineral Metabolism,* ed 1. Kelseyville, Calif, American Society of Bone and Mineral Research, 1990, pp 18–22.
32. National Institutes of Health Consensus Development Conference Statement on Osteoporosis (Vol 5, No. 3, 1984). *JAMA* 1984; 252:799–802.
33. Parfitt AM, Drezner MK, Glorieux FH, et al: Bone histomorphometry: Standardization of nomenclature, symbols and units. Report of the ASBMR Histomorphometry Nomenclature Committee. *J Bone Miner Res* 1987; 2:595–610.
34. Peck WA, Woods W: The cells of bone, In Riggs BL, Melton LJ III (eds): *Osteoporosis: Etiology, Diagnosis, and Treatment*. New York, Raven Press, 1988.
35. Posner A, Betts F, Blumenthal NC: Bone mineral composition and structure, in Simmons DJ, Kunin AS (eds): *Skeletal Research, An Experimental Approach* New York, Academic Press, 1979.
36. Riggs BL, Hodgson S, O'Fallon W, et al: Effect of fluoride treatment on the fracture rate in postmenopausal women with osteoporosis. *N Engl J Med* 1990; 322:802–809.
37. Riggs BL, Melton JL III: Involutional osteoporosis. *N Engl J Med* 1986; 314:1676–1686.
38. Riggs BL, Melton JL III: *Osteoporosis: Etiology, Diagnosis, and Management*. New York, Raven Press, 1988.
39. Rizzoli RE, Somerman M, Murray TM, et al: Binding of radioiodinated parathyroid hormone to cloned bone cells. *Endocrinology* 1983; 113:1832–1838.
40. Rodan GA, Rodan SB: Expression of the osteoblast phenotype, in Beck W (ed): *Bone and Mineral Research,* ed 2. Amsterdam, Elsevier, 1984, pp 244–285.
41. Rubin CT, Lanyon LE: Osteoregulatory nature of mechanical stimuli: Function as a determinant for adaptive remodeling in bone. *J Orthop Res* 1987; 5:300–310.
42. Smith DC, Khairi MRA, Johnston CC Jr: The loss of bone mineral with aging and its relationship to risk of fracture. *J Clin Invest* 1975; 56:311–318.
43. Smith EL, Gilligan C, McAdam M, et al: Deterring bone loss by exercise intervention in pre and postmenopausal women. *Calcif Tissue Int* 1989; 44:312–321.
44. Storm T, Thamsborg G, et al: Effect of intermittent cyclical etidronate therapy on bone mass and fracture rate in women with postmenopausal osteoporosis. *N Engl J Med* 1990; 322:1265–1271.
45. Teitelbaum SL: Skeletal growth and development, in *Primer on the Metabolic Bone Diseases and Disorders of Mineral Metabolism,* ed 1. Kelseyville, Calif, American Society of Bone and Mineral Research, 1990, pp 7–11.
46. Termine JD, Belcourt AB, Conn KM, et al: Mineral and collagen-binding proteins of fetal calf bone. *J Biol Chem* 1981; 256:10403–10408.
47. Watts N, Harris ST, Genant H, et al: Intermittent cyclical etidronate treatment of postmenopausal osteoporosis. *N Engl J Med* 1990; 323:73–79.
48. Wong GL: Skeletal effects of parathyroid hormone, in Peck W (ed): *Bone and Mineral Research,* ed 4. Amsterdam, Elsevier, 1987, pp 103–130.

PART XIV

SPINAL MICROSURGERY

43

*Microsurgical Lumbar Nerve Root Decompression Utilizing Progressive Local Anesthesia**

Stephen D. Kuslich, M.D.

PURPOSE

During the past 15 years I have had the opportunity to evaluate several thousand patients with low back pain and sciatica. Of these, more than 600 have undergone surgical decompressions. The following report will summarize my experience in a consecutive series of 291 patients with lumbar disc hernia and/or localized stenosis. These patients were evaluated prospectively, and rating was accomplished by persons other than the author.[12]

Since the result of any surgical procedure is dependent upon many factors other than the type of operation, this chapter will also discuss the other elements that influence the outcome. These include patient selection, patient education, positioning, anesthesia, surgical technique, and postoperative follow-up. Finally, I will include thoughts on nomenclature, qualifications of surgeons, and preferred diagnostic procedures.

HISTORY

In order to put this topic into perspective, the following section will summarize the medical literature that forms the foundation of microsurgical lumbar nerve decompression.

Although Goldthwaith[8] and later Danforth and Wilson[4] expressed some opinions about the lumbar disc as a possible cause of sciatica, credit must be given to Mixter and Barr, who in 1934 published the paper that began the modern era of lumbar surgery for discogenic nerve root compression.[13] Since that time numerous articles published in many countries have established the fact that laminectomy (or laminotomy) is a useful procedure for the relief of sciatica due to a herniated disc. A personal review of the English language literature concluded that in a combined series of over 15,000 patients, the overall success rate was 77%.[12] The reasons for failure have been described in several articles including the classic paper by Pheasant.[14]

*Reprinted in part from Williams RW, McCulloch JA, Young PH (eds): *Microsurgery of the Lumbar Spine*. Rockville, Md, Aspen, 1990, pp 139–147. Used by permission.

Casper[3] in Germany and Yasargil[21] in Switzerland reported separate series of lumbar nerve decompressions utilizing the operative microscope during the late 1970s. Both authors claimed impressive results in comparison to standard laminectomy.

Williams was the first to report his experience with microsurgical nerve root decompression in this country.[19] Since that report, several other publications have appeared on the subject.[7, 9, 11, 20] In general, the procedure has received widespread approval. Four articles have compared the procedure with standard laminectomy.[2, 10, 16, 20] Judging from the frequency of publication and the numerous presentations at medical symposia on the subject, I think that it is safe to conclude that microsurgical nerve root decompression is growing in popularity and may soon replace standard laminectomy as the procedure of choice for extruded lumbar disc hernias with and without spinal stenosis.

From a purely technical standpoint, the operating microscope offers several advantages over traditional methods. These include better lighting, larger magnification, and a better angle of view, i.e., directly in line with the anteroposterior axis of the patient. These factors may result in several side benefits:

1. Smaller incisions
2. Shorter operation and anesthetic times
3. Less bleeding
4. Less perineural scaring
5. Less chance of iatrogenic nerve injury
6. Shorter hospital stays
7. Less postoperative pain and required analgesics
8. Earlier return to normal function and work
9. Lower cost of care
10. "Marketing advantages" for the surgeon

Aside from the increased learning time and the theoretical disadvantages of smaller incisions, there appear to be no absolute contraindications for the use of the operating microscope in virtually all cases of lumbar nerve compression. In spite of the protestations of a few prominent surgeons such as Fager,[5] the often-quoted exceptions of the migrated disc fragment and multilevel compression are not contraindications. This is because we now appreciate that the pathology can be precisely defined preoperatively by appropriate scanning technology and the length of the incision increased to whatever size is necessary to accomplish the decompression. The days of "spinal exploration" are over. The limitation of "microdiscectomy" to those cases with 1-in. incisions and no bone removal, as originally defined by Williams, does not appear to be rational or correct.

To the best of this author's knowledge, no article has been published that demonstrates any documented, significant disadvantages to the microsurgical decompression of lumbar nerves, although several theoretical problems are sometimes mentioned in publications on the subject.[1, 5]

NOMENCLATURE

The following terms have been used to describe the operative procedures considered here:

1. Microdiscectomy
2. Microlaminectomy
3. Micro-lumbar-discectomy
4. Microsurgical lumbar nerve decompression

The first term, "microdiscectomy," is perhaps the most commonly used. I believe that it is inappropriate because the surgeon rarely if ever performs a total discectomy. There are, in fact, many instances when the compressed nerve roots may be adequately decompressed without any disc removal at all. In these instances, the surgeon simply unroofs the compressive posterior structures in order to free up the nerve.

The second term, "microlaminectomy," is also a poor choice. The opening or removal of the lamina is only a small portion of the typical operation. In fact, it is rarely necessary to perform even a complete hemilaminectomy, much less a total laminectomy, in order to decompress a nerve compressed by a herniated disc.

The term "micro-lumbar-discectomy" was coined by Williams. While it is more descriptive than the former terms, it is similarly incomplete and misleading.

I prefer the term "microsurgical lumbar nerve decompression" because it correctly defines both the intent and the actual technical features of the operation. This term has sufficient accuracy to be used in preoperative consent forms. Perhaps more important, it retains certain options on the part of the surgeon to perform whatever bone, soft-tissue, and disc removal that may be necessary at the time of actual surgery.

The author is aware that several experienced surgeons have opted for the use of loupes over the use of the true surgical microscope. I am also aware that there are certain advantages to this choice. The term "microsurgery," however, is not appropriate when describing these procedures.

RATIONALE FOR THE USE OF LOCAL ANESTHESIA

Several types of anesthesia may be used for lumbar nerve decompression. By far the most commonly used is general inhalation anesthesia. Spinal and epidural anesthesia are employed less commonly.

While a medical student at the University of Minnesota during the mid-1960s I had the opportunity to operate with a very skilled Minneapolis surgeon, Dr. Daniel Moos. Dr. Moos was well known in this region for his exceptional ability to perform cholecystectomy with local anesthesia. He operated with the utmost skill and careful technique, slowly infiltrating the tissue planes as he dissected the region of the gallbladder and common bile duct. I noticed that his patients suffered little intraoperative pain. More important, however, the patients experienced little postoperative pain. I noted that his patients spent fewer days in the hospital and were able to regain normal eating and bowel function much sooner than similar patients who had been given a general anesthetic.

In 1979 I visited Dr. Robert Williams and learned his technique of microsurgical removal of a herniated lumbar disc. When I returned to Minneapolis, I began to use the procedure in selected cases. As my expertise in the technique increased, I decided to attempt the procedure and use the local anesthetic technique that I had learned from Dr. Moos. I have chosen to label the anesthetic "progressive local anesthetic" because each tissue layer is successively infiltrated as the operation proceeds from the skin to the disc.

FACTORS INFLUENCING SUCCESS RATES IN LUMBAR SURGERY

The successful conclusion of any operative procedure is dependent upon the concordance of several factors, including the following:

1. The correct diagnosis
2. The appropriate patient
3. The proper operation
4. The skill of the surgeon

The Correct Diagnosis

No discussion of a surgical technique can be complete without mention of the methods used to diagnose the problem. As we read the literature concerning surgery for herniated discs, we must notice a recurring conclusion that the most important factor governing the overall success and failure rates is the proper selection of cases. Only those patients who have the proper mix of organic and functional indicators should be offered this operation.[6]

Although exceptions exist, in the main, candidates for microsurgical lumbar nerve decompressions of any type must present with the following characteristics:

1. Leg pain should be predominant. While it is true that in rare cases of a central sequestered disc causing mainly back pain, fragment removal will lead to resolution of the back pain, most cases of central disc herniation with back pain predominating do not respond well to "decompression." Operating for back pain rather than leg pain is one of the most important reasons for the occurrence of failed back syndrome.

2. An adequate trial of conservative treatment should be tried prior to the consideration of surgery.

I do not believe that precise time limitations are appropriate here since many patients with severe pain and large disc hernias should be offered immediate surgery for humanitarian reasons. On the other hand, the surgeon should be aware that many if not most herniated discs spontaneously resolve with simple nonsurgical methods or no treatment at all. In general, patients should not be offered any operation prior to a 4- to 6-week trial of nonsurgical treatment.

3. Appropriate imaging studies must confirm the presence of nerve compression in correlation with the clinical history and physical examination. Cases with disc hernia simply stretching the nerve rather than compressing it usually do not require surgery of any kind.

Experience in the interpretation of computed tomographic (CT) scans, magnetic resonance imaging (MRI), and myelograms will assist the surgeon in identifying those patients who are unlikely to respond to conservative measures.

It is now a rare case indeed in which a patient with sciatica cannot be accurately diagnosed. Modern imaging technology should not only provide the surgeon with the exact diagnosis, including an appreciation of the multiple pathologic conditions, but should also indicate the exact extent of surgery needed to fully decompress the nerve. In addition, the surgeon must consider and plan for any instability that might result from the pathology or the surgical decompression.

I have found that preoperative flexion-extension lateral radiographs of the lumbar spine and "complete" CT scans, including sagittal-plane foraminal views, are necessary to appreciate the details of pathology that must be thoroughly understood in order to obtain consistently good results.

In spite of the current enthusiasm for MRI, I have found that a good quality CT scan is the best overall study to define nerve root compression and plan the surgical procedure. This is particularly true in older patients, who are likely to have bony stenosis with or without disc hernia. MRI is excellent for the diagnosis of disc degeneration and hernia, but it is inferior to CT in the appreciation of bony stenosis.

In cases in which previous surgery has been performed on the lumbar spine, I prefer a water-soluble myelogram followed by CT scanning with the dye in place in order to differentiate the nerve and dura from surrounding disc and scar tissue. Occasionally, myelography, CT, MRI, and even discography are needed. Electromyographic (EMG) testing is rarely useful because of the very high incidence of false-positive and false-negative reports.

The Appropriate Patient

The psychosocial or "functional" characteristics of the patient must be considered. In general, the presence of one or more of the following factors adversely affects the results of any lumbar operative procedure:

1. Depression
2. Chemical dependency
3. Litigation whose outcome depends upon the continuance of disabling pain
4. Family stress such as divorce, poverty, or physical abuse
5. Job dissatisfaction
6. Low educational level
7. Religiosity
8. Hostility toward present or past physicians and surgeons

In addition to the standard history, I have found the following techniques to be of great value in terms of objectively identifying the functional components of a patient's pain problem:

1. Analysis of the pain drawing[15]
2. Waddell testing[18]
3. Analysis of work history
4. Detailed drug and alcohol history

I do not use the Minnesota Multiphasic Personality Inventory (MMPI) or similar tests because I find them unnecessary, time-consuming, and costly. In addition, they offend the patient, who infers that the surgeon believes the pain "to be in his head."

Unless the operation is considered an emergency, sufficient time and effort should be expended to resolve the above issues prior to the performance of a surgical procedure. It is not at all unusual to have the "pain" resolve after the psychosocial issues have been adequately managed.

The author would be less than honest, however, if he

were to imply that resolution of the above problems were anything but exceedingly difficult. Their appropriate management usually involves a significant expenditure of time and effort by a team of professionals working in concert with the physician.

The Proper Procedure

Nerve compression syndromes may present at any time along the continuum of the process of degenerative disc disease. A detailed understanding of the natural history of the condition as well as the ability to correctly diagnose the various features of the individual patient's problem is essential to the success of the surgical procedure. The diagram in Figure 43–1 illustrates the interplay of the various factors involved in lumbar nerve root compression, and planning for a procedure to relieve sciatica secondary to lumbar nerve compression must take into account these features of the disease process.

CT and MRI are invaluable in determining the nature, degree, and specific sites of nerve root compression. Myelography only demonstrates compression in the central spinal canal. The nerve may also be compressed or stretched in the foraminal or extraforaminal zones. Relief of sciatic pain can only result when all areas of compression are recognized and corrected. Fortunately, it is usually possible to adequately decompress these areas with the aid of the operating microscope without producing instability at the motion segment. Unfortunately, the ability to accomplish this feat requires a lengthy learning and practice experience.

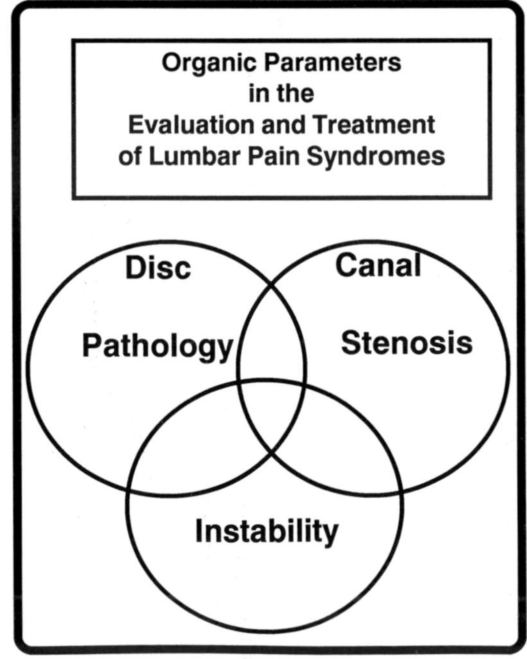

FIG 43–1.
This diagram shows the interrelationships among the various types of pathology associated with lumbar nerve root compression. If possible, all of the significant pathology should be corrected in order to ensure a good long-term result.

The Skill of the Surgeon

It is assumed that only properly trained and experienced surgeons would venture into the field of spinal microsurgery. As each year passes, it is increasingly apparent that the field of spinal surgery is becoming a defined if not a boarded specialty. The need for the "occasional" spinal surgeon to operate on the lumbar spine is now rare due to the following important factors:

1. The current medicolegal climate
2. The increasing availability of fully trained spinal surgeons from both orthopedic and neurosurgical residency and fellowship programs
3. The increased sophistication of patients and third-party payers who have come to recognize that the "failed back syndrome" can be avoided by means of appropriately applied case selection criteria and skillfully performed surgery

My technique of surgery has been published.[11] It involves a gradual and careful dissection of the involved motion segment, with progressive injections of small volumes of local anesthetic used only when and where needed. A few essential details of the procedure are provided below in order to provide a basis for evaluating the results of a series of patients so treated.

AUTHOR'S SURGICAL TECHNIQUE

Preoperative Preparation

Once the patient has given consent for the surgical procedure, our nurse practitioner spends about 20 minutes in preoperative teaching. We usually have a family practitioner or internist perform a history and physical examination prior to the procedure. This medical report complements the spinal and neurologic examination of the surgeon and is of considerable benefit in recognizing possible complicating factors that may interfere with a successful outcome. The patient is kept with nothing to eat or drink from midnight to the time of surgery. We provide him with a small bottle of chlorhexidine gluconate (Hibiclens) for a skin-cleansing shower the morning of the procedure. Patients are admitted 2 hours prior to the procedure. Two grams of cetazolin (Kefzol) or other broad-spectrum antibiotics is given intravenously in the preparation room before the patient enters the surgical suite.

Positioning

I use the Heffington frame, which places the patient in a kneeling-sitting position. This reduces intra-abdominal and intraspinal venous pressure and thereby attenuates intraoperative bleeding. I have tried the more severe flexion positions such as the Tarlov position but found that they make the operation more difficult. The use of simple rolls and laminectomy frames are sufficient, but they are not as comfortable for the awake patient and do not provide the degree of venous decompression afforded by the Heffington- or Andrews-type frames.

Anesthesia and Surgical Exposure

If necessary, the patient is given an intravenous dose of midazolam (Versed) for sedation, but never enough to interfere with the ability to cooperate and answer questions. Figure 43–2 demonstrates the relationship of the surgeon, the anesthetist, and the patient during the operation. In actual practice, we use a face-to-face binocular scope so that the assistant has the same view as the surgeon. Figure 43–2 shows the optional monocular attachment, which is much less satisfactory. I perform the exposure of the lamina without the aid of the microscope and prefer to use the scope only for the more delicate portions of the procedure.

I inject about 20 cc of 1% lidocaine (Xylocaine) with 1 : 100,000 epinephrine in the midline dermis of the lumbar spine along the line of the planned incision.

Once the skin and subcutaneous fat have been retracted and the bleeders cauterized, I incise the lumbar fascia just lateral to the supraspinous ligament and, if necessary, use a little more local infiltration. I then place some lidocaine (Xylocaine) between the spinous process and the paravertebral muscle (Fig 43–3) and a little more at or near the facet joint. This provides sufficient anesthesia for muscle retraction provided that the retraction is done gently.

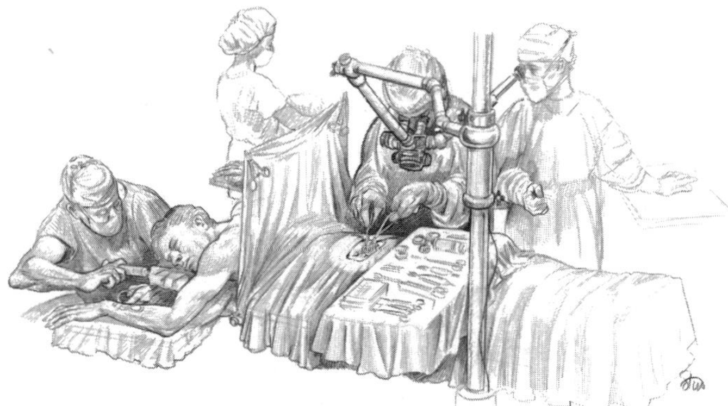

FIG 43–2.
The patient is positioned in the kneeling-sitting position on the Heffington frame while awake or only slightly sedated by intravenous agents. The patient is then able to report sensations of pain and its relief during the procedure. Sometimes we allow the patient to visualize part of the disc removal by looking at the television monitor attached to the surgical microscope. In appropriate patients, this experience is very exciting and comforting. In actual practice, we use a binocular scope for the surgeon and assistant, with the assistant standing on the side opposite the surgeon. The less adequate monocular scope is shown here.

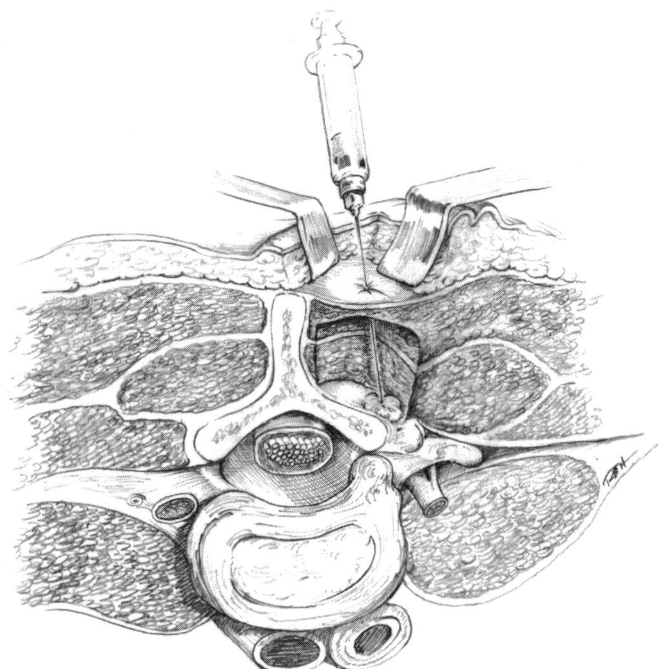

FIG 43–3.
Infiltration of the space between the spinous process and the paravertebral muscles to allow retraction of the muscles.

At this point, I bring the operating microscope into the field. It has been draped with a transparent, custom-made plastic sheet to allow the surgeon the opportunity to touch the microscope, adjust the focus and position, and regulate the amount of magnification. I use a lens with a 300- or 350-mm focal length.

The further details of the operation depend upon the exact pathology to be corrected. If the ligamentum area is large and there is no bony stenosis, I remove only the ligamentum flavum with a no. 6700 Beaver blade. Otherwise, I remove whatever amount of bone is necessary to achieve safe and adequate exposure of the epidural contents. My results do not support the contention that stingy bone removal improves the final outcome of the operation. On the contrary, too little exposure usually results in frustration, increased operating time, and greater risk of nerve injury. I found that it was necessary to remove some bone in 55% of my patients operated on for herniated discs. Of course, cases of spinal stenosis always require bone removal. In cases of pure foraminal stenosis, the nerve is approached lateral to the facet joint. Once the nerve is identified, I remove the offending bone or disc tissue until the nerve is free from compression or stretch.

Once the epidural fat and the nerve root have been exposed and identified, I turn up the magnification somewhat and gently probe the epidural space with a small no. 4

Penfield dissector in an attempt to reproduce the back and leg pains that most closely resemble patient's preoperative complaints. Patients vary a great deal with regard to sensitivity to pain from various epidural structures, but there is seldom any question about the true origin of back and leg pain when the disc hernia and the compressed nerve root are gently stroked.

It is very important to be able to reproduce the referred pain; otherwise the surgeon must be suspicious that the wrong space has been entered. If one exposes the incorrect level inadvertently, there is no great harm done. I suggest simply placing an instrument into the epidural space and retaking the radiograph. Then one simply extends the incision up or down to the correct level. Avoiding even one operation at the wrong level is worth the time and effort involved.

The offending nerve root may be anesthetized in several ways. The surgeon may use a 30-gauge needle to inject ½ cc of plain lidocaine (Xylocaine) into the nerve sleeve, or if the nerve is exquisitely tender, I recommend inserting the needle into the subarachnoid space just above the level of compression and injecting about 3 cc of local anesthetic at that site. This degree of spinal anesthesia will produce only a sympathetic and sensory block. Motor function and perineal sensation will usually be little affected by this injection.

Figure 43–4 illustrates the technique of nerve sleeve infiltration. These maneuvers will allow adequate pain relief to retract the nerve root gently to the midline and thereby provide sufficient exposure to visualize the disc as well as the area above and below the disc space. The surgeon is then able to thoroughly explore the epidural space and determine the need to remove more ligamentum flavum, bone, or disc.

The outer portion of the annulus is tender in about a third of cases. If necessary, I use a 22-gauge needle to infiltrate the annulus with local anesthetic (Fig 43–5). I then remove the disc tissue according to the nature of the pathology. If the herniation is free in the epidural space, I simply remove the loose piece and any necessary debris in the disc space. In cases of extruded but contained discs, it is necessary to pierce the thin outer annular membrane in order to gain access to the offending material.

The nucleus itself is never tender, and therefore anesthetic is not necessary. The vertebral end plate, however, is sometimes sensitive, and it is difficult to completely anesthetize. I may choose to proceed with the disc removal in spite of the minor pain or have the anesthetist inject some intravenous fentanyl (Sublimaze) at this point. Frequently, I will inject 1 cc or 2 of local anesthetic into the nucleus (Fig 43–6), which after a few minutes will diffuse into the annulus and end plate to provide sufficient pain relief for disc debridment.

I do not perform a radical disc removal but instead choose to remove only loose and degenerated portions of the disc. The amount of disc removal is still an open question. My experience, discussions with other surgeons, and reading of the literature have led me to believe that it is never possible to remove more than 20% to 30% of the disc. Overly ambitious attempts to remove a great deal of disc tissue increase the likelihood of nerve or great-vessel injury. Until a safe and effective disc debridement tool is available (and we are in the process of developing one), subtotal or total disc removal is neither possible nor indicated in most cases of herniated disc. Sometimes, I suture the outer portion of the annulus back together, although I do not know whether this is necessary.

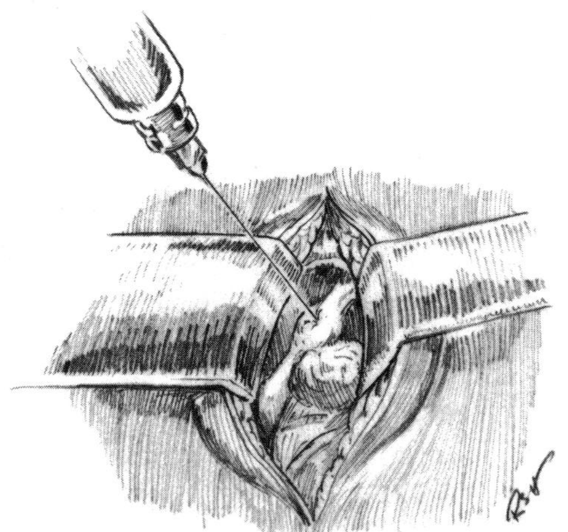

FIG 43–4.
Once exposed, the nerve root is stimulated by gentle pressure. Sciatica may then be routinely relieved by injecting 0.5 mL of local lidocaine under the nerve sleeve with a 30-gauge needle proximal to the herniation.

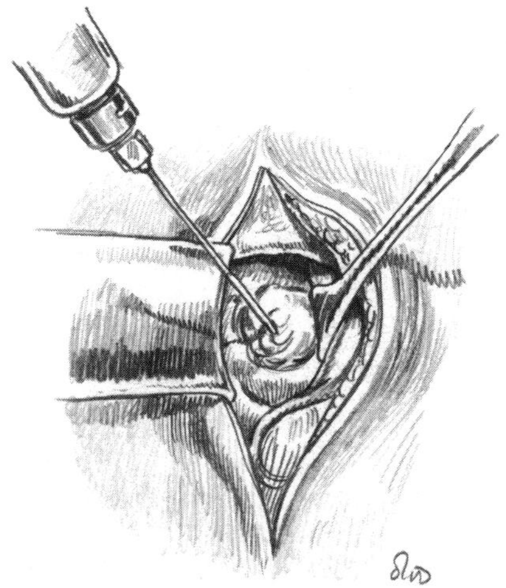

FIG 43–5.
The outer margins of the annulus is sometimes tender. It may be anesthetized by the injection of several milliliters of local anesthetic into its outer fibers.

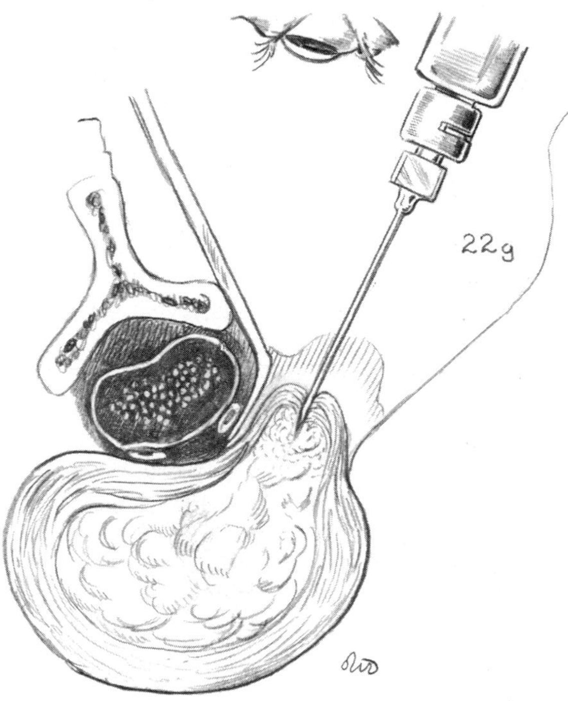

FIG 43–6.
The nucleus pulposus is never sensitive. However, the end plate and annulus may cause considerable pain when stimulated. In those cases, the disc is infiltrated with several milliliters of anesthetic before proceeding with removal of the herniated disc material.

I would not normally expose the entire foraminal zone since I trust the sagittal CT views to inform me of compression at that site. I routinely remove the medial third of the overlying superior articular facet because I believe that its retention might lead to lateral recess stenosis should the disc bulge again in the future.

Spengler has nicely demonstrated that limited disc excision and selective foraminotomy result in very high, long-term success rates, even without the use of microsurgical techniques.[17]

To complete the operation, I irrigate with antibiotic solution, deposit 2 cc of betamethasone (Celestone) into the epidural space, and cover the laminotomy site with either the removed ligamentum flavum or a medium-sized piece of fat obtained from the area of the incision. My studies of the effect of various dural coverings, including Gelfoam, did not show any difference in the final result. There is good evidence, however, that the use of medium-sized pieces of fat does decrease postoperative scarring between the muscle and the dura. I have not used large pieces of fat derived from separate incisions.

I close over a medium Hemovac drain with standard suture technique.

Postoperative Care

The patient usually experiences immediate relief of the sciatica. If not, I worry that I have not corrected the pathology. There are occasional instances where it is necessary to wait a few days to get relief.

The patient is allowed to walk as soon as possible, but I restrict sitting, stooping, and bending for several weeks in order to allow the annular tissues to heal. I prescribe daily straight leg raising exercises for several months.

The patient is allowed to leave the hospital in 1 or 2 days, depending upon circumstances. It is not uncommon for patients to require no postoperative analgesics when this surgical technique is used, but sometimes I will prescribe aspirin or acetaminophen (Tylenol) with or without codeine. The need for other, more potent medications is rarely observed and indicates that the patient is habituated or that the pathology has not been corrected.

We see the patient in the clinic in about 2 weeks. At that time I make recommendations about work capabilities depending upon circumstances. Self-employed individuals usually return within 2 weeks, whereas heavy laborers, especially when the injury was "work related," usually require a month or two before returning to work.

In general, the time to return to work and sports activities is governed by nonsurgical factors such as pain tolerance, job demands, overall fitness level, and basic motivation of the patient (Table 43–1).

ADVANTAGES OF LOCAL ANESTHESIA

I have found that the use of local anesthesia provides several advantages to the patient and surgeon:

1. The surgeon is able to be sure that the proper nerve is being decompressed since the offending nerve is first stimulated to produce the clinically significant pain, and second, anesthetization of the offending nerve ought to result in complete relief of the sciatica. This occurrence assures the surgeon and the patient that the correct level and nerve have been decompressed.

2. The surgeon is able to learn a great deal about the origin of low back pain and sciatica. This knowledge will lead to a greater practical understanding of the causes of low back pain and sciatica.

3. The use of local anesthesia with the patient fully awake or slightly sedated allows for a safer operation. Any changes the patient reports, in terms of pain or other sensations, can be immediately communicated to the surgeon. As a consequence of this knowledge, the surgeon is far less likely to injure nerve roots and other tissues during the exposure and performance of the decompression.

Furthermore, since the patient is able to report sensations such as nausea, light-headedness, chest pain, dyspnea, etc., changes in physiologic parameters can be appreciated earlier, and corrective action can be taken before a crisis develops.

For example, vasovagal phenomena, which occasionally occur during spinal surgery, are frequently presaged

TABLE 43–1.

Results of a Personal Series of Patients

Total patients	291
Time frame	1980–1987
Available for long-term follow-up	245
Follow-up time	6 mo (minimum)–7 yr
Complications	
None	218 (89%)
Infection	4 (1.6%)
Reherniation	16 (6.5%)
CSF leak	7 (2.9%) Most occurred in the first 100 patients)
Percent leg pain relief at last follow-up, average	85%
Findings at surgery	
No pathology	1
Protrusion	29
Contained and extruded	121
Sequestered	87
Other	7 (Pure stenosis, tumor, etc.)
Final rating, average	8.1 out of possible 10.0
Operative site	
L2–3	1%
L3–4	2%
L4–5	45%
L5–S1	52%
Operation time (min)	
Average	100
Maximum	240
Minimum	35
Preoperative duration of leg symptoms (wk) (Statistics skewed by several patients with a very long history of pain)	
Average	35
Minimum	1
Maximum	254
Preoperative duration of back symptoms (wk)	
Average	68
Minimum	1
Maximum	254
Occupation type	
Light	80
Moderate	95
Heavy	70
Final rating vs. stenosis	
None	8.0
Mild	8.2
Moderate	8.5
Severe	5.8
Time in hospital postoperatively (days)	
Average	2.4
Maximum	12
Minimum	1
SD	1.4
Time for return to employment (wk)	
Average	5.1
Maximum	28
Minimum	1
SD	4.2
Returned before 9 wk	80%

by light-headedness and nausea, even before hypotension and bradycardia develop. The condition is effectively treated by atropine without interruption of the operation.

Since the patient is able to feel pressure caused by positioning on the operating table, appropriate repositioning can be accomplished before pressure sores and nerve palsies develop.

The patient is able to breathe for himself and contract muscles in the abdomen and extremities. These functions prevent the development of atelectasis and venous stasis, respectively, thereby reducing the incidence of pneumonia and thromboembolic phenomena.

4. We have noticed that patients who have local anesthesia do better than those who awaken from a general anesthetic in a confused and disoriented state. They are able to experience the production and elimination of sciatica during the procedure. They are able to feel as though they are part of the team that is correcting the problem. Once they have mustered the courage to be involved in the actual operation, they are able to experience the exhilaration of successfully conquering the problem since the sciatic pain is usually relieved immediately following the operation.

This psychological phenomenon is a real and powerful adjunct to the total therapeutic effect of the operation.

5. Finally, our recent analysis of cost-of-care data indicates that microsurgical nerve root decompression using local anesthesia is significantly less costly than standard laminectomy using general anesthesia.[16]

CONCLUSIONS

Microsurgical lumbar nerve decompression using progressive local anesthesia is a valuable technique that offers the potential for safer and more accurate decompression of nerves that are compressed by herniated discs and/or bony stenosis. This anesthetic technique provides the patient with satisfactory intraoperative pain relief while reducing the overall morbidity and mortality.

The low morbidity probably results from improved visualization of the anatomy, reduced bleeding, and more careful handling of the nerves. Appropriate selection of cases and proper technique are much more important than the length of the surgical incision.

REFERENCES

1. An H, Balderstom RA, Rothman RA: Microdiscectomy: A critique, in Williams W, McCulloch J, Young P (eds): *Microsurgery of the Lumbar Spine*. Rockville, Md, Aspen, 1990.
2. Andrews DW, Lavyne MH: Retrospective analysis of microsurgical and standard discectomy. *Spine* 1990; 15:329–335.
3. Casper W: A new surgical procedure for lumbar disc herniation causing less tissue damage through a microsurgical approach. *Adv Neurosurg* 1977; 4:74–77.

4. Danforth M, Wilson P: The anatomy of the lumbosacral region in relation to sciatic pain. *J Bone Joint Surg* 1925; 7:109.
5. Fager CA: Microsurgical intervention for lumbar disc disease: A critique, in Williams W, McCulloch J, Young P (eds): *Microsurgery of the Lumbar Spine*. Rockville, Md, Aspen, 1990.
6. Frymoyer JW, Cats-Baril W: Predictors of low back pain disability. *Clin Orthop* 1987; 221:89–98.
7. Goald HJ: Microlumbar discectomy: Followup of 147 patients. *Spine* 1978; 3:183–185.
8. Goldthwait JE: The lumbosacral articulation. An explanation of many cases of lumbago, sciatica and paraplegia. *Boston Med Surg J* 1911; 164:365–372.
9. Hudgins WR: The role of microdiscectomy. *Orthop Clin North Am* 1983; 14:589.
10. Kahanovitz N, Viola K, McCulloch J: Limited surgical discectomy and microdiscectomy: A clinical comparison. *Spine* 1989; 14:79–81.
11. Kuslich SD: Microsurgical lumbar nerve root decompression utilizing progressive local anesthesia, in Williams W, McCulloch J, Young P (eds): *Microsurgery of the Lumbar Spine*. Rockville, Md, Aspen, 1990.
12. Kuslich SD: Unpublished data, 1989.
13. Mixter WJ, Barr JS: Rupture of the intervertebral disc with involvement of the spinal canal. *N Engl J Med* 1934; 221:210–215.
14. Pheasant HC: Sources of failure in laminectomies. *Orthop Clin North Am* 1975; 6:319–329.
15. Ransford AD, Carrins C, Mooney V: The pain drawing as an aid to the psychologic evaluation of patients with low back pain. *Spine* 1976; 1:127–134.
16. Schwartz D, Ulstrom C, Chowins J, et al: Lumbar disc herniation: How does the choice of treatment affect the cost of care? *Minn Med* 1988; 71:489–491.
17. Spengler G: Lumbar discectomy: Results with limited disc excision and selective foraminotomy. *Spine* 1982; 7:604–607.
18. Waddell G, et al: Nonorganic physical signs in low back pain. *Spine* 1980; 5:117–125.
19. Williams R: Microlumbar discectomy: A conservative surgical approach to the virgin herniated lumbar disc. *Spine* 1978; 3:175–182.
20. Wilson DH, Harbaugh R: Microsurgical and standard removal of protruded lumbar disc: A comparative study. *Neurosurg* 1981; 8:422–427.
21. Yasargil MC: Microsurgical operation of herniated lumbar disc, in Wullenweber R, Brock M, Hamer J, et al (eds): *Advances in Neurosurgery. Lumbar Disc, Adult Hydrocephalus,* vol 4. New York, Springer-Verlag 1977, p 81.

44

*The Tissue Origin of Mechanical Low Back Pain and Sciatica as Identified by Spinal Microsurgery**

Stephen D. Kuslich, M.D.

The past several decades have witnessed an explosion of knowledge in the area of low back pain and sciatica. Advances in diagnostic radiology are responsible for a quantum leap forward in our ability to visualize the anatomy and pathology of the spine. Epidemiologic studies have demonstrated that certain anatomic, genetic, and social factors significantly contribute to the development of pain and disability in this category of patients. Treatment regimens based upon this new knowledge promise to reduce suffering and disability while lowering the cost of care.

In spite of these optimistic factors, several questions and controversies remain to be solved, including the following:

- What tissues are responsible for the pain?
- Why is one person disabled while another is able to continue productive labor when both are apparent victims of the same "disease"?

This chapter will discuss the above questions from the point of view of a surgeon who has spent the past 10 years evaluating patients and performing surgery, when necessary, with the aid of the operating microscope and local anesthesia. This experience has provided a unique opportunity to draw conclusions that might help answer some of the remaining issues in this field of medical science. Do these opinions represent the final word in this complex and constantly changing arena? Of course not, but I hope that they will provide a new and challenging viewpoint from which others may derive some benefit.

If one defines rehabilitation as a process of treatment that begins with a diagnosis and ends with the restoration of maximum abilities, then the topics of tissue pathology and their correction fall within the domain of the rehabilitative art. In keeping with the theme of this book, the current chapter provides a surgeon's perspective on the topic of the tissue origin of lumbar pain syndromes. It seems reasonable and obvious that we might be more successful in our rehabilitative efforts if we know more about those tissues that are capable of causing pain and those that are not.

WHERE IS THE PAIN COMING FROM? A REVIEW OF THE PREVIOUS LITERATURE

The modern era of lumbar spine surgery began with the publication of a paper by Mixter and Barr in 1934 on the subject of disc herniation.[8] This pivotal work established two important principles that have stood the tests of time and peer review: (1) herniated discs are a common cause of low back pain and sciatica, and (2) decompression by laminotomy and partial disc excision relieves the leg pain reliably and permanently in a majority of patients.

During the past 56 years these principles have been reconfirmed by numerous scientific studies.[10, 13] Unfortunately, simple disc hernia causing pure sciatica is a fairly uncommon condition when compared with the number of patients who present with back pain and back pain–sciatica combinations. Laminectomy and discectomy or, more precisely, laminotomy with partial disc excision is very effective in properly selected cases of pure sciatica. Those procedures are much less effective in cases of low back pain and combined leg and back pain. In fact, a careful review of the literature will indicate that operations aimed at decompressing bulged discs in patients with back pain alone may produce results less satisfactory than with conservative treatment or no treatment at all.[3]

Because of these facts, many authorities have concluded that the disc is a minor contributor to the problem of low back pain in general. During the past two decades, the idea that the disc is the principal cause of back pain has been regarded with some skepticism if not complete disbelief.[17] Some authors refer to "the dynasty of the disc" as if it were a bygone era, having been replaced by a new regime based upon an enlightened awareness of several other potential causes of low back pain. I am convinced that the disc *is* the principal tissue responsible for the production of low back pain. Additionally, I think that direct

*Reprinted in part from by Williams RW, McCulloch JA, Young PH (eds): *Microsurgery of the Lumbar Spine*. Rockville, Md, Aspen, 1990, pp 1–7. Used by permission.

evidence derived from in vivo studies of human spines can explain some of the apparent discrepancies in the discogenic theory of low back pain and sciatica. The data provided in the following section will attempt to establish the correctness of these opinions.

What other tissues might be involved in the production of low back pain and sciatica? Theories abound to answer this question. Muscles, fascia, subcutaneous fat nodules, the facet joint and facet joint capsule, spinal ligaments, and even vertebral bone itself have been proposed as possible tissues of origin. Much of the evidence supporting these tissues as causes of low back pain consists of anecdotal reports and "deductive reasoning" based on anatomic studies showing pain fibers in various tissues of the spine. Prior to the advent of computed tomography (CT) and magnetic resonance imaging (MRI), plain radiography, and myelography constituted the most commonly used diagnostic techniques. Given the inadequacies of these diagnostic methods, we can now appreciate the reasons for the often-quoted opinion that "in most cases, we are unable to determine the true cause of low back pain."

The available clinical and neuroanatomic evidence indicates that there must be some relationship between these pain syndromes and the process of degenerative disc disease. The exact relationship, however, remains unclear.

In 1948, Hirsch performed an experiment on 16 cases of low back pain unresponsive to conservative measures. Without any anesthesia, he placed needles into the posterior of the annulus. He found that he could reproduce the clinical discomfort by thus stimulating certain discs. Furthermore, he was able to completely obliterate the low back pain and improve spinal mobility by the injection of as little as ½ cc of 1% procaine (Novocaine). In some cases where the disc puncture itself was painless, he was able to reproduce the pain by applying pressure within the disc by the injection of saline.[4]

Smythe and Wright performed studies in humans in which nylon threads were placed around various tissues of the lower part of the back. After the patient had awakened from anesthesia, the threads were pulled to stimulate the tissue. The authors concluded that the annulus and the nerve sleeve are the primary sources of clinical back and leg pain.[12]

While some controversy exists regarding the overall utility of discography, there is little doubt that stimulation of the pathologic disc can induce pain syndromes that closely resemble the painful conditions seen in clinical practice.[2, 6, 7]

In 1948, Falconer et al. published their observations made during exploration of a small number of lumbar spines under local anesthesia.[1] Murphy reported similar results in his small series of surgical cases similarly treated.[9] Once again, these authors concluded that the annulus and the nerve are the tender tissues.

Spurling and Granthum in 1940 stated that "we have repeatedly had patients who complained of pain in the back during operation with local anesthesia when the annulus fibrosus is manipulated."[14]

Similarly, in 1950 Wiberg, operating on some 200 patients by using local anesthesia of the skin and muscles only, reported that "in most subjects, firm pressure on the posterior surface of the vertebral body causes no pain. . . . On the other hand, touching the disc itself caused pain of lumbosacral distribution in nearly all cases."[16] Unfortunately, this tediously obtained knowledge is not widely known or appreciated.

Roffe subsequently performed elegant dissections of the region. By means of special staining techniques, he was able to identify a rich nerve supply to the outer part of the annulus as well as the posterior longitudinal ligament.[11] These nociceptive fibers are connected to the central nervous system via the sinovertebral nerve, which was described in detail as early as 1850 by von Luschka.[15]

We have recently presented our study on the origin of spinal pain based on our experience with microsurgical operations using local anesthesia.[5] The following section will summarize the salient points of that investigation.

THE ORIGIN OF MECHANICAL LOW BACK PAIN AND SCIATICA: AN IN VIVO STUDY OF PAIN RESPONSE TO TISSUE STIMULATION DURING MICROSURGICAL OPERATIONS ON THE LUMBAR SPINE UNDER LOCAL ANESTHESIA

Over the past decade, I have had the opportunity to operate on more than 600 cases of disc hernia and lumbar spinal stenosis. The following report outlines our methods and the results in a carefully studied subgroup of those cases.

Methods

We prospectively evaluated 193 consecutive patients with herniated lumbar discs and/or spinal stenosis during the 3-year period from September 1987 to September 1990. All patients underwent decompression operations using progressive local anesthesia. This technique involved the infiltration of 1% lidocaine into the skin and subcutaneous space and thereafter into each successive layer of tissue as needed.

We touched, stretched, or applied pressure to each tissue with a surgical instrument. We used an operating microscope in order to clearly define the tissue being stimulated. Table 44–1 lists the tissues tested.

TABLE 44–1.
Tissues Tested for Pain Sensitivity by Mechanical Stimulation

Skin
Fat
Fascia
Supraspinous ligament
Interspinous ligament
Spinous process
Muscle
Lamina
Ligamentum flavum
Facet capsule
Facet synovium
Epidural fat
Nerve root dura
Nerve root
  Compressed
  Uncompressed
Annulus fibrosus
  Central
  Centrolateral
  Lateral
Nucleus

Results

We asked the patients to report any painful sensation in terms of severity, location, and similarity to the preoperative pain. Table 44–2 summarizes the pain sensitivity of the various tissues of the lumbar region. Table 44–3 summarizes the tissue origin of clinically significant low back and leg pain. The following paragraphs provide a more detailed explanation of our findings.

TABLE 44–2.
Sites of Actual Pain Production

Always
  Skin
  Compressed nerve root
Often
  Outer rim of the annulus fibrosus
  Vertebral end plate
  Tissues in the anterior epidural space, e.g., anterior dura and posterior longitudinal ligament
Rare
  Supraspinous and interspinous ligament
  Facet capsule
  Muscle at the attachment to bone
Never
  Ligamentum flavum
  Lumbar fascia
  Lamina
  Spinous process
  Facet synovium
  Uncompressed nerve root
  Uninflamed dura
  Facet cartilage

TABLE 44–3.
Referred Pain From Anatomic Structures

Low back pain
  Annulus fibrosus, outer layers
  Anterior epidural tissues when inflamed
  Facet capsule, occasionally
  Vertebral end plate, occasionally
Buttock pain
  Compressed nerve root and annulus simultaneously
Sciatica
  Compressed, stretched, or inflamed nerve root

Lumbar Fascia

The lumbar fascia consists of a glistening, white, moderately tense fibrous tissue overlying the lumbar paravertebral musculature. In most cases the fascia may be touched or even cut without anesthetic. In occasional cases we were able to produce some level of low back pain by stimulation along the central tissue connecting the spinous processes. This tissue is the so-called supraspinous ligament. I emphasize, however, that this occurred in rare cases only. Traction or cautery directed at the location of blood vessels or nerves piercing the fascia sometimes produced a sharp and localized discomfort.

Muscles

Gentle pressure never produced pain. Forceful stretching at the base of the muscles, especially at the site of blood vessels or nerves or at their attachment to bone, usually produced a localized low back pain. This pain varied with the amount of pressure and stretch applied. The pain was described as "sharp" and rarely simulated the deep, dull ache of lumbago. We were unable to observe any evidence of gross pathologic changes in the muscle and concluded that the pain was probably derived from local vessels and nerves rather than the muscle bundles themselves.

Normal Nerve Root

The normal, uncompressed or unstretched nerve root was completely insensitive to pain. It could be handled and retracted without any anesthetic. Forceful retraction over an extended period of time resulted in mild paresthesias, but never any significant pain.

Compressed Nerve Root

Stimulation of the compressed or stretched nerve root consistently produced the same sciatic distribution of pain that the patient had experienced preoperatively. In spite of all that has been written about other tissues in the spine causing leg pain, we were never able to reproduce the patient's sciatica except by finding and stimulating a stretched, compressed, or swollen nerve root. Sciatica could be produced by either pressure or stretch on the caudal dura, on the nerve root sleeve, on the ganglion, or on the nerve distal to the ganglion, depending upon the site of compression. The ganglion was somewhat more tender than other parts of the nerve root, but the difference was not dramatic. In general, the closer one stimulated to the site of compression or tension, the greater the pain response. This pain could always be eliminated by the injection of ½ cc of 1% lidocaine (Xylocaine) via a 30-gauge needle beneath the nerve sleeve proximal to the site of compression.

Scar Tissue

Another interesting finding involved operations on patients who had undergone prior laminectomies. In those cases there was always some degree of perineural fibrosis. The scar tissue itself was *never tender*. The nerve root, however, was frequently very sensitive. In addition, we concluded that the presence of scar tissue compounded the nerve pain by fixing the nerve in one position and thus increasing the susceptibility of the nerve root to tension or compression.

Annulus Fibrosus

About two thirds of patients responded with pain at this site. In those patients, stimulation always produced back pain that was similar to the low back pain suffered preoperatively. Likewise, the application of local anesthesia obliterated the pain. We had more difficulty producing buttock pain, but sometimes we were able to produce it by the application of pressure on the nerve root and outer part of the annulus simultaneously. Otherwise, the reproduction of true, clinically significant buttock pain was rarely possible by the stimulation of any other tissue. Stimulation of a disc hernia lateral to the foramen sometimes resulted in the sensation of buttock pain.

The annulus was exquisitely tender in about one third of cases, moderately tender in one third, and insensitive in the remaining third of patients operated on for a herniated disc and/or stenosis. Perhaps certain individuals are more richly innervated than others, or alternatively, perhaps there exists some chemical or mechanical irritant that sensitizes certain discs to become painful. Our observations did not clarify this point. They did, however, provide an explanation for the observations made by other authors that some individuals with disc protrusion are asymptomatic while other patients are acutely tender.

Referral of pain depended upon the exact site of the annulus being stimulated. The central portion of the annulus and the posterior longitudinal ligament produced central back pain. Stimulation to the right or left of center of the posterior longitudinal ligament directed pain to the side of the back being stimulated. This observation correlates with the finding of back pain on one side or the other when a "bulge" is noted on CT on that side of the midline.

The Posterior Longitudinal Ligament

We observed that the posterior longitudinal ligament was intimately connected to the posterior, central portion of the annulus. It was frequently tender and produced central low back pain. Because of its close proximity to the annulus, we were not able to differentiate its specific role as well as we would have preferred. In general, when the posterior portion of the annulus was tender, the posterior longitudinal ligament was also sensitive.

The Vertebral End Plate

Pressure or curettage of the vertebral end plate frequently resulted in a deep, rather severe low back pain. It was usually more severe and sharper in quality than the preoperative discomfort.

The Facet Joint

The tissues around the facet capsule were sometimes sensitive to forceful stimulation by means of a needle or Cobb elevator during efforts to mobilize the paravertebral muscle. The pain, however, was described as sharp and localized to that region. Its quality did not match the preoperatively perceived deep, dull pain of clinical low back pain syndrome. The capsule was sometimes tender, and when it was, it referred pain to the back or very rarely the buttock, never the leg. It could always be blocked by a few cubic centimeters of local anesthetic injected around the facet. It was never necessary to inject into the joint itself. The facet synovium was never sensitive. The facet articular cartilage was never tender.

One further observation regarding the facet joint may be of interest to the reader. In those cases where a trefoil-shaped central canal produced a tight lateral recess, we observed that the undersurface of the superior articular facet and its joint capsule frequently came into intimate contact with the posterior surface of the disc. We were able to produce low back pain by applying pressure to the disc at this site in many cases. Could it be that repeated contact between the superior facet and the disc causes an irritation that the patient interprets as low back pain and the physician interprets as facet syndrome? Figure 44–1 demonstrates this concept. We offer this as another possible cause of low back pain and a reason for the effectiveness of facet injections in certain cases of low back pain.

Other Tissues

The ligamentum flavum, epidural fat, posterior dura, nucleus, lamina, and spinous processes were insensitive to local mechanical stimulation. Forceful stretch of the interspinous ligament occasionally produced localized central low back pain. The surface of bone, even at the level of the periosteum, was insensitive. The spinous processes, laminae, and facet bone could be removed with a rongeur without anesthetic. We did not test for deep bone pain by means of increasing the marrow hydrostatic pressure.

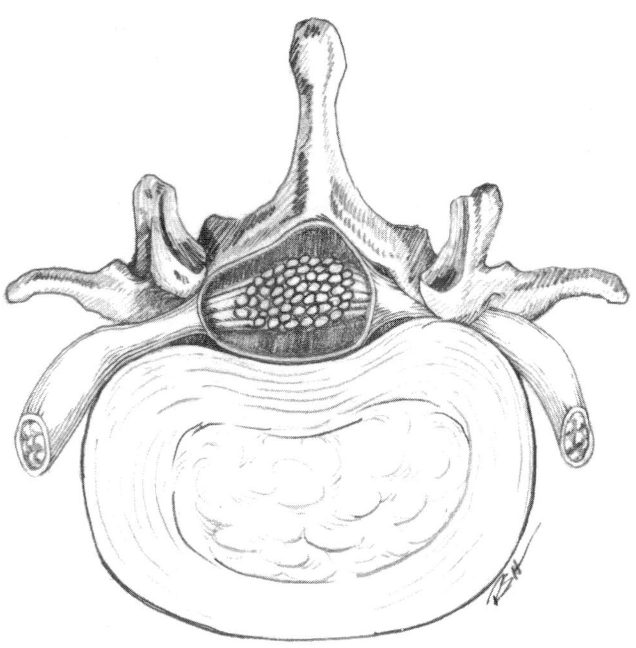

FIG 44–1.
This diagram shows the posterior part of the annulus and the superior articular facet to be in contact. This may be a cause of backache in the patient with this type of anatomy.

In summary then, Figure 44–2 illustrates the only two sites of clinically significant pain production in the lumbar spine: the outer part of the disc, which causes back pain, and the nerve root, which causes sciatica.

CONCLUSIONS

1. Operative exploration of the lumbar spine by using a progressive local anesthetic technique provides a unique opportunity for the surgeon to learn about the tissues that are responsible for the mechanical pain syndromes seen in clinical practice.

2. The spinal surgeon has the opportunity to define the true origin of pain in vivo.

3. Sciatica can only be produced by direct pressure or stretch upon an inflamed, stretched, or compressed nerve root. No other tissues in the spine are capable of producing leg pain.

4. Proximal infiltration of the nerve by using a 30-gauge needle and ½ cc of 1% lidocaine completely relieves the sciatica and allows for painless retraction of the nerve root.

5. The facet synovium is never the site of back or leg pain.

6. The facet capsule is sometimes tender, but its true significance in the area of low back pain and sciatica probably involves its ability to compress or irritate other sensitive local tissues such as the nerve root or the outer portion of the annulus of the disc.

7. The nucleus is never tender.

8. In spite of all that has been written about muscles, fascia, and bone as a source of pain, these tissues are really quite insensitive.

9. These observations cast doubt upon the effectiveness of several commonly used forms of therapy for spinal pain, e.g., massage, ultrasound, electrical stimulators, exercises, magnets, toe tickling, manipulation, muscle relaxants, anti-inflammatory medicines, psychotherapy, and even some surgical procedures. Perhaps we should be spending more time learning how to effectively treat the true sources of spinal pain and less time massaging, manipulating, heating, and cooling tissues that have little to do with the production of low back pain and sciatica.

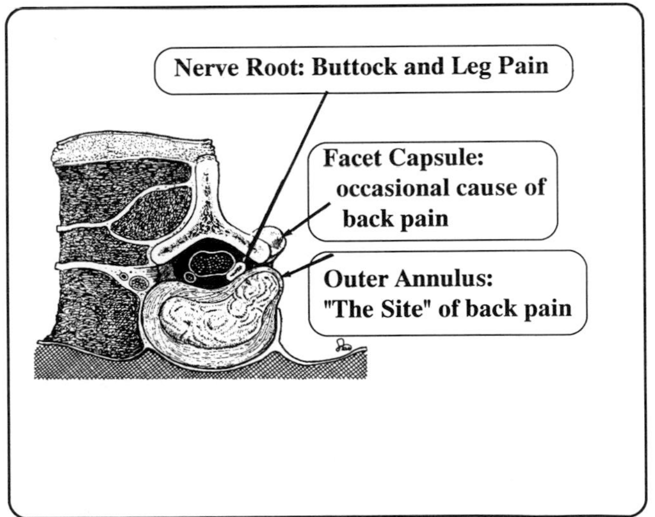

FIG 44–2.
Conclusions of the study: primary sources of low back pain and sciatica.

Acknowledgment

The author is indebted to his coworkers Cynthia L. Ulstrom, R.N., and Cami J. Michael, P.A., for assistance in the design, performance, and analysis of this research project.

REFERENCES

1. Falconer MA, McGeorge M, Begg AC: Observations on the cause and mechanism of symptom production in sciatica and low back pain. *J Neurol Neurosurg Psychiatry* 1948; 11:13–26.
2. Fernstrom U: A discographical study of ruptured lumbar intervertebral discs. *Acta Chir Suppl* 1960; 258:9–59.
3. Frymoyer J: Back pain and sciatica. *N Engl J Med* 1988; 318:291–300.
4. Hirsch C: An attempt to diagnose the level of disc lesion clinically by disc puncture. *Acta Orthop Scand* 1948; 18:132–140.

5. Kuslich SD: The origin of low back pain and sciatica. Presented at the American Academy of Orthopaedic Surgeons Annual Meeting, New Orleans, 1990.
6. Lindblom K: Diagnostic puncture of intervertebral discs in sciatica. *Acta Orthop Scand* 1949; 17:231–239.
7. Lindblom K: Technique and results in myelography and disc puncture. *Acta Radiol* 1950; 34:321.
8. Mixter W, Barr JS: Rupture of the intervertebral disc with involvement of the spinal canal. *N Engl J Med* 1934; 211:210–215.
9. Murphy F: Experience with lumbar disc surgery. *Clin Neurosurg* 1973; 20:1–8.
10. Nachemson A: The lumbar spine: An orthopaedic challenge. *Spine* 1976; 1:59–71.
11. Roffe PG: Innervation of the annulus fibrosus and posterior longitudinal ligament. *Arch Neurol Psychiatry* 1940; 44:100.
12. Smyth MJ, Wright V: Sciatica and the intervertebral disc. An experimental study. *J Bone Joint Surg [Am]* 1958; 40:1401–1418.
13. Sprangfort EV: The lumbar disc herniation: A computer aided analysis of 2,504 operations. *Acta Orthop Scand Suppl* 1972; 142:1–95.
14. Spurling GR, Grantham EG: Neurologic picture of herniations of the nucleus pulposus in the lower part of the lumbar region. *Arch Surg* 1940; 40:375–388.
15. von Luschka, H: *Die Nerven des menschlichen Wirbelkanales*. Tübingen, Germany, Laupp & Siebeck, 1850.
16. Wiberg G: Back pain in relation to the nerve supply of the intervertebral disc. *Acta Orthop Scand* 1950; 19:211–221.
17. Wyke B: The neurology of low back pain, in Jayson MIV (ed): *The Lumbar Spine and Back Pain,* ed 2. Turnbridge Wells, England, Pitman, 1980, pp 265–339.

45

*Percutaneous Procedures: Percutaneous Disc Excision, Arthroscopic Microdiscectomy, and Laser Disc Decompression**

Stephen H. Hochschuler, M.D., and Richard D. Guyer, M.D.

The concept of a percutaneous approach for the surgical treatment of a herniated disc is quite appealing. Despite the fact that percutaneous discectomy is a procedure that at this point has limited applicability, the indications will broaden with experience and new technology. As with any patient with a herniated disc, the conservative approach should be the first line of treatment. However, if this proves ineffective, then a percutaneous discectomy procedure should be considered. In this chapter, we will discuss percutaneous discectomy, arthroscopic microdiscectomy, and laser disc decompression.

HISTORY OF THE PROCEDURES

Valls and associates first described the posterior lateral approach in 1948.[32] Thereafter, Craig (1956) described the approach for vertebral body biopsies.[5] In 1951 Hult described a series of 30 patients who had relief of both low back pain and sciatica after fenestration of the annulus and nucleus via an open retroperitoneal approach.[13] In 1975, Hijikata described a procedure in which a 5-mm cannula was inserted by the posterior lateral approach percutaneously, the disc space was entered, and thereafter modified pituitary rongeurs and other instruments were used to decompress the disc space.[11] He described a 72% satisfied patient population. A similar technique has been utilized by Kambin and Schaffer, who have had an 87% success rate in 100 prospective cases[17] and 88% in their second 100 patients.[29]

Other approaches have also been described. Friedman in utilizing a 10-mm cannula described a true lateral approach that was fraught with complications.[8] More recently, Onik et al. utilized the surgical nucleotome and described a technique using a 2.8-mm cannula to introduce a 2-mm suction, cutting, and irrigating device.[23] The initial success rate of a multicenter study was reported as 75%.[24]

Unfortunately, clinical results utilizing the surgical nucleotome for percutaneous lumbar discectomy have varied from center to center. Some reports such as that by Kahanovitz et al. noted a success rate of approximately 50%.[14] Nevertheless, in the properly selected patient, the proper procedure might still prove efficacious.

The use of lasers for percutaneous disc decompression is still in the early stages. In 1986 Ascher et al. began using the neodymium-YAG laser for lumbar disc decompression and in 1988 changed to an Nd-YAG laser with a greater wavelength.[1] In a series of more than 200 patients, they reported that 75% did not need to undergo conventional, open surgery. The KTP (potassium-titany-phosphate) laser is also being used for lumbar disc decompression.[6]

MECHANISMS OF PAIN RELIEF

Traditionally the relief of sciatica was thought to be due to mechanical resolution of nerve compression. However, it has been speculated that inflammatory agents, autoimmune mechanisms, as well as neural mechanisms may be involved. It is known that the majority of patients with sciatica experience symptom resolution with appropriate conservative care including a short course of rest, anti-inflammatories with or without epidural steroids, physical therapy, and education. Such results are not dependent upon the size of the herniation because large extruded discs can be resolved conservatively. It is difficult to explain to patients how a ruptured disc can respond conservatively based on present knowledge. Certainly it is known that the herniation does not undergo any significant physical change within the first 2 or 3 months of resolution of the patient's symptoms. But then why does the sciatica disappear? Is it strictly a mechanical deformation, or is it related to some biochemical changes? It appears now, as more evidence is provided by investigators, that the latter may be the case.

Among those who proposed mechanical etiologies, it was shown in 1951 by Virgin that vertical compression causes the disc to bulge.[33] One could then deduce that this also could compress the nerve. Brown et al. in 1957 demonstrated disc bulging with lateral bending and flexion.[3] Nachemson in 1960 and 1965 found progressive annular

*Published in part in Hochschuler SH: Percutaneous discectomy. *Spine State Art Rev* 1990; 4:467–474. Used by permission.

bulging with increased loading and in his in vivo discometry study found that sitting increased intradiscal pressure by 40%, bending and lifting increased the pressure by 100%, and forward flexion and rotation should increase intradiscal pressure by 400%.[21, 22]

Hult in 1951 reported on a series of 30 patients on whom he performed retroperitoneal anterolateral fenestration of the disc, with relief of sciatica and back pain.[13] In 1974, Markolf and Morris carried out a study in cadaver spines and found that an annular fenestration markedly decreased the disc's compressive stiffness and caused an increased "creep" and relaxation of the disc as well.[19] In younger specimens, however, nuclear material tended to plug the annular fenestration, and nearly normalized the compressive behavior. Hampton et al. in 1989 reported on experimental fenestration in 10 dogs and found that at 3 to 12 weeks fibrous tissue was forming in the fenestration itself.[9] Kambin and Brager in 1987 measured the intradiscal pressure with extension before and after arthroscopic microdiscectomy and found that it decreased from 181 mm to 19.4 mm after arthroscopic microdiscectomy.[15] Sakamoto et al. reported a 40% pressure reduction in patients undergoing arthroscopic microdiscectomy and found this to remain up to 21 months.[28]

Additionally, removal of the compressing disc fragments appears to be important in relieving sciatica. In well-selected patients, open surgery should relieve sciatica in 85 to 95% of patients. Arthroscopic microdiscectomy, in contrast to other percutaneous procedure techniques, allows removal of the offending fragment from the inside out. This has succeeded for Kambin and Schaffer in greater than 85% of their series of 100 patients.[17]

There has been an increasing trend toward implication of inflammatory agents producing sciatica. Saal et al. in 1990 reported a thousand-fold increase in phospholipase A_2 (PLA_2) in patients with herniated discs.[26] This enzyme is responsible for the production of arachidonic acid, which leads to the production of leukotrienes and prostaglandins, which then promote an inflammatory reaction. They injected PLA_2 into mice paws and found that it was extremely inflammatory and produced edema.[27] They felt that the local production of inflammatory mediators could cause nerve inflammation and swelling, thus altering electrophysiologic function. Prostaglandins and leukotrienes have been shown to cause sensitization of small neurons, which also enhances pain generation. Intravascular permeability and response to inflammatory mediators could result in "venous congestion" and intraneural edema. They also speculated that further insult or mechanical deformation in the neural elements could magnify the degree of nerve injury. The extremely high levels of PLA_2 could help explain the mechanism of action of corticosteroids to inhibit this enzyme and also the mechanism of action of chemonucleolysis to cause degradation of inflammatory PLA_2 in the nuclear matrix along with the proteoglycans. It is also known that there may not be any appreciable change in the disc herniation as demonstrated by postchemonucleolysis scans, yet the patient still has relief. Results with percutaneous discectomies can also be related to the irrigation and removal of inflammatory mediators such as PLA_2. It is felt that sciatica may arise from biochemical sources as much as from altered anatomy.

Other biochemical mechanisms have been suggested as well. In 1990 Pedrini-Mille et al. in a rabbit study found that the production of neuropeptides such as substance P and vasoactive intestinal peptide (VIP) could promote increased synthesis of proteases causing degradation of the spinal motion segment.[25] Yamagisha et al. in 1991 demonstrated that interleukin-1 could stimulate the production of metaloproteinase in the disc as well as increase prostaglandin release.[35] Wehling et al. in 1991 also demonstrated both experimentally and clinically that the persistence of radicular pain after an appropriate nerve block was felt to be the basis of centrally generated activation of nocioceptive mechanisms.[34] These mechanisms of central information storage may serve as an explanation for the persistence of radicular pain in patients despite surgical decompression of the nerve root. These findings cast doubt on the validity of the classic peripherally stimulated concept of pain development and nocioception in lumbar radiculopathy in all cases. They explain that neuronal excitation triggers sets of events that extend over time from milliseconds to hours to days. The short-term response is manifested by action potential neurons independent of de novo protein synthesis, while long-term changes require alteration in gene expression. Immediate early genes are thought to be part of the stimulus transcription cascade that couples extracellular neurotransmitters to nuclear events, thus affecting the expression of secondary target genes over a long period of time.[34]

It is generally accepted that 85% to 95% good results can be expected after surgical decompression, but then why do the remaining 5% to 15% of patients have continued sciatica? Hudgins in 1990 presented a series of more than 400 consecutive patients undergoing laminectomy/discectomy and found that approximately 85% had relief of sciatica.[12] Further, it was reported by Bush in 1991 that of 164 patients with ruptured discs, only 14% required surgery.[4] He also noted that 62 of 84 patients with a large ruptured disc had diminution in the size of the herniation.

In summary, the mechanisms of pain relief remain an enigma to surgeons who are proponents of laminectomy/discectomy as well as those who are strict proponents of decompressions such as suction discectomy. In percutaneous procedures, there are two mechanisms that appear to be involved: the first is the reduction of intradiscal pressure, and the second involves the removal of offending disc material that may also affect the biochemical alterations invoked by a rupture. Finally, the mechanisms are complex, and even in the best of hands with the best selection criteria, 85% to 95% success rates may be expected with open surgery, but that still leaves a significant number of failures. Considering the limited morbidity and very good results, less invasive procedures appear to be far superior for appropriately selected patients.

INDICATIONS

The advantages of percutaneous discectomy over other surgical procedures are multiple. Despite the fact that chymopapain had proved to be a successful treatment modality, several reported cases of anaphylaxis and neurologic complications caused both the patient and the surgeon some hesitancy in its utilization. Subsequently, despite the fact that it is a reasonable treatment alternative, it is not widely utilized at this time. It is to be noted, however, that some investigators are reinstituting the use of low-dose chymopapain. The results of these procedures are still being evaluated.

In contrast to a simple laminectomy/discectomy, percutaneous discectomy has the theoretical advantage of decreased perineural fibrosis as well as a decreased incidence of epidural bleeding. In addition, the approach does not compromise ligamentous stability, nor does it prohibit future surgical intervention through virgin tissue if necessary. It is performed as an outpatient procedure, is less expensive, and does not require the use of general anesthesia. It is thought that the incidence of significant reherniation is diminished secondary to the establishment of a fenestration in the posterolateral aspect of the annulus that affords egress of any future disc material preferentially through this site rather than into the spinal canal. In fact, Hijikata demonstrated in two postoperative discograms that indeed the fenestration remained patent at 4- and 9-month intervals.[11]

Who is a candidate for percutaneous discectomy?

The ideal patient presents with a history of lumbar radicular syndrome (i.e., back pain and leg pain), with the leg pain being worse than the back pain. Ideally, the patient should be one who has not had previous surgery at this disc level, although Davis reported an 80% success rate in this subgroup of patients.[7] Prior to any type of operative intervention, including percutaneous discectomy, a thorough trial of conservative modalities must be undertaken. At our institute, this includes analgesics, nonsteroidal anti-inflammatories, muscle relaxants, and a thorough trial at physical therapy that might include William's flexion exercises, McKenzie extension exercises, various modes of traction therapies, etc. Bed rest, when appropriate, is utilized, but not for prolonged periods. A course of epidural steroid injections is likewise often undertaken in an attempt to ameliorate the sciatica.

On physical examination the patient should demonstrate clear-cut evidence of lumbar radicular syndrome. One would like to find evidence of sensory, motor, or reflex changes, positive root tension signs, and a lack of histrionics. The clinical findings should be corroborated by objective, diagnostic studies. We most commonly use either computed tomography (CT) or magnetic resonance imaging (MRI). Electromyographic (EMG) testing has likewise been of assistance. It is quite important not only to ascertain the disc level involved but indeed to also demonstrate that the herniated disc remains in continuity and that one is not dealing with a free fragment lying within the spinal canal. The importance of this is self-evident in that the posterolateral approach can not afford access to such a fragment. In those cases where it remains doubtful as to the exact pathology, myelography with a postmyelographic computed axial tomographic (CAT) scan can prove helpful. In addition, discography with postdiscography CT scanning is likewise utilized when indicated.

CONTRAINDICATIONS

Percutaneous discectomy is to be avoided in patients presenting with cauda equina syndrome. In addition, it plays no present role in the treatment of spinal stenosis, tumors, or sequestered discs. Relative contraindications include previously operated spines, significantly high-riding iliac crests, and significant psychological problems. The reason for the aforementioned is that percutaneous discectomy is performed under local anesthesia and requires considerable patient cooperation, which is difficult for most patients and might prove impossible for an individual with significant psychological problems. In addition, most investigators feel that the technique should only be utilized for a herniated disc. Nevertheless, Hijikata reported satisfactory results in a subgroup of patients with back pain consistent with degenerative disc disease.[10]

ANATOMY

Perhaps the best description of the surgical anatomy is that published by Kambin in 1988.[18] It is to be noted that the lumbar spinal nerve exits the neuroforamen along the inferior aspect of the pedicle and thereafter migrates anteriorly and distally across the intervertebral disc space (Fig 45–1). Thereafter the nerve descends anteriorly to the transverse process below (Fig 45–2). Fully understanding the anatomy is crucial to the successful performance of percutaneous discectomy. The "safe zone," therefore, is a triangular target that is inferior and posterior to the exiting nerve root. The approach should be medial to the nerve root itself. The safe or target zone should be that portion of disc just lateral to the superior facet of the inferior ver-

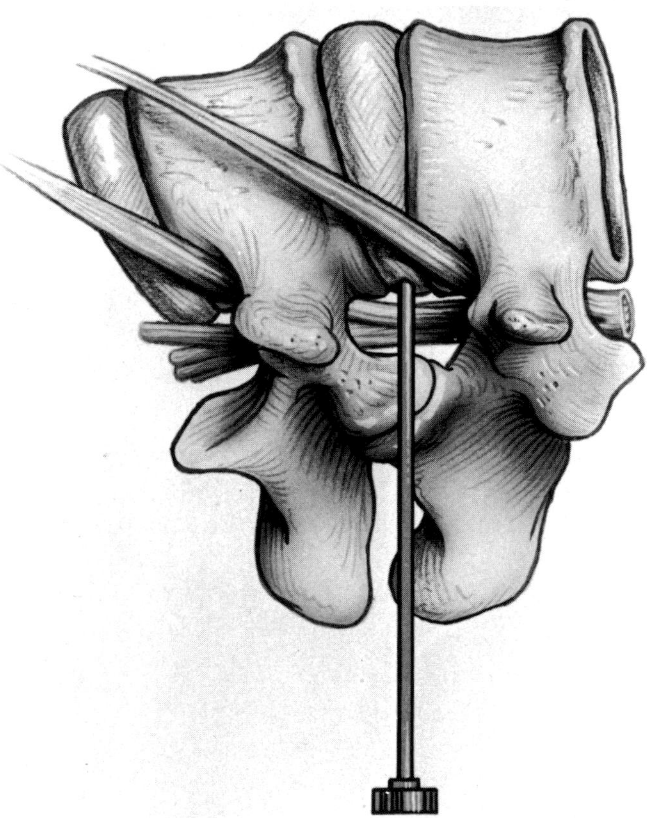

FIG 45–1.
The path of the lumbar spinal nerve root as it exits the neuroforamen.

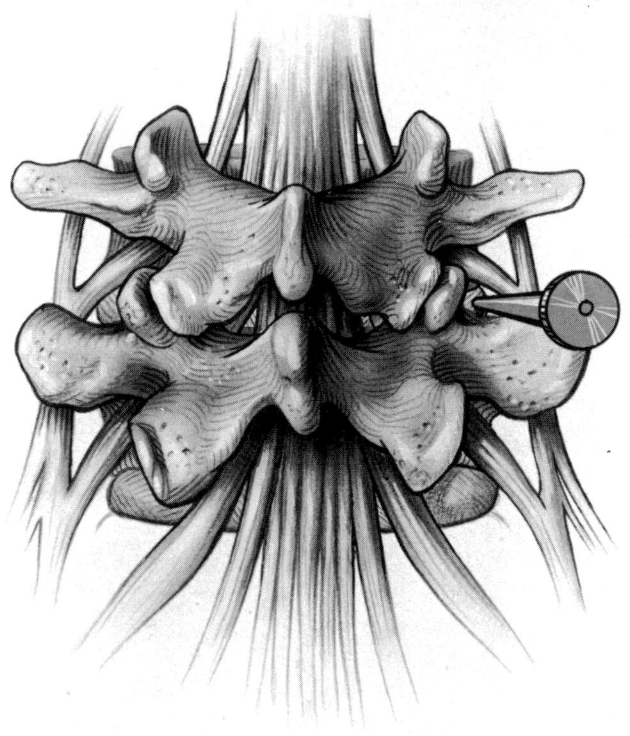

FIG 45–2.
The relationship of the exiting spinal nerve root to the transverse process.

tebral body, just cephalad to the end plate of the inferior vertebral body, and posterior and medial to the exiting nerve root. The iliac arteries and veins as well as the sympathetic nerve root fibers are located anterior to the vertebral body and therefore would not be violated with the correct operative approach (Fig 45–3). In utilizing the posterolateral approach, it is generally agreed that a point somewhere between 8 and 12 cm lateral to the midline should be used as the point of entry. One should approach the disc from the involved side. The direction of the probe would be at approximately 45 degrees, parallel to the disc space. This trajectory will penetrate subcutaneous tissue, fascia, and quadratus lumborum muscle, thereafter pass between the transverse processes and the contiguous vertebrae, and then penetrate the psoas major muscle prior to entering the disc space itself. One needs to vary the approach slightly for the L5–S1 interspace in that it is not possible to approach it in a parallel fashion in most instances.

ANESTHESIA

It is generally accepted that percutaneous discectomy should be performed under local anesthesia. As the technique evolves, however, and various satisfactory means are established to identify the spinal nerve roots, general anesthesia might be utilized sometime in the future.

Most surgeons performing percutaneous discectomy utilize monitored anesthesia care (MAC). At the Texas Back Institute we utilize a combination of fentanyl and midazolam (Versed). It is important that the patient be comfortable but responsive and able to respond if indeed the instruments are violating the exiting spinal nerve.

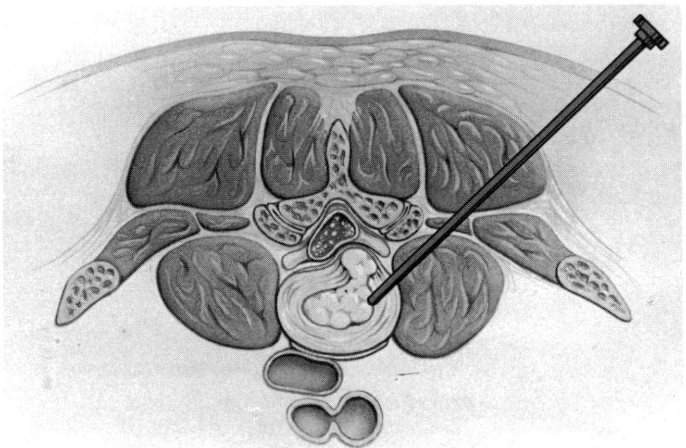

FIG 45–3.
Axial view of the probe pathway when performing percutaneous discectomy. The probe point of entry is between 8 and 12 cm lateral to the midline.

Lidocaine is utilized in the skin and the subcutaneous tissue in addition to anesthetizing the fascia. One must be cautious, however, to not penetrate too deeply with the lidocaine and anesthetize the exiting spinal nerve. Once the disc space itself has been successfully entered, stronger sedation might be utilized to make the patient more comfortable.

TECHNIQUE

The patient is positioned in either a lateral or prone position with the abdomen decompressed. The procedure is preformed under sterile conditions. Prophylactic antibiotics are utilized. Depending on the technique utilized, the procedure is performed on either an inpatient or outpatient basis with proper preoperative and postoperative instructions having been administered.

As mentioned previously, various techniques have been described for percutaneous discectomy including Jacobsen's lateral approach using a larger cannula, which was fraught with significant complications.[8] This approach seems to have been generally abandoned. The posterolateral approach as initially described by Hijikata is the approach utilized for both automated percutaneous discectomy as well as the more traditional technique described by Hijikata[11] and advocated by Kambin. The difference in the two procedures seems to be the size of the operating sleeve utilized as well as the size of the instruments. In addition, the positioning of the instruments themselves that is advocated by these two groups is also somewhat different.[16, 17, 20] Surgical Dynamics has advocated the utilization of small probes measuring approximately 2 mm and 2.9 mm and positioning the instrument in the center of the disc as demonstrated on anteroposterior and lateral x-ray control. Kambin has advocated utilization of a larger sleeve measuring approximately 6.5 mm and positioning of the discectomy equipment in the posteromedial aspect of the disc itself, not the central portion. He believes that the larger fenestration with the 5-mm instruments affords a more adequate decompression of the disc itself as well as allows a larger portal of exit for future potential herniations. In addition, he feels that placement of the dissecting instruments in the posteromedial aspect of the disc allows one to more effectively decompress the area where the herniation has occurred. Proper instrument placement is a very important component of this procedure since it directly influences success or failure. Hijikata reports one case of a poor result where too much disc was taken anteriorly as noted by postoperative discography, but when a second procedure was performed in which the instruments were placed in a more posterior position, a good result was attained.[10]

Arthroscopic microdiscectomy utilizes the same approach as percutaneous discectomy but incorporates modified arthroscopic instruments including scopes, automated suction punches, automated cutters, and a series of curets. The instruments are utilized through the Kambin 6.5-mm sleeve. A bilateral technique can be utilized to allow visualization during discectomy.

Laser discectomy is performed from the same approach as for percutaneous discectomy and arthroscopic microdiscectomy procedures, but laser energy is used to remove disc tissue. Various lasers are being studied for this application. One of these systems utilizes a side-cutting probe. This system is smaller than the Surgical Dynamics system, thus being less invasive but not affording as large a fenestration. The clinical results of this approach are being evaluated in a multicenter trial at the time of this writing.

It is to be noted that when a percutaneous procedure is performed, bi-planar image intensification is mandatory. One must be absolutely certain of the positioning of one's dissecting instruments prior to performing the discectomy itself. Usually 1 to 3 g of disc material is extracted.

POSTOPERATIVE CARE

A successful procedure will usually be noted by the patient immediately postoperatively, although in some instances patients have noted gradual improvement over the ensuing several days. Patients may experience some back discomfort associated with settling and inflammation, although this is usually minor. They are generally discharged with a minor pain medication as well as anti-inflammatory medication and thereafter progress into a gentle aerobic exercise and stretching program. Over the ensuing several weeks, a strengthening program is instituted. The patient is schooled in proper body mechanics and cautioned as to any excessive strenuous activities for the initial 6-week period. In general, the patient is returned to a sedentary-type occupation within a week to 10 days postoperatively and to more strenuous labor within a 4- to 6-week period.

In the event of an unsuccessful result, conservative modalities are once again utilized including anti-inflammatories, physical therapy, and epidural steroids. If this does not prove efficacious, open operative intervention may be indicated but is usually not undertaken prior to 6 weeks.

COMPLICATIONS

There have been few complications associated with percutaneous procedures. However those that occur can be significant. There have been reports of postoperative infection.[2, 10] One investigator advocates the use of a lavage cocktail of methylprednisolone (Depo-Medrol), lidocaine, and gentamicin (40 mg of gentamicin, 40 mg of Depo-Medrol, and 2 cc of bupivacaine [Marcaine], 0.5%).[31] In addition, several investigators,[2] including the authors, utilize prophylactic antibiotics. Other reported complications include hematoma formation, for which some have used Gelfoam and others a single-tube Hemovac.[17, 31] Finally, nerve root injury has been described as well as vascular injury.[17, 30] Consequently, although complications are infrequent, they can indeed occur, and the procedure should be treated with respect.

RESULTS

As mentioned previously, successful results vary from 50% to 87%. There is concern in regard to potential overutilization of percutaneous techniques. The procedure should be used within strict parameters as outlined earlier. The procedure itself can prove to be quite efficacious when discriminately applied.

THE FUTURE

We believe that there is a future for percutaneous discectomy and one will see the evolution of various techniques utilizing previously proven arthroscopic technology as well as many new and innovative variations. Schreiber et al.,[30] as well as others, have described the use of discoscopy with elongated arthroscopic instruments. The development and evolution of spinal operating arthroscopes is occurring. The concept of laser percutaneous discectomy is being addressed. Some investigators have been developing percutaneous fusions as well as percutaneous lumbar intervertebral disc replacements. The exact role of lumbar myeloscopy for the treatment of an extruded fragment by perhaps employing a laser through the fiberscope will in itself evolve. The future is bright and will probably follow a developmental course similar to that of operative knee arthroscopy.

REFERENCES

1. Ascher PW, Holzer P, Sutter B: Laser denaturation of the nucleus pulposus of herniated intervertebral discs, in Kambin P (ed): *Arthroscopic Microdiscectomy. Minimal Intervention in Spinal Surgery*. Baltimore, Urban & Schwarzenberg, 1991, pp 137–140.
2. Blankstein A, Rubinstein E, Ezra E, et al: Disc space infection and vertebral osteomyelitis as a complication of percutaneous lateral discectomy. *Clin Orthop* 1987; 225:234–237.
3. Brown T, Hansen RJ, Torra AJ: Some mechanical tests on the lumbosacral spine with particular reference to the intervertebral disc: A preliminary report. *J Bone Joint Surg [Am]* 1957; 39:1135.
4. Bush: Presented at the International Society for the Study of the Lumbar Spine. Heidelberg, Germany, May 1991.
5. Craig FS: Vertebral body biopsy. *J Bone Joint Surg [Am]* 1956; 38:93.
6. Davis JK: Laser-assisted percutaneous lumbar discectomy. KTP/532 clinical update in neurosurgery. San Jose, Calif, Laserscope, 1990.
7. Davis WG: Clinical experience with automated percutaneous lumbar discectomy, in Onik G, Helms LA (eds): *Automated Percutaneous Lumbar Discectomy*. San Francisco, Radiology Research and Education Foundation, 1988, pp 111–117.
8. Friedman WA: Percutaneous discectomy: An alternative to chemonucleolysis. *Neurosurgery* 1983; 13:542–547.
9. Hampton D, Laros G, MacCarron R, et al: Healing potential of annulus fibrosus. *Spine* 1989; 14:398–401.
10. Hijikata S: Percutaneous nucleotomy. *Clin Orthop* 1989; 238:9.
11. Hijikata SA: A method of percutaneous nuclear extraction. *J Toden Hosp* 1975; 5:39.
12. Hudgins WR: Micro-operative treatment for lumbar disc disease, in Youmans JR (ed): *Neurological Surgery*. Philadelphia, WB Saunders, 1990.
13. Hult L: Retroperitoneal disc fenestration in low back pain and sciatica. *Acta Orthop Scand* 1951; 20:342–348.
14. Kahanovitz N, Viola K, Watkins R, et al: A multicenter analysis of automated percutaneous discectomy. Presented at the North American Spine Society, Quebec City, Canada, June 1989.
15. Kambin P, Brager MD: Percutaneous posterolateral discectomy: Anatomy and mechanism. *Clin Orthop* 1987; 223:145.
16. Kambin P, Gellman H: Percutaneous lateral discectomy of the lumbar spine: A preliminary report. *Clin Orthop* 1983; 174:127.
17. Kambin P, Schaffer JL: Percutaneous lumbar discectomy: Review of 100 patients. *Clin Orthop* 1989; 238:24–34.
18. Kambin P: *Surg Rounds Orthop* Dec 1988.
19. Markolf KL, Morris JM: The structural components of the intervertebral disc. A study of their contributions to the ability of disc to withstand compressive forces. *J Bone Joint Surg [Am]* 1974; 56:675–687.
20. Mooney V: Percutaneous discectomy. *Spine State Art Rev* 1989; 3:103–112.
21. Nachemson A: In vivo discometry in lumbar discs with irregular myelogram. *Acta Orthop Scand* 1965; 36:418.
22. Nachemson A: Lumbar intradiscal pressure. *Acta Orthop Scand Suppl* 1960; 43:104.
23. Onik G, Helms C, Ginsberg L, et al: Percutaneous lumbar discectomy using a new aspiration probe. *Am J Neuroradiol* 1985; 6:290.
24. Onik G, Maroon J, Helms C, et al: Automated percutaneous diskectomy: Initial patient experience. *Radiology* 1987; 162:129–132.
25. Pedrini-Mille A, Weinstein JJ, Found EM, et al: Stimulation of dorsal root ganglia and degradation of rabbit annulus fibrosus. *Spine* 1990; 15:1252–1256.
26. Saal JS, Franson RC, Dobrow R, et al: High levels of inflammatory phospholipase A_2 activity in lumbar disc herniations. *Spine* 1990; 15:674–678.
27. Saal JS, Franson RC, Saal JA, White AH: Human disc PLA_2 is inflammatory. Presented at the North American Spine Society. Keystone, Colo, August 1991.
28. Sakamoto T, Yamakawa H, Tajima T, et al: A study of percutaneous lumbar nucleotomy and lumbar intradiscal

pressure. Presented at the International Symposium on Percutaneous Nucleotomy, Brussels, Belgium, March 1989.

29. Schaffer JL, Kambin P: Percutaneous posterolateral lumbar discectomy and decompression with a 6.9-millimeter cannula. Analysis of operative failures and complications. *J Bone Joint Surg [Am]* 1991; 73:822–831.
30. Schreiber A, Suezawa Y, Leu H: Does percutaneous nucleotomy with discoscopy replace conventional discectomy? *Clin Orthop* 1989; 238:35–42.
31. Shepperd JAN, James SE, Leach AS: Percutaneous disc surgery. *Clin Orthop* 1989; 238:43.
32. Valls J, Ottolenghi EC, Schajowicz F: Aspiration biopsy in diagnosis of lesions of vertebral bodies. *JAMA* 1948; 136:376–382.
33. Virgin WJ: Experimental investigation into the physical properties of the intervertebral disc. *J Bone Joint Surg [Br]* 1951; 33:607.
34. Wehling P, Toole TR, Zieglgansberger W: The persistence of radicular pain after lumbar nerve root infiltration: A clinical study and experimental observations on the same phenomenon? Presented at the International Society for the Study of the Lumbar Spine, Heidelberg, Germany, May 1991.
35. Yamagisha M, Nemoto O, Kikuchi T, et al: Ruptured human disc tissues produce metalloproteinase and interleukin-1. Presented at the International Society for the Study of the Lumbar Spine, Heidelberg, Germany, May 1991.

46

Rehabilitation After Microdiscectomy

Pamela R. Snyder, B.S., P.T.

It is a paradox that if a person is not a surgical candidate, a high emphasis of treatment is placed on conditioning, education, self-management, ergonomics, and psychosocial intervention. However, the postsurgical patient is generally not provided with the same selection of options. Is this perhaps based on the premise that surgery is an ultimate treatment? Although the general characteristics of the surgical vs. the nonsurgical patient may differ somewhat, treatment still needs to be individualized. This is accomplished through the evaluation and treatment of the whole person. The sophistication of the microdisectomy technique presents an interesting challenge to provide a corollary level of care by the physical therapist—a level based on objective, scientific principles combined with refinement and precision.

REVIEW OF THE LITERATURE

The philosophies of treating postoperative back pain patients range from "optimistic nihilism" (letting the patient progress independently with minimal guidelines) to "aggressive intervention" (providing comprehensive reconditioning and educational programs). Clearly some guidance is necessary in determining how much intervention is appropriate.

The following citations found in the literature are early intuitive approaches to the problem:

Sawyer reviewed the role of the physical therapist relative to back school, exercise, and general postoperative care with an emphasis on activity. No results were given.[28]

Williams advocated no lifting, bending, or sitting in the car for 1 month; resumption of light duties and basic sports, with nonmanual workers returning to work at 5 to 8 weeks; maximum lift of 22 lb from 9 to 24 weeks; and gradual resumption of running, skiing, and lifting up to 55 lb at 6 months.[35]

Young indicated that 65% of his patients returned to full home activities at 2 weeks and 95% by 1 month, with 28% returning to work after 1 month, 76% after 2 months, and 90% after 4 months.[36]

Casper reported a study performed in Germany that indicated that 60.6% returned to work after 3 months and 90% returned after 6 months. He noted that patients in the United States take three times less time to return to work. This variation raises questions related to the social and economic structure under which benefits are administered.[6]

There are only a few scientific studies that have attempted to evaluate postoperative care.

Naylor reported that routine postoperative care appeared adequate and no specific program was indicated. However, this was not a controlled prospective study.[23]

Alaranta et al. performed a controlled, prospective study comparing comprehensive care to variable care provided at various facilities. They reported *no* significant difference in terms of surgical results between postoperative patients undergoing a comprehensive rehabilitation program of 2 weeks' duration 1 month postoperatively vs. a group undergoing variable programs at normal-care facilities. These results were based on 1-year follow-up evaluations. The apparent discrepancy in expected outcomes may have been due to the lack of an individualized approach and only 2 weeks of treatment without intermittent follow-up. This study was useful in that it reported a statistical difference in total sick leave between groups in light vs. heavy occupations. It also reported a lower success rate if a person had sick leave greater than 2 months and recommended evaluation of vocational and psychosocial factors at that point.[1]

Although the citations and studies to date have provided some useful information, they have not addressed the need for *individualizing* postoperative treatment. Active intervention requires a biomechanical and physiologic understanding of the specific pathology and how these factors will function.

BIOMECHANICAL CONSIDERATIONS

Postoperative rehabilitation must consider the fact that the spine may be biomechanically altered through the degenerative process as well as the surgical process.

Discogenic Changes

Farfan proposed that torsion is a factor in disc herniation. Forced rotation of 2 to 3 degrees may damage the annulus, with the highest stress obtained first in the outermost fibers and failure occurring at the posterolateral angles. Tensile stress in conjunction with torsional stress produced by axial rotation makes the annulus more vulnerable. This stress is reduced if compression is simultaneously increased to compensate; up to a 20% difference in torque strength is produced. He also reported that removal of a 2-cm portion of the posterior of the annulus produced a 25% decrease in torque strength.[10]

Gracovetsky has described the theory of spinal locomotion.[14, 15] This functional theory of the spine permits a determination of safe loads that can be loaded and transported. It also predicts the conditions of load transfer through a joint. Axial compression in combination with sagittal bending and lateral bending creates fissures in the annulus that may allow the nucleus to herniate. Axial torque increases these stresses, and radial fissures result. These combinations of forces are encountered in daily life.[14]

Butler et al. addressed the relationship between facet joint osteoarthrosis and disc degeneration and concluded that disc degeneration occurs first. This may lead to mechanical changes in the loading of the facet joints and result in facet osteoarthritis.[5]

Strength

Kahanovitz et al. measured abdominal and back strength and endurance and found a 30% loss of normal strength in postoperative patients. He concluded that more intensive physical therapy is necessary to improve the postoperative strength in the surgical patient.[18]

A quantitative study of trunk muscle strength and fatigability found that the trunk strength of patients suffering from backache for less than 1 month was significantly lower than in a control group without back pain. The patients with low back pain also exhibited a greater fatigability of trunk flexors.[32]

Postsurgical Changes

Panjabi et al. observed that injury to the annulus and removal of the nucleus significantly altered the main motions and coupled motions of the spinal unit. The clinical consequences of a posterolateral injury to the disc, asymmetrical movement, and loading may produce cartilage degeneration, osteoarthritis, and facet atrophy.[24]

Goel et al. investigated the biomechanical effects of discectomy and concluded that translational and rotational instability at the injury level is less with subtotal discectomies.[12, 13] Extension exercises were advised for treatment since extension appears to be the most stable loading mode after subtotal discectomy. Lateral bending and rotation should be avoided. Their results suggested that the detrimental effects of motion could be modulated by the patient learning to either inhibit or facilitate the muscles.[12]

Hurme and Alaranta reported that overall outcome satisfaction and results may be related to surgical pathology. A disc protrusion predicted poorer results than a prolapse or extrusion.[16]

Ryan and Zwerling indicated that postsurgical patients are at greater risk of injury than nonsurgical patients are.[25]

These studies suggest that the treatment protocol should accomodate the individual's pathology. Therefore, it is of theoretical and practical importance to address the factors of individual strength, mobility, endurance, ergonomics, and biomechanics.

PSYCHOSOCIAL CONSIDERATIONS

Additional research has led us to recognize that psychological, vocational, and financial considerations are important factors in the rehabilitation equation.[3, 8, 9, 16, 33]

Waddell et al. reported that psychological and physical factors interact and combine to determine the surgical outcome.[33]

Dvorak and associates reported that poorer results may be related to psychosocial factors, including age of greater than 50 years and working disability of more than 4 months. They also noted a difference in coping mechanisms between patients without complaints vs. those with complaints or those on a pension. Their comprehensive review of the literature emphasized the need for psychological testing in conjunction with preoperative screening.[8, 9]

PRECAUTIONS

Before any active treatment is initiated, postoperative precautions need to be emphasized. It is imperative to have an understanding of the surgical pathology because a primary concern of the physician is the rate of recurrent herniation.

McCullough has stated that every discectomy series, standard or microdiscectomy, carries approximately a 5% recurrence rate regardless of postoperative activity limitations. The majority of these will occur within 9 months.[35]

Sprangfort reported that the recurrence of back pain and sciatica is related to the process of disc degeneration and is perhaps inevitable and unavoidable.[31]

The exact cause of recurring disc herniation is enigmatic. Consideration for the biomechanical changes occurring postoperatively in conjunction with the implementation of a specific program related to those changes could potentially have an effect. This needs further investigation and provides the basis for an interesting study.

THE NEW APPROACH TO REHABILITATION

The physical therapist must elevate herself to a new level of involvement with microdiscectomy patients. A multidisciplinary approach is critical and should be *individualized*. The ultimate goals are maximizing function and minimizing the risk of reinjury by addressing the biomechanical, physiologic, and psychosocial needs placed on a person through work, home, and recreational activities. The therapist needs to be interested in the "whole" person. Early and accurate diagnosis of patients' physical and psychosocial profiles will greatly determine whether the treatment program will be effective. Our goals need to change from the "traditional" approach to the "active intervention" approach:

- Traditional goals
  - Increase strength
  - Increase mobility
  - Decrease pain
- Active intervention goals
  - Initiate team approach
  - Maximize function, physical and emotional
  - Minimize reinjury
  - Create self-assurance in activity progression
  - Promote self-management
  - Improve endurance
  - Address vocational and psychosocial needs
  - Implement ergonomic intervention

Initiation of the Team Approach

We attempt to approach this constellation of variables by following a comprehensive, precision-oriented approach. Our approach is not conventional, nor is it limited to the postoperative period. Ideally, it begins with the patient's initial involvement with the physician.

Kuslich has defined rehabilitation as the process of progressing the patient from the diagnosis through a return to maximal function (see Chapter 45). We have attempted to maximize the efficiency of this process by incorporating a *team approach into the initial visit*. The physical therapist performs the initial history and physical examination and discusses the data with the orthopedic surgeon. The physician then performs further physical tests, reviews scans, etc., and determines the diagnosis. At this point, we estimate the function, mobility, strength, and cardiovascular status of the patient. A psychosocial profile and prognosis are then established.

The patient becomes a member of the team. Individualizing the program by explaining the problem, the plan, and the projected outcome will help to ensure success. The goals and amount of intervention will vary depending upon the outcome of the initial profile evaluation. Misconceptions regarding etiology, diagnosis, treatment, and prognosis are corrected at the time of the initial interview. These factors are reinforced on subsequent visits.

PROGRAM COMPONENTS

Preoperative Teaching

If surgery is indicated, *preoperative teaching* is considered vital for both the patient and family. An attempt is made to relate the patients' pathology to the anatomy by using a spine model and correlating this with radiographic studies. Patients prefer to hear this from the surgeon.[34] Deyo and Diehl reported that the main reason for patient dissatisfaction is a failure to receive an adequate explanation of the problem.[7]

Back School

Back school is an effective approach in efficient management of patients.[17] It promotes compliance and self-management in patients with both acute and chronic pain.[2] Back education begins in the preoperative phase or shortly postoperatively. Anatomy, body mechanics, exercise progression, and work and leisure activities are addressed. Stress management is addressed as indicated. These sessions are generally 1 hour in length and include audiovisual and written materials as well as group participation. The most effective form of beneficial treatment in back care is education followed by an exercise program.[29] Ergonomics and sports-related activities may need to be addressed on an individualized basis.

Immediate Postoperative Period

The goal of the surgeon postoperatively is to minimize the risk of scar tissue formation and the chance of recurring disc herniation. Ninety-degree straight leg raising is recommended because this alters the position of the cauda equina nerve roots and allows dynamic movement to occur without stressing the healing annulus. Flexion activities are minimized. Williams states that "if patients perform the 90 degree sitting straight leg raise daily for the rest of their lives, recurrent sciatica secondary to lateral recess neural fibrosis will not occur."[35]

Cold may be used in the initial postoperative phases. General physiologic principles indicate that cold decreases local metabolic activity, decreases muscle spindle activity, and slows nerve conduction velocity to provide longer relief of pain and muscle spasms.

Cardiovascular Conditioning

Lack of endurance can compromise the results of surgery and the rate of return to work. Endurance contributes to the frequency and intensity of performance. Patients are encouraged to initiate walking activities 1 to 2 weeks postoperatively and progress to 30 to 45 minutes as tolerated. Aerobic activities such as swimming, walking, or biking are encouraged as a maintenance program.

Job-specific endurance training should be initiated if a person is returning to medium or heavy manual work activities. A muscular endurance training program involving 16 sessions increased endurance time 248% for symmetrical lifting tasks and 46% for asymmetrical tasks. The frequency of handling increased 44% and 34%, respectively.[11] This can be a tool to minimize reinjury.

The author believes that endurance training is a key component in maximizing function. This step needs to be emphasized just as much if not more than strengthening.

Strengthening Programs

It has been established that a postsurgical patient presents with greater muscular weakness than a nonsurgical patient.[18] It has also been established that a person is weaker after 1 month of back pain.[32] As the biomechanical alterations are addressed and an individualized exercise program is established, function can be restored.

Stabilization exercises, a specific type of strengthening, were "designed to develop isolated and co-contraction muscle patterns to stabilize the spine in neutral position."[26] The concept theoretically works by minimizing repetitive torsional stresses to the spine. Precise repetition of movements are emphasized. Saal has described a specific comprehensive approach to overall strengthening.[26, 27] These exercises can be initiated postoperatively because they are individualized (progressing from basic to advanced techniques) and minimize the potential of exceeding range or stress limits. The length of a supervised program is dependent upon pathology, strength, mobility, and learning ability. The ultimate goal is progressing to a home program, which should be continued indefinitely.

Strengthening programs using free weights, Nautilus, resistive weight equipment, etc., should be closely monitored and may not be appropriate or necessary for everyone.

Rehabilitation can potentially contribute to not only the obvious direct goal of increased strength and increased function but also the less obvious goals of reducing reinjury.

Work Hardening

Work Hardening programs are discussed in detail elsewhere in this book. The concept deserves some mention here. The emphasis of work hardening is to emphasize job simulation activities in a structured productivity-oriented program. The goal extends to match a person's physical and physiologic needs with work opportunities. This is achieved by addressing ergonomic and biomechanical concerns specific to the patient's workplace. The program incorporates not only strengthening, reconditioning, and job simulation but also the educational component in terms of injury prevention, self-management, and dealing with the fear of reinjury.

The effectiveness of work-hardening programs have been established in the literature.[19, 20] A preliminary study performed on the initial 80 patients completing the Minnesota Lumbar Spine Clinic's (MLSC) work-hardening program and followed for 6 months after completion further established the positive role in returning a patient to work (Table 46–1). Isometric strength for arms, legs, and torso

TABLE 46–1.
Work-Hardening Program at the Minnesota Lumbar Spine Clinic

Average age	37 yr
Average time off work	8 mo
Average duration of pain	12 mo
Average number sessions	19
Diagnosis	
Degenerative disc disease	23%
Disc bulge/herniation	57%
Soft-tissue strain	15%
Other	5%
Released to return to work	100%
Full-time	86%
Part-time	5%
Light duty	9%
Job search	15%

doubled to quadrupled in 1 month. Functional lifting and carrying activities increased three to five times when compared with the initial baseline evaluation.

Patients after microdiscectomy actually exhibited a greater improvement in strength and returned to higher levels of functioning than did nonsurgical patients with low back strain.

Lifting

A worker is three times as likely to sustain a low back injury if exposed to heavy manual handling tasks.[30] A great amount of work has been reported to identify elements of lifting style. But in addition to style, the speed of the lift and acceleration are critical. Movement and load relationship are significantly influenced by the lifting speed. A higher moment occurs at each load level when lifting at increasing velocity. Moments are less when lifting with a leg-lifting technique than when lifting freestyle. Analysis of a lifting style may determine where specific strengthening or endurance issues need to be addressed.[4]

OVERVIEW

The author is currently evaluating the effectiveness of individualizing rehabilitation. Preliminary results indicate that self-management skills and endurance are significant components. An example of program progression relative to work classification is outlined in Table 46–2. The purpose of the study is to determine what factors can be affected relative to recurring back pain, reinjury, and return to work. In addition to the physical changes, we are also seeing the potential influence of compensation relative to a return to work, as outlined in Figure 46–1. Theoretically, self-employed patients return to work much faster than do injured workers receiving compensation. It has not been established whether this could be influenced by rehabilitation.

TABLE 46–2.
Postmicrodiscectomy Program

Work Classification	Sedentary	Light	Medium	Heavy
Back school	*	*	*	*
Stabilization exercise	Basic	Basic	Advanced	Advanced
Cardiovascular conditioning	*	*	*	*
Job analysis	*	*	2–3 mo PO	2–3 mo PO
Work hardening			2 mo PO	2 mo PO
Functional capacity evaluation			3 mo PO	3 mo PO
Lifting		25 lb in 4–8 wk	35 lb in 6–8 wk 50 lb in 8–12 wk	35 lb in 6–8 wk 55 lb in 8–12 wk

*Initiated postoperatively (PO)

SUMMARY

Theoretical and research-based data have established the following conclusions:

- The disc is weakened by torsional stress.
- Biomechanical changes can result from degenerative disc disease and surgery.
- Back and abdominal muscles may be weakened secondary to low back pain and surgery.
- Psychosocial factors play a critical role in recovery.
- The reason for the recurrence rate is not clearly established.
- Ongoing research is critical.

Every patient does not need every component, but each component must be considered. To often, important aspects are forgotten or lose significance because a comprehensive approach is not a feature of a practice. The abstract goals of refinement and precision can be attained by meticulous attention to physical and psychosocial detail, minimal intervention when indicated, and maximally directed intervention when justified.

There are theoretical, philosophical, and hard scientific reasons why therapy can positively affect the recovery of the microdiscectomy patients. The role has gone beyond that of strengthening and mobilizing. The challenge of lumbar spine care presents the therapist as a professional with the opportunity to truly contribute to the patient's function and potentially decrease the risk of injury.

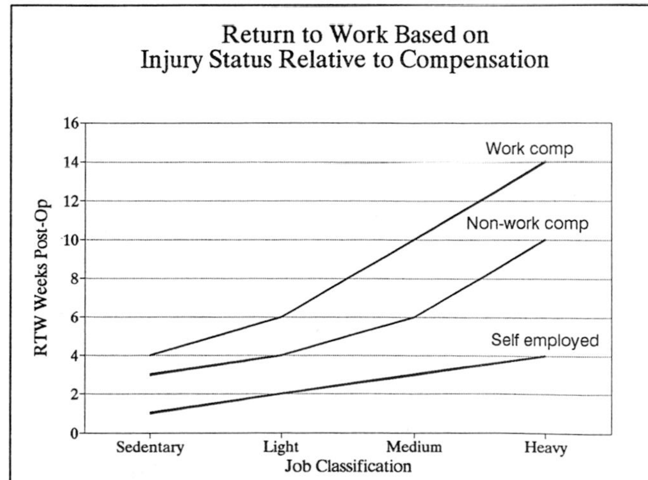

FIG 46–1.
The relationship of the number of weeks before returning to work and compensation in each of the job categories.

REFERENCES

1. Alaranta H, Hurme M, Einola S, et al: Rehabilitation after surgery for lumbar disc herniation: Results of a randomized clinical trial. *Int J Rehabil Res* 1986; 9:247–257.
2. Berquist-Ulman M: Acute low back pain in industry. *Acta Orthop Scand Suppl* 1977; 170:1–117.
3. Biering-Sorensen F, Thomsen C: Medical, social and occupational history as risk indicators for low-back trouble in a general population. *Spine* 1986; 11:720–725.
4. Buseck M, Schipplein OD, Andersson GBJ, et al: Influence of dynamic factors and external loads on the moment at the lumbar spine in lifting. *Spine* 1988; 13:918–921.
5. Butler D, Trafimow JH, Andersson GBJ, et al: Discs degenerate before facets. *Spine* 1990; 15:111–113.
6. Caspar W: Results of microsurgery, in Watkins RG (ed): *Microsurgery of the Lumbar Spine,* Rockville, Md, Aspen, 1990, pp 227–231.
7. Deyo RA, Diehl MS: Patient satisfaction with medical care for low-back pain. *Spine* 1986; 11:28–30.
8. Dvorak J, Gauchat M-H, Valach L: The outcome of surgery for lumbar disc herniation I. *Spine* 1988; 13:1418–1422.
9. Dvorak J, Valach L, Fuhrimann P, et al: The outcome of surgery for lumbar disc herniation II. *Spine* 1988; 13:1423–1427.
10. Farfan H: Biomechanics of the lumbar spine, in Kirkaldy-Willis WH (ed): *Managing Low Back Pain,* ed 2, New York, Churchill Livingstone, 1988, pp 25–27.
11. Genaidy AM, Bafna KM, Sarmidy R, et al: A muscular endurance training program for symmetrical and asymmetrical manual lifting tasks. *J Occup Med* 1990; 32:226–233.

12. Goel VK, Goyal S, Clark C, et al: Kinematics of the whole lumbar spine. *Spine* 1985; 10:543–554.
13. Goel VK, Nishiyama K, Weinstein J, et al: Mechanical properties of lumbar spinal motion segments as affected by partial disc removal. *Spine* 1986; 11:1008–1012.
14. Gracovetsky S: Response of the intervertebral joint to compression and torsion, in *The Spinal Engine*. New York, Springer-Verlag, 1988, pp 238–239.
15. Gracovetsky S, Farfan H: The optimum spine. *Spine* 1986; 11:543–573.
16. Hurme M, Alaranta H: Factors predicting the result of surgery for lumbar intervertebral disc herniation. *Spine* 1987; 12:933–938.
17. Jackson CP, Klugerman M: How to start a back school. *J Orthop Sports Phys Ther* 1977; 10:1–7.
18. Kahanovitz N, Viola K, Gallagher M: Long-term strength assessment of postoperative diskectomy patients. *Spine* 1989; 14:402–403.
19. Kuhn MP, Kneidel TW: Work hardening: A two-year experience. *Indust Rehabil Q* 1990; 3:1–45.
20. Mayer TG, Gatchel RJ, Mayer H, et al: A prospective two-year study of functional restoration in industrial low back injury: An objective assessment procedure. *JAMA* 1987; 258:1763–1767.
21. Mitchell RI, Carmen GM: Results of a multicenter trial using an intensive active exercise program for the treatment of acute soft tissue and back injuries. *Spine* 1990; 15:514–521.
22. Nachemson A: Advances in low back pain. *Clin Orthop* 1985; 200:266–278.
23. Naylor A: The last results of laminectomy for lumbar disc prolapse: A review after ten to twenty-five years. *J Bone Joint Surg [Br]* 1974; 56:17–29.
24. Panjabi MM, Krag MH, Chung TQ: Effects of disc injury on mechanical behavior of the human spine. *Spine* 1984; 9:707–713.
25. Ryan J, Zwerling C: Risk for occupational low-back injury after lumbar laminectomy for degenerative disc disease. *Spine* 1990; 15:500–503.
26. Saal JA: Rehabilitation of sports-related lumbar spine injuries. *Phys Med Rehabil* 1987; 1:613–638.
27. Saal JA, Saal JS: Nonoperative treatment of herniated lumbar intervertebral disc with radiculopathy. *Spine* 1989; 14:431–437.
28. Sawyer MW: The role of the physical therapist before and after lumbar spine surgery. *Orthop Clin North Am* 1983; 14:649–659.
29. Sikorski JM: A rationalized approach to physiotherapy for low-back pain. *Spine* 1985; 10:571–579.
30. Snook SH, Campanelli S, Hart H: A study of three preventive approaches to low back injury. *J Occup Med* 1978; 20:478–481.
31. Sprangfort EV: The lumbar disc herniation; a computer-aided analysis of 2504 operations. *Acta Orthop Scand Suppl* 1972; 142:1.
32. Suzuki N, Endo S: A quantitative study of trunk muscle strength and fatigability in the low-back-pain syndrome. *Spine* 1983; 8:69–74.
33. Waddell G, Morris E, DiPaola MP, et al: A concept of illness tested as an improved basis for surgical decisions in low-back disorders. *Spine* 1986; 11:712–719.
34. Wallace LM: Surgical patients' preferences for preoperative information. *Patient Educ Counsel* 1985; 7:377–387.
35. Williams RW: Perioperative management of the lumbar microsurgical patient, in Watkins RG (ed): *Microsurgery of the Lumbar Spine*. Rockville, Md, Aspen, 1990, pp 156–158.
36. Young P: Microsurgery of the lumbar spine: A 4-year experience, in Watkins RG (ed): *Microsurgery of the Lumbar Spine*. Rockville, Md, Aspen, 1990, p 221.

PART XV

PSYCHOLOGICAL FACTORS IN SPINAL DYSFUNCTION

47

Psychological Screening of Spine Surgery Candidates

Andrew R. Block, Ph.D.

Back pain is one of the most significant health problems in America since it affects somewhere between 70%[18] and 85%[51] of all individuals at some time in their lives. It is also the leading symptomatic cause of hospitalization and accounts for 2.8% of all hospital discharges.[10] Fortunately, 80% to 90% of individuals suffering back pain recover within 6 weeks regardless of the treatment administered.[46, 57] However, major problems for the health care system are created by the small percentage of patients who do not have such sanguine outcomes. For example, a well-conducted study by Leavitt et al. found that 25% of the industrial claims for low back pain are responsible for 87% of the total medical costs incurred.[30] Similarly, Spitzer found that 7.4% of all industrial back pain claims were responsible for 86% of the total costs.[49]

Many patients with protracted back pain go on to be considered for surgery. However, surgery is no panacea. Although according to Spitzer only 1% of individuals experiencing back pain require such invasive procedures, the outcome of surgery is highly variable.[49] For example, in a randomized study of 126 patients, there were no striking differences between operated and conservatively treated patients 1 year after surgery.[60] Similarly, Dzioba and Doxey in reviewing results of 116 randomly selected worker's compensation patients who underwent lumbar surgery found that 43.2% had poor results and 50% had moderate to good results.[14] These and other similar results led Spengler et al. to a conclusion regarding discectomy that typifies discussions of lumbar spine surgery in general: "Although lumbar discectomy is a common operation, valid indications for operative treatment of a patient who has herniation of a lumbar disc are still elusive, and the results of such treatment have been inconsistent."[47]

There are, of course, numerous explanations for the inconsistent results seen in lumbar surgery. One explanation rests on the fact that there are "no universally accepted criteria for scoring the presence, absence, extent, or importance of the results of a particular medical finding or diagnostic procedure."[43] Additionally, a growing body of research suggests that even if medical diagnostic tests strongly confirm the presence of an identifiable surgical lesion, the patient's psychological status can have a significant influence upon surgical outcome. It is the purpose of this chapter to review the current knowledge on psychological factors affecting the outcome of lumbar spine surgery and present a program for presurgical psychological screening of patients with back pain.

PERSONALITY FACTORS

Patients being evaluated for spine surgery undergo some of the most sophisticated medical evaluation procedures available. A plethora of technological devices can pinpoint pathophysiologic basis for pain in ways unimaginable a few years ago. However, such evaluative procedures ignore the simple fact that patients are much more than surgical lesions. The pain from injuries is experienced by patients who vary widely in personality and coping mechanisms. These individual differences in patients' psychological makeup can account for a large portion of the variation in surgical outcome.

Individual psychological differences among spine surgery candidates have been most thoroughly investigated in the area of "personality." Personality has been defined as "deeply ingrained patterns of behaviors, which include the way one relates to, perceives and thinks about the environment and oneself."[1] Personality can be elucidated through objective psychological testing using devices such as the Minnesota Multiphasic Personality Inventory (MMPI)[9] and the Millon Behavioral Health Inventory (MBHI).[35] The MMPI contains a number of scales that identify personality traits of potential significance in patients with back pain. Table 47–1 describes the major clinical MMPI scales.[2]

Table 47–2 lists studies correlating personality (as assessed by the MMPI) with the results of spine surgery. Column 4 of the table describes medical outcome measures, which can be broken into two broad categories—clinical and surgical outcome. Clinical outcome is usually determined through a combination of self-report and physician rating.[8] The most frequent indicators of clinical outcome are some variant on the Stauffer and Coventry criteria: medication use, pain relief, work status, and pain-related restrictions in nonwork activity.[50] As can be seen, most of these medical outcome data are based either on

TABLE 47–1.

Minnesota Multiphasic Personality Inventory: Overview of Clinical Scales

Scale No.	Description
1	HS (hypochondriasis): concern about health and somatic functioning
2	D (depression): low morale, moodiness, and feelings of hopelessness and sorrow
3	Hy (hysteria): tendencies toward somatic complaints or denial of emotional distress
4	Pd (antisocial): reflects impulsivity, low frustration tolerance, poor social adjustment, and anger
5	Mf (masculinity-femininity): identification with the stereotyped masculine or feminine role
6	Pa (paranoia): elevation suggests paranoid characteristics; the absence of elevation does not preclude the presence of these characteristics
7	Pt (psychasthenia): anxiety, low self-confidence, low self-esteem, excessive sensitivity, and moodiness
8	Sc (schizophrenia): disorganized thinking, feeling of alienation, isolation or social withdrawal, and general anxiety
9	Ma (hypomania): reflects expansiveness, high energy level, and high activity level
10	Si (social introversion): discomfort in interpersonal relations

global physician ratings or else on patient self-reports of pain and function. Surgical outcome measures—those determining successful resolution of the surgical lesion—vary widely from global ratings of "surgical success" to more specific examinations of lesions confirmed at surgery.

The general conclusion to be drawn from these studies is that certain personality traits correlate strongly with poor clinical outcome. The most consistent findings are seen with high scores on the hysteria scale (scale no. 3) and, to a lesser extent, high scores on the hypochondriasis scale (scale no. 1). Patients with such MMPI scores are often characterized as displaying heightened sensitivity to pain, denial of affect, unrecognized needs for affection, general dissatisfaction with life, and "conversion" of psychological turmoil into physical complaints.[21] The studies included in Table 47–2 suggest that caution should be exercised when lumbar spine surgery is considered for patients with high scores on the hysteria and also the hypochondriasis scales of the MMPI. Because their personality traits may predispose such patients toward excessive physical symptoms and a negative attitude toward treatment, good clinical outcomes may be more difficult to obtain.

In most of the studies listed in Table 47–2, depression is not consistently related to surgical outcome. However, a depressed affect is frequently seen in patients with back pain. Studies examining the existence of depression in patients with chronic back pain report prevalence rates ranging from 10% to 66%.[11]

Studies have shown that for most back-injured patients, depression is a reaction to the pain rather than a cause of pain.[23] Depression is associated with many symptoms similar to those created by pain, including sleep loss, appetite disturbance, impaired concentration, and social withdrawal. Thus, depression may worsen the functional disabilities engendered by back injuries. Consideration of antidepressant medication prior to surgery may therefore promote more rapid surgical recovery. One note of caution is in order concerning the application of presurgical personality testing. The studies listed in Table 47–2 are both correlational and retrospective in nature. Further, MMPI scores account for only about 25% to 30% of the variance in clinical outcome. It is therefore not justifiable to deny surgery to a patient with operative indications simply because of his MMPI scores. Rather, such results suggest that patients who are poor psychological risks should undergo further psychological evaluation and perhaps receive psychotherapy prior to surgery. One must also examine physical and additional psychological factors that could influence the outcome. Future prospective research utilizing objective measures of clinical outcome is needed to more clearly delineate personality issues associated with surgical outcome.

PERSONALITY DISORDERS

While MMPI research shows several personality traits that can affect the surgical outcome, this questionnaire is not specifically designed to assess "personality disorders." Such disorders exist when "personality traits are inflexible and maladaptive and cause significant functional impairment or subjective distress."[1] Fishbain et al. studied 182 patients with chronic pain, 90.1% of whom had back or neck pain, and found that 58.4% of patients fit a personality disorder diagnosis.[16] A previous study had reported a personality disorder prevalence rate of 37% among chronic pain patients.[39] The most frequent diagnosis, passive aggressive personality disorder (PAPD), was found in 14.9% of the total chronic pain population studied.[28] Significantly, 24.7% of male worker's compensation patients fit the criteria for this personality disorder vs. 0% of noncompensation male patients.

PAPD and personality disorders in general may present significant management problems for the surgeon, particularly in the postsurgical rehabilitation phase. PAPD falls under a general class of personality disorders in which the patient appears anxious and fearful. The specific diagnostic criteria for PAPD are given in Table 47–3.[1] It is not difficult to imagine how PAPD may affect rehabilitation. If an individual with PAPD feels that he is being pushed too hard to improve, one can expect either active resistance or minimal compliance, as well a tendency to denigrate the health care team. The surgeon should there-

TABLE 47–2.
Studies Relating MMPI to Lumbar Surgery Outcome

Authors	Subjects	Evaluation Interval	Medical Outcome Data	MMPI Results*
Cashion and Lynch (1979)[8]	78 patients undergoing hemilaminectomy, no previous surgery	1 yr	Global ratings: good outcome = pain relief + return to work (n = 48) vs. bad outcome (n = 30)	Significant differences (no statistics given) between good and bad outcome on scales Hs, D, K, F, Es
Doxey et al. (1988)[12]; Dzioba and Doxey (1984)[14]	116 worker's compensation patients. No previous operations. 74 received surgery; 42 did not	12 mo	4-point global rating of orthopedic outcome based on ratings of pain and function	Poor outcome for surgical patients correlated with Hs, "nonorganic physical pain," non-English proficiency, pain location In nonsurgery patients poor outcome correlated with Hs (+.48), Hy (+.36)
Kuperman et al. (1979)[28]	37 discectomy patients, no previous surgery	1 yr	Global rating (4-point scale) based on residual pain and ability to work	Hs, Hy, D each correlated with outcome between −.27 and −.33 Hs + Hy + D correlated with outcome −.58 (no significance values reported)
Long (1981)[32]	44 patients, various surgery, referred because "nonorganic" factors contributed	6–18 mo postoperatively	Retrospective global dichotomy (success vs. failure) based on neurosurgeons' records, (examined for pain relief, resumption of normal activities)	Hy significantly higher in failure group
Sorenson and Mors (1988)[45]	57 discectomy patients (1st surgery)	6 and 24 mo postoperatively	Visual analog rating of pain level. Patients' ratings of health status regarding back	Correlated with "poor outcome": Hs = .37; D = .37; Hy = .47
Spengler et al. (1990)[47]	84 discectomy patients (1st surgery)	≥1 yr	Stauffer and Coventry (1972) criteria—3-point global rating scale based on pain relief, return to function, analgesic use, and return to work	Hs + Hy significantly associated with poor outcome
Turner et al. (1986)[55]	106 laminectomy patients (25 had previous surgery)	1 yr	Stauffer and Coventry criteria—3-point global rating	Hs correctly predicted outcome for 83% of patients Pain assessment index of MMPI predicts outcome
Uomoto et al. (1988)[56]	129 laminectomy patients (surgery history unclear)	1–4 yr postsurgery	Stauffer and Coventry criteria—3-point global rating	In discriminate analysis, MMPI correctly predicted outcome for 69.7% MMPI scales adding significance to discriminant function: Hs, P <.0001; K, P <.0003; L, P <.0003
Wiltse and Rocchio (1975)[62]	130 chemonucleolysis patients (no previous surgery)	1 yr after injection	5-point global rating scale of symptomatic "success," "organic recovery"	Symptomatic success most strongly predicted by Hs + Hy (accounting for 36.2% of variance). Not predicted by physical findings

*See Table 47–1 for scale descriptions.

fore be alert for the presence of PAPD (especially in worker's compensation patients). Other personality disorders found less commonly in lumbar surgery candidates are presented in Table 47–4. Since personality disorders, by definition, represent maladaptive patterns of dealing with difficult situations, the treatment regimen should be adjusted to avoid eliciting these behavioral patterns.

BEHAVIORAL FACTORS

Although it is the goal of the surgeon to relieve back pain, the studies reviewed in the previous section, especially the Stauffer and Coventry criteria, make clear that a positive surgical outcome involves more than simple pain relief.[50] Rather, one hopes for improvement in functional behaviors related to pain: the ability to work and enjoy

TABLE 47–3.
Diagnostic Criteria for Passive Aggressive Disorder

A pervasive pattern of passive resistance to demands for adequate social and occupational performance, beginning by early adulthood and present in a variety of contexts, as indicated by at least five of the following:

1. Procrastinates, i.e., puts off things that need to be done so that deadlines are not met.
2. Becomes sulky, irritable, or argumentative when asked to do something he does not want to do.
3. Seems to work deliberately slowly or to do a bad job on tasks that he really does not want to do.
4. Protests without justification, that others make unreasonable demands on him.
5. Avoids obligations by claiming to have "forgotten."
6. Believes that he is doing a much better job than others think he is doing.
7. Resents useful suggestions from others concerning how he could be more productive.
8. Obstructs the efforts of others by failing to do his share of the work.
9. Unreasonably criticizes or scorns people in positions of authority.

recreational activities, a decrease in narcotic consumption, and improved sexual activity. In other words, back pain has behavioral concomitants that ought to improve as pain subsides. However, Fordyce has pointed out that such "pain behaviors" may be influenced or controlled by factors in addition to underlying pathophysiology.[17] Patients may receive financial gain for continued pain complaints.

TABLE 47–4.
Personality Disorder Descriptions

Disorder	Descriptions*
Paranoid	Unwarranted tendency to interpret the actions of people as deliberately demeaning or threatening
Schizoid	Indifference to social relationships and a restricted range of emotional experience and expression
Schizotypal	Deficits in interpersonal relatedness and peculiarities of ideation, appearance, and behavior
Antisocial	Irresponsible and antisocial behavior (beginning as a conduct disorder before the age of 15 yr)
Borderline	Instability of mood, interpersonal relationships, and self-image
Histrionic	Excessive emotionality and attention seeking
Narcissistic	Grandiosity (in fantasy or behavior), lack of empathy, hypersensitivity to the evaluation of others
Avoidant	Social discomfort, fear of negative evaluation, and timidity
Dependent	Dependent and submissive behavior
Obsessive-compulsive	Perfectionism and inflexibility
Passive-aggressive	Resistance to demands for adequate social and occupational performance

*Behaviors are pervasive and enduring patterns exhibited in a wide range of important social and personal contexts.

Pain complaints may serve as an excuse to avoid difficult situations or as a means of gaining attention. That is, these functional "pain behaviors" may be influenced by environmental reinforcement. When the receipt of rewards (or perceived rewards) are contingent upon the patient's continued disability, the surgical outcome may suffer.

Cairns and Pasino have shown how powerful such reinforcers may be.[7] In their classic study, patients with chronic pain being treated in a pain unit were rewarded with praise and staff attention for improvement in specific functional behaviors such as walking around a track or riding a stationary bicycle. In this study, patients only showed improvement in specifically rewarded exercises, and when reinforcement was stopped, behavioral improvements ceased.

Fordyce et al. have applied a behavioral approach to patients whose status was less than 2 weeks after back injury.[18] The patients were subjected to one of two treatment regimens: one group was allowed to cease activity whenever pain increased, and a second group was encouraged to be as active as possible, continually pushing for activity increases despite pain increases. Results showed dramatic functional improvements in the more active group, whereas the group allowed to cease activity demonstrated almost no improvement.

These studies, based on a behavioral approach, point to the importance of patient-staff interaction. The health care team must be trained to systematically praise and reward "well behaviors" such as activity increases, pain medication decreases, and talk about non–pain-related subjects. Pain complaints, poor attitude, and other "pain behaviors" can be decreased by extinction, i.e., ignoring such behaviors as much as possible.

MARITAL INTERACTION

Attention and reward for pain behavior may come not only from health care providers but also from the patient's family. Family members may directly reinforce disability by discouraging the patient to be active and bringing him medication when the pain increases. Further indirect reinforcement may occur, as when the patient can avoid unpleasant responsibilities or undesired sexual activity due to pain complaints. The influence of such reinforcement was demonstrated in a study involving patients with chronic pain who were interviewed and asked to rate their current pain level twice during the interview.[6] The interview was structured such that observers were present throughout the process. During half the interview, the observer was the patient's spouse, and during the other half, the observer was a ward clerk. Patients were also asked to assess how much reinforcement their spouse provided for pain behavior by rating the spouse's likelihood of engaging in certain reactions such as bringing the patient medications, taking over household responsibilities due to pain, calling the doctor, etc. Results showed that pain complaints varied depending on who was observing and on the nature of the spouses' responses. Patients whose spouses were relatively "nonsolicitous" in responding to pain complaints reported higher levels of pain when the ward clerk was observing than when their own spouse was observing. The patients with "solicitous" spouses displayed just the opposite pattern: they reported more pain when spouses were present than when the ward clerk was present. In other words, based on a history of perceived reinforcement, the presence of the spouse could act as a cue for the patient to display greater pain behavior. It should be noted that no attempt was made to control or verify whether patients were actually receiving spousal reinforcement for pain. Rather, it was the perception of reward and punishment that determined how patients responded in the presence of the spouse.

Besides direct reinforcement of pain behavior, spouse responses can indirectly affect the clinical outcome. In many cases, spouses (especially wives) of patients with back pain are highly dissatisfied with their marriages and are depressed themselves.[41, 44] Spouses with general dissatisfaction have been shown to be particularly pessimistic and to attribute the patient's pain to psychological problems.[3] Further, such spouses have poorer outcome expectancies for patients.[4] Sexual difficulties are also common.[36] It is easily assumed, therefore, that maritally dissatisfied or depressed spouses may provide little encouragement to the patient, thus leading to higher pain levels and possibly diminishing surgical recovery. Support for such an assumption is provided by a study of patients with myofascial pain in which high levels of marital conflict were found to be associated with more intense pain.[15]

VOCATIONAL FACTORS

Reward for pain behavior may be more overt than mere attention. It has long been speculated that financial considerations may play a large part in maintaining pain behavior. Since many patients receive worker's compensation payments or legal settlements based on their injuries, it may seem valid to assume that such financial factors influence pain behavior independent of any underlying lesion. There does appear to be a large body of evidence demonstrating the general effect of financial incentives and, more specifically, worker's compensation on patients with back pain. Hudgins compared clinical outcomes at 1 year postlaminectomy for 76 worker's compensation patients vs. an equal number of noncompensation patients.[24] Of the compensation patients, only 10 reported complete pain relief, and 14 were unimproved as compared with the noncompensation group in which 31 reported complete relief and 4 were unimproved. All noncompensation patients were working at 1 year postinjury vs. only 24% of the compensation group. Other studies have shown that worker's compensation patients with chronic low back pain do not respond as well as do noncompensation patients to multidisciplinary treatment.[5] Such results have led Frymoyer and Cats-Baril to posit "compensability" as the third strongest predictor of excessive disability in back patients—just behind psychological factors (i.e., high hysteria scores on the MMPI) and physical findings at 6 months postinjury.[19,20]

The above studies on compensation for back injury would seem to imply that many patients are malingering—consciously manufacturing symptoms for financial gain. This is, of course, not a new notion and corresponds roughly to the term "compensation neurosis," first coined by Kennedy: "A state of mind, born out of fear, kept alive by avarice, stimulated by lawyers and cured by verdict."[26] However, Leavitt and Sweet have shown that malingering is much less common than might be expected in patients with back pain.[29] In their study, 105 orthopedic surgeons and neurosurgeons completed a questionnaire that listed 40 clinical behaviors that might be associated with malingering in patients with back pain. Physicians were asked to rate the importance of each behavior in their forming an opinion concerning the presence of malingering. Four clinical behaviors were endorsed by 70% or more of the surgeons as being very important or extremely important in forming such an opinion. These included weakness to manual muscle testing not seen in other activities (81.2%), disablement disproportionate to objective findings (81.2%), pain not following an organic pattern (79.1%), and overreaction during examination (70.8%). The surgeons were also asked to estimate the magnitude of malingering in their practices. Most surgeons (58.6%) felt that malingering occurred in fewer than 5% of their back pain patients.

Not only is malingering uncommon, but outcome studies comparing compensation and noncompensation patients have produced mixed results, with many showing no difference in response to treatment between the two groups.[13] Further, Mendelson demonstrated that compensation patients are no different from noncompensation patients on measures of pain severity, pain description, and psychological disturbance.[34]

The mixed results may be accounted for by the fact that financial reward itself is not the critical factor in determining differences in outcome between compensation and noncompensation patients. After all, in most states, injured workers only receive weekly pay benefits equal to two thirds % of their preinjury wage while on temporary total disability. Even with tax breaks, the net income is rarely greater than 85% of the preinjury wage.[40]

Worker's compensation patients, however, may have two characteristics that make them likely to respond poorly to surgery. First, due to their injuries, these patients frequently are not working when initially evaluated. The amount of time a patient has been nonfunctional has been clearly shown to affect treatment outcome. Dworkin et al. examined relationships among compensation, litigation, and employment status (time off work) with short- and long-term treatment responses in a series of 454 patients with chronic pain.[13] Compensation benefits and time off work both predicted a poorer short-term outcome in univariate analyses; however, when time off work and compensation status were jointly used to predict the outcome in multiple regression analyses, only time off work was a significant predictor. In additional analyses, only the length of time off work significantly predicted long-term treatment outcome, whereas compensation and litigation did not.

Mayer et al. have coined the term "deconditioning syndrome" to describe the decreased functional ability and increased pain associated with prolonged disuse of spinal joints and muscles.[33] The study of Dworkin et al. suggests that the length of time a patient has been out of work prior to surgery may adversely affect the treatment outcome by creating this deconditioning syndrome.[13]

A second reality among worker's compensation patients is that many are not satisfied with their jobs. In a landmark study, Bigos et al. followed 3,020 aircraft employees for 4 years and prospectively examined factors that predicted the occurrence of a job-related back injury.[2] Job dissatisfaction—expressed as "I hardly ever enjoy the tasks involved in my job"—was found to be the strongest predictor of back injury. In fact, the most dissatisfied workers were 2.5 times more likely to incur a back injury than were employees with greater levels of job satisfaction. Only a history of previous back injury was equivalent to job dissatisfaction in predicting such injuries. In dissatisfied employees, there may be limited incentives for improvement since a return to function may mean a return to undesirable employment.

In summary, patients receiving worker's compensation are sometimes found to respond poorly to surgery and conservative care. The surgeon must take this fact into account. However, it is perhaps more critical to examine the length of time out of work and job dissatisfaction in patients being considered for surgery.

COGNITIVE FACTORS

Patients vary widely in the methods they use to handle or cope with their back pain. Further, they may have widely divergent expectations about the course of their injury and about the outcome of surgery. Such differences, falling under the general heading of cognitive factors, can have a significant influence upon surgical outcome.

Coping

Coping has been defined as "the thoughts and behaviors people use to manage their pain or emotional reactions to the pain so as to reduce emotional distress."[54]

Rosenstiel and Keefe constructed and validated the Coping Strategies Questionnaire (CSQ), which has been applied to patient's with low back pain in a number of studies.[42] This questionnaire initially examines six different types of cognitive strategies: diverting attention, reinterpreting pain sensations, coping self-statements (exhorting oneself to be strong), ignoring pain sensations, praying or hoping, and catastrophizing (believing that the injury is the beginning of a disaster). One behavioral strategy, increasing activity level, is also examined. Patients also rate how much they believe they can control and decrease their pain.

Gross gave the CSQ to 50 patients undergoing lumbar laminectomy.[22] Patients also completed measures of psychological adjustment preoperatively and postoperatively. The results indicated that individuals scoring high in active coping and suppression (combining the coping self-statements, cognitive distraction, and increased activities dimensions) showed better presurgical adjustment than did individuals low on this scale. Further, a lack of control over pain and catastrophizing were associated with poor presurgical adjustment. The CSQ was predictive of pain ratings and surgical satisfaction in an interview conducted an average of 41 days postinjury. Most predictive of positive outcome was the dimension of self-reliance (i.e., a patient's belief that he could decrease pain as well as a tendency to avoid praying and hoping).

In an intriguing study by Ressor and Craig,[38] 80 patients with chronic low back pain (mean chronicity, 8.8 years) completed a series of questionnaires concerning their pain, including the CSQ, and were also subjected to the direct behavioral observation of pain.[25] Patients were also examined to determine whether their pain behaviors and complaints were congruous or incongruous with their medical conditions. Three criteria were used to determine congruity: nonorganic signs,[59] inappropriate symptoms,[58] and nonanatomic or exaggerated pain drawings.[37] Significant cognitive differences were revealed between medically congruent and incongruent patients. Catastrophizing as assessed by the CSQ was much higher among the medically incongruent patients. The sense of control over pain, as assessed by a cognitive interview, was poorer among the medically incongruent patients. Interestingly, these incongruent patients also had poorer tolerance for an induced pain stimulus than did the congruent group.

Several other studies have found the CSQ to be predictive of treatment outcome for chronic low back pain. Turner and Clancy subjected patients with chronic low back pain to cognitive-behavioral or operant treatment.[54] They found that decreased catastrophizing as a result of treatment was related to decreased pain intensity, as well as to decreased physical and psychosocial impairment. A somewhat similar study using the CSQ reported that high levels of perceived pain control predicted a significant reduction in pain at the 6-month follow-up.[48] This last finding on the importance of perceived control of pain receives further validation from a recent study by Toomey et al. with a different assessment device, the Pain Locus of Control scale.[52] Among patients with myofascial pain, they found that patients' belief in their ability to control pain was associated with reports of less intense and less frequent pain episodes.

In summary, CSQ research on patients with low back pain indicates that the way in which patients perceive, interpret, and cope with pain can affect the clinical outcome of both surgical and postsurgical rehabilitation. Presurgically, patients scoring high on active coping and suppression are better adjusted psychologically, whereas those scoring high on loss of control display worse psychological adjustment. A sense of self-reliance and avoidance of dependence on external factors are associated with good surgical outcome. A lack of control over pain and, to a lesser extent, catastrophizing are associated both with poorer outcome in conservative care and with a greater tendency to display medically incongruent symptoms.

The CSQ is not the only questionnaire developed to assess patient cognitions concerning low back pain. Other less researched instruments (investigating similar cognitive dimensions) include the Cognitive Errors Questionnaire,[31] the Pain Beliefs and Perceptions Inventory,[61] and the West Haven–Yale Multidimensional Pain Inventory.[27] Whichever method of cognitive assessment is chosen, the surgeon should exercise caution in the surgical decision when the patient tends to rely on external factors, deny his own ability to achieve or participate in treatment or pain control, or catastrophize or believe that the physical condition will inevitably worsen.

SUMMARY AND CONCLUSIONS

The current chapter has reviewed the growing literature on psychological factors influencing the outcome of back surgery and postsurgical rehabilitation. While many of the studies reviewed are correlational in nature and some are retrospective, taken together they demonstrate that personality, emotional, behavioral, vocational, marital, and cognitive factors need to be assessed in order to maximize the patient's opportunities to benefit from treatment. Table 47–5 provides a summary of the most critical, empirically validated factors that should be examined in spine surgery patients. By evaluating such factors, the spine surgeon can improve the probability of a sanguine clinical outcome. Further, presurgical psychological evaluation may improve the prognosis for postsurgical outcome and rehabilitation by allowing for early psychological intervention to deal with issues that could hinder progress. Additional prospective research is needed to explore and refine the examination of psychological factors that can predict surgical outcome.

TABLE 47–5.
Presurgical Psychological Screening

Factor	Probable Effect on Outcome
Personality	
Hysteria and hypochondrias (MMPI scales HY, HS)	Heightened attention to pain Decreased motivation Decreased self-responsibility
Depression (MMPI scale D)	Symptoms of depression mimic and increase the effects of pain; the patient is less able to see progress or positive assets
Personality disorders (especially passive aggressive personality)	Enduring maladaptive traits create behaviors that are eccentric, erratic, anxious, or resistant
Behavioral	
Marital	
Overprotection by spouse	Discourages functional improvement; reinforces pain behavior
General marital dissatisfaction	Spouse less optimistic and provides less encouragement for improvement
Vocational	
Worker's compensation status	Patients may receive greater income while disabled
Time off work	Deconditioning syndrome (increasing disability and avoidance of pain make improvement difficult)
Work attitude	Job dissatisfaction decreases motivation and goals
Cognitive	
Catastrophizing	Diminished ability to resist setbacks Pessimism about outcome leads to hopelessness, poorer motivation
Perceived lack of control	Diminished self-responsibility for improvement. Poorer expectations

REFERENCES

1. American Psychiatric Association: *Diagnostic and Statistical Manual of Mental Disorders,* ed 3, revised. Washington, DC, American Psychiatric Association, 1987.
2. Bigos SJ, Battie MC, Spengler DM, et al: A prospective study of work perceptions and psychosocial factors affecting the report of back injury. *Spine* 1991; 16:1–6.
3. Block AR, Boyer SL: The spouse's adjustment to chronic pain: Cognitive and emotional factors. *Soc Sci Med* 1984; 19:1313–1317.

4. Block AR, Boyer SL, Silbert RV: Spouse's perception of the chronic pain patient: Estimates of exercise tolerance, in Fields HL, et al (eds): *Advances in Pain Research and Therapy,* vol 9. New York, Raven Press, 1985, pp 897–904.
5. Block AR, Kremer E, Gaylor M: Behavioral treatment of chronic pain: Variables affecting treatment efficacy. *Pain* 1980; 8:367–375.
6. Block AR, Kremer EF, Gaylor M: Behavioral treatment of chronic pain: The spouse as a discriminative cue for pain behavior. *Pain* 1980; 9:243–252.
7. Cairns D, Pasino JA: Comparison of verbal reinforcement and feedback in the operant treatment of disability due to chronic low back pain. *Behav Ther* 1977; 8:621–630.
8. Cashion EL, Lynch WJ: Personality factors and results of lumbar disc surgery. *Neurosurgery* 1979; 4:141–145.
9. Dahlstrom WG, Welsh GS, Dahlstrom LE: *An MMPI handbook,* vol 2. Minneapolis, University of Minnesota Press, 1975.
10. Deyo RA, Tsui-Wu J: Descriptive epidimiology of low back pain and its related medical care in the United States. *Spine* 1987; 12:264–268.
11. Doan BD, Wadden NP: Relationships between depressive symptoms and descriptions of chronic pain. *Pain* 1989; 36:75–84.
12. Doxey NC, Dzioba RB, Mitson GL, et al: Predictors of outcome in back surgery candidates. *J Clin Psychol* 1988; 44:611–622.
13. Dworkin RH, et al: Unravelling the affects of compensation, litigation and employment on treatment response in chronic pain. *Pain* 1985; 23:49–59.
14. Dzioba RB, Doxey NC: A prospective investigation in the orthopedic and psychologic predictors of outcome of first lumbar surgery following industrial injury. *Spine* 1984; 9:614–623.
15. Faucett JA, Levine JD: The contributions of interpersonal conflict to chronic pain in the presence or absence of organic pathology. *Pain* 1991; 44:35–44.
16. Fishbain DA, et al: Compensation and non-compensation chronic pain patients compared for DSM-III operational diagnoses. *Pain* 1988; 32:197–206.
17. Fordyce W: *Behavioral Methods in Chronic Pain and Illness.* St Louis, Mosby–Year Book, 1976.
18. Fordyce W, et al: Acute back pain: A control group comparison of behavioral vs. traditional management models. *J Behav Med* 1986; 4:127.
19. Frymoyer JW, Cats-Baril W: Predictors of low back pain disability. *Clin Orthop* 1987; 221:89–97.
20. Frymoyer JW, et al: Risk factors in low back pain. *J Bone Joint Surg [Am]* 1988; 65:213.
21. Graham JR: *The MMPI-2: Assessing Personality and Psychopathology.* New York, Oxford University Press, 1990.
22. Gross AR: The effect of coping strategies on the relief of pain following surgical intervention for lower back pain. *Psychosom Med* 1986; 48:229–238.
23. Gunsa A, Viking-Freibergs V: Psychological events are both risk factors in, and consequences of, chronic pain. *Pain* 1991; 48:271–278.
24. Hudgins WR: Laminectomy for treatment of lumbar disc disease. *Tex Med* 1976; 72:65–69.
25. Keefe FJ, Block AR: Development of an observation method for assessing pain behavior in chronic low back pain patients. *Behav Ther* 1982; 13:636–375.
26. Kennedy F: The mind of the injured worker: Its affect on disability periods. *Compensation Med* 1946; 1:19–24.
27. Kerns RD, Turk DC, Rudy TE: The West Haven–Yale Multidimensional Pain Inventory. *Pain* 1985; 23:345–356.
28. Kuperman SK, Osmon D, Golden CJ, et al: Prediction of neurosurgical results by psychological evaluation. *Percept Motor Skills* 1979; 48:311–315.
29. Leavitt F, Sweet JJ: Characteristics and frequency of malingering among patients with low back pain. *Pain* 1986; 25:357–364.
30. Leavitt SS, Johnston TL, Beyer RD: The process of recovery: Patterns in industrial back injury: 1. Costs and other quantitative measures of effort. *Ind Med Surg* 1971; 40:7.
31. LeFevbre MF: Cognitive distortion and cognitive errors in depressed psychiatric and low back pain patients. *J Consult Clin Psychol* 1981; 49:517–525.
32. Long C: The relationship between surgical outcome and MMPI profiles in chronic pain patients. *J Clin Psychol* 1981; 37:744–749.
33. Mayer TG, et al: A prospective short-term study of chronic low back pain patients utilizing novel objective functional measurement. *Pain* 1986; 25:53–68.
34. Mendelson G: Compensation, pain complaints and psychological disturbance. *Pain* 1984; 20:169–177.
35. Millon T, Green C, Meagher R: The MBHI: A new inventory for the psychodiagnostician in medical settings. *Prof Psychol* 1979; 10:529–539.
36. Muruta T, Osborne D: Sexual activity in chronic pain patients. *Psychosomatics* 1978; 19:531–537.
37. Ransford AO, Cairns D, Mooney V: The pain drawing as an aid to the psychological evaluation of patients with low-back pain. *Spine* 1976; 1:127–134.
38. Reesor KA, Craig KD: Medically incongruent chronic back pain: Physical limitations, suffering and ineffective coping. *Pain* 1988; 32:35–45.
39. Reich J, Tupen JP, Abramowitz SI: Psychiatric diagnosis of chronic pain patients. *Am J Psychiatry* 1987; 150:471–475.
40. Report to the Governor: *Major Issues in the Indiana Worker's Compensation System.* December 1990.
41. Romano JM, Turner JA, Clancy SL: Sex differences in the relationship of pain patient dysfunction to spouse adjustment. *Pain* 1989; 39:289–296.
42. Rosenstiel AK, Keefe FJ: The use of coping strategies in chronic low back pain patients: Relationship to patient characteristics and current adjustment. *Pain* 1983; 17:33–44.
43. Ruby TE, et al: Quantification of biomedical findings of chronic pain patients: Development of an index of pathology. *Pain* 1990; 42:167–182.
44. Schwartz L, Slater MA, Birchler GR, et al: Depression in spouses of chronic pain patients: The role of patient pain and anger, and marital satisfaction. *Pain* 1991; 44: 61–68.
45. Sorenson LV, Mors O: Presentation of a new MMPI scale

to predict outcome after first lumbar diskectomy. *Pain* 1988; 34:191–194.

46. Spengler DM, et al: Back injuries in industry: A retrospective study. *Spine* 1986; 11:241.
47. Spengler DM, Ouelette EA, Battie M, et al: Elective discectomy for herniation of a lumbar disc. *J Bone Joint Surg [Am]* 1990; 12:230–237.
48. Spinhoven P, Lissen ACG: Behavioral treatment of chronic low back pain. I. Relation of coping strategy used to treatment outcome. *Pain* 1991; 45:29–34.
49. Spitzer WO: Scientific approach to the assessment and management of activity-related spinal disorders. *Spine* 1987; 12(suppl):1.
50. Stauffer RN, Coventry MB: Anterior interbody lumbar spine fusion: Analysis of Mayo Clinic series. *J Bone Joint Surg [Am]* 1972; 54:756–789.
51. Taylor H, Curren HM: *The Nuprin Pain Report*. New York, Louis Harris, 1985.
52. Toomey TC, et al: Relationship between perceived self-control of pain descriptions and functioning. *Pain* 1991; 45:129–134.
53. Turner J: Comparison of group progressive relaxation training and cognitive—behavioral group therapy for chronic low back pain. *J Consult Clin Psychol* 1982; 50:757–765.
54. Turner JA, Clancy S: Strategies for coping with chronic low back pain: Relationship to pain and disability. *Pain* 1986; 24:355–364.
55. Turner JA, Herron LD, Weiner P: Utility of the MMPI pain assessment index in predicting outcome after lumbar surgery. *J Clin Psychol* 1986; 42:764–769.
56. Uomoto JM, Turner JA, Herron LD: Use of the MMPI and MCMI in predicting outcome of lumbar laminectomy. *J Clin Psychol* 1988; 44:191–197.
57. Waddell G: A new clinical model for the treatment of low back pain. *Spine* 1987; 12:632–644.
58. Waddell G, Bircher M, Finlayson D, et al: Symptoms and signs: Physical disease or illness behavior? *Br Med J* 1984; 289:739–741.
59. Waddell G, McCulloch JA, Kummell EG, et al: Nonorganic physical signs in low-back pain. *Spine* 1980; 5:117–125.
60. Weber H: Lumbar disc herniation: A controlled prospective study with ten years of observation. *Spine* 1983; 8:131–140.
61. Williams DA, Thorn BE: An empirical assessment of pain beliefs. *Pain* 1989; 36:351–358.
62. Wiltse LL, Rocchio PD: Preoperative psychological tests as predictors of success of chemonucleolysis in the treatment of low-back syndrome. *J Bone Joint Surg [Am]* 1975; 57:478–483.

48

Individual/Group Psychological Treatment for Chronic Back Pain

David T. Hanks, Ph.D.

There is no question that chronic back pain is a persistent, prevalent problem that costs our federal and state governments as well as insurance companies millions of dollars each year. Unfortunately, a sizable number of people who have chronic back pain do not become significantly improved. Many assume a role of permanent disability. Making matters worse, the etiology of chronic back pain is not well understood.

In 1965, Melzack and Wall published a novel theory of pain that expanded the traditional somatosensory model to include psychological factors.[16] Their multimodal theory essentially proposed that the pain experience results from an interaction of physiologic mechanisms with psychological mechanisms, such as the sensory discriminative, affective, motivational, and cognitive evaluative systems of the individual. This conceptualization of pain moved us from understanding the phenomena of pain as a purely physiologic event to include the person's experience of pain. With rising acceptance of this model over the ensuing years, multidisciplinary treatment approaches have been developed to more comprehensively address the complexities of treating the person with chronic pain. Today, multidisciplinary treatment approaches are well accepted.

A cure of chronic back pain is rare. The focus of most treatment is consequently to improve the patient's functioning and experience of pain in spite of the persistence of pain. Moreover, problems such as depression, anxiety, anger, and fear often develop as a result of persistent pain. Fortunately, these issues can improve even though the pain per se does not. The same is generally true with physical function. Individuals who have experienced pre-existent psychological problems and injure their backs frequently report exacerbations of their emotional distress. Consequently, psychological factors are generally viewed as important to the contribution, development, maintenance, and exacerbation of the pain experience. Psychological intervention has likewise become an accepted and necessary part of its treatment.

It is the purpose of this chapter to provide a basic overview of current psychological approaches in treating the person with chronic back pain and to briefly review what is known about psychological treatment effectiveness.

PSYCHOLOGICAL MODELS

Psychoanalytic Approaches

Freud and his followers were some of the earliest writers to propose a link between psychological variables and pain.[9] Physical problems such as pain that could not be attributed to known organic findings were thought to have resulted from an unconscious conflict between forbidden wishes, or desires, and their anticipated consequences. The conflict could become converted into a physical form such as pain and thereby serve as an unconscious symbolic solution to the conflict. Defenses of repression and denial would often maintain the physical solution and prevent the individual from becoming consciously aware of the actual source of the problem, i.e., the underlying conflict. Once the conflict was resolved, the need for a physical solution would diminish and thus result in eventual elimination of the physical symptom. So the theory goes.

More recent psychoanalytic authors have proposed that pain patients are avoidant and have fantasies of running away from stressful situations,[10] are plagued with aggressive urges whose inhibition results in muscular tension and pain,[1] and that they use pain to balance feelings of anger and subsequent guilt. Moreover, pain patients are often viewed by these theorists as having needs to suffer and be punished with concomitant difficulties accepting success.[5] Finally, Blumer and Heilbronn consider pain to be an essential variant of an underlying depressive disorder.[3]

As mentioned, the psychoanalytic conceptualization regarding the treatment of pain must therefore address the underlying conflicts and presumed depression in order for improvement to occur. Unfortunately, the research evidence used to support these theories and treatment models has been largely anecdotal or so poorly designed and controlled from a research perspective that any number of competing hypotheses could account for the reported findings.[20] Ironically, many physicians continue to believe in the concept of psychogenic pain based on these psychoanalytic theories. This may be particularly so when organic findings are considered insufficient to account for the reported degree of pain.

Operant Approaches

Fordyce and his colleagues ushered in a new era in the treatment of people with chronic back pain that was developed from theories grounded in learning research.[8] Moreover, the behaviorist's values for empiricism, quantification, and greater scientific scrutiny have lent more credibility to these theories.

Treating the person with chronic back pain, according to the operant model, relies on the analysis and systematic manipulation of purported external reinforcers of pain behaviors with the goal of reducing or extinguishing the targeted pain behavior. Medication consumption, complaining, grimacing, guarding, physical activity or a lack of it, etc., are all considered pain behaviors and subject to modification. Attention from significant others, social activity, rest, etc., are classified as reinforcers and are often utilized to increase the frequency of well behaviors and decrease the occurrence of pain behaviors. Because controlling external contingencies is such a critical component to this approach, much of this kind of work has been carried out in hospital settings.

As might be imagined, an extensive amount of research has been conducted on both operant theory and treatment. Space limitations prevent a comprehensive review of these data, but the reader is referred to excellent articles by Turk and Flor[20] and Keefe and Bradley,[11] for this material. Likewise, experimental design and statistical problems aside, it is generally held that the operant approach is more effective than no treatment or attention control conditions for some patients with chronic back pain.[20] However, it is not well known which kinds of patients are best suited for an operant approach. Further, since most operant-based treatment occurs within a multidisciplinary program context, it is not known which of the operant components account for the majority of positive changes measured.

Generalization and maintenance of change remains questionable as well over the long term, even though most patients studied are significantly better in the targeted behaviors at the conclusion of treatment. In an effort to increase generalizability, spouses and/or significant others have been included in the treatment and trained to respond to the pain behaviors in a manner consistent with staff. However, as Block noted, the value of including others in the treatment has yet to be demonstrated, although it is clear that their reactions to the patient with pain are highly important.[2] Nonetheless, Fordyce and his followers are to be credited with making the study and treatment of pain more objective and in promoting the use of straightforward behavioral techniques in helping patients with chronic back pain.

COGNITIVE BEHAVIORISM

Cognitive behaviorists differ from the traditional, often labeled radical behaviorists in their acceptance of thought and feelings as behavior that can be modified and lead to changes in overt behavior. Further, this type of conceptualization of behavior seems more encompassing of what we normally consider as the experience of pain and allows the clinician more possible areas of intervention. It should also be noted that the cognitive behavioral model is an interactive model whereby change in one particular dimension of behavior is believed to result in a change in other dimensions of behavior. As a result, cognitive behaviorists attempt to help people modify useless thoughts and feelings as well as overt behaviors in an effort to more comprehensively change a person's experience of pain.

For example, many patients with chronic pain experience depression and a profound sense of helplessness and hopelessness. Thoughts, feelings, and behaviors as they relate to these symptoms can be altered with education, information, analysis and change of inappropriate cognitions, allowance for grieving the physical losses associated with pain, and a variety of skills and management techniques for stress, relaxation, and pain.

The cognitive behavioral group has also spawned a significant amount of research. Turk and Flor,[20] Keefe and Bradley,[11] and Tan[19] generally report significant improvements in the measured areas in patients treated with the cognitive behavior therapy methods over no treatment and attention/expectancy controls. Turk and Flor also suggest a cost advantage to the cognitive behavioral model over the operant model because this technology can be implemented in group and outpatient settings.[20]

More recently, research has been undertaken by Fernandez and Turk[6] and Keefe et al.[12] to further refine our understanding of the specific contribution of certain cognitive coping strategies to changing pain experience. This is a logical next step in identifying necessary and sufficient factors of change inasmuch as the cognitive behavioral techniques are generally held to be useful. These authors have essentially agreed and concluded that cognitive coping strategies such as distraction, external focus of attention, imagery, reframing, etc., can affect the perception and experience of pain as compared with control conditions. Although no specific strategy has been found to be superior, the imagery techniques are generally noted to be more effective. Unfortunately, the majority of studies reviewed in this area have involved acute pain manipulated in laboratory settings, which certainly limits generalizability to the usual patient seen in chronic pain programs.

SYSTEMS THEORY

Although no writings could be found that specifically relate this set of theories to chronic back pain, several authors have discussed physical health issues. Minuchin et al., in particular, have extensively studied patients with anorexia nervosa and bulimia.[17] Patients with these difficulties often live in families that can be described as exhibiting significant degrees of enmeshment, overprotection, role rigidity, and lack of effective conflict resolution. The systems theory holds that symptoms often develop in response to family organizational imbalances such as hierarchical confusion and blurring of role boundaries. Symptoms also often serve the function of rebalancing the family organization (homeostasis) and stabilizing roles and interactions, but now around the symptom. As such, a physical health problem can coincidentally occur in a family whose organization is as described above and later serve as a purpose to continue the enmeshment, rigidity, and overprotection that may have originally developed for other reasons. Likewise, symptom change would not likely occur until the presumed underlying organizational dysfunction is addressed and the family interactions are reorganized in more adaptive ways.

Fisch et al. disagree that symptoms serve a particular function for a family but instead believe that a symptom may develop for one particular reason and become maintained essentially by the attempted solutions utilized to resolve the original problem.[7] When an attempted solution fails to achieve a desired result, people most often will continue with basically "more of the same" class of attempted solutions, thereby further crystallizing the problem. Change can therefore only occur when novel solutions are used that result in different interactions around the old problem. Repetitious and multiple medical procedures for chronic back pain, for example, may well fit this type of problem description.

More recently, DeShazer has developed a model of brief solution-focused treatment as opposed to the brief problem-focused treatment of Fisch et al.,[7] among others. Essentially, therapy in this regard begins by examining and highlighting exceptions to general rules and having the person continue to do those things that are more likely to bring about improvement. If walking or the use of cognitive distraction, for example, helps attenuate the experience of pain, then homework assignments follow in this direction. Observation and identification of other variables that help to continue improvement pursue this same line of intervention in subsequent treatment sessions.

Unfortunately, no research based on these assumptions could be found for chronic pain. One problem in subjecting the systemic theories to traditional inquiry is the underlying assumption of circular causality, which does not lend itself well to investigation by the traditional scientific method. The scientific method is a linear model. In fact, a number of the systemic theorists have gone so far as to propose that we reject the traditional scientific model all together because it in itself is merely an illusion of truth and contributes to the myth that truth can be discovered by a method that essentially does not fit experienced reality.

ECLECTIC

A number of multidisciplinary treatment programs fall into this category since they often blend techniques from a wide variety of theoretical sources. Most often, core treatment ingredients will include such things as exercise or physical therapy; operant conditioning in terms of staff withdrawal of attention toward pain behaviors and the reinforcement of well behaviors; cognitive strategies to challenge maladaptive thoughts; self-control techniques such as relaxation, self-hypnosis, stress management, biofeedback, and assertiveness training; medication management; education; group and individual treatments ranging from supportive techniques to uncovering and historical approaches; goal setting; and measurement. Research into the efficacy of multicomponent treatments has generally provided support for their being effective in terms of improving function in a variety of areas.[2, 11, 13, 20] Enthusiastic endorsement for this kind of treatment approach, however, is qualified by similar design and statistical objections generally true of most research in this field, e.g., a lack of adequate control groups, heterogeneity of samples, nonsimilar methods of measurement, lack of standardization, etc. Moreover, while significant improvements may indeed be obtained, at the conclusion of treatment as many as one third of patients apparently fail to maintain gains at long-term follow-up.[14, 17, 18, 20]

WHAT DO WE KNOW?

From the foregoing, research and methodologic flaws aside, it seems that general support can be found for the statement that a variety of psychological techniques do indeed help many persons with chronic back pain improve their mental and physical functioning. Multimodel treatments, particularly those that include behavioral-based treatment interventions, continue to receive support for their efficacy. Likewise, multimodel or multicomponent treatment programs appear to fare better than do single-treatment programs. To date, no single-treatment component has been shown to be superior to another single-treatment component. Some kind of treatment is generally believed to be better than no treatment at all. Most patients are better in measured targeted behaviors at the conclusion of treatment. Likewise, most treatment components emphasize with equal importance exercise, increased functional ability, increased cognitive and behavioral skills, improved ability to relax, work with family, and education and skills practice. Unfortunately, many patients appear to lose the gains achieved at the end of treatment as time passes. Follow-up is a relatively ill-defined domain and often not given attention in a number of treatment programs. Although we do not know which treatments work best with which kinds of patients or in what contexts, it seems reasonable to assume that many patients at the completion of treatment can do more in spite of feeling lousy.

Once patients leave treatment, it seems clear that something needs to occur to help them maintain their gains. Along these lines, a national organization has developed to provide a support and informational network for people with chronic back pain. One study conducted by Mayer and Gatchel seems to support the value of follow-up.[15] Their results suggested that patients could indeed maintain gains across longer follow-up periods when a core part of the treatment also included a follow-up program. Intuitively, structured follow-up is an appealing idea. Most people admittedly tire of "a program for life," and periodic reinforcement of skills through "booster sessions" may help curtail the relapse phenomenon. Also appealing is the notion that help after treatment falls to those who know the problems better that anyone, other patients with chronic pain. Thus, structuring follow-up to include participation in a group and meeting away from the medical setting may help.

Certainly, these tentative conclusions and hypotheses give those of us in the field of treating people with chronic back pain reason to continue. I would also like to make the point that theoretical developments over the course of years have essentially allowed us to return to respecting the importance of the patient's experience with pain and also to finding as many ways as possible to affect this experience from a variety of vantage points. As is often true in the field of psychotherapy in general, a relationship with a person who cares and is willing to help seems critical. It may not be that the particular techniques delivered, in terms of attempting to intervene in altering the experience of pain, are so important as that someone is willing to assist the person with pain in finding alternate ways to manage and cope with the experience. In reality, having persistent pain can be a difficult problem to deal with. Often these people feel alone and without resources to cope. They are fellow human beings who, for the most part, respond to this type of problem much like the rest of us. We can all probably recall working on a difficult problem with the assistance of someone who accepts our experience. Even though the problem was not completely resolved, that caring person's efforts gave us hope and helped us to renew our motivation and belief in ourselves. Certainly, using any variety of techniques cannot help but be augmented by respecting the person who has the problems, respecting the value of his experience, and assisting with finding as many ways as possible to live fully in spite of chronic pain. After all, living with a disability is as much "attitude" as anything else.

REFERENCES

1. Alexander F: *Psychosomatic Medicine*. New York, WW Norton, 1950.
2. Block A: Multidisciplinary treatment of chronic low back pain: A review. *Rehabil Psychol* 1982; 27:51–63.
3. Blumer D, Heilbronn M: Chronic pain as a variant of depressive disease. The pain prone disorder. *J Nerv Ment Dis* 1982; 170:381–406.
4. DeShazer S: *Keys to Solutions in Brief Therapy*. New York, WW Norton, 1985.
5. Engel G: Psychogenic pain and the pain-prone patient. *Am J Med* 1959; 26:899–918.
6. Fernandez E, Turk D: The utility of cognitive coping strategies for altering pain perception: A meta-analysis. *Pain* 1989; 38:123–135.
7. Fisch R, Weakland J, Segal L: *The Tactics of Change*. San Francisco, Josey-Bass, 1985.
8. Fordyce WE, Fowler E, Lehmann J, et al: Operant conditioning in the treatment of chronic pain. *Arch Phys Med Rehabil* 1973; 54:399–408.
9. Freud S: Fragment of an analysis of a case of hysteria, in *Standard Edition of the Complete Words of Sigmund Freud*, vol 7. London, Hogarth Press, 1953.
10. Grace WJ, Graham DT: Relationship of specific attitudes and emotions to certain bodily diseases. *Psychosom Med* 1952; 14:243–251.
11. Keefe FJ, Bradley L: Behavioral and psychological approaches to the assessment and treatment of chronic pain. *Gen Hosp Psychiatry* 1984; 6:49–54.
12. Keefe FJ, Crisson J, Urban B, et al: Analyzing chronic low back pain: The relative contribution of pain coping strategies. *Pain* 1990; 40:293–301.
13. Linton SJ: A critical review of behavioral treatments for chronic benign pain other than headaches. *Br J Clin Psychol* 1982; 21:321–337.
14. Maruta T, Swanson D, McHardy M: Three year follow-up of patients with chronic pain who were treated in a multidisciplinary pain management center. *Pain* 1990; 41:47–53.
15. Mayer TG, Gatchel R: *Functional Restoration of Spinal Disorders: The Sports Medicine Approach*. Philadelphia, Lea & Febiger, 1988.
16. Melzack R, Wall PD: Pain mechanism: A new theory. *Science* 1965; 150:971–979.
17. Minuchin S, Baker L, Rosman B, et al: A conceptualiza-

tion model of psychosometric illness in children. *Arch Gen Psychiatry* 1975; 32:1031–1038.

18. Stith WJ, Ohnmeiss DD, Carranza CB, et al: Rehabilitation of patients with chronic low back pain. *Spine State Art Rev* 1989; 3:125–138.
19. Tan SY: Cognitive and cognitive behavioral methods for pain control: A selective review. *Pain* 1982; 12:201–228.
20. Turk D, Flor H: Etiological theories and treatments for chronic back pain. II. Psychological models and interventions. *Pain* 1984; 19:209–233.

PART XVI

CHIROPRACTIC REHABILITATION OF THE SPINE

49

Chiropractic Rehabilitation

John J. Triano, M.A., D.C.

UTILIZATION AND SOCIAL IMPACT OF CHIROPRACTIC SERVICES

The magnitude of the socioeconomic problem caused by spine-related disorders has been well described.[16] In spite of a heavy emphasis on both clinical and fundamental research over the past 30 years, the overall lifetime prevalence of back pain continues unabated.[20] For the United States, the number of persons disabled by back pain has increased 14 times faster than the growth rate of the population.[41, 42]

Chiropractic health care delivery for spine pain has ranked third in patient utilization after the family physician and the orthopedist[17] for severe back pain. Short-term benefits of treatment using manipulation in the conservative management of painful episodes has been evident in a number of studies reviewed elsewhere.[58] Recent reports by Wolk,[67] Hadler et al.,[19] and Meade et al.[39] imply that early aggressive intervention with the high-velocity, low-amplitude manipulation used by chiropractors may have improved outcomes evident as late as 2 years after the cessation of treatment. A similar consequence has been noted for surgical interventions that have been studied.[13, 30, 64]

The rate for using services provided by chiropractic physicians from 1974 to 1982 was 7.5%.[50] Generalized to North America alone, an estimated 18 million patients per year are seen by chiropractors. With the possible exception that a higher percentage of chiropractic users are between 18 and 50 years of age,[50] they represent a typical cross section of the adult population.[44] Chief complaints for which services commonly are requested involve all of the musculoskeletal system[11] (Tables 49–1 and 49–2).

While only about 4% fail to return to their preinjury status after 6 months, these patients are responsible for the majority of back-related health care costs. The preponderance of evidence from studies of medication, manipulation, back school, and physical therapy shows that when any of these conservative treatments cease, the natural course of ongoing disability reasserts itself for these cases.[20] Clearly, new treatment options are needed in order to improve upon these long-range clinical outcome statistics.

A brief review of the available information on clinical outcome experience from using manipulative treatment may help convey the context from which chiropractic rehabilitation practice has developed. Descriptive studies on the frequency and duration of treatment for spine disorders under management with manipulative procedures have been carried out. The clinical characteristics of these patients are essentially the same as for those who seek nonmanipulative care.[44, 66] If the severity of injury is similar for a population of patients, the natural history and course of the condition can be expected to be the same. In a prospective study, 241 consecutive cases were classified as entrapment or mechanical or muscular complaints. Resolution or stabilization with significant improvement of symptoms was attained in 89.6% within 6 weeks of commencing intervention.[55] A maximum of 22 treatment sessions was required. Reporting on 3943 cases, Phillips and Butler[45] found a mean of 12.5 (±13.1) treatments. Separately, Phillips[43] reported a mean of 9.02 treatments for 871 people with spine-related complaints. Patients fit all categories from acute to subacute to chronic. Symptoms had been present for less than 30 days in 57%, 60 to 180 days in 11%, and longer than 180 days in 22%. The mean length of case management was 11.4 days. Twenty-four percent of patients attended for a week or less, while 56% received care for up to 30 days. One hundred three cases[18] of lumbosacral pain were treated by using up to four sessions of manipulation and were followed from 1 to 3 years. Recurrence of symptoms appeared in only 11.7% during that time.

Wolk[67] studied 17,198 worker's compensation claims for diagnosis-related group (DRG) code no. 243. Comparisons of total cost including all prescribed outpatient and physician-performed procedures and the duration of care were made. Overall, a significantly higher frequency of treatment was noted for the chiropractic providers using manipulative procedures at a lower total cost[67] than for other methods. Manipulative services on work-related back disorders averaged 29 office-based procedures per patient. The average temporary total disability period under chiropractic management was 39 days as contrasted with 58 days for other approaches. Conclusions from the study suggest that a more aggressive in-office intervention early

TABLE 49–1.
Distribution of Complaints Seen by Chiropractors

Region	% of Cases
Low back and pelvis	44.6
Thorax	7.8
Neck	19.8
Extremities	11.0
Other	16.8
Total	100.0

TABLE 49–2.
Chronicity of Patients Treated by Chiropractors Using Definitions From the Quebec Study (1987)[16,29]

Chronicity	% of Cases
Acute	26.5
Subacute	19.2
Chronic	35.4
Recurrent	18.9
Total	100.0

in the course of treatment may ultimately result in reducing the frequency of disabling injury and the necessity for more extensive inpatient procedures. Thus the main focus of practice for most chiropractors continues to rely upon the traditional manual methods of passive care. However, for the smaller percentage of sufferers who fail to respond as expected, other methods must be available.

The chiropractic profession has responded to this need in managing patients at risk for becoming chronic. Advanced understanding of the progression of acute pain to chronic[43] deconditioning syndromes,[32] illness behavior,[52] and the risk of physician dependence has resulted in more providers actively specializing in preventive and rehabilitative practice. The Chiropractic Rehabilitation Certification Board and the Chiropractic Rehabilitation Association are among those organizations developing guidelines for ethical and sound practices.

Rehabilitation centers supplying secondary care are becoming increasingly common. Their primary purpose is to provide a vehicle for successful transition of patient care from relying upon passive treatment interventions to active patient participation. The factors that enter into consideration of appropriateness include (1) duration of the painful episode, (2) the number of previous episodes, (3) response to acute intervention, (4) anticipated future physical activity, (5) patient motivation, and (6) training of the physician and staff. Once therapeutic necessity has been determined, success of the rehabilitation plan will be determined primarily by the latter three elements.

STAGES OF TREATMENT AND NATURAL HISTORY

Therapeutic intervention should be aimed at achieving specific objectives. The development of treatment goals may require some compromise between what the attending physician believes can be realized and the expectations or desires of the patient.[53] Traditionally, chiropractic intervention can be viewed as being divided into the general phases of primary acute care, rehabilitation, and maintenance care. Controversy has surrounded the later and has served to confound the understanding of chiropractic therapeutic goals. Maintenance strategies have arisen empirically and consist of long-range plans for the use of periodic passive treatments in one of two circumstances. In the experience of the attending physician, either the patient is susceptible to future impairment from recurrent subclinical spine lesions,[41] or repeated withdrawal of treatment has been associated with renewal of symptoms. The cost-benefit of maintenance, like other prophylactic therapy, has often been questioned and cannot be readily settled through standard clinical research methods.[15] As currently applied, maintenance care is either preventive or supportive in the scope of its objectives.[52] Its aims in prevention are to reduce the incidence and prevalence of impairment and to promote optimal performance. As a means of supportive care, the objective is to sustain previous therapeutic gains that, empirically, tend to otherwise progressively deteriorate if treatment is withdrawn. Maintenance is clearly inappropriate when it interferes with other appropriate primary care or when treatment risks outweigh the benefits.

Table 49–3 lists the conceptual progression for therapeutically necessary care and the general objectives of each. Often it is unnecessary to proceed beyond the primary-care phase. Moreover, an uncomplicated case should

TABLE 49–3.
Treatment Phases: Short-Term Goals

- Primary care
  - Acute care
    - Promote anatomic rest
    - Reduce muscle spasm
    - Reduce inflammation
    - Relieve pain
  - Remobilization
    - Expand pain-free motion
    - Minimize deconditioning
- Rehabilitation
  - Rehabilitation training
    - Improve strength/endurance
    - Increase physical capacity
  - Life-style adaptation/education
    - Train in spine mechanics
    - Temper psychological responses
    - Minimize work/environment risk of reinjury

reach complete resolution in advance of the time expected to reach the same point by natural history alone.

Primary Care

When the patient is exhibiting acute distress, efforts to reduce soft-tissue and joint stresses are made so that inflammation and swelling will diminish. A short term of reduced mobility that limits the joint-loading effects of gravity may be warranted. Passive forms of treatment, including manual and palliative procedures, are used with deference to the type of mechanical lesion present. Table 49–4 gives a partial listing of the therapeutic options available. Once pain and discomfort are controlled, the area is remobilized with low-speed, minimal-load exercises directed at improving flexibility without being mechanically stressful. As range of pain-free motion is improved, a gradual increase in exertion can be introduced. Finally, rehabilitation for strength and endurance can begin.

Reaching the rehabilitation phase as rapidly as possible and minimizing dependence upon passive forms of treatment will bring the best result. Prolonged limited activity is related to the risk of returning to the preinjury status. Often complete resolution of pain is not possible until the patient begins to focus on increasing the number and kind of activities in which he participates. Even then, some residual pain can be expected but may be offset by the benefits of increasingly productive function.

Clearly, the duration and intensity of in-office treatment for the uncomplicated case should not extend beyond the time frame observed in reports of the untreated course. As a set of minimal standards, attention to how the patient is progressing in comparison helps to set an upper boundary on the time a patient should be followed without modification of the treatment plan.

Each episode of back pain can be described as acute, subacute, chronic, or recurrent. Definitions for each category appear to be loosely based upon the duration of work absence and relative clinical improvements and are listed in Table 49–5. Recurrent episodes of back pain are not listed separately here since there is little justification for treating them in a fashion dissimilar from acute cases. On one fact there is agreement: of those who remain disabled from work more than 6 months, more than half will still be disabled at the end of a year.

TABLE 49–4.
Passive Treatment Options

High-velocity manipulation
Joint mobilization
Muscle "energy"
Soft-tissue massage
Stretching and flexibility exercises
Cryotherapy
Hydrotherapy
Electrotherapy
Transcutaneous electrical nerve stimulation (TENS)
Spray and stretch
Acupuncture
Other

TABLE 49–5.
Stages of Episode Time Course

Stage	Quebec Study[29] (1987)	Frymoyer[16] (1988)	Mayer & Gatchel[32] (1988)
Acute	0–7 days	0–6 wk	0–8 wk
Subacute	7 days–7 wk	6–12 wk	8–16 wk
Chronic	>7 wk	>12 wk	>16 wk

Whether the patient's pain is a first acute episode, a recurring pattern, or a flare from a chronic back, a substantial reduction in symptom severity should be expected within 10 to 14 days. An accompanying expansion in activities of daily living normally follows. The overriding concern is the focus upon the patient's rate of improvement in comparison to that predicted by natural history. Some variation can be expected from case to case due to reinjury, work habits, life-style, or psychosocial factors. A systematic interview that includes family members will often reveal influences competing with the treatment objectives. After correcting these factors, a trial therapy should be implemented again. Patients persisting without substantial improvement and who have no underlying complications warrant consideration for rehabilitation. Patients at risk for becoming chronic generally present common warning signs.[61] They include (1) stationary symptoms of somatic pain for 3 to 4 weeks, (2) functional impairment, (3) chemical dependency used recreationally or for pain control, and (4) emotional distress, including possible family disruption. The presence of these indicators should signal the physician to move quickly away from passive care as the primary emphasis of treatment.

Rehabilitation

Patient Assessment

The main features of assessment are the evaluation of patient motivation and physical capability and a screening for evidence of somatization or symptom amplification syndromes. Evaluation of the kind described here is necessary when a patient's response to appropriate acute care has been impaired. Where a patient is seeking to return to a materials handling or physically demanding job, it may also be helpful in determining the suitability of activity restrictions. A more comprehensive review of instruments available for use in patient assessment has been reported elsewhere[49, 57] and is beyond the scope of the present discussion. An application of this technology will be described.

The initial evaluation should generate a performance baseline and lead to the development of distinct, quantifiable objectives for the rehabilitation program to achieve. These objectives, however, should not be produced in isolation. Therapeutically necessary care should consciously strive to restore the preinjury status by contrasting the existing functional ability with the requirements of activity expected in the patient's personal life. That is, they must be job relevant. In principle, this amounts to estimating critical work-related demands and setting them as the therapeutic goal. While optimization of physical performance may be desirable, continuation of care past the treatment goal is considered elective care.

Patient Motivation and Illness Perception

Estimating the patient's motivation and screening for psychosocial factors that may be complicating recovery is accomplished through interviews that may include members of the family. A panel of questionnaires is available to quantify aspects of pain severity, activities of daily living, and illness behavior (Table 49–6). From a comparison of questionnaire instruments for validity, reliability, and responsiveness to clinical change, a series of self-reporting and physician-administered instruments are recommended that provide information useful in screening and treatment planning. They also offer advantage by being convenient and quickly administered.

The Oswestry questionnaire provides a simple means to quantify the perceived impact of the disorder on the patient's life-style. The Roland-Morris scale is administered shortly afterward as a means to test the sincerity of responses by posing similar questions about the same activities but with different phrasing. While the scores from each cannot be directly related to one another, consistency in the relative severity reported can be anticipated.[2] Significant disparity in responses are used as only one indicator suggesting that the examination and performance tests also should be inspected for evidence of internal inconsistency.

The Waddell chronic disability and illness behavior instruments[62,63] serve well to focus attention on any inappropriate reactions the patient may be using to express distress. The pain drawing diagram[46] is also used to give graphic representation of the location and intensity of pain. The clinical impression gained from this panel of tests is further verified during a regional examination by including tests for nonorganic signs.

Job Analysis

The job or activity analysis is an important part of an evaluation to guide the setting of treatment goals. A number of job evaluation methods are available that vary in complexity and comprehensiveness.[31] The task of activity analysis is to document the physical requirements, including the joint locations under stress and the relative intensity of the loads. Physical stress checklists provide a valid means of conducting either a direct survey or a recall history of job task or recreation physical factors. The United States Department of Labor has used such information to classify physical demands of jobs.[6] Two checklists are recommended that can be combined in simple questionnaire form for convenience. Common tasks (e.g., pressing, grasping, crouching, bending, lifting, etc.) are offered for the hands, arms, legs, feet, and trunk. The maximum and average frequency of occurrence along with the weights or forces encountered are then obtained.[23] It is also important to inquire about the body postures and the speeds that are used as the job tasks are performed.

Quantitative information from the activity analysis is used to compare with patient performance under close simulation of job tasks, where possible. If the job task cannot be adequately approximated, then normative data for regional joint function can be used,[36, 37] but with some loss in relevance.

Physical Performance

The ideal measure of performance would quantify activity during the conduct of the actual job task. Often this is not possible. As a result, a series of approximations are used that begin with isometric strength evaluations in postures simulating the job task. Standardized positions are added, and isolated regional function is assessed dynamically. Dynamic strength testing can be performed in a number of different ways (Table 49–7). Each method has advantages and disadvantages, and there is no clear evidence to indicate that one method is superior to another. The more important question, for the present, is whether test results are interpreted within the constraints specific to

TABLE 49–6.

Selected Instruments Validated for Quantifying Patient Perception of Pain and Activities of Daily Living

Outcome Variable	Instrument
Pain	Visual Analog Scale[4, 10]
	McGill Pain Score[60]
	Back Pain Scale[28]
Disability	Sickness Impact Profile[12]
	Roland-Morris Scale[19]
	Million Subjective Index[34, 40]
	Oswestry Disability Score[14]

TABLE 49–7.

Muscle Strength Testing Methods

Psychophysical
Isometric
Isotonic
Isokinetic
Isoinertial

each methodology. A detailed review of the application of each method is available elsewhere.[49, 57]

Psychophysical strength estimates[51] and isometric strength measures are the basis for work standards adopted by National Institute for Occupational Safety and Health (NIOSH)[7, 25] and have the largest base of normative data for various occupations. For that reason, they are the cornerstones from which other test measures are referenced.

The psychophysical procedure is the most versatile (Fig 49–1). Through its methods, the actual work-related exertions can be simulated very closely. Unfortunately, they are time-consuming and are often reserved for confirming studies where patient motivation is challenged. Isometric measures, performed by using sagittally symmetrical postures, may be successfully approximated up to 70% of materials handling tasks.[7] For injury to the lumbar spine, routine test procedures evaluate several postures (Fig 49–2). They include (1) the simulated work posture, (2) the whole-body lift strength using a knees-bent posture, (3) leg strength, and (4) upright-standing extensor and flexor trunk strengths (Fig 49–3). For complaints of the upper part of the body, NIOSH standard arm lift tests are added. Results from these tests are contrasted with the activities and demands drawn from the job analysis and again with normative data from a healthy population when it is available. Computerized biomechanical analysis may also be carried out to estimate joint compressive stresses. Jobs using rapid and significantly asymmetrical movements or tasks that are performed with high frequency must be considered carefully since isometric tasks will underestimate the stresses that arise in practice.[24]

Beyond a comparison to the job analysis, measures of absolute strength of a muscle group are probably not very

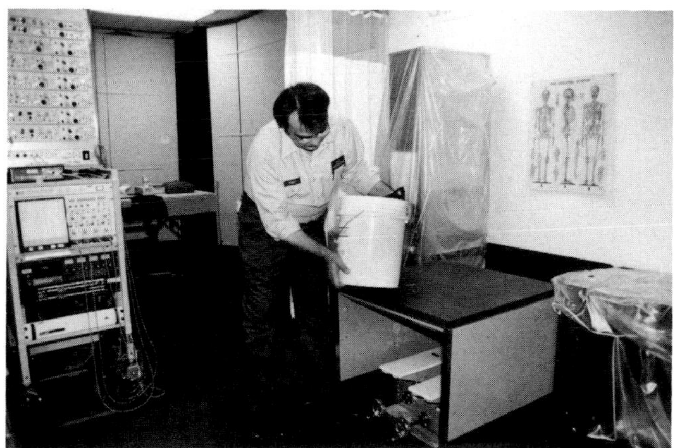

FIG 49–1.
Psychophysical testing simulates work task postures, loads, and speeds by using false-bottomed containers with weight limits set by the patient's perception of effort. (Courtesy of the National College of Chiropractic Clinics.)

important. However, the reciprocal ratio of strengths between agonist and antagonist muscle groups[1, 22, 56] is more useful. For isometric trunk strengths, the normal mean values are listed in Table 49–8. These relationships remain valid for slow-speed isokinetic measures.[3] These ratios fall when impairment is present[27, 33, 35, 38, 59]; however, a thorough analysis of discriminability for these measures has not been carried out.

Instrumented dynamic measures (Figs 49–4 and 49–5) serve to estimate function of the joint regions being tested. It is difficult to directly relate results to work tasks. However, comparisons to normative data are feasible. Moreover, if the activities to be carried out by the patient involve significant speed or asymmetry, relative reciprocal function at varying speeds can be tested.

Biomechanical Modeling

The accurate estimate of spinal stress is an invaluable aid to understanding the relative risk[21] for a given task because of its ability to estimate the compressive forces at the major musculoskeletal joints. The standards for risk to the spine from a lifting, lowering, pushing, or pulling job task are based upon information on the susceptibility of the lumbar vertebrae to compression.[7] Information from the model can be used both in planning therapy and as an interactive part of patient education.

The rudimentary information necessary to conduct a model analysis is available from the isometric strength evaluations. By obtaining a static photograph during the exertion, posture can be quantified and added to the exertional force measures to yield the data required as input to the computer model. Results are automatically contrasted to NIOSH healthy population data with respect to acceptable risk factors (Fig 49–6).

Therapeutic Goal Setting and the Job Stress Rating

Determining the appropriate treatment goals can be difficult. Long-term goals set the objective for performance when recovery has been reached. Short-term goals reflect desired improvement in individual skills that, together, will produce the long-term effects. The baseline performance determined from the various assessment methods described gives insight into the relative fitness of the patient to meet expected long-term activity demands. In principle, resolution of differences between the estimated fitness and the expected activity becomes the therapeutic goal for the rehabilitation program. Specific short-

TABLE 49–8.
Mean Trunk Strength Ratios

Extension/flexion	1.3
Side bending	1.0
Rotation	1.0

A

B

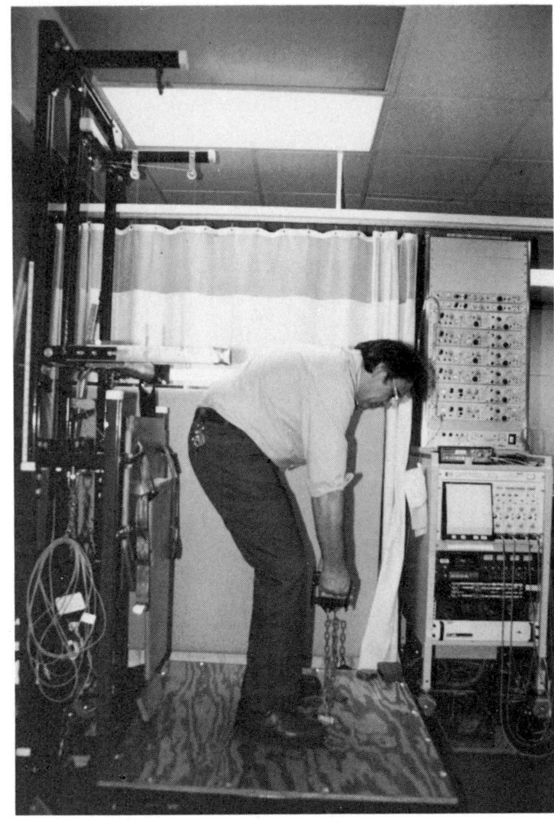

C

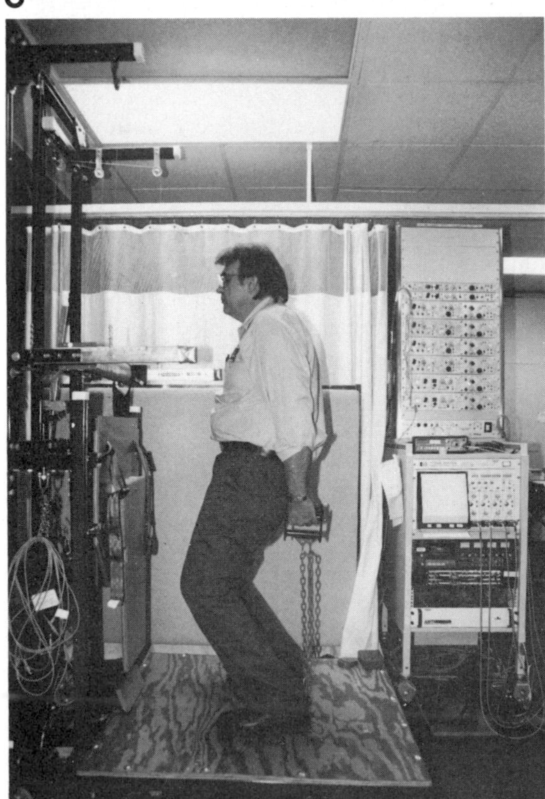

FIG 49–2.
Testing of whole-body lift capacity is performed by simulating the work environment **(A)** and in standardized postures **(B** and **C).** (Courtesy of the National College of Chiropractic Clinics.)

A

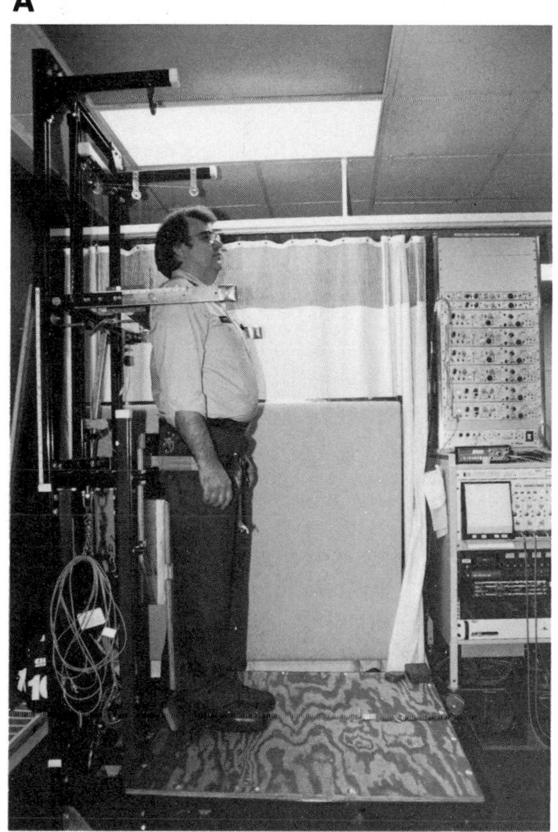

B

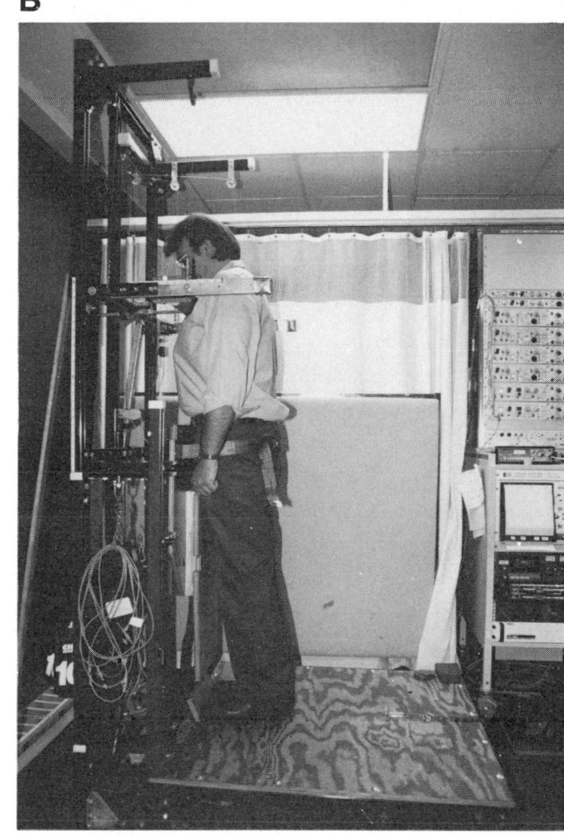

FIG 49–3.
Upright trunk isometric strengths in attempted flexion (**A**) and extension (**B**) exertions are used to quantify extensor/flexor reciprocal ratios. (Courtesy of the National College of Chiropractic Clinics.)

term goals addressing understanding of body biomechanics, flexibility, strength, comfort, and endurance should be specified.

The regional examination provides estimates of the flexibility needed to be gained. Biomechanical modeling assists in concepts and specific points to be included in educational programs as well as making recommendations on job site modifications that might be helpful. Reciprocal strength ratios, both isometric and dynamic, can focus strength training to specific muscle groups and identify directional limitations to be corrected.

A straightforward comparison of measured performance can be made with job task demands by establishing a ratio, the Job Stress Rating (JSR), between their quantitative descriptions.

$$\text{JSR} = \frac{\text{Job demand}}{\text{Performance}}$$

Normative data rather than individual measurements may also be used where appropriate.[26] The value of these numerical comparisons comes from the safety factor that is incorporated into interpretation of the result. For occasional exertions, a safe load would require up to 50% of the worker's isometric strength. Tasks arising frequently are considered safe at levels not to exceed 20% of capacity. The reserve strength preserved by the calculation accounts for observations that individuals operating at or near their maximum are likely to be injured.[5, 8] Once the performance limits of a patient are known, the JSR allows a quick determination of functional goals that can be used to guide rehabilitation therapy. For example, some airlines limit their reservation clerks to lifting baggage weighing up to 125 lb, a load that is likely to be encountered only occasionally. If after treatment for acute injury the maximum work-related lift test yields a sincere effort registering 142 lb, the JSR would be 0.88. Even for a healthy individual, repeated exertion at this level is likely to be risky. To achieve a desirable safe limit, the rehabilitation objectives should be set to achieve a work-related lift capability of 250 lb. Such a level of performance is readily met by using proper biomechanics of the legs and back to carry the load.

Therefore, through the use of quantified therapeutic goals and a written treatment plan, the patient is given an easily monitored program to follow. Goal setting itself is

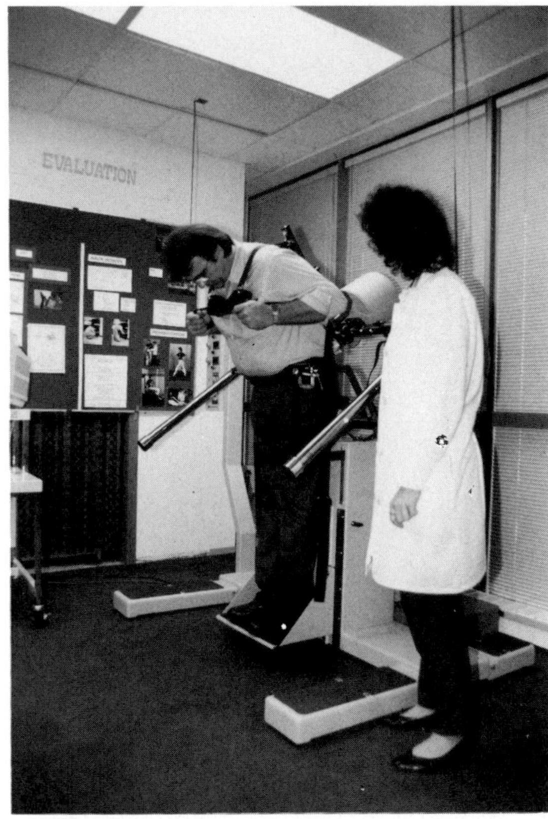

FIG 49–4.
Evaluation of isolated regional motion parameters including position, velocity, and torque. (Courtesy of the National College of Chiropractic Clinics.)

useful in dealing with the illness conviction[53] and pain-related behavior that many express. As gains are made toward treatment goals, a sense of confidence and improved self-image is supported.

TREATMENT PROTOCOLS

There are nearly as many preferences in exercise programs available as there are health care providers using them. What is more important, however, is the recognition that early return to activity[12] promotes recovery. Program design should balance its components based on the needs of the patient. Its elements should address (1) the dissuasion of pain-related behavior, (2) education on body biomechanics, and (3) supervised training for flexibility with stability, strength, and endurance. For patients already demonstrating signs of chronicity, this will require more than handing out a simple list of exercises to be performed at home.

Pain Behavior

Pain behavior and illness conviction are best managed with a conceptual shift in thinking about pain. The care giver must switch focus from inquiry and attention to the

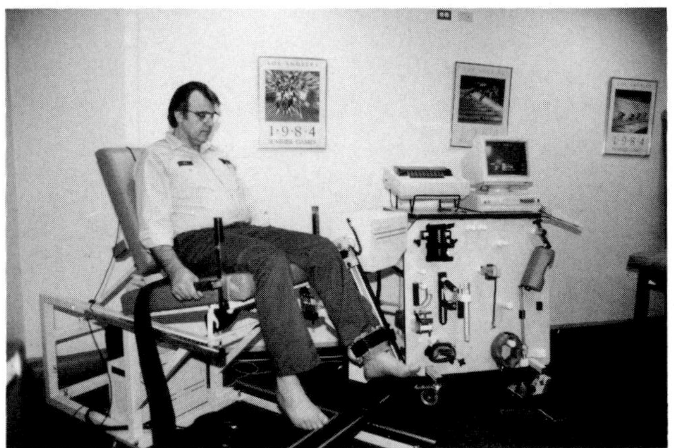

FIG 49–5.
Isolated extremity function evaluation. (Courtesy of the National College of Chiropractic Clinics.)

patient's level of discomfort to what the patient is able to do.[53] An understanding that movement is safe and helpful, even if not completely comfortable, needs to be emphasized. When psychosocial factors predominate in the assessment, referral for counseling should be made. However, lesser psychosocial effects arise from ongoing pain itself. Focusing upon rehabilitation as a means to improve the quality of life and to reduce suffering can result in a significant reduction in secondary somatization.

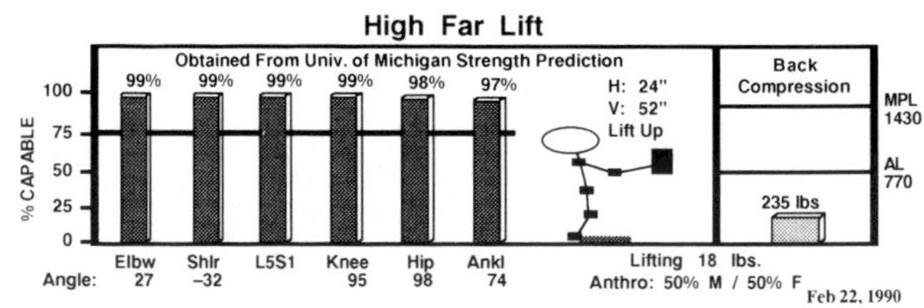

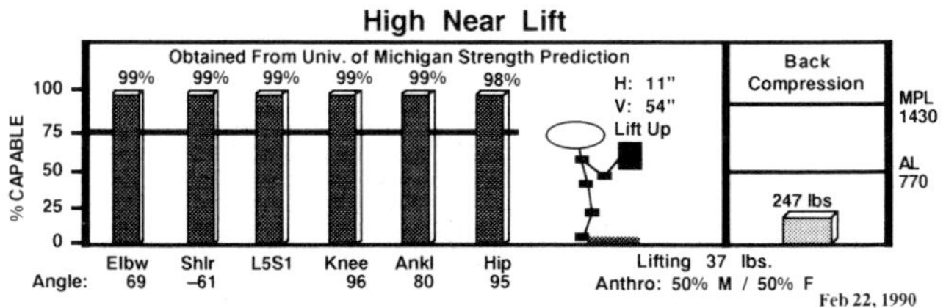

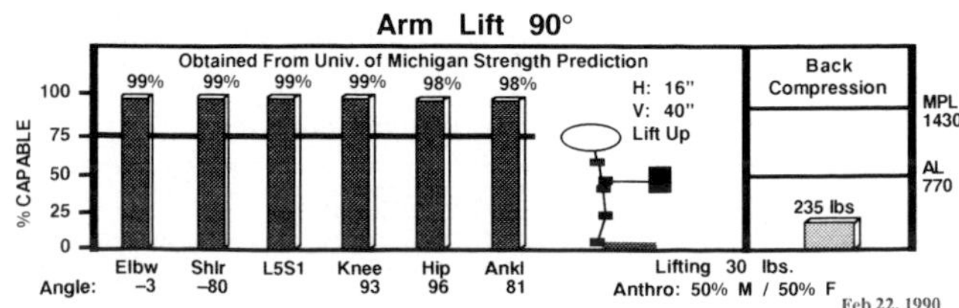

FIG 49–6.
Biomechanical modeling derived from measured posture and exertions during lift task evaluations. (Courtesy of Promatek Medical Systems, Inc.)

Patient Education

Educational instructions should be given to promote safe habits. The job and biomechanical analyses help steer topics toward specific activities and conditions in which the person is likely to find himself. However, a general explanation of function and stressors should be attempted with terms familiar to the patient. Topics to be included are the classic bending, lifting, pushing, and pulling movements; entry and exit from vehicles; sitting; yard work; recreation; personal care; and sexual activity.[54, 65] Emphasis should be placed on personalizing the activities commonly experienced by the patient.

Exercise Training

Flexibility and Stability

The long-term goal of rehabilitation is to restore the patient to preinjury function with reduced chances of recurring episodes. Repetitive microtrauma superimposed on a previous injury will lead to advanced degeneration.[47] Spinal stabilization is designed to teach trunk muscle recruitment in an effort to control and reduce flexion and torsional stresses on the joint segments. Through the use of voluntary muscles, pain-free regional postures are maintained while the patient carries out normal daily activities. The necessary posture and combination of muscle actions determined experimentally are specific for each case. Once a comfortable position is found, the patient is assisted in rehearsing progressively more complex tasks while keeping the spine in its neutral, pain-free position.

Strength and Endurance

Early during recovery stretching, within the pain-free range of motion, isometric exercises may be used to limit the effects of deconditioning.[6] Once the patient has successfully passed the remobilization phase of treatment, progressively increasing loads throughout the full range of motion is initiated. These may be accomplished through the use of free weights, weight stack machines (Fig 49–7), or the same computerized isokinetic or isoinertial machines that aid in the assessment of function (see Figs 49–4 and 49–5). The usual exercise training plan begins with direct supervision of assigned exercise tasks three to five times per week intermixed with rest periods when educational material can be given. A number of progressive-resistance protocols are available and are summarized by Christensen[9] as well as Saal and Saal.[48] The combination of multiple sets of repetitions with increasing or decreasing increments of weight results in benefits for both strength and endurance. The maximum exertion is increased weekly over a course of 4 to 12 weeks for the typical case. Computerized instruments may be used in an analogous fashion. They offer immediate feedback and may help maintain user interest; however, their use is not essential to a good clinical outcome.

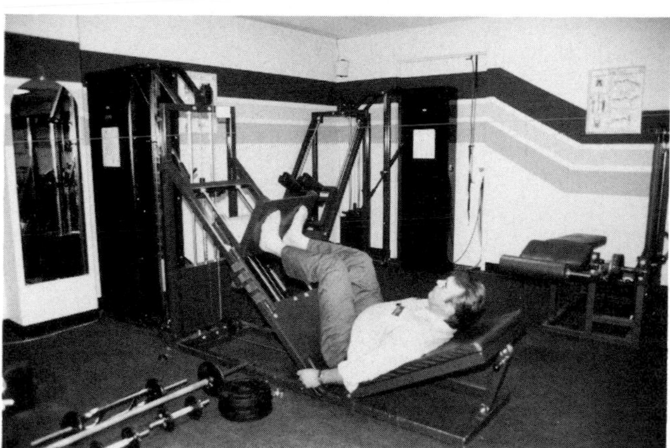

FIG 49–7.
Regional exercise training for strength and endurance of muscle groups involved in job-related critical tasks. (Courtesy of the National College of Chiropractic Clinics.)

Persons who fail to comply with the treatment schedule or who are insincere in their efforts should be discharged from care. The remaining patients are reassessed near the completion of the treatment plan to determine the outcome.

CONCLUSIONS

Rehabilitation practice is not a simple or uncomplicated process. Service that meets patient needs requires intense commitment of staff time and expertise to individualize assessment and rehabilitation protocols. The assessment scheme outlined here can be accomplished in one 2-hour session. The treatment regimen may last from 4 to 12 weeks depending upon the severity of impairment and the presence of complications. To be meaningful, treatment results must be linked to goals that are related to expected activities in which the patient will engage when recovered.

While a large segment of the population will experience spine-related complaints, only a small percentage will deteriorate sufficiently to require rehabilitation. Those who do are responsible for a significant cost in human suffering and health care expense. A gratifying aspect of engaging in a practice that focuses on these few patients comes from the improved quality of life and wider benefits that can be seen from even modest gains in patient performance.

REFERENCES

1. Baltzopoulus V, Brodie D: Isokinetic dynamometry applications and limitations. *Sports Med* 1988; 8:101–116.
2. Barlow D, Hayes S, Nelson R: *The Scientist Practitioner*. New York, Pergamon Press, 1984, pp 112, 124.
3. Beimborn D, Morrissey M: A review of the literature related to trunk muscle performance. *Spine* 1988; 13:655–662.

4. Bergquist-Ullman M: Acute low back pain in industry: A controlled prospective study with special reference to therapy and vocational factors. *Acta Orthop Scand Suppl* 1977; 170:1–117.
5. Cady LD, Bischoff DP, O'Connel ER, et al: Strength and fitness and subsequent back injuries in fire-fighters. *J Occup Med* 1979; 21:269–272.
6. Campbell MK: Rehabilitation of soft tissue injuries, in Hammer W (ed): *Functional Soft Tissue Examination and Treatment by Manual Methods*. Rockville, Md, Aspen, 1991, pp 277–291.
7. Chaffin D, Andersson G: *Occupational Biomechanics*. New York, John Wiley & Sons, 1984, p 246.
8. Chaffin DB, Park SK: A longitudinal study of low-back pain as associated with occupational weight lifting factors. *Am Ind Hyg Assoc J* 1973; 34:513–525.
9. Christensen KD: *Chiropractic Rehabilitation*. volume 1, *Protocols*. Ridgefield, Wash, Chiropractic Rehabilitation Association, 1991, p 45.
10. Coxhead CE, Inskip H, Meade TW, et al: Multicentre trial of physiotherapy in the management of sciatic symptoms. *Lancet* 1981; 1:1065–1068.
11. Cramer G, McGregor M, Triano J, et al: A feasibility study to conduct a randomized clinical trial in chiropractic—Part III: Ability to generalize. *J Manip Physiol Ther,* in press.
12. Deyo RA, Diehl AK, Rosenthal M: How many days of bed rest for acute low back pain? A randomized clinical trial. *N Engl J Med* 1986; 315:1064–1070.
13. Dvorak J, Velach L, Fuhrimann P, et al: The outcome of surgery for lumbar disc herniation. I. A 4–17 year's follow up with emphasis on somatic aspects. *Spine* 1988; 13:1418–1422.
14. Fairbanks JC, Davies JB, Mbaot JC, et al: The Oswestry low back pain disability questionnaire. *Physiotherapy* 1980; 66:271–274.
15. Feinstein AR: Problems, pitfalls and opportunities in long-term randomized trials. *Drug Res* 1989; 39:980–985.
16. Frymoyer J: Magnitude of the problem, in Weinstein J, Weisel S (eds): *The Lumbar Spine*. Philadelphia, WB Saunders, 1990, pp 32–38.
17. Frymoyer J, Pope M, Clements J: Risk factors in low-back pain. An epidemiological survey. *J Bone Joint Surg [Am]* 1983; 65:213–218.
18. Guifu C, Zonmin L, Zhenzhong Y, et al: Lateral rotary manipulative maneuver in the treatment of subluxation and synovial entrapment of lumbar facet joints. *J Tradit Chir Med* 1984; 4:211–212.
19. Hadler NM, Curtis P, Gillings B, et al: A benefit of spinal manipulation as adjunctive therapy for acute low-back pain: A stratified controlled trial. *Spine* 1987; 12:703–706.
20. Haldeman S: Presidential Address, North American Spine Society: Failure of the pathology model to predict back pain. *Spine* 1990; 15:718–724.
21. Keyserling W, Herrin G, Chafin D: Isometric strength testing as a means of controlling medical incidents on strenuous jobs. *J Occup Med* 1980; 22:332–336.
22. Kibler WB, Chandler TJ, Uhl T, et al: A musculoskeletal approach to the preparticipation physical examination. Preventing injury and improving performance. *Am J Sports Med* 1989; 17:525–531.
23. Koyl FF, Marsters-Hanson P: *Age, Physical Ability and Work Potential* (unpublished contract report). Washington, DC, Manpower Administration, U.S. Department of Labor, 1973.
24. Kroemer K: Testing individual capability to lift materials: Repeatability of a dynamic test compared with static testing. *J Safety Res* 1985; 16:1–7.
25. Kroemer K: *The Assessment of Human Strength, Safety in Manual Materials Handling*. National Institute for Occupational Safety and Health, DHEW Publication No. 78-185, 1978, pp 39–45.
26. Kvalseth TO: *Ergonomics of Workstation Design*. London, Butterworths, 1983.
27. Langrana N, Lee C, Alexander H, et al: Quantitative assessment of back strength using isokinetic testing. *Spine* 1984; 9:287–290.
28. Leavitt F, Garron DC, Whisler W, et al: A comparison of patients treated by chymopapain and laminectomy for low back pain using a multidimensional pain scale. *Clin Orthop* 1980; 46:136–143.
29. LeBlanc F: Scientific approach to the assessment and management of activity-related spinal disorders. *Spine* 1987; 12:16–21.
30. Lehmann T, Spratt K, Tozzi J, et al: Long-term follow-up of lower lumbar fusion patients. *Spine* 1987; 12:87–104.
31. Lytel RB, Botterbusch KF: *Physical Demands Job Analysis: A New Approach*. Materials Development Center, University of Wisconsin, Madison, 1981.
32. Mayer T, Gatchel R: *Functional Restoration for Spinal Disorders: A Sports Medicine Report*. Philadelphia, Lea & Febiger, 1988.
33. Mayer T, Gatchel RJ, Kishino N: A prospective short-term study of functional restoration in industrial low back pain injury. An objective assessment procedure. *JAMA* 1987; 258:1763–1767.
34. Mayer T, Gatchel RJ, Mayer H, et al: A prospective two year study of functional restoration in industrial low back pain injury. An objective assessment procedure. *JAMA* 1987; 258:1763–1767.
35. Mayer T, Smith S, Keeley J, et al: Quantification of lumbar function. Part 2: Sagittal plane trunk strength in chronic low-back pain patients. *Spine* 1985; 10:765–772.
36. Mayer TG: Using physical measurements to assess low back pain. *J Musculoskel Med* 1985; 2:44–59.
37. Mayer TG, Gatchel RJ, Kishino N, et al: Objective assessment of spine function following industrial injury. *Spine* 1985; 10:482–493.
38. McNeill T, Warwick D, Andersson G, et al: Trunk strengths in attempted flexion, extension, and lateral bending in healthy subjects and patients with low-back disorders. *Spine* 1980; 5:529–534.
39. Meade TW, Dyer S, Browne W, et al: Low back pain of mechanical origin: Randomized comparison of chiropractic and hospital outpatient treatment. *Br Med J* 1990; 300:1431–1437.

40. Million R, Hall W, Nilsen K, et al: Assessment of progress of the back pain patient. *Spine* 1982; 7:204–212.
41. National Center for Health Statistics: *Prevalence of Selected Impairments, United States, 1971*. Hyattsville, Md, DHHS Publication No. (PHS) 75-1526, Series 10, No. 99, 1975.
42. National Center for Health Statistics: *Prevalence of Selected Impairments, United States, 1981*. Hyattsville, Md, DHHS Publication No. (PHS) 87-1587, Series 10, No. 159, 1986.
43. Phillips R: A survey of Utah chiropractic patients. *J Am Chiropract Assoc* 1981; 15:113–128.
44. Phillips R: *Physician Selection in Low Back Pain Patients* (dissertation). Salt Lake City, University of Utah Department of Sociology, 1987.
45. Phillips R, Butler R: Survey of chiropractic in Dade County, Florida. *J Manip Physiol Ther* 1982; 5:83–89.
46. Rainsford AO, Cairns D, Mooney V: The pain drawing as an aid to the psychologic evaluation of patients with low back pain. *Spine* 1976; 1:127–132.
47. Saal JA, Saal JS: Rehabilitation of the patient, in White A, Anderson R (eds): *Conservative Care of Low Back Pain*. Baltimore, Williams & Wilkins, 1991, pp 25–29.
48. Saal JS, Saal JA: Strength training and flexibility, in White A, Anderson R (eds): *Conservative Care of Low Back Pain*. Baltimore, Williams & Wilkins, 1991, pp 65–77.
49. Sapega AA: Muscle performance evaluation in orthopedic practice. *J Bone Joint Surg [Am]* 1990; 72:1562–1574.
50. Shekelle P, Brook R: A community-based study of the use of chiropractic services. *Am J Public Health* 1981; 81:439–442.
51. Snook S: Psychophysiological indices—what people will do, in Drury C (ed): *Safety in Manual Materials Handling*. Buffalo, NY, National Institute for Occupational Safety and Health, DHEW Publication No 78-185, 1978, pp 63–67.
52. Sportelli L: American Chiropractic Association statement on maintenance care (letter). Arlington, Va, May 1990.
53. Sullivan MD, Turner JA, Romano J: Chronic pain in primary care identification and management of psychosocial factors. *J Fam Pract* 1991; 32:193–199.
54. Triano J, Cramer G: Patient information: Anatomy and biomechanics, in White A, Anderson R (eds): *Conservative Care of Low Back Pain*. Baltimore, Williams & Wilkins, 1991, pp 45–57.
55. Triano J, Hondras MA, McGregor M: Differences in treatment history for acute, subacute, chronic and recurrent spine pain. *J Manip Physiol Ther* 1992; 15:24–30.
56. Triano J, Schultz AB: Correlation of objective measure of trunk motion and muscle function with low-back disability ratings. *Spine* 1987; 12:561–565.
57. Triano J, Skogsberg D, Kowalski M: The use of instrumentation and laboratory procedures by the chiropractor, in Haldeman S (ed): *Modern Developments in the Principles and Practice of Chiropractic*. E Norwalk, Conn, Appleton-Lange, 1992.
58. Triano JJ, Hyde TE: Nonsurgical treatment of sports-related spine injuries: Manipulation, in Hochschuler S (ed): *The Spine in Sports*. Philadelphia, Hanley & Belfus, 1990, pp 246–255.
59. Thorstensson A, Arvidson A: Trunk muscle strength and low back pain. *Scand J Rehabil Med* 1982; 14:69–73.
60. Turner JA, Clancy S: Comparison of operant behavioral and cognitive behavioral group treatment for chronic low back pain. *J Consult Clin Psychol* 1988; 56:261–266.
61. Valfors B: Acute, subacute and chronic low back pain clinical symptoms, absenteeism and working environment. *Scand J Rehabil Med Suppl* 1985; 11:1–90.
62. Waddell G: A new clinical model for the treatment of low back pain. *Spine* 1984; 2:632–644.
63. Waddell G, Main CJ: Chronic low back pain, psychologic distress and illness behavior. *Spine* 1984; 9:209–213.
64. Wever H: Lumbar disc herniation: A controlled prospective study with ten years of observation. *Spine* 1983; 8:131–140.
65. White AW: *Back School and Other Conservative Approaches to Low Back Pain*. St Louis, Mosby–Year Book, 1983.
66. Wickes D: *Demographic Characteristics and Presenting Complaints of Initial Visit of Patients at Lombard Chiropractic Clinic*. Unpublished internal report, 1980.
67. Wolk S: *Chiropractic Versus Medical Care: A Cost Analysis of Disability and Treatment for Back-Related Workers' Compensation Cases*. Boston, American Public Health Association, Boston, 1988.

PART XVII

INDUSTRIAL MEDICINE OF THE SPINE

50

Epidemiology of Industrial Low Back Pain

Gunnar B.J. Andersson, M.D., Ph.D.

The epidemiology of low back pain (LBP) has attracted increasing interest over the last several years. The importance lies in the ability to predict the magnitude of the problem and the resultant demand on medical and other resources, as well as in determining the natural history of back problems and studying the association between LBP and individual, work-related, and other factors.

It must immediately be conceded that the epidemiology of back pain is, at best, approximate. This is because there is a lack of general agreement in diagnosis, because pain is difficult to study epidemiologically, and because there are often no objective signs of back pain. For that reason, it has been suggested that epidemiologic research be restricted to studies of sciatica or disc herniations where the definitions are more stable.[35] Another problem is that the data sources are of variable quality. The best sources, such as insurance and hospital data, are difficult to access and cover only part of the problem. For a more thorough discussion of these problems, refer to Wood and Badley,[78] Worrall and Appel,[79] and Andersson.[3] Other sources rely on questionnaires and interviews that have questionable validity and reliability. Further, the intermittent nature of back symptoms make cross-sectional prevalence studies difficult, and retrospective studies have problems in terms of recall.[13, 16, 69]

In studies of relationships between back pain and occupational risk factors, there is also a problem of measuring exposure. Further, the so-called healthy worker effect, which allows healthy workers to stay in the same occupation while workers with back pain have to leave the job and move to less demanding jobs, will influence the job-specific prevalence. Compensation issues enter into this as well since it is more likely for subjects to relate low back pain to an injury if this results in compensation.[40] It is also important to stress here that epidemiologic data does not prove causality and that all data must therefore be viewed with caution.[66]

The purpose of this chapter is to present current knowledge about the prevalence of LBP and sciatica and its relationship to individual and work factors. Emphasis will be on data from the United States.

PREVALENCE OF BACK PAIN INCLUDING SCIATICA

Prevalence is defined as the number of people in a given population who have back pain and/or sciatica at a particular time. The time period can be short (now or point prevalence) or longer and defined by the period of observation such as a 1-month prevalence. Prevalence can be determined by a single survey and is different from incidence, which is a measure of the number of people without back pain and/or sciatica who will develop such pain over a defined period. Incidence requires following a population over time.

Prevalence data in the United States stem primarily from the National Health and Nutrition Examination Surveys performed in 1970–1974 (NHANES I), and 1976–1980 (NHANES II) (Table 50–1). In NHANES I, the prevalence of self-reported symptoms was 17%, while 1% were estimated as having or having had a disc disorder.[22] The peak prevalence occurred in the 40- to 50-year-old age group. In NHANES II, the cumulative lifetime prevalence of LBP lasting for at least 2 weeks was 13.8%, while 1.6% reported that they had ongoing or previous sciatica.[26] The peak prevalence of LBP in NHANES II was in the 55- to 64-year-old age group, while the prevalence of sciatica peaked in the 45- to 54-year-old age interval (Fig 50–1). Eighty-four percent of those with LBP had consulted a health care professional, 30.9% had been admitted to a hospital because of back pain, and 11.6% had undergone surgery. The NHANES data, while interesting, are difficult to evaluate. The studies were not designed specifically with LBP in mind. The high percentage of hospital admissions and surgery among those with pain complaints indicate that a more severely affected subset of back pain sufferers was identified than has often been the case in other studies.

Data from different publications of the U.S. National Center for Health Survey indicate that back problems are the most frequent cause of activity limitations among people below the age of 45 years, that the rate of visits to physicians caused by LBP is second only to heart problems among chronic disorders, that back pain is the fifth most

TABLE 50–1.
Back Pain in the United States Based on NHANES I and II*

	NHANES I†	NHANES II
Study population	6913	27,801
Prevalence of back pain (%)	17.7	13.8
Disc disorder (%)	1	2.0

*Data from Cunningham LS, Kelsey JL: *Am J Public Health* 1984; 74:574–579; and Deyo RA, Tsui-Wu Y-J: *Spine* 1987; 12:264–268.
†NHANES = National Health and Nutrition Examination Survey.

frequent reason for hospitalization, and that it is the third ranking reason for surgical procedures.[3]

The U.S. data compare quite well with data obtained from national data bases in other countries. The only exceptions are the frequencies of hospitalizations and operations, which in the United States are greater. Swedish data indicate that 12.5% to 13.5% of all sickness absence has a back diagnosis.[34, 59] In 1987, 8% of the adult Swedish population was sick-listed, at some time, with a back diagnosis. Lee et al. report a 4.4% prevalence of "serious back and spine trouble" in Canada, a figure quite similar to that reported for chronic back pain in the United States, Sweden, and Finland.[54]

Cross-sectional studies confirm the national surveys and the insurance statistics. Frymoyer et al.[29, 30] reported a lifetime prevalence of 70% in Vermont, similar to that reported from Denmark,[13] Sweden,[68, 72] and the Netherlands.[75] In these studies, point prevalence rates vary from 12% to 35%, the difference reflecting primarily the way the information was obtained.

PREVALENCE OF OCCUPATIONAL LOW BACK PAIN

While the data reported above reflects the overall problem, the industrial problem is equally disturbing. In the United States it is estimated that about 2% of the working population have a compensable back injury each year and that the number of injuries exceed 400,000 annually, thus contributing about 1.5% of all workmen's compensation injuries. Most of these injuries are diagnosed as sprains and strains[51] with an average incidence of 0.75 sprains and strains per 100 workers in 1979. This incidence is quite variable geographically. Incidences as high as 4.2% have been reported from certain counties in Washington in 1985.[76] In Canada the yearly incidence of low back injury resulting in work absence was 1.4% in 1981,[1] while in England rates of 4.5% have been reported for cross-sectional studies covering a range of occupations.[2]

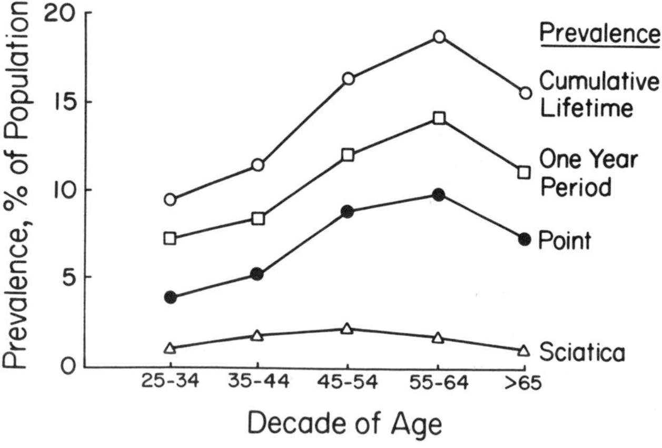

FIG 50–1.
Prevalence of low-back pain and sciatica episodes lasting for at least 2 weeks. (Adapted from Deyo RA, Tsui-Wu Y-J: *Spine* 1987; 12:264–268.)

PREVALENCE OF SCIATICA AND DISC HERNIATIONS

Sometimes sciatica is defined broadly as "pain in the leg," while others have specific requirements, some even requiring structural or operative confirmation. Clearly, this leads to significant differences between studies. The studies reported here were all carefully designed with clear definitions of sciatica. Kelsey and associates performed two case-control studies in Connecticut: one in the early seventies and one in 1979–1981.[39–48] An increased risk of disc herniations was found in workers with sedentary occupations, drivers of motor vehicles, and workers in jobs with heavy lifting and twisting. Other risk factors identified were smoking and a lack of physical exercise. Heliovaara et al. studied the prevalence of sciatica in a large Finnish population (Table 50–2).[35–37] Men were more frequently affected than women, and the prevalence rate was highest in the 45- to 64-year-old age group. Disability due to lumbar disc syndrome was present in 3.5% of men and 4.5% of women. The prevalence for true disc herniations was 1.9% for men and 1.3% for women.

Operations for disc herniations are more common in men than women.[37, 53, 64] Almost 97% are about equally distributed at the L4 and L5 levels (Fig 50–2). An increasing mean age at surgery is associated with an increasing

TABLE 50–2.
Prevalence of Lumbar Disc Syndrome (Sciatica) by Sex (Age Adjusted) in a Finnish Population (n = 8000)*

Diagnosis	Men (%)	Women (%)
Lumbar disc syndrome	5.3	3.8
Herniated nucleus pulposus		
Definite	1.9	1.3
Probable	0.2	0.2
Sciatica		
Definite	1.9	1.3
Probable	1.3	1.0

*Based on data from Heliovaara.[36]

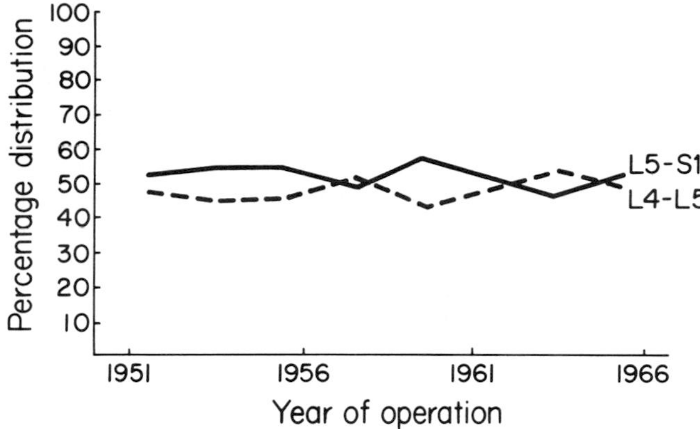

FIG 50-2.
The incidence of L4-5 and L5-S1 disc herniations over the review period. (Adapted from Spangfort EV: *Acta Orthop Scand Suppl* 1972; 142:1.)

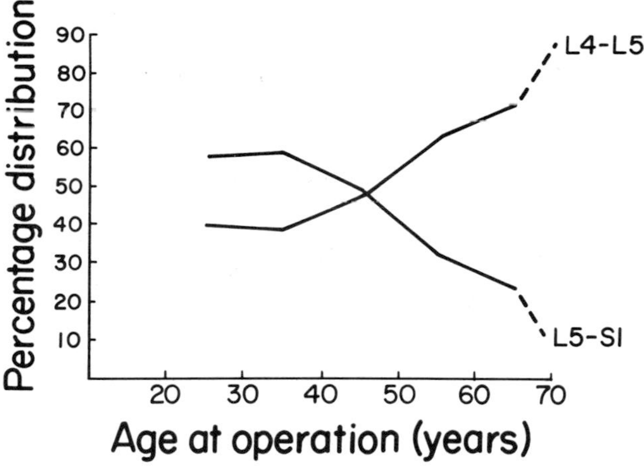

FIG 50-3.
The level of herniation by age at surgery (percent distribution). (Adapted from Spangfort EV: *Aeta Orthop Scand Suppl* 1972; 142:1.)

incidence of herniations in the cranial direction (Fig 50-3). The most frequent age at surgery is just over 40 years. Heliovaara et al. performed a case-control study in a sample of 57,000 Finnish women and men.[37] The relative risk was higher for men, motor vehicle drivers, metal workers, construction workers, nurses, and very tall subjects of both sexes (Table 50-3).

Overall, in the United States there are some 258,000 back operations performed annually, i.e., over 100 per million inhabitants. The number of people operated on for disc herniations has been variably estimated at 450 to 900 per million. The corresponding numbers are 100 for Great Britain, 200 for Sweden, and 350 for Finland.

TABLE 50-3.
Multivariate Relative Risk of Herniated Intervertebral Disc or Sciatica: Case-Control Studies*

Factors	RR of HNP†	RR of Sciatica (Including HNP)
Sex		
Women	1.0	1.0
Men	1.6	1.3
Occupation		
White collar	1.0	1.0
Men		
Motor vehicle drivers	2.9	4.6
Metal workers	3.0	4.2
Construction	2.4	3.1
Women		
Nurses	2.2	1.5
Housewives	0.4	0.8
Height		
Men (>180 cm)	2.3	
Women (>170 cm)	3.7	

*Based on data from Heliovaara.[36].
†RR = relative risk; HNP = herniated nucleus pulposus.

FACTORS INFLUENCING THE PREVALENCE OF LOW BACK PAIN AND SCIATICA

In the preceding section a number of occupations and individual factors have been mentioned that are associated with an increased prevalence of back pain. As discussed, these associations are difficult to establish, and therefore caution must be made in evaluating data. This is, of course, the case both for individual and occupational factors. Environmental factors have received comparatively little attention.

Occupational Factors

The seven most frequently discussed occupational factors are listed in Table 50-4. The six physical work factors have been experimentally associated with the development of injuries in spinal tissues. The seventh, "psychological and psychosocial work factors," is probably more related to back pain disability than to an actual back injury.

There is presently an enormous body of data implicating physically heavy work as increasing the risk of back pain, sciatica, and disc herniations. Most investigators are using sickness absence and injury reports as their sources

TABLE 50-4.
Occupational Factors Associated With an Increased Risk of Low Back Pain

Heavy physical work
Static work postures
Frequent bending and twisting
Lifting, pushing, and pulling
Repetitive work
Vibrations
Psychological and psychosocial factors

and thus reflect not only back pain but also disability caused by back pain, but some are based on questionnaires, interviews, and even disc hernia operations. Several countries report similar data. A few U.S. reports are discussed here.

Klein et al., using occupational safety and health data, found significantly higher rates of back sprain/strain among workers in heavy industries and workers with physically demanding occupations[51] (Tables 50–5 and 50–6). These data were confirmed by Frymoyer and Pope for the State of California.[28] Herrin et al. related injury rates to predicted spine compression forces in 55 industrial jobs.[38] Back pain was twice as common if the predicted disc compression was above 6800 newtons (1500 lb).

Static work postures include primarily long-term sitting, which appears to increase the risk of LBP[56] and in combination with driving increases the risk of disc herniation.[42, 46]

Frequent bending and twisting are usually associated with lifting when reported as causes of back injuries. Keyserling et al., however, found LBP to be associated with asymmetrical postures in a car assembly plant even when lifting was not performed.[49] Lifting is a well known triggering event for back pain.*

Repetitive work increases sickness absence in general. LBP is no exception in this respect. Unfortunately, it is unclear to what degree the physical component of work or the psychological stress of repetitive and often paced work is responsible.

LBP is more frequent in drivers than in controls, which implicates vibrations (perhaps in combination with the sitting posture). Kelsey and Hardy found truck drivers to have a fourfold increased risk of disc herniations, while simple car commuting increased the risk by a factor of 2.[46] Other studies indicate an increased risk of LBP with whole-body vibration.[19, 23, 30, 62] Heliovaara et al. found that the risk of being hospitalized for a herniated nucleus pulposus in Finland was particularly high for professional motor vehicle drivers.[37] Other studies of vehicle drivers have disclosed that radiographic changes occur over time.[27]

*References 12, 18, 30, 40, 51, 55, 56, 71.

TABLE 50–5.
1979 Ratios (Claims per 100 Workers) of Compensation Claims for Back Strains/Sprains in 26 States by Industry*

Industry	Claims per 100 Employees
Construction	1.6
Mining	1.5
Transportation	1.2
Manufacturing	1.0
Agriculture	0.9
Services	0.7
Wholesale/resale trade	0.6
Government (state and local)	0.2
Finance	0.2
Total	0.7

*Adapted from Klein BP, Jensen RC, Sanderson LM: *J Occup Med* 1984; 26:443–448.

TABLE 50–6.
1979 Ratios of Compensation Claims in 26 States Due to Strains/Sprains of the Back by Occupation*

Occupation	Claims per 100 Workers
Miscellaneous laborers	12.3
Garbage collectors	11.1
Warehousemen	9.3
Miscellaneous mechanics	5.6
Nursing aides	3.6
Nonspecific laborers	3.4
Material handlers	3.4
Lumbermen	3.3
Practical nurses	3.3
Construction laborers	2.8

*Adapted from Klein BP, Jensen RC, Sanderson LM: *J Occup Med* 1984; 26:443–448.

Psychological and psychosocial work factors have received increasing attention because of the effect on low back disability. Monotony has been identified as a risk factor for back pain,[12, 71] as has poor work satisfaction.[11, 57, 71] Bigos et al.[18] and Battie et al.[9] concluded that psychological work factors were more important than physical work factors as risk indicators of LBP.

Individual Factors

Eight individual factors have been particularly discussed in the context of LBP (Table 50–7). Of those eight, only age and sex have a major direct influence. LBP often begins early in life. Back pain in schoolchildren is more frequent than previously thought but is usually mild and short in duration. Balague et al. studied 1715 schoolchildren in a Swiss community.[5] Overall, 35% had a history of previous LBP, and the 1-week prevalence was

TABLE 50–7.
Individual Factors Often Discussed as Potential Risk Factors in Low Back Pain

Factor	Importance
Age	Certain
Sex	Probable (age dependent)
Posture	Low (severe only)
Anthropometry	Low (extremes only)
Muscle strength	Low (work related)
Physical fitness	Low (work related)
Spine mobility	Low
Smoking	Probable

16%. As many as 14% had actually sought medical advice at some time. Because serious conditions can be the cause of back pain in children, those few children with severe back pain require a careful diagnostic workup.

The highest prevalence rates for back pain in the adult population appear to be in the 35- to 55-year-old age span. Differences exist in this respect, however, depending on sex and type of injury. Women appear to have higher prevalence rates with advancing age,[15, 72] perhaps as a consequence of osteoporosis (Fig 50–4). Men, on the other hand, have a higher risk of sickness absence (disability) for work-related injuries when in their twenties.[51, 65]

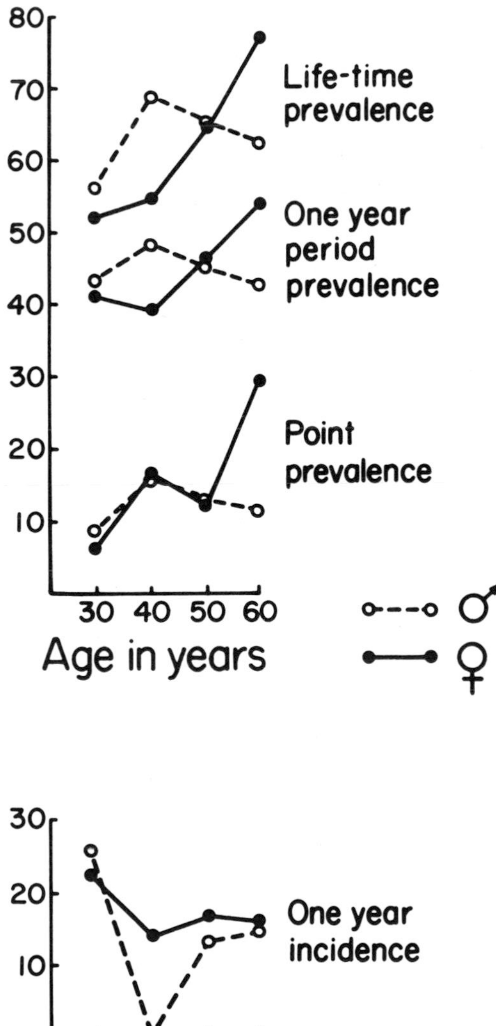

FIG 50–4.
Lifetime, 1-year period, and point prevalence of low back pain in a Danish community along with the 1-year incidence. (Adapted from Biering-Sorensen F: *Dan Med Bull* 1982; 29:289.)

Operations for disc herniations are most frequent in the early forties and about twice as common in men as in women.[36, 64] Overall, the prevalence rates of back pain for women and men are similar.

Postural deformities are of minor importance as risk factors for LBP and sciatica. Advanced scoliosis (exceeding 60 degrees) is associated with an increased risk,[52] while the more common, less advanced scoliotic deformities are not. Lordosis and kyphosis are probably without significance but occur frequently in patients suffering from back pain, perhaps because of muscular spasm. Leg length inequality has been found to be associated with back pain in a few studies,[31, 63] but the majority of investigations conclude that no association was present.[3]

There is no strong correlation among height, weight, body build, and LBP.[3, 14, 15, 42, 68, 72] Tallness has been found to be associated with back pain in some studies, as has severe obesity.[25] Battie, in a review of the literature, found that seven studies reported an association between LBP and tallness while eight did not.[6] Only Biering-Sorensen's[14] and Gyntelberg's[32] studies are prospective, the first finding no association while the second did. Heliovaara and Battie et al. both found a positive correlation between tallness and the risk of disc herniation.[7, 35]

Poor strength in abdominal and back muscles is a frequent observation in patients with back pain, particularly chronic pain. Most investigators believe that the strength loss is secondary, but there is some evidence that poor strength is a risk factor when job requirements are significant.[20, 49] Battie et al. did not find isometric strength as such to be a risk factor, i.e., without relation to job demands strength is probably not a risk factor.[7] This supports previous studies by Biering-Sorensen (1984).[14]

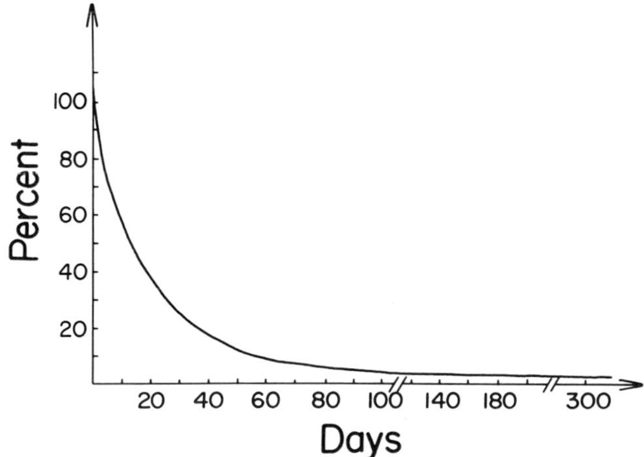

FIG 50–5.
The normal recovery curve following an acute low back episode. (Adapted from Andersson GBJ, Svensson HO, Oden A: *Spine* 1983; 8:880–884.)

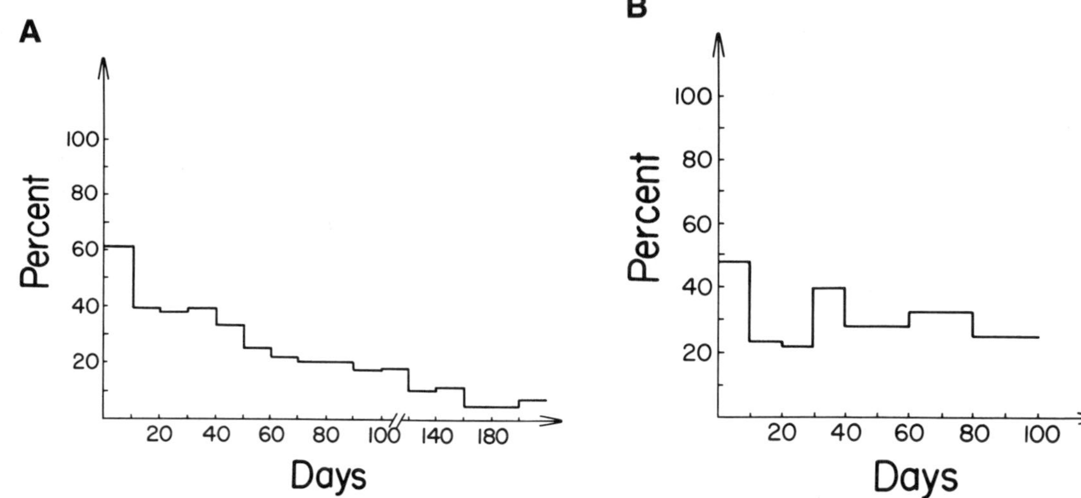

FIG 50–6.
A, the intensity of work recovery for low back pain. Over 60% return to work in 10 days. Of those absent at 10 days, another 40% return to work in the next 10-day period, etc. **B,** the intensity of work recovery for sciatica. About 48% return to work in the first 10 days. Of those absent at 10 days, another 23% return to work in the next 10-day period, etc. (Adapted from Andersson. GBJ, Svensson HO, Oden A: *Spine* 1983; 8:880–884.)

Physical fitness appears not to be associated to a risk of back pain as such,[8, 74] but it is a positive factor hastening recovery after a back pain episode.[24, 60] Spine mobility is another factor often discussed as a potential risk, but with low probability of association with back pain.[10, 12] Interestingly, Biering-Sorensen found that reduced spine mobility in subjects with previous back pain indicated increased future risk, while in "back-healthy" subjects the opposite was true, i.e., those with more spine mobility had an increased risk for future LBP.[15]

Smoking has been found to be associated with back pain by so many investigators that its relationship is almost certain.* Physiologic and mechanical factors may both be contributing to this relationship. Smokers cough, bronchitis causes repetitive strain, and smoking decreases the oxygen tension in discs and increases the risk of disc degeneration.

NATURAL HISTORY OF LOW BACK PAIN AND SCIATICA

The recovery rate for uncomplicated LBP is excellent. Independent studies from, for example, Sweden[4, 21] and Canada[67] indicate that 70% recover in a few weeks and 90% by 6 to 8 weeks (Fig 50–5). The natural history can be positively influenced by exercise both in the acute[21, 60] and chronic stages.[58] Risk factors for chronicity include the presence of adverse psychological and physical work factors, psychological factors per se, social factors, compensation and litigation, and the use of passive treatment modalities. Sciatica has a slower recovery rate than localized back pain, particularly when caused by a herniated disc (Fig 50–6). Even then, however, spontaneous recovery is common. Hakelius found that 50% of patients with sciatica improved by 4 weeks and 90% by 90 days.[33] Surgery appears to hasten recovery from disc herniation, but long-term function is minimally influenced, as is the risk of recurrence and residual neurologic deficits.[77]

Unfortunately, recurrences of LBP and sciatica are common and reported to occur in as many as 85%.[12, 21, 32, 75] Bergquist-Ullman and Larsson reported that 62% of a group of 217 workers with acute LBP had recurrences within 1 year and another 18% within 2 years.[12]

SUMMARY

LBP is one of the most common ailments to man. While usually benign in nature, chronic pain and long-term disability occur with such frequency that the socioeconomic and health care costs as well as the degree of personal suffering are unacceptable. Prevention of back pain must therefore be a first-order priority and should aim at both preventing pain occurrence as such and preventing disability resulting from pain in the lower part of the back with or without sciatica.

*References 16, 17, 25, 29, 30, 36, 42, 61, 71.

REFERENCES

1. Abenhaim LL, Suissa S: Importance and economic burden of occupational back pain: A study of 2500 cases representative of Quebec. *J Occup Med* 1987; 29:670–674.
2. Anderson JAD: Epidemiological aspects of back pain. *J Soc Occup Med* 1986; 36:90–94.
3. Andersson GBJ: The epidemiology of spinal disorders, in

Frymoyer J (ed): *The Adult Spine: Principles and Practice*. New York, Raven Press, 1991, pp 107–146.
4. Andersson GBJ, Svensson HO, Oden A: The intensity of work recovery in low back pain. *Spine* 1983; 8:880–884.
5. Balague F, Dutoit G, Waldburger M: Low back pain in school children. *Scand J Rehabil Med* 1988; 20:175–179.
6. Battie MC: *The Reliability of Physical Factors as Predictors of the Occurrence of Back Pain Reports. A Prospective Study Within Industry* (thesis). University of Goteborg, Sweden, 1989.
7. Battie MC, Bigos SJ, Fisher LD, et al: Anthropometric and clinical measurements as predictors of industrial back pain complaints: A prospective study. *J Spinal Disorders* 1990; 3:195–204.
8. Battie MC, Bigos SJ, Fisher LD, et al: A prospective study of the role of cardiovascular risk factors and fitness in industrial back pain complaints. *Spine* 1989; 14:141–147.
9. Battie MC, Bigos SJ, Fisher LD, et al: Isometric lifting strength as a predictor of industrial back pain. *Spine* 1989; 14:851–856.
10. Battie MC, Bigos SJ, Fisher LD, et al: The role of spinal flexibility in back pain complaints within industry: A prospective study. *Spine* 1989; 14:851–856.
11. Bergenudd H, Nilsson B: Back pain in middle age; occupational workload and psychologic factors: An epidemiologic survey. *Spine* 1988; 13:58–60.
12. Bergquist-Ullman M, Larsson U: Acute low back pain in industry. A controlled prospective study with special reference to therapy and confounding factors. *Acta Orthop Scand Suppl* 1977; 170:1.
13. Biering-Sorensen F: Low back trouble in a general population of 30-, 40-, 50-, and 60-year old men and women. Study design, representativeness and basic results. *Dan Med Bull* 1982; 29:289.
14. Biering-Sorensen F: Physical measurements as risk indicators for low-back trouble over a one-year period. *Spine* 1984; 9:106–119.
15. Biering-Sorensen F: *The Prognostic Value of the Low Back History and Physical Measurements* (unpublished dissertation). University of Copenhagen, 1983.
16. Biering-Sorensen F, Hilden J: Reproducibility of the history of low-back trouble. *Spine* 1984; 9:280–286.
17. Biering-Sorensen F, Thomsen C: Medical, social and occupational history as risk indicators for low-back trouble in a general population. *Spine* 1986; 11:720–725.
18. Bigos SJ, Spengler DM, Martin NA, et al: Back injuries in industry: A retrospective study. III. Employee-related factors. *Spine* 1986; 3:252–256.
19. Buckle PW, Kember PA, Wood AD, et al: Factors influencing occupational back pain in Bedfordshire. *Spine* 1980; 5:254–258.
20. Chaffin DB, Herrin GD, Keyserling WM: Preemployment strength testing. An updated position. *J Occup Med* 1978; 20:403.
21. Choler U, Larsson R, Nachemson A, et al: *Back Pain* (in Swedish). Spring report 188, Stockholm, ISSSN 05860-1691, 1985.
22. Cunningham LS, Kelsey JL: Epidemiology of musculoskeletal impairments and associated disability. *Am J Public Health* 1984; 74:574–579.
23. Damkot DK, Pope MH, Lord J, et al: The relationship between work history, work environment and low-back pain in men. *Spine* 1984; 9:395–399.
24. Dehlin O, Berg S, Andersson GBJ, et al: Effect of physical training and ergonomic counseling on the psychological perception of work and on the subjective assessment of low-back insufficiency. *Scand J Rehabil Med* 1981; 13:1–9.
25. Deyo RA, Bass JE: Lifestyle and low back pain. The influence of smoking and obesity. *Spine* 1989; 14:501–506.
26. Deyo RA, Tsui-Wu Y-J: Descriptive epidemiology of low-back pain and its related medical care in the United States. *Spine* 1987; 121:264–268.
27. Dupuis H, Zerlett G: *The Effects of Whole Body Vibration*. New York, Springer-Verlag, 1986.
28. Frymoyer JW, Pope MH: Epidemiologic insights into the relationship between usage and back disorder, in Hadler NH (ed): *Current Concepts in Regional Musculoskeletal Illness*. Orlando, Fla, Grune & Stratton, 1987, pp 263–279.
29. Frymoyer JW, Pope MH, Clements JH, et al: Risk factors in low back pain. An epidemiological survey. *J Bone Joint Surg [Am]* 1983; 65:213.
30. Frymoyer JW, Pope MH, Costanza MC, et al: Epidemiologic studies of low-back pain. *Spine* 1980; 5:419–423.
31. Giles LGF, Taylor JR: Low-back pain associated with leg length inequality. *Spine* 1981; 6:510.
32. Gyntelberg F: One year incidence of low back pain among male residents of Copenhagen aged 40–59. *Dan Med Bull* 1974; 21:30.
33. Hakelius A: Prognosis in sciatica: A clinical follow-up of surgical and nonsurgical treatment. *Acta Orthop Scand Suppl* 1970; 129:1–76.
34. Helander E: Back pain and work disability (in Swedish). *Socialmed Tidskr* 1973; 50:398–404.
35. Heliovaara M: Body height, obesity, and risk of herniated lumbar intervertebral disc. *Spine* 1987; 12:469–472.
36. Heliovaara M: *Epidemiology of Sciatica and Herniated Lumbar Intervertebral Disc*. Helsinki, The Research Institute for Social Security, 1988, pp 1–147.
37. Heliovaara M, Knekt P, Aromaa A: Incidence and risk factors of herniated lumbar intervertebral disc or sciatica leading to hospitalization. *J Chronic Dis* 1987; 3:251–285.
38. Herrin GD, Jaraiedi M, Anderson CK: Prediction of overexertion injuries using biomechanical and psychophysical models. *J Am Ind Hyg Assoc* 1986; 47:322.
39. Kelsey JL: An epidemiological study of acute herniated lumbar intervertebral discs. *Rheumatol Rehabil* 1975; 14:144–159.
40. Kelsey JL: An epidemiological study of the relationship between occupations and acute herniated lumbar intervertebral discs. *Int J Epidemiol* 1975; 4:197.
41. Kelsey JL: Idiopathic low back pain, magnitude of the problem, in White AA III, Gordon SL (eds): *Symposium on Idiopathic Low Back Pain*. St Louis, Mosby–Year Book, 1982.

42. Kelsey JL, Githens PB, O'Connor T, et al: Acute prolapsed lumbar intervertebral disc. An epidemiologic study with special reference to driving automobiles and cigarette smoking. *Spine* 1984; 9:608–613.
43. Kelsey JL, Githens PB, Walter SD, et al: An epidemiologic study of acute prolapsed cervical intervertebral disc. *J Bone Joint Surg [Am]* 1984; 66:907–914.
44. Kelsey JL, Githens PB, White AA, et al: An epidemiologic study of lifting and twisting on the job and risk for acute prolapsed lumbar intervertebral disc. *J Orthop Res* 1984; 2:61–66.
45. Kelsey JL, Golden AL: Occupational and workplace factors associated with low-back pain. *Spine State Art Rev* 1988; 3:7–16.
46. Kelsey JL, Hardy RJ: Driving of motor vehicles as a risk factor for acute herniated lumbar intervertebral disc. *Am J Epidemiol* 1975; 102:63.
47. Kelsey JL, Ostfeld AM: Demographic characteristics of persons with acute herniated lumbar intervertebral disc. *J Chronic Dis* 1975; 28:37.
48. Kelsey JL, Pastides H, Bigbee GE Jr: *Musculo-Skeletal Disorders: Their Frequency of Occurrence and Their Impact on the Population of the United States*. New York, Prodist, 1978.
49. Keyserling WM, Herrin GD, Chaffin DB: Isometric strength testing as a means of controlling medical incidents on strenuous jobs. *J Occup Med* 1980; 22:332.
50. Keyserling WM, Punnett L, Fine LJ: Postural stress of the trunk and shoulders: Identification and control of occupational risk factors, in *Ergonomic Interventions to Prevent Musculoskeletal Injuries in Industry*. Chelsea, Mich, Lewis, 1987, pp 11–26.
51. Klein BP, Jensen RC, Sanderson LM: Assessment of worker's compensation claims for back strains/sprains. *J Occup Med* 1984; 26:443–448.
52. Kostuik JP, Bentivoglio J: The incidence of low back pain in adult scoliosis. *Spine* 1981; 6:268–273.
53. Kozak LJ, Moien M: *Detailed Diagnoses and Surgical Procedures for Patients Discharged From Short-Stay Hospitals. United States, 1983*. Washington, DC, Vital and Health Statistics 13, No 82, 1985.
54. Lee P, Helewa A, Smythe HA, et al: Epidemiology of musculoskeletal disorders (complaints) and related disability in Canada. *J Rheumatol* 1985; 12:1169–1173.
55. Lloyd MH, Gould S, Soutar CA: Epidemiologic study of back pain in miners and office workers. *Spine* 1986; 11:136–140.
56. Magora A: Investigation of the relation between low back pain and occupation. III. Physical requirements: Sitting, standing and weight lifting. *Ind Med Surg* 1972; 41: 5–9.
57. Magora, A: Investigation of the relation between low back pain and occupation. 5. Psychological aspects. *Scand J Rehabil Med* 1973; 5:191.
58. Mayer TG, Gatchel RJ, Kishino N, et al: Objective assessment of spine function following individual injury: A prospective study with comparison group and one-year follow-up. *Spine* 1985; 10:482–493.
59. Nachemson A: *Back Pain: Etiology, Diagnosis, and Treatment*. Stockholm, The Swedish Council on Technology Assessment in Health Care, 1991.
60. Nachemson AL, Eek C, Lindstrom IL, et al: Chronic low back disability can be largely prevented: A prospective randomized trial in industry. Presented at the 50th Annual Meeting of the American Academy of Orthopaedic Surgeons, Las Vegas, 1989.
61. Pentinnen J: *Back Pain and Sciatica in Finnish Farmers*. Helsinki; Publications of the Social Insurance Institution, ML:71, 1987.
62. Riihimaki H, Wickstrom G, Hanninen K, et al: Predictors of sciatic pain among concrete reinforcement workers and house painters—a five year follow-up. *Scand J Work Environ Health* 1989; 15:415–423.
63. Rush WA, Steiner HA: A study of lower extremity length inequality. *AJR* 1946; 56:616–623.
64. Spangfort EV: The lumbar disc herniation. *Acta Orthop Scand Suppl* 1972; 142:1.
65. Spengler DM, Bigos SJ, Martin NA, et al: Back injuries in industry: A retrospective study. I. Overview and cost analysis. *Spine* 1986; 11:241–245.
66. Spitzer WO: Strategies for surgical investigators, in Troidl H, Spitzer WO, McPeek B, et al (eds): *Principles and Practice of Research*. New York, Springer-Verlag, 1986.
67. Spitzer WO, LeBlanc FE, Dupuis M, et al: Scientific approach to the assessment and management of activity-related spinal disorders: A monography for clinicians. Report of the Quebec task force on spinal disorders. *Spine* 1987; 12(suppl 7):1–59.
68. Svensson H-O: *Low Back Pain in Forty to Forty-Seven Year Old Men: A Retrospective Cross-Sectional Study* (thesis). University of Goteborg, Sweden, 1981.
69. Svensson HO: Low-back pain in 40–47 year old men: Some socioeconomic factors and previous sickness absence. *Scand J Rehabil Med* 1982; 14:54–59.
70. Svensson H-O, Andersson GBJ: Low back pain in forty to forty-seven year old men. I. Frequency of occurrence and impact on medical services. *Scand J Rehabil Med* 1982; 14:47.
71. Svensson H-O, Andersson GBJ: Low back pain in forty to forty-seven year old men: Work history and work environment factors. *Spine* 1983; 8:272.
72. Svensson H-O, Andersson GBJ, Johansson S, et al: A retrospective study of low back pain in 38- to 64-year-old women. Frequency and occurrence and impact on medical services. *Spine* 1988; 13:548–552.
73. Svensson HO, Vedin A, Wilhelmsson C, et al: Low back pain in relation to other diseases and cardiovascular risk factors. *Spine* 1983; 8:277.
74. Troup JDG, Foreman TK, Baxter CE, et al: The perception of back pain and the role of psychophysical tests of lifting capacity. *Spine* 1987; 12:645–657.
75. Valkenburg HA, Haanen HCM: The epidemiology of low back pain, White AA III, Gordon SL (eds): *Symposium on Idiopathic Low Back Pain*. St Louis, Mosby–Year Book, 1982, pp 9–22.
76. Volinn E, Lai D, McKinney S, et al: When back pain be-

comes disabling: A regional analysis. *Pain* 1988; 33:33–39.
77. Weber H: Lumbar disc herniation: A controlled prospective study with ten years of observation. *Spine* 1983; 8:131–140.
78. Wood PHN, Badley EM: Epidemiology of back pain, in Jayson M (ed): *The Lumbar Spine and Back Pain*. London, Churchill Livingston, 1987, pp 1–15.
79. Worrall JD, Appel D: The impact of workers compensation benefits on low back claims, in Hadler NM (ed): *Current Concepts in Regional Musculoskeletal Illness*. Orlando, Fla, Grune & Stratton, 1987, pp 281–298.

51

Rehabilitation of the Heavy Manual Laborer

Kathleen S. Botelho, P.T., Sherlyn Fenton, O.T.R./L., Valerie Shaw Jones, O.T.R./L., Nancy Meedzan, B.S.N., and Patricia McGauley Meyers, O.T.R./L.

The incidence of low back pain and the cost of its treatment has gained attention from the entire medical field and from health care reimbursement systems. The intensity of this problem has prompted medical practitioners to develop and implement specialized protocol and programs. Heavy manual laborers account for 63% of low back–injured workers.[30] Moreover, statistics show that the heavier one's job demands are, the more difficult it is to achieve a return-to-work status.[7] There is no standard definition classifying the heavy manual laborer; therefore the term *material handler* is commonly interchanged to describe an individual who must rely on physical capacity to accomplish job demands. Very often care givers and laymen mistakenly perceive strength as the primary factor required to accomplish job tasks; however, the rate and duration demands are equally significant components. This chapter outlines one facility's approach to providing rehabilitation for the back-injured material handler.

Liberty Mutual Insurance Company, the country's largest underwriter of workermen's compensation insurance, began developing a center to address the needs of this population in 1913. Based on this long experience in treating industrial injuries, the rehabilitation team has learned that a multidisciplinary approach is the most effective means to reduce disability and assist clients in returning to productive independent lives. Three types of rehabilitation services are available: an acute-care clinic, general rehabilitation, and the Liberty Mutual Back Education and Rehabilitation (LIMBER) program.

ACUTE-CARE CLINIC

The acute-care program is equipped to treat 90% of all types of industrial injuries, with cases of acute cardiac conditions and severe surgical procedures being directed to an area hospital. Often workers with heavy job demands come to the clinic with acute back symptoms. A thorough physical examination is performed, and diagnostic testing may be recommended. During the initial clinic visit, workers experiencing low back pain view a film demonstrating proper body mechanics and activities to avoid during the acute phase of low back pain.[3, 25] Components of wellness such as proper nutrition and exercise are also addressed to minimize the effects of low back injury.[10]

The protocol for treating an acute back injury begins with the application of ice. The client is advised to utilize this modality for the first 24 to 36 hours postinjury. Immediately following this period, the application of heat to the injured area is recommended.[23] To expedite the home treatment process, clients are issued ice packs, hydrocollator packs, and medication when appropriate.[2, 8, 28, 37] The client is scheduled to return to the clinic in 3 to 4 days for reevaluation. Depending upon the residual symptoms, the client is either maintained on bed rest, referred to physical therapy or occupational therapy, or sent back to work on regular or adjusted duty at the clinic physician's discretion.[26]

When workers are referred for physical therapy, they are evaluated for objective and subjective findings. A tailored treatment program is developed to implement these data, and progress is carefully monitored by the treating therapist. Clients are assessed on an ongoing basis to allow the treatment plan to be adjusted to the client's progress. The typical treatment plan for the heavy manual laborer emphasizes education and exercise to improve musculoskeletal flexibility and restore normal muscle balance and strength. Modalities are used to decrease inflammation, edema, or muscle spasm.[23] Exercises that address postural awareness and specific problem areas are also taught during the therapeutic treatment and are incorporated into a home program. It is essential for this exercise regimen to be augmented with education that links posture to the use of proper body mechanics in everyday life including tasks that require manual handling. Occupational therapy plays a key role in this educational process.

A client is referred to occupational therapy for proper body mechanics training and work hardening, which may include job simulation. The effects of an injury to the manual laborer span far beyond job demands. The client's whole daily routine is affected by loss of function. Therefore issues of home management, personal roles, and recreational activities are also incorporated into the therapy. Instruction and training varies from one to many sessions according to individual needs and physician recommendations. Work simplification techniques are taught and reviewed in reference to activities of daily living and work-related tasks.[14, 27] Most clients are familiar with some principles of proper body mechanics. However, they may require reinforcement and practice to incorporate proper posture and body positioning in all aspects of daily life.[7]

Following the acute phase of an injury, a client may participate in a work-hardening and exercise program that simulates job tasks, thus better preparing the worker to face the return to work demands.

GENERAL REHABILITATION

The goal of the general rehabilitation program is to provide a multidisciplinary treatment approach to enhance the quality of a client's life through a functional restoration program. Injured workers are referred to the rehabilitation program from a variety of sources. The worker's attending physician may directly refer an individual, or clients treated in the acute-care program may also be recommended. When a policy holder's employee is injured, a claims adjuster is automatically assigned, and a rehabilitation nurse intervenes when warranted by the severity of the injury.

Once referred to the center, an orthopedic evaluation is scheduled, and at this time the program coordinator orients the client to the facility's treatment program, transportation, lodging, policies, emergency procedures, and any other pertinent issues. After the physician has approved the patient's participation in the program, therapeutic evaluations are scheduled. Due to the strenuous nature of these assessments, rest periods are incorporated into evaluations schedules for optimal client performance during each discipline's session. During the multidisciplinary evaluations, strength, flexibility, and endurance are measured to determine physical and functional capacity. An essential adjunct of this evaluation process is the physical examination by the internist, who outlines health problems including possible cardiac risk factors and makes recommendations for individual workers. These recommendations are addressed by the cardiac nurse, a member of the rehabilitation team, through a functional health patterns evaluation emphasizing risk factors and exploring personal wellness.[1] A comprehensive cardiac evaluation is performed and may include checking the client's blood cholesterol level, monitoring daily blood pressure before and after exercise, and providing instruction in the areas of nutrition, weight reduction, and smoking cessation. These educational sessions may be presented in a group or individual setting depending on the client's specific needs and abilities.

Prior to entering an exercise program, all clients over the age of 35 years undergo an exercise stress test performed by a cardiologist. The protocol for testing is based on the Guidelines for Exercise Testing and Prescription according to The American College of Sports Medicine.[1] Recommendations and appropriate referrals are made when a client has positive stress test findings and there is need for further testing, i.e., thallium stress testing. These clients may be cleared by the cardiologist to participate in a rehabilitation program while adhering to cardiac precautions during exercise. A four-channel telemetry monitoring system is available to monitor the client's heart rate and rhythm while exercising. This can be a very important aspect of treatment, especially for a client with known heart disease. The use of a telemetry monitoring system alleviates the client's fear of exercising and facilitates the rehabilitation process. When cardiac abnormalities are detected as the client's treatment program becomes more demanding, this is immediately addressed by the cardiac nurse. Teaching is ongoing for all cardiac patients, including medication information, cardiovascular anatomy, the physiology of heart disease, and aspects of healthy living. To promote wellness, a daily class called "Healthy Lifestyles" is presented that consists of either a half-hour walk or a class on health-related issues pertinent to the heavy manual laborer.

The goal of general fitness is to reverse the effects of inactivity following a back injury. There is a significant reduction in aerobic capacity after 2 weeks of decreased activity.[32] Muscle atrophy is also likely to be present. For manual laborers this is a major barrier to returning to work since strength is essential to accomplishing job demands. The fitness program addresses cardiovascular fitness as well as muscle strength and endurance in an attempt to restore balance to the kinematic chain of the body while considering orthopedic and medical contraindications.

The client's baseline aerobic capacity is determined from results of the exercise stress test or submaximal exercise test. Strength assessment involves establishing a ten-repetition maximum for the trunk and upper and lower extremities and utilizing range-adjustable, variable-resistive equipment. Results from strength testing in conjunction with aerobic capacity are used to establish a fitness baseline and exercise prescription. The deconditioned material handler frequently presents with disproportional trunk musculature. The normal ratio of 2:1 trunk extensor muscles to abdominal muscles is often reversed secondary to inactivity.[16] This imbalance is directly addressed by using a resistive equipment circuit for whole-body strengthening while providing trunk stability. This equipment plays a major role in that muscle groups are challenged with minimal pain due to seating design and isolation of fluid movement. Optimal fitness for the material handler should require a level elevated beyond that of job demands to account for possible post-training deconditioning.[5] Achievement of this higher goal, enhanced by the visual feedback of daily charting, instills a feeling of accomplishment that decreases the worker's fear and increases confidence for a successful return to work.

The physical therapy component of the program involves a thorough evaluation, including subjective reports and objective measures to assess the entire body. The heavy manual laborer often presents with musculoskeletal imbalances that may be related to specific job tasks. Objective measures are obtained by using standard evaluation devices such as a digital inclinometer to determine the trunk range of motion (ROM).[16, 22, 24] Special tests such as the Thomas test and straight leg raises are used to assess muscle shortening, dural signs, or other soft-tissue tightness.[12] The client also undergoes a thorough standard postural assessment performed while sitting and again while standing to determine structural alignment problems. If alignment or postural deviations are noted, further assessment in the supine and/or prone position is indicated. Gross sensation testing is performed to detect impairments in proprioception, touch, and temperature. Gait is observed and deviations noted to help clarify the clinical picture.

Objective findings and subjective reports during specific activities are examined to determine the best approach to address the client's individual problems. Treatment goals are established by taking into account the client's pathology, musculoskeletal deficiencies, and job demands as well as personal objectives and vocational goals.

ROM, joint mobility, strength, and posture are addressed in a physical therapy treatment plan and serve as the building blocks for the rehabilitation program. Proper body alignment and flexibility are important prerequisites for building muscle strength in areas of general fitness and in occupational therapy for work-hardening exercises. This is particularly important in the rehabilitation of heavy material handlers since unaddressed strength deficits may lead to reinjury or a new injury upon returning to work.

The primary emphasis of most treatment programs is exercise, including active ROM, stretching, general flexibility exercises, progressive resistive exercises (PREs) to extremities, gait, and postural activities.[29] The use of modalities is deemphasized and only used when needed to prepare soft-tissue problem areas for exercise. Clients are instructed in individualized home exercise and walking programs that encourage a carryover of rehabilitation into their life-style.

The therapist assesses client performance through observation of monitored sequencing, substitution, and movement patterns during exercise and functional activities. Educating the client in spinal anatomy, physiology, the mechanics of injury, and basic treatment principles increases client understanding and compliance. As the client begins to incorporate this new knowledge and acquired skills, less supervision is required, and the emphasis is placed on strengthening, activities of daily living (ADL), and work-related tasks in fitness and occupational therapy.

When the heavy material handler begins occupational therapy, a functional capacity evaluation is performed. Subjective reports include the client's assessment of ADL, pain perception, functional tolerances, and job description. A subjective ADL checklist addressing personal, home, automobile, and recreational management is compiled to represent a level of dysfunction. To assess pain perception, the client is asked to mark all areas of discomfort on a schematic drawing of the human body. Perceived functional tolerances for sitting, standing, lying supine, walking, and driving are reported. The job description provides a subjective task analysis and is completed by the client and the employer. The two job descriptions as well as other pertinent job information are then compared to establish the client's occupational therapy and vocational goals. There are occasions when further contact with the employer is beneficial for clarification of specific job duties.

Objective testing involves static and dynamic components. A dynamometer is used to test static grip strength at three handle positions, and these results are compared with normative data.[19] Dynamic testing includes progressive isoinertial lifting evaluation (PILE), which is used as an indication of the worker's endurance and effort.[20] Another component of dynamic testing is the maximum-effort test, which evaluates lifting at three levels, carrying, pushing, pulling, and squatting.[4, 15] This information is extrapolated into a physical demand level (PDL), which represents the worker's functional capacity.[13]

The occupational therapist's evaluation process initiates therapeutic rapport between the client and therapist to better design a treatment program addressing the worker's individual needs. Initially, the heavy laborer's program incorporates nonspecific tasks but then progresses to components of job simulation and work hardening. The primary components of the heavy material handler's program include repetitive lift, carry, pull, climb, reach, and forward trunk flexion tasks. These nonspecific job tasks emphasize strength, endurance, and flexibility. A combination of these components is emphasized as the client progresses to job simulation.

For the heavy material handler, a work-hardening program may include shoveling, wearing a tool belt, stocking, clearing the loading dock by using various hand trucks and pallets, carrying weighted loads while climbing up ladders (tools, roofing shingles, etc.), pushing a wheelbarrow up an inclined surface, or walking on scaffolding or beams. The work-hardening program focuses on worker's performing job components at the actual speed, force, rate, and duration required for the job.

When a worker is injured, he often goes through

stages of loss. Vocational, family, and personal roles as well as attitudes are all influenced by the client's ability to function.[31, 33] Clients learn how to utilize coping skills to effectively manage the situations that occur. Many people with physical limitations are not cognizant of their internal strengths and may require professional psychological support as an adjunct to their therapeutic services to explore alternative perspectives concerning their extraordinary circumstances. Psychologists and psychiatrists may provide services to aid clients in the management of stress reactions, situational and biological depression, and chronic pain syndromes.

These counseling services may be presented in either a group setting or on an individual basis. Treatment approaches range from relaxation training to therapeutic drug administration and monitoring. It is common for the entire team to discuss a client's behavior to gain insight into emotional progression, regression, or subtle inconsistencies. If symptom magnification is questioned, the team supports their suspicions with objective data and conferences with the client to design and facilitate the elimination of secondary gains.[34–36] Once this is achieved, the client has a clearer path toward the road to recovery while the staff is better able to provide quality personalized treatment through the benefits of team communication, which helps to reestablish treatment goals.

From this holistic viewpoint, psychology addresses the many specific problems of the heavy manual laborer. The more pertinent issues that may require intervention are the feelings of inadequacy concerning the ability to complete job demands required for a return to work, fears of injury to self and coworkers, and apprehension regarding fulfilling family and financial obligations.[13]

Many rehabilitation clients discover that returning to their previous job may not be an option upon discharge. There are occasions when a worker's physical capacity remains limited, his emotional state impedes function, the company's employment status is restricted, or the company does not provide adjusted or permanent light-duty placement.[17, 21] In such cases, vocational counseling may be initiated. When vocational counseling is incorporated as part of the multidisciplinary program, the process is begun by the counselor gathering a thorough work history. This service focuses on the client's transferable skills, education, aptitudes, financial incentives, job goals, and obstacles to employment. The vocational counselor consults with the other therapeutic disciplines to ensure that the client's physical, functional, and emotional capacities are compatible with vocational interests, explorations, and goals established during client sessions.

LIMBER

The most recent addition to the treatment center is the Liberty Mutual Back and Rehabilitation Program, known as LIMBER. This functional restoration program was developed to meet the needs of the subacute back-injured worker who would benefit from group dynamics while participating in an intensive program. Although participants represent a wide variety of occupations, this program directly addresses the rehabilitation needs of the heavy material handler. Through its multidisciplinary approach, this short-term aggressive program is designed to maximize function and has the capability of returning clients to regular or modified work.

Candidates are referred to the program by the same mechanism as general rehabilitation. The client's attending physician, who is involved in the referral process, is updated on progress and discharge status. If the client does not have an attending physician, one may be assigned at the center. The criteria for admission to the program is as follows:

1. Disability due to low back pain of at least 4 months' duration.
2. Not a candidate for surgery at the time of admission.
3. No substance abuse, i.e., alcohol or prescription or street drugs.
4. Postoperative clients may be appropriate once they have been cleared by the attending physician for an aggressive treatment program. In general, clients should be at least 3 months postlaminectomy or at least 6 months postfusion. Individual cases may vary.

There may be instances when further diagnostic studies or therapeutic blocking procedures are recommended by the treatment team prior to admission or during the program.

The functional restoration program incorporates a multidisciplinary team, including occupational therapy, physical therapy, general fitness, psychology, vocational counseling, nursing, and physician consultation. Quantitative functional evaluations (QFE) are performed by the entire rehabilitation team upon admission, at midprogram, at discharge, and at follow-up. Based on the team's evaluations, a consensus determines the worker's appropriateness for LIMBER. Clients approved for the program who would benefit from a preliminary stretching and strengthening program, participate in a 1- to 2-week preprogram before beginning the core program. Clients not appropriate for the program at the time of referral may be recommended to a contingency program and then reconsidered at a later date.

The core program is a 4-week structured schedule that requires participants to attend full 8-hour days. The first week of the core program is unique in that it includes a strong educational component focusing on the etiology, anatomy, pathology, clinical course, treatment, and progress of low back pain.

The anatomy and physiology course provides fundamental principles that the other lectures build upon. Presented by a physical therapist, this lecture emphasizes spinal anatomy and physiology and its application with regard to body mechanics and posture. Occupational therapists utilize videotaping of individual clients performing daily tasks. This tape is then viewed in a group setting where proper body mechanics are presented by the occupational therapist and reviewed with the worker. Visual feedback facilitates the transitional process of applying proper body mechanics to tasks ranging from ADL to heavy material handling. The class presented on general fitness emphasizes the correlation between fitness level and low back injury and the effectiveness of rehabilitation.[5, 20] The importance of a total fitness program is discussed and focuses on strength, endurance, flexibility, and aerobic fitness. The worker's individual recreational and fitness interests are also explored. A class in wellness, presented by the cardiac nurse, provides basic knowledge of the cardiovascular system for the client to identify the significance of individual risk factors in order to facilitate life-style changes. To exemplify this message, a film is presented portraying a father and son with multiple cardiac risk factors and their eventual experience with heart disease. The remainder of this class instructs clients in proper nutrition, weight reduction diets, as well as information on smoking cessation. An occupational therapist presents the week's final class, which focuses on completing ADL by utilizing adaptive equipment, adjusted positioning, and work simplification techniques. These methods minimize the effects of pain while maximizing independent function.[9, 14, 18]

A typical day begins with a client attending physical therapy for general flexibility exercises. The goal of these exercises is to begin to use proper biomechanical positions through increased ROM in order to minimize recurrent injuries.[5, 6, 11] This is performed in a group format incorporating full-body flexibility exercises modified according to client's needs. Occupational therapy directly follows, and participants begin the first of two sessions incorporating ten workstations designed to facilitate and increase strength, flexibility, and endurance through nonspecific job-simulated tasks. The progression of these functional capacities is addressed through grading the tasks according to resistance and repetitions.[20] The heavy manual laborer is expected to increase resistance at a uniform rate of twice a week. When strength plateaus, the worker continues to increase repetitions to maximize endurance.

The next session is psychology, which addresses psychosomatic responses within a supportive group atmosphere. There are three groups presented, two of which are didactic and one that is interactive. This is an educational experience increasing awareness of psychophysical functions, and workers learn to enhance individual coping skills and to manage stress and pain responses. Through the group process, workers explore and discover their internal resources and are given the opportunity to exchange newfound views. There are two group processes that we introduce to our clients, relaxation group and support group. Relaxation group provides instruction and practice, through a variety of methods, to relieve muscular tension and psychological stress and ultimately minimize pain perception. By utilizing these techniques, relaxation encourages the body's natural healing process. The support group is an interactive experience where the workers are able to discuss pertinent issues on such topics as pain, fear of reinjury, family roles, and return-to-work attitudes. This group also provides workers with the opportunity to express their experiences within the program and give each other feedback and support. Additionally, the participants meet on an individual basis to discuss progress, problems, and personal concerns. Further psychological services or referrals are available on a per diem basis to ensure a strong supportive structure in the transitional process of rehabilitation.

The final morning session is general fitness and includes either a strengthening or cardiovascular program. The strengthening program utilizes nine adjustable progressive-resistance machines that isolate individual muscle groups. Clients begin their individualized strengthening program at a weight determined by the results of a ten–maximum-repetition test. The resistance is increased once the clients exceed ten repetitions at their current weight. Twice a week, clients do an easy weight program consisting of only one set of ten repetitions at their current weight. The cardiovascular program begins with a 20-minute aerobic workout at 60% to 80% of the client's age-predicted maximum heart rate.[4] Clients utilize a variety of aerobic exercise equipment based on physical comfort and preference. Workout time is increased weekly.

Workers need to strengthen their large muscle groups in order to maintain proper biomechanical positions throughout their fitness and functional restoration programs. Strengthening is achieved through basic gravity-resistive exercises uniformly progressed to a more challenging level while addressing trunk and lower-extremity deficits. Although the group completes exercises simultaneously, the exercises are adjusted according to individual capabilities. Clients are monitored closely for progress and proper execution of these exercises. The workers then return to occupational therapy to complete ten workstations incorporating job-specific simulated tasks. The group is then engaged in physical restoration sessions. Time is allotted throughout the day for individual vocational, psychological, and wellness counseling.

During the 4-week core program the entire treatment team meets weekly to review each worker's program in order to address and implement appropriate correspondence and treatment. The workers participate on an individual basis in this meeting. During this time they receive input from the team regarding all aspects of their program, and they have the opportunity to discuss their impressions, issues, and concerns in an open forum.

Following completion of the core program, the need for a postprogram is determined. The heavy manual laborer may remain in a postprogram for 1 to 2 weeks that emphasizes job simulation in preparation for returning to a specific job. Vocational counseling services continue when the worker's regular job or adjusted positions are not available.

Upon program completion, workers are given individualized home programs. General fitness guidelines are based on client interest and ability. Information on walking, biking, and health club equipment is provided. Occupational therapy maintains that workers understand the importance of proper body mechanics, stretching, and strengthening to maximize their functional status. Clients are asked to write down two tasks performed in their daily routine that incorporate the positions and techniques learned from participating in the workstations. These lists are reviewed with the worker upon their 3-month reevaluation. Physical therapy provides workers with individualized stretching and strengthening exercises addressing their physical capabilities. The physical therapy department is presently developing a video to assist workers with their home exercise program. It is the intent of the psychology department that workers utilize coping and relaxation skills as warranted in their daily lives.

The follow-up program was designed to prevent as well as detect evidence of recurrent deconditioning that may lead to further disability. The treatment team recommends weekly telephone calls by the worker to the center for the first 5 weeks after discharge and a 3- and 12-month QFE.

Long-term monitoring of the heavy manual laborer is part of the follow-up program. Participant information is collected for 3 years. Recurrent episodes of low back pain, days lost from work, visits to practitioners, medications, and surgical procedures are recorded. The program teaches skills for initiating life-style changes that workers maintain throughout their lives. All workers participating in our clinic and general rehabilitation programs are discharged with an established aftercare plan. This plan, under the supervision of the participant's attending physician, may include returning to the worker's previous job, adjusted employment, vocational retraining, and/or continued vocational services.

Due to a cohesive staff sharing good communication skills, a client's administrative, psychological, and medical issues are recognized and timely referrals made to the appropriate disciplines within this facility. There is also access to diagnostic and surgical procedures when needed.

As insurance company and the medical provider, we feel that the worker ultimately benefits from the advantages of this unique system. Unlike other medical facilities whose length and type of care is often governed by the guidelines of third-party payers, our programs are developed, supported, and enhanced company-wide. It has been our observation that as heavy material laborers experience the company's investment firsthand, they tend to take a more active role in rehabilitation programs, thus facilitating the return-to-work process.

REFERENCES

1. American College of Sports Medicine: *Guidelines for Exercise Testing and Prescription*. Philadelphia, Lea & Febiger, 1986.
2. Bell GR, Rothman RH: The conservative treatment of sciatica. *Spine* 1984; 9:54–56.
3. Bergquist-Ullman M, Larsson V: Acute low back pain in industry—a controlled perspective study with special reference to therapy and vocational factors. *Acta Orthop Scand Suppl* 1977; 170:1.
4. Blankenship K: *Work Capacity Evaluation and Industrial Consultation*. Macon, Ga, American Therapeutics, 1985.
5. Cady LD, Bischoff DP, O'Connell ER, et al: Strength and fitness and subsequent back injuries in firefighters. *J Occup Med* 1979; 21:269–272.
6. Carson J: Stretching away from back pain injury. *Occup Health Saf* 1983; 52:235–238.
7. Caruso LA, Chan DE, Chan A: The management of work-related back pain. *Am J Occup Ther* 1987; 41:112–116.
8. Deyo RA: Conservative therapy for low back pain—distinguishing useful from useless therapy. *JAMA* 1983; 250:1057–1062.
9. Ganz SB: Back smart; Self-help. *Arthritis Information Magazine* 1988; Aimplus, pp 42–43.
10. Hebert L, Miller G: *Taking Care of Your Back*. Augusta, Me, IMPACC, 1984.
11. Himmelstein J, Andersson G: Low back pain: Risk evaluation and preplacement screening. *Occup Med* 1988; 3:255–269.
12. Hoppenfeld S: *Physical Examination of the Spine and Extremities*. New York, Appleton-Century-Crofts, 1976.
13. Isernhagen S: *Work Injury: Management and Prevention* Rockville, Md, Aspen, 1988.
14. Johnson C: Managing spinal pain with body mechanics. *Advice Occup Ther* 1988; 4:1–7.
15. Kamon E, et al: Dynamic and static lifting capacity and muscular strength of steel mill workers. *Am Ind Hyg Assoc J* 1982. 43:853–857.
16. Keeley J, Mayer TG, Cox R, et al: Quantification of lumbar function, part 5: Reliability of range of motion measures in the sagittal plane and an in vivo torso rotation measurement technique. *Spine* 1986; 11:31–35.
17. Magliozzi LA, LeClair PH: Pain centers, transcutaneous electrical nerve stimulation, vocational rehabilitation—a

panacea? Presented at the Liberty Mutual Back Pain Symposium, Boston, March 1981.
18. Mason F: Bending and reaching, Self-help. *Arthritis Information Magazine* 1988; Aimplus, pp 40–41.
19. Mathiowetz V, Kashman N: Grip and pinch strength: Normative data for adults. *Arch Phys Med Rehabil* 1985; 66:16–21.
20. Mayer TG, Gatchel RJ: *Functional Restoration for Spinal Disorders, the Sports Medicine Approach*. Philadelphia, Lea & Febiger, 1988.
21. McManus LA: Evaluation of disability insurance savings due to beneficiary rehabilitation. *Soc Secur Bull* 1981; 44:19–26.
22. Mellin G: Measurement of thoracolumbar posture and mobility with a Myrin inclinometer. *Spine* 1986; 11:759–762.
23. Michlovitz S, Wolf S: *Thermal Agents in Rehabilitation*. Philadelphia, FA Davis, 1988.
24. Million R, Hall W, Nilsen KH, et al: Assessment of the progress of the back-pain patient. *Spine* 1982; 7:204–212.
25. Nachemson AL: Work for all. *Clin Orthop* 1983; 179:77–85.
26. Quinet RJ, Hadler NM: Diagnosis and treatment of backache. *Semin Arthritis Rheum* 1979; 8:261–287.
27. Rodgers S: *Working with Backache*. Fairport, NY, Perinton Press, 1985.
28. Rowe ML: *Backache at Work*. Fairport, NY, Perinton Press, 1983.
29. Schraun DA: Resistance exercises, in *Therapeutic Exercise*. New Haven, Conn, Elizabeth Licht, 1965.
30. Snook S: *Low back pain*. Hopkinton, Mass, Liberty Mutual Insurance, 1989.
31. Stith W, Ohnmeiss DD, Carranza CB, et al: Rehabilitation of patients with chronic low back pain. *Spine State Art Rev* 1989; 3:125–137.
32. Taylor HL, Henschel A, Brozek J, et al: Effects of bed rest on cardiovascular function and work performance. *J Appl Physiol* 1949; 2:233–239.
33. Viney L, Westbrook M: Patient's psychological reactions to chronic illness: Are they associated with rehabilitation? *J Appl Rehabil Counsel* 1982; 13:38–44.
34. Waddell G, Main CJ, Morris EW, et al: Chronic low-back pain, psychological distress, and illness behavior. *Spine* 1984; 9:209–213.
35. Waddell G, Main CJ: Assessment of severity in low back disorders. *Spine* 1984; 9:204–208.
36. Waddell G, McCulloch JA, Kummell E, et al: Nonorganic physical signs in low back pain. *Spine* 1980; 5:117–125.
37. Wiesel SW, Cuckler JM, DeLuca F, et al: Acute low back pain: An objective analysis of conservative therapy. *Spine* 1980; 5:324–330.

52

Exercise Physiology and Fitness

G. Mitch Bogdanffy, M.S.

Low levels of habitual physical activity and the inability to attain physical fitness have become the most serious threats to the overall health of Americans. Inadequate activity is a major factor in the development of several diseases, including cardiovascular disease, non–insulin-dependent diabetes mellitus, musculoskeletal dysfunctions, osteoporosis, arthritis, and a variety of psychosomatic anomalies such as ulcers and general chronic fatigue syndrome.[11, 12, 51] These disuse disorders have been collectively termed *hypokinetic disease*.[13] Recently, the United States has witnessed an increased participation and awareness of leisure time activities, which in turn may help to explain the steady decline in cardiovascular disease.[26, 68] This occurrence may, however, be race and socioeconomic specific.[28–30] The exact role that exercise plays in both the prevention and rehabilitation of back pain and disability remains unclear at this time.[48, 70] The pathophysiology of the majority of cases of back pain is not known. Chronic back pain is recognized as a multidimensional syndrome resulting from differing etiologies, socioenvironmental factors, predispositions, and personalities.[76] The vast scope of this anomaly requires a multifaceted approach to its treatment. While few controlled studies have been initiated, active exercise has been suggested to offer the best approach in both prevention and rehabilitation.[20, 32, 36, 42] In a recent multicenter study, empirical and traditional strategies were tested.[60a] Five clinics utilizing a three-phase treatment plan were instituted. The sequence of treatments involved pain relief and mobilization, followed by increased movement and muscle strengthening along with cardiovascular exercise and simulated work-specific conditioning. The control group consisted of seven centers following a more traditional approach of passive modalities. The results of this large-scale study demonstrated a more rapid return to work and substantial cost savings in the experimental group. The experimental group followed a regimen more commonly used in sports medicine to accelerate the recovery process in order to return to competition as soon as possible. The most common indications for prescribing exercise to the patient with back dysfunction in theory are to decrease pain, strengthen weak muscles, decrease mechanical stress to spinal structures, and improve general fitness to prevent subsequent injury.[57] In addition, specific exercises have been suggested to help stabilize hypermobile segments, improve posture, and increase mobility.[48] However, no data currently exist to support the concept of voluntary muscular control of the paravertebral muscles on intersegmental motion.[47] In addition, it appears that limited–range-of-motion exercises may produce a carryover effect in an untrained range.[40] In a study of 96 persons with chronic low back pain, psychological and physiologic measures were taken to determine the effects of exercise training.[57] Additionally, greater overall physical fitness was significantly correlated with less physical dysfunction or pain. Fitness accounted for 23% of the variance in physical dysfunction and 17% of the variance in depression. Interestingly, of the physiologic components, strength correlated best with both physical and psychological dysfunction. In another report, the preventive effects of exercise on subsequent back injuries was investigated.[17] A graded effect was demonstrated in that on follow-up, the least-fit group experienced a 7.1% injury rate; the average-fit group, 3.2%; and the most-fit group, a 0.8% back injury rate. It could not be determined from the current analysis which of the five fitness parameters contributed the most to the reduction in back injuries; however, of the five components, three were indices of cardiovascular fitness.[17] These results support the contention that workers with greater physical work capacities are more fatigue resistant and recover more rapidly. Perhaps the latter parameter is of greatest consequence. In another population-specific study, maximum oxygen uptake ($\dot{V}O_2$ max) estimates were not predictive of future back injuries.[8] However, selection criteria excluded those employees at cardiovascular risk. In this study, smoking was a stronger predictor than aerobic capacity of future back injuries. Aerobic capacity and self-reported low back pain as assessed by the visual analog scale and low back pain disability index were evaluated in 245 subjects, 71% of whom were males.[45] The subjects were followed for 30 months. Results indicated no significant differences between groups, inpatient, outpatient, and control, at pretreatment evaluation. When analyzed at 3 and 30 months' follow-up all groups were combined, and again no relationship existed between changes in

Vo_2 and pain index or low back pain disability index. Neither inpatient nor outpatient intervention delineated the type of physical exercise program (i.e., cardiovascular, resistance training, mobilization, stabilization, or flexibility). From this prospective, it has been demonstrated that physiologic adaptation is specific to the imposed demands of the training stimulus.[72, 73] For instance, unless cellular respiration occurs, no change in muscle metabolic activity will occur, and therefore there would be no change expected in Vo_2. While the effects of physical exercise and fitness on back pain and dysfunction are scant, numerous studies exist on the benefits of exercise training and fitness on weight loss and cardiovascular risk reduction.[2] Exercise may exert its most profound effect in this low back pain population through behavior modification.[2, 3, 11, 26] It is generally believed that active exercise has the potential to have an impact on back pain sufferers in the following ways: (1) strengthened bones, ligaments, and muscles; (2) improved nutrition to joint cartilages and intervertebral discs; (3) enhanced oxidative capacity of skeletal muscle; (4) improved neuromotor control and coordination; (5) increased mechanical efficiency; and (6) improved cardiovascular and respiratory function.[65] Another important factor related to the psychosomatic interrelationship is that of enhanced neuropeptide release and function. Endurance exercise produces increased β-endorphin release in cerebrospinal fluid. Endorphins appear to modulate pain receptors, which have been shown to be reduced in persons with chronic back pain.[57] Workers engaged in physically demanding occupations necessitate improved physical working capacities.[4] Sustained and repetitive work load demands must be met by a corresponding level of physical work capacity.[5, 58] Several factors, both internal and external, confound this relationship. However, for optimal performance, an equilibrium is essential. Physical work performance encompasses the following components: energy output, including aerobic and anaerobic metabolic processes; neuromuscular function, including strength and technique; as well as psychological factors, including motivation and tactics. Together, this complex psychosomatic interrelationship must consider both the worker's actual and perceived stress or distress.

Directly, sympatheticoadrenomedullary activity has been quantified physiologically by excretion of the cholinergic amines such as epinephrine, which is released by the adrenal cortex directly into the systemic circulation, and local release of norepinephrine. Increased release of these counterregulatory hormones is responsive to any one or combination of the aforementioned factors, internal and external. Heavy industrial labor has reported a nearly tenfold increase in epinephrine and fourfold increase in norepinephrine.[4] These values have been reportedly higher in soldiers during combat. Physical training, particularly endurance training, decreases this hypersympathetic response.[15]

The correlation between aerobic capacity and specific physical work requirements was investigated in 78 young male Brazilian workers.[18] It was found that of the 11 jobs these workers performed, a high correlation between job energy requirements and mean aerobic capacity existed. In addition, the average job metabolic rate was 35% of the estimated capacity. The jobs that were the most demanding yielded an energy expenditure above 5.0 kcal/min, with an average heart rate of 110 beats per minute. This chapter discusses the role of physical work capacity (PWC), with an emphasis on its physiologic basis and a rationale for prevention and rehabilitation of the industrial worker.

PHYSICAL WORK CAPACITY

The term *physical work capacity* recently has been used in the context of athletic performance and has been used interchangeably with a variety of acronyms such as aerobic capacity, *or* power, cardiovascular endurance and maximal oxygen uptake (Vo_2max). Figure 52–1 demonstrates all the parameters that have an impact on PWC. Classically, PWC was used in association with physical labor workers in a traditional sense.[4] Whichever the application, this value takes into account two principal factors. The first parameter, central or cardiac output, describes the delivery of substrate (glucose and fat) and oxygen to the working skeletal muscle. The second parameter, peripheral or arteriovenous O_2 (a-vo_2) difference, involves the extraction of substrate and oxygen by the working muscle.[15, 81, 82] This phenomenon is known as the Fick principle and can be expressed as the equation $Vo_2 = Q$ (cardiac output) × a-vo_2 difference. This value, Vo_2, is expressed in absolute measures of liters per minute or, more conveniently adjusted to body weight, in milliliters per kilogram per minute (Vo_2 mL/kg/min). The test for determination of Vo_2max most commonly is performed on either a treadmill or bicycle ergometer.[59, 60] Treadmill graded-exercise testing will elicit approximately a 10% greater value than leg cycle ergometry. Additionally, leg cycle ergometry will yield greater values than arm ergometry.[1] This response is explained in the additional muscle mass recruited during walking and jogging.[1, 3] Respiratory gas exchange through open circuit spirometry is generally the preferred method. Oxygen uptake can, however, be predicted from the peak exercise during the graded exercise test protocol with a reasonable degree of accuracy.[4, 5] Generally, males will produce 10% to 20% greater Vo_2max values than females when expressed relative to body weight. It appears that Vo_2max decreases after the age of 25 years by approximately 9% each decade of life. However, it is unclear as to

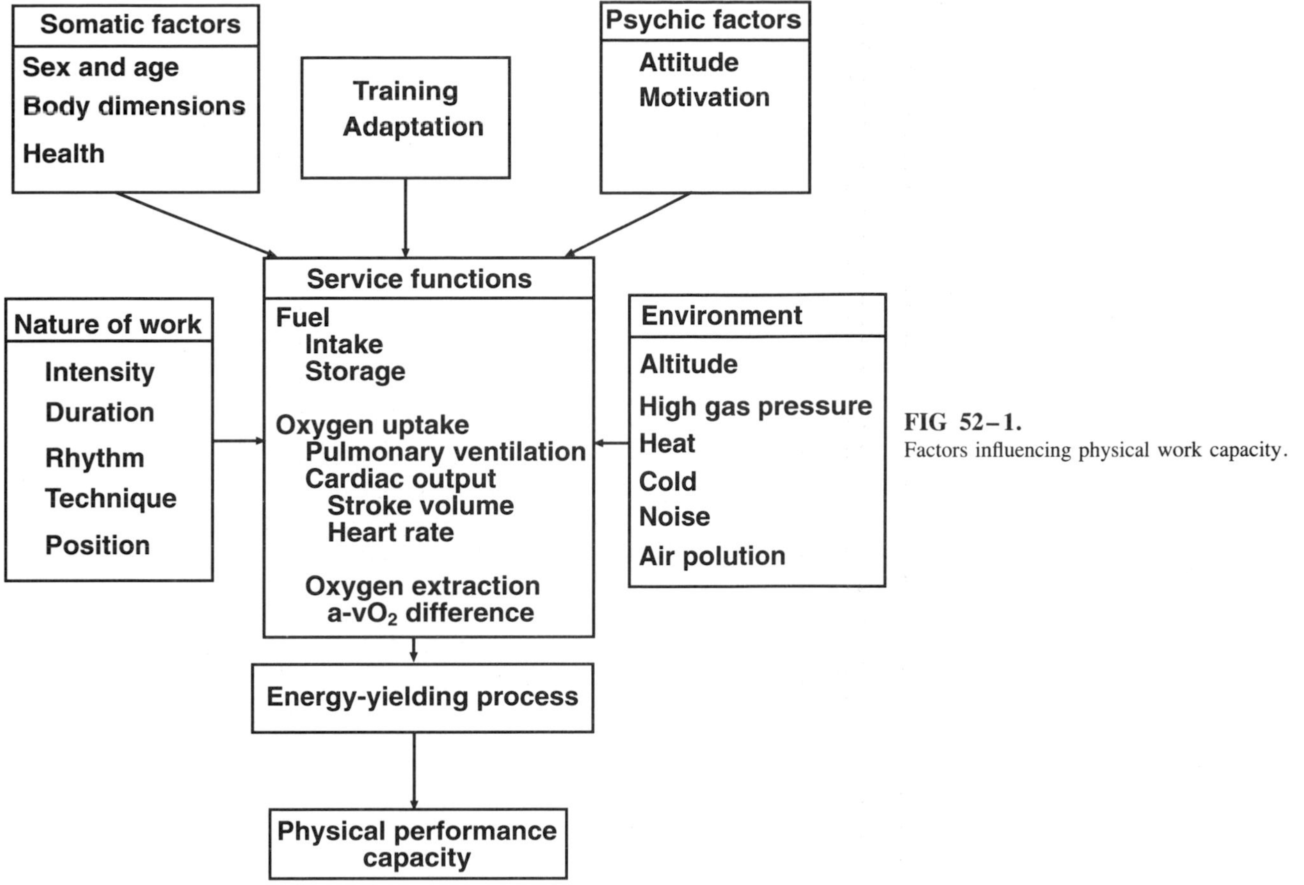

FIG 52–1.
Factors influencing physical work capacity.

whether this is a result of the natural aging process or a consequence of reduced physical activity.[2] External factors affecting Vo_2max are altitude exposure (hypoxia), air pollution, heat, and humidity. This value, which represents the ability to perform work for sustained periods of time, can be very low in deconditioned persons due to prolonged bed rest (20 mL/kg/min) and very high (greater than 80 mL/kg/min) in elite endurance athletes. Workers suffering back pain and with pathology such as herniated intervertebral discs have PWC values of 27 mL/kg/min.[14] While this measure may be genetically set within limits, it has been observed to increase on the order of 20% to 30%. More important than the worker's upper limit may be the greatest percentage of this upper limit that he maintains throughout the workday. As an example, the employee possessing a high Vo_2max but unable to maintain a high percentage of this value will fatigue quickly. Consequently, fatigue may result in poor body mechanics and predispose the individual to back injury. In contrast, the individual with a lower Vo_2max but trained specifically to enhance this system will be able to accomplish more work with less effort and resist fatigue. Hence this worker has developed a greater working efficiency explained by the equation efficiency = external work/internal work.

METABOLISM

The ability to perform physical work relies on three principal metabolic systems, two of which are anaerobic. Anaerobic energy production occurs in the absence of oxygen. High-intensity work requires high power output and utilizes phosphogens stored within muscle. Once adenosine triphosphate (ATP) is broken down to adenosine diphosphate (ADP), creatine phosphate donates a phosphate, and ATP is formed.[78] The second anaerobic system is fast glycolysis.[16] Work at high intensities lasting longer than 30 seconds relies on the breakdown of glycogen stored within the specific muscle fibers recruited. Glycolysis proceeds with the resultant formation of lactate in the absence of oxygen. Under non–steady-state conditions in which the oxygen supply does not keep up with energy demand, increased hydrogen ion accumulation decreases muscle pH. Muscle contraction will cease under these conditions. Since muscle glycogen represents a relatively small endogenous energy reserve (approximately 300 to 400 g), aerobic metabolism is necessary for prolonged work, usually greater than 3 minutes.[39, 44] It should be mentioned that lactate is formed at rest and during submaximal work; however, because production and removal are in equilibrium, hydrogen ions do not accumulate, and thus muscle pH is stable. During prolonged work such as that experienced by an industrial laborer over the course of an 8-hour day, aerobic metabolism provides the necessary energy. Oxidative metabolic pathways include the tricarboxylic acid cycle (also referred to as the Krebs' or citric acid cycle) and the electron transport chain. While the peak metabolic power output of this system is low, the total endogenous energy reserve is large.[46] The ability to utilize this pathway during submaximal exercise throughout the worker's day is essential with regard to the total substrate pool.[61] Oxygen availability is required for these processes to occur. To the industrial worker, maximizing this system is of primary concern. Intricately linked together with local metabolic processes are hormonally mediated responses as a result of sympathetic discharge. The degree of discharge varies in direct proportion to both the intensity and the muscle mass engaged in the work. Elevated plasma norepinephrine levels from sympathetic nerve terminals are observed. Catecholamine responses to exercise (epinephrine and norepinephrine) are attenuated as a response to physical training. More efficient synchronization and recruitment of neural pathways together with enhanced central and peripheral metabolic characteristics may account in part for this observation. Improved metabolic capacity of the worker will enable him to work more efficiently and with less specific and general fatigue. Table 52–1 provides a summary of the metabolic processes.

SKELETAL MUSCLE FIBER COMPOSITION

Skeletal muscle is a heterogeneous tissue that composes the greatest proportion of the human body. Its major functions are to support the skeleton and produce coordinated movements such as locomotion and various lifting tasks. Neural input to muscle via motor nerves form motor units yielding distinct functional characteristics.[16, 25, 74] Human skeletal muscle can be divided into three major types.[23, 27, 67] Type I fibers demonstrate slow contraction time, possess high oxidative capacity, and are fatigue resistant. In contrast, type IIb fibers develop rapid tension and have a fast contraction time. These fibers contain high levels of myofibrillar adenosine triphosphatase (ATPase). However as a result, these fibers fatigue quickly.[24] Type IIa fibers have fast contraction times; however, they do not appear to fatigue as quickly as type IIb fibers.[6] The metabolic characteristics of type IIa fibers have been shown to possess moderate levels of both oxidative and glycolytic enzymes. Human skeletal muscle has varying percentages of these fiber types. In addition, the distribution of these fibers varies within each muscle group and among individuals. It has been definitively determined that individuals possessing a predominance of type I over type IIb fibers excel in endurance-oriented activities.[6, 7, 24] Conversely, a dominance of type IIb fibers naturally selects individuals with greater explosive power. From this standpoint, the worker required to carry out a sustained energy output over the course of an 8-hour day would conceivably be predisposed to premature fatigue. These employees theoretically may be more vulnerable to back injury. In turn, workers required to lift heavy objects who possess a predominance of type I fibers could be at risk. The plasticity of type IIa fibers appears to respond to physical training both aerobically and anaerobically.[37, 38] Table 52–2 presents the characteristics of motor units composing human skeletal muscle.

PHYSICAL TRAINING ADAPTATIONS OF SKELETAL MUSCLE FIBERS

The training effects of aerobic exercise are well documented.[7] Mitochondria and capillary density increase as well as skeletal muscle myoglobin consequent to endurance training. There is a direct correlation between these parameters and oxidative enzymes, specifically succinate dehydrogenase and malate dehydrogenase.[43, 56] The effects of resistance training on muscle mitochondria and capillary supply is not as well defined. At this time, it has been suggested that because resistance training causes an increase in contractile protein (hypertrophy), dilution may occur.[40] The number of capillaries per fiber either remains the same or decreases.[22, 55] In terms of endurance, this would be disadvantageous. The effects of resistance train-

TABLE 52–1.
Characteristics of the Major Energy-Producing Systems*

System	Substrate	O_2 Required	Speed of ATP Mobilization	Total ATP Production Capacity
Anaerobic metabolism, ATP-CP† system	Stored phosphagens	No	Very fast	Very limited
Glycolysis	Glycogen, glucose	No	Fast	Limited
Aerobic metabolism (TCA† cycle, electron transport chain)	Glycogen, glucose, fats, protein	Yes	Slow	Essentially unlimited

*From the American College of Sports Medicine: *Guidelines for Exercise Testing and Prescription*. Philadelphia, Lea & Febiger, 1991, p 12. Used by permission.
†ATP-CP = adenosine triphosphate–creatine phoshate; TCA = tricarboxylic acid.

TABLE 52–2.
Characteristics of Motor Units in Human Skeletal Muscle*

Characteristic	Type I	Type IIa	Type IIb
Contraction time	Slow	Fast	Fast
Oxidative capacity	High	Moderate	Low
Myofibrillar ATPase† activity	Low	High	High
Stored phosphagens	Low	High	High
Glycolytic capacity	Low	Moderate	High
Fatigability	Low	Low	High

*From the American College of Sports Medicine: *Guidelines for Exercise Testing and Prescription*. Philadelphia, Lea & Febiger, 1991, p 16. Used by permission.
†ATPase = adenosine triphosphate

ing on increasing intramuscular stores of ATP and creatine phosphate have been demonstrated. While this does not increase the muscle's ability to generate force, it does increase the ability to sustain force. Glycolytic enzymatic adaptations have not been as intensively investigated. Short-term repeated isokinetic contractions have demonstrated increased activities of phosphofructokinase and lactate dehydrogenase.[79] Neural adaptation within skeletal muscle has been identified and mainly focuses on activation of the motor unit. The initial increases in strength are largely attributed to greater recruitment of motor units. Efficiency in performing tasks that require high energy output throughout the day are met primarily by neuromuscular patterning and, hence, coordinated movements. Once maximum efficiency has been attained, increases in both muscular strength and endurance are required. The metabolic characteristics of all muscles innervated by type I, IIa, and IIb motor units can be enhanced by physical training.[10] In fact, it has recently been demonstrated that with the proper intensity, duration, and frequency of the physical training stimulus, type IIb fibers take on more oxidative characteristics.[15, 73] This would result in a greater capacity to resist fatigue by utilizing a more abundant energy reserve. Consequently, less lactic acid would be produced, and muscle pH would remain within a desirable range.[27] The ability to exert force rapidly in addition to performing repetitive movements requiring enhanced endurance capacity is necessary in reducing the risk profile of the worker.

EXERCISE TESTING AND SPECIFIC TRAINING OF THE LUMBAR FLEXORS AND EXTENSORS

Specific lumbar muscular weakness has been identified as a contributing risk factor in individuals susceptible to low back injury.[54, 75, 79] These muscle groups collectively include the low back extensors, multifidus, longissimus, iliocostalis lumborum, erector spinae, and several synergists, all working in concert.[19] Lumbar flexors include the rectus abdominus, internal and external obliques, and transversalis. Identification of weakness in these muscle groups has been made possible through several commercially available dynamometers. Torques can be recorded throughout the lumbar range of motion isometrically, isotonically, and isokinetically by isolating the lumbar spine.[49, 52, 53, 83] Evaluation can be made in the sagittal and coronal planes. Pelvic stabilization and axial alignment are essential in obtaining reliable data.[31, 77] An evaluation of these muscle groups has been made in order to determine peak torque as well as dynamic muscular endurance.[66] Testing can be performed in the sitting and standing postures.[54] Values obtained have demonstrated a population-specific relationship along with a sex dichotomy. Several reports have indicated lower peak torques in patients with low back pain; however, stratification into specific diagnoses has rarely been made.[71] This would appear to make interpretation rather difficult from a clinical perspective. However, in one study, men were able to produce between 39% and 57% greater torque for the abdominals and low back extensors than women, respectively.[52] When normal individuals were collectively compared with patients with chronic low back pain, this range increased to 48% and 82%. In another study, women demonstrated greater muscular endurance than men.[66] The relationship between torque, velocity, and power with a constant resistive load was evaluated in an attempt to develop predictive models for performance within specific percentile distributions.[66] Clinical implications suggest that manual material handling can be determined within this data base with respect to torque and velocity. Although few studies reporting outcome on postsurgical patients exist, an interesting study involving 20 postoperative discectomy patients reported a 30% strength reduction.[50] The ability to quantify isolated lumbar extension and flexion strength has made it possible to accurately measure the effectiveness of various rehabilitative interventions where strength and muscular endurance deficiencies exist. The lumbar strength range of motion and pain rating were studied in 21 females and 40 males stratified into three diagnostic groups[71]: 18 with lumbar strain, 20 with herniated lumbar discs, 9 with degenerated lumbar discs, and 14 with a variety of diagnoses. After a 10-week training program of dynamic exercise, significant changes were observed in all dependent measures. It has been demonstrated that isometric training of the lumbar extensors throughout the lumbar range of motion is as effective as dynamic exercise.[41] Training frequency effects on lumbar extension isometric strength have indicated that 1 day per week elicits the same gains as 2 and 3 days per week.[80] This finding is in contrast to those reported for peripheral musculature.[9] In fact, training once every other week yielded significant results, but not to the same magnitude as one, two, or three times per week. The clinical significance here is that because normal daily activities do not encounter overloads, the lumbar extensors become weak.[49] The low training frequency initially may be adequate in increasing strength. Longer periods of recovery may be necessary initially when progressively overloading this muscle group. Limited–range-of-motion strength training may also have some carryover effect in strength training of the lumbar extensors. This may be beneficial in patients restricted in certain ranges of motion. More studies are needed with regard to the proper training dosage in patients with back dysfunction. It should be emphasized that adjusting for body weight is necessary since relative scores should be used for comparison.[21] Perhaps one of the primary goals in this population is weight loss. It has also been suggested that other variables such as activity level and age be considered when explaining individual variation. Recently, it has been proposed that fiber-type characteristics may be a predisposing risk factor in developing low back pain, and a protocol to test this hypothesis has been suggested.[32] Testing for fresh strength followed by a submaximal lumbar extension training period and then a repeat test for remaining strength may identify premature fatigability. Individuals losing a larger percentage of their initial strength may possess higher percentages of type IIb fibers. These skeletal muscle fibers characteristically fire quickly with high power output but fatigue rather quickly. On the other hand, type I fibers resist fatigue due to their greater capillary-to-fiber ratio and a more highly developed mitochondrial density. These individuals, when retested, would conceivably maintain or even gain strength on retesting. Hypothetically, this latter group, when performing repetitive lifting tasks over the course of an 8-hour day, may have a selective protection against back injuries. Translating this energy efficiency into biomechanical terms, these workers would be less likely to substitute poor lifting technique. The fact that back injuries occur in the latter part of the day may be due to either local or general fatigue. Lifting heavy objects properly requires moving the load as close as possible to the center of gravity. Bending at the knees with an alternate stance has also been suggested to decrease the high stresses on the annular fibers of the intervertebral discs. Muscular strength and endurance are perhaps the two most important physical characteristics to be developed by the industrial worker. Proper body mechanics are required in order to minimize the stress on soft-tissue structures of the spine. In fact, the loads transmitted to the lumbar spine are increased dramatically when objects are moved away from the body's center of gravity. When heavy loads are lifted properly and repeatedly, the bone mineral content will increase as a protective adaptation in addition to changes observed in muscle, ligament, tendon, and fascia. The effects of physical activity, both occupational and recreational, on the vertebral bodies and intervertebral discs of eight postmortem young men demonstrated a statistically significant positive relationship.[69] This report indicated that while both the vertebral body and intervertebral disc increase load-bearing capacities, discs appear to lag behind in the adaptation cascade. It was concluded that the discs are most vulnerable to injury in the early months after starting a physically demanding job or new recreational activity.

EXERCISE TRAINING INTERVENTIONS

The emphasis of this chapter has been, to this point, on the development of general functional capacity from a preventive standpoint. This is essential; however, from a rehabilitative perspective, identification of the specific musculoskeletal anomalies is necessary in order to gain effective restoration of functional capacity.[63] At times, this can be a relatively difficult task. Evaluation to identify dysfunction precedes treatment. This would include a complete history, recording clinical signs and symptoms, and psychological and physiologic testing when indicated. Included within the assessment should be both a static and dynamic analysis and any information gained from occupational activities that may be related to the injury. Once all pertinent information is collected, therapeutic interventions can be prescribed.

The primary goal initially is to decrease the pain enough so that functional movement can be performed. Passive treatments may be necessary to accelerate the healing process. At this time, various pain management strategies are introduced, such as transcutaneous electrical nerve stimulation (TENS), thermotherapy, cryotherapy, and neuromuscular electrical stimulation.[64] This phase, while ideally lasting less than 2 weeks, is critical in decreasing inflammation and pain as well as establishing control and patient self-confidence. At this time, education with regard to anatomy, pathophysiology, and body mechanics is emphasized. In the next phase of the rehabilitative process, the injured worker takes a more active role in recovery. Decreased use of modalities for pain relief is encouraged; neuromuscular mobilization, stabilization exercises, and the use of unloading techniques may be incorporated.[42] These exercises provide the appropriate stimulus to enhance the local muscular endurance necessary to tax the cardiovascular system. Cardiovascular exercise can be very helpful in reducing pain, anxiety, mild depression, and stress, all of which are a consequence of back dysfunction.[47, 57] Resistive exercises can be implemented for the antigravity muscles and to correct postural imbalances. Once control and biomechanical efficiency are established, the overload principle can be initiated. Generally, intensity is the variable most closely monitored in relation to duration and frequency. The American College of Sports Medicine has set forth guidelines for the development and maintenance of cardiovascular health.[2] Once the rehabilitative process is complete, these recommended guidelines are appropriate. In order to prevent future back injuries these guidelines should be followed throughout life. At this time, it appears prudent to strengthen all structures of the spine, including those supporting the spine such as the hip and leg musculature. Particular emphasis should be placed on proper lifting body mechanics, but this is beyond the scope of this chapter.

Circuit weight training and super circuit weight training have been shown to improve both cardiovascular as well as muscular strength. When compared with a standard jogging program, increased Vo_2max values were of similar magnitude.[32] Circuit weight training also improved body composition in terms of decreasing the percentage of body fat and increasing lean body mass.[33] The benefits to the worker are improved overall metabolic function. The vast majority of injured workers are overweight. It appears that a frequency of 3 days per week is adequate in terms of promoting strength and cardiovascular improvement.[35] More frequent exercise may be necessary to decrease body fat. Isotonic resistance training programs yield similar strength improvements when compared with isokinetic training.[34] However, strength gains are specific to the velocity of movement. Isokinetic strength training does not appear to cause the muscle hypertrophy that isotonic exercise does, possibly due to elimination of the eccentric component.[66]

INTENSITY

The determination of exercise intensity is most accurately derived from information acquired during a formal graded-exercise test. Patients with back injuries and pain generally have low physical work capacities. Once the pain has been reduced, the patient can be given a functional capacity test to establish a baseline that can be used as a motivational tool while monitoring progress with subsequent testing. Table 52–3 has been suggested for determining exercise intensity. Under steady-state conditions, measuring the heart rate will accurately reflect exercise intensity. The Borg scale for rating perceived exertion during exercise has been frequently used as well.[62] While more subjective, its advantage is that individuals taking β-blockers will display attenuated heart rate responses inaccurately reflecting work demand. The perceived exertion rating can be used along with heart rate measures in order to establish an accurate relationship. During the early phase of the worker's rehabilitation, the intensity should be kept low. Developing a comfortable range of motion is of primary concern. Once pain control has been established and the worker has become familiar with the type of exercise, the duration can be established. Due to the fact that poor aerobic capacity is common in patients with back pain, a multimodal exercise program may be necessary. The use of a variety of aerobic exercise modes such as leg cycle ergometry, arm ergometry, treadmill walking, and stairmaster activities may be needed to develop local muscular endurance. Weight loss is often a confounding problem. Table 52–3 presents an intensity classification of exercise based on 20 to 60 minutes of endurance training.

TABLE 52–3.

Intensity Classification of Exercise Based on 20 to 60 Minutes of Endurance Training*

HR† max (%)	Vo_2max of HR Reserve (%)	Rating of Perceived Exertion	Classification of Intensity
<35	<30	<10	Very light
35–59	30–49	10–11	Light
60–79	50–74	12–13	Moderate
80–89	75–84	14–16	Heavy
≥90	≥85	>16	Very Heavy

*Adapted from American College of Sports Medicine: *Med Sci Sports Exerc* 1990; 22:265–274.
†HR = heart rate.

MODE

The exercise type is based upon what the worker tolerates with the least amount of discomfort and will prepare him to return to work. The greater the muscle mass involved in the work, the greater the metabolic effect. This is particularly important from the standpoint that the majority of individuals with low back pain are overweight. Consistent exercise training will increase the resting metabolic rate and allow more effective weight loss. Weight loss should not exceed 1 kg/wk. Caloric expenditure is accelerated during exercise and during the postexercise recovery period.

FREQUENCY

The minimum frequency needed to improve Vo_2 has been determined to be 3 days per week.[2] Training 2 days per week does not appear to be adequate to cause a change in oxygen uptake. Frequencies greater than 5 days per week do not cause any added value. However, due to the low physical work capacities (Vo_2) evident in the patient with a low back injury, daily aerobic exercise is often necessary in order to accomplish enough work. Increased exercise frequency may be equally as important from a psychological perspective. The development of positive exercise behavior remains a primary focus in this population. The major emphasis is on increasing the volume of work done and to do it in as comfortable a manner as possible.

DURATION

Aerobic conditioning should initially last 15 minutes as tolerated by the patient. This may require the use of two or possibly three different exercise modes, in which case 5 minutes with each would suffice. The recommended minimum duration of exercise for developing and maintaining cardiovascular fitness is 20 minutes. It should be emphasized that the training adaptation is specific to the muscle groups involved in the work. Jobs that use predominantly upper-body work must be trained specifically with this objective in mind. Self-reported exercise behaviors indicate that individuals with herniated lumbar discs have reduced exercise time by more than 75%.[14] In addition, exercise frequency is reduced from 2.5 times per week to 0.5 times per week. The below-average Vo_2max values (28.9 mL/kg/min) exhibited by this group is a consequence of the aforementioned.

SUMMARY

Exercise is an important aspect of the rehabilitative process and the primary focus of preventing back injuries and pain. Workers requiring a high energy output must be able to physically produce the work efficiently. Exercise training programs must be designed specifically to enhance those physiologic systems stressed by the worker within the requirements of tasks to be performed. General conditioning serves the purpose of raising the energy-producing potential of the worker, thus providing a residual to recruit during emergency situations of high demand. Specific exercise conditioning plays a primary role in strengthening weak links in an organized structure. Efficient biomechanical movements are necessary in order to decrease abnormal stresses placed on the intervertebral discs. In addition to active participation in a formally administered exercise program, the worker will develop confidence and self-assurance that he has control over himself and increase the quality of life during leisure time activities.

REFERENCES

1. American College of Sports Medicine: *Guidelines for Exercise Testing and Prescription.* Philadelphia, Lea & Febiger. 1991, pp 11–33.
2. American College of Sports Medicine: Position stand on the recommended quantity and quality of exercise for developing and maintaining cardiorespiratory and muscular fitness in healthy adults. *Med Sci Sports Exerc* 1990; 22:265–274.
3. American Heart Association Committee on Exercise: *Exercise Testing and Training of Apparently Healthy Individuals: A Handbook for Physicians.* New York, American Heart Association, 1972, p 106.
4. Åstrand PO, Rodahl K: *Textbook of Work Physiology: Physiological Bases of Exercise.* New York, McGraw-Hill, 1977, pp 449–477.
5. Åstrand PO, Saltin B: Oxygen uptake during the first minutes of heavy muscular exercise. *J Appl Physiol* 1961; 16:971–976.
6. Barnard RJ, Edgerton VR, Farukawa T, et al: Histochemical, biochemical, and contractile properties of red, white and intermediate fibers. *Am J Physiol* 1971; 220:410–414.
7. Barnard RJ, Edgerton VR, Pefer JB: Effect of exercise on skeletal muscle I: Biochemical and histochemical properties. *J Appl Physiol* 1971; 28:401–414.
8. Battie MC, et al: A prospective study of the role of cardiovascular risk factors and fitness in industrial back pain complaints. *Spine* 1989; 14:141–147.
9. Berger RA: Comparison of static and dynamic strength increases. *Res Q* 1962; 33:329–333.
10. Bergstrom J, Hultman E: Muscle glycogen synthesis after exercise: An enhancing factor localized to the muscle cells in man. *Nature* 1966; 210:309–310.
11. Blair SN, Kohl HW, Paffenbarger RS, et al: Physical fitness and all-cause mortality: A prospective study of healthy men and women. *JAMA* 1989; 262:2395–2401.
12. Blair SN, Paffenbarger RS: Physical activity and risk of cancer. *Med Sci Sports Exerc* 1987; 19:570.
13. Bortz WM: The disuse syndrome. *West J Med* 1984; 141:691–694.
14. Brennan GP, Ruhling RO, Hood RS, et al: Physical characteristics of patients with herniated intervertebral lumbar discs. *Spine* 1987; 12:699–702.
15. Brooks GA, Fahey TD: *Exercise Physiology: Human Bioenergetics and Its Applications.* New York, John Wiley & Sons, 1984, pp 701–717.
16. Burke RE, Edgerton VR: Motor unit properties and selective involvement in movement, in Wilmore T (ed): *Exercise and Sport Science Review.* New York, Academic Press, 1975, pp 31–81.
17. Cady LD, Bischoff DP, O'Connell ER, et al: Strength and fitness and subsequent back injuries in firefighters. *J Occup Med* 1979; 21:269–272.
18. Chaffin DB, DeAraujo Couto H: Correlation of aerobic capacity of Brazilian workers and their physiologic work requirements. *J Occup Med* 1986; 28:509–513. 1986.
19. Daniels L, Worthingham C: *Muscle Testing Techniques of Manual Examination.* Philadelphia, 1980, pp 37–44. WB Saunders,
20. Davis JE, Gibson T, Tester L: The value of exercises in the treatment of low back pain. *Rheumatol Rehabil* 1979; 18:243–247.
21. Delitto A, Grandell EC, Rose S: Peak torque-to-body weight ratios in the trunk: A critical analysis. *Phys Ther* 1988; 69:138–143.
22. Dudley GA, Djamil R: Incompatibility of endurance and strength training modes of exercise. *J Appl Physiol* 1985; 59:1446–1451.
23. Eberstein D, Goodgold J: Slow and fast twitch fibers in human skeletal muscle. *Am J Physiol* 1968; 215:535–541.
24. Edstrom L, Kugelberg E: Histochemical composition, contraction speed and fatiguability of rat soleus motor units. *J Neurol Sci* 1973; 20:177–198.
25. Edstrom L, Nystrom B: Histochemical types and sizes of

fibers of normal human muscles. *Acta Neurol Scand* 1969; 45:257–269.

26. Ekelund LG, Haskell WL, Johnson JL, et al: Physical fitness as a predictor of cardiovascular mortality in asymptomatic North American men: The Lipid Research Clinic's Mortality Follow-Up Study. *N Engl J Med* 1988; 319:1379–1384.
27. Essen B, Haggmark T: Lactate concentration in type I and type II muscle fibers during muscular contraction in man. *Acta Physiol Scand* 1973; 89:374–383.
28. Farrell SW, Kohl HW, Bogdanffy GM: Incidence and reasons for medical referral in a worksite health promotion program. *Amer J Health Promotion* 1989; 3:6–10.
29. Farrell SW, Kohl HW, Rogers T: The effect of ethnicity in cardiovascular fitness. *Med Sci Sports Exerc* 1986; 18:529.
30. Farrell SW, Kohl HW, Rogers T, et al: Cardiovascular fitness and maximal heart rate differences among ethnic groups. *Med Sci Sports Exerc* 1987; 19:582.
31. Fix C, et al: Comparison of two methods of pelvic stabilization on isometric lumbar extension strength (abstract 114). *Med Sci Sports Exerc* 1990; 22:519.
32. Gettman LR, Ayres JJ, Pollock ML, et al: Physiologic effects of circuit strength training and jogging. *Arch Phys Med Rehabil* 1979; 60:115–120.
33. Gettman LR, Ayres JJ, Pollock ML, et al: The effect of circuit weight training on strength, cardiorespiratory function, and body composition of adult men. *Med Sci Sports* 1978; 10:171–176.
34. Gettman LR, Culter LA, Strathman J: Physiological changes after 20 weeks of isotonic vs. isokinetic circuit training. *J Sports Med Phys Fitness* 1980; 20:265–274.
35. Gettman LR, Pollock ML, Durstine JL, et al: Physiological responses of men to 1, 3, and 5 days per week training programs. *Res Q* 1976; 47:638–646.
36. Glisan BJ, Stith WJ, Kiser S: Physiology of active exercise in rehabilitation of back injuries. *Spine State Art Rev* 1989; 3:139–149.
37. Gollnick PD, Armstrong RB, Saltin B, et al: Effect of training on enzyme activity and fiber composition of human skeletal muscle. *J Appl Physiol* 1973; 34:107–111.
38. Gollnick PD, Armstrong RB, Saubert CW IV, et al: Enzyme activity and fiber composition in skeletal muscle of untrained and trained men. *J Appl Physiol* 1972; 33:312–319.
39. Gollnick PD, Armstrong RB, Sembrowich WL, et al: Glycogen depletion patterns in human skeletal muscle fibers during prolonged work. *Pflugers Arch* 1973; 344:1–12.
40. Gonyea WJ, Ericson GC: An experimental model for the study of exercise-induced skeletal muscle hypertrophy. *J Applied Physiol* 1976; 40:630–633.
41. Graves JE, Pollock M, Leggett S, et al: Non-specificity of limited range of motion lumbar extension strength training (abstract 13). *Med Sci Sports Exerc* 1990; 22:519.
42. Grimby G, Hook O: Physical training of different patient groups. *Scand J Rehabil Med* 1971; 3:15–25.
43. Hermansesn L, Wachtlova M: Capillary density of skeletal muscle in well-trained and entrained men. *J Appl Physiol* 1971; 30:860–863.
44. Holloszy JO: Biochemical adaptations to exercise: Aerobic metabolism. *Exerc Sport Sci Rev* 1986; 1:45–51.
45. Hurri H, Mellin G, Korhonen O, et al: Aerobic capacity among chronic low back pain patients. *J Spinal Disorders* 1991; 4:34–38.
46. Ivy JC, Costil DC, Maxwell BD: Skeletal muscle determinants of maximized aerobic power in man. *Eur J Appl Physiol* 1980; 44:1–8.
47. Jackson CP, Brown MD: Analysis of current approaches and a practical guide to prescription of exercise. *Clin Orthop* 1983; 179:46–54.
48. Jackson CP, Brown MD: Is there a role for exercise in the treatment of patients with low back pain? *Clin Orthop* 1983; 179:39–45.
49. Jones A, Pollock M, Graves J, et al: *Safe, Specific Testing and Rehabilitation Exercise for the Muscles of the Lumbar Spine*. Santa Barbara, Calif, Sequoia Communications, 1988, pp 69–74.
50. Kahonovitz N, Viola K, Gallagher M: Long-term strength assessment of postoperative diskectomy patients. *Spine* 1989; 14:402–403.
51. Kohl HW, Moorefield DL, Blair SN: Is cardiorespiratory fitness associated with general chronic fatigue in apparently healthy men and women (abstract 31): *Med Sci Sports Exerc* 1987; 19:56.
52. Langrana NA, et al: Quantitative assessments of back strength using isokinetic testing. *Spine* 1984; 9:287–290.
53. Langrana NA, Lee CK: Isokinetic evaluation of trunk muscles. *Spine* 1984; 9:171–175.
54. Linton SJ: The relationship between activity and chronic back pain. *Pain* 1985; 21:289–294.
55. MacDougall D, Sale G, Elder G, et al: Untrastructural properties of human skeletal muscle following heavy resistance training and immobilization (abstract). *Med Sci Sports Exerc* 1976; 8:72.
56. Max SR: Disuse atrophy of skeletal muscle: Loss of functional activity of mitochondria. *Biochem Biophys Res Commun* 1972; 46:1394–1398.
57. McQuade KJ, Turner JA, Buchner DM: Physical fitness and chronic low back pain: An analysis of the relationships among fitness, functional limitations, and depression. *Clin Orthop* 1988; 233:198–204.
58. Mitchell JH: Cardiovascular physiology of dynamic and static exercise. *Dallas Med J* 1976; 62:502–506.
59. Mitchell JH, Blomquist G: Maximal oxygen uptake. *N Engl J Med* 1971; 284:1018–1022.
60. Mitchell JH, et al: The physiological meaning of the maximal oxygen intake test. *J Clin Invest* 1958; 37:538–597.

60a. Mitchell RI, Carmen GM: Results of a multicenter trial using an intensive active exercise program for the treatment of acute soft tissue and back injuries. *Spine* 1990; 15:514–521.

61. Morgan TE, Cobb LA, Short FA, et al: Effects of long-term exercise on human muscle mtochondria in Pernow B, Saltin B, (eds): *Muscle Metabolism During Exercise*. New York, Plenum, 1971, pp 87–95.
62. Mihevic PM: Sensory cues for perceived exertion: A review. *Med Sci Sports Exerc* 1981; 13:150–163.

63. Muller EA: Influence of training and of inactivity on muscle strength. *Arch Phys Med* 1970; 51:449–463.
64. Nordin M, Kahanovitz, Verderame R: Normal trunk muscle strength and endurance in women and the effect of exercises and electrical stimulation. Part I: Normal endurance and trunk muscle strength in 101 women. *Spine* 1987; 12:105–111.
65. Nutter P: Aerobic exercise in the treatment and prevention of low back pain. *Spine State Art Rev* 1987; 2:137–145.
66. Pearson DR, Costill DL: The effects of constant external resistance exercise and isokinetic exercise training on work-induced hypertrophy. *J Appl Sports Sci Res* 1988; 2:39–41.
67. Pefer JB, Barnard RJ, Edgerton VR, et al: Metabolic profiles of three fiber types of skeletal muscle in Guinea pigs and rabbits. *Biochemistry* 1972; 14:2627–2633.
68. Petters RK, et al: Physical fitness and subsequent myocardial infarction in healthy workers. *JAMA* 1983; 249:3052–3056.
69. Porter RW, Adams MA, Hutton WC: Physical activity and the strength of the lumbar spine. *Spine* 1990; 14:201–203.
70. Roos R: Active treatment for patients with low back pain. *Patient Fitness* 1988; 1:5–15.
71. Russell SG, et al: Changes in isometric strength and range of motion of the isolated lumbar spine following eight weeks of clinical rehabilitation. Presented at the North American Spine Society Meeting, Monterey, Calif, August 1990.
72. Saltin B, Nazar K, Costill DC, et al: The nature of the training response, peripheral and central adaptation to one-legged exercise. *Acta Physiol Scand* 1976; 96:289–305.
73. Savard G, Kiens B, Saltin B: Central cardiovascular factors as limits to endurance; with a note on the distinction between maximal oxygen uptake and endurance. in *Fitness, Exercise Benefits, Limits and Adaptations*. 1988, pp 162–180.
74. Siva REP, McComas AJ: Fast and slow twitch units in human muscle. *J Neurol Neurosurg Psychiatry* 1971; 34:118–120.
75. Smidt G, et al: Assessment of abdominal and back extensor function: A quantitative approach and results for chronic low back patients. *Spine* 1983; 8:211–219.
76. Stith WJ, Ohnmeiss DD, Carranza C, et al: Rehabilitation of patients with chronic low back pain. *Spine State Art Rev* 1989; 3:126–136.
77. Stokes IA, Gookin DM, Reid S, et al: Effects of axis placement on measurement of isokinetic flexion and extension torque in the lumbar spine. *J Spinal Disorders* 1990; 3:114–118.
78. Taylor AW, Essen B, Saltin B: Myosin, ATPase in skeletal muscle of healthy men. *Acta Physiol Scand* 1974; 91:568–570.
79. Thorstensson A, Arvidson A: Trunk muscle strength and low back pain. *Scand J Rehabil Med* 1982; 14:69–75.
80. Tucci J, et al: Effect of reduced training frequency and detraining on lumbar extension strength (abstract 105). *Med Sci Sports Exerc* 1990; 22:518.
81. Wilmore JH, Norton AC: *The heart and Lungs at Work V: A Primer of Exercise Physiology*. Fullerton, Calif, Beckman Instruments, 1978, pp 1–14.
82. Wilson PK, Bell C, Norton AC: *Rehabilitation of the Heart and Lungs*. Fullerton, Calif, Beckman Instruments, 1980, pp 4–8.
83. Zeh J, et al: Isometric strength testing: Recommendations based on a statistical analysis of the procedure. *Spine* 1986; 11:43–46.

53

*Nutrition And Obesity**

Mary Lynn Mayfield, R.N., B.S.N.

The goals of rehabilitation of the individual who has suffered a back injury include building strength and stamina to enable the person to return to a productive and active life-style. The best nutritional preparation for the individual with a back injury is a well-balanced diet.

The patient beginning a rehabilitation program will in all likelihood still be in the healing process following the injury. When tissues are being repaired, more amino acids, carbohydrates, fats, vitamins, minerals, water, and oxygen are needed than during the normal breakdown and buildup of mature tissue. However, painful injuries are stressors.[46] Much of the disability imposed by stress is nutritional.[48] Yet, when the body is stressed, digestion and absorption of nutrients are impaired. If the stress is prolonged, the nutrient stores are also depleted.[16] Many back-injured patients have been off work and/or engaging in reduced physical activity for long periods of time while trying to cope with their physical injury; in addition, emotional, social, and economic circumstances seem to follow in the wake of the injury. When spinal surgery is required, this is a major stressor.

There are approximately 50 nutritional factors that must be continuously available to the cell to sustain life. Some of the biological compounds are synthesized by the cell from simple compounds or nutrients from outside sources.[30] A basic diet plan that can be effective in supplying these nutrients is the food guide pyramid, which was recently adopted by the U.S. Department of Agriculture as its primary device for educating the public[44] (Fig 53–1).

As long as the recommended number of servings from the variety provided in each group is supplied and cooking and handling are properly done, adequate nutrition will be attained. The dietary intake should provide a caloric distribution of approximately 55% from carbohydrates, 30% from fat, and 15% from protein (Table 53–1).

If these nutrients are not being supplied by the diet, then the question arises whether the patient should take supplements during periods of stress and healing. The answer should probably be yes. The injured patient, because of inactivity, will need to reduce caloric intake to avoid weight gain. Reduced caloric intake means a reduced supply of nutrients.

Taking a balanced vitamin/mineral supplement, not in mega doses, but in amounts comparable to the recommended daily allowance (RDA) may be necessary.[48] The delivery of nutritional substances to tissue in repair depends upon the availability from exogenous and endogenous sources, diffusion rates across capillaries, and the distance substances must travel to reach their points of use.[32] Due to the biochemical and metabolic changes after injury, the requirement for particular nutrient substances such as proteins, vitamins, and minerals is increased.[27]

Central to any discussion of the reparative responses by tissues in the spine is the topic of DNA synthesis and cell replication in the formation of epithelial, connective (cartilage, bone), muscle, and nervous tissue.[28] The tissues to be healed involve primarily connective tissues, of which collagen is most abundant. In fact, collagen is the most abundant protein in the body and accounts for over 60% of all proteins. It is the major organic component of the structural and supportive system of the body.[17, 28] Bones, discs, ligaments, tendons, and joint cartilage are classified as connective tissues. They provide mechanical support, transmit forces, and maintain the structural integrity of the body.[17] Collagen serves as the matrix on which bone is formed. Following an injury, collagen forms a scar by connecting the separated tissues together. The material that holds cells together is largely made of collagen; this function is especially important in the walls of arteries and capillaries.[48] Whether a tissue repairs with a scar as in the skin or whether it repairs with a tissue resembling the parent tissue (bone, tendon, synovial membrane, etc.), the response is cellular in the sense that either fibroblasts (which produce the scar) or specific cells (osteoblasts, chondrocytes, etc.) must be present at the local site in order to synthesize the components of the repair tissue.[28]

Collagen synthesis depends on a large number of factors, the final common denominator of all of them being circulation-infusion of the tissue to be healed. Platelets, thrombin, inflammatory cells, amino acids, vitamins, and

*Published in part in Mayfield ML, Stith WJ: The effect of nutrition on the spine in sports, in Hochschuler SH (ed): *The Spine in Sports*. Philadelphia, Hanley & Belfus, 1990, pp 54–67. Used by permission.

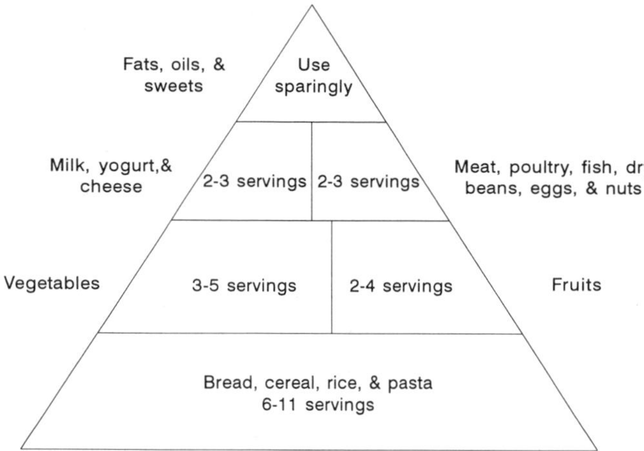

FIG 53–1.
Food group pyramid. (Adapted from United States Department of Agriculture: *Home and Garden Bulletin No. 249: Food Group Pyramid.* Washington, DC, Government Printing Office, 1990.)

minerals all reach the tissue via the microcirculation.[37] This can present a problem after injury to the cartilaginous disc since it only receives nutrition through the movement of fluid in and out of the disc space after physical activity.[23, 42]

There are no studies showing the relationship between diet and the healing of injuries to the back. However, there have been studies on the role of nutrition in wound healing and the effect of nutrient deficiencies on the human body. From this research we can make the supposition that perhaps certain nutrients, when supplied in supplemental amounts, may accelerate or at least prevent delays in the healing of back injuries.

In particular, protein deficiency delays wound healing and produces a wound with diminished tensile strength. The presence of all the essential amino acids is necessary for the synthesis of proteins such as collagen, which is a component of the majority of the spinal tissues to be healed.[13, 49] Specific amino acids identified as having an influence on wound healing include cysteine, a sulphur-containing amino acid that is thought to be an essential component of the intracellular procollagen molecule and may be required for fibroblastic proliferation. After injury, the requirement for nonessential amino acids such as arginine may increase, so a dietary supplement may be needed.[25, 36] Studies have shown that disuse after injury results in muscle atrophy reflected in an increase in urinary nitrogen content. This muscle catabolism causes a protein loss of 8 g/day.[6] Food has to replace the protein lost after injury to ensure adequate levels of protein for new tissue formation. The quality of protein is important. Animal protein must be included; for example, milk, eggs, meat, and/or cheese ensure a balance of amino acids.[11]

TABLE 53–1.
Dietary Goals for the United States

Current Diet	Recommended Diet
Fat, 42% of calories	Fat, 30% of calories
Protein, 12%	Protein, 12%
Complex carbohydrates, 22%	Complex carbohydrates, 48%
Sugar, 24%	Sugar, 10%

NUTRITIONAL FACTORS

Vitamin A

Vitamin A deficiency has been shown to retard epithelialization, closure of wounds, the rate of collagen synthesis, and the cross-linking of newly formed collagen. Another way in which vitamin A may be used in wound healing relates to its suppressive action on certain infections probably mediated by the influence of the vitamin on the thymus gland. Patients who have had prolonged interference with food intake or gastrointestinal absorption are at risk of developing vitamin A deficiency.[25, 27, 41, 49] Vitamin A is also required for bone remodeling. Some of the cells in bone formation are packed with sacs of degradative enzymes that can destroy the structure of bones. With the help of vitamin A, these cells release their enzymes. Vitamin A also helps maintain the nerve cell sheaths.[48] Only animal foods such as, milk, butter, cheese, liver, and egg yolk contain vitamin A. Dark green leafy and yellow vegetables as well as yellow fruits contain β-carotene, the precursor of vitamin A.

Vitamin B

B-complex vitamins serve as cofactors or coenzymes (small protein molecules that associate with enzymes to promote their activity in chemical reactions) in a variety of enzyme systems necessary for normal protein, fat, and carbohydrate metabolism. Although the mechanism by which the B-complex vitamins affect wound healing is poorly understood, it appears that a serious deficiency of these vitamins would interfere with repair. Deficiencies of pyridoxine, pantothenic acid, and folic acid are believed to have major effects on antibody formation and white blood cell formation.[25, 32, 37] Some of the B-complex vitamins, known as stress vitamins for their role in healing nerves, are thiamine (B_1), niacin (B_3), pyridoxine (B_6), cyanocobalamin (B_{12}), folic acid, and pantothenic acid.[48] Meat, milk, whole-grain cereals, and breads are food sources of B vitamins.

Vitamin C

The best understood of the vitamins is vitamin C (ascorbic acid), which in deficiency causes scurvy, notable for abnormal wound healing. Vitamin C has an important role in collagen formation. The amino acid used in abundance to make collagen is proline. After proline is added to the chain of amino acids, an enzyme hydroxylates it (adds an OH group) to make hydroxyproline. Vitamin C is essential for the hydroxylation step to occur. Vitamin C is also an antioxidant (a body guard for oxidizable substances), and because of its antioxidant property, it is sometimes added to food to protect important constituents. In the cells and body fluids, it helps to protect other molecules, and in the intestines, it protects ferrous iron. It also promotes the absorption of iron, important for its role in the production of red blood cells to carry oxygen in the blood. Vitamin C is also involved in the metabolism of several amino acids. The adrenal glands contain a high concentration of vitamin C, and during emotional or physical stress, they release larger quantities of the vitamin with the hormones epinephrine and norepinephrine. Vitamin C is also needed for the synthesis of thyroxin, which regulates the rate of metabolism.[48] There is no convincing evidence that wound healing is accelerated by the administration of vitamin C when tissue levels are normal. However, seriously ill or injured patients may develop ascorbic acid deficiency rapidly because it is not stored in appreciable amounts. Consequently, large doses of 1 to 2 g of ascorbic acid daily may be administered on the possibility of aiding in wound healing.[25, 32, 37, 41, 49] Citrus fruits, tomatoes, potatoes, and leafy green or yellow vegetables are the best food sources of vitamin C.

Vitamin D

Vitamin D is required for normal absorption, transport, and metabolism of calcium and phosphorus. Vitamin D is important for normal bone growth and healing.[32, 37, 41, 49] Fortified milk is the best food source, and exposure to sunlight brings about the synthesis of vitamin D.

Calcium

There is much information about the critical role of minerals in wound healing. We know that sodium, potassium, calcium, phosphorus, and chloride are essential for a wide variety of tissue functions including many necessary for tissue repair.[25, 32] Calcium regulates the transport of ions in and out of cell membranes. It is essential for muscle action and is required in many enzyme systems that are important in collagen remodeling. Vitamin D and calcium work together in the formation of bones. Calcium wastage is uniformly associated with inactivity, and both the mineral content and matrix of bone deteriorate. Bed rest results in a calcium loss of 1.54 g/week.[15] The Sky Lab astronauts lost appreciable amounts of calcium while in space.[6] Milk products are the outstanding source of calcium in the diet as well as salmon with bones, sardines, and dark green leafy vegetables.

Magnesium, Manganese, and Copper

Magnesium activates a number of enzymes involved in energy-producing cycles as well as protein synthesis. Its presence is required in all stages of healing, particularly collagen formation. Calcium and magnesium also antagonize each other in normal muscle contraction: calcium acts as a stimulator, while magnesium acts as a relaxer. Vegetables, dry beans, and seeds are good sources of magnesium. Manganese and copper are critical cofactors in collagen metabolism. Copper is also a catalyst in the formation of hemoglobin and helps to maintain the sheath around nerve fibers. Connective tissue synthesis would suffer in the presence of deficiencies of any of the minerals.[32, 36, 37] Seeds, nuts, legumes, and whole grains are good sources of manganese. Organ meats, shellfish, whole grains, legumes, and nuts are the best sources of copper.

Iron

Divalent ionic iron is required for effective collagen synthesis. It has been reported many times in the past that severe anemia seems to interfere with wound healing; however, there is debate about whether the interference in wound healing is due to anemia or to hypovolemia, vasoconstriction, trauma, and elevated blood viscosity impairing oxygen transport.[32, 36]

Of all the nutrients, the iron allowance is the most difficult to provide in the diet. Men and boys with their caloric requirements can easily meet their iron needs, but it is difficult for women and girls. Lean meats, deep green leafy vegetables, and whole-grain cereals and breads are the best sources of iron.

Zinc

Clinical evidence of impaired healing due to a deficiency of the trace elements mentioned above may be lacking. However, there have been many investigations into the role of zinc in wound healing. It is clear that zinc deficiency has adverse effects on the rate of epithelialization and the rate of gain of wound strength and that it decreases collagen strength. Zinc is an important cofactor in a variety of enzyme systems responsible for cellular proliferation such as the biosynthesis of RNA, DNA, and collagen. Zinc deficiency may also interfere with wound healing because it is needed in the metabolism of vitamin A. There is controversy as to whether administering supplemental zinc can accelerate healing to an above-normal rate. As noted earlier, excessive amounts of zinc may displace copper, which is needed in covalent cross-linkages in young collagen. Zinc deficiency is rare but may occur in patients who have suffered severe injury, infection, disorders of the digestive tract, or prolonged unsupplemented intravenous hyperalimentation. Oral zinc sulfate corrects zinc deficiency readily.[32, 36, 41, 49] As with many nutrients, the absorption and utilization of zinc is influenced by the composition of the diet as a whole. Excessive intake of fiber such as bran can reduce the absorption of zinc. Meat is a good source of zinc and enhances its absorption and utilization by the body.[11]

The injured patient in rehabilitation will need food to meet the energy demands of exercise. Carbohydrates, fats, and protein are the primary sources of energy to the body; however, fats and carbohydrates are the two major energy sources used during exercise. Either source can be predominant, depending upon the duration and intensity of the exercise, the degree of prior physical conditioning, and the composition of the diet in the days prior to the exercise. It is assumed that the average person will use a certain number of kilocalories from protein and then use the remaining kilocalories from carbohydrates and fats to meet energy needs.[48] Work performed under anaerobic conditions will favor fat oxidation, whereas work performed under aerobic conditions will be supported mainly by carbohydrate oxidation.[3] In the past, protein has been promoted for enhancing physical activity and supplying extra energy. The RDA for protein intake is 0.8 g/kg of body weight. Proteins are extremely complex nitrogenous compounds consisting of amino acids. Amino acids supply the materials for repair, growth, and building of new tissue. Intakes above requirement are either burned for energy to support activity or converted to fat. Excess protein is wasted protein since carbohydrates and fats can supply adequate energy.[48] Provided that the energy intake is sufficient to maintain body weight, the normal dietary intake of protein is adequate.[14] This is particularly true since the protein intake of the average American diet exceeds the recommended protein requirement.[5] If patients in rehabilitation base their diet on the food guide pyramid plan presented in Figure 53–1[44] and their dietary intake follows the recommended distribution of nutrients (see Table 53–1), they will be able to meet the energy demands for exercise.

OBESITY AND WEIGHT CONTROL

A particular concern in rehabilitation and a very common problem after spinal injury is obesity. In many instances, the obesity preceded the injury and may have even contributed to its occurrence. We know that too much fat is associated with loss of endurance[40] and that there is a greater incidence of work-related injuries toward the end of the workday. It has been shown that excess weight adds stress to the spine. For every pound of excess weight added to the waistline, 5 lb of additional pressure are placed on the spine. This occurs because the muscles of the abdomen are not properly supporting the vertebrae of the lower part of the back. The "rubber tire" syndrome, which pulls the spine forward, causes increased tension in the lower back musculature and also stretches the ligaments that hold the spine together.[19]

The association of obesity with musculoskeletal morbidity or low back pain has been addressed in several investigations.[4, 47] Most of these studies come to conflicting conclusions.[33, 34] Similar studies describing the association of obesity with acute lumbar herniated nucleus pulposus are conflicting.[22, 26] However, Hannigan et al. in a study of patients who underwent surgical treatment for the relief of sciatica confirm an earlier study by Weir that obese patients are overrepresented among patients with acute sciatica.[20, 45]

Table 53–2 shows acceptable weight ranges for most adults.[43] An individual's ideal weight is generally found within the range for his sex and height.[47] If someone has been obese since childhood, it may be difficult to reach or to maintain weight within the acceptable range. Generally speaking, a person's weight should not exceed what it was at age 20 to 25 years.

Obesity also affects normal body mechanics by making it more difficult to sit, stand, and walk. Obesity, defined as 20% to 30% over proper weight, increases the time required to recover from an injury. Fat tissue is a stress on the body even when a person is not injured. It decreases the flow of blood carrying nutrients for healing

TABLE 53–2.
Suggested Weights for Adults*

Height†	Weight (lb)‡	
	19–34 yr	≥ 35 yr
5′0″	97–128	108–138
5′1″	101–132	111–143
5′2″	104–137	115–148
5′3″	107–141	119–152
5′4″	111–146	122–157
5′5″	114–150	126–162
5′6″	1118–155	130–167
5′7″	121–160	134–172
5′8″	125–164	138–178
5′9″	129–169	142–183
5′10″	132–174	146–188
5′11″	136–179	151–194
6′0″	140–184	155–199
6′1″	144–189	159–205
6′2″	148–195	164–210
6′3″	152–200	168–216
6′4″	156–205	173–222
6′5″	160–211	177–228
6′6″	164–216	182–234

*Adapted from United States Department of Agriculture: *Home and Garden Bulletin No. 232*. ed 3. Washington, DC, Government Printing Office, 1990.

†Without shoes.

‡Without clothes; the higher weights in the range generally apply to men, who tend to have more muscle and bone; the lower weights often apply to women, who have less muscle and bone.

to the injured area.[35] Obesity also makes rehabilitation more difficult for the back-injured patient since poor endurance and cardiovascular fitness, often associated with obesity, may hinder full participation in therapy.[40]

The patient entering a rehabilitation program has an excellent opportunity to start a successful weight loss program because of the increased activity and exercise encountered during rehabilitation.

The ideal method of weight loss is decreasing caloric intake while increasing energy expenditure, i.e., reducing caloric intake by 500 to 1000 calories/day and simultaneously adding an energy expenditure of 300 to 500 calories/day.[40] Starvation or extremely low-calorie diets are not recommended[18] because of the effect on the metabolic rate.[7] It is not clear what metabolic adaptations are responsible, but studies have shown that there is a reduction in the resting or basal metabolic rate when calories are greatly restricted. The findings of Mole et al. suggest that there are benefits to incorporating moderately intense, daily exercise into a regimen of caloric restriction to enhance the loss of body fat.[29] Aerobic exercise in particular lowers glycogen stores and, when accompanied by a low-fat diet, mobilizes the body's fat deposits for fuel.[9] Exercise alone, without caloric restriction, is probably insufficient to yield significant fat loss except in individuals who are extremely motivated to commit themselves to prolonged workouts over a long period of time.[38]

It is the combination of caloric restriction, low dietary fat, and increased aerobic physical activity that reduces body fat. Exercise is one of the few factors positively correlated with successful long-term maintenance of body weight.[10]

Low dietary fat is an important element in weight reduction. Several studies suggest that dietary fat is processed more efficiently, i.e., requires less energy to metabolize than other constituents of the diet.[39] Increased oxygen consumption after ingesting food was first reported by Seguin and Lariosier in 1789, and Rubner in 1902 noted that both carbohydrates and protein had greater effects upon heat production than did fat.[30] The American Heart Association diet is an excellent reference in designing a low-fat diet.[1] However, the low-fat diet was not developed by the American Heart Association but originated during the 1950s by Pritikin, who was not a doctor. The average American consumes 40% to 50% of his calories from fat sources. Many health authorities recommend cutting this down to 30% (see Table 53–2). In Pritikin's program for diet and exercise, it is recommended that fat in the diet be restricted to 5% to 10%. A diet high in fat suffocates tissues by depriving them of oxygen, contributes to atherosclerosis and gout by raising the level of cholesterol and uric acid in the tissues, impedes carbohydrate metabolism, and can foster diabetes.[35] It is recommended that saturated fats (animal products) be limited and polyunsaturated fats be substituted when possible.[5, 35]

The typical dairy-vegetarian diet combining vegetable sources of protein, grains, beans, nuts, and seeds with dairy products and eggs is generally low in fat and has twice as much dietary fiber as the normal American diet, and vegetarians do appear to be leaner.[24]

In a weight loss program it is wise to choose high-fiber foods as often as possible. High-fiber foods are filling. Fiber holds food in the stomach longer, slows down calorie absorption, prevents a rapid rise in blood sugar, and staves off hunger.[24] Wheat bran is an insoluble fiber that speeds up elimination. Oats and fruits such as apples are soluble fiber that bind with fats like cholesterol and carry them out of the body.[2] About one third of the calories in high-fiber foods are excreted undigested as food residue.

Complex carbohydrates are also a very important part of a weight loss program. They are starchy foods (potatoes, rice, pasta, bread, some vegetables, and fruits) that have the reputation for resulting in weight gain. Actually, they fulfill both the psychological and physical need for food. They fill the stomach, "stick to your ribs," while providing something to chew. In the case of fruits, they can satisfy a sweet craving without overloading calories. If the carbohydrates come from whole grains, fruits, and vegetables, bulk and bowel regularity are provided by noncaloric fiber.[8]

An increase in water consumption should be an important part of any weight loss regimen. Water is essential to performance of functions vital to maintaining life such as digestion, excretion, and cooling. Everything in the body occurs in a water medium, and an individual can only survive a few days without water. The kidneys need water to remove wastes such as uric acid, urea, and lactic acid, and if there is not enough water, the kidneys can be damaged. Water is also vital to digestion and metabolism. It acts as a medium for various enzymatic and chemical reactions in the body and carries nutrients and oxygen to the cells through the blood; water also lubricates joints. This is particularly important in musculoskeletal problems, arthritis, and athletics. Water is even required for breathing since the lungs must be moistened to facilitate the intake of oxygen and excretion of carbohydrates. Each individual loses approximately a pint of liquid each day just exhaling.

Proper water intake is the key to weight loss. If those who are trying to lose weight do not drink enough water, the body cannot metabolize the fat, and fluid is retained, which keeps weight up and thus destroys the weight loss efforts.

If the kidneys are overloaded, they put part of their load on the liver. The liver is charged with metabolism of fat and will be unable to do its work if it has had to take on part of the load from the kidneys.

The minimum amount of water a healthy person should drink is ten 8-oz glasses a day. Overweight people should drink an extra glass for every 25 lb exceeding their normal weight.[31]

Simple carbohydrate foods to avoid are white flour, white rice, refined sugar, sugar-coated cereals, processed fruit products, and overcooked vegetables. These are foods in which milling, refining, processing, and cooking have removed much of the fiber, vitamins, minerals, and starch; what is left is a little starch and a lot of sugar.[12]

In the rehabilitation of patients with back injuries, nutrition for healing and stress management, meeting energy requirements for exercise, and weight maintenance or weight loss should be emphasized. Optimal nutrition is gained by patients following a regimen of eating from the food group pyramid daily. Additional dietary guidelines are presented in Table 53–3. The patient should adhere to dietary guidelines that provide 5% of calories from carbohydrates, 12% from protein, and 30% from fat. Following a sound dietary plan will provide nutrients for healing, energy, and weight control to enable the patient to return to a productive life-style.

TABLE 53–3.

Dietary Guidelines for Americans: Suggestions for Food Choices*

1. *Eat a variety of foods.* Include the following foods every day: fruits and vegetables; whole-grain and enriched breads and cereals and other products made from grains; milk and milk products; meats, fish, poultry, and eggs; dried peas and beans.
2. *Maintain healthy weight.* Increase physical activity; control overeating by eating slowly, taking smaller portions, and avoiding "seconds"; eat fewer fatty foods and sweets and less sugar, drink fewer alcoholic beverages, and eat more foods that are low in calories and higher in nutrients.
3. *Choose a diet low in fat, saturated fat, and cholesterol.* Choose low-fat protein sources such as lean meats, fish, poultry, and dry peas and beans; use eggs and organ meats in moderation; limit intake of fats on and in foods; trim fats from meats; broil, bake, or boil—do not fry; limit breaded and deep-fried foods; read food labels for fat content.
4. *Choose a diet with plenty of vegetables, fruits, and grain products.* Substitute starchy foods for foods high in fats and sugars; select whole-grain breads and cereal, fruits and vegetables, dried beans, and peas to increase fiber and starch intake.
5. *Use sugars only in moderation.* Use less sugar, syrup, and honey; reduce concentrated sweets such as candy, soft drinks, and cookies; select fresh fruits or fruits canned in light syrup or their own juices; read food labels—sucrose, glucose, dextrose, maltose, lactose, fructose, syrups, and honey are all sugars. Eating less sugar also helps to reduce dental caries.
6. *Use salt and sodium in moderation.* Learn to enjoy the flavors of unsalted foods; flavor foods with herbs, spices, and lemon juice; reduce salt in cooking; add little or no salt at the table; limit salty foods like potato chips, pretzels, salted nuts, popcorn, condiments (soy sauce, steak sauce, and garlic salt), some cheeses, pickled foods and cured meats, and some canned vegetables and soups; read food labels for sodium or salt contents, especially in processed and snack foods; use lower-sodium products when available.
7. *If you drink alcoholic beverages, do so in moderation.* For individuals who drink, limit all alcoholic beverages (including wine and beer) to one or two drinks per day. One drink is defined to be 12 oz. of beer, 3 oz. of wine, or 1.5 oz. of distilled spirits. Pregnant women should not use alcohol at all. If you drink, do not drive.

*From U.S. Department of Agriculture, U.S. Department of Health and Human Services; *Nutrition and Your Health, Dietary Guidelines for Americans,* ed 3. (Washington, DC, Government Printing Office, 1990).

REFERENCES

1. American Heart Association: *American Heart Association Diet:* Austin, Tex, American Heart Association. Austin, Texas.
2. Anderson J, Sieling B, Chen W: *Professional Guide to HCF Diets.* Lexington, Ky HCF Diabetes Research Foundation, 1981.
3. Askew E: Role of fat metabolism in exercise. *Clin Sports Med* 1984; 3:605–621.
4. Bergenudd H, Nilsson B, Uden A, et al: Bone mineral content, gender, body posture and build in relation to back pain in middle age. *Spine* 1989; 14:577–579.
5. Berger SM: *How to be Your Own Nutritionist.* New York, William Morrow, 1987, pp 62–74, 113–118.
6. Bortz W: The disuse syndrome. *West J Med* 1984; 141:691–694.
7. Bray G: Effect of calorie restriction on energy expenditure in obese patients. *Lancet* 1969; 2:397–398.
8. Brody J: *Jane Brody's Good Food Book.* New York, WW Norton, 1985, pp 20–25, 129.
9. Bielinkski R, Schutz Y, Jequier E: Energy metabolism during the post-exercise recovery in man. *Am J Clin Nutr* 1985; 42:69–82.
10. Brownell K, Marlett G, Lichtenstein E, et al: Understanding and preventing relapse. *Am Psychol* 1986; 41:765–782.
11. Burchill P: Wound care: Body builders. *Community Outlook* 1986; 19–28.
12. Davis M, Eshelman E, McKay M: *The Relaxation and Stress Reduction Workbook.* Oakland, Calif, New Harbinger Publications, 1982.
13. Dickhaut S, Delee J, Page C: Nutritional status: Importance in predicting wound healing after amputation. *J Bone Joint Surg [Am]* 1984; 66:71–75.
14. Dohm GL: Protein nutrition for the athlete. *Clin Sports Med* 1984; 3:595–604.
15. Donaldson CL, Hulley SB, Vogel SM, et al: Effect of prolonged bedrest on bone mineral. *Metabolism* 1970; 19:1071–1084.
16. Fox A, Fox B: *DLPA.* New York, Pocket Books, 1985, pp 40–45.
17. Gamble J: *The musculoskeletal system.* New York, Raven Press, 1988, pp 57, 58, 81.
18. Grandjean A: Nutrition for swimmers. *Clin Sports Med* 1986; 5:65–76.
19. Hall H: *The Back Doctor.* New York, Berkley Books, 1980, pp 232–233.
20. Hanningan W, Elwood P, Henderson JP, et al: Surgical results in obese patients with sciatica. *Neurosurgery* 1987; 20:896–899.

22. Heliovaara M: Body height, obesity and risk of herniated lumbar intervertebral disc. *Spine* 1987; 12:469–472.
23. Holm S, Nachemson A: Variations in the nutrition of the canine intervertebral disc induced by motion. *Spine* 1983; 8:866–874.
24. Jennings-Sauer C: *Living Lean by Choosing More*. Dallas, Taylor Publishing, 1989, pp 80–82.
25. Keithley J: Wound healing in malnourished patients. *Am Op Room News J* 1982; 35:1094–1099.
26. Kelsey J: An epidemiological study of acute herniated lumbar intervertebral discs. *Rheumatol Rehabil* 1975; 14:144–150.
27. Levenson S, Seiffer E: Dysnutrition, wound healing, and resistance to infection. *Clin Plast Surg* 1977; 4:375–388.
28. Mankin H: The articular cartilages, cartilage healing, and osteoarthrosis, in Cruess R, Rennie W (eds): *Adult Orthopedics*. New York, Churchill Livingstone, pp 163–270.
29. Mole PA, Stern JS, Schultz CL, et al: Exercise reverses depressed metabolic rate produced by severe caloric restriction. *Med Sci Sports Exerc* 1989; 21:29–33.
30. Oscai LB, Miller WC: Dietary-induced severe obesity: Exercise implications. *Med Sci Sports Exerc* 1985; 18:6–9.
31. Perry LR: *Are You Drinking Enough Water?* Los Angeles, Foundation for Athletic Research and Education–International Sports Medicine Institute, 1990.
32. Pollack S: Wound healing: A review. III Nutritional factors affecting wound healing. *J Dermatol Surg Oncol* 1979; 5:615–619.
33. Pope M, Bevins T, Wilder D, et al: The relationship between anthropometric, postural, muscular and mobility characteristics of males ages 18–55. *Spine* 1985; 10:644–648.
34. Pope M, Rosen J, Wilder D, Frymoyer J: The relation between biomechanical and psychological factors in patients with low-back pain. *Spine* 1980; 5:173–178.
35. Pritikin N: *The Pritikin Program for Diet and Exercise*. New York, Grosset & Dunlap, 1979, pp 9–14.
36. Ruberg R: Role of nutrition in wound healing. *Surg Clin North Am* 1984; 64:705–714.
37. Schrock T, Cerra F, Hawley P, et al: Wounds and wound healing. *Dis Colon Rectum* 1982; 25:1–15.
38. Segal K, Pi-Sunyer X: Exercise and obesity. *Med Clin North Am* 1989; 73:217–236.
39. Simoppoulos A: Nutrition and fitness. *JAMA* 1989; 261:2862–2863.
40. Smith N: Nutrition and the athlete. *Orthop Clin North Am* 1983; 14:387–396.
41. Smith R: Recovery and tissue repair. *Br Med Bull* 1985; 41:295–301.
42. Urban J, Holm S, Maroudas A, et al: Nutrition of the intervertebral disc. *Clin Orthop* 1982; 170:296–302.
43. United States Department of Agriculture: *Home and Garden Bulletin No. 232: Suggested Weights for Adults* Washington, DC, Government Printing Office, 1990.
44. United States Department of Agriculture: *Home and Garden Bulletin No. 249: Food Group Pyramid*. Washington, DC, Government Printing Office, 1990.
45. Weir B: Prospective study of 100 lumbosacral discectomies. *J Neurosurg* 1979; 50:283–289.
46. Weiss M, Troxel R: Psychology of the injured athlete. *Athletic Training* 1986; 154:104–109.
47. White A, Panjabi M: *Clinical Biomechanics of the Spine*. Philadelphia, JB Lippincott, 1978, pp 329–336.
48. Whitney E, Hamilton E: *Understanding Nutrition*. St Paul, Minn, West Publishing, 1987.
49. Williams C: Wound healing: A nutritional perspective, in *Nursing*, ed 7. Philadelphia, Bailliere Tindall, 1986, pp 249–251.

54

Business Considerations in Establishing a Work Rehabilitation Center

Tommy Clark, M.B.A.

MARKETING A WORK HARDENING PROGRAM

A product or service has four basic stages to its life—introduction, growth, maturity, and decline. In my opinion, work hardening is approaching the end of the introductory stage and entering a period of rapid growth. It is therefore an appropriate time to examine the service of work hardening to make sure its purpose is meaningful in terms of the society it serves. This process of self-examination is a fundamental component of marketing.

What is marketing and why do we need it anyway? Marketing is one of the most necessary and basic processes at work in our society today. It is the link between society's needs and wants and the producers who try to fulfill them. Without marketing, producers would not know what consumers wanted, and consumers would not know what producers had. Actually, marketing was first introduced in Japan around 1650 by a merchant named Mitsui. The man who westernized the concept is more widely know as the inventor of a mechanical harvester. Cyrus McCormick brought the basic tools of marketing to the West in the mid-1800s—market research, customer satisfaction, and pricing policies. Since then, marketing has grown and expanded into the foundation for all consumer activity in the free world. It is common to confuse marketing with selling or advertising because while both selling and advertising are components of marketing, it is much, much more. In the book *Marketing Myopia,* Levitt has drawn a sharp contrast between the two:

> Selling focuses on the needs of the seller; marketing on the needs of the buyer. Selling is preoccupied with the seller's need to convert his product into cash; marketing with the idea of satisfying the needs of the customer by means of the product and the whole cluster of things associated with creating, delivering and finally consuming it.

At this point in the product life cycle of work hardening, rather than focus on traditional elements of marketing such as advertising and promotion, the critical issues surrounding work hardening are much more fundamental. Work-hardening programs must first concern themselves with what society needs, how best to deliver it, and who is going to buy it. These are the issues I hope to shed light on in this chapter.

Although there are many different marketing concepts that can be applied across an endless spectrum of products and target markets, the concept that seems to best enhance the appropriate approach to a work-hardening program is the *societal marketing concept*. The societal marketing concept holds that the organization's task is to determine the needs, wants and interests of target markets (the consumer) and to deliver the desired satisfactions more effectively and efficiently than competitors in a way that preserves or enhances the consumer's and society's well-being or, in more simple terms, (1) determine who the customer is, (2) find out what he needs, and (3) satisfy that need better than anyone else. Although the terms may be simple, the task of determining those fundamental elements necessary to create a successful work-hardening program represents a formidable endeavor.

First we identify our customer. For many products, the customer is fairly easy to identify. Men normally choose their own golf clubs, and women normally choose their lipstick. On the other hand, the purchase of work-hardening therapy involves a decision-making "unit" consisting of more than one person. Consider the purchase process:

1. The patient is injured and selects (or is referred to) a primary-care physician for treatment.
2. That primary-care physician may refer the patient to a specialist.
3. The specialist (or the primary-care physician) may decide to refer the patient into a work-hardening program.
4. The patient has the ultimate choice of accepting or not accepting the recommendation.
5. Assuming the patient enters the program, the in-

surance company is then notified in order to get authorization for payment of the services.
6. Behind the scenes, there may be other influencers such as the spouse or an attorney.

Thus we can distinguish several roles that different people might play in the purchase decision:

Initiator.—The initiator is the person who first thinks of the idea of purchasing a product or a service. In this case, the initiator will most likely be the physician; however, it could also be the insurance company, a rehabilitation consultant, the company the patient works for, or for that matter, the patient himself.

Gatekeeper.—A gatekeeper is one who has the power to control the flow of information from producer to consumer. In this case, if the physician or someone else does not tell the patient about work hardening, he is unlikely to seek it out. The primary gatekeeper in work hardening is clearly the physician.

Influencer.—An influencer is a person whose views or advice carries some weight in making the final decision. In this case, an influencer might be the spouse, attorney, or perhaps a friend.

Decider.—The decider is the person who ultimately determines some key part of the buying decision: whether to buy, what to buy, and where to buy it. In the case of work hardening, deciders include the physician or the rehabilitation consultant, the insurance company, and the patient, who can ultimately decide whether or not to accept delivery.

Buyer.—The buyer is the person who makes the actual purchase. In the case of work hardening, if you define "makes the actual purchase" as payment, the insurance company is clearly the primary buyer. However, we must also recognize that under this definition, business is the *ultimate* buyer.

User.—The user is the person who ultimately consumes or uses the product or service. In this case, the patient is the user.

Who then, is the customer? Recognizing these different roles in the purchase process is critical in the management of the marketing efforts. In an attempt to embrace the basic tenets of marketing—determining the customer's needs and meeting them—we must recognize the complexity of this purchase process and assume that we have multiple customers. The following are the *goals* each potential "customer" would hope to achieve through a work-hardening program:

1. The *physician* is the primary link between the work-hardening program and a patient referral. One might say that the process of getting a patient into work hardening starts with the physician. Therefore, the physician is an initiator, gatekeeper, and influencer within the purchase process, three very key roles concentrated in one person. What is it that a physician expects to achieve by referring a patient into a work-hardening program? Generally speaking, the referrals that come into work hardening from physicians are prolonged, chronic cases that have failed to successfully respond to other treatment methods. The physician views a work-hardening program as a concentrated effort to break the destructive cycle of an injury, get the patient better, and return him to a productive life-style with a reduced risk of reinjury. In brief, the physician expects *patient improvement*.

2. The *insurance company* plays the role of both a decider and a buyer. Clearly insurance companies have significant influence over where the patient goes for treatment, how much is spent, and in some states, whether the treatment is purchased at all. Again, the insurance company plays a critically important role in the purchase process. What does an insurance company expect from the program? While there is no doubt that patient improvement is an important goal for insurance companies, you can be sure that they want the most cost-effective treatment plan to achieve it. They want what they are paying for—an outcome that mitigates the overall cost of the injury. The particular outcome necessary to accomplish this may be different from state to state depending on workermen's compensation laws; however, generally speaking, it will involve a safe, early, and prolonged return to work and/or reaching maximum medical improvement as defined by the state.

3. The *patient* is a decider in that he can refuse to accept delivery of the service (which shows up in a program statistic called "noncompliance"), and he is also the end user of the service. So, what is it that the patient expects from a work-hardening program? The truth is, different patients probably expect different things; however, universal goals might be such things as feeling better (reduced pain or pain management), overcoming the fear of reinjury, and returning to a productive life-style while recognizing that at this point there will likely be a severe disruption in their life.

4. Another customer is *business*. Although in many states companies have very little to say about the treatment of an injured patient, as the ultimate "buyer" of the service, I would expect their role to increase over time. What, then, would industry expect from a work-hardening program? To answer this, we must recognize that companies have both a financial and emotional motive for seeing an injured patient get better. Undoubtedly, companies are interested in seeing the injured patient get better; however, they also recognize that an injured patient represents a significant financial exposure. The company's agenda would

be similar to the insurance company's: restore the injured patient to a productive life-style by the most cost-effective treatment plan possible.

This examination of the purchase process and the "customer's" needs makes it clear that there is an extremely varied agenda when it comes to a work-hardening program. Is it possible, in a complex market like this, to focus on just one customer and ignore the others? Say, for instance, focus one's marketing efforts strictly on physicians? Ask the question another way. Is it possible to respond to the needs of only one of these "customers" and ignore the needs of the others? Will a particular program succeed in the long term if it "makes the patient better," which satisfies the physician's expectations of work hardening, but ignores the cost/benefit aspect of the program so critical to the insurance companies and industries? The answer is obviously no. If one is to successfully compete in the marketplace, it is imperative that the product be designed to respond to the specific needs of the whole *customer group* and society's needs in general.

Fundamentally, the "product" of work hardening is a service as opposed to some other type of product such as durable goods. A service is a benefit that one party can offer another that is essentially intangible and does not result in the ownership of anything. Most "medical" treatments fall in this category of product. Now that the variety of needs and expectations involved with the customer group have been explored, the single most important and comprehensive service provided by the program must be selected as the "product." Is it return to work? Is it making the patient better? Is it cost containment for the insurance company?

To determine this, one needs to understand the different levels of a product. The most fundamental level is the *core product,* which answers the question, what is the buyer really buying? The secondary level is the *tangible product,* which includes the components of quality, features, packaging, and brand name. And finally there is the *augmented product,* which is made up of other benefits and features. Therefore, we must determine which services provided by work hardening represent the core product, the tangible product, and the augmented product. Only then will we know how to design our product and present it to the marketplace.

To determine the core product, let's look at the service by definition. What service is the *buyer* (we defined the buyer as the insurance company and secondarily as industry) really *buying?* In this case, what the buyer is really buying is the expectation that the service of work hardening will "pay for itself" by reducing the overall cost of the injury by a dollar amount equal to or greater than the cost of the service. They are buying a form of therapy that, unlike other traditional therapies, must by definition be cost-effective. This is not to say that patient improvement is unimportant. On the contrary, it is only pointing out that the "niche" work hardening has carved out for itself is more of a cost-benefit than a patient care service, and that is how its success or failure will be judged. In fact, selecting the cost-benefit to the buyer as a core product works well since it is the only one of the services provided by work hardening that is comprehensive. That is to say, in order for the service to be cost-effective and reduce the overall injury costs, certain other components are implicit. Patients *must* be improved, they *must* return to a productive life-style, and they *must* be reasonably conditioned against reinjury. Otherwise, the core product, as we have defined it, simply cannot be delivered.

The selection of cost containment as a core product draws into sharp focus one of the major problems in marketing a work-hardening program—verification. The cost management of a work-related injury is often left to a number of parties and is complicated by fragmented accounting and many times clouded by emotional and legal issues that have little to do with the result of the medical treatment. By choosing cost containment as a core product rather than patient improvement, work hardening has positioned itself to be objectively vs. subjectively measured. For this reason, a fundamental component of successfully marketing a program must be a credible program evaluation system and a case management process that allows outcome analysis on an after-the-fact basis.

This brings us to the tangible product. The tangible product is the more visible, commercially exploitable component containing such elements as packaging, brand name, features, quality, and styling. Charles Revson of Revlon, Inc., distinguished between the core and tangible product: "In the factory, we make cosmetics; in the stores, we sell hope." The tangible products of a work-hardening program might be things such as the type of equipment utilized, the design or locations of the clinics, the quality or accreditation of the program, the multidisciplinary nature of the treatment plan, the frequency or nature of the reports, or the brand name associated with the program. The tangible aspects of a product, unlike the core product, can be plural and measured in subjective terms. The tangible products are the "icing on the cake." In markets with relatively generic products, tangible components are often the most visible points of differentiation among competitors.

The augmented products of a work-hardening program may include such things as patient follow-up or extended care, "graduation" awards, and program reports. They are largely viewed as extra benefits or values added.

Marketing, as we have already discussed, is a process through which society's needs are determined and producers meet those needs. We have carefully examined the needs of our target market group as well as the components of the product. It is now time to look into structuring the product to meet those needs and promoting it in the marketplace.

Since work hardening is a people-based service, we start the design of our program by understanding that service products are fundamentally very different from physical products. Four primary characteristics of services are (1) intangibility, (2) inseparability, (3) variability, and (4) perishability. Second, the design of a work-hardening program must start with the treatment definition of a particular program. In other words, at what stage of the injury recovery does the program administer care—acute, subacute, or chronic.

First, since services are intangible in that they cannot be seen, felt, tasted, or heard prior to purchase, once must realize that the consumer has to have faith in the provider of the service. For providers of work hardening, this means that increasing the tangibility of the service will help patients understand the treatment and will result in their being more confident and enthusiastic about the program. Tangibility can be added in a variety of ways such as brochures and pamphlets, orientation videos introducing the program, taking a potential candidate through the clinic to let him see the facility, or even showing him photographs of other patients in treatment. Another way of providing tangibility would be to discuss the benefits of the service with the patient prior to entry in the program. Discussing such things as feeling better, getting back to work, and overcoming the pain associated with back injuries helps to make the product more tangible and should help to motivate the patient as well.

Second, unlike a physical product that exists on its own, a service is inseparable from its source. This has implications for staffing a program to make sure that patients are receiving consistent treatment from day to day. It is absolutely critical to the success of a program that the quality of the program be maintained day after day at all patient levels. Obviously, the larger a program intends to become, the more staff intensive the quality level becomes. In addition to staff, there should be clear, concise treatment protocols. While work-hardening treatment should be highly individualized to the functional capacity goals of the individual patients, there should be consistent, objective measures to ensure a smooth progression through the program.

Variability simply means that there can be a significant difference in people-based services depending on who provides them. Variability in work-hardening programs should be addressed in four ways: (1) personnel selection, (2) training, and (3) protocols, and (4) quality control to ensure compliance. Even though there may be a shortage of physical and occupational therapists, every effort should be made to hire only those applicants who have good clinical experience and good motivational skills. Training should be formalized, provided to every employee, and address every facet of the program from patient care to reports. Finally, frequent audits of the program should be conducted by daily observation by the therapists, by patient charts, and by patient surveys as well. To the extent that the treatment is found to be lacking, corrections should be implemented immediately.

Perishability speaks to the perishable nature of the service. Unlike a tangible product, it cannot be stored. Therefore, a patient who fails to show up for the program has forever used up that treatment time allocated for him. While perishability is less of a problem when there is surplus demand and patients can be substituted on short notice, most work-hardening programs will rarely have that luxury. For that reason, patient noncompliance is a critical problem that must be dealt with swiftly for three reasons: (1) the motivation of the patient group depends on the perception that all patients are treated equally and no one is given special treatment; (2) noncompliant patients should be discharged so that treatment time and resources initially reserved for them can be transferred to motivated patients; and (3) insurance companies should not be made to pay for sporadic patient care that will not result in the success that a full-treatment program should.

An integral component of the program (product) design has to do with where in the progress of the injury the program is designed to begin patient care—acute, subacute, or chronic. This is one of the most important determinants as to how the program will be designed. "Work hardening" is widely defined in today's marketplace and runs the gambit from being an extension of physical therapy administered in the acute or subacute phase of the injury all the way to comprehensive, interdisciplinary programs that treat the total patient in the most chronic phase of the injury. Often these comprehensive programs begin to treat patients 12 to 18 months postinjury, a time when the patient is physically *and* emotionally deconditioned. Determining the point at which the program will deliver patient care has major implications for staffing, treatment protocols, clinic design and location, and outcome evaluation.

At this point, it is worth summarizing what has been covered to this point:

1. We have examined the purchase process and therefore determined who the "customers" of a work-hardening program are.
2. We have examined the needs and wants of the customer group.
3. We have discussed the design of the product to meet those needs and wants.

With that foundation, we should now look at how best to introduce and promote our product to the marketplace. I believe that there are only three fundamental ways to effectively promote a work-hardening program:

1. First and foremost is education. With work hardening in its infancy, the market for work-hardening programs must be more fully developed before individual clinics can realize their full potential. The fact is, although there may be an extremely large potential market of people who could benefit from work-hardening services, the served market is limited in size at this point because there are only a few physicians, nurses, insurance companies, and businesses that are familiar with the treatment benefits. Therefore, educating the referral sources about work hardening and its benefits will tremendously increase the access to the potential market. This educational process should be directed at the entire "customer group" and can be handled through in-service programs, continuing education programs, personal calls, and to a limited degree, direct mail and newsletters.

2. Second is building relationships with referral sources through personal contact. Building relationships is important so that the work-hardening program is viewed as an extension of the patient care available through the referral source rather than a substitute. The referral source, if a physician, must first believe that the work-hardening program provides the patient with a beneficial service and, second, must be assured that he will remain as the primary-care physician. This means that the contact person with the referral source must be sensitive to these issues and maintain consistent, reliable communication with the referral source and others in the case management team such as the insurance company, the rehabilitation counselor, the patient's company, and perhaps even the patient's family. Perhaps the most important element in building this relationship is the successful delivery of the product—deliver good patient care in a cost-effective manner that results in an early and safe return to work. If the product is delivered, the entire customer group—the patient, the referral source, the insurance company and the patient's company—is served.

3. Finally and to a lesser degree, direct mail and newsletter promotions help to promote awareness of work-hardening programs. However, it should be recognized that particularly with physicians, direct mail often goes unnoticed. This means that while some undoubtedly gets through, the average physician actually reads only a small amount of the "bulk" mail sent to him. The cost-effectiveness of mail campaigns will need to be judged in each individual market.

In general, it should be recognized that soliciting referrals for work hardening is a highly personal endeavor. Solicitations should be made in a professional manner that will develop a trust between the referral source and the program, and that trust must be preserved by a successful outcome and good communication.

In summary, a work-hardening program can be successfully marketed if the program is well designed to meet the needs of its particular target market and the wants and needs of that market are served. However, if one is to enter the field of work hardening for the long term, it is critical to recognize that the real product that must be delivered is cost containment. To deliver anything less will result in a failure to deliver the core product and a dilution of the program to its nonessential components.

SUGGESTED READING

Kotler P: *Marketing Management: Analysis, Planning and Control,* ed 5. Englewood Cliffs, NJ. Prentice-Hall.

PART XVIII
PREVENTION PROGRAMS

55

Pre-employment Screening

Charles K. Anderson, Ph. D.

Ergonomics is the discipline that maximizes the assets of the work force by optimizing the interaction between the worker and the workplace. The ergonomist considers how workers are able to work best and then designs the workplace to optimize their capabilities, trains them to perform efficiently and safely, and carefully places the right worker into the right job. These practices make jobs easier and safer and workers more productive.

Employers have many goals concerning their workers, including reducing injuries, retaining high-quality workers, and increasing productivity. These goals are critical to profitability, particularly in light of skyrocketing worker's compensation costs, slim profit margins, and tight labor pools in some areas. Given the physically demanding nature of many jobs, it is logical to conclude that one way to address these goals is to ensure that new employees will be physically capable of performing their jobs.

This chapter focuses on pre-employment screening to match new workers with the demands of the job. In the United States the issue of pre-employment screening is associated with many legal concerns. The key question is how can job performance be predicted? To answer this question, one must consider the legal requirements and all the components involved with designing a test valid to assess physical demands for a particular job.

In 1985 a project was undertaken to develop a physical ability screening battery that would address several goals: decrease the number and severity of injuries, decrease turnover, and increase productivity; generate a battery of physical tests that are inexpensive, safe, and reliable and that could be implemented on a uniform basis; have defined scores reflecting the physical demands of the job; and fulfill the legal requirements. From this, a physical ability test battery that yielded a physical fitness score called the "job match factor" (JMF) was developed. The JMF evaluated an individual's combined strength and endurance relative to the job requirements. Newly hired workers with a "marginal" JMF may well be physically fit in comparison to the work force as a whole, but they just meet the minimum standard of fitness for grocery warehouse work. This report summarizes the process involved in designing and evaluating the pre-employment screening battery for this population.

LEGAL ISSUES

The legal requirements for a screening program are defined in Title VII of the Civil Rights Act, the Age Discrimination in Employment Act (ADEA), and the Rehabilitation Act of 1973. The federal government published the Uniform Guidelines of Employee Selection Procedure in 1978 as a means to clearly delineate the standards for a screening battery. The ADEA and the Rehabilitation Act have very similar specifications, although there are no equivalent guidelines published. In essence, the screening battery must be job related, predictive of performance, and fair to members of any race, sex, or ethnic group.

VALIDATION

A prospective validation study needed to be designed and conducted to provide evidence regarding the predictiveness of the test battery. There can be costly discrimination suits filed against employers who use screening batteries that have not been validated according to the guidelines specified in the pertinent employment practice legislation. Back radiographs are an example of an unvalidated pre-employment test. The prospective validation study protects the employer when such suits arise and serves as a foundation for evaluating the potential effectiveness of the battery.

JOB ANALYSIS

A job analysis was performed with the intent of identifying the heaviest tasks in terms of strength requirements and to quantify the average and peak metabolic requirements.

Strength Requirements

The strength requirements were assessed through three mechanisms. The first was on-site observation coupled with computerized biomechanical modeling of the heaviest tasks. The second mechanism was a study of the warehouse case movement reports. The concern here related to the frequency of encountering the heaviest cases. The third mechanism was a survey of the workers regarding the frequency of encountering cases in various weight ranges.

Biomechanical Analysis

The heaviest tasks were identified through an on-site analysis of the forces exerted on the job when lifting, pushing, or pulling. Additionally, the hand positions relative to the ankles and the postures in which the forces were exerted were recorded for further analysis with a computerized biomechanical model. Tasks for which it was estimated by the model that fewer than 75% of the female population would have sufficient strength to perform were considered for simulation with the strength tests. Similarities in the critical tasks allowed them to be grouped into lifts at floor level and lifts at the midchest level.

Case Movement Report

A key concern of the Equal Employment Opportunity Commission (EEOC) is to document the frequency with which a job candidate could be expected to encounter the heaviest loads, particularly those being used to justify the level at which pass/fail criteria are set. One way to collect information on the frequency of encountering loads in various weight ranges was to study the case movement reports. These listed the product weight and number of items moved per period of time. This information was considered along with the number of workers moving the cases to assess the frequency of handling by each worker.

Worker Surveys

Workers were asked how often they encountered objects in the various weight ranges so as to obtain the perspective of the individuals handling the loads. The choices were "daily, weekly, less than monthly, or seasonally." These data corroborated the frequency profiles found with the movement reports.

Metabolic Requirements

The strength requirements focused on the occasional heavy exertions. Even though there were cases as heavy as 100 lb, the typical case weight was 20 to 30 lb. A significant endurance requirement can arise even when a low-to-moderate weight is lifted repeatedly. Because of the large overall amount of weight handled, it was important to document the endurance needed or the metabolic requirements of the jobs.

The metabolic requirements for the jobs were determined by collecting 115 shifts of heart rate data. The data were collected by having incumbent selectors, loaders, and drivers wear heart rate monitors during a typical shift. These incumbents were later given a maximal treadmill stress test with oxygen uptake being recorded. The heart rate data collected on the job were then converted into metabolic demand.

Early studies of drivers indicated that the average metabolic requirement was nominal for this group. Observation of the job revealed that there were frequent "breaks" while driving to the next stop interspersed between short bouts of manual handling while unloading cases at a stop. Hence, a further metabolic analysis of drivers was not pursued.

VALIDATION

Retrospective Validation

A group of 238 incumbent workers were given a physical ability test, and their previous injury experience and productivity were related to their test results.[1] A retrospective validation study can be performed quickly and gives a rough indication of the potential effectiveness of screening but does not indicate whether screening will be predictive of future performance.

Prospective Validation

The results of the retrospective work indicated that it would be worthwhile to design a study that would meet legal requirements. Six hundred sixty-five newly hired personnel underwent a series of physical tests. The workers were classified as full case selectors, hand-stack loaders, or hand-unstacker delivery drivers. Hand stacking and unstacking are differentiated from loading and delivering done with full pallets. The selectors and loaders were given two strength tests and an endurance test. Drivers underwent only the two strength tests.

Test Description

Isometric strength tests were selected because of their effectiveness and low costs. The first test focused on arm strength. The individual pulled up against a stationary bar at midchest height. The force of the pull registered on a strength monitor. The second test involved pulling against a stationary bar located near floor level. Three trials were conducted by using the method recommended by Chaffin.[3]

A step test was used to assess endurance. The individual stepped up and down on a bench for 3 minutes at a controlled pace. If this did not impose an adequate work load to illicit a significant heart rate response, another 3-minute bout was performed at a faster pace. Up to three bouts were conducted. The pulse rate at the end of the last bout completed along with the individual's weight, age, and sex was used to predict the aerobic capacity adjusted for body weight.

Data Collection

The data collected for each newly hired person included general demographic information, time worked, productivity, and injury experience. If an injury occurred, the date of injury, body part involved, type of injury, days lost or restricted, and the incurred workmen's compensation costs were recorded. Productivity was defined as the number of cases handled during a 1-week period as the percentage of the local warehouse standard for the week. This information was collected for an 8-week period. This time frame was selected because it was felt that a worker should reach the standard performance level in 8 weeks and the probation period typically ended at this time.

Injuries were classified as contact or musculoskeletal in nature. Contact injuries included lacerations, abrasions, bruises, fractures, and other injuries that occurred by coming in contact with something. Musculoskeletal injuries were primarily strains, sprains, and repetitive trauma disorders. These were divided into those involving the back and those that did not. Incidents that were due to the environment (such as inhalation of carbon monoxide or a foreign body in the eye) rather than a worker's performance were not included in the study.

RESULTS

The relation between the physical ability test results and each of the performance indices, risk of workmen's compensation injury, retention for at least 8 weeks, reaching the standard performance by the eighth week, and average productivity during the eighth week, were analyzed.

Injury Experience

The injury incidence rate was analyzed by company and warehouse. One center had an unusually high injury rate and was excluded from the study. The remaining 15 warehouses were divided into two groups: those that experienced significant growth during the study and those that did not. The rapid-growth warehouses had a workmen's compensation injury rate 62% greater than the typical warehouses. The consensus of management from the various warehouses was that the typical growth locations had a slow rate of new workers into the warehouse whereas the four rapid-growth locations had very little time for training the large number of newly hired personnel.

Among the typical growth warehouses, the injury experience was analyzed based on the JMF. These data are presented in Figure 55–1. There was a trend of decreasing incidence with increasing JMF. JMF and injury rates were studied by age group. It was found that the injury rate increased with age.

Another way to consider the results is in terms of the projected reduction in injuries if the battery had been implemented. This was done by calculating the injury rate for newly hired persons above a defined JMF. Table 55–1 presents the performance level based on the JMF, the projected percentage of injuries that would have been prevented if the battery had been implemented, and the percentage of newly hired workers who performed at the particular JMF level. Had performance at the marginal JMF level been required, the injury rate would have been reduced by 10.4%, and 91% of the newly hired workers performed at this marginal level. In the rapid-growth warehouses, no clear relationship between injury rate and JMF was noted. Due to the small group size, no conclusions could be made concerning the effect of age on the injury rate.

Endurance Capacity

Table 55–2 presents the aerobic capacity in each age group. Endurance, as measured by aerobic capacity, decreased with age. However, it was noted that incumbent employees aged 35 years or more had a greater aerobic capacity than did the newly hired workers of the same age. This demonstrates that individuals increased their capacity

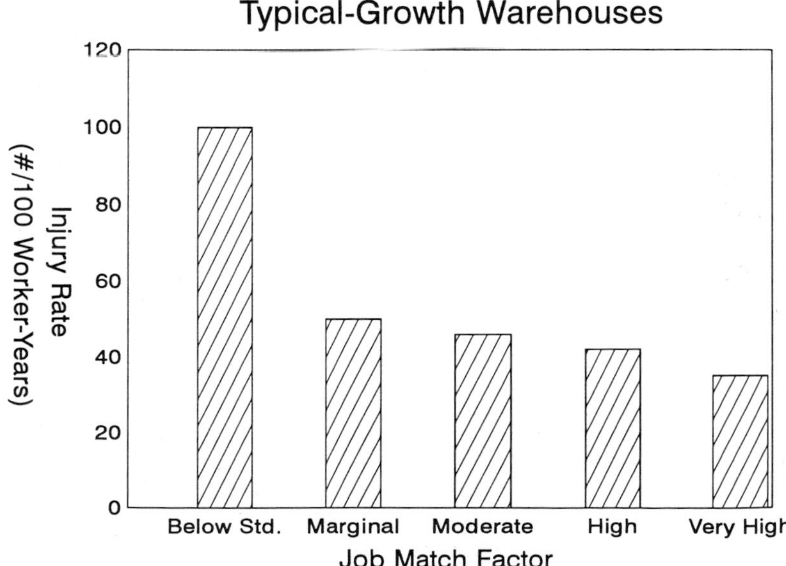

FIG 55–1.
The injury rate in each of the job match factor categories in the typical growth warehouses (those with a slow rate of new workers being hired).

TABLE 55–1.

Projected Decrease in Worker's Compensation Injuries and the Associated Pass Rate for a Range of Cutoff Levels in Terms of Job Match Factor

Cutoff Level	Projected Reduction in Worker's Compensation Injuries (%)	Pass Rate (%)
No testing	—	100
Marginal	10.4	91
Moderate	14.1	76
High	18.2	56
Very high	23.0	32

when exposed to physically demanding work over a period of time. It should also be noted that stronger workers tend to be "bulkier" due to greater muscle mass associated with greater strength. This may put them at a disadvantage when measuring endurance since they must move more body weight.

Retention

There was a increasing likelihood of retention for newly hired personnel with a greater JMF: those performing at the marginal JMF level were 3% more likely to stay at work, and those with a very high JMF were 15% more likely to stay.

Productivity

The projected improvement in the percentage of newly hired workers reaching standard productivity with the marginal requirement implemented was 5%. If only job candidates with a very high JMF were hired, this figure would have risen to 21%.

ADVERSE IMPACT FOR MINORITY GROUPS

Sex

Physical ability testing can be anticipated to have an adverse impact for females. Women will probably pass the battery at a rate of less than 80% of the pass rate for men. Therefore the EEOC requires a consideration of test fairness for women. In this warehouse study, there were only five women applicants, so the test battery and JMF could not be analyzed in this group.

The EEOC allows evidence of test fairness from other studies to be used when it is not feasible to conduct a study for the group in question. There are at least three studies that show significant correlations for both males and females on physical ability test batteries.[2, 4, 5] The tests and the pass/fail criteria were selected independent of sex. They entail basic abilities, strength, and endurance, which were required of anyone performing the warehouse jobs, regardless of sex. The pass/fail criteria were directly deduced from the job, not from a statistical analysis of the data, which were almost completely collected for males. For example, the strength requirements for lifting was based on the weight of cases, which was obviously the same regardless of if a male or female was lifting them. The metabolic requirements were adjusted for body weight, which puts the generally lower-weight female on equal ground with the generally heavier male.

TABLE 55–2.

Average Aerobic Capacity for Males by Age Group

Age Group (yr)	Average Aerobic Capacity (mL/kg$^{2/3}$)
<20	203.8
20–24	196.2
25–29	182.9
30–34	176.2
>34	157.9

Age

Strength capacity was roughly equivalent for newly hired workers under 20 years of age and those over 35 years; but older job candidates tended to have a lower aerobic capacity in general. Older newly hired workers did have a lower pass rate for aerobic capacity than did young ones; however, the difference did not exceed the guidelines used by the EEOC. Similar patterns were seen at the other threshold levels; hence there was no indication of adverse impact for older workers.

Race/Ethnic Group

The pass rates and validity were analyzed by ethnic group and race for those groups with sufficient sample size. Individual studies were performed for whites, blacks, and Hispanics. There was no evidence suggesting differences among these three groups. Furthermore, there was no evidence suggesting different trends in predictiveness for the three groups.

SUMMARY

Based on the test battery designed for the grocery warehouse workers, newly hired personnel with greater JMF scores had fewer injuries and greater employment retention and were more likely to reach the productivity standard. As this example demonstrates, with careful workplace analysis, tests designs relevant to work tasks, and precise data collection and analysis, it is possible to design a pre-employment screening test battery that meets legal requirements and can be effective in reducing injuries and increasing productivity in jobs with heavy physical requirements.

REFERENCES

1. Anderson C: Strength and endurance testing for pre-employment placement, in Kroemer K (ed): *Manual Material Handling: Understanding and Preventing Back Trauma*. Akron, Ohio, American Industrial Hygiene Association, 1989, pp 73–78.

2. Arnold JD, Rauschenberger JM, Soubel WG, et al: Validation and utility of a strength test for selecting steelworkers. *J Appl Psychol* 1982; 67:588–604.
3. Chaffin D: Ergonomics guide for the assessment of human static strength. *Am Ind Hyg Assoc J* 1975; 36:269–272.
4. Herrin GD, Kochkin S, Scott V: *Development of an Employee Strength Assessment Program for United Airlines. Technical Report*. Ann Arbor, University of Michigan Center for Ergonomics, 1982.
5. Reilly RR, Zedeck S, Tenopyr ML: Validity and fairness of physical ability tests for predicting performance in craft jobs. *J Appl Psychol* 1979; 64:262–274.

56

Ergonomics

Anna Bodenhamer, O.T.

Ergonomics is the study of the worker in relation to the workplace and emphasizes fitting the workstation to the worker rather than forcing the worker to fit the station. Human characteristics and environmental factors are considered. In the past, the layout and dimensions of workstations were designed without considering the worker at all; instead, they were more likely based on equipment cost and what was considered efficient space utilization. However, soon the costs and severity of workplace injuries gained notice. Between 1957 and 1976, the awards from the Security Disability program for back pain increased 2800%, which was 14 times the population growth.[4] Due to the incidence and associated costs of injuries, prevention began gaining attention. Snook felt that many industrial injuries were due to a poor fit between the worker and the workstation, poorly designed workstations, or poorly designed job tasks.[10] Three approaches to this problem were identified: carefully selecting workers, training workers to use safe lifting techniques, and designing the job to fit the worker. Based on a series of studies, Snook felt that the third approach was the most effective in reducing injuries.[10] Yu et al. reported that redesigning the job site was probably the most effective approach but should probably be combined with worker selection.[12] It has been reported that 79% of all manual material handling injuries are to the lower part of the back.[10] Ergonomists evaluate the workstation, the worker, and the job task in its environment to create a safer and more productive workplace. Ergonomics can be applied to the prevention of injuries as well as in redesigning the workstation when a problem area is identified. Utilizing ergonomic principles to evaluate employees for proper job placement can also help prevent injuries.

Ergonomists consider the dimensions and demands of the workstation and fit this to the workers to make the worker and machine interface more compatibly. This allows the worker to be more comfortable with the workstation, which can help increase productivity and decrease the risk of injury. Each station cannot be fitted to any one particular worker; therefore, the station is designed to fit a large percentage of workers by using anthropomorphic data. The National Institute of Occupational Safety and Health (NIOSH) has generated guidelines based on these measurements.[9] Their guidelines specify tasks that could be performed by individuals ranging from the 75th percentile (or lower) of males to the 25th percentile (or greater) of females.

More work is being done to identify factors related to low back pain and injury in the workplace. Some of the contributing factors are driving, vibration, cumulative trauma, bending, lifting, and getting in and out of a vehicle.[5, 8, 12] As more information of this kind becomes available, ergonomists will have more criteria with which to design increasingly safer workplaces.

JOB ANALYSIS

To evaluate the workstation, a job analysis must be performed for each job task or job description. This involves a detailed analysis of each part of the workstation. First, one must become familiar with the job task and the work process involved. A generalized recommendation will not work for all job tasks. An understanding how the workstation operates must be included in the recommendations to prevent making changes that would slow or interrupt productivity. Many times the solution can create new problems; therefore, the recommendations must be evaluated and reevaluated carefully. This should include an objective evaluation that considers specific topics such as the amount of weight lifted, the repetitiveness of tasks, the body mechanics required to move objects, the height of workstations, and all other items required for the workers to perform their tasks. Talking with workers is usually very beneficial. They are the "frontline" and are the ones most familiar with the details of the job tasks. Additional insight can be gained by the evaluator performing the task. A thorough work job analysis includes evaluating the overall work environment, psychosocial issues, and physical demands.

Work Environment

When evaluating the work environment, all areas that concern physiologic functioning must be reviewed (visual, auditory, temperature, tactile, etc): light, heat, cold, humidity, surface areas for walking and working, obstacles (such as objects on the floor, equipment overhead, confined spaces, slippery or wet surfaces), chemical hazards from contact or inhalation, temperature changes, figure-ground recognition, color discrimination, fine and gross motor motions required, indoor and outdoor work locations, space restrictions, workstation location (proximity to break rooms, restrooms, coworkers, supervisors), noise levels, proximity to moving machinery, and mandatory or optional protective clothing/devices worn. When specifically dealing with industrial back injuries, which are frequently related to lifting, lifting while twisting or bending, carrying items while in an awkward posture, slipping or falling, or fatigue (which may vary with heat and humidity), environmental factors associated with these particular topics are very carefully evaluated. Also, one needs to note the frequency and duration of breaks the workers take during the workday because this can be related to worker fatigue and boredom.

Psychosocial Issues

Psychosocial issues have often been overlooked in the past. Many industries have not considered this as an area closely related with the workplace. Studies have found an increasingly important factor regarding workplace injury rates to be rooted in psychosocial issues. Boredom and job dissatisfaction have been found to increase the risk of low back pain. Several studies reported that workers who are unhappy with their jobs, who are bored, or whose job lacks a need for concentration remain off work longer following an episode of low back pain.[1, 11] Workers who "hardly ever" enjoyed their jobs were 2.5 times more likely to report a back injury than those who "almost always" enjoyed their jobs.[3] It has also been reported in a study of female workers that psychological variables directly associated with low back pain are dissatisfaction with the work environment, fatigue at the end of the day, and a higher degree of worry.[11] The negative or strained relationship between an injured worker and supervisors or coworkers also correlates with an increased risk of low back pain and illness. A positive relationship tends to correlate with decreased lost-time injuries on the job. The family situation can also affect job productivity and injury rates. When the stress level at home is high, workers tend to be less productive and more prone to injury at work. They are also more likely to fall into the "injured" or "sick" role, which prolongs the rehabilitation process. Positive work and home environments are more likely to result in a faster, more complete recovery than if these factors are negative. When a worker feels that the employer is on his side and is willing to work toward correcting the workplace problems, he will be a more positive and ultimately a more productive worker.

Physical Requirements

The physical requirements of the job encompasses all the physically demanding activities including manual material handling tasks, motions, and postures required (sitting, standing, walking, climbing, crawling, pushing/pulling, reaching, bending, twisting, driving, manipulating objects, operating machinery, and using tools). Each activity is broken down into individual steps and analyzed piece by piece to assess stressors that may be involved. For example, unloading a pallet of boxes consists of lifting from different levels, carrying each box to its destination, placing the box, and returning to get the next box. This job task requires more than just lifting; one must also be able to grasp and hold an object, walk, bend or stoop, see, feel, hear (if motorized equipment is nearby), use cognitive judgment to plan the move, etc.

Heavy labor jobs are designed to fit a stronger population. The workstation would be designed to fit anthropomorphic measures associated with this group. The heights of workstations would tend to be designed to fit a taller population. An ergonomic problem may arise if the job demands are changed due to technology or assistive devices so that a weaker and possibly smaller population is assigned to the workstations. The workstations may be too tall for these shorter workers and possibly lead to workers having problems with the upper extremities and cervical spine. A good example of a limited workstation is a United States Air Force jet. The cockpit design is based on the anthropomorphic guidelines for the male population. There are strict height and weight requirements for pilots. This helps to keep production costs lower by not having to allow for variation in pilot size. However, it also limits the population who can operate the jet. In the industrial workplace many factories were originally built with only one population in mind, generally a larger, stronger, male population. Changes in technology and the work force composition have led to ergonomic problems in some factories. The key to workstation design is to design for the extremes and for adjustability. If the workstation can be adjusted, this will prevent potential future problems with a changing work force. It also allows for a better worker-workstation fit with the current work force.

Ergonomic evaluation is being utilized more often in the area of injury prevention. The traditional use of ergonomics was after a problem had been recognized through the occurrence of an injury. Recently, training sessions or industrial back schools have become more popular in industry. This education involves an analysis of the workplace and the jobs tasks being performed. After the educator has become familiar with the job requirements at a particular work site, then workers are taught specific techniques to work in a safe and efficient manner. This teaching is also used in rehabilitation programs for workers who have already experienced an injury. The worker's job can be evaluated while he is in therapy, which allows for close monitoring and more detailed training to enable a safe return to work. The specific job training can help reduce the risk of reinjury and actually result in a safer worker than a noninjured worker who has had no training.

PRE-EMPLOYMENT SCREENING

Another use of ergonomic evaluation involves pre-employment screening for potential employees. This is also used to place current employees. Preplacement screening involves ergonomically evaluating the specific job tasks and then testing the potential employee to place him in a specific job role. The test must be job specific to prevent the problem of discrimination from arising. This allows the employer to more accurately assess the worker's ability to perform the job tasks to ensure that physical capabilities match job demands. The ergonomic evaluation is a must when evaluating for job placement. The test must be job specific to each of the jobs being filled. Many different types of test can be utilized. Dynamic and static tests have been used. Dynamic testing entails having the worker perform true-life activities as performed on the job during a typical workday. This might include lifting boxes, carrying objects, climbing, or walking. Static testing using a force gauge has been used and is reported to correlate with dynamic strength.[7] According to Chaffin, dynamic strength testing has too many variables to allow an accurate assessment of an individual's true dynamic strength. Static testing can be controlled and is therefore more consistent and can be standardized for general testing purposes. However, it is criticized for not being "real-life."

The ergonomist must evaluate the job and design static tests simulating work postures. The information can then be compiled to test the existing employees and determine strength guidelines for a particular job. New employees must then meet these guidelines when tested for that particular job. The role of static strength testing in a population performing a wide variety of tasks was not found to be beneficial.[1] Employees can be trained by the ergonomist to perform job tasks by using proper and efficient body mechanics to decrease the chance of injury.

EFFECTIVE IMPLEMENTATION

A well-trained ergonomist can provide valuable input to workstation design. However, this is only a part of what is required to make the workplace safer. The best-designed workstation may still produce injury if those using it are not properly trained and willing to implement this training on a daily basis. The success of an injury prevention program relies as heavily upon worker acceptance as the quality of the program itself. For the program to be successful, the employer and the workers must support it. Isernhagen stressed the importance of employer support and recommended that employers demonstrate support by attending safety meetings, talking directly to employees in a positive manner, and noticing safe behavior in the workplace.[6] She also noted the importance of the supervisors truly having a "safety-first" attitude in the long term.

SUMMARY

Ergonomics is the study of the relationship of the worker and the workplace. It is concerned with preventing injuries by designing workplaces and better matching workers with job demands, as well as with retraining injured workers. Ergonomic evaluations are a necessary part of any rehabilitation program. This provides a better understanding of the job requirements of the injured worker and thus allows the rehabilitation team to better prepare the individual for returning to work.

With the increasing costs associated with low back pain and back injuries, more emphasize is being placed upon prevention programs. These include employee education and redesigning the workplace to create an environment in which injury is less like to occur. Also, more care is being given to placing workers in job roles that they are physically capable of performing. More work is needed to better identify factors contributing to industrial back injuries and what type of preplacement screening, if any, proves to be valuable in reducing injuries. As more knowledge is gained in the area of biomechanics and muscle performance, more changes may be made to create a safer working environment.

Some employers have been hesitant to invest in the equipment and/or space necessary to provide well-designed workstations and assistive devices (conveyor belts, carts, hoists, etc.) due to their expense. However, if these devices can help to reduce the injury rate, they would prove to be well worth the investment.

Although one generally thinks of heavy lifting tasks when discussing job-related injuries, seated workplaces are also receiving attention with regard to injuries. This is not so surprising with the rapidly increasing number of computer-related jobs. Although problems dealing with heavy industrial lifting were recognized much earlier than desk-related problems, the specific guidelines for designing these workstations have been much slower in development. This may be due at least in part to the differences in the tasks being evaluated. There is much more variability related to a lifting task than with seated tasks. In lifting there are variations in the amount of weight, the reach required to move the weight, carrying postures, bending postures, the shape of the objects being lifted, the lifting repetitiveness, and the lift duration. When dealing with seated jobs, which are more static in nature, there are fewer variables and more standardized variables to deal with.

As the work force, job demands, and information concerning the causes for injury in the workplace continue to change, the ergonomist will continually play a role in the prevention of low back injury.

REFERENCES

1. Battie MC, Bigos SJ, Fisher LD, et al: Isometric lifting strength as a predictor of industrial back pain reports. *Spine* 1989; 14:851–856.
2. Bergquist-Ullman M, Larsson U: Acute low back pain in industry. *Acta Orthop Scand* 1977; 170:1–117.
3. Bigos SJ, Battie MC, Spengler DM, et al: A prospective study of work perceptions and psychosocial factors affecting the report of back injury. *Spine* 1991; 16:1–7.
4. Cats-Baril WL, Frymoyer JW: The economics of spinal disorders, in Frymoyer JW, et al (eds): *The Adult Spine*. New York, Raven Press, 1991, pp 85–106.
5. Damkot DK, Pope MH, Lord J, et al: The relationship between work history, work environment and low-back pain in men. *Spine* 1984; 9:395–399.
6. Isernhagen SJ: General program parameters. *Spine State Art Rev* 1991; 5:471–478.
7. Keyserling WM, Herrin GD, Chaffin DB: Isometric strength testing as a means of controlling medical incidence of strenuous jobs. *J Occup Med* 1980; 22:332–336.
8. Kumar S: Cumulative load as a risk factor for back pain. *Spine* 1990; 15:1311–1316.
9. National Institute for Occupational Safety and Health: *Work Practices for Manual Lifting*. Cincinnati, NIOSH US Public Health Service, Publication 81-122), 1981.
10. Snook SH: The design of manual handling tasks. *Ergonomics* 1978; 21:963–985.
11. Svensson HO, Andersson GB: The relationship of low-back pain, work history, work environment, and stress. A retrospective cross-sectional study of 38- to 64-year old women. *Spine* 1989; 14:517–522.
12. Yu T, Roht LH, Wise RA, et al: Low back pain in industry. An old problem revisited. *J Occup Med* 1984; 26:517–524.

57

Industrial Back School

Michael S. Melnik, M.S., O.T.R.

A chapter on back injury prevention in industry in a text directed primarily toward orthopedic surgeons reflects the changes in attitude that have taken place over the last decade regarding back care. Health professionals are recognizing the efficacy of prevention, and as a result, the time, effort, and dollars being channeled into this area continue to grow.

This chapter will examine the costs and causes of back injuries and the variety of approaches used to prevent these injuries, as well as the myths and misconceptions surrounding prevention. It will explore industry's role in the injury prevention process, including the variables that have an impact on program success and the components of a comprehensive program.

EXAMINING THE COSTS OF BACK INJURIES

The latest statistics indicate that the costs for back injuries have reached well into the billions of dollars. These costs are an accumulation of direct and indirect costs associated with an injury. Medical management and disability payments, worker's compensation, lost production, replacement costs, and costs associated with processing an injury combine to make even a minor injury costly. The amount that employers spend on workmen's compensation insurance has nearly doubled over the last decade.[46] Liberty Mutual Insurance, the nation's largest workmen's compensation carrier, pays out $1 million dollars a day on back injury claims.[10] According to the Bureau of National Affairs, in any given year an estimated 10 million employees in the United States encounter back pain serious enough to affect work performance.[6] Compensation costs and the laws regulating this system vary widely between states. Many companies are forced to relocate or start businesses in states where the financial impact of injuries is not as great. Others choose to remain "home" and struggle with the ever-increasing costs. Some high-risk industries, such as construction, may pay as much as 10% of its payroll into the compensation system.[46]

There is more to the costs of a back injury than its financial impact. The hidden costs of a back injury are experienced through pain and suffering. The physical and psychological effects of an injury can be severe, particularly when they lead to chronic pain and disability. Whether viewed from an economic or a personal perspective, back injuries are costly.

Despite the magnitude of the problem, the literature on back injury prevention programs is sparse. Articles that have measured effectiveness in a "controlled" manner are even more difficult to find. "Back schools" vary dramatically depending on the implementer and the industry. They range from relatively simple educational programs to those that follow a more comprehensive approach.[6, 28, 36, 43, 45] While several programs have reported substantial injury reductions and impressive cost savings,[6, 28, 36] the variations between program methods make it difficult to identify a single "best" method for reducing back injuries.

CAUSES OF BACK DISORDERS

Unsafe Conditions–Unsafe Acts

While the list of risk factors that contribute to back disorders is extensive, it can be broken down into two basic categories: unsafe conditions and unsafe acts. An unsafe condition is an environment that forces or encourages employees to use their bodies in a way that increases the risk of a back disorder. Unsafe work conditions respond well to engineering and design controls. The National Institute for Occupational Safety and Health (NIOSH) guidelines were developed to define unsafe conditions and offer corrective measures and are the basis for many workplace ergonomics programs.[32]

Unsafe work conditions include jobs requiring the following:

1. Repetitive lifting of heavy/awkward loads
2. Repetitive lifting from floor height
3. Lifting and twisting
4. Prolonged sitting/driving
5. Prolonged standing
6. Static forward bending
7. Repetitive/constant work at arms' reach
8. Exposure to vibration

Unsafe "acts" refer to the unsafe work methods an individual chooses even when safer alternatives are available. Unsafe acts can place workers at risk in even the safest conditions. An example involves an individual choosing to perform an activity manually when an assistive device has been made available and the individual has been instructed in its use. Unsafe acts can be caused by ignorance about safe procedures as well as attitude, stress, and depression.[6, 16, 22–25] Unsafe conditions are the focus of many industrial safety programs. Numerous guidelines have been developed by NIOSH to address these conditions. In many cases, however, meeting these guidelines requires an initial "safe act" by the employee to be effective. Lock-out, tag-out programs require employees to disconnect the power source to a machine during repairs to create a "safe condition." Despite training in this area and enforcement by the Occupational Safety and Health Administration (OSHA), employees can still be observed circumventing these policies and in the worst scenarios losing life or limb. Construction workers are required to secure themselves or "tie off" when working near the edge of a building, yet it is not uncommen to hear complaints about this policy from employees despite the fact that it could save their lives.

Traditionally, lifting has been identified as "the incident" associated with a back injury. There is an abundance of literature available on lifting[7, 17, 32, 33, 35]; however, the literature identifies several factors that need to be considered:

1. Predisposition to injury[37, 38, 40, 48]
2. Workplace design[3, 11, 19, 20]
3. Level of physical fitness[2, 4, 8, 14, 41]
4. Stress[25]
5. Attitude[6, 16, 23–25]
6. Smoking[18, 29]
7. Work style/body mechanics[7, 17, 26, 27, 32–35, 50]
8. Financial compensation for an injury[5, 12, 21, 47]

Lifting, particularly at jobs with very high physical demands, certainly contributes to injuries. In other situations, however, identifying a single lift as the culprit may be similar to identifying a specific meal that led to the development of a cavity or the last cigarette smoked as the one that caused the heart attack. Back injuries have been defined as disorders associated with lifting, and the solutions to this problem have developed around that mind set. For years the literature on contributing factors to injuries has been underutilized by those who provide injury prevention services to industry. For example, information that identifies the relationship between depression and risk of injury was published nearly 3 decades ago,[23, 24] yet few back schools recommend employee assistance programs as a part of their programs. In the same light, the literature indicates that a "smoking cessation" program may, in some instances, be more effective in reducing back injury costs over time[18, 29] than a 30-minute class on lifting.

WHAT AFFECTS PROGRAM SUCCESS?

One need only examine attitudes and human nature to realize the difficulties encountered in implementing an injury prevention program. If people are resistant to policies and procedures that demonstrate a direct bearing on their loss of life, what will be their motivation to expend energy toward a program that may prevent something as seemingly innocuous as a back disorder? Back disorders affect as much as 80% of the population. One would assume that a disorder this prevalent would generate a great deal of preventive attention. Back disorders unfortunately suffer from an "image problem." Many minor back disorders resolve themselves within a week to 10 days. This ability of the back to spontaneously "recover" perpetuates a belief that it is easier to "wait it out" for a week in pain than to invest unnecessary energy toward prevention. The "quick-fix" approach so readily available in the community feeds the myth that there is no relationship between an individual's action and the condition of his back. Grocery stores and pharmacies are filled with pills for back pain relief, billboards promote back rehabilitation services with the same zealousness as McDonald's and the airwaves are full of commercials calling for anyone who thinks that he may have been hurt at work to dial 1-800 "Law-Suit" for a free consultation. This emphasis on action after the injury makes the promotion and implementation of prevention a monumental task.

When developing a program for injury prevention it is imperative that industry recognize all the variables that can have an impact on success. These include attitudinal shifts, increased awareness, new policies directed at safety, a safer working environment, and a commitment from management.

Attitudinal Shift

To gain insight into attitudinal problems contributing to a company's injury problem two very simple questions should be asked.

1. Do the employees feel that they are recognized/respected by management/supervisors?
2. Do the employees and supervisors contribute in some manner to the decisions that are made in this facility?

The literature is beginning to identify the need to enlist support at all levels for a program to experience success.[44, 49] Companies that have successful programs make communication and empowerment a priority.[49] In many companies individuals work at isolated workstations and are unable to communicate even with their coworkers due to noise. Isolation and a lack of recognition can foster negative attitudes. Strained relationships between supervisors and employees can lead to turf battles and may cost industry billions of dollars.[22] The "human-factor" portion of an injury prevention program is critical in achieving success.

Increased Awareness

Educated decisions require education. It needs to be recognized that for most employees getting hurt is not a conscious decision but working safely is. One of the best examples of a program that has experienced a great deal of success is the DuPont "STOP" (Safety Training Observation Program.)[43] The premise of the program is to keep an employee aware through a variety of ongoing educational programs. In some companies each supervisor meeting ends with the supervisors being asked to complete the following sentence: "this company would be a safer place to work if. . . ." Their responses are then prioritized, and plans of action are generated.

Development of Policies

Policies for safe work behaviors such as the use of assistive devices, team lifts, and good housekeeping can substantially reduce the risk of back injuries. If it were true that all employees would work as hard as they could, there would be no need for productivity standards. If it could be assumed that each employee would work as safely as possible, the need for safety-related policies would also not exist. Unfortunately, in both cases compliance is generated by understanding the rules and the repercussions for not following these rules. It is up to the injury prevention specialist to work with the company and its employees to come up with policies and procedures that are not only effective but enforceable as well.

Safer Work Environment

The ergonomic approach has had a great impact on the reduction of back injuries. By altering the environment, work styles can be limited to those that lessen the employee's risk of injury.[30, 31, 39]

Ongoing Commitment

Eventually the hype that follows a back school subsides, and things return to "normal." An injury prevention program needs to become something that is viewed in the same light as productivity standards and quality control. It is the presence of activities over time that allows safe work behaviors to become safe work habits.

COMPONENTS OF A COMPREHENSIVE PROGRAM

Injury prevention specialists are frequently approached by industry to provide brief programs to teach people how to lift. While it is uncommon for patients to dictate their own treatment, this scenario is all too common when industry searches for solutions to back injury problems. Like a physician treating a patient, injury prevention must be targeted toward activities that will have the greatest impact on the problem. A truly comprehensive back injury prevention program is developed after a thorough investigation of the risk factors. It is clear that some industries may benefit from nontraditional approaches to injury prevention. These may include the initiation of a human relations program to address communication problems in the plant, smoking cessation classes, implementation of an employee assistance program, and development of incentive programs. These activities combined with the following components provide industry with a comprehensive approach to back injury prevention:

1. Meeting with management—It is important to get a time and dollar commitment from management and meet with a representative from management on an ongoing basis to measure program success and to develop strategies for future activities.
2. Meeting with supervisors—In general, the most sophisticated and effective safety programs in industry are carried out by supervisors. If supervisors do not buy into the program or are not committed to its success, the effectiveness will be substantially reduced. An initial meeting with the supervisors allows the injury prevention specialist to address concerns and questions and provides the supervisors with ownership of the program.
3. Development of a task force.—The development of a task force or "focus group" to be the watchdog over the program provides the employee and supervisor populations with an additional degree of program ownership. Companies need to recognize that while management is paying for the program, it belongs to the employees and supervisors. Many large organizations, particularly the auto industry, have begun utilizing these groups not only for safety but also to make positive changes in quality and productivity.
4. Worksite evaluation.—A thorough evaluation of the workplace by the injury prevention specialist familiarizes him with the work environment and the employee population. If this consultant will be providing instruction on safe work practices, he must be knowledgeable about what takes place in the plant. Pictures need to be taken to customize educational programs, and the consultant should, where possible, work with the employees at their jobs. Talking with employees concerning their jobs and recognizing and noting their ideas and concerns increases their investment in the program.

This visit also begins the process of evaluating the need for ergonomic adaptations or redesign. A worksite evaluation can be completed with the assistance of the plant superintendent, a plant engineer, and supervisors and employees from their respective departments. Input from all levels will give the injury prevention specialist a broader perspective of the facility's condition.

5. Educational programs.—Educational programs, or "back schools," have traditionally been the method of choice for injury prevention in industry. If proper emphasis is placed on this aspect of prevention, it can be a very effective tool. To be most effective, all levels of employees from management to hourly personnel must be targeted for training. In addition, consideration should be taken when choosing the program content and instructional methods for each group.

BACK SCHOOL PROGRAM CONTENT

Management Class

Key concepts to be addressed in the management session include the following:

1. Establishing management's goals in the program and ensuring that these goals are measurable and attainable
2. Establishing management's role in keeping the program alive
3. Discussing the development of a medical management policy within the company (if not already in existence)
4. Setting a timetable for the implementation of various activities

Supervisor Class

The goal of these sessions is to help the supervisors become on-site "safety directors" for their departments. Educational background, communication skills, work load, and attitude toward the program will influence a supervisor's level of participation.

Supervisors sessions need to address the following:

1. Ergonomics.—While supervisors do not need to become ergonomic experts, they will benefit from being able to recognize work environments that increase an employee's risk of injury.

2. Body mechanics.—Just as a supervisor is expected to address an employee who is incorrectly tooling a product, a supervisor can also be expected to recognize and address employees when they are working in a manner that increases their risk of injury.

3. Program maintenance.—Supervisors need to learn how to keep the employees involved in the injury prevention process. Program success will be affected by whether or not the employees view this as a team effort or a dictatorship.

4. Communication.—The supervisors need to be assured that they will not be "hung out to dry" with this program. The injury prevention specialist should remain readily available to the supervisors throughout the program.

5. Injury management.—The supervisor should be well-versed in how to respond to an injury when it does occur. A supervisor's handling of an incident should be based more on policy than personality. Supervisors also need to be familiar with effective ways of managing an employee who is returning to work following an injury.

Employee Classes

A back class should not be expected to alter employee behavior. Long-term changes come from ongoing education and reinforcement in the workplace. "Back school" needs to be identified to the participants as the "orientation" to an ongoing injury prevention program. It is a session that allows the employees, through increased knowledge, to become active participants in the injury prevention process.

Typical back schools address the following topics:

1. General anatomy
2. Common causes of back disorders
3. Common disorders/treatment
4. Methods for protecting the back (home/work activities)
5. Exercises for a healthy back

Back schools last anywhere from 30 minutes to 3 hours and generally use one of the methods described below.

"BACK SCHOOL" METHODS

Videos/Manuals

The popularity of this method is based in part on the ease with which it is implemented. Fill the room, dim the lights, show the video, and the company's training needs have been met. Many of OSHA's regulations can be met through this medium. The power of video training and the sophistication of video production has made this one of the most common forms of safety training to date. There are numerous programs on the market that offer both video training programs and written support materials in the area of back injury prevention. While these programs meet certain needs, their limitations need to be recognized:

1. Audience participation is limited unless there is a live instructor to complement the video.

2. Videos are unable to take into account the wide variety of learning styles and educational levels of the viewers.

3. Informational videos, unless very professionally produced, have difficulty maintaining audience interest.

4. Retention and application of material following a viewing are questionable.

5. Handouts or manuals may not be appropriate for the educational level of the reader, may not accommodate language barriers that exist, and may have limited applicability to the actual job demands of the reader.

It is for these reasons that numerous companies and injury prevention specialists use audiovisuals and manuals in conjunction with one of the following methods.

Lecture/Discussion

This is the most common form of "back school." It generally involves a therapist presenting a class on "how to take care of your back." The standard back school makes the following assumptions:

1. The audience wants to know this information.
2. The information presented is pertinent to this audience.
3. The information is presented in a way that the audience can understand.
4. The information presented will be reinforced over time so that the concepts presented will be learned.

In many instances some of these assumptions will prove to be false. To be effective a presenter must recognize the variables affecting presentation and prepare accordingly. Too often this type of program is viewed as something that can stand alone and prevent injuries. The literature indicates that many people do not learn and retain practical skills in this manner.[9] Despite the inherent limitations, programs utilizing this approach have claimed success following this type of training.[6]

Lecture/Discussion/Participation

This is a variation of lecture/discussion and provides laboratory time in the class for the employees to practice the techniques presented. While this offers "hands-on" training, the length of practice time is insufficient for altering long-standing work habits.

Interactive Training (Hands-On Training in the Work Environment)

In this format the instructor and the employees work together in the work area to address potential causes of back injuries and to practice preventive techniques. It is the recognition of real situations and the problem solving that follows that makes this type of training effective.

FOLLOW-UP ACTIVITIES

It is at this point, following completion of the educational components, that a comprehensive "back school" actually begins. Prevention must be viewed as a process rather than a single act. Follow-up activities include the following:

1. Review sessions.—These are sessions that address employees' questions and concerns and review the key points of the initial education program. These ongoing sessions demonstrate management's commitment to the program.

2. Ongoing task force/focus group meetings.—These provide the supervisors and employees with ownership over the future direction of the program.

3. Development of an effective medical management/return-to-work program.—A comprehensive injury prevention program must address the need to "prevent" back injuries from becoming long-term, chronic problems. By developing a claims review process, a company can begin to identify methods for cost control. Early return to work is becoming a more viable option for companies and has demonstrated the potential for providing significant savings[13, 42]

4. Development of warm-up/stretching programs.—This allows the employees to take increased responsibility for their condition. Care must be taken in the implementation of a program of this type. It is important to educate the participants as to why this is important, and the stretching activities should be customized to address the muscle groups that are overutilized as well as those that are underutilized on the job.[1]

5. Ongoing consultation.—Periodic visits to a work site by the injury prevention specialist allow for ongoing dialogue and problem solving.

6. Program evaluation.—It is important to periodically evaluate the program to determine effectiveness. Changing the course to increase effectiveness is far more productive than allowing a program to run itself into the ground.

WHO IS QUALIFIED TO PROVIDE INDUSTRIAL INJURY PREVENTION SERVICES?

There are numerous professions who have identified themselves as "the professionals" qualified to provide this type of service. These include physical therapists, occupational therapists, chiropractors, rehabilitation consultants, physicians, nurses, and exercise physiologists. All of these groups possess educational backgrounds that qualify them to talk about back care. Unfortunately there is an illusion that because of their education these groups are "capable"

58

The Psychology of Prevention

Edwin F. Kremer, Ph.D.

RISK FACTORS

Job Characteristics

A substantial amount of research has characterized at-risk populations for back injury.[35] Although there is little debate regarding the need for large-sample prospective studies,[5] the available literature, which is largely retrospective, provides a clear direction in preventive measures.[11, 34, 64, 70] Further, there is evidence that some prevention programs based on this literature have resulted in a dramatic reduction of injury and compensation claims.[33, 66]

Table 58–1 outlines the characteristics of the at-risk population and prevention strategy by category. As can be seen in the Table 58–1, risk factors such as lifting, carrying, pulling, pushing, and twisting indicate the development and teaching of the most biomechanically efficient techniques for accomplishing any particular physical activity as a prevention strategy.[6, 18–20, 52, 68, 73, 74] Although there is debate as to whether or not there is a single correct lifting technique,[28, 55] it is plausible to assume that adoption of a single biomechanically sound strategy for lifting would be an improvement over a laissez-faire approach.

Beyond increasing the efficiency of the worker, it would also be necessary to apply the current knowledge of ergonomics to the work situation. This would entail workstation design, development of assistive devices, and engineering to minimize vibration. Despite successful engineering efforts, however, there can be little impact on risk if the individual worker does not utilize available equipment or techniques. A number of authors have found, for example, that even when lifting aids were available, nursing personnel utilized them only 25% of the time.[43, 61, 71] Thus, injuries might more often be the result of doing a safe job in an unsafe manner than an inherent lack of safety on the job.[44]

The observation that employees with less tenure are at greater risk for injury[2, 6, 25, 33] could reflect either a lack of experience or selectively more physical demands for low-seniority workers. Regardless of the precise reason for the relationship, the relevance for prevention would be to intensify the injury prevention efforts on this group.

Worker Characteristics

As can be seen in the second section of Table 58–1, there are a number of worker characteristics that are demonstrated risk factors. Less-fit individuals in occupations as diverse as fire fighting[8] and bus driving[56] have a greater incidence of back injury.[17, 20] Cigarette smokers have a greater incidence of back injury in both retrospective[20, 53] and prospective[5] studies. Further, back pathology is correlated with the amount of smoking.[20]

A number of researchers report a relationship between stress and back injury.[20, 53, 56] These findings, although retrospective and methodologically weak, are consistent with a broader literature relating stress to accident and illness.[27, 32, 47, 51] As Hansen[27] has shown, distractibility secondary to distress is a plausible mechanism for the increased incidence of injury. Reducing stress as it relates to injury is a complicated matter reflecting the fact that the concept of stress itself represents a nexus of a substantial number of variables that are largely interactive.[31] Further, opportunity for control is diminished by the fact that morbidity is predicted equally well by the level of stress at work and the level of stress outside of work.[51] Also, there appears to be individual differences in susceptibility to environmental stress. Melamed et al.[47] examined the relationship between work and environmental stress and accidents. Although the level of work/environmental stress was related to the incidence of accidents, the more sensitive variable was subjective annoyance. That is, sensitivity to environmental stress rather than the stressor was the more potent predictor.

For back injury per se, in the absence of literature demonstrating a robust relationship between stress precisely defined and the incidence of injury, it would not be terribly productive to mount injury prevention programs based on stress reduction. Rather, the more prudent approach would be to reduce stress by increasing the worker's sense of control over the job through ergonomics and back school. A complementary approach would be to focus on fitness programs as described later in this chapter. This approach relies on the fact that programs designed to treat stress-related disorders routinely include regular exer-

TABLE 58–1.
Characteristics of the At-Risk Population and Prevention Strategies

Characteristics	Studies	Prevention Strategy
Work or job characteristics		
Lifting, carrying, pulling, pushing, twisting	Bigos et al.[6]	Ergonomics
	Frymoyer et al.[18–20]	
	Johnston[33]	
	Owen[52]	Back school
	Shim & Mensink[66]	
	Svensson[68]	
	Venning et al.[73]	
	Videman et al.[74]	
Driving	Frymoyer et al.[20]	Ergonomics
Nondriving vibrational exposure	Frymoyer et al.[20]	Ergonomics
Newer employees	Astrand[2]	Back school
	Bigos et al.[6]	
	Greenwood[25]	
	Johnston[33]	
Worker characteristics		
Behavioral medicine, or life-style		Health promotion programs
Fitness	Cady et al.[8]	
	Frymoyer et al.[20]	
	Patterson et al.[56]	
	Frymoyer[17]	
Cigarette smoking	Frymoyer et al.[20]	
	Owen & Damron[53]	
	Bigos & Battie[5]	Health promotion programs
Stress	Frymoyer et al.[20]	Health promotion programs
	Owen & Damron[53]	Ergonomics
	Patterson et al.[56]	Back school
Psychological characteristics		
Neuroticism, worry, tension	Frymoyer et al.[20]	
	Owen & Damron[53]	
	Astrand[2]	
Depression	Frymoyer et al.[20]	
	Frymoyer & Cats-Baril[18]	
	Mechanic and Angel[46]	
Hypochondriasis	Frymoyer et al.[21]	
	Pope et al.[60]	
	Frymoyer & Cats-Baril[18]	
Hysteria	Frymoyer et al.[21]	
	Frymoyer & Cats-Baril[18]	

cise as a means of enhancing an individual's control and the resistance of the organism.[24] Such an approach to stress is theoretically intelligible and, at the same time, attacks variables such as lifting, twisting, cigarette smoking, etc., which already have a defined empirical relationship to back injury. Further encouraging such an approach, Svensson et al.[69] found that the correlation between back pain and perception of stress dropped out when an analysis of covariance was applied to these data. Factors such as smoking and high physical activity at work did not.

The final section of Table 58–1 lists psychological risk factors for back injury.[2, 18, 20, 21, 46, 60, 69] In each case, the data are retrospective and do not allow any determination of whether these psychological measures are predictive of or a consequence of the back injury. The better speculation at this point would be that these changes are a consequence of the back injury. Some time ago, Sternbach and Timmermans[67] found that psychological changes of hypochondriasis, depression, and hysteria resolved following a reduction of pain through surgical intervention. Gatchel et al.[22] reported the same findings following treatment in a functional restoration program. Similarly, Levenson et al.[39] found that the magnitude of hypochondriasis, depression, and hysteria increased as time since the injury increased. In addition, Sedlak[65] reported the same relationship between the affective dimension of the McGill Pain Questionnaire, anxiety, and chronicity. Given these various findings, these psychological risk factors would appear to be the result of injury rather than its cause.

This posture apparently contradicts earlier work by

Hirschfeld and Behan[4, 29, 30] and Weinstein,[77] whose accident process model contended that certain personality types when vocationally challenged beyond their capability initially became dysphoric and less productive. An accident and subsequent injury secondary to their own carelessness, etc., became a socially acceptable reason for low or no productivity, and the dysphonic mood resolved. The present argument need not be construed as an outright rejection of the accident process model but, rather, suggests that psychological factors probably account for too small a portion of the variance when compared with more potent variables such as lifting, driving, smoking, etc. Again, as with the stress variables discussed above, this line of reasoning would encourage focus on the prevention strategies of ergonomics, back school, and health promotion programs rather than screening for psychological variables.

Psychological factors, although not demonstrated primary risk factors, have been shown to be secondary and tertiary risk factors. Secondary risk factors refer to a failure to respond to acute treatment of back injury. Numerous studies have variously identified anxiety, depression, hypochondriasis, and hysteria as significant risk factors.* Tertiary risk factors refer to a failure to respond to treatment for chronic pain. Again, various researchers have found hypochondriasis, depression, and hysteria to be related to treatment failure.[3, 36, 59] Because this chapter is focusing on primary risk factors, these secondary and tertiary factors will not be considered.

PSYCHOLOGY OF PREVENTION

In view of the risk factors reviewed above, there are three obvious points of attack to effect prevention: the worker, the job, and the interaction of the two. The various chapters in this section dealing with prevention will address these three points and elucidate the available technology. The success of this technology in reducing back injury, however, depends sensitively on a psychology of learning and incentive motivation. The worker must have an opportunity to learn new work and life-style habits as well as be motivated to consistently utilize new habits once acquired. Similarly, management must be motivated to provide resources for the worker and to provide incentives to facilitate the workers' level of motivation. The balance of this chapter examines learning and motivation variables involved in the habit-change prevention efforts of back school and health promotion programs.

The Back School

As Leonard has noted, the back school concept has developed over the past decade as an inexpensive approach to low back injury prevention.[38] Generally, the school teaches workers the anatomy and physiology of the spine, proper nutrition, stress reduction, body mechanics, physical fitness, and the role of posture in preventing back injuries. In reality, each school would necessarily alter focus as a function of the idiosyncrasies of the target job. A failure to have an impact on the injury rate could well reflect a problem of learning (including instruction) and/or incentive-motivation rather than inadequacy of the approach. Indeed there are sufficient data demonstrating a decreased number of injuries, workmen's compensation claims, and lost days due to injury following back school implementation[33, 66] that failure of effect would point to the qualitative or quantitative aspects of the intervention rather than the intervention per se.

The challenge of back school efforts is to change lifetime habits in a group of workers who might be indifferent or resistant to the effort and who might also have been less than overwhelmingly successful at previous formal instructional efforts. Thus, each program must contain (1) components for learning the new motor skills to the point where they occur automatically under appropriate stimulus conditions and (2) components that help the worker appreciate the relevance of these skills to his safety.

Learning/Instruction Variables

Instruction through lecture and demonstration is an integral part of each of these programs. Alavosius and Sulzer-Azaroff, however, have shown that instruction by itself has little impact on behavior.[1] Practice with feedback is critical to the successful integration of the new skills. Not only is feedback important, but the density or schedule of feedback also determines how rapidly change will occur. Continuous reinforcement is much superior to intermittent schedules for targeted health care routines. Formal programs have provided for continuous reinforcement in different ways. Shim and Mensink[66] provide for practice and peer feedback immediately after the lecture/demonstration aspect of their program for health care workers. This feedback component was carried over to the work setting by training peer "back care leaders" to provide instruction and reinforcement on each of the wards. Johnston[33] described a program that targeted workers particularly "at risk" and varied the density of feedback as a function of risk. In each case, however, the feedback was immediate and direct. Other researchers suggest training supervisors and team leaders[72] as well as coworkers and clients[43, 72] in appropriate techniques for feedback.

In addition to the initial learning sessions there must be provision for periodic refresher courses. Alavosius and Sulzer-Azaroff found that even when target behaviors were well learned in the initial training sessions, a 7-month follow-up revealed increased variability in performance.[1] Park and Chaffin reported results consistent with this.[54] This learning component has variably taken the form of

*References 12, 13, 37, 41, 49, 58, 63, 75, 79.

periodic in-service training, signs, and slogans as well as rigorous evaluation and reinstruction of injured workers.[7, 33, 66]

The fact that refresher courses are necessary has important implications for prevention program design. Theoretically, if correct performance becomes self-reinforcing as Venning[72] contended, then one would expect the correct technique to become stronger over time rather than more variable. The fundamental assumption here, however, is that correct performance is seen as positive by the individual worker. Obviously, in a climate of strongly negative work-related attitudes this assumption would be a poor one,[71] and attention would have to be directed to morale issues as part of the prevention program. Work-related attitudes aside, another potential source of performance variability would be insufficient initial training to effect the necessary level of behavior change. McKechnie described a back injury prevention program for nursing staff.[45] Questionnaire evaluation of comprehension indicated that only 58% could correctly describe the proper standing posture, only 76% could identify improper lifting techniques, and only 82% could correctly identify a basic back exercise. Against such a baseline of performance, deterioration over time would be anticipated. Thus, the duration and intensity of instruction for back care prevention should be criterion based rather than simply a standard package that might be impeccable in terms of instructional design but fail to accommodate individual variability in learning ability and motivation. Indeed, a number of researchers have found that back injury is associated with fewer years of education[2, 46] and poorer performance on tests of cognitive ability.[2] Frymoyer and Cats-Baril[18] identified education as a more potent predictor of back disability than pain, fitness level, or lawyer involvement. Clearly, then, particular care must be taken to determine exactly what the individual worker has acquired in instructional sessions.

Even when target behaviors are well learned, they do not necessarily generalize to the work site without specific efforts to ensure that they do so. Carlton[9] found that even though food service personnel instructed in body mechanics performed better on a novel task than did personnel not instructed, there was no difference between the groups when surreptitiously observed in the work environment. Efforts to ensure generalization in prevention programs typically involve training at the bedside for nursing[33] and demonstrating concrete field applications in factory work.[7]

Motivation Variables

The individual worker must be able to see the relevance of the prevention effort if he is to be expected to apply new strategies to the work site. As Button and Pater[7] have noted, many employees fail to be motivated by a strictly academic approach. Shim and Mensink[66] used a "walkabout" to provide direct relevance of the instructional unit to individual work areas and activities.

Broad-based institutional support is critically important, and all levels of management and labor should be committed to the prevention effort.[26] In the absence of such a commitment, the prevention program can be easily undermined. For example, in nursing injury prevention programs, if the use of assistive lifting devices is recommended but such devices are unavailable or in poor repair, there will be little motivation for their use. Similarly, prevention techniques that cannot be applied given space restraints or "buddy" programs in the context of understaffing all erode motivation so as to make the balance of the prevention program (i.e., instruction) worthless.

The job itself must be possible to do safely if the worker is to be motivated to use prevention strategies. Liles and Mahajan[40] demonstrated that the vast majority of lifting injuries and number of days lost per injury in their study population were in jobs that had action limit ratios making the job inherently unsafe. The action limit is defined by the National Institute of Occupational Safety and Health (NIOSH) guide as the average weight of lift that can be safely handled by 99% of the male and 75% of the female workers. The action limit ratio takes frequency into account as well as load. Since the NIOSH guide was published in 1981,[50] the necessary information for appropriate worker-job matching or job redesigning has long been available. This line of reasoning would place primary responsibility for injury prevention on management. Worker-initiated prevention strategies become relevant only when the inherent risk of a job is brought within NIOSH guidelines either by redesign, appropriate screening,[48] or provision of a conditioning program.[23]

Intrinsic motivation is preferable when the employee sees prevention behavior as related to professional competence[71] or simply in his or her own best interest. When this fails, however, external incentive-motivation through a system of rewards and punishments (withdrawal of rewards) as typically found in safety programs might be necessary. Griffiths[26] reported a safety program implemented by Air Product Companies in Europe following consultation with safety advisors from DuPont, an organization that has distinguished itself in the field of industrial safety. Under this program, back injury lost-time accidents decreased from an average of approximately 20 per year to approximately 1 per year. There were several DuPont principles incorporated into their program that bear on the issue of motivation. First, safety is viewed at the same level of importance as finance, sales, and production. Second, it is a line management responsibility with defined goals, reporting, and accountability. Third, management is responsible for the safety of its employees, and finally, safety is a condition of employment. Thus, even if the company's commitment to the employee cannot inspire the individual worker to work safely, the potential punishment of loss of employment would probably suffice for incentive-motivation.

Health Promotion Programs

As identified risk factors for back injury, modification of health behaviors related to fitness, smoking, and stress management should, at least theoretically, reduce risk. Unfortunately, unlike back school approaches, there has not been any appreciable evaluative research to support the efficacy of the health promotion approach as they relate directly to back injury. Further, as Warner et al. have noted, much of the research in this area is methodologically unsophisticated.[76] Thus, there is no empirical basis for strongly promoting fitness as a preventive measure for back injury. The obvious need, then, is for well-designed evaluation research in this area.

The major difficulty with health promotion programs is incentive-motivational. Simply put, those who are most likely to participate are nonsmokers, those who are more knowledgeable about the benefits of exercise, and those already fit and already engaged in an exercise program.[10, 16, 78] Obviously, these would also be the workers with the least risk of back injury. The challenge, then, is to motivate the smoking, poorly fit worker who does not appreciate the benefits of exercise. This challenge is compounded by the fact that the reinforcing effect of life-style changes promoted in fitness programs are much delayed and slow in coming.[42]

As regards the conceptual model of incentive-motivation, there are several program characteristics that could enhance participation. Table 58–2 outlines these learning and motivation variables. The task within learning is to provide sufficient reinforcers or incentives to bridge the delay between health behavior and the inherent positive consequences, e.g., reduced illness, greater energy, improved mood, etc. Similarly, alternative sources of motivation must be generated to support the health behaviors until the effects of the program are sufficient to motivate the individual worker. Part of this effort will entail engineering participation to minimally tax whatever level of motivation exists.

TABLE 58–2.
Learning and Motivation Variables in Health Promotion Programs

- Learning
  - Reinforcers
    - Periodic reinforcement
    - Social reinforcement
    - Material reinforcement
- Motivation
  - Minimize effort
    - Location in worksite
    - Available during work hours
  - Organizational support
    - Adequate facilities
    - Consistent health policies

There are a variety of strategies for reinforcing healthful behavior. Feldman suggested that work site programs with periodic contact with health professionals provide many opportunities to reinforce target behaviors.[15] Moreover, self-monitoring or record keeping that is designed by utilizing appropriate behavioral technology allows the worker to see his progress toward the goal and has inherent reinforcing properties.[62]

Social reinforcement is likely greater when the program is located within the workplace. The population is relatively stable, and supervision can be trained to provide reinforcement. Competition among teams, shops, divisions, etc., offers social reinforcement from team members.[15]

Finally, Feldman reported a number of material reinforcers that have been used in various company-based health promotion programs.[15] These include money, show tickets, trading stamps, books, T-shirts, release time, and lottery tickets. Theoretically, at least, these material reinforcers should only be necessary until the beneficial and reinforcing effects of health behavior are realized.

A consistent finding in program adherence is that participation is a function of convenience. Workers are more likely to participate if the program is on-site at the workplace, is offered during work hours, and minimizes any waiting time.[15, 42] Beyond minimizing required effort so as not to tax marginally motivated behavior, participation can be enhanced by allowing workers to participate in program planning.[42] Finally, organizational support in the form of adequate exercise facilities, consistent health policies within the workplace, nutritious food in the cafeteria, etc.,[14] minimizes the effort required by the individual worker to effect life-style changes.

SUMMARY

The principles of successful safety programming outlined by Griffiths captures the essence of injury prevention: both labor and management must each take responsibility for their respective roles.[26] Management must provide an ergonomically safe work environment with the opportunity to learn appropriate body mechanics and injury prevention techniques. Management also has the responsibility of providing a consistent policy and promoting a healthy life-style. In turn, labor has the responsibility to consistently learn and use risk-reducing strategies and devices. Further, labor has the responsibility to participate in fitness programming. The technology of back injury prevention in terms of back school, ergonomics, and physical conditioning is well established. Whether injuries occur or not will be contingent on whether labor and management are sufficiently motivated to implement available technology. The incentive for management lies in an overall cost savings, which means that outcome research expressed in terms of cost-effectiveness is critically important. Unfortunately, it is woefully lacking.[76] The incentive for labor is more obscure. The fact that many injuries occur because workers have not used available safety devices[43, 61, 71] suggests that injury prevention itself is not a sufficient incentive. It might well be the case that the DuPont imperative of safety as a condition of employment is a necessary condition for back injury prevention.

REFERENCES

1. Alavosius MP, Sulzer-Azaroff B: Acquisition and maintenance of health-care routines as a function of feedback density. *J Appl Behav Anal* 1990; 23:151–162.
2. Astrand NE: Medical, psychological and social factors associated with back abnormalities and self reported back pain: A cross sectional study of male employees in a Swedish pulp and paper industry. *Br J Ind Med* 1987; 44:327–336.
3. Barnes D, Smith D, Gatchel RJ, et al: Psychosocioeconomic predictors of treatment success/failure in chronic low-back pain patients. *Spine* 1989; 14:427–430.
4. Behan RC, Hirschfeld AH: The accident process: II. Toward more rational treatment of industrial injuries. *JAMA* 1963; 186:91–96.
5. Bigos SJ, Battie MC: Preplacement work testing and selection considerations. *Ergonomics* 1987; 30:249–251.
6. Bigos SJ, Spengler DM, Martin NA, et al: Back injuries in industry: A retrospective study II. Employee-related factors. *Spine* 1986; 11:252.
7. Button R, Pater R: Pretraining is essential tool for fall and back injuries. *Occup Health Saf* 1988; 57:23–25.
8. Cady LD, Bischoff DP, O'Connell ER, et al: Strength and fitness and subsequent back injuries in firefighters. *J Occup Med* 1979; 21:269.
9. Carlton RS: The effect of body mechanics instruction on work performance. *Am J Occup Ther* 1987; 47:16–20.
10. Conrad P: Who comes to work site wellness programs? A preliminary review. *J Occup Med* 1987; 29:317–320.
11. Dereberey JV, Tullis WH: Low back pain exacerbated by psychosocial factors. *West J Med* 1986; 144:574–579.
12. Deyo RA, Diehl AK: Psychosocial predictors of disability in patients with low back pain. *Spine* 1988; 15:1557–1563.
13. Dzioba RB, Doxey NC: A prospective investigation into the orthopaedic and psychologic predictors of outcome of first lumbar surgery following industrial injury. *Spine* 1984; 9:614–623.
14. Everly GS, Feldman RH (eds): *Occupational Health Promotion: Health Behavior in the Workplace*. New York, John Wiley & Sons, 1985.
15. Feldman RHL: Strategies for improving compliance with health promotion programs in industry. *Health Educ* 1983; 14:21–25.
16. Fielding JE: Health promotion and disease prevention at the work site. *Annu Rev Public Health* 1984; 5:237–265.
17. Frymoyer JW: Helping your patients avoid low back pain. *J Musculoskel Med* 1984; 1:65–74.
18. Frymoyer JW, Cats-Baril W: Predictors of low back pain disability. *Clin Orthop* 1987; 221:89–98.
19. Frymoyer JW, Pope MH, Clements JH, et al: Risk factors in low back pain. An epidemiologic survey. *J Bone Joint Surg [Am]* 1983; 65:213–218.
20. Frymoyer JW, Pope MH, Costanza MC, et al: Epidemiologic studies of low-back pain. *Spine* 1980; 5:419–423.
21. Frymoyer JW, Rosen JC, Clements J, et al: Psychologic factors in low-back-pain disability. *Clin Orthop* 1985; 195:178–184.
22. Gatchel RJ, Mayer TG, Capra P, et al: Quantification of lumbar function. Part 6: The use of psychological measures in guiding physical functional restoration. *Spine* 1986; 11:36–42.
23. Genady AM, Bafna KM, Sarmidy R, et al: A muscular endurance program for symmetrical and asymmetrical manual lifting tasks. *J Occup Med* 1990; 32:226–233.
24. Genest M, Genest S: *Psychology and Health,* Champaign, Ill, Research Press, 1987.
25. Greenwood JG: Back injuries can be reduced with worker training, reinforcement. *Occup Health Saf* 1986; 55:26–29.
26. Griffiths DK: Safety attitudes of management. *Ergonomics* 1985; 28:61–67.
27. Hansen CP: A causal model of the relationship among accidents, biodata, personality and cognitive factors. *J Appl Psychol* 1989; 74:81–90.
28. Herbert L, Miller G: Newer heavy load lifting methods help firms reduce back injuries. *Occup Health Saf* 1987; 56:57–60.
29. Hirschfeld AH, Behan RC: The accident process: I. Etiological considerations of industrial injuries. *JAMA* 1963; 186:84–90.
30. Hirschfeld AH, Behan RC: The accident process: III. Disability, acceptable and unacceptable. *JAMA* 1966; 197:125–129.
31. Holroyo KA, Lazarus RS: Stress, coping and somatic adaptation, in Goldberger L, Breznutzs (eds): *Handbook of Stress*. New York, Free Press, 1982.
32. Israel BA, House JS, Schurman SJ, et al: The relation of personal resources, participation, influence, interpersonal relationships and coping strategies to occupational stress, job strains and health: A multivariate analysis. *Work Stress* 1989; 3:163–194.
33. Johnston B: Back care program eases strain on backs and budgets. *Dimens Health Serv* 1987; 64:41–42.
34. Kelsey JL, Golden AL: Occupational and workplace factors associated with low back pain. *Occup Med* 1988; 3:7–16.
35. Kirkaldy-Willis WH (ed): *Managing Low Back Pain,* ed 2. New York, Churchill Livingstone, 1988.
36. Lawlis GF, Mooney V, Selby DK, et al: A motivational scoring system for outcome prediction with spinal pain rehabilitation patients. *Spine* 1982; 7:163–167.
37. Lee PWH, Chou SP, Lieh-Mak F, et al: Psychosocial fac-

tors influencing outcomes in patients with low-back pain. *Spine* 1989; 14:838–842.

38. Leonard SA: The role of exercise and posture in preventing low back injury. *AAOHN J* 1990; 38:318–322.
39. Levenson H, Glenn N, Hirschfeld JL: Duration of chronic pain and the Minnesota Multiphasic Personality Inventory: Profiles of industrially injured workers. *J Occup Med* 1988; 30:809–912.
40. Liles DH, Mahajan P: Using NIOSH lifting guide decreases risks of back injuries. *Occup Health Saf* 1985; 54:57–60.
41. Long CJ: The relationship between surgical outcome and MMPI profiles in chronic pain patients. *J Clin Psychol* 1981; 37:744–749.
42. Lovato CY, Green LW: Maintaining employee participation in workplace health promotion programs. *Health Educ Q* 1990; 17:73–88.
43. Marchette L, Marchette B: Back injury: A preventable occupational hazard. *Orthop Nurs* 1985; 4:25–29.
44. Matheson LN: *Work Capacity Evaluation: Interdisciplinary Approach to Industrial Rehabilitation,* ed 1. Anaheim, Calif, Employment Rehabilitation Institute of California, 1984.
45. McKechnie MR: Preventing back injuries: An application of the nursing research process. *Occup Health Nurs* 1985; 33:552–557.
46. Mechanic D, Angel RJ: Some factors associated with the report and evaluation of back pain. *J Health Soc Behav* 1987; 28:131–139.
47. Melamed S, Luz J, Najenson T, et al: Ergonomic stress levels, personal characteristics, accident occurrence and sickness absence among factory workers. *Ergonomics* 1989; 32:1101–1110.
48. Morris A: Identifying workers at risk to back injury is not guesswork. *Occup Health Saf* 1985; 54:16–20.
49. Murphy KA, Cornish RD: Prediction of chronicity in acute low back pain. *Arch Phys Med Rehabil* 1984; 65: 335–337.
50. National Institute for Occupational Safety and Health: *Work Practice Guide for Manual Lifting*. National Institute for Occupational Safety and Health Publication No 81-122. Cincinnati, NIOSH Public Health Service, 1981.
51. Niemcryk SJ, Jenkins CD, Rose RM, et al: The prospective impact of psychosocial variables on rates of illness and injury in professional employees. *J Occup Med* 1987; 29:645–652.
52. Owen BD: The lifting process and back injury in hospital nursing personnel. *West J Nurs Res* 1985; 7:445–459.
53. Owen BD, Damron C: Personal characteristics and back injury among nursing personnel. *Res Nurs Health* 1984; 7:305–313.
54. Park K, Chaffin D: Prediction of load lifting limits for manual materials lifting. *Professional Saf Am Soc Saf Eng* 1974; 20:44–48.
55. Parnianpour M, Bejjani FJ, Pavlidis L: Worker training: The fallacy of a single, correct lifting technique. *Ergonomics* 1987; 30:331–334.
56. Patterson PK, Eubanks TL, Ramseyer R: Back discomfort prevalence and associated factors among bus drivers. *AAOHN J* 1986; 34:481–484.
57. Pavett C: Evaluation of the impact of feedback on performance and motivation. *Hum Relations* 1983; 36:641–654.
58. Phillips BV, Bee DE: Determinants of postoperative recovery in elective orthopedic surgery. *Soc Sci Med* 1980; 14:325–330.
59. Polatin PB, Gatchel RJ, Barnes D, et al: A psychosociomedical prediction model of response to treatment by chronically disabled workers with low-back pain. *Spine* 1989; 14:956–961.
60. Pope MH, Rosen JC, Wilder DG, et al: The relationship between biomechanical and psychological factors in patients with low-back pain. *Spine* 1980; 5:173–178.
61. Prezant B, Demers P, Strand K: Back problem, training experience and lifting aids, in Asfour SS (ed): *Trends in Ergonomics/Human Factors VI*. Amsterdam, Elsevier, 1987.
62. Rimm DC, Masters JC: *Behavior Therapy*. New York, Academic Press, 1974.
63. Rosen JC, Grubman JA, Bevins T, et al: Musculoskeletal status and disability of MMPI profile subgroups among patients with low back pain. *Health Psychol* 1987; 6:581–598.
64. Schmidt AJM, Arntz A: Psychological research and chronic low back pain: A standstill or breakthrough. *Soc Sci Med* 1987; 25:1095–1104.
65. Sedlak K: Low-back pain: Perception and tolerance. *Spine* 1985; 10:440–444.
66. Shim M, Mensink N: A back care program for health care workers. *Occup Health Saf* 1989; 66:24–26.
67. Sternbach RA, Timmermans G: Personality changes associated with reductions in pain. *Pain* 1975; 1:177–181.
68. Svensson HO: Low back pain in forty to forty-seven year old men. II. Socio-economic factors and previous sickness absence. *Scand J Rehabil Med* 1982; 14:55–60.
69. Svensson HO, Anders V, Wilhelmsson C, et al: Low-back pain in relation to other diseases and cardiovascular risk factors. *Spine* 1983; 8:277–285.
70. Turk DC, Flor H: Etiological theories and treatments for chronic back pain. II. Psychological models and interventions. *Pain* 1984; 19:209–233.
71. Venning PJ: Back injury prevention among nursing personnel: The role of education. *AAOHN J* 1988; 36:327–332.
72. Venning PJ: Back injury prevention: Instructional design features for program planning. *AAOHN J* 1988; 36:336–341.
73. Venning PJ, Walter SD, Stitt LW: Personal and job-related factors as determinants of incidence of back injuries among nursing personnel. *Occup Med* 1987; 29:820–825.
74. Videman T, Nurmimen T, Tola S, et al: Low-back pain in nurses and some loading factors of work. *Spine* 1984; 9:400–404.
75. Villard HP, Imbeault J, Duguay M: Low-back pain: A psychosomatic clinical study. *Psychother Psychosom* 1986; 45:78–83.
76. Warner KE, Wickizer TM, Wolve RA, et al: Economic

implications of workplace health promotion programs: Review of the literature. *J Occup Med* 1988; 30:106–112.
77. Weinstein MR: The concept of the disability process. *Psychosomatics* 1978; 19:94–97.
78. Wier LT, Jackson AS: Factors affecting compliance in the NASA/Johnson Space Center fitness programme. *Sports Med* 1989; 8:9–14.
79. Wiltse LL: Psychological testing in predicting the success of the low back surgery. *Orthop Clin North Am* 1975; 6:317.

PART XIX

DEVELOPMENT OF A SPINE REHABILITATION CENTER

59

General Considerations

Stephen H. Hochschuler, M.D.

In 1977 the concept of a back institute was pursued by myself and another spine specialist. The vision was to be an academically oriented private practice, thus affording academicians who would have preferred staying in a university setting an opportunity to have the benefits of both an academic and private practice experience. It became obvious that in order to have a successful practice addressing the conservative and surgical management of spinal disorders, a multidisciplinary approach would be required. Originally, the disciplines were spine surgery, physical therapy, occupational therapy, psychology, and patient education. As the patient population grew and more facets of the complexity of back pain were recognized, so too was the need to incorporate the expertise of other disciplines. These other specialties include conservative-care physicians, general surgeons, neurologists, neuroradiologists, anesthesiologists, dolorologists, and exercise physiologists. In order to remain up to date with current knowledge, provide education, and contribute to developments in spine care, a research foundation was established. From our experience gained from building the Texas Back Institute, this chapter was written to outline the components and organization of a spine center. These areas include the following:

- Prevention
  - Pre-employment screening
  - Industrial back school
  - Ergonomic analysis and consulting services
- Conservative care
  - Physical therapy
  - Occupational therapy
  - Psychology
  - Exercise physiology
- Work rehabilitation
- Diagnostic services
- Surgery
- Educational and informational services
  - Patient education
  - Continuing medical education
  - Spine fellowship program
- Research and new product development
  - Publishing (books and journals)
  - Management

PREVENTION

The problem of back pain and related expenses is thought to cost American society approximately 80 billion dollars per year. It is the contention of many people in the field of spine disorders that much of this could be avoided with proper prevention programs. This includes appropriate ergonomic analysis of the workplace, education in proper body mechanics and lifting techniques, as well as appropriate seating and desk configurations. It is also important to exercise at the workplace itself. The interrelationship of stress and back pain needs to be addressed, and the whole concept of making the workplace a more friendly environment will tend to reduce health care costs in general and back pain problems specifically. Many companies have started to utilize pre-employment screening, education and training programs, and preventive devices such as back supports. In addition, it becomes very important to match the worker to the job and not put a worker in a position of manual labor that places considerable stress on the back when indeed the worker is not conditioned for such. In addition, continued periodic monitoring of employees' spine status, much like one monitoring the heart with periodic electrocardiograms, will likely evolve.

Another branch of prevention and cost containment associated with low back injuries involves the development of computerized knowledge-based artificial intelligence systems to provide more information as to the type of work most commonly associated with injury and to track back care once an insult has occurred. It is hoped that this, combined with the proper rehabilitative services after injury, will prevent further insult.

CONSERVATIVE CARE

Most injuries involving the spine are self-limiting, but it is important that the individual, once injured, be properly trained in all aspects of good spinal health including proper body mechanics as well as the role of exercise. This should include aerobic and anaerobic conditioning, stretching, strengthening, and first aid.

Just as a diabetic is given responsibility to help maintain his good health, so too the patient with back pain is instructed in proper back health. In most instances, the patient signs a contract stipulating his commitment to follow prescribed protocols and thus buys into the whole rehabilitative process. Treatment is provided through a multidisciplinary team approach. Naturally, not every patient requires physical therapy, occupational therapy, and psychological services. A basic screening process takes place and the appropriate treatment plan determined.

Physical therapy services include the traditional approaches to spine therapy, but the treatment program itself is individualized based on the patient's diagnosis. Therefore, whether Williams flexion, McKenzie extension, Paris protocols, medical exercise training, or other protocols are utilized depends entirely on the diagnosis and patient's response to treatment. The focus is not merely on the spine, but on rehabilitation of the entire patient. This is particularly important for patients whose activity level has been greatly decreased for a period of time due to back pain.

Occupational therapy services include such functions as job placement, coordinating the patient's most recent functional physical capabilities assessment and job requirements, developing work simulation activities, and helping to arrange for the patient's ongoing educational opportunities in regard to cross-training, when indicated.

Psychological services are becoming increasingly more important. Many back pain sufferers experience frustration in all areas of life. Psychological services include group and individual psychotherapy, biofeedback, behavior modification, and well-being programs. It is to be noted that behavior modification has proved to be an effective adjunct for weight reduction programs. Indeed, the present fad of liquid diets per se, has not proven to be nearly as efficacious as when combined with proper behavior modification. Problems of sexual dysfunction and marital discord are associated with back injury and often with a significant psychological overlay. Proper attitude and support systems in these areas can accelerate the back sufferer's recovery.

Exercise physiology interacts in a conjoint fashion with both physical therapy and occupational therapy. Exercise and aerobic conditioning have played a very important role in treating patients who have developed depression. We have found that the concept of wellness and fitness is most holistically embodied in the training of exercise physiologists. The addition of this discipline in the treatment of back pain has been beneficial.

WORK REHABILITATION

The need for a specialized treatment approach directed toward returning injured workers back to the work force was recognized very early in our development. This eventually led to the creation of a rehabilitation center for injured workers. A prototype model was developed over a 4-year period, and extensive procedural manuals were organized to facilitate appropriate patient tracking and help coordinate outcome studies. This type of documentation is required to meet the guidelines for certification by the Commission of Accreditation of Rehabilitation Facilities (CARF). Once all the treatment and documentation procedures were developed, this program was replicated in other parts of the country.

DIAGNOSTIC SERVICES

The challenge of properly diagnosing back pain, particularly in patients with very chronic pain and those who have previously undergone spine surgery, brought about the need for diagnostic specialists. For several years now, myelography and discography have been performed on an outpatient basis at our institute. A well-equipped diagnostic center also allows epidural steroid injections, facet injections, facet rhizotomies, differential spinals, Pentothal studies, and other diagnostic/therapeutic procedures to be performed on outpatients.

Case managers coordinate all studies and are responsible for the comprehensive compilation of the patient's diagnostic and therapeutic history. This information is reviewed periodically to ensure that the patient is progressing satisfactorily with treatment and, if not, what actions (such as changes in therapy, diagnostic procedures, or possibly surgical intervention) need to be taken.

SURGERY

Surgical care is deemed appropriate only when conservative modalities have not proved effacacious and the patient meets surgical selection criteria. It is essential to good surgical patient care to remain up to date on procedures and devices. One way of doing this is to become involved with the spine societies, participate in multicenter trials evaluating new devices, and be involved in development efforts. Some items currently being developed and investigated are various instrumentation systems, percutaneous spinal procedures, new bone graft substitutes, and an artificial disc prosthesis.

With a large number of spine surgeons in the group, we have had the opportunity to subspecialize in areas of cervical, lumbar, adult, or pediatric deformity, tumor/oncology, and trauma. Each surgeon is integrally involved with ongoing research in his area of interest, teaching projects, and participation in the various subspecialty societies of the spine.

EDUCATIONAL AND INFORMATIONAL SERVICES

Patient education takes on many forms. The two main thrusts of our patient education efforts have been on back school and presurgical teaching. Booklets dealing with general topics in back pain, anatomy, nutrition, and exercise are frequently given to patients. Also, reprints are available on recreational activities such as golf, running, and cycling for patients with interests in these specific areas.

The *back school* is taught in a group setting and deals with topics of anatomy, body mechanics and lifting techniques, nutrition, relaxation techniques, and the importance of exercise. The sessions are taught by nurses, occupational therapists, physical therapists, and psychologists. The *presurgical teaching program* has led to the development of a collection of videotapes in English as well as Spanish. This has taken a tremendous amount of time and financial commitment but has proved very effective. The prospective surgical patient views the appropriate tape with a nurse-educator present to answer questions. A consent form is reviewed and signed that states that the patient has had the opportunity to view the tape, that he understands the surgical procedure and had the opportunity to ask questions, and that these questions were satisfactorily answered. This is documented by the nurse clinician. The patient's family is also involved. All are made aware that surgical intervention does not mean cure. The hope is that the pain perception will diminish, but the reality is that it will not become nonexistent. In addition, the patient must commit to the rehabilitation process prior to undergoing surgery and, wherever possible, must lose the appropriate amount of weight as well as stop smoking. Medication policies are reviewed prior to the surgical endeavor. The emphasis, therefore, is on patient commitment to the entire treatment process, and the surgeon is no longer deemed a magician.

In order to continually provide quality service, all members of the health care team must stay abreast of current treatment issues and techniques. *Continuing education* is also very important in stimulating intellectual growth and interaction throughout the organization. A weekly conference is held for employees and others interested in the treatment of patients with back pain. Special workshops are held that deal with new surgical techniques, and other courses train therapists in specialized spine treatment methods.

Persons in each discipline are encouraged to attend specialty meetings in their areas. It is important for professionals to not only attend major conferences but also participate by presenting their research work.

Through a *spine fellowship* program the organization has the opportunity to train surgeons in operative techniques, treatment decision making, rehabilitation, and research. This program not only teaches the fellows but also stimulates our physicians with a continuous barrage of challenges as to procedural methods and helps to develop new ideas. Each fellow is required to participate in a research project and must be present on a frequent basis at the weekly meetings.

RESEARCH AND NEW PRODUCT DEVELOPMENT

The Texas Back Institute Research Foundation was developed to further spine education and to help advance basic science and clinical research as well as help in the area of new product development. It is felt that the 1990s will stress the importance of cost containment in relation to all aspects of medicine, especially spinal problems. Outcome studies will become quite important in regard to fiscal expenditures. Through research and technological efforts, patient tracking and evaluation methods are being developed to assess treatment outcome. In order to adequately evaluate the efficacy of new procedures, we have become involved with prospective, multicenter studies.

PUBLICATIONS

In order to promote education to both the professional and lay communities, the role of the research foundation was expanded to include publication of books and journals. This addition provided us the opportunity to develop and disseminate educational materials dedicated to the spine and low back care.

MANAGEMENT

Interwoven among these different aspects of the organization is a very sophisticated management team. The development of a management team that realizes the goals of the care providers and understands the health care arena can be difficult. Open communication between management and physicians is not easily achieved. The system itself takes constant nurturing, and there must be a fine balance between the business and the academic aspects. The goal must be for excellence and quality care for the patient. By keeping this in mind one is able to balance most of the elements of a very dynamic organization.

SUMMARY

The development of a back institute is an ongoing, long-term process not to be undertaken without careful planning. As has been our experience, the organization must be flexible enough to accommodate the changing needs of the patient population and health care environment. There is no doubt that research and technology will improve our understanding of low back pain, develop better diagnostic procedures, distinguish beneficial from useless treatments, and develop new treatments. This will result in changing the approach to low back pain, and thus the components and organization of a back institute will also change.

60

Back School

David F. Fardon, M.D.

Back school is the most important contribution to spine care of this century. Eighty percent of adults have problems with back pain.[21] Although most episodes of back pain resolve in 2 or 3 months,[94] 20% to 50% recur.[5, 55, 95] While operations have cured the few whose disorders were amenable, most back pain cannot be cured surgically. Back school offers relief to all back pain sufferers and prevention to those not yet afflicted.

The predecessors and early examples of back school date well back into medical history, but the term *back school* and the widespread familiarity of concepts signified by the term began in the 1970s. By 1980 there were hundreds of back schools, and now there are thousands.[116] The majority of spine surgeons prescribe back school for a large percentage of their patients.[37, 119]

WHAT IS BACK SCHOOL?

Something called "back school" is so popular that one is accessible practically everywhere. But if the concepts have been around since before the term, what is new that is unique, and what exactly does "back school" mean?

White defined back school, in its narrow sense, as an educational and training facility that teaches back health care and body mechanics to individuals, but he goes on to expand the definition to include back-related industrial health, perisurgical hospital care, and various other public education efforts for nonpatients.[115]

At one end of the spectrum, we find back school programs that incorporate conditioning techniques often described as functions of a "pain clinic"[10, 54, 92, 104] that offer care of neck disorders, osteoporosis, and other spine-related disorders and provide hospital care, sports rehabilitation, work hardening, and industrial injury prevention. At the other end, we find the self-operated, sound-slide program tucked in the corner of a physical therapy unit with the patient watching a prepackaged presentation that will be the only manifestation of the "back school" into which he has enrolled.

Suppose one spine surgeon works with a therapist who teaches exercise, body mechanics, health, and nutrition to back patients, follows the surgical patients through surgery and guides their rehabilitation, assesses jobs and the patients' capacities to perform them, and assists with whatever modifications are needed for the patient to return to a productive life but does not have a "facility" or a program called "back school." Suppose another surgeon has an employee who gives a one-time instruction in exercise and has each patient watch a prepackaged sound-slide program that they promote as "back school." Who really has a back school?

History sometimes clarifies meaning. The principles of exercise to maintain health, particularly health of the spine, were expressed by Nicholas Andry, the father, or at least the namer, of modern orthopedics.[60] In 1825 in France, Jacques Malthieu Delpech established an elaborate facility to care for spine patients through supervised exercise and attention to posture. Delpech had both indoor and outdoor facilities, promoted general health, fitness, and nutrition, and used a pool and numerous sophisticated exercise machines to assist his efforts.[60, 89]

In the mid-20th century, Henry Fahrni made popular the concept of teaching back health.[31, 32] In the early 1970s, Zacrisson-Forsell established the Swedish back school at Danderyd Hospital and thus began the worldwide teaching of back health under the term "back school."[118] Hamilton Hall's Canadian Back Education Unit in Toronto brought back school to North America in 1974.[50] Soon followed Arthur White's California back school in San Francisco[115] and Nancy Selby's Spine Education Unit in Dallas,[100] both of which expanded the concept into industrial education and prevention programs. Soon after, individual practitioners in smaller cities found back schools useful.[3, 9]

During the 1980s, back schools expanded services to offer the different programs discussed below, included the talents of various specialists, and applied the latest technological advances. Nowadays, some back schools have indoor and outdoor facilities, promote general health, fitness, and nutrition, and use a pool and numerous sophisticated exercise machines to assist their efforts.[53]

"Back school," we must accept, is a generic term that refers to a variety of programs of varying depth and a wide range. Later in this chapter we will consider that range. For now and for the purpose of considering effectiveness, we will consider back school within White's narrower definition as an educational facility that teaches back health care and body mechanics to individuals, with occasional reference to the qualification added by Jackson and Klugerman, whose definition added the clause "in a cost-effective manner."[58]

DOES BACK SCHOOL WORK?

Several studies document that instructional courses may be beneficial treatment for diseases other than back pain.[29, 51, 59, 69, 78, 111] Bergquist-Ullman and Larsson in 1977 reported successful treatment of back patients by a back school in a Volvo factory.[5] Others followed with similar assertions.[34, 46, 50, 63, 103, 120] Some researchers, however, have reported that back school was of qualified value or no benefit.[6, 67, 70, 106] Two concepts help explain such contraindictions: the problem with definition of the term "back school" and difficulties with outcome assessment.

One of the studies that reported poor results described their back school as a single 45-minute teaching session to patients who were instructed not to exercise.[106] The "back school" of another study that reported poor results consisted of a single 4-hour instruction, a format to which they had reverted because of poor attendance at a previous attempt at a multisession course.[6]

Outcome assessment is particularly difficult for back schools. Few studies related to spine care are adequately controlled.[8, 21, 84, 92] To assess the effect of a multivariate treatment regimen like back school upon a heterogeneous group like patients with back pain would strain even the most carefully constructed protocol. Even when a positive effect seems to exist, the causal links may be hard to define and could be such nonspecific factors as the influence of authority figures, promotion of self-sufficiency, or an avenue for "escape" into wellness.[34, 40] The widespread endorsement of back school by spine surgeons is due to the inherent good sense of it rather than documented effectiveness.

WHAT IS THE ESSENCE OF BACK SCHOOL?

We said that back school is this century's most important contribution to spine care, and then we said that we cannot define back school or prove that back school works. What, then, is there about back school that makes it so valuable?

Back school focuses the patient upon his role as guardian of his own health, with particular attention to his spine. Back school shifts the focus of responsibility from the doctor/therapist to the patient.

In 1919, Arthur Keith stated, "the sooner the patient ceases to rely on outside help, and the sooner he comes to realize that progress depends on his own effort, the quicker and the better will be the ultimate result. . . ."[60] While Keith and a few others espoused such a philosophy, that was not the dominant message from generations of practioners anxious to sell their services to a dependent public. Nor was it the mood engendered in the following era when safe anesthesia, transfusions, antibiotics, and other advances of modern medicine encouraged patients to assume passive roles while miracle cures were attempted.

The advent of disc surgery brought a cure for sciatica to a few but encouraged passive compliance to treatment by the multitude with nonsurgical back pain. The decades of the disc were also decades of heat, massage, and ultrasound. Back school represents a shift of focus that brings the patient a more realistic attitude toward acceptance of health care and the confidence and tools to deal with those problems he can handle himself.

Back school focuses the professional upon his role as mentor. In modern society, self-care has become popular and profitable. The patient is besieged with data and advice about health—most of it either bad or beside the point. Information is not enough. The patient needs someone with the judgment to select health information and sort and deliver it in ways that are pertinent to his problem and acceptable to his use.

Physicians have marvelous new scientific ways to diagnose and treat back pain. While that is good, it also widens the gap between the way the patient relates his symptoms to his life and the way his doctor relates his symptoms to scientific understanding. Back school is the bridge over that gap. Back school demands that the physician extend to make his science relevant and comprehensible, and it demands that the patient extend to grasp the knowledge and apply it to his life. Those who work in back schools are the guides across that bridge. One of the essential elements of back school is therefore that it demands that health care professionals seize and expand their roles as educators.

VARIATIONS OF BACK SCHOOLS

It is easier to define some of the twists and tangents that back schools have taken than it is to define an "average" or "standard" back school program. Everyone's personal needs and experiences drive their own ideas of what a standard back school is or should be. The descriptions that follow represent mainstream concepts but do not define the terms unique to each circumstance.

Standard Back School

The course is presented in three to five sessions of 2 to 4 hours each, given at weekly intervals. The subject is low back pain.

Everyone is accepted. Whether physician referral is required or not depends upon local law, custom, billing circumstances, and preference of the directors. Most schools require physician referral. It is recognized that back school may not succeed for patients with severe pain, limited comprehension,[50] drug dependence, or severe psychiatric disturbance[34]; however, all who can comply with the program are accepted.

Class sizes vary from 1 to 12. Not all phases of the program are done in the same groups. Individual attention is required for evaluation and some phases of exercise and body mechanics instruction, whereas lecture demonstrations that deal with topics such as nutrition are presented to larger groups.

Patients are assigned tasks and expected to maintain prescribed programs during the days between sessions. Their progress is assessed at each session. They are encouraged to call as needed and to return for a routine evaluation session 3 to 6 months later.

Standard "Short" Course

Some patients whose economic and social circumstances demand it may take the same comprehensive program offered in the standard course in a compressed course over a 3- to 5-day period. Such a schedule demands more of the patient and is more difficult for the therapist to implement.

Neck Course

The principles of a back school apply to neck care. Most of the details are different, so the therapist must prepare special programs. The space and equipment requirements are not much greater, the format can be quite similar, and the same personnel can provide the care. Whether one calls such an effort a "neck school" seems of little import, but application of the concept can be quite rewarding.

Since many patients have neck and back pain, a *combined course* may be designed in which both problems are addressed in five or six sessions.

Work Hardening

Work hardening is discussed more exhaustively elsewhere in this text. However, the programs ordinarily referred to as "back school" and those referred to as "work hardening" so overlap that it is not possible to thoroughly discuss back school without some discussion of work hardening.

Among the patients who are treated at every back school are some who are so deconditioned or who must face such a great discrepancy between what life expects of them and what they can deliver that a four-session self-help course is insufficient. Some of those patients could benefit by a more prolonged, supervised effort at physical, psychological, and social readjustment.

The elements of a standard back school should either precede or be incorporated into the care of each patient who undergoes work hardening. The back school may remain separate and distinct, it may be an incorporated adjunct of a work-hardening facility, or the back school may offer work hardening for certain patients.

Pain Clinic

The term *pain clinic* can, like *back school*, mean many things. In general, the pain clinic treats a greater variety of disorders with the common problem of chronic pain. Many pain clinics emphasize behavior modification and psychological adaptation,[42] focal injections, and drug withdrawal. Pain clinics may involve representatives of as many as 13 disciplines.[104]

Many patients who are referred to pain clinics suffer from back pain. The elements of a standard back school should be included in the treatment of each pain clinic patient with back pain, either as a separate course or as an integrated part of the pain clinic regimen. Likewise, many back schools incorporate some of the psychological and drug avoidance programs of the pain clinic.

Osteoporosis

People can learn a great deal about how to prevent the progression and complications of osteoporosis. The nutrition, health, exercise, and injury prevention strategies needed for osteoporosis care fit well into the capacities of a functioning back school. Since many patients with osteoporosis suffer from spine complications, referral sources overlap. To treat osteoporosis, back schools need little additional space, equipment, or personnel, but special programs are essential.

Evaluation

Many back schools possess the personnel and equipment needed to provide services for industrial adjustments and settlement of legal disputes. Calculation of physical impairment, assessment of work capacity, job analysis, and pre-employment advice may all become functions of the back school that chooses to develop in those areas.

Sports Medicine Center

Rehabilitation of the spine-injured athlete requires a combination of the unique knowledge of the back school therapist and the unique knowledge of the athletic trainer/therapist. This may be accomplished if the back school therapist establishes a liaison with the athletic trainer/therapist, if the back school develops a special program for spine-injured athletes, or if the sports rehabilitation center incorporates a modified back school into its facility.

Hospital Back School

Many hospitals offer outpatient physical therapy services that include back school. As such, there may be little difference between a hospital back school and a standard back school.

However, some hospitals offer back schools for the needs of certain hospitalized patients, and some back schools offer special programs that they take into the hospitals to fulfill those needs. Examples include programs for surgical patients, adjuncts to drug withdrawal and chronic pain management, and programs for patients who have become debilitated and deconditioned by prolonged illness.

Industrial Back School

Many large industries have their own physical therapy and medical facilities for which back school is a logical adjunct. Many back schools take the messages of good back health to industry. They analyze job sites and advise employees and safety officers. They either personally instruct employees or set up self-sustaining teaching programs within the industry's health and safety department.

Public School Back School

If back school is good for everyone, why should not everyone have it? One study showed that 21-year-olds with decreased spinal mobility have more back pain.[76] Could citing such studies and teaching the remedies to schoolchildren catch the back pain problem at its beginning? White and others have begun to introduce back health education into the public school system.[66, 116] Back schools are a community's best source for consultation and implementation of such efforts.

GOALS OF A BACK SCHOOL

Each back school should establish its mission. For most, the major goal is to serve patients—to relieve pain and restore function and to help them avoid harmful, expensive, or unnecessary treatment. But, in so doing, others are served as well. Each school should define the extent of responsibility that it wishes to accept.

Usually, families and dependents benefit if the patient benefits. Sometimes that is not true, or some people may not believe it to be true at the time. In some cases, families must become involved in order to help the patient. The back school must set its limits of such involvement.

Back schools may serve the business community. They can evaluate, teach, advise, or treat employees of local industries. The school must decide what sort of programs it wants to offer and the extent to which it wishes to serve corporations or other groups.

Back schools may serve insurance companies or health provider organizations. They must decide to what extent they wish to offer services and modify their programs to suit such entities.

Back schools serve physicians. They improve the results of the physician/surgeon's care. They provide diagnostic feedback. They relieve the physician of the burden of the time to properly educate his patients, and they relieve him of the burden of excessive demands from overly and unproductively dependent patients. Each back school should plan the ways in which those goals should be accomplished and what it should demand of the physicians.

Back school may serve science. Back school is a place where patients with one of the world's great unsolved health problems gather. Properly designed studies implemented through back schools could contribute to knowledge about back pain.

Back school serves society. If successful, it reduces the cost of back care. It educates the public about the prudent and rational use of medical resources. It correlates back health with other pertinent health care topics and teaches general health as well as spine health. Each school needs to plan how aggressively it wishes to influence society by contacts with politicians, schools, and public forums.

When one tries to assess outcome, to ask "Are we succeeding or are we failing?" questions can be asked from the viewpoint of each recipient of service, and the answers may vary. Then, the back school must decide which answers are most important.

GOAL SETTING FOR PATIENTS IN A BACK SCHOOL

Unless the patient sees where the back school program will lead him, the experience may occur as though in a vacuum. Many patients will say how helpful back school is during the time they are attending but will retain and apply little and thus not profit from the experience. Goal setting avoids that pitfall.

For the patient to set goals, the therapist must do an evaluation. He gathers information about the diagnosis and treatment from the referring physician, from back school intake forms, and from personal interviews and performs a physical examination to assess flexibility, strength, permissible level of activity, and whether the patient should be restricted to a primarily flexion or extension regimen.

The patient is asked to demonstrate his current knowledge of body mechanics. Going through an obstacle course where he is asked to perform various tasks gives the patient the opportunity to demonstrate the link between his spinal disorder and tasks of his ordinary life. The therapist makes practical observations of the patient's physical disability. He may record a score of the patient's knowledge of body mechanics. The score may be compared with that achieved when the test is repeated later in the course.

For most patients, a skilled therapist can obtain adequate information from such a history, physical, and body mechanics test to set goals for the standard back school experience. For more difficult patients and for more extensive treatment programs such as work-hardening and pain clinic regimens, more data may be needed, as from treadmill examination, computerized assessment of back strength and motion, and psychological testing. Such data may help the back school that wishes to assess the results of its efforts.

Many back school patients are in poor condition and

are at high risk for coronary artery disease. Some have their functional capacities limited more by cardiac tolerance than by back pain. Most back schools request that such patients have cardiac evaluations through the usual medical channels. Some, however, find it more convenient and inexpensive to the patient and more efficient for the school to provide a treadmill examination for each patient.[96] Such programs require the consultation of a cardiologist.

Most important for psychological assessment is that the therapist be empathetic with the patients and yet recognize pain as a behavior as well as a symptom. In the setting of the standard back school, psychological assessments must be made rather quickly and upon a diverse group of patients. Psychological testing can help recognize those patients whose disturbed mental status will interfere with the program and provide clues as to how each patient is likely to handle pain and respond to treatment.

A therapist who is familiar with the application of certain psychological tests to the back school may administer, score, and interpret them rather easily. White recommends a battery of tests that include a social readjustment rating scale, a brief psychological screening test, a personal concerns inventory, a pain drawing, and a pain scale.[115] Each back school can select from a larger number of such tests.

Many tests reflect physical capacity and practical function as well as psychological status. Such tests as the Oswestry Back Pain Disability Questionnaire,[22, 33] the Evans-Kagan Functional Rating Scale,[30] the Sickness Impact Profile[4, 22, 41] with its Roland-Morris modification,[94] the Million Questionnaire,[79] the Waddell Disability Index,[112] and the McGill Pain Questionnaire[77] are all reasonably brief and offer the back school therapist both information about the patient's current abilities and an index by which to measure future progress.

For more extensive psychological testing and for more prolonged efforts to modify behavior and change life-style, the back school needs a consultant psychologist. Many back schools have full-time psychologists, and many more have consulting arrangements with a psychologist for selected patients. For such consultation to be successful, the psychologist must understand the programs of the back school and have experience with chronic back pain. In facilities that provide prolonged treatment programs, the psychologist may help the patient set goals, whereas in the standard back school the therapist and patient usually set the goals.

Machines may aid physical assessment beyond the scope of the ordinary physical examination. Isometric trunk strength testing,[97] quantitative assessment of strength through various motions of lifting,[14] and simultaneous measurements of angular position, angular velocity, and torque against constant resistance[74] are all possible with machines that are available at reasonable cost to most back schools. The information gained from such machines may be used to assess present status, set goals, and gauge progress. As we collect more normative data for various job requirements and accumulate more experience with such machines, we should be able to realistically predict a patient's potential capability and set accurate goals.[88]

Whether or not a back school should choose to use quantitative back strength and motion machinery depends upon the goals of the school, the demands of the patients, the willingness of the personnel to become skilled with the machines, and the budget of the school. That the technology of such machinery has evolved rapidly may dissuade the back school that is trying to adhere to Jackson's inclusion of reasonable cost in the definition of a back school.[58] On the other hand, the machines may be used for treatment as well as assessment, and the costs may not be excessive if spread over a large volume.

Those who would include sophisticated testing machinery in their back schools must understand the limitations of the machines. The back school director must expend considerable effort to compare various machines and select the ones that best suit his program. The market is in flux, so no advice can substitute for a careful investigation of what is currently available at the time and for the purpose of a school's need. Once committed, the therapists must keep up with new information and changes in technology.

Back schools that employ machines must guard against a dependency on the glamour of machinery by both the patients and the therapists lest the essential changes wrought by back school—the patient's grasp of the guardianship of his own health and the professional's acceptance of the role of educator—be lost to a passive dependency on machinery.

The medical records, interview, forms and tests, physical examination, body mechanics examination, psychological evaluation, and results of machine testing produce a profile that the therapist can present to the patient as a summation of current resources. Resources thus include physical capacity, social and economic circumstances, and outside support from family and employer. The variable of time must be applied to all such resources, so the therapist and the patient must weigh the effects of the natural history of the underlying problem, aging, and any other anticipated changes.

Evaluation and goal setting can be quite complex, as is appropriate for long-range reconditioning programs.[72] For the standard back school, the therapist must simplify and exert judgment.

The patient and therapist must compare the patient's resource profile with his demand profile. There are general demands common to almost all patients such as pain reduction, improved function, avoidance of excessive cost, and avoidance of harmful treatment. While back schools must keep mindful of these goals, it is more important for the patient that these goals be translated into specifics.

Levels of fitness, knowledge of body mechanics, pounds of weight loss, cessation of smoking, freedom from analgesics and tranquilizers, reduced reliance on health professionals, and reduced demands upon family can be considered in quantifiable terms and agreed upon as goals. The patient may choose to reinstate items from a list of daily living activities that have been forsaken due to back pain. With the therapist's guidance, the patient may work for improvement in specific areas of social maladjustment or psychological distress.

Most difficult for many patients is the issue of return to work. Goal setting about work requires a most careful assessment of the physical and personal resources of the patient, adjusted for future change, vis-à-vis the demands of the previous job and the potential for any job modification or change to a different job. The problem is so difficult that it leads many back schools to all but ignore the issue. Certainly, if a return to the previous job were the only criterion of success or failure of a back school, back school success rates would suffer. To ignore the issue, however, is to avoid the central problem for many patients and to avoid what may be one of the most therapeutic tools available.[83]

The therapist may have to consult with the patient's family, employer, attorney, or vocational rehabilitation counselor before goals about work are agreed upon. The patient who has a realistic goal that all involved parties understand is more likely to succeed. During this process of goal setting, the therapist and some patients may conclude that a more extensive program such as work hardening or psychological support is needed. It is better to make that determination at this stage and integrate the efforts of back school than to lead the patient into another failure by taking him through a back school that is insufficient for his needs.

Goal setting for the athlete who wishes to return to his sport is a variation on the theme of returning to work. Returning to the same sport at the same level may or may not be a realistic goal. The therapist may need to consult with the coach, trainer, sports psychologist, and the athlete's family. A decision not to return to the sport does not constitute a failure if the program achieves other goals.[36]

The back school experience may fail to satisfy the patient for various reasons—physical, psychological, or social. Most often, the failure is because the initial goals were improper or not well understood.

WHAT BACK SCHOOLS TEACH

Certain topics are common to most back school programs, albeit tailored to the specific course and patient. Anatomy, general health, nutrition, and psychological and social aspects of back pain may be presented as lectures, whereas other topics such as first aid, body mechanics, relaxation, and exercise should be supplemented by demonstration and supervised application.

First Aid

First aid for back pain is a good opening topic. It establishes the theme of self-reliance and begins to build the confidence needed to participate in the other features of the program.

Unlearning misconceptions and misinformation may be as important as some learning. Except for the very short term, bed rest is not a successful treatment for back pain. The therapist who cites personal experience and explains good scientific studies such as that of Deyo et al.[24] will convince patients to seek a cure out of the bed.

Body positioning to relieve pain may be demonstrated by assuming a "rest position" in recumbency with the knees and hips flexed over pillows or specially designed cushions. This posture reduces pressure in the disc[82] and relieves tension on the roots of the sciatic nerve. Patients can practice this posture and feel its effects as they listen to the lectures in the back school.

Depending upon the individual problem and the preference of the therapist, certain patients may be taught to do extension posturing. While many patients have been helped by a supervised "McKenzie" regimen,[28, 75] many do not persist with the recommended self-care aspects of the program. For others, the benefits of extension posturing can be made available for the first time through a self-care program in the back school.

Mobilization and its forceful extension, manipulation, are ancient, widespread, generally harmless, and often successful techniques.[48, 85] One common drawback, as commonly practiced, is that these techniques are coupled to a passive role of the patient and dependence upon the healer. Patients can learn some of these techniques and apply them alone or with the assistance of family or friends. Self-mobilization of the facet joints by lying with one's side over a pillow, painful side up, while rotating the hip forward and shoulder back is easy to learn.

The benefits of traction are debatable.[13, 44, 68, 113] Few claim more than short-term relief, but if traction is uncoupled from dependency on healers and provided at minimal cost, short-term relief is reason enough to include it for the self-care of some patients.

Ice or heat, appropriately applied, relieve back pain. Therapists teach practical hints for safe and inexpensive home applications of thermal treatments.

Over-the-counter medications such as acetaminophen, aspirin, and ibuprofen have risks and benefits that the self-caring patient needs to understand beyond advertising messages.

Some patients use elastic abdominal binders, corsets, and other orthotic devices to achieve comfort and self-reliance. As weight lifters have long believed, an abdominal support does seem to increase lifting ability.[52] Back school patients learn how to use them properly and how to avoid the loss of lordosis and other problems that some believe to be associated with their use.[56]

Transcutaneous electrical nerve stimulation (TENS) offers a noninvasive, nonaddictive approach to pain control that can be self-managed. However, TENS has not passed scientific scrutiny of effectiveness,[25] but many patients seem to benefit from its use. Back school therapists can teach patients how to use TENS.

Posture and Applied Body Mechanics

Props to simulate various work, recreation, and daily living activities may be arranged to constitute an "obstacle course" for evaluation. They may also be used to teach posture and body mechanics. Therapists may discuss the principles in lectures and demonstrate with slides or videotapes and then ask patients to demonstrate that they understand.[115]

Patients learn from lectures and demonstrations how posture affects the lower part of the back.[27] They practice standing, sitting, lying, walking, driving, crouching, reaching, lifting, leaning, twisting, pushing, pulling, carrying, climbing over, climbing under, dressing, and bathing. Sex is discussed but, alas, not demonstrated.

Basic differences may exist for patients with predominantly posterior disease, who must avoid extension, from those with other back disorders. Fine tuning for individuals depends upon age, strength, and skills. There are variations among individuals, pathology may change, and individuals do not always follow theory.[26] Patients should therefore seek understanding rather than memory, and therapists should be ready to adapt to variations.

Job requirements make lifting mechanics especially important to some patients. Sophisticated machinery may help the patient analyze his technique and the modifications to protect his back.[87]

Recreation is important to health. The therapist who gives attention to recreation bonds with the patient, gains trust, and diffuses the spectrum of concern from the emotionally loaded subject of job fitness. The therapist can gather for the patient special training and technique information about such activities as golf,[110] biking,[101] running,[93] swimming,[86] racquet sports,[38] horse riding,[91] weight training,[39] and aerobics.[99]

The back school may keep mechanical aids to various tasks for demonstration. The patient learns how to modify clothing, shoe wear, bedding, and home and work environments to protect his back.

Patients learn the virtues of various chairs and ways to adjust them. Attention is given to the type and location of backrests, inclination of the seat pan, height of the chair, armrests, and other adjustable features.[1] The therapists should know where special chairs and other aids can be purchased and offer that information to patients.

Paperback books with illustrated details of body mechanics, posture, and various self-care measures are commercially available in bookstores at minimal cost.[35, 49, 100] While written for the public, such books are good sources of detail for those who are establishing a back school, and they provide good reference material for patients at the back school. A nice service of a back school is to stock a library of good written-for-the-public books and tapes on back and neck care, exercise, diet, nutrition, and pain and stress control.

General Health and Nutrition

A problem with nutrition for most North Americans means a need for weight reduction. The deleterious effects of obesity upon back pain are so obvious that they hardly require explanation. The problem, however, needs to be placed in proper context. Many obese patients have been told and come to believe that their excess weight is the sole cause of their back pain. Relief from the burden of that concept may lead them to ignore the weight problem. Weight reduction for obese patients must be included as one of many essential goals.

Most obese patients have been on numerous diets. A different diet book is a best seller practically every month. The patient needs some sense distilled from all these books and help to obviate the frustration of failure from one more fad diet. Back school therapists should be ready to offer solid information about weight reduction, recommend rational books on the subject, and be able to refer patients to reputable dietitians or weight reduction centers in the community.

Obesity is not the only problem with nutrition. People with chronic pain, those who have been through surgery, and those with drug dependencies may be truly malnourished. Others such as athletes may have unusual demands upon their diets.[73]

People who smoke cigarettes have more back pain[43, 108] and are more likely to have osteoporosis.[20] Whether the link is coughing, interference with microcirculation, or just a reflection of multifaceted inattention to health is unknown. Regardless, back schools should offer relief from back pain as one more reason to quit smoking and offer advice or referrals for help with breaking the addiction.

Sometimes in order to deal with drug and alcohol dependency the therapist must communicate with the patients' physicians and seek their cooperation. The therapist's explanation of why analgesics and tranquilizers make chronic pain worse does little good for the patient whose physician writes prescriptions for benzodiazapines or codeine derivatives to relieve pain or muscle spasm. Yet, the addicted patient cannot be allowed to ignore the problem.

The patient who is using addictive drugs to control back pain will have little hope of recovery until the addiction is broken. It may be easiest to explain the problem in an emotionally unloaded classroom setting. Patients can accept the explanation that analgesic and tranquilizing medications lower the pain threshold without feeling like they are being chastised or accused. Patients must dispel the notion that they can cease taking the medicines when the pain is relieved and accept the idea that withdrawal of addictive medicine is an essential part of the cure.

For many patients, such an impersonal presentation suffices. For some, however, the therapist must enlist the cooperation of the patients' doctors. The physician may prescribe alternative medications such as nonsteroidal anti-inflammatories or tricyclic antidepressants and allow the therapist to use physical modalities and reassurance to help withdrawal symptoms. Some patients need consultation with a psychologist, dolorologist, or addiction specialist.

Anatomy and Physiology

Deyo found that the most common criticism leveled by patients with low back pain at their physicians was that there had been no adequate explanation of the problem.[23] Yet the patients who seem to understand the least about their back problem are those who have been to the most doctors.[18] Although he may risk contributing to the confusion, the back school therapist has the opportunity to enlighten those who want to understand.

Perhaps due to habit derived from the traditional order of medical curricula, many back schools begin their instruction with explanations of anatomy and pathology. That may not always serve well. A beginning that offers some relief, such as through first aid and some of the exercise and body mechanics techniques, gains the patient's trust more than dazzling him with the jargon of science.

The patient may become more appropriately curious about the anatomy and may readily understand how it applies to his life after beginning to practice some of what has been learned at back school. When the therapist shows the patient with spinal stenosis how the spinal canal of the demonstration skeleton becomes smaller when the facet joints extend, flexion posturing will make sense in a visual way that is not boggled by alien vocabulary.

In talking with patients about pathologic anatomy, it is important that the therapist be especially sensitive to misconceptions patients may harbor about their diagnoses. Covington cited the example of a patient who had been afraid to bend his back for 10 years because his doctor had told him to limit his back motion after surgery.[18] Relative terms in the gray zones of normal such as "bulging disc," "arthritis," and "stenosis" must be used carefully and care taken to be sure that patients are not harmed by a little knowledge. Common misconceptions of "slipped disc" and "deterioration" should be dispelled. Such misunderstandings may be especially difficult to avoid for those patients who obtain secondary gain when the seriousness of their condition is exaggerated by the terms applied to it. As Spengler and Guy suggested, some lawyers can take any information and misuse it to everyone else's detriment.[105]

The therapist who explains pathology and the effects of surgery should also explain how tissues heal and how the anatomy will respond favorably to the efforts the patient makes in response to what is learned in back school. Explanations of what is diseased or removed are balanced by pointing out the reserve capacity and alternative strengths of the body. If a patient's disc has been "removed," he should understand what is left to absorb the forces that cross the disc. If a fusion has been done, he should see what motion remains from unfused segments and how well the loss of lumbar motion can be compensated by hip motion.

Psychology and Social Interaction

Most patients accept a classroom discussion of how psychological factors may cause low back pain. Some patients misinterpret and come to believe that the therapist thinks that the pain is somehow imagined or feigned. For those who want or need personal and extensive psychological help, the back school should have a means of securing it, but for many, some clues to recognizing psychological factors and some practical self-help measures will suffice.

Frequently, psychological disturbance accompanies low back pain.[5, 43, 71, 109] One study showed that the stress of change in life events, not necessarily psychiatric illness, is a factor that precedes the onset of low back pain.[19] People accept that fatigue, worry, nervousness, and tension cause headache, and most have little problem with the analogy that those same stresses contribute to back pain.

The therapist can teach and lead demonstrations of simple relaxation techniques such as contrast relaxation exercises, meditation, visual imagery, and deep relaxation. Audiotapes are useful supplements. While such efforts are rudimentary when compared with what those with more severe problems of this type can gain from a psychologist or through biofeedback, many patients with back pain find them helpful.

Some patients can discover how their emotions relate to back pain by keeping a diary that relates events, feelings, and back pain. While a detailed analysis of such efforts is beyond the scope of most back schools, the therapist can introduce the idea and encourage patients to confront sources of frustration in more successful ways.

Beyond the search for psychological factors as a source of pain lies the recognition of contraproductive behavior in response to pain. One may use pain to avoid responsibility, protect oneself from rejection, justify demands for care, excuse the abuse of drugs or alcohol, or seek financial gain.[42] The therapist can teach patients to recognize such behavior in a relaxed format by exposition of the concept of "pain games"[107] but must be careful to be nonjudgmental and hold carefully to the role of the patient's advocate.

Back school personnel should confront contraproductive pain behavior and try to convince the patient that health is more valuable than the gains that they receive from such behavior. In 1975, Mooney discussed the importance of this aspect of the care of patients with low back pain.[81] Psychological confrontation and conditioning techniques have become integral parts of comprehensive back pain management programs. Back schools that are not prepared to offer such services must recognize when they are needed and refer the patient.

Social circumstances may affect the back school experience as much as psychological makeup. Mention of the importance of family relationships, legal ramifications of the back pain problem, and vocational fitness introduces topics that may be central to some patients.

The support of the patient's spouse is critical. Efforts to lose weight, stop smoking, exercise, and curtail pain behavior are much more likely to succeed if the spouse cooperates. In some cases, the patient can anticipate that his family will be part of the problem rather than part of the solution. If these factors are introduced in a lecture, individuals who have reason to be concerned about such problems are more likely to confide their concerns to the therapist, later. The therapist may need to involve the spouse in the program or enlist outside help.

Some patients who are involved in lawsuits find it difficult to get well. Improvement may jeopardize the outcome of the suit, or they may have been led by their attorney or spouse to believe that it will. An open discussion of these influences in group presentation makes it easier to confront the issue with the individual. The therapist may have to intervene with the attorney or spouse, or it may be best to delay the back school program until after settlement of the legal issues.

At the very least, legal entanglements should be recognized as a source of stress. Open recognition may defuse the situation and lead to a tacit understanding between the therapist and patient that allows for improvement even if not verbalized as such.

For some back schools, work capacity is the most important social issue and focus of their most valuable services. In those situations, the personnel may do sophisticated testing of job demands and patient capabilities and make careful, individualized judgments. When such care is not given, discussions about work should be qualified by recognition that only general guidelines can be offered, and room must be made for many exceptions.

In general, patients may be advised that work that subjects them to a lot of vibration may be more difficult to sustain without back pain.[12, 62, 116, 117] Likewise, frequent and heavy lifting increases the risk of back pain,[108, 114] and twisting may contribute to back pain.[61] Monotony may also be a risk factor for work-related back pain.[108] Those to whom such disadvantages apply must weigh them against the social and economic value of work and the observation that, in general, work seems to be good for back pain.[83] The back school should encourage the often difficult search for an opportunity for the no longer employed to return to "mechanically kind" work and should exhort itself and its students to exert political and community influence for such opportunities to be made available.

Exercise

Julius Wolff proved about bones what every weight lifter knows about muscles—that their size, strength, and form reflect the stresses that have been applied to them. Bierling-Sorenson showed that weak trunk endurance, decreased range of lumbar motion, and tight hamstrings predispose to low back pain.[7] It stands to reason, then, that controlled stress, i.e., exercise, may influence the form and function of the lower part of the back and help control back pain. Medical researchers have not come forth with well-controlled scientific data to prove that reasoning.[57] The therapist should therefore accompany efforts to induce patients with back pain to exercise with lucid explanations of why exercise should help.

Those who doubt the value of exercise may note that some who advocate exercise zealously endorse an extension posturing exercise regimen while others endorse flexion exercises and that sometimes members of one camp impugn the other. Is the success of "opposite" exercise regimens because the body's capacity to heal is so great that success is achieved regardless of the imposed circumstances? Are apparent successes best ascribed to the healing powers and transmitted enthusiasm of the therapist rather than the method? Perhaps the success of both methods depends on proper fit of the prescribed regimen to the particular pathologic anatomy.[102]

One approach to convince patients about exercise is for them to consider the alternative. No one has trouble understanding that prolonged inactivity leads to increasing weakness and stiffness. The alternative of no exercise is therefore not tenable. At the other extreme, no one can argue with the patient who says that exercise could make him hurt, even do harm. The safe and effective middle ground can be demonstrated graphically by a curve that shows the efficacious effects of exercise within a prescribed range and the dangers outside that range (Fig 60–1).

Exercise is closely allied with other aspects of the back school curricula. Stress control and weight reduction are commonly held benefits of exercise. Saal has shown a way that back school personnel can make rational judgments about a patient's ideal posture and put them to practical use in the design of an exercise program.[98]

The goals of exercise are increased flexibility, increased strength, and increased endurance. As mentioned in the discussion of psychology, one may also do certain exercises to achieve relaxation.

Abdominal muscle strengthening exercises have been basic in most active therapy for preventing back pain. Although it has been pointed out that there is no evidence that abdominal strengthening can reduce lordosis or improve posture,[57] the alternative of weak abdominal musculature has obvious deleterious effects upon the body's ability to distribute stresses in a way to avoid injury to the lower part of the back.

Pelvic tilts, modified sit-ups, and isometric contractions of the abdominal musculature are safe and inexpensive ways to strengthen abdominal musculature. More sophisticated means to strengthen the abdominal muscles through isometrics at distinct positions through the range of motion may lead to more rapid gains.[97]

Lumbar extensor strengthening may also be learned as an isometric exercise. As with flexor strengthening, machines may be used to facilitate training and measure progress. People can gain strength with as little as one training session per week.[47]

Back patients should not limit strength training to their trunk muscles. Strong arms and legs maintain balance and control, thereby preventing undue stresses from being transmitted to the back. Exercising the various muscle groups in sequence may avoid injury from overuse and fatigue and keeps the program interesting.[80] The wall slide exercise is a particularly safe way to strengthen gluteal and quadriceps muscles without the risk of back injury and has become the cornerstone of at least one major industrial back injury prevention program.[115]

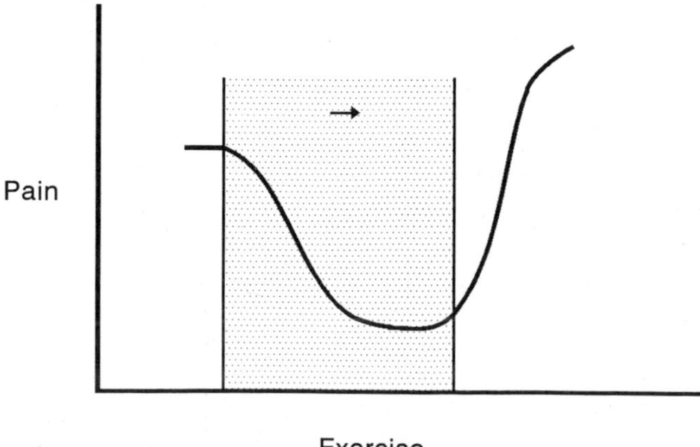

FIG 60–1.
Relationship of the level of exercise to pain.

Traditional exercises for flexibility include gentle attempts to stretch the hamstrings and flex the lower part of the back. One cannot effectively stretch the hamstrings without tension on the sciatic nerve, so for those who have sensitive sciatic nerve roots, hamstring stretching must be done slowly and cautiously. The therapist can correlate the rationale of various hamstring stretching exercises with the teachings of anatomy and help each patient arrive at the method and vigor suited to him.

Recumbent knee-to-chest stretching flexes the lumbar muscles and stretches the facet capsules. The coincident increase in intradiscal pressure is less than with seated or standing flexion movements. The addition of gentle rocking movement in the flexed posture may apply further stretch to the facet capsules and sacroiliac ligaments.

Whether stress to the annulus, as must occur with twisting exercises such as leg-overs, is harmful or helpful depends upon the health of the annulus and its attachments and the control with which the exercise is done. Using the principle that healthy tissue becomes stronger in response to stress, one may reason and teach that such exercises may actually strengthen discs. That there is some risk of reducing the strength of a damaged annulus by these or any stressful exercises cannot be denied.

McKenzie cited poor posture with frequent lumbar flexion and loss of extension capability as a cause of much back pain.[75, 106] He popularized a program of exercises that emphasize flexibility through extension posturing. Some believe that extension may force a posteriorly displaced but contained nucleus to move anterior into a less pain-provocative location. Others have doubted that the latter occurs[65] and stated that although a trial of these exercises may have predictive value through provocation, surgery is not prevented by such a regimen.[64]

Whether or not the nucleus moves or surgery is prevented, the popularity of McKenzie's teachings has renewed emphasis on the importance of maintaining a normal range of extension of the lumbar spine. For those in whom there is no contraindication, extension exercises should be part of a balanced program of exercise leading to a self-care maintenance regimen.[56]

Of all the scientific studies that indicate that exercise helps back pain, the most convincing are those that gauge the effect of endurance exercises. Endurance exercise increases endorphins, and higher levels of endorphins are associated with greater pain tolerance.[17, 90] General fitness and endurance training have been shown to result in a decreased incidence of back pain.[15, 16] Industrial fitness programs may reduce disability and health care costs of low back pain through aerobic training.[11]

While great progress through endurance training takes longer than the duration of a standard back school curriculum, the back school instructors should cite studies and examples to convince the patient of the importance of fitness. They should consider the relative merits of walking, running, aerobics, biking, swimming, and other endurance training methods. Each patient should choose and embark upon such a regimen. Safety factors, including pre-exercise evaluation and intraexercise monitoring, should be part of the instruction.

Distinct from general endurance training that leads to increased cardiorespiratory capacity and higher pain threshold, the concept of specific muscle endurance training should be introduced. Inadequate trunk muscle endurance may predispose to back pain in a more important way than absolute strength or flexibility.[56] Patients who are engaged in a work-hardening program designed to allow them to return to a physically stressful job may find endurance training for specific muscles to be especially important.

WHAT A BACK SCHOOL NEEDS

Personnel

Whatever else a back school does or does not have, it must have people who are healers, people who are empathetic, understanding, and yet sophisticated about what they do and tough about applying it. With that, the back school will succeed, and without that, it will fail—regardless of buildings, machines, equipment, or programs.

The back school must have one or more therapists who can evaluate patients, set goals, prescribe a course, and supervise implementation. In most cases, these will be registered physical therapists.

The therapist must have the patience and personality to be able to deal effectively with patients, employers, insurers, physicians, and attorneys. She must be willing to become involved in the community so that she knows what organizations are available to help the patients; understands the habits of the patients' physicians; knows the available sources of exercise, diet centers, orthotic aids, special chairs, and home adaptations; and is confident in her ability to refer to reputable consultants.

Assistant therapists, or trainers, may implement much of the program. Since they act under the supervision of the physical therapist, they do not need to possess the same educational credentials, but it is important that they also have the personal attributes that allow them to gain the confidence of the patients and work with them effectively.

Back schools generate enough records and engage in enough correspondence that secretarial assistance is necessary. For smaller programs, those duties may be combined with those of a receptionist.

Special programs require specialized personnel. For an industrial education program, someone must call on industrial health officers and executives to sell the program, and someone with the appropriate skills must analyze and present the programs to the industry.

Work-hardening programs may require full-time psychologists or vocational rehabilitation counselors. An occupational therapist with special training and interest in spine care may have a special place in such programs.[96]

The back school director manages the budget, purchasing, personnel, and other business. The director may be the therapist, a physician, a business manager, or a board. Some back schools operate without profit because of support from a university, industry, government, or medical group. For schools that are not so endowed, the income from a back school may support those who work there but is seldom sufficient to attract uninvolved investors.

Programs

The back school needs written goals and plans. A name, a logo, a letterhead, and a brochure provide identity. It should have detailed outlines of each program, including written narratives of the lectures. Slides or movies should be prepared or purchased. Each back school should write a manual for its patients or assemble a notebook of information to give to each patient. In lieu of a self-prepared manual, the school may purchase a commercially available back school kit or select a self-help book and add in the information that is of local significance or uniquely important to the school.

Space

With the right dedication and some imagination, the right person can provide an effective back school in very little space.[2] An expanded range of programs and a large volume of patients, however, require more room.

Unless the back school shares space with another facility, it will need its own waiting room, reception area, and bathrooms. The secretary/receptionist needs a desk if not an office. The therapists and other personnel require some personal office space. The therapist needs a physical examination room.

Group classes are held in a lecture room of sufficient size to project slides or movies. The lecture room can serve as a limited exercise area if the patients are allowed to recline on exercise mats with special cushions during the lectures and later the cushions are removed for floor exercises. Large mirrors along one wall help with posture training.

The body mechanics training/obstacle course area

must be large enough to contain the needed equipment and to accommodate patients being tested and patients being trained. If work hardening is included, this may be extended into an occupational readiness laboratory in a large room, preferably with access to the outdoors.

A library or area in which books and tapes are stored for patients to use may be combined with a rest and refreshment area and, perhaps, used for patients to complete forms and written tests.

Exercise machines require space. If trunk machines and a series of muscle-strengthening machines for comprehensive strength training are included, a lot of space will be required. For vigorous exercise programs, a locker room may also be necessary.

More elaborate facilities may include a pool, a track, and outside conditioning equipment.

Some space needs to be dedicated to storage. Security must be provided for the audiovisual equipment and medical records.

Not least important, the back school should be a cheerful place. The decor should reflect optimism and health. Appropriate colors, textures, lighting, and artwork influence the way patients and therapists feel and make important contributions to the success of the school.

Equipment

The minimum exercise equipment consists of floor mats only. Optional but very useful equipment includes trunk flexion and extension and torsion strengthening machines, computerized quantitative trunk strengthening machines, a series of strengthening machines for the various muscle groups, a stationary bicycle, and a treadmill.

TABLE 60–1.

Equipment for Home Body Mechanics Training and Testing (Obstacle Course)

Various chairs—good, bad, adjustable
Steps with rail
Grocery cart, shelves, sacks, groceries
Refrigerator, stove, sink
Cabinets, high and low
Telephone
Clothing basket, washing machine
Ironing board, clothesline
Suitcase, flight bag, briefcase, purse
Plants, pots
Standing block
Reading desk
Step stool
Extension mirror
Bathtub
Bathroom sink and cabinet
Baby high chair, crib, doll, infant seat
Bed, bedspread, pillows
Car or half-car, infant car seat
Golf clubs, racquets

A large number of items may be assembled in a reasonable space in order to simulate most activities of daily living and many forms of work (Tables 60–1 and 60–2).

Audiovisual equipment includes audio and video cassette tapes and players; carousel slide projectors with remote control; a large projection screen; a camera (and perhaps, a video recorder) for preparation of lecture material; a collection of self-prepared, borrowed, and commercially purchased slides for presentation; models of spines; and poster graphics of anatomy.

Tables are needed for examination and treatment such as the application of ice packs. The therapist selects tools for examination such as inclinometer, scales for height and weight, and routine physical examination and emergency resuscitation equipment.

Forms and Administrative Supplies

The number of forms is determined by the number and type of programs offered. Some that are common to most back schools are listed in (Table 60–3).

CAVEATS

Etiologies May Change

Back school should not be a tunnel. A patient should not be dismissed from consideration of invasive treatment because he has been labeled as a "back school patient." Previously contained discs may extrude further and be best treated by excision. Overly vigorous exercise may precipi tate tendinitis that would be relieved by local injection. In-

TABLE 60–2.

Equipment for Industrial Body Mechanics

Hoe, shovel, sandbox (filled with kitty litter)
Broom, rake, gravel bed
Wheelbarrow, buckets
Mower
Workbench and tables—various heights
Tunnel or low overhead obstacle
Table crafts, hand saw, hammer, nails
Nail pegboard and pegs
Balance beam, foot and ankle balance board
Ladders, stairs, scaffold
Sawhorses
Trash cans, buggies, bins
NIOSH* boxes
Wood boxes, wire moving boxes
Lumber, tar rolls
Clothing bundles, sewing machine
Dollies
Conveyor belt
Industrial vacuum cleaner
High shelves and file cabinets
Sled
Copier and stand
Typewriter, computer terminal

*NIOSH = National Institute for Occupational Safety and Health.

TABLE 60–3.
Administrative Forms

History and physical
Pain drawing
Selected psychological or outcomes testing forms
Progress chart and forms
Standard thank you/acceptance to referral source
Standard request for medical records
Standard summation report to referral source
Diploma for patient
Daily plans for patients in various programs
Attendance record and recall file
Charge ticket
Brochure

flammation from overstretching of a scarred nerve root might recover faster after injection of an epidural steroid. The therapist should be attuned to such possibilities and quick to repeat the examination of a patient whose symptoms change.

Don't Be Holistic

Back school therapists should be educators. They should exert mature judgment about therapeutic claims and recommend to their patients only those things that make good sense. That some fragment of the rhetoric of quacks rings true does not constitute a reason for endorsement. An effort to be comprehensive and useful in all possible ways should not preclude discretion. While it is important to keep an open mind, one must not allow one's brain to fall out.[45]

Don't Be Part of the Problem

Just as there are medication addicts, there are education addicts. Some patients, like some students, would like to stay in school indefinitely. Overtreatment only reinforces illness behavior.[105] If it would do more for the patient to return to work or settle a legal dispute than to prolong back school, then that course should be selected. The ultimate success of a back school depends upon its ability to provide quality programs to patients who need and want the help that they offer.

REFERENCES

1. Andersson GB, Murphy RW, Ortengren R, et al: The influence of back rest inclination and lumbar support on lumbar lordosis. *Spine* 1979; 4:52–58.
2. Attix EA, Nichols J: Establishing low back school. *South Med J* 1981; 74:327–331.
3. Attix EA, Tate MA: Low back school: A conservative method for the treatment of low back pain. *J Miss State Med Assoc* 1979; 20:4–9.
4. Bergner M, Bobbitt RA, Pollard WE, et al: The sickness impact profile: Validation of a health status measure. *Med Care* 1976; 14:57–67.
5. Bergquist-Ullman M, Larsson U: Acute low back pain in industry. *Acta Orthop Scand Suppl* 1977; 170:1–117.
6. Berwick DM, Budman S, Feldstein M: No clinical effect of back schools in an HMO—a randomized prospective trial. *Spine* 1989; 14:338–344.
7. Bierling-Sorensen F: Physical measurements as risk indicators for low back trouble over a one year period. *Spine* 1984; 9:106–119.
8. Block R: Methodology in clinical back pain trials. *Spine* 1987; 12:430–432.
9. Blusk K: Back school. *Am Corr Ther J* 1979; 33:23–25.
10. Bonica JJ: Organization and function of a pain clinic. *Adv Neurol* 1974; 4:433.
11. Boone DW, Russell ML, Morgan JL, et al: Reduced disability and health care costs in an industrial fitness program. *J Occup Med* 1984; 26:809–816.
12. Buckle PW, Kember PA, Wood AD, et al: Factors influencing occupational back pain in Bedfordshire. *Spine* 1980; 5:254–258.
13. Burrios C, Ahmed M, Arrotegui JI, et al: Clinical factors predicting outcome after surgery for herniated lumbar disc: An epidemiologic multivariate analysis. *J Spinal Disorders* 1990; 3:205–209.
14. Butler L, Mayer T, Gatchel R: Changes in lifting capacity in the industrially injured patient with chronic low back pain in response to functional restoration treatment. Presented at the Fifth Annual Meeting of the North American Spine Society, Monterey Calif, 1990.
15. Cady LD, Bischoff DP, O'Connell ER, et al: Strength and fitness and subsequent back injuries in fire fighters. *J Occup Med* 1979; 21:269–272.
16. Cady LD, Thomas PC, Karwasky RJ: Program for increasing health and physical fitness of fire fighters. *J Occup Med* 1985; 27:110–115.
17. Colte E, Wardlaw S, Frantz A: The effect of running on plasma beta-endorphin. *Life Sci* 1981; 28:1637–1640.
18. Covington EC: Psychiatric aspects of chronic back pain. *Semin Spine Surg* 1989; 1:35–42.
19. Craufurd DIO, Creed F, Jayson MIV: Life events and psychological disturbance in patients with low back pain. *Spine* 1990; 15:490–494.
20. Daniell HW: Osteoporosis of the slender smoker. *Arch Intern Med* 1976; 136:298–304.
21. Deyo RA: Conservative therapy for low back pain—distinguishing useful from useless therapy. *JAMA* 1983; 250:1057–1062.
22. Deyo RA: Measuring the functional status of patients with low back pain. *Arch Phys Med Rehabil* 1988; 69:1044–1045.
23. Deyo RA: Patient satisfaction with medical care for low back pain. *Spine* 1986; 11:28–30.
24. Deyo RA, Diehl A, Rosenthal M: How many days of bedrest for acute low back pain? *N Engl J Med* 1986; 315:1065–1070.
25. Deyo RA, Walsh NE, Martin DC, et al: A controlled trial of transcutaneous electrical nerve stimulation (TENS) and exercise for chronic low back pain. *N Engl J Med* 1990; 322:1627–1634.

26. Dillin WH: Conservative management in acute back pain and sciatica. *Semin Spine Surg* 1989; 1:18–27.
27. Dolan P, Adams M, Hutton W: Commonly adopted positions and their effect on the lumbar spine. *Spine* 1988; 13:197–201.
28. Donelson R: The McKenzie approach to evaluating and treating low back pain. *Orthop Rev* 1990; 19:681–686.
29. Egbert LD, Battit GE, Welch CE, et al: Reduction of postoperative pain by encouragement and instruction of patients. *N Engl J Med* 1964; 270:825–827.
30. Evans JH, Kagan A: Development of functional rating scale to measure treatment outcome of chronic spinal pain patients. *Spine* 1986; 11:277–281.
31. Fahrni WH: *Backache Relieved*. Springfield, Ill, Charles C Thomas, 1966.
32. Farhni WH, Orth M: Conservative treatment of lumbar disc degeneration: Our primary responsibility. *Orthop Clin North Am* 1975; 6:93–103.
33. Fairbank JJ, Couper J, Davies J, et al: The Oswestry Low Back Pain Disability Questionnaire. *Physiotherapy* 1980; 66:271–273.
34. Fardon DF: Back School. Presented at the First Annual Meeting of the North American Lumbar Spine Association, Vail, Colo, June 1984.
35. Fardon DF: *Free Yourself From Back Pain*. Englewood Cliffs, NJ, Prentice-Hall, 1984.
36. Fardon DF: Herniation of lumbar disc in a football athlete with spinal stenosis, in Hochschuler SH (ed): *The Spine in Sports*. Philadelphia, Hanley & Belfus, 1990, pp 293–299.
37. Fardon DF, White AH, Wiesel SW: Lumbar diagnostic terms and conservative treatments favored by spine surgeons in North America. Presented at the First Annual Meeting of the North American Spine Society, Bolton's Landing, NY, July 1986.
38. Feeler LC: Racquet sports, in Hochschuler SH (ed): *The Spine in Sports*. Philadelphia, Hanley & Belfus, 1990, pp 143–151.
39. Feeler LC: Weight lifting, in Hochschuler SH (ed): *The Spine in Sports*. Philadelphia, Hanley & Belfus, 1990, pp 132–142.
40. Fisk JR, DiMonte P, Courington SM: Back schools—past, present, and future. *Clin Orthop* 1983; 179:18–23.
41. Follick MJ, Smith TW, Ahern DK: The sickness impact profile: A global measure of disability in chronic low back pain. *Pain* 1983; 21:67–76.
42. Fordyce WE: *Behavioral Methods for Chronic Pain and Illness*. St Louis, Mosby–Year Book, 1976.
43. Frymoyer JW, Pope MH, Costanza MC, et al: Epidemiologic studies of low back pain. *Spine* 1980; 5:419–423.
44. Gillstrom P, Ehrnberg A: Longterm results of autotraction in the treatment of lumbago and sciatica: An attempt to correlate clinical results with objective parameters. *Arch Orthop Trauma Surg* 1985; 104:294–298.
45. Glymour C, Stalkov D: Engineers, cranks, physicians, magicians. *N Engl J Med* 1983; 308:960–963.
46. Grant PH, Hall H: Effect of early intervention by the Canadian Back Institute on costs and time loss after back injury. Presented at Fourth Annual Meeting of the North American Spine Society, Quebec, July 1989.
47. Graves JE, Pollock ML, Foster D, et al: Effect of training frequency and specificity on isometric lumbar extension strength. *Spine* 1990; 15:504–509.
48. Haldeman S: Spinal manipulative therapy. *Clin Orthop* 1983; 179:62–70.
49. Hall H: *The Back Doctor*. New York, McGraw-Hill, 1980.
50. Hall H, Iceton JA: Back school—an overview with specific reference to the Canadian Back Education Units. *Clin Orthop* 1983; 179:10–23.
51. Healy KM: Does preoperative instruction make a difference? *Am J Nurs* 1968; 68:62.
52. Hochschuler SH, Guyer RD, Ohnmeiss DD, et al: The effects of wearing an abdominal support belt on the amount of weight lifted by low back patients. Presented at the Fifth Annual Meeting of the North American Spine Society, Monterey, Calif, August 1990.
53. Hochschuler SH, Rashbaum RF: Texas Back Institute programs. Personal communication, Plano, Tex, 1990.
54. Holzman E, Turk DC: *Pain Management: A Handbook of Psychological Treatment Approaches*. New York, Pergamon, 1966.
55. Horal J: The clinical appearance of low back disorders in the city of Gothenburg, Sweden. *Acta Orthop Scand Suppl,* 1969; 118:1–109.
56. Jackson CP: Physical therapy for lumbar disc disease. *Semin Spine Surg* 1989; 1:28–34.
57. Jackson CP, Brown MD: Is there a role for exercise in the treatment of patients with low back pain? *Clin Orthop* 1983; 179:39–45.
58. Jackson CP, Klugerman M: How to start a back school. *J Orthop Sports Phys Ther* 1988; 10:1–7.
59. Kaye RL, Hammond AH: Understanding rheumatoid arthritis—evaluation of a patient education program. *JAMA* 1978; 239:2466–2467.
60. Keith A: *Menders of the Maimed*. Huntington, NY, Robert E Krieger, 1975.
61. Kelsey J, Githens P, White A: An epidemiologic study of lifting and twisting on the job and risk for acute prolapsed lumbar intervertebral disc. *J Orthop Res* 1984; 2:61–66.
62. Kelsey JF, Hardy RJ: Driving of motor vehicles as a risk factor for acute herniated intervertebral disc. *Am J Epidemiol* 1975; 102:63–73.
63. Klaber-Moffett JA, Chase SM, Portek I, et al: A controlled, prospective study to evaluate the effectiveness of a back school in the relief of chronic low back pain. *Spine* 1986; 11:120–122.
64. Kopp JR, Alexander H, Torocy RH, et al: The use of lumbar extension in the evaluation and treatment of patients with acute herniated nucleus pulposus. *Clin Orthop* 1986; 202:211–218.
65. Korenko P, Boumphrey F, Bell G, et al: McKenzie extension exercises in the treatment of acute disc prolapse: A prospective study. *Orthop Trans* 1985; 9:509.
66. Kunse P, White AH: Instruction of preventive back care in the public school system. Presented at the Second Annual

Meeting of the North American Spine Society, Banff, Alberta, Canada, June 1987.
67. Lankhorst GH, vandeStadt RJ, Vogebar TW, et al: The effect of Swedish Back School in chronic idiopathic low back pain. *Scand J Rehabil Med* 1983; 15:141–145.
68. Larsson V, Choler V, Lidstrom A, et al: Autotraction for treatment of lumbago-sciatica. A multicenter controlled investigation. *Acta Orthop Scand* 1980; 51:791–798.
69. Levine PH, Britten AF: Supervised patient management of hemophilia. *Ann Intern Med* 1973; 78:195–201.
70. Lindquist S, Lundberg B, Wilkmark R, et al: Information and regime at low back pain. *Scand J Rehabil Med* 1984; 16:113–116.
71. Magora A: Investigation of the relation between low back pain and occupation. V. Psychological aspects. *Scand J Rehabil Med* 1973; 5:191–196.
72. Mayer TG, Gathchel RJ, Kishinon KJ, et al: Objective assessment of spine function following industrial injury. *Spine* 1985; 10:482–493.
73. Mayfield ML, Stith WJ: The effect of nutrition on the spine in sports, in Hochschuler SH (ed): *The Spine in Sports*. Philadelphia, Hanley & Belfus, 1990, pp 54–67.
74. McIntyre DR, Glover LH, Seeds RH, et al: The characteristics of preferred low back motion. *J Spinal Disorders* 1990; 3:147–155.
75. McKenzie RA: *The Lumbar Spine: Mechanical Diagnosis and Therapy*. Waikanae, New Zealand, Spinal Publication, 1981.
76. Mellin G: Decreased joint and spinal mobility associated with chronic back pain in young adults. *J Spinal Disorders* 1990; 3:238–243.
77. Melzack R: The McGill Pain Questionnaire: Major properties and scoring methods. *Pain* 1975; 11:277–299.
78. Miller LV, Goldstein J: More efficient care of diabetic patients in a county hospital setting. *N Engl J Med* 1972; 286:1388–1391.
79. Million R, Hall W, Nilsen KH, et al: Assessment of the progress of the back pain patient. *Spine* 1982; 7:204–212.
80. Mitchell RI, Carmen GM: Results of a multicenter trial using an intensive active exercise program for the treatment of acute soft tissue and back injuries. *Spine* 1990; 15:514–521.
81. Mooney V: Alternative approaches for the patient beyond the help of surgery. *Orthop Clin North Am* 1975; 6:331–334.
82. Nachemson A: Disc pressure measurements. *Spine* 1981; 6:93–97.
83. Nachemson A: Work for all. *Clin Orthop* 1983; 179:77–85.
84. Nachemson A, LaRocca H: Editorial. *Spine* 1987; 12:427–429.
85. Ohenbacher K, DiFalio R: Efficacy of spinal manipulation/mobilization therapy. *Spine* 1985; 10:833–837.
86. Paris SV: The spine and swimming, in Hochschuler SH (ed): *The Spine in Sports*. Philadelphia, Hanley & Belfus, 1990, pp 117–124.
87. Parnianpour M, Nordin M, Kahanovitz N, et al: The triaxial coupling of torque generation of trunk muscles during isometric exertions and the effect of fatiguing isoinertial movements on the motor output and movement patterns. *Spine* 1988; 13:982–992.
88. Parnianpour M, Nordin M, Sheikhzadeh A: The relationship of torque velocity and power with constant resistive load during sagittal trunk movement. *Spine* 1990; 15:629–643.
89. Peltier LF: The "back school" of Delpech in Montpellier. *Clin Orthop* 1983; 179:4–9.
90. Puig M, Laorden M, Miralles F: Endorphin levels in cerebrospinal fluid of patients with post-operative and chronic pain. *J Anesthesiol* 1982; 57:1.
91. Rashbaum RF: Soft tissue trauma in equestrian participation, in Hochschuler SH (ed): *The Spine in Sports*. Philadelphia, Hanley & Belfus, 1990, pp 180–191.
92. Raskob GE, Lofthouse RN, Hall RD: Methodological guidelines for clinical trials in evaluating new therapeutic approaches in bone and joint surgery. *J Bone Joint Surg [Am]* 1985; 67:1294–1297.
93. Regan JJ: Back problems in the runner, in Hochschuler SH (ed): *The Spine in Sports*. Philadelphia, Hanley & Belfus, 1990, pp 111–115.
94. Roland M, Morris R: The natural history of low back pain. Development of guidelines for trials of treatment in primary care. *Spine* 1983; 2:141–144.
95. Rowe ML: Low back pain in industry. A position paper. *J Occup Med* 1969; 11:161–169.
96. Russell GS, Dreisinger TE: Personal communication, Columbia, Mo, 1990.
97. Russell GS, Highland TR, Dreisinger TE, et al: Changes in isometric strength and range of motion in the isolated lumbar spine following eight weeks of clinical rehabilitation. Presented at the Fifth Annual Meeting of the North American Spine Society, Monterey, Calif, 1990.
98. Saal JA: Dynamic muscular stabilization in the nonoperative treatment of lumbar pain syndromes. *Orthop Rev* 1990; 19:691–700.
99. Sachs BL: Aerobic sports activities and the spine, in Hochschuler SH (ed): *The Spine in Sports*. Philadelphia, Hanley & Belfus, 1990, pp 175–179.
100. Selby N: *My Aching Back*. Los Angeles, The Body Press, 1988.
101. Sheets CG, Hochschuler SH: Considerations in cycling for persons with low back pain, in Hochschuler SH (ed): *The Spine in Sports*. Philadelphia, Hanley & Belfus, 1990, pp 125–131.
102. Sikorski J: A rationalized approach to physiotherapy for low back pain. *Spine* 1985; 10:571–579.
103. Simmons JW, Dennis MD, Rath D: The back school. *Orthopedics* 1984; 7:1453–1456.
104. Spengler DM: Chronic low back pain—the team approach. *Clin Orthop* 1983; 179:71–76.
105. Spengler DM, Guy DP: Industrial low back pain: A practical approach, in Weinstein JN, Wiesel SW (eds): *The Lumbar Spine*. Philadelphia, WB Saunders, 1990, pp 869–871.
106. Stankovic R, Johnell O: Conservative treatment of acute low back pain—a prospective randomized trial: McKenzie

method of treatment versus patient education in "mini back school." *Spine* 1990; 15:120–123.

107. Sternbach RA: Varieties of pain games. *Adv Neurol* 1974; 4:423–430.
108. Svensson HO, Andersson GB: Low back pain in forty to forty-seven year old men. *Spine* 1983; 8:272–276.
109. Svensson HO, Vedin A, Wilhelmsson C, et al: Low back pain in relation to other diseases and cardiovascular risk factors. *Spine* 1983; 6:277–285.
110. VanderLaan VK, Gaines RW: The spine in golf, in Hochschuler SH (ed): *The Spine in Sports*. Philadelphia, Hanley & Belfus, 1990, pp 207–217.
111. Vickery DM, Kalmer H, Lowry D, et al: Effect of a self-care education program on medical visits. *JAMA* 1983; 250:2950–2956.
112. Waddell G, Main CJ: Assessment of severity in low back disorders. *Spine* 1984; 9:204–208.
113. Weber H, Ljungren A, Walker L: Traction therapy in patients with herniated lumbar intervertebral discs. *J Oslo City Hosp* 1984; 34:61–70.
114. White AA, Gordon SL: Synopsis: Workshop on low back pain. *Spine* 1982; 7:141–149.
115. White AH: *Back School and Other Conservative Approaches to Low Back Pain*. St Louis, Mosby–Year Book, 1983.
116. White AH: Back school: State of the art, in Weinstein JN, Wiesel SW (eds): *The Lumbar Spine*. Philadelphia, WB Saunders, 1990, pp 770–792.
117. Wilder DG, Woodworth BB, Frymoyer JW, et al: Vibration and the human spine. *Spine* 1982; 7:243–254.
118. Zacrisson-Forsell M: The back school. *Spine* 1981; 6:154–106.
119. Zindrick RM: The tabulator—results from questionnaire number 3. *NASS News* 1990; 4:2.
120. Zucherman JF, White AH: The "back school" approach to low back pain. *J Musculoskel Med* 1984; 1:13–22.

61

Work Hardening

Catherine B. Carranza, O.T.R.

Work hardening, the most recent development in rehabilitation, has gained the attention of many insurance companies, employers, and medical health care providers. Although uncertainty still exists concerning what constitutes a true work-hardening program, many health care providers are beginning to promote this treatment method. In general, a work-hardening program is an interdisciplinary treatment approach bringing together the skills and interests of all those involved with an injured worker, including health care providers, employers, and sometimes family members. With the increasing interest in this treatment method, guidelines are being established to standardize the definition and implementation of work-hardening programs.

THE ROOTS OF WORK HARDENING

"Work hardening," "functional restoration," and "industrial rehabilitation," are terms often associated with rehabilitation for the injured worker. While the general term "work hardening" has been established, its definition may be sufficiently descriptive to encompass the expertise required for successful evaluation and treatment of the injured worker. Work hardening has two primary sources. In 1923, the Vocational Training and Employment Federal Industrial Rehabilitation Act required that occupational therapy be available in every general hospital dealing with industrial accidents or illness. As early as the 1950s, the May T. Morrison Center for Rehabilitation in San Francisco and the Workmen's Compensation Convalescent Centre in Malton, Canada, provided a "work therapy" program. Many of the concepts and components from these programs are still accepted and utilized today. Although traces of significant impact from the profession of occupational therapy have been found over the years, occupational therapists today are known to be instrumental in the development and practice of work hardening.

Guidelines for work hardening were established by the American Occupational Therapy Association (AOTA), Inc., in 1986. Thereafter, in 1988, the Commission on Accreditation of Rehabilitation Facilities (CARF) and the National Advisory Committee on Work Hardening, composed of a multidisciplinary team, defined work hardening, and its first standards were published in 1990.[5] Today, more than 100 work-hardening programs are accredited in the United States.

AOTA guidelines and CARF's definition of work hardening reflect the same goal: returning an injured worker to a productive life-style. AOTA recognizes that the occupational therapy model of work hardening demonstrates the expertise of preventive and injury management concepts. CARF endorses an interdisciplinary approach to the evaluation and treatment of an injured worker. No single discipline could fully provide the comprehensive and holistic approach to injury management needs; thus, an interdisciplinary approach is employed. Turk and Stieg described the treatment team as follows:

> An interdisciplinary team ideally consists of a core group of individuals who (a) share a common conceptualization of the chronic pain patient; (b) synthesize the diverse sets of information based on their own evaluations, as well as those of outside consultants, into an intelligent differential diagnosis and treatment plan for each patient; (c) work together to formulate and implement a comprehensive rehabilitation plan based on the available data; (d) share a common philosophy of disability management; and perhaps most important, (e) act as a functional unit whose members are willing to learn from each other and modify, when appropriate, their own opinions based on the combined observations and expertise of the entire group.[14]

In a typical work-hardening setting, the core team members include physicians, occupational therapists, physical therapists, psychologists, vocational specialists, exercise physiologists and/or physical trainers, and a case manager consultant. The worker and his family members are a vital part of the team. Clinic staff members (receptionists and billing personnel) are also key individuals since they usually have the initial contact with the worker and interface with all those involved with his treatment.

Although each team member has a distinct background and training, the worker must understand the necessity for involving all the disciplines. For the sake of clarification and to promote confidence in the team effort, the "program manager" (who oversees the medical attention given the worker) explains the role of each team member. The occupational therapist focuses on activities of daily living, work performance, and the feasibility of returning to work safely, or he may function as the case manager and act as a liaison between the employer, insurance carrier, and medical provider. The physical therapist emphasizes the musculoskeletal system as it pertains to muscular flexibility, posture, and biomechanics. The psychologist will deal with issues such as coping with the inability to work and its effects on family relationships. The exercise physiologist or trainer concentrates on endurance and strength conditioning. The vocational specialist addresses employment modification or career redirection. Many private practitioners, hospital-based programs, and rehabilitation facilities promoting work-hardening services are asked what the components of a work hardening program are. Some models are described below.

OCCUPATIONAL THERAPY MODEL

This model typically focuses on the independence of activities of daily living. Although the training for an occupational therapist emphasizes function and activity-oriented tasks, the holistic approach to treatment places much emphasis on home and work performance. Knowledge of biomechanics, the neuromuscular system, physiology, vocation, psychosocial interactions, and cognitive skills all concern the occupational therapist in a work-hardening program. Training emphasizes ergonomics, or work design modification, and therefore may allow the therapist to play an active role in work site analysis. An occupational therapist who serves as a case manager may be a mediator in communication with the interdisciplinary team as well as with employers.

Equipment suitable for an occupational therapy model may include various isometric and isokinetic machines as well as hand dynamometers. Work-simulated props such as the Baltimore Therapeutic Equipment (Baltimore Therapeutic Equipment, Inc., Baltimore) and the Lido Workset (Loredan, Davis, Calif) help duplicate requirements of the worker's job. Functional pulleys, theraband systems, and exercise equipment are also commonly found in this industrial setting. Physical disabilities in the hands and back are the areas most frequently encountered in the occupational therapy model.

PHYSICAL THERAPY MODEL

This model may be employed in the acute recovery stage and later lead into work simulation. The initial focus is on flexibility, strength, and pain management through such modalities as cryotherapy, thermotherapy, ultrasound, and transcutaneous electrical nerve stimulation (TENS). The physical therapist may educate the patient in ways to counteract stress encountered in sustained postures and how to deal with acute pain if it occurs. A physical therapist brings expertise in physiology, neuromuscular systems, biomechanics, and pain management to the injury management arena. Job analysis may or may not be a part of this model; however, pre-employment screening appears to be a growing area. The physical therapy model is most valuable in uncomplicated cases where the major barrier to a return to work is physical deconditioning secondary to injury.[7] Typically, exercise equipment such as Cybex and Eagle (Cybex, Ronkonkoma, NY), or Hydrofitness (Hydrofitness, Belton, Tex) is used, as are weights, exercise bikes, and treadmills. Patients with back pain are most frequently treated in this model.

PSYCHOLOGY MODEL

Psychologists evaluate and counsel the worker during adjustment to an injury. This discipline is essential because the injured worker must face many issues ranging from financial problems to family conflicts. The psychologist may spend a great deal of time helping the worker and his family adjust to the loss of employment and cope with injury and pain, possible financial problems, and possible change of vocation and related training. By placing a strong emphasis on family support systems and "self-image" dynamics, the psychologist attempts to build the worker's confidence in preparation for returning to employment. Coping with stress and pain are two primary factors addressed in this model, which makes it frequently perceived by the insurance carrier as a "pain program." The psychophysical model, another multidisciplinary approach, utilizes the same team members mentioned earlier. Patients with back pain are the most frequent participants in the psychology model.

VOCATIONAL SPECIALIST MODEL

When the injured worker has no job waiting, he must seek a new place of employment or train for a new career; either of these changes can be frustrating for the injured worker. The vocational specialist generally provides services only in those cases requiring vocational redirection secondary to an unsafe job or a physical inability to return to the same type of work. Although the vocational specialist is sometimes a consultant to the team, this discipline must be involved early in the evaluation and treatment stage so that the patient has employment when he is physically ready.

EVALUATION TOOLS: AN OVERVIEW

Many types of evaluations are available to assess the physical and functional status of an injured worker. A menu or a package of different assessments may be based on the time required to perform (2, 4, 6 hours), on individual components of the assessment such as posture tolerance (sitting, standing, crawling, or climbing), or on the ability to perform other designated tasks. Some tasks can easily be evaluated through functional obstacle courses.

Some common evaluations include dynamic or isometric lift assessments. Dynamic measurements may include isoinertial or psychophysical evaluations, allowing the patient more control of the weight to be handled, expression of pain factors, and establishment of maximum acceptable work loads in repetitive lifting tasks.[13] Isometric assessments are static in nature and include the National Institute of Occupational Safety and Health (NIOSH) *Work Practices Guide for Manual Lifting*.[12] Isometric testing is one of the most established assessments for screening, and many commercial devices promote isometric measurements as valid tools. Although both assessments have normative industrial data, each should be questioned concerning its applicability for a given situation.

Mayer and Gatchel note that in order for a physical capacity measurement to be effective it should be valid, accurate, reproducible, reliable, and relevant; assess the effort put forth by the patient; and have a normative data base available for comparison.[10] Controversy continues over the value of emerging high-technology testing devices, and careful evaluation of the equipment and the provider's needs is required before time and money are invested in these machines. A normative data base providing a benchmark for normal performance required for the physical demand characteristics of the job is essential. Mayer and Gatchel also indicate that the test should be shown to have a demonstrated ability to predict injury and recurrence.[10] When evaluating the patient's effort while performing various assessments, factors such as inconsistency of pain, deconditioning, guarding secondary to fear of injury, or conscious malingering may be noted to help determine physical and psychological traits.

Other components of the functional physical capabilities assessment (FPCA) include evaluating muscular and cardiovascular endurance. Although many methods assess endurance, the aerobic measurement is the most reliable. Work and power consumption, easily normalized to body weight, can also be gauged since distance and repetitions can be controlled. The bottom-line question of whether the patient can endure an 8-hour day performing physical work points out that muscular strength and endurance are absolutely essential, even more so than increased aerobic capacity, to reduce the chance of reinjury.[6]

Another objective measurement is flexibility. The ability to function throughout various ranges is absolutely necessary. Range-of-motion measurements may be administered via goniometric, fingertip-to-floor, or tape measure methods. The EDI-320 (Cybex, Ronkonkoma, NY) and other such computerized tools are frequently used today.

Various types of computerized muscle measurement devices assess trunk and abdominal strength and endurance. Although the isokinetic equipment may be expensive, the data provide visual feedback to the patient and therapist and address the reproducibility of patient effort.

Psychosocial assessments are essential to determine pain associations, motivation, and other characteristics that may have an impact on the patient's interest in returning to work. The Minnesota Multiphasic Personality Inventory (MMPI), Millon Behavioral Health Inventory (MBHI), Sickness Impact Profile (SIP), and the Beck Depression Inventory (BDI) are commonly used assessments in work-hardening programs. Although the MMPI is cumbersome, it has been identified as a potential predictor of treatment outcome and change in a variety of patient populations.[3] The possible reactions identified by this assessment include hysteria, depression, and hypochondriasis, all commonly found in patients with chronic back pain and disability.[9] The MBHI provides a measure of psychological function and predicts the patient's style of relating to health care personnel and compliance with treatment.[11] The SIP is a short inventory that measures health status and the impact of a medical problem on daily functions.[2] Finally, the BDI focuses on manifestations such as insomnia, weight change, sexual dysfunction, and anhedonia.[1]

The activities of daily living assessment is usually administered by a licensed occupational therapist. A comprehensive work and home assessment, it requires an interview with the patient to address issues such as mechanism of injury, work productivity, work history, and physical demand characteristics of the job. In addition, the therapist will ask questions to gauge the patient's ability to perform activities of daily living such as dressing independently, getting into and out of a car, driving, shopping, and taking care of children (if applicable).

Typically activities of daily living or a work/home assessment is conducted as an initial screening device. A follow-up interview with the employer is essential to confirm work issues and the potential for future employment. Not only can this be used as a tool to compare notes with the patient's report, but it also provides the employer an opportunity to get involved with the interdisciplinary team. He can help build the patient's confidence and enhance work simulation by loaning job simulation props. Having initial contact with the employer will also provide information concerning job availability. Knowing this early will give the rehabilitation team a head start in vocational direction: whether the worker should pursue work simulation directly related to the old job site, prepare to seek employment elsewhere, or consider a new vocation. Addressing this issue early allows a better chance of having a job available for the worker after treatment is complete, thus reducing the cost of care associated with continued unemployment.

Vocational assessments are important because there is

a good chance that the worker's previous job is no longer available. In some states, vocational rehabilitation is mandatory, and intensive vocational counseling occurs in the early stages of treatment. Vocational intervention can be provided on a selective basis, and criteria for this intervention must be established, particularly for a patient who has a job available but has no intention of returning to it. This can sometimes be an uncomfortable position when the main focus is to return the worker to the original job in order to close or settle the case. Criteria can be set for workers (1) who have no job waiting; (2) who have a job but question what the job entails, which may, in turn, lead to a doubtful return; and (3) whose attending physician has recommended that the worker not return to the original job secondary to physical limitations. Many vocational evaluations are available for use in work hardening, including academic and aptitude testing. Below is a brief list of vocational assessments:

- Wide Range Achievement Test (WRAT)[8]
  - Range of school levels including kindergarten to college
  - Basic subjects in reading, spelling, and arithmetic
  - Intellectual functioning level at basic skills
- Wechsler Adult Intelligence Scale (WAIS-R)[16]
  - Evaluates intellectual functioning, which can aid in determining the patient's ability to integrate in the program
  - Evaluates cognitive ability
  - Evaluates behavioral data in relation to basic psychologic functioning, i.e., coping skills
- Bennett Mechanical Comprehension Test (BMCT)
  - Measures the ability to perceive and understand the relationship of physical forces and mechanical elements in practical situations
  - Appropriate for a variety of jobs and for engineering training and trade schools
- Valpar Work Samples[15]
  - Standardized work samples
  - Includes range-of-motion tolerances, problem solving, simulated assembly, trilevel measurements, and the ability to apply basic skills necessary to perform tasks at varying levels of difficulty, i.e., dexterity, eye-hand coordination, and the use of hand tools
- Crawford Small Parts Dexterity Test (CSPDT)[4]
  - Measures fine eye-hand coordination and dexterity
  - Predicts suitability to jobs relating to wiring of intricate devices, electronics, engraving, assembly, and office machines.

"Career inventory interest tests" can also be used to assess career interest and assist with vocational direction and motivation.

COMPONENTS OF WORK HARDENING: AN OVERVIEW

The components of work hardening include many areas, all of which play an integral role in the program. Outlined below are some of the primary components that may be identified as quality components by the consumer or purchaser of work hardening.

Interdisciplinary Team.—As mentioned earlier, the expertise of occupational and physical therapists, psychologists, vocational specialists, and exercise physiologists or trainers are all integral components of a program addressing the many facets of the low back–injured worker.

Education.—Promoting the patient's understanding and willingness to assume responsibility for his success or failure is important. Courses usually include anatomy, body mechanics, nutrition, work-related issues, stress management, and vocational intervention classes such as resume writing.

Intensive Conditioning.—Total-body conditioning is the key to success for overall fitness. Flexibility, strength, and endurance are major factors in reaching total-body conditioning. Active exercise and stretching promote disc nutrition and healing, thereby encouraging "wellness" and a faster recovery. Specialized conditioning targeting skills necessary for a particular occupation is also addressed.

Work Simulation.—One must accurately simulate the physical demand characteristics of the patient's job to assess his ability to return to work. Performing activity-oriented tasks not only conditions the patient in a specific posture but also builds confidence in his ability to perform the task.

Vocational Intervention.—Vocational intervention is absolutely necessary when a worker has no job waiting for his return. The patient may become very frustrated if he completes a rather intense work rehabilitation program only to find that no job is available. Vocational evaluation and counseling can be administered by a certified vocational evaluator, occupational therapist, or vocational rehabilitation specialist.

Case Management.—Case management can be performed by a rehabilitation nurse or occupational therapist and is necessary to establish communication with the employer, insurance carrier, physician, and others involved with the patient. The case manager also coordinates the components of the patient's care. There may also be an insurance case manager who communicates to treatment providers and employers. Case management is the nucleus of the program, and communication aids strongly in yielding positive outcomes and healthy relationships among the rehabilitation team and all others involved with the injured worker.

Other Vital Components.—Other components that are perceived as necessary for work hardening include (1) an effective program monitoring and evaluation system; (2) ongoing research to evaluate entrance screening criteria, assessment tools, and clinical outcomes and report the results to others working in rehabilitation; (3) effective screening that does not exclude patients in active litigation; (4) projected time frames of treatment with objective documentation and efficient reporting systems; (5) reasonable fees that are compatible with services available and do not exceed the market value; and (6) results—return-to-work outcomes that provide efficient case resolution and thereby reduce medical costs.

WORK HARDENING: FLOW PROCESS MODEL

Since projected time frames of program completion may vary, treatment flow must be closely monitored to identify "red flags" that warn of potential problems.

BRIEF OVERVIEW OF THE CONSUMER

While the ultimate goal of returning the injured worker to employment is generally agreed upon by those involved in the patient's case, this general goal may be interpreted differently by these parties. The employer wants the worker to return to his job without restriction, the insurance carrier seeks case settlement, the physician wants improved function, the therapist desires to improve the patient's physical and functional capacity as well as coping skills, the worker wishes to get rid of the pain, and the adjuster works toward closing the file. Although each team member wants the worker to return to work, many factors have an impact on the final outcome of work hardening. Some elements to be considered are how early work hardening is undertaken, how long the patient has been receiving medical care, the difficulties encountered in litigation, and of course, the motivation of the patient prior to entering the program. If the team expects positive results from work hardening, participants must be appropriately screened and closely monitored.

The consumer will play an even more integral role as changing laws require careful monitoring by insurance carriers to prevent abuse by expensive work-hardening programs that do not produce good results. For instance, in Texas, the patient may choose the first physician he sees for treatment, the second choice must be approved by the insurance carrier, and the third physician (if necessary) is selected by the insurance carrier. Again, this will reinforce early intervention. Another factor to be considered when addressing consumer needs is the self-insured employer or a company that has not subscribed to workers compensation coverage and who has a genuine interest in containing health care costs. The increasing number of self-insured employers may increase in-house work-hardening programs, which would have an impact on the existing market. In summary, if consumers (providers) want to be part of the rehabilitation team, they need to know why and when work hardening is appropriate.

FUTURE TRENDS OF WORK HARDENING

After reviewing the literature in the field of injury prevention and management, the author feels that the following will be the future in this area:

1. Industrial work-hardening programs will surface as a new market and promote cost containment, wellness, and early intervention.
2. Occupational therapists will become more competitive in work hardening, pursuing private practice, and consulting with various companies.
3. The Commission on Accreditation of Rehabilitation Facilities (CARF) will continue to bring awareness of standards and regulations for work hardening to the federal and state governments, and more programs will apply for CARF accreditation.
4. Accident prevention training programs will become components of work-hardening programs and will be increasingly used by employers.
5. Industrial fitness programs will evolve with different philosophies and strategies of evaluating and treating injured workers as athletes.
6. Much emphasis will be given to research and results from established programs.
7. The work hardening concept will be broadened to an increasing number of disabilities.

SUMMARY

Work hardening has been around for a long time. Its roots are well planted in today's medical arena. Education of the consumer and an effort toward progressive change in the product will be key factors in the success of these programs. Aggressive and innovative approaches in the areas of injury prevention, industry work hardening, and health promotion will be continually redefining the role of work hardening.

REFERENCES

1. Beck AT: *Beck Depression Inventory*. 1962.
2. Bergner M, Bobbit RA, Carter WB, et al: The Sickness Impact Profile: Development and final revision of a health status measure. *Med Care* 1981; 19:787–805.
3. Capra P, Mayer TG, Gatchel R: Adding psychological scales to your back pain assessment. *J Musculoskel Med* 1985; 2:41–52.
4. Crawford JE, Crawford DM: *Crawford Small Parts Dexterity Test*. Psychological Corp, 1946.
5. Commission on Accreditation of Rehabilitation Facilities: *Standards Manual for Organizations Serving People with Disabilities*. Tuscon, Commission of Accreditation of Rehabilitation Facilities, 1990.
6. Glisan B, Stith WJ, Kiser S: Physiology of active exercise

in rehabilitation of back injuries. *Spine State Art Rev* 1989; 3:139–152.

7. Isernhagen S: *Work Injury, Management and Prevention*. Rockville, Md, Aspen, 1988, p 198.
8. Jastak JF, Jastak S: *Wide Range Achievement Test—WRAT R2 '78 Edition*. Jastak Assoc, 1984.
9. Keefe FJ: Behavioral assessment and treatment of chronic pain: Current status and future directions. *J Consult Clin Psychol* 1982; 50:896–911.
10. Mayer T, Gatchel R: *Functional Restoration for Spinal Disorders: The Sports Medicine Approach*. Philadelphia, Lea & Febiger, 1988.
11. Millon T, Green CJ, Meagher RB: *Millon Behavioral Health Inventory,* ed 3. Minneapolis, Interpretive Scoring System, 1982.
12. National Institute for Occupational Safety and Health: *Work Practices Guide for Manual Lifting*. Cincinnati, NIOSH US Public Health Service Publication 81-122, 1981.
13. Snook S: *The Design of Manual Handling Tasks*. Hoplanton, Mass, Liberty Mutual Insurance, 1978.
14. Turk D, Stieg R: Chronic pain: The necessity of interdisciplinary communication. *Clin J Pain* 1987; 3:163–167.
15. Valpar International Corporation, Tuscon.
16. Wechsler D: *Wechsler Adult Intelligence Scale (WAIS),* revised edition. Psychological Corp, 1981.

62

The Future of Spinal Health Care Rehabilitation

Vert Mooney, M.D.

The future of spinal rehabilitation can be classified into three perspectives. The first view is evolving understanding of the controllable factors of soft-tissue inflammation and repair. The second view is focused on techniques of rehabilitation that will be important in the future. Finally, a third perspective is the social/political aspects of spinal rehabilitation and the residual disability.

BASIC FACTORS OF REPAIR

First we will look at emerging understanding of the healing process. Principles of soft-tissue repair must be similar whether we look at the strained ligament of the knee or a low back injury. The basic principle must be related to inflammation and repair of soft tissues. Certainly all studies point out that varying degrees of tissue inflammation accompany all soft-tissue injuries. Tissue inflammation will alter functional activity. Altered function leads to a cessation of some activity and modification of others. The resulting series of events is substitution of muscle activities, subsequent alteration of strength balance, and eventually some decrease in flexibility. The same process occurs whether the injury is acute, an acute exacerbation of a chronic condition, or chronic.

What do we know of mechanisms that stimulate repair following postinjury inflammation? Changing the inflammatory process in connective tissues requires inciting an appropriate cellular and/or matrix tissue response. Growing experience in clinical medicine and attempts at the use of modifiers are becoming more accepted. Potential modifiers include anti-inflammatory medications, which may be oral or injectable, and physical techniques such as thermotherapy and cryotherapy. There is even an emerging potential for electrical field induction and rehabilitative exercises.

A current example of a specific inflammatory modifier are the nonsteroidal anti-inflammatory drugs (NSAIDs). These pharmacologic agents enter into the inflammatory cycle in a variety of ways to stabilize cell membranes and dampen the effect of arachidonic acids. There is no evidence that NSAIDs speed the process of healing, but they do apparently retard inflammatory reaction and associated pain. Less pain allows more effective exercise and reactivation. This is a very complex issue, but available chemical and pharmacologic manipulation will be available in the future. There are a multitude of growth factors that have been discovered, and all of these have the potential to speed the process of inflammation[31] (Fig 62–1).

Examples of other modifiers of inflammation repair are the biological effects of electrotherapeutic currents. High-voltage pulsed galvanic stimulation has been used to eliminate edema from the inflammatory cascade, reduce fluid loss to the interstitium, and increase lymphatic flow as well as circulation in capillary beds.[23, 28] These techniques should facilitate the resolution of edema. In the future, investigators will be able to project the correct timing of the intervention and also the threshold dose. Electrotherapy can apparently orient collagen organization. The use of 1-Hz alternating current has been shown to improve the healing rate of ligaments.[18] Pulsed electromagnetic fields have been shown to improve blood supply in areas of chronic injuries such as rotator cuff tendinitis and thus offer a potential to enhance the rate of healing in chronically injured soft tissues such as fascia.[6] Currently researchers are working with direct current, capacitive coupling, and electromagnetic fields. Most of the work has been performed in animal models because of the great difficulty of comparative work in humans wherein similar lesions must be documented. Nonetheless it has been demonstrated that pulsed electromagnetic fields will enhance the rate of bone repair after fusions.[24]

The most important controllable stimulus of soft-tissue repair is therapeutic exercise. Certainly it has been well demonstrated that muscles will strengthen with increasing stress. Skeletal muscle fibers respond to overloading by increasing their structure and functional capability. Specificity of training means that a specific stimulus elicits specific structural changes in the skeletal muscle. Whether strength or endurance is necessary, they can specifically be enhanced by training. For instance, endurance training can double the oxidative capacity of the muscle and increase the percentage of fibers classified as highly oxidative in the limbs.[30] On the other hand, muscle hypertrophy and increased muscle strength are produced by high-tension/low-frequency skeletal muscle contraction.[12] Strengthening

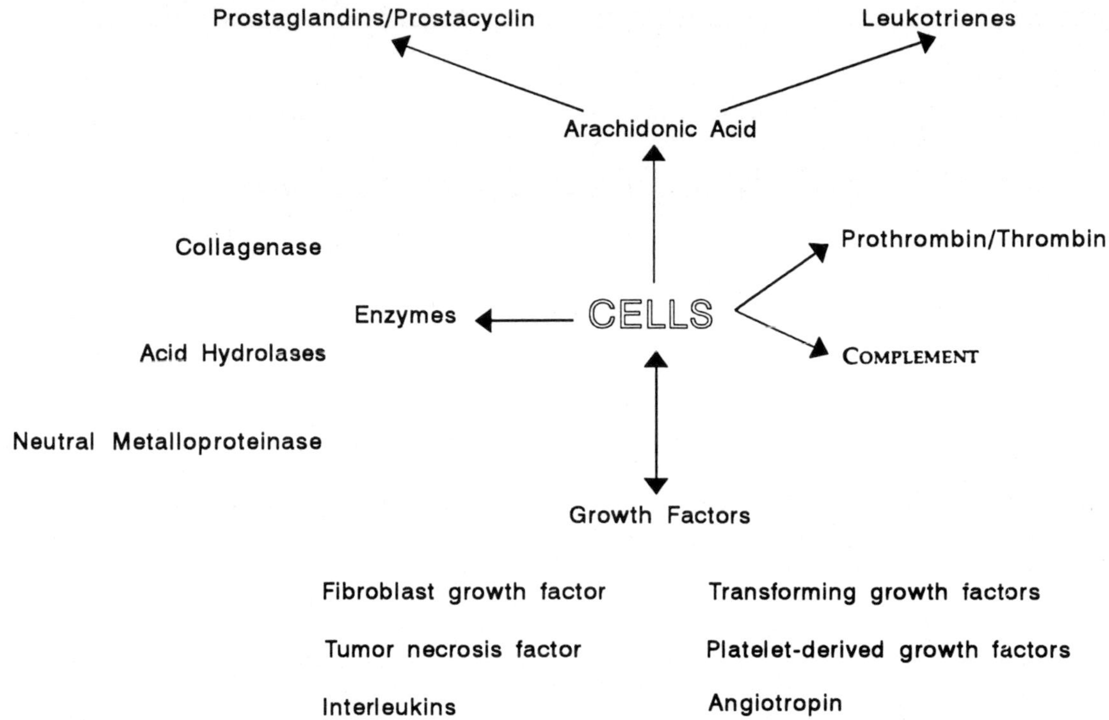

FIG 62–1.
Modulators of inflammation and tissue repair.

training programs will increase the total muscle mass by increasing the number of myofibrils per fiber. Type II fibers, or fast-twitch fibers, respond to this type of stimulation more than type I fibers, the endurance muscle fibers. It has been demonstrated that although training can increase the size of various fibers, it will not basically change the composition of fast- vs. slow-twitch fibers.[15] Thus, when exercises are prescribed for the deconditioned individual, both endurance and strength must be stimulated by appropriate approaches. Greater understanding of training routines will emerge largely from sports medicine. With this clinical research background, greater efficiency in chronic back pain care by exercises can be expected in the future.

Probably a more important aspect of tissue response to therapeutic exercise is the concept of a Wolff's law of soft tissue. Wolff's law essentially means that mechanical forces "tell" tissues to respond with additional tissue to defend against that force. Certainly, therapeutic exercise has demonstrated that the ligament-bone junction is increased in strength.[7] In addition, progressive exercise increases the strength of the ligaments themselves.[33] This again supports the view that progressive exercises should be of benefit to the strength of connective tissue. At this point we do not quite understand the source of stimulus to increase the strength of soft tissues. It is thought that mechanical loading that creates soft-tissue strain has a direct effect on cells.[8] This could involve a direct effect on almost any of the components of the cell either internally or externally. There seems to be little doubt, however, that loading of soft connective tissue plays an important role in cellular control of the matrix. Loading therefore represents a critical entity and may explain most of the soft-tissue pathology in circumstances of overload. It is the most controllable therapeutic modality available.

TECHNIQUES OF SPINAL REHABILITATION

A significant principle of musculoskeletal rehabilitation has emerged over the past several years largely based on sports medicine. This principle essentially comes down to the use of functional testing to document progress through rehabilitation. An adjacent principle is that consistency of performance provides the most important insight into the ability of the patient/client to cooperate with the rehabilitation program. An inability to provide consistent performance, however, must not be misconstrued to necessarily mean malingering or dishonesty on the part of the patient. The inability to make a reasonable and enthusiastic effort in the area of physical performance may just as well be on the basis of fear and ignorance as a desire to magnify the significance of impairment.

Documentation of performance for the spine is far

more complex than with the extremities. Right-to-left comparisons are the hallmark of functional definition in rehabilitation of the upper and lower extremities. The slight predominance of the dominant upper extremity also provides insight as to functional performance. The first standardized test for functional performance was the JAMAR grip test.[4] This simple mechanical isometric test device, first proposed in the 1950s, is quite reliable. Nonetheless, it has been pointed out that standardization of testing is necessary to provide valid cross-population results.[13] Even with the extensive history available with this piece of simple and inexpensive equipment, normative values are still inconsistent. Such variations as hand position, altered instruments, small numbers of subjects in various age subgroups, and even differences in professional testing groups are a source of inconsistency.[19] We must recognize that even with the 35-year experience with the JAMAR grip strength testing device it was not felt reliable enough to be a standard for use in the American Medical Association (AMA) *Guides to the Evaluation of Permanent Impairment*.[11] This is a serious problem in the consideration of objective testing when used as a definition for deviation from normal and for a mechanism to identify levels of impairment in comparable populations. The lack of acceptance of even this simple tool to establish levels of relative impairment emphasizes that we must look at objective testing of function basically only as a way to monitor the progress of rehabilitation. For the spine, functional testing using any sort of sophisticated measuring device will not emerge as a reliable statement of disability and impairment for purposes of job placement, job return, and awards for job incapacity. Nonetheless, tools that can measure lumbar function still are necessary to guide progress in rehabilitation. Let us therefore turn to tools that can be used to measure performance.

Functional performance of the spine can essentially be evaluated on the basis of strength, endurance, coordination, and perhaps range. The question mark related to range is that even though it is the easiest of the characteristics to measure, it probably is the least important. We must recognize that multiple strategies are available to us that will allow us to substitute for absent lumbar range. These alternative motion locations may not impair performance at all. On the other hand, the other three characteristics, although more complex to measure, have much more to do with performance. Muscle strength is the capacity to produce torque or work by voluntary contraction. Muscle endurance is the ability to maintain torque or work over a period of time. Finally, coordination in this context is defined as adjustment or action of muscles in producing movements and maintaining the quality of motor output. Quality of motor output from the back injury standpoint means the ability to defend against the unguarded moment of sudden overload.

Certainly it was recognized early that the lack of trunk muscle strength and endurance is a factor in the cause of low back pain, and therefore the implication is that improvement in trunk strength should correlate with improvement in back pain. It has been demonstrated that asymptomatic individuals are stronger than individuals with low back pain.[1] Also, it has been demonstrated that improvement in trunk strength correlates with improvement in function and even ultimately with reduction of the pain complaint.[21] Whether these studies and many others are reliable depends on our perception of the best way to measure muscle strength. Historically, isometric (static) tests were the first to emerge because the equipment was simple and available.[9] Isometric testing does have the capacity of repeatability in a simple manner. The simplicity of the isometric test equipment used in studies such as Chaffin's is counterbalanced by the lack of significant repeatability due to the failure to isolate position and contributing musculature. Moreover, it does not reflect real-world performance. Indeed, isometric testing without complete isolation of the torso has the capacity to create injury on its own in that movement against a rigid object may overload the weak link and create additional soft-tissue strain. In comparison with isokinctic testing, isometric testing has a higher incidence of test-related injuries in the usual test without constraint of position.[20] Thus, in the context of spinal rehabilitation some caution should be entertained in using nonisolated isometric testing. It does give a needed objective statement of performance but may not be a reliable projection of what the individual actually can do and may carry with it a liability for additional injury.

Due to the deficits of nonconstrained isometric testing of trunk function, alternative systems of evaluation have emerged. Obviously it is important to objectively measure function. For a comparison of one individual to another, some method by which a number is created must be developed. In addition, to achieve reliable objective testing variables, the complex maneuver of trunk performance must be controlled. The isokinetic method of muscle testing has emerged. It controls at least the rate of performance, and attempts to measure torque during this performance. It seems to be a well-accepted method of testing muscle performance in that it is taught in most physical therapy schools. Isokinetic testing earlier was applied to the extremities in various areas of sports medicine and more recently has been applied to the lumbar spine.[22] This equipment initially was produced by Cybex (Lumex Corp., Ronkomkoma, NY), but later several other manufacturers produced similar devices. The initiation of computerized isokinetic testing into the area of lumbar and trunk rehabilitation brings in the issue of expense and complexity of equipment. It is a reliable principle that commercially available equipment is necessary for comparable complex measurements. It is certainly inappropriate for a rehabilitation center to be constantly distracted by the technical problems related to equipment, maintenance, and adjustment that are typical of home-made equipment. Moreover, if the measurements of function are to be compared with anything other than the individual's performance one day to the next, consistent equipment must be available. Consistent equipment really means that it must be manufactured in quality control conditions and sold at a profit so that the company can afford to make more of the same equipment. The question emerges, of course, as to how complex and expensive the system can tolerate the equipment to be. In the use of spinal isokinetic test equipment, with progressive patient experience and thus many comparisons available, enlarging questions emerge as to its reliability. For instance, such questions as the relationship of gravity to isokinetic testing in any but the horizontal plane emerges. The initial burst of energy inherent in the use of isokinetic lumbar test equipment may have serious problems in analysis. This phenomenon known as "overshoot" measures inertial forces rather than true torque and thus gives confusing data as to early peak torque. Finally, such issues as calibration, filters of electronic data, and the use of inertial corrections must be brought into consideration and universally applied if data are to be comparable.[35] Once again we need to reflect on the limitations of the JAMAR hand-held grip meter. It has greater simplicity and far longer clinical experience and is even applied to a simpler physiologic question, yet it is not a universal test. It therefore seems unlikely that isokinetic test equipment with all the inherent flaws noted above will be able to emerge as a universally applied test tool. Nonetheless, this type of measurement as part of a broader array of test equipment can certainly monitor progress in function. It can give an objective statement of torque and can point out such factors of performance wherein the trunk extensors (normally stronger than the trunk flexors) are now weaker or equal to the trunk flexors in the injured back. It can suggest patient level of cooperation. Are there other factors of trunk performance that can be measured? Probably a more important test than trunk torque or strength is trunk muscle endurance.

It is generally assumed that local muscular fatigue predisposes an individual to injury.[2] Also, it has been demonstrated that trunk extensors are more resistant to fatigue than trunk flexors and that males have less endurance than females.[32] It has also been shown that isometric testing of the duration needed to hold a position of horizontal unsupported posture will predict potential risk for back trouble.[5] Thus, measures of endurance and methods to improve this are important. Although isokinetic equipment has the potential to measure an endurance deficit by noting decreasing torque over an increasing number of repetitions, this is not a true physiologic maneuver.[17] The physiologic maneuver by which fatigued muscles are allowed to rest, regain capacity, and thus allow overall continued performance is known as substitution. This is best demonstrated by a tool that can simultaneously measure movement in the sagittal, lateral, and rotatory planes. The only commercial equipment available that can monitor this aspect as well as speed and torque (isoinertial testing) is equipment from Isotechnologies known as the Isostation B-200 (Isotechnologies, Hillsborough, NC). This equipment thus measures the velocity of performance over a set resistance. The combination of testing three-dimensional motion and controllable resistance allows a much broader picture of spine motor performance. In situations where fatigue develops after multiple repetitions, it was noted that not only did the speed of performance diminish but deviations in position also occurred during flexion and extension.[27] Under the circumstances of testing to exhaustion with a resistance 70% of maximum isometric extension, normal subjects decreased not only their speed and torque but also the range of motion in the primary motion strategy (sagittal in this case) while increasing motion in the transverse and coronal planes. This points out that the reduction in functional capacity of primary muscles performing a required task is compensated for by secondary muscle groups. The spine therefore may be loaded in an off-balance, more injury-prone pattern. Fatiguing muscles are less able to compensate for any perturbation of load or position in the trunk. Also, there is probably greater stress to the passive (ligamentous) elements of the spine with stretching of the viscoelastic material. Thus, this equipment can monitor efficient and effective rehabilitation mechanisms that have the goal of reducing fatigue and enhancing the strength of the muscles being substituted.

One of the criticisms of Isotechnologies' equipment is that in an effort to provide a wide array of data, reliability is diminished. For instance, in an effort to allow rotation and lateral movements simultaneously with sagittal flexion/extension, the subject is only minimally restrained. Also, in keeping with the other types of computerized test equipment, the degree to which the buttock and thigh muscles contribute to performance cannot be estimated or defined. Some equipment such as that manufactured by Loredan (Loredan, Davis, Calif) allows a choice of position, either sitting or standing. At this time no research identifies which equipment provides more reliable information or is more useful in predicting future performance.

Another view of the reliability problem is that the only way to clearly identify variabilities in lumbar performance is to completely isolate the spine from any other contributing segment. The Medx (Medx Corp., Ocala, Fla) group has proposed to do this. Their equipment only tests isolated lumbar extension isometric strength with special restraints designed to do this. (Another machine recently introduced tests torso rotation.) This equipment places extremely tight restraints on the seated subject with the pelvis fixed. The subject is precisely counterbalanced so that gravity forces can be totally discounted. Seated in the constrained position, the hips are flexed at greater than 90 degrees, which allows the limit of extension to be past the verticle. A range of 72 degrees is offered to test the subject, and testing is accomplished only from full flexion to full extension. In a test to evaluate reliability, following an initial practice session reliability coefficients were computed as ranging from 0.94 to 0.98 in a group of 136 normal men and women. One day of pretesting was required to gain familiarity with the equipment. This equipment offers a curve of performance with seven isometric points equally distributed along the 72-degree range.[16]

Great effort is made to control the pelvis when testing with the Medx equipment. If the pelvis is free to move during lumbar extension, it will rotate as the hamstrings, gluteal, and adductor muscles contract. The need to stabilize the pelvis and lower extremities to eliminate pelvic movement and isolate the lumbar area during lumbar testing has been recognized for some time.[32] The success of isolating lumbar motion by this equipment also allows a very accurate statement of flexion/extension range. Because of its unique ability to isolate spine function, this equipment is likely to emerge as most reliable for spine testing.

Due to acceleration at the beginning and deceleration at the end of movement, dynamic strength tests may not be appropriate for quantifying strength through a range of motion. Weakness in a specific area of lumbar extension may go undetected as an individual goes through a dynamic test. In addition, dynamic strength is influenced by the speed of movement, which brings into controversy whether isokinetic testing (control of the speed of movement) is the ideal way of measuring human function. Also, as the speed of movement increases such as at 120 degrees per second, kinetic forces may become so severe that they give an inaccurate measure of true strength and thus influence the shape of the strength curve.[26] These problems justify measuring strength in an isometric manner at multiple positions in the arc of function. One additional advantage is offered for multiple-point isometric testing in that with motion obliterated, the adverse effects of impact loading when the speed of the body does not match the test equipment can be avoided.

Medx equipment is used for training as well as testing, which also makes it somewhat unique among the various types of computerized test equipment. Usually training is accomplished on different equipment than the test equipment. By using very slow rates, dynamic training will increase measured extensor strength between 60% and 100% in normal subjects with training as infrequently as once a week. Using equipment such as this that so specifically isolates the torso reinforces our knowledge that when a muscle is trained at a given angle, its strength increases from 15 to 20 degrees at either side of that point.[14] Obviously lumbar extensor strength varies greatly through the full range of motion, and therefore single-point or limited-range testing for training is inadequate.

The experience with the Medx equipment brings up several questions in terms of the efficiency and effectiveness of spine rehabilitation. Although their data suggest that once-a-week exercise is enough, how long should it be performed? It seems to have been established that strength increases during the first 3 to 5 weeks of resistance training are due to neuromuscular factors.[25] It also has been demonstrated that muscle hypertrophy becomes the predominant factor in strength increases after that time. It seems to be agreed that lumbar extensor muscles exist in a state of some disuse and weakness even during normal conditions, but much more so during episodes of back pain. Therefore, significant efforts toward strengthening extensors must be undertaken. So far no published data correlate the loss of pain, return to work, and maintenance of a pain-free status to duration and percent increase in exercise strength. We still do not know whether frequent exercise over a short period or infrequent but more intense therapy is better.

Emphasis on isometric testing through a full range brings up the question of coordination. This is the third leg of the platform for enhanced trunk performance and the most difficult to test. On the other hand, it must be the maneuver by which improvement of function, whether tested by isometric performance, isokinetic performance, or isoinertial performance, must be achieved. All tests that have evaluated performance during rehabilitation note rapid increased performance in those individuals making a significant effort to produce consistent and maximum effort. It is not possible for muscles to become strengthened on the basis of increased numbers of myofibrils (hypertrophy) for perhaps 6 weeks. Thus, improved performance must be on the basis of neurologic integration and better control. How do we enhance coordination, and indeed how do we test it?

One way of testing coordination is in the form of various types of obstacle courses. Because no commercially available piece of equipment challenges the wide array of testing maneuvers necessary, no comparative data are available. Maneuvers such as crawling, pushing, pulling, stair climbing, and lifting overhead and the duration of standing and sitting in one position are all parameters that relate to neuromotor control. Various exercises that relate to the ability to hold prescribed postures have been advocated and are useful measurements of increasing performance. The so-called stabilization programs require intricate positioning and holding a position by using a wide array of neuromotor control mechanisms that can monitor the ability of an individual to carry out neuromuscular control maneuvers with greater finesse.[34]

The most important parameter of neuromuscular control in a practical sense is the ability to do day-to-day activities. In this sense it brings up the concept of work hardening. In this situation the combination of strength, endurance, and neuromotor control as well as range of motion are all summarized in activities of daily living. Rehabilitation has really become a form of reactivation wherein the individual is placed into settings where work activities such as materials handling are reproduced over and over again so that the individual can accomplish this with the regularity and ease of performance that he did apparently routinely until the occasion of injury at work or at home. Such challenges as shoveling sand, plumbing a house, and lifting suitcases are used as treatment/test maneuvers. The duration with which one can perform this activity and the speed at which they can do the performance are the measures of increased function. In an effort to compare one day with the next and one individual with another, however, this performance must be done according to standardized protocols. These protocols would include such maneuvers as lifting from floor to knuckle height either frequently or infrequently. Other maneuvers such as pivoting at the waist, push and pull of some standardized object, over-the-shoulder lifting, and various aerobic endurance exercises are available for standardized protocols. It would of course be necessary to perform aerobic exercises in some standardized maneuver such as on a treadmill or on a bicycle ergometer. In this setting, however, other than aerobic test equipment, the only specialized devices necessary are essentially tools of normal activity.

Coordination, perhaps best summarized as sports skills, is partially inherited, partially trained, but certainly not a skill that can be rapidly changed. The role of an effective spinal rehabilitation program is to return the individual to previous levels of performance—not to create a super athlete. Thus, some understanding of previous levels of performance are necessary. In the workmen's compensation situation, this probably is related to fully understanding the job to be accomplished. An on-site evaluation may be necessary to fully comprehend the complexity of the job. Thus, in a practical sense work simulation is the goal of testing and enhancing neuromuscular coordination. We all have the capacity to strengthen musculature over a long period of time, but the strengthening of overall performance could far better be created by developing alternative strategies when certain muscles fatigue. As yet we do not have a tool that totally summarizes this type of performance. Perhaps in the future a tool that summarizes speed and acceleration and has the ability to carry out progressive resistance and real-world performance will be available. The Lido (Loredan, Davis, Calif) lift device comes closest to this ideal. It seems clear that speed of performance is the ultimate definition of normalcy and of the ability to function at the maximum with the least opportunity for failure due to physical stress at an unguarded moment.

SOCIAL/POLITICAL ASPECTS OF SPINAL REHABILITATION

In a recent study by Deyo and Tsui-Wu, it was clearly demonstrated that education and job income were the strongest predictors for continued disability due to back pain.[10] In this study over 1500 persons from a wide array of educational backgrounds, job activities, and severity of back disability were surveyed. Very significant differences ($P < .001$) correlated fewer disability days to greater levels of education of the worker, no matter what the job. This was regardless of the severity of the back pain or sciatica. Thus, knowledge of a patient's education level may be clinically useful in estimating the prognosis of the patient with back pain. Certainly this information has to be taken into account in conducting clinical trials of back pain treatment. Also, in the major prospective study trying to identify factors that create prolonged disability—the Boeing study—work dissatisfaction was the most significant factor in identifying those most likely to have continuing back pain.[3]

Against the backdrop of socioeconomic factors as related to back pain, we have the history of a greater potential for reinjury once the back problems have been documented. The most dramatic presentation of this phenomenon was a recent paper that pointed out the reinjury risk of postlaminectomy postal workers.[29] In this study 32 postal service workers were matched against similar job categories, age, and sex. The potential for reinjury was demonstrated in that at an average of 5.6 years following surgery there was a 25% reinjury rate in postal workers as compared with a 6% injury rate in controls. What we do not know in the study, which is typically the flaw in this type of study, is the nature of the presurgical and postsurgical treatment. To what degree were the increased incidents of reinjury due to deconditioning and a failure of patients to maintain a level of postinjury concern for the weak link in their back. Without question, a postsurgical patient is at greater risk due to the surgically created weak link. When there is a concern for a continued exercise program for strength, reinjury in industry does not occur at any higher rate than in the population as a whole.[21] These two studies bring up the discrepancy in care available to the American worker. (Back rehabilitation generally has to be in reference to workmen's compensation injuries in that this is the only entity that financially covers significant rehabilitation programs.) If the postlaminectomy postal workers had gone through a valid work-hardening program, would they have had a better record of continued healthy behavior? Unfortunately, the postal workers are a poor population on which to evaluate efficacy of care. The rewards for disability are so high in the government services, especially the postal services, that motivation to return to work are quite limited. As we are aware, the states vary considerably as to their workmen's compensation laws and the amount of disability payment. The same is true with social security disability and verterans' benefits. No uniform system of payment or even evaluation has emerged.

We cannot escape the reality that far more significant factors than purely the soft-tissue injury related to back pain are at play in the effectiveness of spinal rehabilitation. Patient attitude is probably the most important. The complexity of achieving the rewards of disability payment is also a factor. How does society identify the severity of the problem? Many institutions are currently struggling with this dilemma. For instance, in the state of California new legislation has recently been passed that tries to speed the process of rehabilitation and return to work or adjudication of disability claims by forcing earlier milestones of decision making. On the other hand, in California the total mechanism by which a definition of disability is accomplished is by the medical report often of a nontreating physician. By the regulations of the state, the level of disability is defined by a formula based on the appearance of various adjectives in the medical report such as minimal, moderate, constant, intermittent, etc. No functional testing is accepted as a means to define the limitation. Other states try to resolve the problem by various maneuvers such as basing the entire level of disability on the medical diagnosis, regardless of postdiagnosis care (Minnesota). Some states merely identify the duration of off time as the criteria on which disability is defined (Florida). Actually the majority of states now use the AMA guidelines as the standard by which impairment is evaluated. The AMA guidelines have severe limitations in that the only functional test used for the spine is range of motion. They do incorporate considerations of pain and diagnosis also and thus do make an effort to balance various factors by somewhat complex formulas. Bad as they are, they seem to be the only accepted guideline.

SUMMARY

What is the future of spinal rehabilitation? All factors point to simpler methods of testing of function as the method by which progress can be identified and even the relationship of individual impairment to the population as a whole. These will be various work performance testing maneuvers such as the ability to lift progressive weights to a standard height. I believe that in the future there will be less and less testing using specialized computerized equipment due to reliability factors and the diversity of the concept noted above. On the other hand, it will be recognized that spinal treatments in the form of modalities such as ultrasound, hot packs, massage, etc., are maneuvers to generate income for the providers and offer no potential to more rapid resolution of the problem. Due to increasing competitiveness for at least efficient medical care, those centers that focus on measurement of function as the criteria of progress rather than evaluation of pain will be the more accepted health care provider. Unhappily, continuing growth of litigation will be the major barrier to progress in effective medical care.

Due to the fact that spinal function is such a complex mechanism and soft-tissue injury cannot be clearly defined by any current test in the great majority of patients with back and leg pain, the potential for disagreement is ever available. Inasmuch as liability for back pain in the socially disgruntled individual is perceived as the responsibility of the employer or society, energy to prove the severity of the injury and the liability of the employer will be translated into legal action. This will become an increasingly destructive maneuver in business competition. The only solution essentially is to develop mechanisms to allow greater employee responsibility and job satisfaction. Healthy behavior after the onset of back pain is best manifested by a willingness to proceed into a progressive exercise program that may indeed be uncomfortable but is the only maneuver of which we are aware that has the potential to hasten the progress of soft-tissue repair. This is no small problem in that economic competitiveness depends on the absence of rewards for prolonged off time or the payoff of the "injured" worker. To solve this problem there may be an attempt to remove back pain as a compensable injury as is the case in Germany. Until then, a focus on function is the basic principle for an early return to work or to conclude litigation.

REFERENCES

1. Addison R, Schultz A: Trunk strength in patients seeking hospitalization for chronic low back disorders. *Spine* 1980; 5:539–544.
2. Asmussen E: Muscle fatigue. *Med Sci Sports* 1979; 11:313–321.
3. Battie M, Bigos SJ, Spengler DM, et al: Back injuries in industry: No. 3, Employee related factors. *Spine* 1986; 11:252–256.
4. Bechtol CD: Grip test: Use of a dynamometer with adjustable handle spacing. *J Bone Joint Surg [Am]* 1954; 36:820.
5. Biering-Sorensen F: Physical measurements as risk indicators for low back trouble over a one year period. *Spine* 1984; 9:106–119.
6. Binder A, Parr G, Hazleman B, et al: Pulsed electromag-

netic field therapy of persistent rotator cuff tendinitis: A double-blind controlled assessement. *Lancet* 1984; 1:695–698.
7. Cabaud HE, Chatty A, Gildengorin V, et al: Exercise effects on the strength of the rat anterior cruciate ligament. *Am J Sports Med* 1980; 8:79–86.
8. Carter DR, Wong M: The role of mechanical loading histories in the development of diarthrodial joints. *J Orthop Res* 1988; 6:804–816.
9. Chaffin DB, Park KS: A longitudinal study of low back pain as associated with occupational weight lifting factors. *Am Ind Hyg Assoc J* 1973; 34:513–525.
10. Deyo RA, Tsui-Wu Y: Functional disability due to back pain: A population based study indicating the importance of socio-economic factors. *Arthritis Rheum* 1987; 30:1247–1253.
11. Engelberg A: *Guides to the Evaluation of Permanent Impairment,* ed 3. Chicago, American Medical Association, 1988.
12. Faulkner JA: New perspectives in training for maximum performance. *JAMA* 1968; 205:741–746.
13. Fess EE: A method for checking JAMAR dynamometer calibration. *J Hand Surg [Am]* 1987; 12:28–31.
14. Gardner GW: Specificity of strength changes of the exercised and nonexercised limb following isometric training. *Res Q* 1963; 34:98–101.
15. Gollnick PD, Armstrong RB, Saubert CW, et al: Enzyme activity and fiber composition in skeletal muscle of untrained and trained men. *J Appl Physiol* 1972; 33:312–319.
16. Graves JE, Pollock ML, Carpenter DM, et al: Quantitative assessment of full range of motion isometric lumbar extension strength. *Spine* 1990; 15:289–294.
17. Hislop HJ, Perrine JJ: The isokinetic concept of exercise. *Phys Ther* 1967; 47:114–177.
18. Kenney TG, Dahners LE: The effect of electrical stimulation on ligament healing in a rat model. *Trans Orthop Res Soc* 1988; 13:107.
19. Mathiowetz V, Kashman N, et al: Grip and pinch strength: Normative data for adults. *Arch Phys Med Rehabil* 1985; 66:69–74.
20. Mayer T, Gatchel R, Kishino N, et al: A prospective short term study of chronic low back pain patients utilizing novel objective functional measurements. *Pain* 1986; 25:53–68.
21. Mayer T, Gatchel R, Mayer H, et al: A perspective two year study of functional restoration in industrial low back injury. *JAMA* 1987; 258:1763–1767.
22. Mayer T, Smith S, Keeley J: Quantification of lumbar function, Part II: Sagittal plane trunk strength in chronic low back pain patients. *Spine* 1985; 10:765–772.
23. Mohr TM, Akers TK, Landry RG: Effect of high voltage stimulation on edema reduction in the rat hind limb. *Phys Ther* 1987; 67:1703–1707.
24. Mooney V: A randomized double-blind prospective study of the efficacy of pulsed electromagnetic fields in interbody lumbar fusions. *Spine* 1990; 15:708–712.
25. Moritani T, DeVries HA: Neurofactors vs. hypertrophy in the time course of muscle strength gain. *Am J Phys Med* 1979; 58:115–130.
26. Murray A, Harrison E: Constant velocity dynamometer: An appraisal using mechanical loading. *Med Sci Sports Exerc* 1986; 18:612–624.
27. Parnianpour M, Nordin M, Brisson P, et al: The effects of isoinertial fatiguing trunk lateral bending on the parameters of motor output and movement patterns (abstract). Presented at the International Society for the Study of the Lumbar Spine, Kyoto, Japan, 1989.
28. Reed BV: Effect of high voltage pulsed electrical stimulation on microvascular permeability to plasma proteins: A possible mechanism in minimizing edema. *Phys Ther* 1988; 68:491–495.
29. Ryan J, Zwerling C: Risk for occupational low back injury after lumbar laminectomy for degenerative disc disease. *Spine* 1990; 15:500–503.
30. Saltin B, Gollnick P: Skeletal muscle adaptability: Significance for metabolism and performance, in Peachey LD, Adrian RH, Geiger SR (eds): *Handbook of Physiology,* section 10, *Skeletal Muscle*. Bethesda, Md, American Physiological Society, 1983, pp 555–631.
31. Schurman DJ, Goodman SB, Lane-Smith R: Inflammation and tissue repair, in Leadbetter WB, Buckwalter JA, Gordon SL (eds): *Sports Induced Inflammation. American Orthopaedic Society for Sports Medicine Symposium,* Park Ridge, Ill, American Academy of Orthopaedic Surgeons, 1990.
32. Smidt G, Herring T, Amundsen L, et al: Assessment of abdominal and back extensor function: A quantitative approach and results of chronic low back patients. *Spine* 1983; 8:211–219.
33. Tipton CM, Schild RJ, Tomanek RJ: Influence of physical activity on the strength of knee ligaments in rats. *Am J Physiol* 1967; 212:783–787.
34. White AH: *Back School and Other Conservative Approaches to Low Back Pain*. St Louis, Mosby–Year Book, 1983.
35. Winter DA, Wells RP, Orr GW: Errors in the use of isokinetic dynamometers. *Eur J Appl Physiol* 1981; 46:397–407.

Index

C

Q

R